# Diagnostic Ultrasound

Text and Cases

*Second Edition*

# Diagnostic Ultrasound
## Text and Cases

*Second Edition*

**Dennis A. Sarti, M.D.**
Clinical Associate Professor of Radiology
Cedars-Sinai Medical Center
UCLA School of Medicine
Los Angeles, California

*Illustrations by* Dennis B. Wisher, R.D.M.S.

YEAR BOOK MEDICAL PUBLISHERS, INC.
Chicago • London

1 2 3 4 5 6 7 8 9 0 YC 91 90 89 88 87

**Library of Congress Cataloging-in-Publication Data**

Diagnostic ultrasound.

   Includes bibliographies and index.
   1. Diagnosis, Ultrasonic.  2. Diagnosis, Ultrasonic—
Case Studies.  I. Sarti, Dennis A.  [DNLM: 1. Ultrasonic
Diagnosis.  2. Ultrasonic Diagnosis—case studies.
WB 289 D536]
RC78.7.U4D52 1987        616.07'543        86–19059
ISBN 0–8151–7537–X

Sponsoring Editors: James D. Ryan, Jr./Kevin M. Kelly
Manager, Copyediting Services: Frances M. Perveiler
Production Project Managers: Carol A. Reynolds/
   Diane K. Purcell
Proofroom Supervisor: Shirley E. Taylor

To Sunny, Marc,
Jennifer, and Jeffrey

# Contributors

**Lawrence W. Bassett, M.D.**
Associate Professor of Radiological Sciences, UCLA School of Medicine; Chief, Section of Mammography, UCLA Medical Center, Los Angeles, California

**Harbinder S. Brar, M.D.**
Clinical Instructor in Obstetrics and Gynecology, Division of Maternal Fetal Medicine, University of Southern California School of Medicine; Postdoctoral Research Fellow, Maternal-Fetal Medicine, Women's Hospital, Los Angeles County— University of Southern California Medical Center, Los Angeles, California

**Catherine Cole-Beuglet, M.D., F.R.C.P.(C.)**
Professor of Radiology, University of California, Irvine; Director of Ultrasound and Computed Body Tomography, University of California, Irvine, Medical Center, Orange, California

**Barbara Carroll, M.D.**
Department of Radiology, Duke University Medical Center, Durham, North Carolina

**Peter L. Cooperberg, M.D., F.R.C.P.(C.)**
Professor of Radiology, University of British Columbia; Chief, Section of Ultrasound, Vancouver General Hospital, Vancouver, British Columbia

**Barbara F. Crandall, M.D.**
Professor of Pediatrics and Psychiatry, UCLA School of Medicine, Neuropsychiatric Institute and Hospital; Director, Prenatal Diagnosis Center, Los Angeles, California

**Greggory R. DeVore, M.D.**
Associate Professor, Department of Obstetrics and Gynecology, University of Southern California School of Medicine, Los Angeles, California

**Richard H. Gold, M.D.**
Professor of Radiological Sciences, UCLA School of Medicine; Professor of Radiological Sciences, UCLA Medical Center, Los Angeles, California

**Frank P. Hadlock, M.D.**
Professor of Radiology, Baylor College of Medicine; Director, Department of Radiology, Jefferson Davis Hospital, Houston, Texas

**Jack O. Haller, M.D.**
Professor of Clinical Radiology, State University of New York—Downstate Medical Center; Director of Pediatric Imaging, Kings County Hospital, Brooklyn, New York

**Janet Horenstein, M.D.**
Assistant Professor, Los Angeles County—University of Southern California Medical Center; Division of Maternal Fetal Medicine, Women's Hospital, Los Angeles, California

**Hedvig Hricak, M.D.**
Professor of Radiology and Urology; Chief, Uroradiology Section; Assistant Chief, Magnetic Resonance Section; University of California, San Francisco, School of Medicine, San Francisco, California

**Hooshang Kangarloo, M.D.**

Chairman, Department of Radiology, UCLA Center for the Health Sciences, Los Angeles, California

**Carolyn Kimme-Smith, Ph.D.**

Adjunct Assistant Professor, Radiological Sciences, UCLA School of Medicine, Los Angeles, California

**William King III, M.D.**

Assistant Professor, Department of Radiological Sciences, UCLA Medical Center, Los Angeles, California

**Frederick W. Kremkau, Ph.D.**

Professor and Director, Center for Medical Ultrasound, Bowman Gray School of Medicine, Winston-Salem, North Carolina

**Faye C. Laing, M.D.**

Professor of Radiology, University of California, San Francisco; Chief, Division of Ultrasound, San Francisco General Hospital, San Francisco, California

**George R. Leopold, M.D.**

Professor and Chairman, Department of Radiology, University of California, San Diego, School of Medicine, San Diego, California

**Michael L. Manco-Johnson, M.D.**

Professor of Radiology and Medicine, University of Colorado School of Medicine; Acting Chairman, Department of Radiology, University Hospital and University of Colorado Health Sciences Center, Denver, Colorado

**Anthony A. Mancuso, M.D.**

Professor of Radiology, University of Florida College of Medicine; Clinical Director of MRI, Shand Hospital, Gainesville, Florida

**Myles Matsumoto, M.D.**

Staff Research Associate, UCLA School of Medicine, Los Angeles, California

**David A. Nyberg, M.D.**

Assistant Professor, University of Washington Medical Center, Seattle, Washington

**Lawrence D. Platt, M.D.**

Professor of Obstetrics and Gynecology, University of Southern California School of Medicine, Los Angeles, California

**Philip W. Ralls, M.D.**

Associate Professor of Radiology, University of Southern California School of Medicine; Chief, Section of Body Imaging and Interventional Radiology, Los Angeles County—University of Southern California Medical Center, Los Angeles, California

**Carol M. Rumack, M.D.**

Associate Professor, Radiology and Pediatrics, University of Colorado School of Medicine; Co-Director of Pediatric Computed Tomography, Ultrasound, and Magnetic Resonance; Acting Chief, Division of Diagnostic Radiology; Director of Pediatric Radiology; University of Colorado Health Sciences, Denver, Colorado

**Dennis A. Sarti, M.D.**

Clinical Associate Professor, Cedars-Sinai Medical Center, UCLA School of Medicine, Los Angeles, California

**Nancy J. Worthen, M.D.**
Assistant Professor, Radiological Sciences, UCLA School of Medicine, Los Angeles, California; Chief, Diagnostic Ultrasound, Harbor–UCLA Medical Center, Torrance, California

**Seymour Zemlyn, M.D.**
Clinical Assistant Professor of Radiology, University of Southern California School of Medicine, Los Angeles, California; Radiologist, Tarzana, California

# Preface to the First Edition

The concept of writing a textbook enters your thoughts fleetingly at first and gradually builds. You discuss the project with others who have accomplished the task and hear, "It was very rewarding, but I'll never do it again." You become cautious but optimistic, for the others all survived. Naively, you make a decision to undertake the project. The mental commitment occurs early on. You have no idea of the time commitment necessary until you are too far along to turn back. It is only at this point that you can decide intelligently whether or not to undertake the project. Alas, it is too late.

Diagnostic ultrasound has undergone numerous recent advances that have consistently and often dramatically improved image quality. This has created difficulties in textbook writing. The time frame necessary from when a case is scanned initially to when it appears in print can be as long as two to three years. This presents a dilemma for the practicing ultrasonographer whose current images are of much better quality and are more informative than those in the textbooks. Information becomes outdated by the time it reaches those for whom it was intended.

However, there has been little change in B-scan image quality since the development of the gray scale. Recent research has been oriented toward a digital scan converter and real-time image improvement. Although the digital scan converter has increased system stability, it has not improved image quality dramatically, if at all. Realtime images presently do not compare with high quality B-scan images. Therefore, the time appears right for an extensive, well-illustrated text in the field.

When developing the groundwork or format for a textbook, an author tries to orient his or her material toward a specific audience. Those who are in most need at the present time for such a book are the practicing ultrasonographers and radiologists who have had no formal training in this specific area. Also, the expanding field of radiology will shortly confront its residents with ultrasonography at the board examinations. It is toward these two groups that this text is specifically oriented with the hope that others, such as medical students, technologists, and referring physicians, may also benefit from it.

Much of the design format for this text came from the suggestions of practicing radiologists who visited the UCLA Ultrasound Laboratory for one- to two-week intervals to acquire further training. While visiting, they often asked to peruse a teaching file or some other organized form of case material. With these requests in mind, we decided to develop this text as an ultrasound teaching file.

The textbook chapters are divided according to organ systems. Each chapter contains two major sections: written text and case material. The written text describes technique, normal anatomy, and pathological states. The initial section of each chapter is primarily the work of the various outstanding contributors, with minor changes by the editors.

The second section of each chapter is comprised of case material compiled and discussed by the editors. Most of the images were obtained from the diagnostic laboratory of the UCLA School of Medicine in Westwood, California, with some from the Harbor General Hospital Campus in Torrance, California. A few of the images were obtained from outside laboratories and will be so noted in the text.

Since diagnostic ultrasound is a visual field, the case material section has been given great attention. The editors have maintained strict control of, and responsibility for, this section for two reasons: (1) the teaching file approach necessitates a uniform presentation; and (2) image quality and extensive labeling are, therefore, more consistent.

Each of the 1192 figures in the text is abundantly labeled. The decision to maintain extensive labeling was both intentional and time-consuming and was accomplished because we felt that the beginning and intermediate ultrasonographer can learn a great deal of anatomy from these images, through the labeling, in addition to the obvious pathology for which each case was presented.

As a project such as this reaches completion, it becomes obvious that the efforts and energies of many individuals are responsible for the end result. Most of the images in this text were performed by, or with the assistance of, technologists who are intelligent, highly motivated, and extremely independent. The excellent technical skills of the following individuals were invaluable in compiling the cases: Gerta Awender, Bob Clark, Fred Gardner, Rosemary Glenny, Janel Parker, Pamela Scarlett, and Kathleen Weber.

Since the text contains a large number of images, photography plays an extremely important role. We have been fortunate to have the assistance of Kim Willis who worked long hours under adverse conditions to accomplish what at many times must have seemed an insurmountable task. Lastly and most importantly, we wish to express a special thanks to Jean Slater who provided the secretarial assistance necessary in this endeavor. In addition to her other duties, which are burdensome, she found the time and energy to complete this project; and she was there to give encouragement at the numerous low points along the way.

DENNIS A. SARTI
W. FREDERICK SAMPLE

# Preface to the Second Edition

The decision to do a second edition of *Diagnostic Ultrasound: Text and Cases* was not an easy one. After doing the first edition, I was well aware of the time and effort necessary. The second edition has been nearly 2 years of nights, weekends, and many 4:30 a.m. empty freeway drives into UCLA. There are several reasons why I decided, against better judgment, to go ahead with the second edition.

First is the tremendous reaction to the first edition of *Diagnostic Ultrasound: Text and Cases.* The numerous positive comments and letters from practicing radiologists, residents, and ultrasound technicians have been overwhelming. One writes a book knowing that only very few books will be successful. To have your efforts so appreciated is a tremendous reward. Second is the feeling of contribution. I was fortunate to be interested in a young, developing field. This book has been my contribution to the field of diagnostic ultrasound. Third is Hooshang Kangarloo, M.D. Hoosh convinced me during several private conversations that I had no choice but to do the second edition.

I have kept the same format for the second edition, with a text section followed by case material. The text sections were written by experts in the field of diagnostic ultrasound. Over 1000 new images have been added to the case section. These are all with black background. The case sections on breast, neonatal brain, and fetal heart have been written by Drs. Bassett, Rumack and Manco-Johnson, and DeVore respectively. The remainder has been written by me with the cases compiled from UCLA, my private office, and the contributors of the text sections.

I would like to thank Helen Thompson, Gloria Bright Siple, and my wife, Sunny. They greatly assisted in compiling the cases and typing the manuscript. Dennis B. Wisher provided the excellent illustrations. I would also like to thank my new publisher, Year Book Medical Publishers, especially James D. Ryan, Jr. They have been most cooperative and encouraging during this undertaking. Finally, I would like to thank my children, Marc, Jennifer, and Jeffrey, for understanding the many hours I couldn't devote to them.

DENNIS A. SARTI, M.D.

# Contents

# 1.
# Physics of Diagnostic Ultrasound

Dennis A. Sarti, M.D.
Carolyn Kimme-Smith, Ph.D.

## Pulse-Echo Technique

Medical imaging in diagnostic ultrasound utilizes the pulse-echo technique. This is different from other forms of medical imaging in that it uses information that is reflected back toward the source that generated the energy. In x-ray or computed tomographic (CT) imaging, transmitted energy is imaged. The x-ray tube is on one side of the patient and the film is on the other side of the patient. Photons are emitted from the x-ray tube into and through the patient and registered on the film. This is considered a transmitted form of imaging. Some experimental work is being done with transmitted ultrasound imaging. However, present-day clinical ultrasound imaging systems use a reflected technique rather than a transmitted technique. The reflected technique consists of pulsing a crystal and sending packets of energy into the patient. This packet of energy is reflected at different interfaces inside the patient. Most of the energy passes through the various interfaces to penetrate deeper into the patient. However, a small percentage of energy at each interface is reflected back toward the transducer. When this reflected wave reaches the transducer it is translated by the transducer as a very small voltage. Therefore, the ultrasound transducer acts as both a transmitter and a receiver of sound. This is made possible by the piezoelectric properties of the transducer, which take effect when a pressure wave compresses the surface of the crystal in the transducer and causes it to give off a voltage on its surface. The piezoelectric effect occurs when the transducer is acting in the receiving mode. The converse or reverse piezoelectric effect occurs when a voltage is applied to the surface of the crystal causing the crystal to expand and give off a pressure wave that passes into the patient if the crystal is in contact with the patient. The reverse piezoelectric effect occurs when the transducer is acting in the transmitting mode.

The transducer pulses energy into the patient for only a very short period of time and follows this pulse with a long silent period so that the transducer can receive returning echos without any interference from other reflected echoes generated by earlier pulses. The pulse of electricity that generates a pulse of ultrasound is usually in the range of 1 to 300 V and lasts less than 1 μsec.[1] The transducer is constructed so that it will vibrate for two to three wavelengths and be damped out almost immediately. Since the transducer stops vibrating in two to three wavelengths, it can then receive returning echoes reflected from inside the patient for the remainder of time it is silent. The time between pulses is long enough that all of the returning echoes, even those from the deepest part of the patient, will have adequate time to return to the surface of the patient and compress the transducer while it is operating in its receiving mode.

Most ultrasound units pulse the transducer at 500 to 3,000 times a second.[1] This is called the pulse repetition frequency. If we use an example of a transducer pulsing at 1,000 times a second, it will be easy to understand the long listening time used in diagnostic ultrasound. As mentioned earlier, a transducer is pulsed for approximately two to three cycles. This lasts only 5–6 $\mu$sec. After that time, the transducer is damped out and is quietly listening for the reflected echoes. For a unit that is pulsing at 1,000 times per second, the time between each pulse is 1 msec. Therefore, the transducer will be vibrating in the transmit mode for 5 or 6 $\mu$sec and listening in the receive mode for approximately 994 $\mu$sec. The transducer is in the receive mode approximately 99.4% of the time.

Let us assume that most patients are no larger than 20 cm thick. A wave traveling from the skin to the deepest portion of the patient and back will travel about 40 cm. Since the velocity of sound in soft tissues is approximately 1,540 m/sec, we can determine the time necessary for ultrasound to make the 40-cm round trip: (40 cm) $\div$ (154,000 cm/sec) = 0.26 msec. Since an ultrasound unit with a pulse repetition frequency of 1,000 would have 1 msec between each pulse, 0.26 msec would be needed for the ultrasound beam to be transmitted from the patient's skin to the deepest portion of the patient and back to the transducer. After that period of time, there should be no more meaningful echoes transmitted through the patient. Since we have used up only about one fourth of the time necessary between each pulse, there is a large amount of time in which no other reflections are occurring.

To summarize, the ultrasound transducer pulses for 5–6 $\mu$sec and is dampened quickly. This is less than 0.6% of the time. It will then receive returning echoes from within the body for approximately 0.26 msec, or 26% of the time. After that there will be a quiet time in which no meaningful echoes return to the transducer until the next pulse. This is approximately 0.74 msec, or 74% of the time. It is easy to see that the transducer transmits for a very short period of time and receives for a long period of time (Fig 1–1). The listening period is long enough that all the echoes within the body will have adequate time to reach the transducer without any interference from reflected echoes from the next pulse. Because of the short pulsing time (0.6%), very little energy is sent into the patient during the time the transducer is on the patient's skin. Because of the long listening period (99.4%), real-time scanning is possible.

## A-, B-, and M-Mode Scanning

The images formed from the echoes received by the transducer may be displayed in three ways. The A-mode (amplitude mode) image was the earliest display form of ultrasound. It consists of an oscilloscope mapping of the received voltage on the y-axis and time on the x-axis. Since the velocity of sound in soft tissue is nearly uniform, the relationship between time and distance is linear. Therefore, the x-axis also rep-

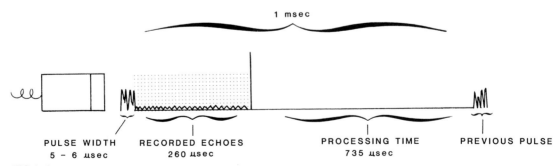

**FIG 1–1.**
*When the time between pulses is 1 msec, the meaningful echoes returning from the patient take up approximately 26% of the time between pulses. After that time is a quiet period before the next pulse, in which no meaningful echoes are returning to the transducer.*

resents distance. In Figure 1–2,A an A-mode display is illustrated, representing a vessel in the body surrounded by soft tissue with bone behind it.

B-mode (brightness mode) imaging yields a two-dimensional cross-sectional spatial representation of the examined tissue on the horizontal and vertical axes. Images are formed by assigning a degree of grayness to voltage amplitude values and displaying these gray levels on an image. For each A-line, the distance from the transducer can be computed from the time it takes for an echo to return. The amount of voltage generated in the transducer by the returning wave is read as a shade of gray and displayed on a television monitor in the position computed from the depth of the returning echo and position of the transducer when the echo was received. The transducer, constrained to move in a single plane, travels over the body of a patient, generating A-lines as it moves. Each pulse fills in another line of gray values. Most noncardiac imaging is B-mode imaging (Fig 1–2,B).

M-mode (motion mode) imaging is used in echocardiology, usually in conjunction with B-mode images, which are generated rapidly enough to image the heart. These are called real-time images. During the generation of M-mode images, the transducer is held still against the body as the heart beats. The movement in the body is imaged by recording the changes of reflecting surfaces over time. One axis of the image represents the distance of reflecting surfaces from the transducer and the other axis represents movement of these surfaces over time (Fig 1–2,C). If the surfaces do not move, M-mode imaging displays straight lines parallel to the face of the transducer. The strength of returning echoes is translated into voltages and the voltage amplitudes are mapped into gray levels, as they are for B-mode images.

**Piezoelectric Properties**

Diagnostic ultrasound transducers make use of certain naturally occurring and artificially produced substances with piezoelectric properties. In 1880 Pierre and Jacques Curie first observed the piezoelectric property in quartz, rochelle salt, and tourmaline. They applied a weight to a crystal and found that a charge was generated in the crystal.[2] The charge was generated because these crystals were anisotropic rather than isotropic. Anisotropic crystals do not have cen-

ters of symmetry, so their properties are different in different directions. When a voltage is applied to a piezoelectric element, the element will expand or contract, depending on the polarity of the voltage. If a piezoelectric element is compressed by a pressure wave such as a reflected sound wave returning from the body, a voltage will be produced across the piezoelectric element. This is called the direct piezoelectric effect.

Piezoelectric properties found application in World War I when Langevin began work on a submarine detector that used an array of quartz crystals. The first medical use of piezoelectric properties in ultrasound was in 1942 by Dussik in Austria. The cerebral ventricles were examined by an A-line instrument based on a metal flaw detector designed by Firestone.[2] Early ultrasound transducers were made from natural piezoelectric materials such as quartz or tourmaline. Modern-day ultrasound transducers are made of ceramic materials, commonly lead zirconate titanate. This is often referred to as PZT.

Ceramic ferroelectric material must be heated to its Curie temperature (328° to 365° C)[3] and placed in a strong electric field (2 kV/mm) applied to each end of the material. The temperature is slowly cooled while the material is under the influence of the strong electric field. This aligns the molecules in the direction of the electric field. Once the material is cooled it has piezoelectric properties. If the ceramic is then reheated above the Curie point, the piezoelectric property will be lost since the molecules will no longer be aligned. For this reason it is important not to autoclave transducers to sterilize them.

Recently, transducers constructed of layers of polyvinyledene fluoride (PVDF) have become commercially available. They are mainly found in high-frequency transducers because their impedance matches that of soft tissue, which results in greater sensitivity.

**The Interaction of Sound with Tissue**

*Frequency*

We are familiar with sound frequency and its relationship to pitch. A high frequency produces a high pitch sound while a low frequency produces a low pitch sound. We can produce sounds by plucking a string

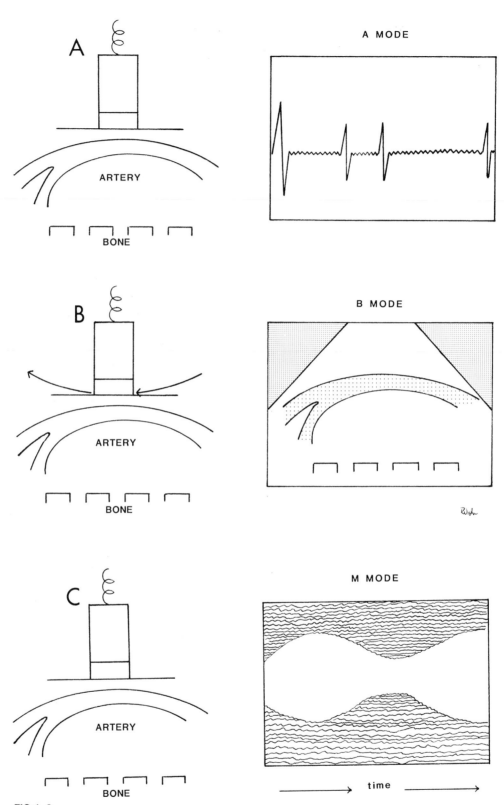

**FIG 1–2.**
*A,* A-mode imaging displays an artery as two amplitude spikes which separate slightly with each pulsation. *B,* B-mode imaging creates a two-dimensional image of the artery on an x-y axis. *C,* M-mode imaging displays only one section of the artery over time. The pulsation of the walls of the artery is shown on the y-axis; time is shown on the x-axis.

on a guitar, so that the string vibrates and transfers its vibration to air and thus to our ears. Similarly, we can ping the edge of a wine glass and produce a high-pitched sound in the air from its vibration. The thinner the glass, the higher the pitch. A medical transducer also works on this principle. A thin piezoelectric wafer is plucked electronically, vibrates, and transfers these vibrations through whatever tissue it is in contact with. The vibrating wafer must be stopped so that it can listen for the reflected echoes returning to it. Just as we may touch the wine glass to stop its ringing, so may we dampen the transducer to create a short pulse of ultrasound. Therefore, by quickly stimulating the wafer with a short burst of energy and then rapidly damping the vibration of the wafer, we are able to produce and send a short pulse of sound into the patient.

These vibrations can be represented by imaging a wave of energy moving through molecules which compress together and move apart. As the wave is transmitted by the molecules, they first crowd together or condense, then recoil from their collisions, leaving the space they once occupied rarefied (Fig 1–3). A cycle consists of the time or distance between successive condensations or rarefactions.

The frequency of the waveform is measured by the number of repetitions or cycles it produces each second. A 2-MHz transducer vibrates at 2 million cycles per second (cps), whereas a 10-MHz transducer vibrates at 10 million cps. The length of one cycle ($\lambda$) determines how far the waveform can travel at its propagation velocity. A wavelength ($\lambda$) can be computed from the formula $\lambda = v/f$, where v is the wave

propagation velocity. This computation is useful in understanding the effects of frequency on resolution. For example, a 2.25-MHz transducer has a wavelength of 0.7 mm. When the waveform emitted from the transducer is dampened after three cycles, the shortest resolution of the transducer is $3\lambda$, or 2.1 mm. The same computation for a 5-MHz transducer would be $\lambda = 0.3$ mm and $3\lambda = 0.9$ mm. We refer to these three cycles as the pulse width of the waveform emitted by the transducer.

Transducer resolution is measured in three directions, axial, lateral (or azimuthal), and slice thickness (or elevation). We will discuss axial resolution in this section because it is mostly dependent on the frequency or wavelength of the transducer and the pulse width. Axial resolution measures how small a structure can be imaged when the structure is parallel to the direction of the sound wave emitted by the transducer (Fig 1–4). If the structure is smaller than $3\lambda$, then the back wall of the structure cannot be distinguished (or resolved) from the front wall of the structure. Thus, the higher the frequency of the transducer, the smaller the structure that can be resolved.

Just as the thickness of the wine glass determines the pitch of sound at which it vibrates, so does the thickness of the transducer's crystal. The velocity of sound in PZT is 4,000 m/sec.[3] To obtain a particular frequency, we first compute what the wavelength would be for that crystal. For example, 3.5-MHz frequency would have

$$\lambda = 4,000 \times 10^3 \text{ mm/sec}/3.5 \times 10^6 \text{ cps}$$

or

$$\lambda = 1.14 \text{ mm}$$

To obtain a 3.5-MHz transducer, we must cut the ceramic exactly $\lambda/2$, or 0.57 mm. This thickness will reinforce vibrations of 3.5 MHz. This is called the "resonant" frequency of the transducer. Just as the diameter, tension, and length of string on a guitar control the pitch, so the thickness of the crystal controls the frequency of a medical transducer.

Frequency bandwidth is associated with audio amplifiers and high-fidelity speakers. It also affects medical ultrasound imaging. We have spoken as though only one frequency were emitted by the transducer. In fact a range of frequencies on each side of the main frequency are sent out of the transducer. This range is the result of two factors.

A pulse of voltage excites the crystal and causes it

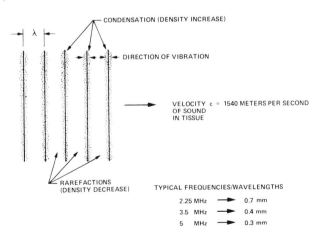

**FIG 1–3.**
*When a pulse passes into a patient, it creates an area of condensation of molecules followed by an area of molecular relaxation. The distance between two consecutive regions of condensation is one wavelength.*

PULSE WIDTH        OBJECTS IN PATIENT        IMAGE ON SCAN

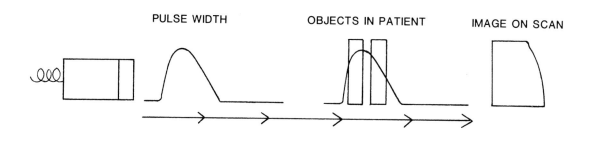

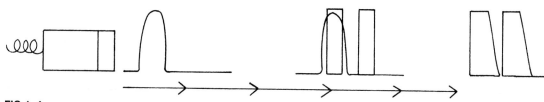

**FIG 1–4.**
*A wide pulse width will not be able to separate two close structures where a smaller pulse width will.*

to vibrate. This short voltage pulse is a mix of many frequencies. Also, the transducer's damping contributes an even greater range of frequencies. These frequencies, particularly those on the high end of the center frequency, contribute additional resolution to the waveform, and so are beneficial. We will be returning to frequency bandwidth later in this chapter when we discuss attenuation, transducer focal zones, and amplifiers.

*Velocity*

Various tissues in the human body have different ultrasound velocities varying from 330 m/sec in air to 4,080 m/sec in skull bone (Table 1–1). However, the velocity of most soft tissues is very close to 1,540 m/sec, and North American medical ultrasound manufacturers use this assumed velocity in their equipment. Blood, brain, kidney, liver, and muscle all differ from 1,540 m/sec by less than 40 m/sec, or 2%. These differences in velocity are independent of frequency in the 2-MHz to 10-MHz range. The velocity of ultrasound in human tissue can be computed from the equation:

$$v = \sqrt{B/\rho}$$

where B denotes bulk modulus and $\rho$ denotes density. Bulk modulus measures the stiffness of tissue. It varies more than the density in tissue and affects tissue velocity the most. As a general rule, the stiffer and more elastic the tissue, the higher the velocity.

Since the velocity of most soft tissues is quite close to 1,540 m/sec, there will be no large measurement errors on B-mode or real-time images when measuring the dimensions of organs. This can be confirmed by computing that a 4-cm gallbladder will be imaged with an error of only 0.8 mm. However, velocity arti-

**TABLE 1–1.**

**Velocity of Sound in Some Common Biological Materials**

| BIOLOGICAL MATERIAL | VELOCITY OF SOUND (M/SEC) |
|---|---|
| Air | 330 |
| Fat | 1,450 |
| Water | 1,480 |
| Human soft tissues (average) | 1,540 |
| Brain | 1,540 |
| Liver | 1,550 |
| Kidney | 1,560 |
| Blood | 1,570 |
| Muscle | 1,580 |
| Lens of eye | 1,620 |
| Skull bone | 4,080 |

facts are occasionally seen behind very large cysts and ascites, where the lower velocity of fluid changes the placement of the diaphragm posterior to the fluid.

## Acoustic Impedance

We are able to see reflected interfaces in body tissues because of differences in acoustic impedance of adjacent tissues. Acoustic impedance of soft tissue is a product of its density and velocity:

$$Z = \rho v$$

Just as velocity is dependent on the density and stiffness of a substance, so is the acoustic impedance. Except for bone and air, most tissue is very similar in density and in velocity (see Table 1–1). Since most soft tissues have very slight differences in density and velocity, it would seem that acoustic impedance does not play a major role. However, even with these slight differences we are able to image the boundaries between many tissues in ultrasound. These boundaries are seen because the ultrasound wave is reflected from the borders, depending on the impedance differences of the two tissues making up the boundary. If there is no acoustic mismatch between the two substances, then no wave will be reflected. It is possible for two tissues of different densities and velocities to have the same impedance. Water and castor oil are examples. However, if there is even a slight mismatch in acoustic impedance between two substances, a small reflected wave proportional to the mismatch will bounce off the interface. The larger the difference in acoustic impedance, the larger the percentage of energy that is reflected from that interface. Since bone and air have large differences in acoustic impedances, any soft tissues in contact with these two substances will give off the largest reflected echoes seen in diagnostic ultrasound. All other soft tissue interfaces give off much smaller reflections.

## Reflection

An ultrasound beam returns to the transducer because it reflects off a structure. But if the structure is a complete reflector, none of the beam will be transmitted to image tissue posterior to the structure. Ultrasound images depend on a balance between reflection and transmission. Several factors control these two phenomena. Reflection requires a large enough smooth surface that the ultrasound beam does not simply split and go around the reflecting object. This usually means that the reflector is 3–8 mm in diameter. The reflected energy is greatest if the surface is perpendicular to the beam direction (or parallel to the face of the transducer). Finally, for the transducer to "see" a difference between the surface and the surrounding tissue, the materials making up the tissues must have different impedance values. The greater the difference in impedance of two tissues, the greater the reflection of an ultrasound beam traversing them. The formula for reflection (R), if $Z_2$ is the impedance of the second tissue, is

$$R = (Z_2 - Z_1) / (Z_2 + Z_1)$$

This equation assumes that the transducer face is parallel to the boundary between the two tissues. If the transducer moves so that this surface is more and more oblique, the reflection back to the transducer decreases and finally is not "seen" by the transducer. There is no specific angle at which the reflection is not detected by the transducer. This angle depends on the impedance mismatch, the sensitivity of the unit, the transducer diameter, and the depth of the reflector.

Ultrasound measurements can consist of two quantities, amplitude or intensity, depending on why the measurements are needed. Amplitude measures the height of the wave and corresponds to the pressure generated by the ultrasound wave in tissue. It can be represented by voltage in the transducer and is used to form the B-mode image. Intensity measurements are proportional to the pressure squared and are used to predict the amount of biologic damage caused by the ultrasound wave in tissue. If an example of reflection is computed with the formula given above, it describes what happens to the amplitude of a wave reflecting off an interface. The percentage of transmitted amplitude tells us how much of the wave is left to image structures deeper than the interface. If we wish to investigate how much intensity is left in the wave to cause possible biologic damage, we use the formula above, squared. Thus a 10% reflection based on amplitude becomes a 1% reflection when intensity is computed, since $R = .10$ and $R^2 = .0100$ result from amplitude and intensity calculations, respectively.

These confusions continue when we discuss the differences in dB values, a measure of attenuation, for amplitude and intensity.

The amount of amplitude in the transmitted ultrasonic pulse is $T = 1 - R$. If R is negative, transmittance is apparently greater than the amplitude of the wave which emerged from the transducer. However, the negative reflection coefficient indicates only that the waveform had a "phase reversal" at the interface, so condensation changed to rarefaction. The wave is transmitted past the interface, with a discontinuity in the waveform when it is at the boundary. For example, the impedance of the kidney is 1.62 and that of fat is 1.35. A boundary formed between kidney ($Z_1$) and fat ($Z_2$) will have a reflectance of $-.09$, or 9%. The transmittance will be 91%, and the waveform will have a phase reversal at the boundary between the kidney and fat. The 9% reflectance will cause the boundaries of the kidneys to be easily imaged, and 91% transmittance will allow more imaging to occur posterior to the kidney. These calculations are performed using amplitude. If intensity is used then 0.81% is reflected and 99.2% is transmitted.

Impedance also accounts for our inability to image the lungs, since air has an impedance of .0004 compared to the 1.63 impedance value of most soft tissues. This mismatch causes the reflection coefficient of a lung–soft tissue boundary to be nearly 1, or 100%. Between bone and fat, 69% of the wave is reflected, so bone also stops most of the ultrasound wave. Between the kidney and the liver, $R = 0.9\%$. Examples are shown in Figure 1–5.

*Refraction*

Refraction is the bending of a light beam or ultrasound beam when it crosses at an oblique angle the surface-surface interface of two materials, through which light or sound waves propagate at different velocities. For example, a straight stick of wood placed halfway into water and at an angle will appear bent, because light waves propagate at different velocities through air and water. The same thing happens to an ultrasound beam passing through various surface interfaces. When the ultrasound beam passes through the interface of two media through which sound propagates at different velocities, and the ultrasound beam strikes the interface at an angle other than 90°, the transmit-

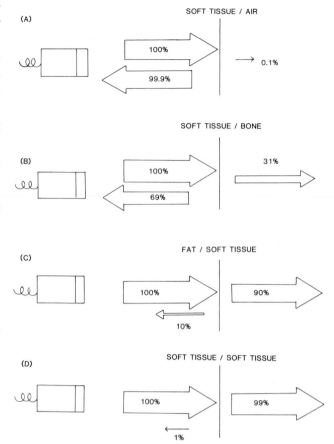

**FIG 1–5.**
*The percentages of sound transmitted and reflected at different interfaces are shown. This is for the amplitude of a wave. Percentages are different if intensities are used. For example, the percentage intensity reflected at a fat–soft tissue interface is 1%, whereas the percentage amplitude reflected at the same interface is 10%.*

ted wave will be refracted. Two things are needed for refraction to occur: (1) the ultrasound beam must pass through the two media with different velocities, and (2) the ultrasound beam must intersect the boundary interface at an oblique angle (Fig 1–6). If the angle of incidence is perpendicular or normal, refraction will not occur. And if the ultrasound beam has the same velocity in the two media, refraction will not occur, even if the angle of incidence is oblique.

Refraction can cause artifacts by bending the ultrasound beam as it travels through the patient. However, this bending is minimal in clinical studies since velocities in soft tissue are quite similar. The greatest distortion of image quality from refraction occurs at the numerous fat–soft tissue interfaces.

The phenomenon of critical angle shadowing is a result of increasing refraction. As the angle of inci-

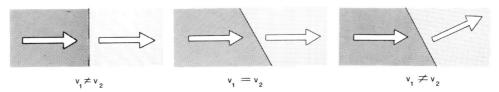

**FIG 1–6.**
*Refraction occurs at an interface only when there is a velocity change between the two media and the ultrasound beam strikes the interface at an oblique angle.*

dence increases away from the perpendicular, there will be slight increase in the amount of refraction at the interface. An angle is finally reached at which the wave is parallel to the interface, and complete refraction occurs (Fig 1–7). The resulting lack of transmission posterior to this site will produce shadowing on the scan. Shadowing is often noted around circular structures such as vessels, the gallbladder, or cysts. Consider an example of throwing a stone into a lake. If the stone is thrown into the lake perpendicular to the lake's surface, which would be the same as a normal angle of incidence, the stone will enter the lake and sink directly to the bottom. If the stone is directed to the lake's surface at an oblique angle of incidence, the stone will still enter the lake's surface. As the angle of incidence increases, finally the stone will be directed parallel to the surface of the lake. The stone will skip over the surface of the lake rather than sinking into the water. The same phenomenon occurs in ultrasound. An ultrasound beam directed into a patient at a normal angle of incidence will refract minimally. Refraction increases as the angle of incidence in-

creases. Finally, the sound beam will literally skip off the surface of the boundary and be completely refracted away from the surface, with no transmission occurring. Critical angle refraction should not be confused with the absorption of ultrasound beams by solid lesions, which results in shadows behind the lesions. Critical angle refraction commonly causes shadows to fall on each side of a curved structure.

## Instrumentation

### Types of Reflectors

We have defined a reflection coefficient as the percentage of the ultrasound beam that is reflected off an interface. In this section we will examine these larger interfaces and smaller reflectors so that we can better understand how edges and boundaries affect an ultrasound image.

SPECULAR REFLECTORS
The word specular means mirror-like. There are no mirror-like interfaces in the body, yet we persist in calling "specular" interfaces that are relatively smooth. For an interface to reflect ultrasound, the two tissues on each side of the interface must have different acoustic impedances.

If small ducts are parallel to the transducer face, they can be imaged even though they are as small as 2 mm. On the other hand, we usually cannot image a kidney stone if it is less than 3 mm in diamter, even though it has a large acoustic mismatch. These examples indicate several characteristics about a specular ultrasound reflector. First, such a reflector must have a large flat surface greater than 3 mm or several $\lambda$ in size. Such reflectors must also have an acoustic mismatch in order for reflection to occur at their surfaces. Finally, the reflecting surface must be nearly perpendicular to the transducer face in order for the

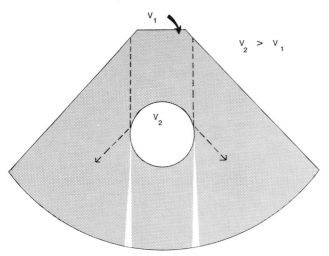

**FIG 1–7.**
*Critical angle shadowing occurs when an ultrasound beam strikes an interface at a very steep angle at which complete refraction and no transmission occur.*

## SPECULAR REFLECTION

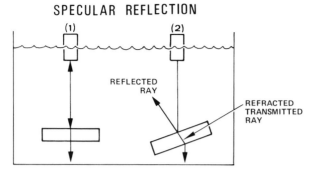

**FIG 1–8.**
*Specular reflectors are large interfaces that must be close to the perpendicular of the beam path in order for the reflected wave to be registered by the transducer.*

## DIFFUSE SCATTERING

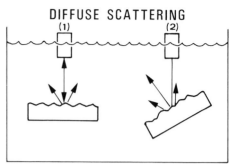

**FIG 1–9.**
*Diffuse reflectors are small, uneven surfaces that send the reflected wave in multiple directions. Some of the wave returns to the transducer.*

reflection to be received by the transducer (Fig 1–8). This last requirement is partially a result of the limited size of the transducer face. Since the transducer is both a transmitter and a receiver of ultrasound, the transducer face must be large enough to receive the returning echo. If the reflecting interface is tipped away from the transducer face, the wave will still be reflected but will miss the transducer surface. Therefore, although reflection occurs at the interface, it will never be registered on the ultrasound transducer. Because of this factor, we do not see specular reflectors that are not almost perpendicular to the transducer face. Reflectivity does occur but is not registered on the transducer surface. When the sides of slanted organs must be seen, compound scans fill in these anatomic borders by scanning closer to the perpendicular of these interfaces. However, compound scanning creates overwriting artifacts, which results in poorer resolution.

### DIFFUSE REFLECTORS

Diffuse or parenchymal reflectors are the result of the ultrasound wave being scattered by small or uneven reflectors (Fig 1–9). The diameters of lobules of the pancreas, liver, breast, and other organs are different and generate different texture patterns ultrasonographically. The amplitude of these scattered signals from small reflectors ($< \lambda$) will increase as the diameter cubed.[5] However, as the frequency decreases and $\lambda$ increases the scattered amplitudes decrease also. This is consistent with the attenuation of the ultrasound wave, which is partly caused by this scattering. As the frequency increases, scattering and therefore attenuation increases. Similarly, very fine cellular

structures such as those in a young, normal spleen do not attenuate ultrasound nearly as much as a young, dense breast full of large glandular lobules. However, scattered echoes are weak and can be imaged only because there are so many of them and they interfere and reinforce each other. Ultrasound units are designed to enhance these low-level parenchymal echoes by emphasizing the low-level signals.

These diffuse reflectors were thought to be isotropic; that is, they radiated energy outward similarly in all directions. Recent work in ultrasonic tissue characterization suggests that the signal scattered backward toward the transducer is mainly related to the impedance mismatch of the scatterers.[6] However, the signal scattered away from the transducer is due to velocity changes. Diffuse reflectors are the result of impedance mismatches which are small compared to specular reflectors. They are thought to be in the range of $2 \lambda$ in diameter or smaller, so that the beam is defracted around diffuse reflectors. The scattering that occurs is not just reflected back to the transducer, but scatters all around the reflectors, bouncing off and being absorbed by the tissues surrounding it. The low-intensity beam that returns to the transducer is therefore due both to the low amplitude of the scattered beam and to the further attenuation of the radiated energy in the surrounding tissue (Fig 1–10).

### Attenuation

While reflection and scattering reduce the amplitude of an ultrasound wave, absorption of the wave contributes even more to the wave's attenuation. Absorption occurs when the mechanical energy in the pulse

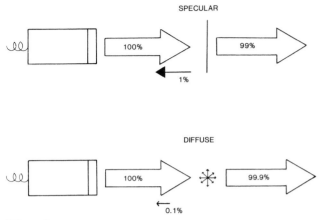

SPECULAR

DIFFUSE

**FIG 1–10.**
*Specular reflectors are large, smooth boundaries that must be nearly perpendicular to the beam path for the ultrasound beam to return to the transducer. Diffuse reflectors are small anatomic packets that weakly reflect in all directions and produce the characteristic parenchymal pattern of various organs.*

FREQUENCY SPECTRUM AT VARIOUS DEPTHS

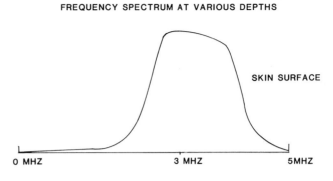

SKIN SURFACE

0 MHZ                3 MHZ                5MHZ

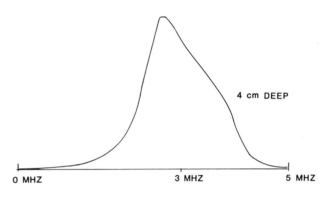

4 cm DEEP

0 MHZ                3 MHZ                5 MHZ

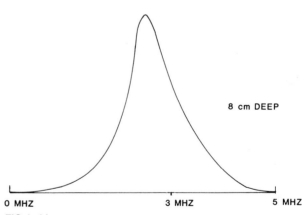

8 cm DEEP

0 MHZ                3 MHZ                5 MHZ

**FIG 1–11.**
*Higher frequency ultrasound is attenuated to a greater degree than lower frequency ultrasound. The body acts as a filter attenuating the higher frequency components of the frequency spectrum the deeper in the patient.*

of ultrasound is converted to thermal energy. This is mainly due to molecular relaxation and friction.[7] Absorption, like scattering, is frequency (f) dependent. However, scattering has an $f^2$ dependence, while most absorption of animal tissue at medical ultrasound frequencies has an f dependency.[8] Small variations in frequency dependence may prove useful for identifying pathogenic tissue, so this relationship is often investigated in tissue characterization experiments.

An ultrasound transducer operates not at a single frequency but at a frequency bandwidth. The wide-frequency bandwidth of the ultrasound wave is also affected by the increased attenuation of high-frequency ultrasound. As the ultrasound pulse travels through tissue, the higher frequencies in the wave packet are attenuated to a greater degree than the lower frequencies. This lowers the center frequency of the ultrasound wave as it passes into the patient and makes it harder to resolve small structures far from the transducer (Fig 1–11).[9]

Because attenuation is exponential in tissue but linear with distance traveled and frequency, it is commonly measured in dB/cm/MHz. The decibel, named after Alexander Graham Bell, is defined as

$$10 \log_{10}\frac{I_1}{I_2}$$

where $I_1$ is the intensity after attenuation and $I_2$ is the intensity before attenuation. If we are measuring voltage or amplitude, then the definition is

$$20 \log_{10}\frac{V_1}{V_2}$$

For example, if a wave equivalent to 2 V enters a patient, but is attenuated to 1 V after traveling 2 cm, then the attenuation is 6 dB. To compute the attenuation coefficient for the tissue traversed by the ultrasound, we must divide 6 dB by the 2 cm that the beam traveled and by the MHz frequency of the ultrasound. We can then use this attenuation coefficient to compute total attenuation for similar tissue for any frequency transducer.

## Dynamic Range

These computations are very useful when deciding which type of ultrasound instrument is needed for specific diagnostic tasks. Each manufacturer's unit will usually have a dynamic range varying from 80 to 110 dB. The dynamic range is the range of signals from the highest amplitude to lowest that the unit can receive and process. The frequency bandwidth of the unit will limit the lower range of signals, or sensitivity of the system, while the transistor types and amplifier design will limit the larger levels that can be processed without distortion. The television monitor can only display up to 30 dB variation in gray levels. However, we have data that range over 50 to 110 dB. Since the sound beam has been attenuated as it passed through the patient's tissue, some of the dynamic range must be used to compensate for this attenuation. We can compute how much attenuation compensation will be needed for our imaging task. If our work is limited to abdominal scans of adults, it is necessary to penetrate about 15 cm with a 3.5-MHz transducer. At 0.8 dB/cm/MHz attenuation, the 3.5-MHz ultrasound pulse, traveling 15 cm and returning 15 cm, will be reduced by $0.8 \times 30 \times 3.5 = 84$ dB. For this imaging task, we would select equipment with the largest dynamic range. If we are imaging a child, then 7 cm of penetration with a 5-MHz transducer gives $0.8 \times 14 \times 5 = 56$ dB. A lower dynamic range unit would be adequate.

The reduction in intensity of a sound beam occurs mainly because of absorption, then because of specular reflection, and finally because of diffuse reflection, or scattering. A crude rule of thumb is that attenuation of sound in soft tissue is approximately 1 dB/cm/MHz. In reality, it is slightly less than this, and 0.8 dB/cm/MHz was used in the example in the preceding paragraph. Ultrasound units must be able to compensate for the normal body attenuation of sound in order to equally represent equal anatomic structures that are at different depths within the patient.

## Time Gain Compensation

Attenuation compensation, or time gain compensation (TGC), is a method whereby the signals received from deep within the patient are altered so that they have the same decibel range as those close to the transducer. For display purposes, this range is 15–30 dB. Therefore, the ultrasound unit has 50–80 dB of dynamic range left to compensate for attenuation. This is usually accomplished by one of two methods.

The first type is the near gain, far gain, slope start, and slope method. The initial reflection and attenuation at the skin of a patient attenuate uniquely, so it must be set at a particular level for each patient. *Near gain* is a level of amplification needed to compensate for this initial loss. If a full bladder or other low attenuation structure intervenes initially, then the TGC can be delayed by the *slope start* setting. The overall attenuation is controlled by the *slope* of the TGC. It is steeper for higher frequency transducers. Presumably, *far gain* can be positioned at the same distance as the last attenuating structure in the patient (Fig 1–12). Unfortunately, sometimes it must be placed earlier in order to increase the slope for very attenuating patients. In this case, enhancement and shadowing will not be as reliable diagnostic signs beyond the position of the far gain distance.

The second method uses five to seven potentiometers mounted as sliders. This method allows the user to design individual TGCs, with each slider representing about 2 cm of tissue. However, care must be taken that each slider is at the same level or higher than the preceding one, since the curve represents total attenuation, not the attenuation of the 2 cm covered by the slider.

## Amplification and Signal Processing

Since the received voltage is often as low as 10–20 $\mu V$, the voltage received from the transducer must be amplified more than the amount that the TGC requires. Furthermore, the voltage consists of a wide band of frequencies, which must be preserved so that axial resolution is maintained. Amplifying broadband frequency signals is more difficult than amplifying narrow band frequencies. Only small amounts of amplification are possible, so several amplifier stages are required for medical ultrasound units. The character-

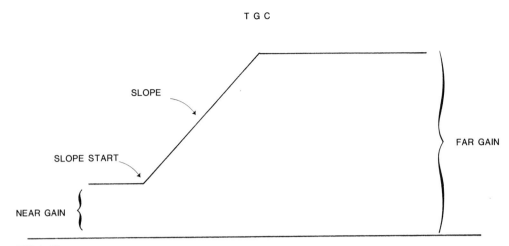

**FIG 1-12.**
*Time gain compensation (TGC) is used to compensate for normal body attenuation. Since higher frequencies are attenuated to a greater degree, the slope will be steeper for higher frequency transducers than for lower frequency transducers.*

istics of these amplifiers will affect the image produced on the B-mode or real-time unit. Several manufacturers preamplify the signal as soon as it is received by the transducer. If this amplifier is logarithmic, small signals are amplified more than larger voltages. Other manufacturers apply the TGC in the first stage of amplification and then gradually amplify the signal in stages until the final stage, which is a logarithmic amplifier.

Some bandpass filtering may accompany this amplification on the theory that the signal should not have frequencies outside the range of the original spectrum of frequencies that went into the patient. Frequencies outside the bandwidth are assumed to contain noise generated by the amplifiers. The signal will also be either full- or half-wave rectified so that all the voltage spikes are positive. The signal may be envelope detected so that small variations are smoothed.

### Analog/Digital Conversion, Digital Scan Conversion Storage

The amplified signal is digitized in one of two methods. It can be demodulated (i.e., rectified and smoothed so that only the peaks of the waves remain) and then the highest value within each sample size detected and digitized. Or it can be rectified (so that all the negative amplitudes are positive), digitized at a fixed high sample rate, and the peak values for the magnification intervals selected and digitized.

The digital scan conversion (DSC) memory is usually arranged in a square array of picture elements (pixels). On a B-mode fixed-arm scanner, potentiometers in the arm send position information back to the scanner for each A-line processed. These $x$, $y$, and $\theta$ coordinates, relative to the centering coordinates established when scanning began, allow each A-line to be placed in the DSC memory in its correct position. The $x$, $y$ coordinates give the location in the A-line of the first waveforms near the transducer, while $\theta$ gives the tilt of the transducer.

When several-A lines go through one pixel, the unit must have some method to decide what value belongs in the pixel. Real-time units always use the last element passing through the pixels. This is called the survey mode of DSC storage. When the largest value is stored instead, this is called the static mode and is used for compound scanning. A few units average the values passing through a pixel in the hopes of reducing the speckled appearance of ultrasound images.

### Gray-Scale Assignment

Digital scan conversion memory allows reliable and reproducible gray-value assignment for each returning wave amplitude. The range of amplitudes in the body can be over 100 dB. Since the highest quality TV monitor can display only 30 dB, some compression of these amplitudes is necessary. For instance, the soft tissue—air interface between the diaphragm and lungs reflects almost all the sound and should be displayed as 0 dB down from the peak intensity. The skin-water interface in a waterpath mammography unit causes the amplitude to drop from 10 V to 100 mV, or −40 dB. If we mapped the 30 dB available on a TV monitor without compression into equal gray levels, we would not have any gray levels left to display soft tissues. Since we want to also display small internal echoes, which are from 10 mV to 100 μV, or −60 dB to −100 dB, we must make uneven assignments between amplitudes and gray-scale values (Fig 1–13).

Most manufacturers amplify the returning signals logarithmically. Small voltages are amplified more than larger voltages. Thus a 1V echo from a tissue-bone interface may only be amplified by 5, while the fine scattering from a neonatal brain at 100 μV may be amplified over 100 times. If the received signal has been log-amplified before the TGC is applied, then the gray-scale assignment can be more nearly linear, since amplitudes have already been compressed to a 30 dB range. However, as tissue characterization imaging becomes more reliable, manufacturers providing quantitative data will prefer to maintain nearly linear amplifiers and compress ultrasound amplitudes just before storage in the DSC memory.

Usually digitization occurs by changing the sample rate with the magnification. Thus at the highest magnification, the highest digitization rate is applied. The signal is peak detected while it is still in analog form, and then the peak signal is digitized and stored. The detected signal is processed through a cascade of resistors which register the boundaries between gray levels. Changes in the resistor levels will change the gray-scale assignment.

The ability to select or even create different gray-scale assignment tables can be a mixed blessing. if certain clinical landmarks are missing, it is a real advantage to rescan at a more logarithmic gray-scale setting, so that texture changes and other faintly visible anatomy can be imaged. However, texture is more dependent on the gray-scale map than on any other instrumentation parameters.[10] If normal texture is imaged with both a logarithmic and a linear gray-scale assignment, the texture will appear very light and uneven with the linear assignment. This is because the small differences in texture echoes must be expanded logarithmically to be visualized in different shades of gray. Since we can resolve only ten gray levels on a 30 dB television monitor, one might ask why more than ten gray levels are offered. The main reason is so that postprocessing the gray level assignment of an acquired image may illustrate the differences in specular reflectors as well as faint anatomic details hidden in texture gray levels. If only 16 gray levels have been saved, then remapping these gray levels will not add information to the image. However, if an image was acquired with 64 or more gray values, then windowing, recompressing, and even linearizing the gray levels down to 16 displayed values will yield new information without rescanning.

## Resolution

Medical ultrasound images do not show as much detail as x-ray images, and so are said to have poorer resolution. As was mentioned at the beginning of this chapter, there are three different resolution measurements in ultrasound images. How good each of these resolutions is depends on how far the object being imaged is from the transducer. We have discussed axial (range or longitudinal) resolution. It is dependent on the frequency, amplification, and the pulse length of the wave packet. As tissue attenuates the high-frequency component of the spectrum of frequencies making up the pulse, axial resolution gets worse the deeper the beam travels into tissue. This is because the center frequency is reduced and because the pulse width gets longer. Furthermore, for very deep penetration, output power and/or gain is usually in-

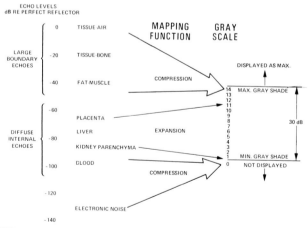

**FIG 1–13.**
*Gray-scale assignment yields maximum diagnostic results when soft tissue echoes are selectively expanded over the majority of gray levels.*

creased by the technologist. This also lengthens the pulse and makes axial resolution worse. However, it remains the best resolution direction in ultrasound and is usually about 2–3 mm. While scanning, we are unconsciously using axial resolution to resolve difficult problems.

Lateral resolution, or the resolution of objects parallel to the face of the transducer, varies from 3 mm to 3 cm, depending on how deep the object is to the transducer. This resolution is also called azimuthal or transverse resolution.

A transducer wafer is usually 1–2 cm in diameter and emits a number of wavelets when pulsed. These wavelets combine, according to Huygen's principle,[11] to form patterns of constructive and destructive interference. As they move farther from the transducer, they constructively interfere at a last peak intensity value in the focal zone and gradually spread apart thereafter. The region where the wavelets constructively and destructively interfere is called the near or Fresnel zone. The far field beyond the last peak intensity is called the Fraunhofer zone. Lateral resolution is determined by the thickness of the beam, which varies according to the depth in the patient. Lateral resolution is best in the focal zone. When we wish to measure a structure with ultrasound, such as a fetal head, we image it so that measurements are in the axial direction rather than in the lateral direction. This is done because axial resolution is better than lateral resolution.

The final direction of resolution is the slice thickness or elevation direction. For a round transducer, this behaves just like lateral direction. If the transducer is split, which occurs in one automated mammography unit and in continuous wave Doppler instruments, then the slice thickness will vary from the lateral direction resolution. This is particularly a problem in phased arrays.

*Transducer Construction*

The major component of a transducer is the piezoelectric element. We have already discussed piezoelectric properties and the construction of a piezoelectric element. In this section we will discuss the thickness and diameter of the piezoelectric element and how these features relate to the ultrasound beam. The thickness of the cut of the piezoelectric element determines the center frequency of the vibrations of the piezoelectric wafer. When the piezoelectric element is struck by a short pulse of voltage, it will vibrate at its resonant frequency, which is determined by its thickness ($\lambda/2$). The formula $\lambda = v/f$ will determine the thickness of the wafer. Since the piezoelectric material is brittle, this thin wafer is fragile and must not be dropped. Remember that the velocity used in the determination of the thickness of the wafer is the velocity of sound in the piezoelectric material, not in body soft tissue. When a short electrical pulse is applied to the piezoelectric wafer, the wafer will ring at its resonant frequency. This vibration will gradually decrease over a period of time until the mechanical oscillations stop completely. The backing material of a transducer will cause the oscillation to stop in three or four cycles.

Damping material, usually tungsten powder embedded in epoxy, is placed behind the piezoelectric wafer. Like placing a hand on the ringing wine glass, this damping material stops the transducer's transmission of sound after the initial packet of sound is transmitted into the patient. Axial resolution (resolution along the direction of the sound beam) is controlled by the thickness of the wafer ($\lambda/2$) and the pulse width.

While the thickness of the piezoelectric wafer determines the frequency of the transducer, the diameter determines the focusing properties of the ultrasound beam generated. Unfocused transducers are no longer used clinically, but we can obtain important information with a short discussion of an unfocused transducer. The focal length of a focused transducer cannot be made longer than the distance of the last maximum intensity point ($r^2/\lambda$) of an unfocused transducer of similar diameter and frequency. We can calculate the focal zone by the formula

$$X_{max} = r^2/\lambda$$

where $X_{max}$ is the distance to the last maximum intensity point and r is the radius of the transducer wafer (Fig 1–14). Thus two 2.25-MHz transducers, one 13 mm in diameter and the other 19 mm in diameter, will have focal distances of 62 mm ($6.5^2/.684$) and 132 mm ($9.5^2/.684$), respectively. How wide the beam will spread in the far field past this point is also determined by the frequency and the diameter of the transducer. As frequency increases, the spreading of the beam in the far field will be more gradual. As the di-

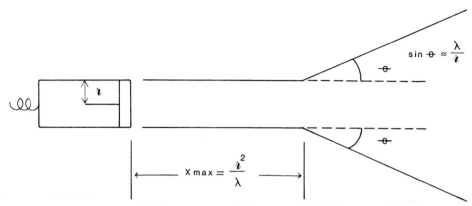

$$\sin \theta \approx \frac{\lambda}{r}$$

$$X\,max = \frac{r^2}{\lambda}$$

**FIG 1–14.**
*The radius (r) and wavelength (λ) of the transducer determine the last maximum intensity point (X max). The beam cannot be focused beyond this point and will spread in the far field according to the formula, sin θ = λ/r.*

ameter of the transducer increases, the spreading of the beam will also be more gradual. Therefore, a high-frequency, large-diameter transducer will have the longest focal zone as well as the least divergence in the far field.

Focused rather than unfocused transducers are used in the clinical setting. Focusing a transducer improves lateral resolution. A transducer can be focused internally or externally. The piezoelectric wafer can be cut in a curved shape so that the vibrations at the periphery of the wafer are closer to the region of interest than those emitted from the center of the wafer (Fig 1–15). This is called internal focusing and is often used in 2.25- or 3.5-MHz transducers. However, as

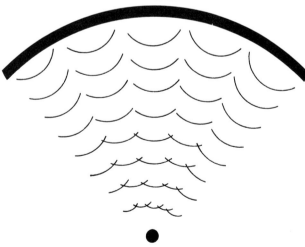

**FIG 1–15.**
*A focused transducer can be constructed by curving the piezo-electric crystal. The vibrations from the periphery of the wafer are closer to the area of interest than those from the center of the transducer.*

mentioned earlier, a 5-MHz wafer is only 0.4 mm thick. This is too delicate to be practical for internal focusing. Therefore, high-frequency transducers are focused externally.

The second way to focus a transducer is to place an external acoustic lens in front of the piezoelectric wafer. The lens material is impedance matched to the piezoelectric crystal, but the velocity of sound in the wafer is different from velocity of sound in the material in front of it, so that refraction occurs and the ultrasound beam is bent inward when it exits the lens. The amount of curvature determines the degree of focusing for that particular transducer. The greater the curvature of the wafer or the lens, the sharper the focus. As focusing increases, the diameter of the ultrasound beam in the focal region decreases. Therefore, increased focusing of a transducer will decrease the diameter of the ultrasound beam and essentially improve lateral resolution. A highly focused transducer will have much better lateral resolution in the focal zone than an unfocused transducer of the same diameter.

Let us consider the construction of a 5-MHz, 19-mm-diameter transducer. Unfocused, this transducer will have a Fresnel zone that ends at 30 cm. Because of attenuation, a 5-MHz transducer can rarely image deeper than 8 cm. Therefore, it is usually focused by an external lens to about 5 cm. This requires a very curved lens for focusing. The focal zone will only be 2–3 cm in length and there will be rapid divergence of the beam once the far field is reached. However, because of the sharp focusing, the lateral resolution of this 5-MHz, 19-mm transducer will be much smaller in diameter in the focal zone than the size of the transducer face.

Let us construct an ultrasound transducer from scratch. First, we must construct the piezoelectric element at high temperature in an electric field and then let it cool. Then we must produce the piezoelectric wafer at λ/2 thickness for whatever frequency we wish to use. Once the correct thickness is determined, we cut the transducer to a diameter that suits our purposes. Assume we are dealing with a 5-MHz, 19-mm-diameter transducer. As mentioned before, the thickness of the wafer is 0.4 mm and the diameter of the wafer is 19 mm. Now we plate the two circular surfaces of the crystal with conductive material. The surface near the patient is grounded and the surface away from the patient carries a 250-V pulse. This plating conducts the short electrical pulse needed to excite the wafer so that it rings at its resonant frequency. A focusing lens is attached to the front of the transducer with a thin layer of epoxy. The lens is covered with a material that differs in velocity appropriately for focusing but has an impedance close to that of the patient's skin. We wish to avoid reflections between piezoelectric wafer, lens, and the patient. These reflections reduce the amount of ultrasound power available for entering into the patient. These reflections can be reduced by using what are called quarter-wave matching layers. The material placed in front of the wafer is cut at λ/4 and attached to the wafer. This series of elements—wafer, damping material, electrodes, and acoustic lens—is placed in a protective casing. This entire complex makes up an ultrasound transducer (Fig 1–16).

## Real-Time Imaging

Real-time imaging is used to study moving parts of the body (such as the heart), to eliminate artifacts in static scans caused by respiration or peristalsis, or to obtain a three-dimensional image by using the observer's eye-brain image analysis talents on rapidly changing sections of anatomy. We previously described the timing considerations in pulse-echo imaging (see Fig 1–1). Real-time imaging uses similar computations to determine how fast and deep a real-time unit can image. We showed earlier that a 20-cm-deep A-line takes 0.26 msec to return to the trans-

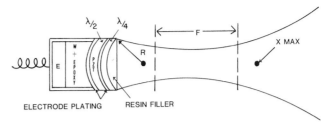

**FIG 1–16.**
*A transducer is composed of a piezoelectric wafer (PZT) cut λ/2 in thickness with electrode plating on each surface. Its backing material is composed of tungsten (W) plus epoxy along with electrical components (E). A quarter wave (λ/4) matching layer may be placed on the wafer. If internal focusing is used, the wafer will be curved with a radius (r) of curvature which produces a focal zone (F) that cannot be extended past the last maximum intensity point (X_{max}).*

ducer. If we only need to image 10 cm, then the wave returns in 0.13 sec. In real-time imaging, each collection of A-lines makes up a frame (as in cine). If we wish to form a flicker-free image, we will need at least 25 frames/sec. If each frame is made up of 100 lines of reflected ultrasound, then 2,500 lines/sec must be generated, received, and processed. This allows 0.4 msec per line. To image at a 20-cm depth, 0.26 msec is needed for sending and receiving and 0.14 msec is available for processing the signal into an image. If processing takes longer, then the frame rate, depth, or lines per frame must be reduced. The formula

$$\frac{\text{frames}}{\text{sec}} \times \frac{\text{lines}}{\text{frame}} \times \frac{\text{depth}}{\text{line}} < 77,000$$

reflects the interrelationship with velocity,[12] but does not include processing restrictions.

This formula represents the problems that real-time imaging has in scanning wide, deep and fast, all at the same time. Many manufacturers will offer a slower frame rate (15 frames/sec) when wider, deeper scans are needed. Some processing options also use a slower frame rate or fewer lines per image. Several manufacturers refresh alternate lines each frame, so that the image changes at 30 frames/sec, but only half the lines are current. Higher frequency real-time transducers cannot penetrate as deep as lower frequency transducers. Since the depth at which they scan is limited, real-time high-frequency transducers may offer more lines per scan or a faster frame rate.

There are two methods of generating a real-time image: the transducer can be mechanically moved, or many small transducers arranged in an array can be fired sequentially. Mechanical real-time transducers usually produce a sector image with a high density of lines and limited field of view near the transducer. The width of the sector can be varied as well as the range on some units.

The best concept for understanding a mechanical real-time transducer is that of a B-scan transducer and a technician with a floppy wrist. Mechanical real-time results from rapid oscillation of transducer (Fig 1–17,A), rotation of several transducers (Fig 1–17,B), or oscillation of an acoustic mirror (Fig 1–17,C). The weight of the transducer has inertia when it is rocked. This problem may be solved in three ways: (1) an acoustic mirror rocking in front of a fixed transducer produces a sector scan; (2) the damping material on the back of the transducer can be reduced or eliminated, so that the short pulse is dependent entirely on several λ/4 matching layers between the transducer and the fluid that the transducer oscillates in; or (3) three transducers mounted together can rotate, each imaging for 120° to produce one frame. This results in three frames per revolution.

Most sectoring transducers are surrounded by a fluid. A plastic or rubber membrane contains the fluid and presses against the patient. Even when the acoustic impedances of the fluid and membrane are carefully selected, some reflection occurs. This reduces the sensitivity of mechanical scanners.

Problems can also develop in single sectoring transducers at the ends of the sector, when the transducer is either slowing down or speeding up as a result of direction changes. If this speed change is not included in the digital scan conversion storage algorithm, then registration errors in the 15° edges of the sector may cause straight edges to curve down at each side of the sector.[13] For this reason, lateral measurement accuracy must be included in quality control procedures of real-time sectoring transducers. This is another reason why it is always better to obtain measurements in the axial rather than lateral direction.

The second type of real-time transducer is the phased array transducer, an electronically steered and focused array of small transducers. To explain this method, we will begin with a linear array of single transducers. Suppose 100 small rectangular wafers are placed in a line about 10 cm long and 1 cm wide. Each piezoelectric element in the array is a rectangle 1 cm by 1 mm. We know from the section on transducer construction that the ultrasound waves emitted

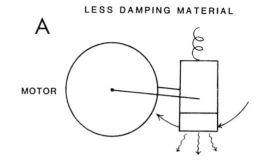

LESS DAMPING MATERIAL

A   MOTOR

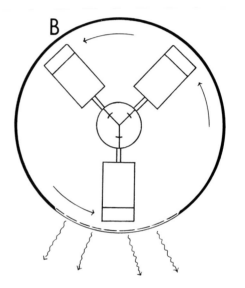

B

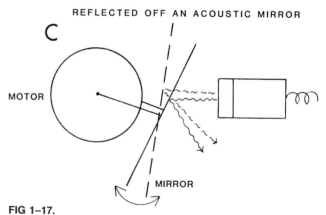

REFLECTED OFF AN ACOUSTIC MIRROR

C   MOTOR

MIRROR

**FIG 1–17.**
*A, mechanical real-time scanning can be produced by rapidly oscillating a transducer back and forth. Less damping material is used so the transducer can change direction more easily. B, real-time scanning is produced when three transducers are rotated continuously in the same direction. Each transducer is functioning only when it passes the small sector open region. C, real-time scanning can be achieved using a stationary transducer and oscillating an acoustic mirror back and forth.*

from smaller diameter wafers will act as though they were in the far field. They will spread out, producing poor images. If ten adjacent elements are fired at once, then, according to Huygen's principle, a columnated ultrasound pulse is formed that will have the focusing characteristics of a $1 \times 1$ cm unfocused transducer. If we now place an acoustic lens on each 1 cm $\times$ 1 mm crystal so that the slice thickness (which was 1 cm thick) is now focused, we can produce a useful medical image by firing sequential sets of ten adjacent elements at a time. Thus elements 1–10 are fired and receive returning waves, elements 2–11 are fired and receive, elements 3–12 are fired, and so on, until finally elements 91–100 are fired and receive. This results in 91 A-lines which are mapped into a real-time rectangular image 9 cm wide.

If we wish to form a steered array with a linear array, we need only put in a sequential delay when firing each of the crystals that previously were fired together. This delay causes an interference pattern (Fig 1–18). The pulses of constructive interference represent the direction of the wave front. Similarly, we can focus the linear array by firing the outside elements

earlier than those in the middle (Fig 1–19). The out-of-phase pulses will constructively interfere at the focal zone. If the focal zone is needed farther from the transducer, the delay in firing is reduced. The firing of phased arrays is controlled by mircoprocessors but depends on a constant tissue velocity.

This process can also be implemented by introducing a delay at the receive end to focus the received reflections. If each depth is processed with a different set of delays, a focus can be formed for each depth. This complex process is called dynamic focusing. Transducers can also be dynamically focused in the transmit mode by reducing the frame rate.[14] If three focal zones are desired, then three A-lines are generated for each line of the frame. Each-A line will be focused for a different zone. On receive, only the data from the focused zone will be used for that part of the image. Focusing can be combined with steering, but processing often takes up more time between lines, so that only 15 frames/sec are generated.

All phased-array scanners have slice thickness focusing by external lenses, so even though they are dynamically focused in the azimuth direction, the elevation direction has a near, focal, and far field. Annular-array scanners try to correct the problem of fixed elevation focus. They consist of two or more rings of

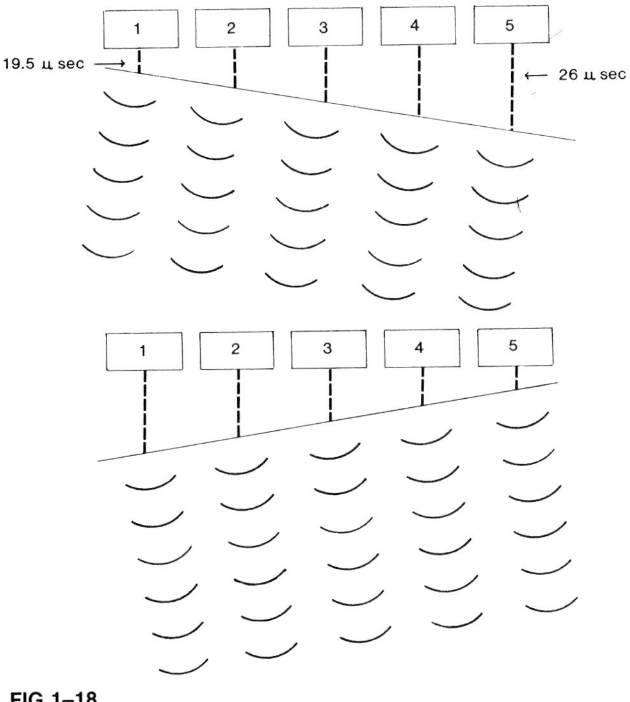

**FIG 1–18.**
*Real-time imaging can be achieved with phased-array systems. As the time sequence of firing the different elements is varied, interference patterns are set up that angle the wave front with respect to the transducer face. This creates an oscillating beam, which results in a real-time image.*

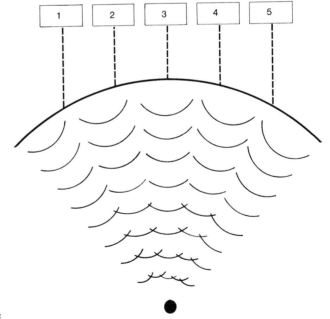

**FIG 1–19.**
*Phased-array systems can be focused by delaying the firing of central elements compared with respect to peripheral ones. The depth of focus can be changed by varying the time sequence.*

small transducers arranged about a center element. By dynamically focusing the rings, both azimuth and elevation can be focused.[15]

When phased-array and mechanical real-time transducers are compared, mechanical sectors usually produce more aesthetically pleasing images, with sharper edges and less artifactual speckle. However, phased-array transducers are more sensitive and can be focused more sharply.

## Artifacts

While some ultrasound artifacts can lead to misdiagnosis, other artifacts can aid diagnosis, since they often give information about tissue characteristics. Examples of artifacts that aid diagnoses are enhancement and shadowing behind lesions. Time gain compensation (TGC) is set with an assumption that attenuation is constant through tissue. When a lesion is imaged that does not have the same attenuation as surrounding tissue, it will either not use up all the gain assigned to it, if it is less attenuating, or it will use up all the gain assigned to it as well as that TGC assigned posterior to the tissue. In the first case, the image will be brighter behind the mass, so it has posterior enhancement. In the more attenuating lesion, the area posterior to the mass will be less echogenic or attenuating. Figure 1–20 shows three echo free masses with (1) no change in attenuation, (2) in-

creased attenuation, and (3) enhanced transmissions. Only (3) is fluid because of enhanced transmission. The others are solid. Echo free does not mean fluid.

### Posterior Shadowing

When the lesion becomes more dense or even calcified, as in the case of renal calculi, the impedance difference between the surrounding tissue and the mass increases. Reflection also contributes to attenuation in the stone and produces a posterior shadow. Sometimes ultrasound transmitted into the mass will be reflected off the back wall of the mass and will be imaged as a reverberation in the shadow.[16, 17]

Shadows also occur when the ultrasound beam encounters air in the body. These shadows are the result of the large impedance mismatch between tissue and air. If due to bowel gas, they will move secondary to peristalsis.[18] Shadows occurring from the skin are due to scars or poor application of coupling gel. Air is trapped between the transducer and skin and causes shadowing. Finally, a shadow may be generated by a linear array when an element is defective. This shadow will occur in the same place on the image wherever the array is placed on the patient.

Critical angle refraction, which looks like a shadow, is the complete loss of the posterior ultrasound beam due to the beam striking an oblique surface which has a higher velocity of sound than the more anterior tissue. Critical angle refraction is most commonly encountered at the capsule surrounding a cyst.

### Posterior Enhancement

Posterior enhancement behind less attenuating tissue is also used diagnostically to differentiate solid from fluid-filled masses. Cysts, hematomas, and abscesses all show posterior enhancement. In the breast, some solid lesions, such as fibroadenoma and medullar carcinoma, may show posterior enchancement because they are less attenuating than the tissue surrounding them.[19]

### Anechoic Masses

Masses are assumed to be solid if they have internal echoes on ultrasound images and show no posterior

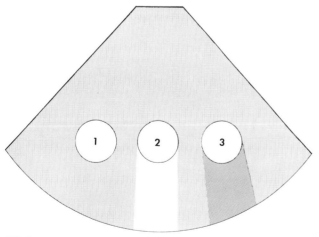

**FIG 1–20.**
*Echo-free masses are not always cystic. Evaluation of the echoes deep to the mass is necessary to determine its nature. Mass 1 has equal echo amplitude deep to it compared to surrounding tissue and therefore is a soft tissue mass. Mass 2 has decreased amplitude deep to it and is an attenuating solid. Mass 3 has enhanced through-transmission and is fluid.*

enhancement. Sonolucent masses only indicate a homogeneous internal structure and do not indicate cysts. In order to determine whether the mass is solid or fluid, it is necessary to evaluate the echoes deep to the mass (Fig 1–21). If enhancement is present, the mass is cystic. If the echoes posterior to the mass are equal to or less than the echoes from adjacent tissue, then the mass is solid. It is always important to evaluate how a mass interacts with the ultrasound beam by evaluating the region directly behind the mass. Occasionally we may see echoes within a mass that are artifacts. These echoes occur if the gain or power is too high. In particular, obstetric scanning with a full bladder may show echoes in the anterior portion of the bladder when the gain is too high. Similarly, cysts tend to fill in with artifactual echoes from anterior to posterior as gain is increased. These echoes are the result of reverberation from the small reflectors anterior to the fluid-filled structure. Because they reflect back and forth between scattering tissue before returning to the transducer, they take a longer time to return than primary scatter. The increased time is calculated as increased distance by the ultrasound unit, so it is mapped posterior to the position of the scatterer. If a cyst is located posterior to the scatterer, the cyst is filled with scatter reverberation echoes in its anterior portion. Since the amplitude of scattered echoes is low compared to reflected echoes, these secondary scattering echoes are only assigned gray level values when the gain is large. If the mass were solid, its interior echoes would overwhelm the secondary scattering echoes. We may also see artifactual echoes in small anechoic regions located in the far field of the scanning transducer. These echoes are due to a partial volume effect, similar to that found in CT imaging when the slice thickness exceeds the diameter of the mass being imaged.[20]

*Phantom Masses*

When a highly reflective border occurs near an anechoic region, reverberations between the reflector and the region will be mapped by the ultrasound unit into the anechoic region. For example, these reverberations create artifactual tumors behind the diaphragm.[21] When the gain is reduced or the direction of the ultrasound beam is changed, the artifactual tumors disappear. This artifact can aid diagnosis if the original tumor is missed. Once the artifactual mass is recognized above the diaphragm, the liver can be more closely examined to identify the true lesion.

Large reflecting surfaces can also create reverberation echoes of sufficient strength to look like tumors in lightly textured posterior structures. When a mass seems to be behind a bowel loop, note whether its size is the same as the more anterior echo. Phantom masses always have the same axial dimensions as the structures that generated them; they can change position when the transducer is moved to a new scanning position.

*Reverberations*

The interface between the transducer and the skin is a large reflector that registers initially as a high-amplitude echo. If the pulse strikes a strong interface such as bone or air close to the skin, a large percentage of the wave will be reflected back to the skin-transducer interface. This returning wave will register as an echo but a large percentage will be reflected back into the patient for a second trip. This occurs because of the large acoustic mismatch between the skin and the transducer. The wave from the second trip encounters the highly reflective bone or air interface and the entire process is repeated. This occurs over and over until the energy of the wave is dissipated. The end result is a series of echoes equidistant and symmetrically decreasing in amplitude (Fig 1–22).

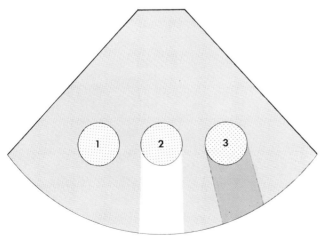

**FIG 1–21.**
*Masses with internal echoes are nonhomogeneous. Their nature is determined by evaluating the echoes deep to the mass. Mass 1 is soft tissue, mass 2 is an attenuating solid, mass 3 is fluid.*

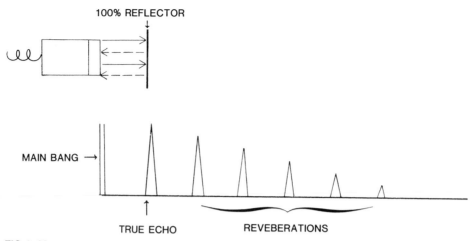

**FIG 1–22.**
*Reverberation artifacts are created when the transducer is close to a highly reflective interface. Nearly all of the pulse returns to the transducer, where it is again reflected for a repeat trip. The result is a series of echoes that are equidistant but steadily decreasing in amplitude.*

Similarly, if the ultrasound beam encounters a hard reflective object, like metal, some of the beam is transmitted, and as it re-reflects within the hard object, a comet-tail of reverberations will result.[16]

### Beam Thickness

Since lateral resolution is usually no better than 3 mm, even in the focal zone, a point target in the far field will look like a line with thickening in the center. The dimensions of the line can be reduced if the gain (and/or output power) is reduced. When a neonatal head or any other curved surface is imaged, the surface on the sides will appear thicker than the top and bottom surfaces because of beam thickness artifact. This is why all measurements should be made in the axial direction, where accuracies to 2 mm are possible, rather than in the lateral direction, where errors of 5 or 6 mm are common.

### Duplication Artifact Secondary to the Abdominal Wall

Besides critical angle shadowing, refraction can also cause the appearance of double gestational sacs and a double head boundary artifact. When the beam encounters the rectus abdominis muscles transversely, the muscle and fat layers refract the beam so that the path is longer and the gestational sac is imaged lateral than its true position (Fig 1–23). A similar scan on the other side of the abdomen images the gestational sac lateral to the true position. The two images are beside each other rather than overlying each other in the correct position.[22, 23] Rescanning in the longitudinal direction will show one gestational sac.

### Organ Boundary Discontinuities

Besides refraction artifacts, velocity changes can also create pseudo-splits in organ boundaries. Normally, changes in tissue velocity from the ultrasound units,

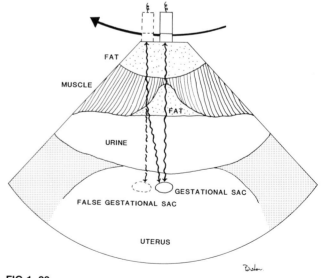

**FIG 1–23.**
*Duplication artifacts can occur secondary to refraction or bending of the beam. Duplication artifacts commonly arise from the anterior abdominal wall.*

assumed to be 1,540 m/sec, do not make more than a 1 or 2 mm difference. When a mass with a markedly different velocity of sound is anterior to an organ boundary, then the boundary may show an artifactual split or discontinuity.[24] Encapsulated liver cysts or tumors with a higher velocity of sound than soft tissue cause refraction of the beam and can also contribute to discontinuities in the diaphragm.[25] Distortions of the beam's lateral resolution have been shown to be significant when the beam passes between the ribs.[26] More recent work has shown that scanning through the cartilage of the ribs can image a pseudo lesion of the liver because of the refraction caused by the higher velocity of sound in cartilage.[27]

*Digital Scan Conversion Memory Mapping Artifacts*

Artifacts due to velocity variations cause incorrect computation of the position of the tissue causing a returned echo. Other incorrect computations internal to the ultrasound unit (not dependent on tissue variations) may also cause artifacts. For example, if the reference voltage established for the scanning arm positioning is unstable,[28] a scalloped artifact similar to what is seen when the transducer is dragged across an unoiled patient can result. For real-time mechanical units with more than one transducer creating sequential frames, interframe, jitter can result if the transducers are not aligned. Even if a single mechanical sector transducer forms half of each frame (the subsequent sweep writes in alternate lines at 15 frams/sec), image jitter may result if the left-to-right sweep does not exactly match the right-to-left sweep. Measurement artifacts can also result in real-time mechanical sector units if the end of the sweep is not as fast as the beginning and middle of the transducer movement.[13] This artifact causes bending of straight interfaces at the sides of the sector, loss of lateral resolution, and caliper measurement inaccuracies for structures measured in the lateral direction.

*Other Real-Time Imaging Artifacts*

All transducers have side lobes that are usually low in amplitude and do not cause problems in properly designed units where sensitivity is adjusted so that side lobe echoes will not be recorded on the image (Fig 1–24). Grating lobes are similar to side lobes, but have

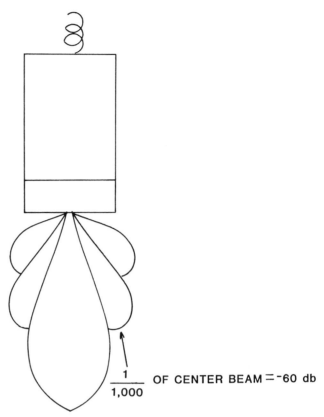

$$\frac{1}{1,000} \text{ OF CENTER BEAM} = {}^{-}60 \text{ db}$$

**FIG 1–24.**
*Side lobes can occasionally cause artifacts. They are usually much lower in echo amplitude than the central beam.*

greater magnitude and only occur in arrays when the separation between elements is too large. Grating lobes (and side lobes, if they are present) create spurious echoes to one side of large reflectors, sometimes creating diagonal septa or linear structures off the diaphragm. They are a defect in the unit's design and can be discovered by a good quality control test of the beam characteristics with a fabric test object. The spurious echoes caused by lobes are static. They do not move on rescanning unless the transducer moves.

Another artifact is responsible for the shimmering echoes seen in real-time units with fast frame rates. These echoes are the result of scattered and reflected echoes from the previous frame which arrived too late to be included in that frame's image. If the frame rate is reduced, the shimmering echoes will disappear.

## References

1. Wells PNT: *Biomedical Ultrasonic.* San Francisco, Academic Press, 1977, pp 164–168.

2. Wicks JD, Howe KS: *Fundamentals of Ultrasonographic Technique.* Chicago, Year Book Medical Publishers, Inc, 1983, pp 1–3.
3. Well PNT: *Biomedical Ultrasonic.* San Francisco, Academic Press, 1977, p 52.
4. McDicken WN: *Diagnostic Ultrasound: Principles and Use of Instruments.* New York, John Wiley & Sons, Inc, 1981, pp 56, 68.
5. Chivers RC: The scattering of ultrasound by human tissues: some theoretical models. *Ultrasound Med Biol* 1977; 3:1.
6. Jones JP, Leeman S: Ultrasonic tissue characterization: A review. *Acta Electronica* 1984; 26:3.
7. Dunn F: *Acoustic properties of biological materials,* in Michaelson SM, Miller MW (eds): *Fundamental and Applied Aspects of Nonionizing Radiation.* New York, Plenum Press, 1975, pp 21–36.
8. Goss SA, Tizzell LA, Dunn F: Ultrasonic absorption and attenuation in mammalian tissues. *Ultrasound Med Biol* 1979; 5:181.
9. Zagzebski JA, Banjavic RA, Madsen EL, et al: Focused transducer beams in tissue mimicking material. *JCU* 1982; 10:159.
10. Kimme-Smith C, Jones JP: The relative effects of system parameters on texture in gray scale ultrasonograms. *Ultrasound Med Biol* 1984; 10:299.
11. Wells PNT: *Biomedical Ultrasonic.* San Francisco, Academic Press, 1977, p 43.
12. Kremkau F: *Diagnostic Ultrasound: Physical Principles and Exercises.* New York, Grune & Stratton, 1980, p 106.
13. Winter J, Kimme-Smith C, King W: Measurement accuracy of ultrasound sector scanner. *AJR* 1985; 44:645.
14. McKnight R: A mixing scheme to focus a transducer array dynamically. *Hewlett-Packard Journal* 1983; 3412:16.
15. Arditi M, Taylor WB, Foster FS, et al: An annular array system for high resolution breast echography. *Ultrasonic Imaging* 1982; 4:1.
16. Ziskin MC, Thickman DI, Goldenberg NJ, et al: The comet tail artifact. *J Ultrasound Med* 1982; 1:1.
17. Thickman DI, Ziskin MC, Goldenberg NJ, et al: Clinical manifestations of the comet tail artifact. *J Ultrasound Med* 1983; 2:225.
18. Burt TB, Knochel JQ, Lee TG: Gas as a contrast agent and diagnostic aid in abdominal sonography. *J Ultrasound Med* 1982; 1:179.
19. Bassett L, Gold R, Kimme-Smith C: *Hand-held and Automated Breast Ultrasound.* New York, Slack Publishers, 1985.
20. Goldstein A, Madrazo BL: Slice-thickness artifacts in gray scale ultrasound. *JCU* 1981; 9:365.
21. Laing FC: Commonly encountered artifacts in clinical ultrasound. *Semin Ultrasound* 1983; 4:27.
22. Muller N, Cooperberg PL, Rowley VA, et al: Ultrasonic refraction by the rectus abdominis muscles: The double image artifact. *J Ultrasound Med* 1984; 3:515.
23. Sauerbrei EE: The split image artifact in pelvic ultrasonography: The anatomy and physics. *J Ultrasound Med* 1985; 4:29.
24. Pierce G, Golding RH, Cooperberg PL: The effects of tissue velocity changes on acoustical interfaces. *J Ultrasound Med* 1982; 1:185.
25. Mayo J, Cooperberg PL: Displacement of the diaphragmatic echo by hepatic cysts: A new explanation with computer simulation. *J Ultrasound Med* 1983; 2:225.
26. Savakus AD, Shung KK, Miller NB: Distortions of ultrasonic field introduced by the rib cage in echocardiography. *JCU* 1982; 10:413.
27. Bonhoff JA, Linhart P: A pseudo lesion of the liver caused by rib cartilage in B-mode ultrasonography. *J Ultrasound Med* 1985; 4:135.
28. Powis RL, Powis WJ: *A Thinker's Guide to Ultrasonic Imaging.* Baltimore, Urban & Schwartzenberg, 1984, p 385.

# 1a.
# BIOLOGIC EFFECTS AND SAFETY

## Frederick W. Kremkau, Ph.D.

The biologic effects and safety of ultrasound imaging in medicine have received considerable attention during the past few years. The public media have dealt with the subject repeatedly with such quotations as the following:

" . . . sparking concern among some doctors who say that it hasn't been proven completely safe."

"Thus far, research has turned up no danger in the technique, . . ."

"Ultrasound: Unsound?"

"Ultrasound technique sparks medical worry."

"How long must ultrasound be on trial?"

"'Safe' form of radiation arouses new worry."

"Limits are advised on viewing fetuses through ultrasound."

"Is ultrasound safe?"

"Ultrasound waves may threaten fetus."

"Caution advised on use of ultrasound."

" . . . insidious dangers on unborn children of invisible ultrasonic waves, . . ."

" . . . a sonogram, or ultrasound, or echogram. Whatever you want to call it, it's safe, . . ."

"Ultrasonics: a safe substitute for x-rays."

" . . . there are questions about the safety of ultrasound."

" . . . critics urge restrictions on its use until more data are available."

"One of the basic principles in modern medicine is that doctors never give up one dangerous procedure without taking on another."

"Armed with complete knowledge of ultrasound's scientifically-established risks, pregnant women can strategically challenge their doctors to prove that this form of diagnostic energy is absolutely essential in their case."

"When parents agree to amniocentesis and ultrasound, they should be aware that their own babies may well be part of the research to determine the possible deleterious effects of these procedures."

"Safe ultrasound video 'movies' made in the comfort of your own home."

"Food and Drug Administration officials candidly admit they cannot say diagnostic ultrasound during pregnancies is safe."

"What scientists and officials are saying is that they really don't know whether ultrasound is dangerous to human fetuses. But they have new clues that suggest we should go easy on its use until we know more, because overuse today is not worth the risk of long-term terrible genetic effects in the future."

Medical journal articles and advertisements have included statements such as the following:

" . . . and to encourage the use of this safe and accurate diagnostic modality."

"Question of risk still hovers . . ."

"The ultrasound debate: safe or subtly harmful?"

"Completely safe . . . no adverse reactions or risks to the patient."

Several review articles on the subject have been published.[1-9] Two textbooks on the subject have been published,[10, 11] and several organizations and institutions have produced monographs.[12-18] The Bioeffects Committee of the American Institute of Ultrasound in Medicine regularly reviews, evaluates, and places in context relevant reports for health professionals who use diagnostic ultrasound.[19]

In this section we will briefly review knowledge regarding mechanisms of action, in vitro studies, in vivo studies, and epidemiology and use this information to develop (1) recommendations for medical practice in view of risk and benefit considerations and (2) suggestions for responses to questions from patients.

## Mechanisms

Heating and cavitation are known mechanisms of action by which ultrasound could produce biologic effects in tissues.[10, 13] Nonthermal, noncavitational mechanisms may exist but have not been identified.[20]

Attenuation in tissue is primarily due to absorption, that is, conversion of ultrasound to heat. Thus, ultrasound produces a temperature rise as it propagates through tissues. The heating produced depends on the applied intensity and frequency of sound (since the absorption coefficient is approximately proportional to frequency). Heating increases as intensity is increased. Superficial heating is increased as frequency is increased. However, at greater depths, heating is decreased at higher frequencies because the increased attenuation reduces the intensity arriving at depth. Heating could only be a relevant mechanism for in vivo biologic effects at intensities above approximately 100 mW/cm$^2$ at diagnostic frequencies.[21, 22] Therefore, for common imaging situations, heating is probably not a relevant mechanism. A potential exception to this, current duplex pulsed-Doppler equipment, is discussed later in this chapter.

Cavitation is the production and motion of bubbles in a liquid medium. A propagating sound wave is one means by which cavitation can occur. Two types of cavitation are recognized to occur. Stable cavitation is the term used to describe bubbles which oscillate in diameter with the passing pressure variations of the sound wave. Streaming of surrounding liquid can occur in this situation and result in shear stresses on suspended cells or intracellular organelles. Transient (collapse) cavitation occurs when bubble oscillations are so large that the bubble collapses, producing pressure discontinuities (shock waves) and localized extremely high temperatures. Transient cavitation has the potential for significant destructive effects. It is the means by which laboratory cell disrupters operate. Recent theory has been developed that predicts that ultrasound could produce transient cavitation under diagnostically relevant conditions in water.[23–25] The occurrence of transient cavitation in water under diagnostic conditions has not yet been observed (although it has been reported to occur with 1 MHz, 1 μsec, 0.1 duty-factor pulses of 14 W/cm$^2$ temporal average intensity).[26] If it does not occur in water under diagnostic conditions, then there will be no need for concern about its occurrence in tissue since tissue has properties (for example, high viscosity) that give it less likelihood for permitting cavitation. If transient cavitation *is* observed in water under relevant conditions, then techniques for its detection under these conditions in tissue will need to be developed and

used. The detection of cavitation in tissues under continuous-wave, high-intensity conditions has been reported.[27] These conditions, however, are not applicable to the pulse-echo diagnostic imaging situation. The occurrence of cavitation or its strength of activity tends to decrease with increasing frequency, decreasing duty factor, or decreasing amplitude or intensity.[20]

## In Vitro Studies

Many studies of biologic effects of ultrasound using in vitro models have been reported. These are summarized in chapter 8 of the monograph published in 1983 by the National Council of Radiation Protection and Measurements[14] and in chapter 4 of Nyborg's and Ziskin's text.[28] End points observed have included plasma membrane permeability; electrophoretic mobility; phagocytic activity; cellular attachment; surface morphology; cell cycle, growth, survival, and lysis; mutation; chromosome aberrations; sister chromatid exchanges; and DNA synthesis. Of all these end points the one that has been studied the most is sister chromatid exchange (SCE). Fifteen reports have appeared,[29, 30] including four reporting positive results and 11 reporting negative results. Many different cell types and experimental conditions were involved in this multitude of studies. It is difficult to come to a conclusion in view of the disparity of the reported results. However, it can be concluded that an effect of ultrasound on SCE is not well established. The most recent report[30] made a noble attempt to closely reproduce the experiments of the initial SCE report.[31] The same ultrasound devices and cell culture facilities used in the 1979 experiment were used in this study as well. Slides were scored by investigators from several institutions. Exposure to ultrasound had no effect on frequency of SCE or on cell cycle progression. An effect of ultrasound on SCE is clearly not established at this time. Even if it were to be shown in the future, the nature and significance of SCE are not well understood and their basis for risk assessment is questionable.[32] In addition, significant differences between in vitro experimental conditions and the clinical imaging situation make it impossible to directly apply such results to clinical risk assessment.[33] Many of the alarming statements that have appeared in the public media have resulted from such an inappropriate application of in vitro data. In vitro results *are* useful in planning in vivo experiments and choosing end points for epidemiologic studies.

## In Vivo Studies

Many studies have been reported that studied the effects of ultrasound on experimental plants and animals. These are reviewed in chapters 6 and 7 of the 1983 monograph[14] published by the National Council of Radiation Protection and Measurements and in chapters 7 and 8 in Nyborg's and Ziskin's text.[28] Plants provide relatively simple systems for study especially where cavitation is involved since they commonly contain gas-filled channels. These will not be considered further in this section. They are reviewed by Miller.[34]

Reported in vivo effects include fetal weight reduction, postpartum fetal mortality, fetal abnormalities, tissue lesions, hind limb paralysis, blood flow stasis, wound repair enhancement, and tumor regression. These effects have occurred at intensities greater than 100 mW/cm$^2$ as described by the American Institute of Ultrasound in Medicine statement on mammalian in vivo ultrasonic biologic effects.[33] Most instruments operate at intensities below this value.[14, 35] A review of the literature on the effects of experimental animal fetuses led to the conclusion that there is no direct evidence that pulse-echo diagnostic ultrasound produces any effect on the fetus.[36]

The in vivo end point that has been studied the most is fetal weight reduction. Several investigators at different institutions have reported effects of ultrasound on rodent fetal weight. A dose-effect dependence of fetal weight has been observed, with a relevant dose parameter being intensity squared times exposure time.[37] Fetal weight reduction has not been observed at intensities less than 100 mW/cm$^2$.

## Epidemiology

Although in vitro and in vivo experimental studies, along with a knowledge of mechanisms, provide helpful information when one is considering bioeffects and safety of diagnostic ultrasound, the most directly applicable results are those from epidemiologic studies.

Here we deal with the subjects of concern, the patients and their offspring. Although epidemiology treats the subjects and end points of most concern, it has serious limitations. Randomization, follow-up, sample size, and other aspects of these studies are difficult to arrange and control properly, thus limiting the value of these studies. Several reports of epidemiology studies have appeared in the literature. None have reported any effect on the end point resulting from ultrasound exposure. The most recent report is that of Stark et al.[38] Apgar scores, gestational age, head circumference, birth weight, length, congenital abnormalities, neonatal infection, and congenital infection, all measured at birth, and hearing, visual acuity and color vision, cognitive function, behavior, and neurologic examination, at 7–12 years of age, were measured in 806 children, 425 of whom had been exposed to diagnostic ultrasound in utero, and 381 matched control children. No statistically significant differences between exposed and unexposed children were found. Although the published epidemiology reports can be faulted on various grounds, they do provide no indication of harm or risk. A review of these reports is included in chapter 5 or the 1983 report of the National Council on Radiation Protection and Measurements,[14] in chapter 10 of Nyborg's and Ziskin's text,[28] and in chapter IV, Section II, of the 1984 report of the National Institutes of Health.[12]

## Risk and Benefit

Information from in vitro and in vivo experimental studies and from epidemiology has yielded no known risk in the use of ultrasound in medical imaging. A thermal mechanism could potentially operate to produce bioeffects in tissues at time-average intensities approaching 1 W/cm$^2$. Some pulsed Doppler devices currently have the capability of operating at such intensities.[35] Nevertheless, currently there is no known risk associated with the use of diagnostic ultrasound. Experimental animal data have helped to define the region in which bioeffects can be observed. However, differences, both physical and biological, between the two situations make it difficult to apply results from one to risk assessment in the other. In the absence of known risk, but recognizing the possibility that bioeffects are occurring but are subtle or delayed, we recommend a conservative approach to the medical use of ultrasound. This approach seeks to minimize (unknown) risk by minimizing exposure presumed to be associated with risk. Exposure is presumed to depend somehow on intensity and exposure time. A prudent approach to the use of ultrasound, therefore, is to use it only for medical indication (thus avoiding the unknown or no-benefit situation), minimizing exposure time during a study, and minimizing exposure intensity if such control is provided by the instrument used. Suggestions for appropriate medical indications have been provided, for example, by the National Institutes of Health 1984.[12] Of particular concern with regard to minimizing output intensity are the more recent pulsed Doppler devices in which care should be taken not to use higher intensities than needed in each study. The American Institute of Ultrasound in Medicine has provided a reasonable statement on the clinical safety of diagnostic ultrasound, as follows:[33]

> No confirmed biological effects on patients or instrument operators caused by exposures at intensities typical of present diagnostic ultrasound instruments have ever been reported. Although the possibility exists that such biological effects may be identified in the future, current data indicate that the benefits to patients of the prudent use of diagnostic ultrasound outweigh the risks, if any, that may be present.

## Conclusion

It is difficult to make firm statements about the clinical safety of diagnostic ultrasound. The experimental and epidemiologic bases for risk assessment are far from complete. However, much work has been done with no evidence of clinical harm revealed. Patients should be informed that there currently is no basis for judging that ultrasound imaging produces any harmful effects in mother or baby. However, unobserved effects *could* be occurring. Thus, ultrasound should not be used indiscriminately, i.e., "just for fun" or "to watch the baby." The American Institute of Ultrasound in Medicine clinical safety statement forms an excellent basis for formulating a response to patient questions and concerns. Prudence in practice is exercised by minimizing exposure time and intensity.

## References

1. Kremkau FW: How safe is obstetric ultrasound? *Contemp Ob Gyn* 1982; 20:182.
2. Kremkau FW: Biological effects and possible hazards. *Clin Obstet Gynecol* 1983; 10:395.
3. Kremkau FW: Safety and long-term effects of ultrasound: What to tell your patients. *Clin Obstet Gynecol* 1984; 27:269.
4. Stewart HF, Moore RM: Development of health risk evaluation data for diagnostic ultrasound: A historical perspective. *JCU* 1984; 12:493.
5. Stewart HD, Stewart HF, Moore RM, et al: Compilation of reported biological effects data and ultrasound exposure levels. *JCU* 1985; 13:167.
6. Dunn F: Selected biological effects of ultrasound, in Repacholi MH, Benwell DA (eds): *Essentials of Medical Ultrasound.* Clifton, NJ, Humana Press, 1982, pp 117–140.
7. Hohler CW: Ultrasound bioeffects for the perinatologist, in Sciarra J (ed): *Gynecology and Obstetrics.* New York, Harper & Row, 1982, pp 1–10.
8. Lele PP: Safety and potential hazards in the current applications of ultrasound in obstetrics and gynecology. *Ultrasound Med Biol* 1979; 5:307.
9. Fry FJ: Biological effects of ultrasound: A review. *Proc IEEE* 1979; 67:604.
10. Nyborg WL: Biophysical mechanisms of ultrasound, in Repacholi MH, Benwell DA (eds): *Essentials of Medical Ultrasound.* Clifton, NJ, Humana Press, 1982, pp 35–75.
11. Williams AR: *Ultrasound: Biological Effects and Potential Hazards.* New York, Academic Press, 1983.
12. National Institutes of Health: *Diagnostic Ultrasound Imaging in Pregnancy* (Publication No 84–667). Bethesda, NIH, 1984.
13. American Institute of Ultrasound in Medicine: *Safety Standard for Diagnostic Ultrasound Equipment.* Bethesda, AIUM, 1981.
14. National Council of Radiation Protection and Measurements: *Biological Effects of Ultrasound: Mechanisms and Clinical Implications* (Report No 74). Bethesda, NCRP, 1983.
15. World Health Organization: *Environmental Health Criteria 22: Ultrasound.* Geneva, WHO, 1982.

16. Food and Drug Administration: *An Overview of Ultrasound: Theory, Measurement, Medical Applications, and Biological Effects.* Rockville, Md, FDA, 1982.

17. National Research Council Canada: *Ultrasound: Characteristics and Biological Action.* Ottawa, NRC, 1981.

18. Health and Welfare Canada: *Safety Code - 13: Guidelines for the Safe Use of Ultrasound (Part I. Medical and Paramedical Applications).* Ottawa, HWC, 1980.

19. American Institute of Ultrasound in Medicine: *Evaluation of Research Reports: Bioeffects Literature Reviews.* Bethesda, AIUM, 1984.

20. Hill CR: Ultrasonic exposure thresholds for changes in cells and tissues. *J Acoust Soc Am* 1972; 52:667.

21. Lele PP: Ultrasonic teratology in mouse and man, in *Proceedings of the Second European Congress on Ultrasonics in Medicine.* Amsterdam, Excerpta Medica, 1975, pp 22–27.

22. Nyborg WL, Steele RB: Temperature elevation in a beam of ultrasound. *Ultrasound Med Biol* 1983; 9:611.

23. Apfel RE: Acoustic cavitation prediction. *J Acoust Soc Am* 1981; 69:1624.

24. Apfel RE: Acoustic cavitation: A possible consequence of biomedical uses of ultrasound. *Br J Cancer* 1982; 45 (suppl V):140.

25. Flynn H: Generation of transient cavities in liquids by microsecond pulses of ultrasound. *J Acoust Soc Am* 1982; 72:1926.

26. Fowlkes JB, Crum LA: Cavitation from short acoustic pulses. *J Acoust Soc Am* 1985; 77(suppl 1):S35.

27. ter Haar G, Daniels S: Evidence for ultrasonically induced cavitation in vivo. *Physics Med Biol* 1981; 26:1145.

28. Nyborg WL, Ziskin MC: *Biological Effects of Ultrasound. Clin Diagn Ultrasound* 16, 1985.

29. Goss SA: Sister chromatid exchange and ultrasound. *J Ultrasound Med* 1984; 3:463.

30. Ciaravino V, Brulfert A, Miller MW, et al: Diagnostic ultrasound and sister chromatid exchanges: Failure to reproduce positive findings. *Science* 1985; 227:1349.

31. Liebeskind D, Bases R, Mendez F: Sister chromatid exchanges in human lymphocytes after exposure to diagnostic ultrasound. *Science* 1979; 205:1273.

32. Jacobson-Kram D: The effects of diagnostic ultrasound on sister chromatid exchange frequencies: A review of the recent literature. *JCU* 1984; 12:5.

33. American Institute of Ultrasound in Medicine: *Safety Considerations for Diagnostic Ultrasound.* Bethesda, AIUM, 1984.

34. Miller DL: The botanical effects of ultrasound: A review. *Environ Exp Botany* 1983; 23:1.

35. American Institute of Ultrasound in Medicine: *Acoustical Data for Diagnostic Ultrasound Equipment.* Bethesda, AIUM, 1985.

36. Carstensen EL, Gates AH: The effects of pulsed ultrasound on the fetus. *J Ultrasound Med* 1984; 3:145.

37. O'Brien WD: Dose-dependent effect of ultrasound on fetal weight in mice. *J Ultrasound Med* 1983; 2:1.

38. Stark CR, Orleans M, Haverkamp AD, et al: Short- and long-term risks after exposure to diagnostic ultrasound in utero. *Obstet Gynecol* 1984; 63:194.

## CASES

Dennis A. Sarti

### Specular and Diffuse Reflectors

There are two major types of ultrasound reflectors within the body. These are specular and diffuse reflectors. Specular reflectors are large (several λ) and have smooth borders. The echoes around the kidney in Figures 1–25, 1–26, and 1–27 are from specular reflectors. The portal vein and diaphragm are also specular reflectors. Diffuse reflectors are smaller and weaker than specular reflectors. Diffuse reflectors represent the parenchymal pattern of various organs seen on ultrasound. The area surrounded by arrowheads in Figure 1–28 is made up of diffuse reflectors. All of the soft, lower-level echoes within the liver in Figures 1–25 through 1–28 are diffuse reflectors.

A specular reflector will be seen when its interface is close to perpendicular to the ultrasound beam. As the ultrasound beam approaches the interface at more oblique angles, the intensity of the registered echo will decrease and finally disappear. Note this finding in the renal capsule in Figures 1–25, 1–26, and 1–27. The renal capsule (arrows) is highest in intensity when it is close to perpendicular to the sound beam. It drops off in intensity and finally disappears as it curves further away. The reason for this phenomenon is the finite size of the transducer. Reflection is still occurring at the interface. However, the reflected echo is not returning to the transducer. Therefore, it does not register on the image.

Such is not the case with the diffuse reflectors. Diffuse reflectors are weaker in intensity but send reflected echoes in all directions. Diffuse reflectors will be registered as long as the output and sensitivity of the unit are high enough. If the diffuse reflectors are extremely weak, they may be hidden in noise and artifact. However, there will always be some echoes reflected back toward the transducer.

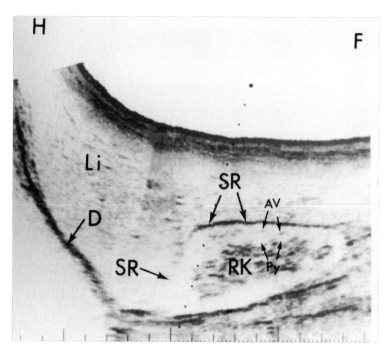

FIG 1–25.

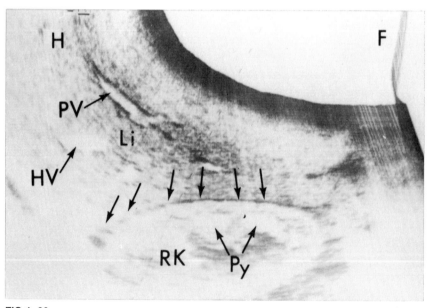

FIG 1–26.

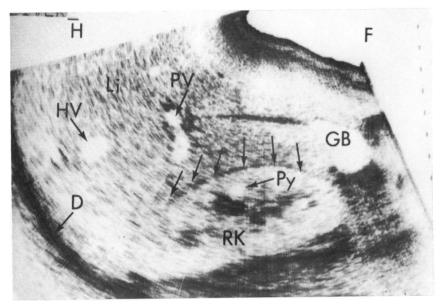

**FIG 1–27.**

Attention to diffuse reflectors is extremely important for high-quality diagnostic images. Specular reflectors may be compared to screams and diffuse reflectors to whispers. If you pay attention to the whispers and turn your unit and eye to see them clearly, you will become an excellent ultrasonographer. Too much attention is paid to the screaming specular reflectors, with a resulting loss in image quality and diagnostic ability. This will be further emphasized when we discuss time gain compensation. Each organ of the body has its own parenchymal pattern created by diffuse reflectors. Various anatomic structures within the organs create small reflectors which yield characteristic parenchymal patterns.

| **Arrows** | = | Specular reflectors |
| **Arrowheads** | = | Diffuse reflectors |
| **AV** | = | Arcuate vessel |
| **D** | = | Diaphragm |
| **F** | = | Foot |
| **GB** | = | Gallbladder |
| **H** | = | Head |
| **HV** | = | Hepatic vein |
| **Li** | = | Liver |
| **PV** | = | Portal |
| **Py** | = | Renal pyramid |
| **RK** | = | Right kidney |
| **SR** | = | Specular reflector |

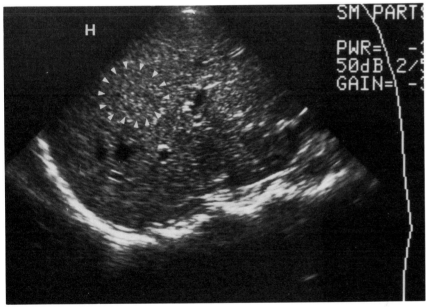

**FIG 1–28.**

## Time Gain Compensation

As an ultrasound wave passes through the body, it is attenuated at approximately 1 dB/cm/MHz. If no attempt is made to compensate for this normal attenuation, echoes deep in the body will not be strong enough to return to the transducer and register on the image. This is especially true of diffuse reflectors since they are weaker than specular reflectors. Because of normal body attenuation, all ultrasound units have the ability to listen to the deeper echoes with amplification compared to those echoes which are nearer the surface. This compensates for normal body attenuation. Although different terminology may be used, this has most commonly been referred to as time gain compensation, or TGC. As the sound beam travels farther into the body, more gain must be used to compensate for the attenuation that is occurring.

Correct adjustment of TGC is essential for high-quality diagnostic images. A common error in scanning is an incorrect TGC. By paying close attention to the diffuse reflectors or whispers, the sonographer can determine whether or not the TGC has been correctly adjusted. Figure 1–29 is a longitudinal scan through the right lobe of the liver in which the diaphragm is well seen. However, the diaphragm is a specular reflector in contact with air. It is a very loud "scream" and should be ignored in the initial evaluation of whether or not this is a technically adequate scan. Instead, the sonographer should concentrate on the "whispers" or diffuse reflectors present within the liver. Note that the near diffuse reflectors (arrowheads) are higher in amplitude than the deep diffuse reflectors (arrows) in Figure 1–29. Therefore, the TGC is not steep enough in this scan to adequately compensate for normal body attenuation. The slope of the TGC should be increased in this scan to correctly adjust for normal body attenuation.

Figure 1–30 is a scan in which the deep diffuse reflectors (arrowheads) are higher in amplitude than the dif-

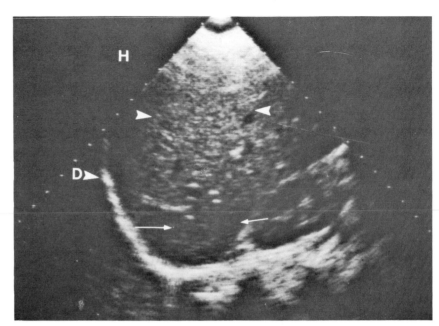

**FIG 1–29.**

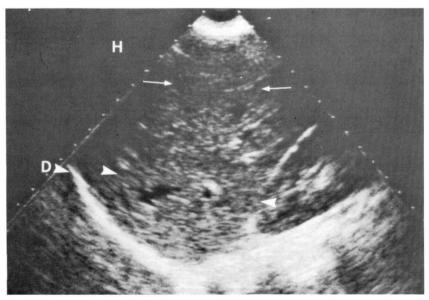

**FIG 1–30.**

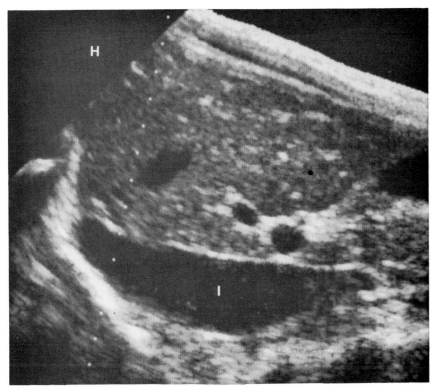

FIG 1–31.

fuse reflectors that are near the skin surface (arrows). Therefore, the TGC slope is too steep in this instance. Always try to evaluate TGC through an area that has diffuse, parenchymal echoes from front to back. This is not always possible but should be attempted. Figure 1–31 is a longitudinal scan in which TGC cannot be evaluated in the deep portion because of the inferior vena cava. Figure 1–32 is a scan in which numerous specular reflectors are present and make evaluation of TGC quite difficult. Remember that diffuse reflectors are the important ones to evaluate. The straight line in Figure 1–32 will be the best region for evaluation of TGC, since only diffuse reflectors are present.

| | | |
|---|---|---|
| **Arrows** | = | Diffuse echoes are too low |
| **Arrowheads** | = | Diffuse echoes are too high |
| **D** | = | Diaphragm |
| **H** | = | Head |
| **I** | = | Inferior vena cava |

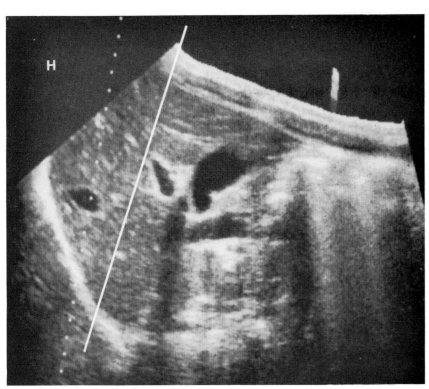

FIG 1–32.

## Time Gain Compensation

Probably the most difficult adjustment on an ultrasound unit is correctly adjusting the TGC. Close attention to the diffuse echoes (whispers) will help in correctly determining TGC. After years of experience, one can easily set a TGC correctly for each patient. However, the novice has difficulty in determining the correct TGC setting. Do not pay attention to specular reflectors. Rather, pay close attention to the diffuse echoes. An easy way to learn how to correctly set the TGC is as follows. First, turn down the output and sensitivity of the unit so that the diffuse echoes are barely visualized. Figure 1–33 is a longitudinal scan in which the diffuse echoes (arrowheads) are barely visualized deep in the liver. The diffuse echoes are not seen in the midportion or near region of the liver. A few specular reflectors are identified, but not the diffuse reflectors. Since the output and sensitivity are adjusted quite low, the diffuse echoes will come in asymmetrically as the sensitivity is slowly increased. In this case, as the sensitivity was slowly increased the diffuse echoes appeared in the deep portion sooner than in the superficial portion. Therefore, the TGC slope was too steep in Figure 1–33. Then readjust the TGC by decreasing its slope.

In Figure 1–34 the diffuse reflectors (arrowheads) are arising first in the superficial rather than deep region. In this instance, the TGC slope is not steep enough. If the output and sensitivity are set quite low, the early appearance of diffuse echoes helps determine whether or not the TGC slope is correct. In this instance (Figure 1–34), the diffuse echoes arose in the superficial region much earlier than in the deep portion.

In Figure 1–35 the diffuse echoes are not arising asymmetrically in the deep or superficial region. This is consistent with a normal TGC slope. By continually changing the TGC slope and observing whether or not the diffuse echoes arise first in the deep or superficial portion, one can slowly reach the correct TGC setting. The

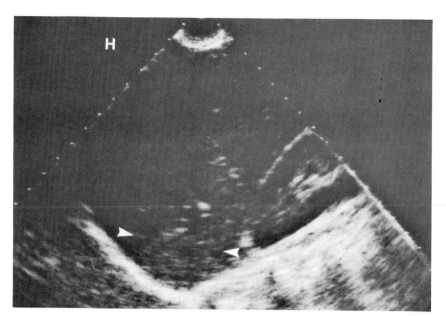

**FIG 1–33.**

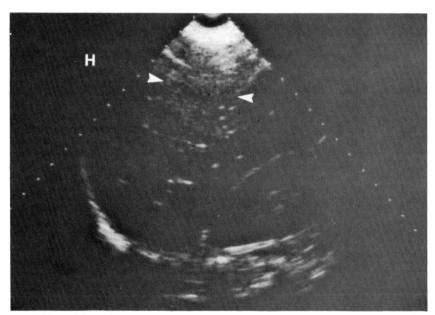

**FIG 1–34.**

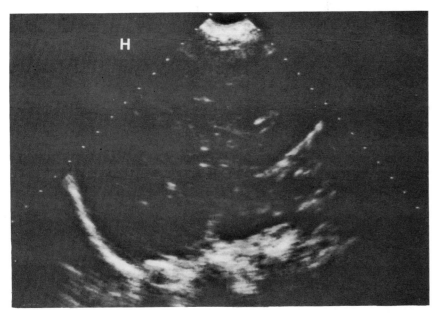

**FIG 1–35.**

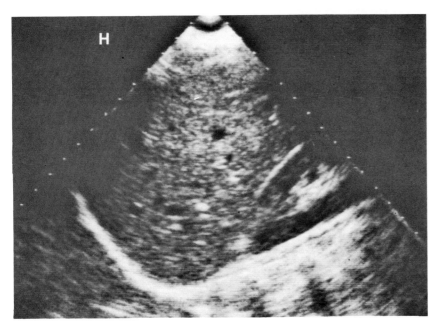

**FIG 1–36.**

scan in Figure 1–35 was made with low output and sensitivity but normal TGC slope. Once this point is reached, the output and sensitivity of the unit can be increased so that an even diffuse parenchymal pattern will be present. This is the case in Figure 1–36. The same TGC slope is used as in the scan shown in Figure 1–35. The only difference is that the sensitivity of the unit has been increased to bring out the parenchymal echoes within the liver. Note that the diffuse reflectors have an even echo amplitude from superficial to deep. The easiest way to learn how to set correctly the TGC is as follows. Turn the output and sensitivity of the unit down until the diffuse reflectors are barely visible. Determine whether the diffuse reflectors are coming in earlier in the superficial or deep region. If they are coming in earlier in one area, readjust the TGC accordingly. Finally, you will reach a TGC at which the diffuse reflectors are coming in evenly both superficially and deeply. Once this TGC is set, the output and sensitivity can be increased so that an even, diffuse parenchymal pattern is present throughout the liver.

**Arrowheads** = Diffuse reflectors appearing too early
**H** = Head

## Time Gain Compensation

Previous cases demonstrated the importance of correctly adjusting the TGC at the beginning of each examination. Most units have a TGC adjustment that changes the TGC slope in its entirety. With these units, the TGC remains a straight line as it changes. Other units have TGC curves that can be individualized. This is performed by means of potentiometers mounted on sliders, with each slider representing a certain depth of tissue. This setup can create highly individual TGC curves but also diagnostic problems in obstetric and abdominal scanning.

Figures 1–37 through 1–40 are scans of the right upper quadrant obtained in the same patient and with a unit whose TGC is controlled by individual potentiometers. The TGC curve is represented by the white line to the right of the image. In Figure 1–37, a potentiometer near the midportion of the TGC curve has been depressed (arrow). This creates a band of decreased echoes in the midportion of the liver (arrow). A low-amplitude metastasis would be missed in this region. Figure 1–38 shows the opposite situation. In Figure 1–38, the potentiometer in the midportion of the TGC has been elevated (arrow). These creates a band of high-amplitude echoes in the midportion of the liver (arrow) which could mask a highly echogenic metastasis. In Figure 1–39, the TGC curve has been altered in the deep portion of the liver (arrow). This has created a region of decreased echogenicity in the liver adjacent to the diaphragm (arrow). This is a very disturbing scan which could be misinterpreted as showing a subdiaphragmatic abscess, hematoma, or other subdiaphragmatic processes. In Figure 1–40 the TGC curve has been correctly adjusted for abdominal scanning. The TGC potentiometers increase steadily through liver tissue. The image in Figure 1–40 demonstrates an even parenchymal pattern to the diffuse echoes within the liver. When using a unit with potentiometers on sliders, it is even more important that the sonographer pay attention to the diffuse

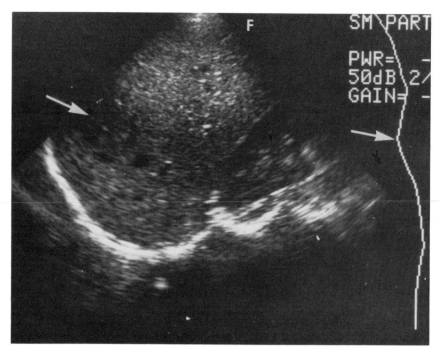

FIG 1–37.

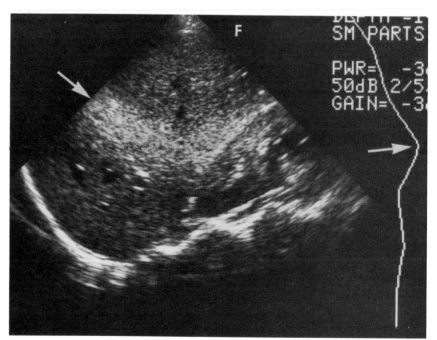

FIG 1–38.

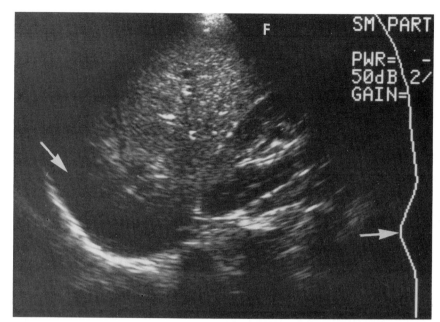

FIG 1–39.

reflectors at all depths throughout the liver. Proper TGC adjustment will yield an even parenchymal pattern to normal liver tissue.

**Arrow** = Variation in TGC
**F**    = Foot

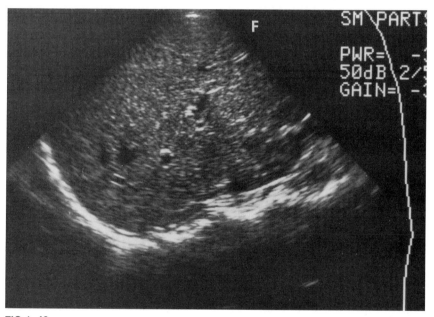

FIG 1–40.

## Compression Curve Assignment

The amount of reflection that occurs at different interfaces varies dramatically within the body. The diaphragm-lung interface reflects nearly all of the sound beam that strikes it. Parenchyma reflects a very small amount of sound and permits nearly all of the sound to pass on to the next interface. The images created on ultrasound scanning do not represent these reflectors in proportion to the amount of reflection that occurs. Emphasis is placed on the low-amplitude reflectors. This region is spread out over the various gray-scale levels. Various curves can be used to assign gray-scale levels to different reflectors in the body. This is called compression curve assignment. These compression curves vary with each unit. The main object in abdominal scanning is to bring out gray-scale differences in the low-amplitude reflectors. Compression curve assignment is critical to high-quality scans. Appropriate gray-scale mapping, gain settings, and scan technique led to the type of spatial and contrast resolution demonstrated in images shown here. Figure 1–41 is a longitudinal scan of the right upper quadrant in which intricate anatomic detail can be seen. The vessels stand out dramatically compared to the diffuse liver parenchymal echoes. Only with this type of technique can subtle, solid abnormalities such as those seen with a slightly more reflective metastasis be appreciated (Figure 1–42). If the TGC compression curve was not correctly assigned in this scan, the echogenic metastasis deep in the liver could easily be missed.

Similarly, the variety of acoustic textures within a gestational uterus (Fig 1–43) requires proper compression curve assignment and scan technique. Only then can subtle differences in acoustic texture be recognized, as is present in Figure 1–44. In this scan, numerous different reflectors are properly assigned varying gray-scale levels. Amniotic fluid is assigned the lowest gray-scale level, followed, in ascending order, by myoma, iliopsoas

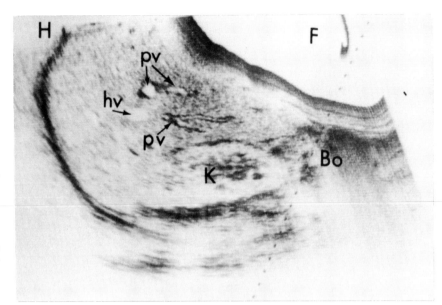

FIG 1–41.

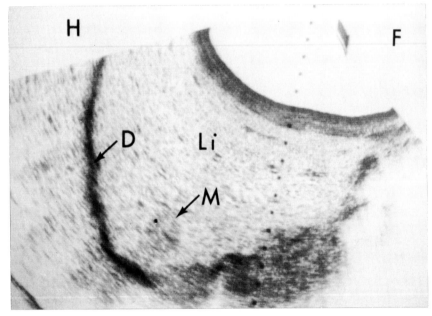

FIG 1–42.

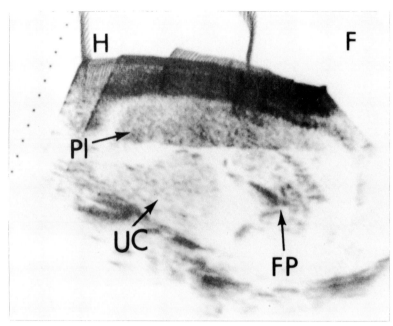

**FIG 1–43.**

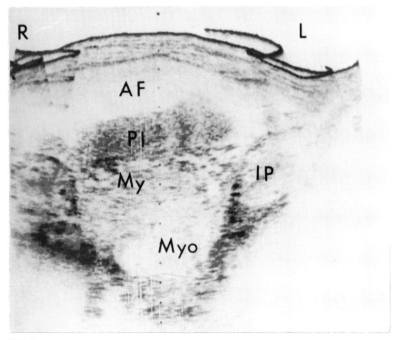

**FIG 1–44.**

muscle, normal myometrium, and placenta. Review this scan closely, viewing each anatomic structure listed and in the order given. By doing so, you will appreciate the importance of correct TGC and gray-scale assignment. Understanding and analyzing the importance of this scan and the anatomic detail it yields will assist you in critically evaluating your own scans.

| | | |
|---|---|---|
| **AF** | = | Amniotic fluid |
| **Bo** | = | Bowel |
| **D** | = | Diaphragm |
| **F** | = | Foot |
| **FP** | = | Fetal parts |
| **H** | = | Head |
| **hv** | = | Hepatic vein |
| **IP** | = | Iliopsoas muscle |
| **K** | = | Kidney |
| **L** | = | Left |
| **Li** | = | Liver |
| **M** | = | Metastasis |
| **My** | = | Myometrium |
| **Myo** | = | Myoma |
| **Pl** | = | Placenta |
| **pv** | = | Portal vein |
| **R** | = | Right |
| **UC** | = | Uterine contraction |

## Beam Profile

In the written section of Chapter 1, the construction of a transducer was discussed in detail. It was mentioned that transducers are focused to improve resolution, especially lateral resolution. This creates a focal zone in which echoes are sharply defined. In the region superficial to the focal zone, the echoes are smaller, less well defined, and lower in amplitude. The echoes in this superficial region usually have a fuzzy appearance. In the region deep to the focal zone, the echoes are wider, thicker, less sharply defined, and slightly lower in amplitude. It is important to know the focal zone of the various transducers you are using. The best diagnostic results are obtained when the anatomic area of interest is scanned in the focal zone of the appropriate transducer. Figure 1–45 is a scan through the liver that was made using a 3-MHZ transducer, 19 mm in diameter. The focal zone is demarcated by arrowheads and is situated in the midportion of the liver. Note the regions superficial and deep to the focal zone. Compare the echoes in these two regions with the echoes in the focal zone. Note how they differ in size and echogenicity. This scan demonstrates an excellent beam profile of a 3-MHZ, 19-mm transducer. This transducer is an excellent one for scanning the liver in its middle and deep portions.

Figure 1–46 is a scan made using a 5-MHz transducer, 13 mm in diameter. The focal zone (arrowheads) is closer to the surface than in the previous case. The near fuzzy region is shorter but the far region is much larger. This transducer would be excellent for examining the anterior half of the liver but would be very poor for examining the deep portion of the liver.

Figure 1–47 is a transverse scan of the testes made using a 5-MHz transducer, 7 mm in diameter. The focal zone starts halfway in the testes and is higher in intensity. The anterior half of the testes are in the fuzzy region. This transducer is focused within the first 1.5 cm, as is shown by the centimeter markers. However, it is still not

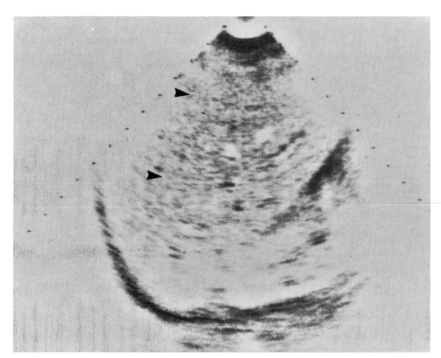

FIG 1–45.

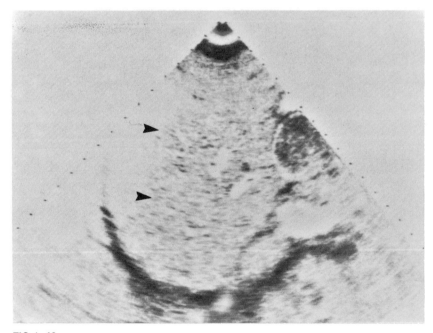

FIG 1–46.

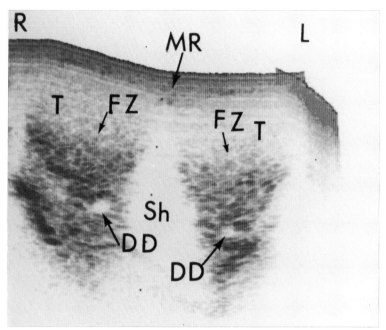

**FIG 1–47.**

adequate in this case to place the entire testes in the focal region. The transducer should be displaced away from the scrotum by means of a water bath or pile of gel in order to place the testes within the focal zone.

Figure 1–48 is a scan made using a 7.5-MHz transducer, 13 mm in diameter, which has a built-in water bath of approximately 2 cm. This transducer has the focal zone (arrowheads) present immediately at the skin surface and down to 2-cm depth. This is an excellent transducer choice for the examination of small, superficial structures.

As can be seen from the above examples, correct transducer choice is necessary for adequate examination of various anatomic regions. The sonographer should choose the transducer with a focal zone that most closely corresponds to the depth of the anatomic area being studied.

| Arrowheads | = Focal zone |
|---|---|
| **DD** | = Ductus deferens |
| **FZ** | = Beginning of focal zone |
| **L** | = Left |
| **MR** | = Median raphae |
| **R** | = Right |
| **Sh** | = Shadow |
| **T** | = Testis |

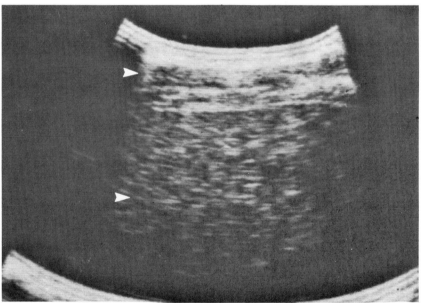

**FIG 1–48.**

## Dynamic Focusing

Figures in the previous section illustrated the focal zone of various transducers. These transducers each had a single piezoelectric element. Only one focal zone was possible for each of the transducers. To change the focal zone, the transducers themselves would have to be changed. In some ultrasound units one can change the focal zone without changing the transducer. These units have numerous piezoelectric elements within a single transducer package and are called array systems. With rapid firing of the elements, these array systems can create real-time images. With timed firing of adjacent elements, these array systems can create images which can be focused at different depths within the patient. This is called dynamic focusing.

Figures 1–49 through 1–52 are scans of the liver and inferior vena cava of the same patient, obtained using a linear-array, real-time transducer with dynamic focusing. The arrow or arrows on the left side of the images indicate the focal zone or zones of the image. In Figures 1–49, 1–50, and 1–51 the focal zone is at a single depth. In Figure 1–52 the focal zone is at various depths. This can only be accomplished by slowing down the frame rate. Compare the sharpness of the echoes from one image to another. Compare the various images in and out of their focal zone. Dynamic focusing is very helpful in studying a large area or an area of interest that continually moves, such as the fetus.

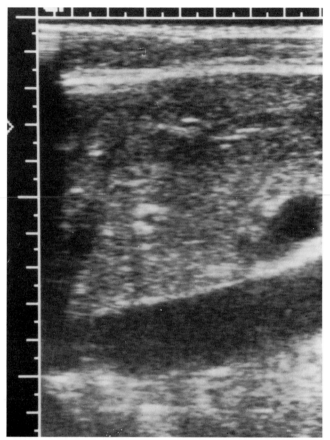

FIG 1–49.

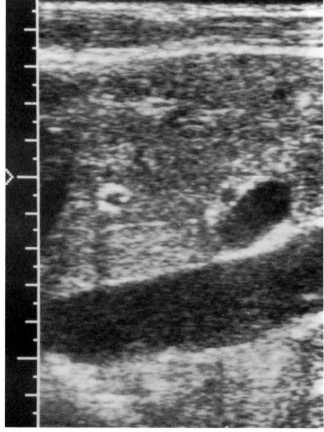

FIG 1–50.

**Arrows** = Focal zone

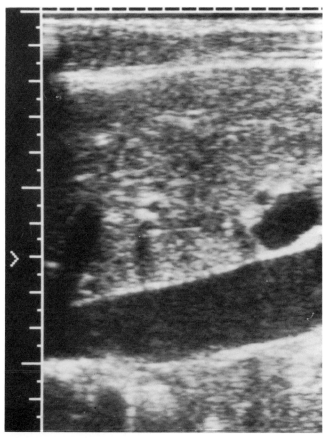

**FIG 1–51.**

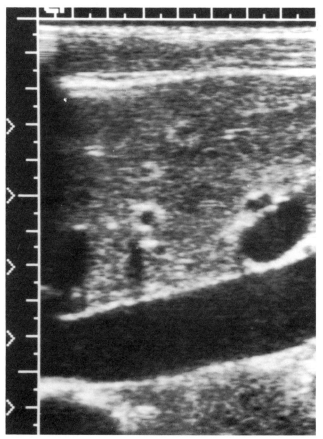

**FIG 1–52.**

## Effects of Areas of Increased Attenuation

Increased attenuation is an important sign of pathology. Depending on the region of the body, however, the appreciation of the increased attenuation may be difficult. Furthermore, the entire path of the sound beam must be appreciated if this sign is to be used as an indicator of disease.

A common entity that may only be recognized by an area of increased attenuation is a benign cystic teratoma within the pelvis. Figure 1–53 demonstrates, in the left adnexal region, an area of increased attenuation that is associated with a deformity of the bladder wall. This could be related to a large gassy area within the colon; however, the rectosigmoid region is identified on the opposite side of the pelvis. Figure 1–54 demonstrates in another case how the posterior wall of a highly attenuative mass may still be visualized with appropriate changes in the gain settings.

Another area where increased attenuation is associated with disease is in cirrhosis of the liver. In Figure 1–55, a small liver surrounded by ascitic fluid should normally have a consistent strong acoustic texture. This liver, however, has been markedly scarred from the cirrhotic process, and the decreased texture in the deeper parts of the liver, a result of the attenuation process, can be appreciated. In the deeper regions of the liver, underlying the gallbladder which counteracts this attenuation by the lower attenuation of the bile, the two processes offset one another and give rise to an apparently normal liver texture.

Therefore, when assessing attenuation, it is important to try to compare organs with similar textures and of the same size. Figure 1–56 is also a scan of a patient with cirrhosis and ascites. The sections of the liver and spleen are similar in size and surrounded by similar amounts of ascites. Therefore, the decreased attenuation seen in the deeper areas of the liver is real and aids in the differential diagnosis of the ascites.

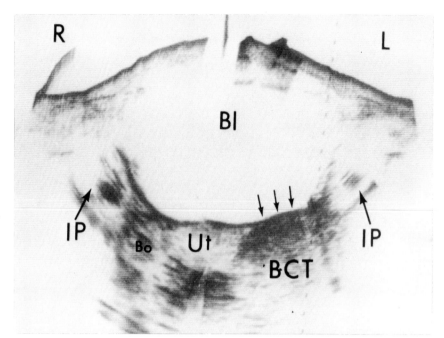

**FIG 1–53.**

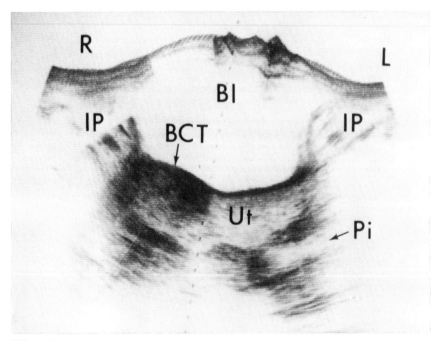

**FIG 1–54.**

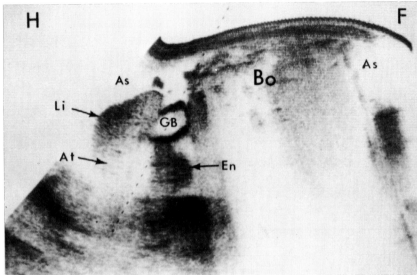

| A | = | Aorta |
| Arrows | = | Bladder wall indentation |
| As | = | Ascites |
| At | = | Attenuation |
| BCT | = | Benign cystic teratoma |
| Bl | = | Bladder |
| Bo | = | Bowel |
| En | = | Enhancement |
| F | = | Foot |
| GB | = | Gallbladder |
| H | = | Head |
| I | = | Inferior vena cava |
| IP | = | Iliopsoas muscle |
| K | = | Kidney |
| L | = | Left |
| Li | = | Liver |
| Pi | = | Piriformis muscle |
| Ps | = | Psoas muscle |
| R | = | Right |
| S | = | Spleen |
| Sp | = | Spine |
| Ut | = | Uterus |

**FIG 1–55.**

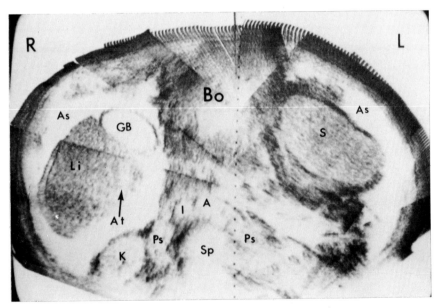

**FIG 1–56.**

## Areas of Increased Attenuation

The TGC is adjusted assuming normal body attenuation. However, there are normal and abnormal regions within the body that will demonstrate increased attenuation compared to the rest of the body. The increased attenuation may be slight and may manifest only as a minimal drop in echo amplitude deep to the structure causing the attenuation, or it may be severe and cause acoustic shadowing deep to the structure. By recognizing the ultrasound findings of increased attenuation, correct diagnoses can be made and interpretative errors avoided.

Fibrous tissue often causes areas of increased attenuation. Scar tissue after surgery can lead to a diagnostic problem. Scars are often difficult to see, yet their effect on attenuation of sound and underlying acoustic texture is dramatic. In Figure 1–57, a small scar in the subcutaneous tissue has caused a dramatic attenuation and shadowing effect which has resulted in a wide area of abnormal texture throughout the underlying liver. In Figure 1–58, the patient has been re-scanned and the scar area was avoided during the scanning process. The more normal hepatic acoustic texture, as well as the clear visualization of interhepatic vascular anatomy, is appreciated. For this reason, when scanning a portion of the body where scars are likely to occur, it is best to hold the transducer between the thumb and index finger and slide the third, fourth, and fifth fingers across the skin to palpate the scar.

Figure 1–59 is a transverse scan of the pelvis which illustrates a relatively nonspecific adnexal mass. This mass could have an extensive differential diagnosis. The presence of an interface within the mass is related to a significant velocity change resulting in shadowing. The shadowing suggests the presence of calcification. This ultrasound finding limits the differential diagnosis of the mass. The findings are highly consistent with benign cystic teratoma, which was found at surgery.

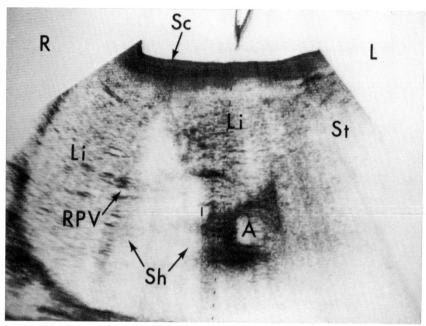

FIG 1–57.

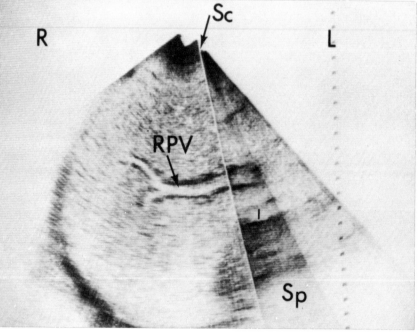

FIG 1–58.

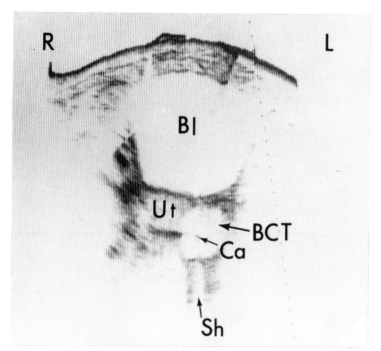

FIG 1–59.

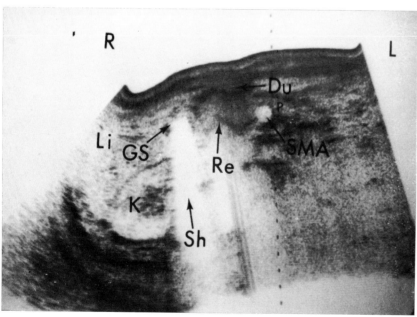

FIG 1–60.

An important aspect of acoustic shadowing related to velocity changes frequently is observed in the gallbladder area. A gallbladder filled with stones may be difficult to outline. The shadowing effects of gallstones lead to a type of shadowing that is often different from the gas-containing structures nearby (Fig 1–60). The area of shadowing deep to the gallstone has no echoes present. The adjacent duodenum has numerous echoes deep to it secondary to reverberation artifacts. Although it is not always diagnostic, it is often helpful to evaluate the shadowed region. This can often give a clue as to whether a gallstone or an air-causing shadow is present.

| A | = | Aorta |
| BCT | = | Benign cystic teratoma |
| Bl | = | Bladder |
| Ca | = | Calcification |
| Du | = | Duodenum |
| GS | = | Gallstone |
| I | = | Inferior vena cava |
| L | = | Left |
| Li | = | Liver |
| P | = | Pancreas |
| R | = | Right |
| Re | = | Reverberation artifact |
| RPV | = | Right portal vein |
| Sc | = | Scar |
| Sh | = | Acoustic shadow |
| SMA | = | Superior mesenteric artery |
| Sp | = | Spine |
| Ut | = | Uterus |

## Enhanced Through-Transmission

Fluid-filled structures do not attenuate
the ultrasound beam to the same degree as normal soft tissue. If the TGC
is adjusted for normally attenuating
soft tissue, what happens when the
sound beam encounters less attenuating fluid? The fluid will permit more
sound energy to penetrate through the
deep structures. This will cause the
echoes deep to the fluid-filled structure to be higher in amplitude than
they would be if the sound beam had
traveled through normally attenuating
soft tissue. Therefore, the diagnosis of
a fluid-filled structure is made by evaluating the echoes deep to the structure. This is more easily done when
soft parenchymal echoes are present
deep to the fluid area. If air or bone is
present deep to the fluid structure, the
diagnosis is more difficult since these
media are such large reflectors they
cannot be dramatically enhanced.

Figure 1–61 is a longitudinal scan
through the right upper quadrant
showing a sonolucent mass adjacent
to the gallbladder. Some soft echoes
are present within the mass, indicating
that it is nonhomogeneous. The important finding is the increased echo
amplitude to the diffuse reflectors
deep to the mass. This indicates
acoustic enhancement and confirms
that the mass is mainly fluid. The
mass was an abscess with some debris. A fluid structure does not have to
be echo free to make the diagnosis of
fluid. However, it must manifest increased through-transmission. Figure
1–62 is the scan of another patient
with a sonolucent mass in the anterior
portion of the liver. The diffuse reflectors deep to the mass are increased
in echo amplitude compared to the
adjacent liver. This finding of acoustic
enhancement confirms the fluid nature
of the mass, which turned out to be
an abscess. Figure 1–63 is the scan
of another patient showing enhancement deep to a mass. The midline
mass has increased through-transmission present. The echoes deep to the
mass are not diffuse reflectors but still
demonstrate increased echo amplitude compared to what would be expected.

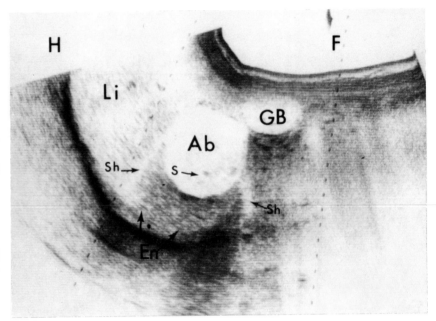

FIG 1–61.

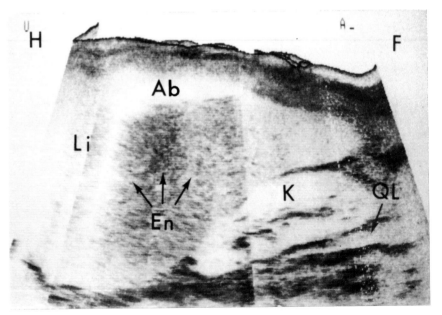

FIG 1–62.

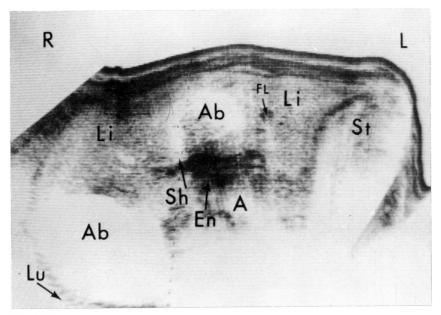

**FIG 1–63.**

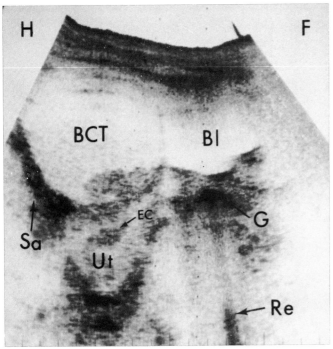

**FIG 1–64.**

Figure 1–64 is a longitudinal scan of the pelvis in a patient with a pelvic mass anterior to the uterus. It is always difficult to evaluate through-transmission in the pelvis because of the numerous high-amplitude echoes arising from bowel gas. Also, the urinary bladder causes a large amount of through-transmission and can lead to confusion. The mass cephalad to the urinary bladder was a benign cystic teratoma but could be called solid by the novice because of the numerous internal echoes. The urinary bladder is a helpful clue in this case. Note the gray-scale echoes of the lower uterine segment and cervix posterior to the urinary bladder. Now compare this echo region with the echoes of the uterine body and fundus posterior to the mass. The echoes of the uterine fundus and body are approximately equal in amplitude to the lower uterus and cervix. The mass has to be a fluid because it is attenuating similarly to the fluid-filled urinary bladder. If the mass were solid, it would attenuate to a much higher degree than the urinary bladder, and the echoes of the uterine body and fundus would be more markedly decreased. Even though the mass has massive internal echoes, it is a mainly fluid-filled structure because of the enhanced through-transmission. The mass transmits sound approximately equal to the fluid-filled urinary bladder.

| | | |
|---|---|---|
| **A** | = | Aorta |
| **Ab** | = | Abscess |
| **BCT** | = | Benign cystic teratoma |
| **Bl** | = | Urinary bladder |
| **EC** | = | Endometrial cavity |
| **En** | = | Acoustic enhancement |
| **F** | = | Foot |
| **FL** | = | Falciform ligament |
| **G** | = | Gas |
| **GB** | = | Gallbladder |
| **H** | = | Head |
| **K** | = | Kidney |
| **L** | = | Left |
| **Li** | = | Liver |
| **Lu** | = | Lung |
| **QL** | = | Quadratus lumborum |
| **R** | = | Right |
| **Re** | = | Reverberation artifact |
| **S** | = | Solid component |
| **Sa** | = | Sacrum |
| **Sh** | = | Shadow |
| **St** | = | Stomach |
| **Ut** | = | Uterus |

## Increased Through-Transmission

Because of decreased attenuation, fluids cause increased through-transmission and increased echogenicity to structures deep to fluid areas. These findings can be helpful in diagnosing masses but can also result in interpretative errors. Difficulty in recognizing certain components of a conceptus may result from the intervening amniotic fluid, as demonstrated in Figures 1–65 and 1–66. In Figure 1–65, because of the overamplification resulting from the intervening amniotic fluid as well as from an inappropriately high gain setting, it is impossible to tell whether the thickened posterior wall of the conceptus represents the placental region or a uterine contraction. In Figure 1–66, the gain settings and time gain compensation have been readjusted, so that the proper acoustic texture of the posterior gestational wall can be analyzed. The texture is seen to be different from that of the anterior placenta and therefore is identified as a uterine contraction.

Most serious interpretative errors in ultrasound occur when sonolucent masses are called cystic. Sonolucent only means that the mass is homogeneous. A sonolucent mass can still be solid. Increased through-transmission is needed to diagnose fluid. Figure 1–67 is an important scan to analyze in detail. Two circular sonolucent areas are present. One demonstrates increased through-transmission, the other does not. The sonolucent mass with increased through-transmission, manifested by increased amplitude echoes deep to the mass, meets the ultrasound criteria for a cyst. The sonolucent mass with no increased through-transmission meets the ultrasound criteria for a homogeneous solid mass. Without the cyst adjacent to it, many would misinterpret the solid mass as a cyst because it is so echo free. This scan is an extremely important one to remember every time you encounter a sonolucent mass.

Increased attenuation and increased through-transmission have been discussed in previous cases. Figure 1–

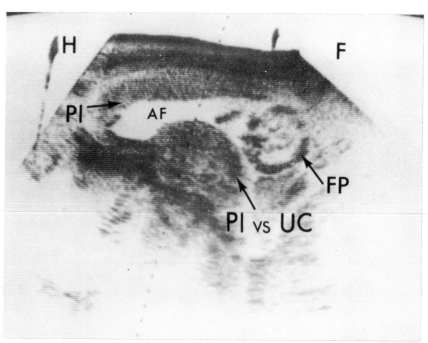

**FIG 1–65.**

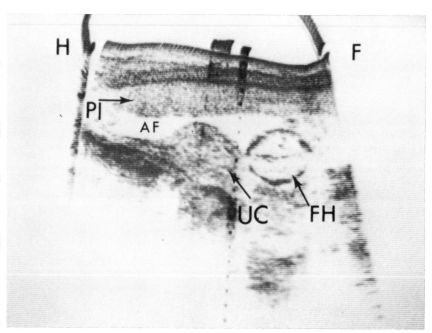

**FIG 1–66.**

Physics of Diagnostic Ultrasound 51

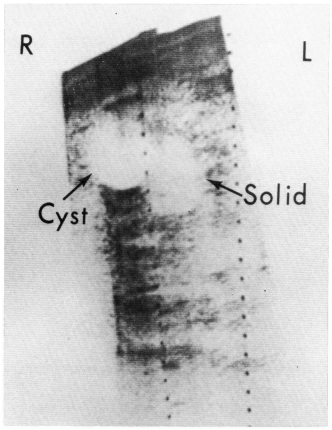

**FIG 1–67.**

68 is a scan in which both are present. This is an excellent scan that will help you understand the importance of evaluating the path that the sound beam must travel to an area of interest. You must evaluate what is in front of a region of interest, in addition to the region itself. Concentrate on the placenta in Figure 1–68. The right and left lateral aspect of the placenta only have soft tissue anterior to them. Posterior are two areas of increased placental echogenicity which are secondary to enhancement from increased through-transmission of the amniotic fluid. In the midline, there is an area of decreased placental echogenicity that is secondary to scar tissue on the surface from a previous cesarean section. The placenta is a consistent, single anatomic structure that has a variable ultrasound appearance in Figure 1–68. The reason for the variable ultrasound appearance is not any anatomic variation in the placenta. The reason is caused by what is anterior to the placenta itself. Every time you examine an area of interest, remember this scan and analyze what is anterior to that area.

**AF** = Amniotic fluid
**En** = Enhancement
**F** = Foot
**FH** = Fetal head
**FP** = Fetal part
**H** = Head
**L** = Left
**My** = Myometrium
**Pl** = Placenta
**R** = Right
**Sc** = Scar
**Sh** = Shadow
**UC** = Uterine contraction

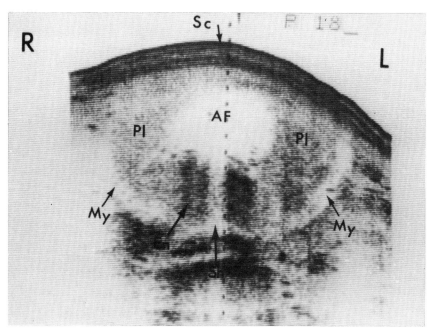

**FIG 1–68.**

## Ultrasound Evaluation of Masses

When a mass is evaluated by ultrasound, attempts are made to determine whether it has increased attenuation, increased through-transmission, or attenuation equal to that of soft tissue. This is not always an easy decision to make. Structures in front of a mass will have an effect on the appearance of the mass itself. The following case is an excellent example. The patient was a middle-aged man with a mass noted on intravenous pyelography. Ultrasound examination was performed to evaluate the mass.

Figures 1–69 and 1–70 are coronal and transverse scans from the initial ultrasound examination. The mass has some soft internal echoes. There is no evidence of increased through-transmission. The echoes deep to the mass are equal in intensity to those that are adjacent to the mass. Because of a suspected solid lesion, CT was performed. Figure 1–71 is a CT scan demonstrating a simple cyst of the right kidney. The straight line represents the scan plane of the initial ultrasound study of Figures 1–69 and 1–70. Note that the sound beam must travel through the fatty central collecting system before passing through the cyst. The increased attenuation of the fatty collecting system cancelled the increased through-transmission of the cyst, so that the renal mass did not demonstrate any sound enhancement when scanned in this plane. After the CT study, the patient again underwent ultrasound scanning, in a plane corresponding to the dotted line in Figure 1–71. Figure 1–72 is the second ultrasound scan, obtained to evaluate the mass without going through the central collecting system. Note the enhanced through-transmission that is now present deep to the mass in Figure 1–72. This indicates its fluid nature. Evaluation of masses is difficult and care must be taken to analyze the structures anterior to the mass.

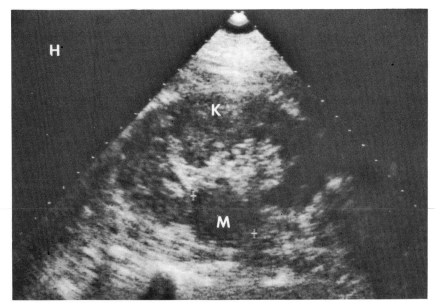

**FIG 1–69.**

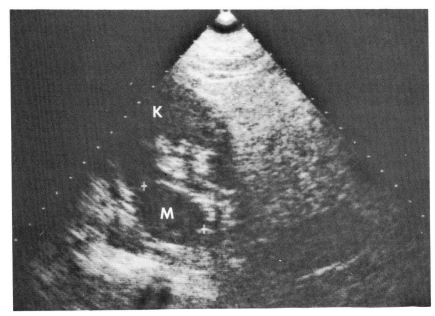

**FIG 1–70.**

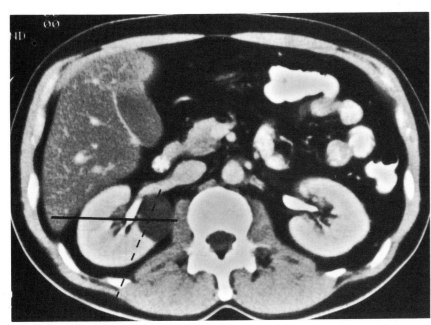

| H | = | Head |
| K | = | Kidney |
| M | = | Renal mass |
| TT | = | Enhanced through-trans-mission |
| **Straight line** | = | Scan plane for Figures 1–69 and 1–70 |
| **Dotted line** | = | Scan plane for Figure 72 |

**FIG 1–71.**

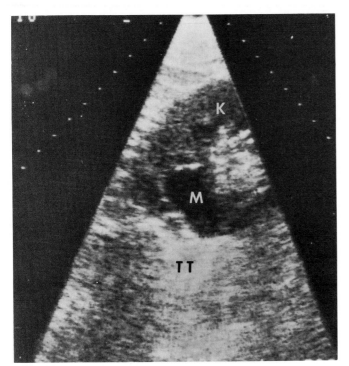

**FIG 1–72.**

## Critical Angle Shadowing

When the sound beam encounters a
specular reflector perpendicular to its
interface, the transmitted wave will
pass straight through the interface. As
the incident beam is tilted slightly off
the perpendicular, the transmitted
wave will be refracted or bent as it
passes through the interface into the
deeper tissue. As the incident beam is
tilted further, the degree of refraction
increases. An angle is finally reached
at which the incident beam completely
reflects off the interface and no sound
is transmitted through the interface to
deeper structures. This is called critical angle shadowing. The analogy of
throwing a stone that skips along the
surface of the lake has been used.
The sound beam similarly reaches an
angle in which it skips off the surface
of the interface, with resulting acoustic
shadowing deep to the interface.

Critical angle shadowing can cause
diagnostic and interpretative problems
on ultrasound images. By being aware
of this phenomenon, and the regions
where it can occur, the sonographer
can avoid diagnostic errors. Critical
angle shadowing usually occurs at a
specular reflector with a curved surface. Figure 1–73 is an example of
critical angle shadowing near the cephalad border of the right kidney. The
renal capsule is a specular reflector
that is markedly curved near the renal
poles. The shadow present at the upper pole of the kidney is secondary to
critical angle shadowing.

A common area for diagnostic problems arising from critical angle shadowing is the proximal portion of the
gallbladder and the cystic duct region.
Since we are usually looking for
acoustic shadowing from gallstones in
this area, the shadowing from the critical angle presents a confusing picture,
as in Figure 1–74. By turning the patient into a decubitus position with the
left side down, the sonographer can
examine the proximal portion of the
gallbladder. Gallstones will usually fall
into the dependent portion. Shadowing
in the cystic duct region when the patient is supine is a common occurrence secondary to critical angle
shadowing.

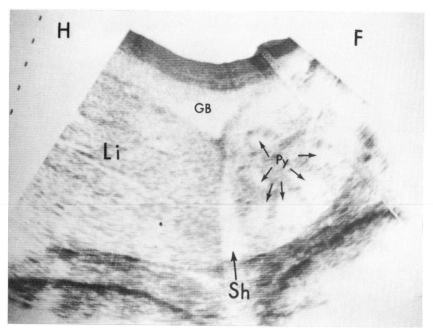

FIG 1–73.

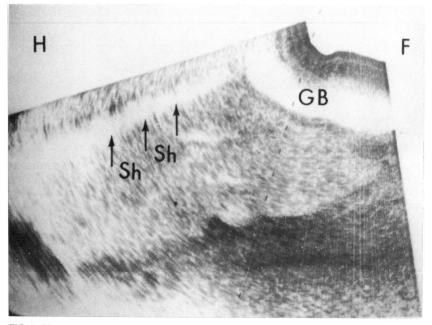

FIG 1–74.

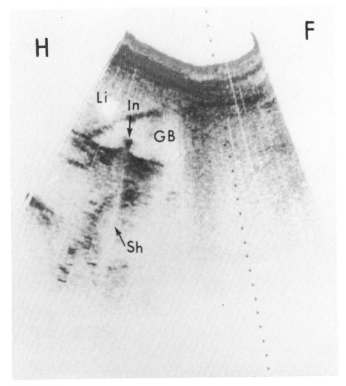

**FIG 1–75.**

Figure 1–75 is a scan of the gallbladder which has an internal echo with acoustic shadowing. The diagnosis of gallstone appears quite likely. However, this is another example of critical angle shadowing occurring from a soft tissue curved surface in the gallbladder. This turned out to be a fold of the gallbladder. When the patient was placed in the decubitus position, the gallbladder unfolded and the internal echoes disappeared. You can see how the diagnosis of gallstone in Figure 1–75 could easily be made.

Figure 1–76 is a longitudinal scan of the pelvis in a patient with a postpartum uterus. There is a drop-off in echoes of the lower uterine segment. This is not secondary to any mass or pathology in the region. It is secondary to critical angle shadowing off the superior urinary bladder wall. This is a typical finding on many pelvic ultrasound examinations. Myomas of the lower uterine segment are often misdiagnosed because of the shadowing in this region.

| | | |
|---|---|---|
| **Bl** | = | Urinary bladder |
| **EC** | = | Endometrial cavity |
| **F** | = | Foot |
| **GB** | = | Gallbladder |
| **H** | = | Head |
| **In** | = | Infolding |
| **Li** | = | Liver |
| **Py** | = | Renal pyramid |
| **Sh** | = | Shadowing |
| **Ut** | = | Uterus |

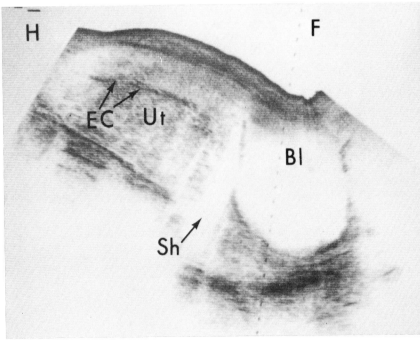

**FIG 1–76.**

## Beam Width Artifact

Since transducers are finite in size and diameter, a problem arises in the size of the echoes created on ultrasound images. In the text discussion of beam profile and focal zone, the characteristics of echoes were noted to be different at different depths within the body. Objects are best visualized in the focal zone because lateral resolution is optimum in this region. However, distortion of true anatomic representation occurs even in the focal zone. Because of beam width characteristics, a dot is represented as a line on the ultrasound image. This is not a true 1-to-1 representation. Most of the time, beam width problems will not cause any diagnostic difficulty. Occasionally they do.

Figure 1–77 is a transverse scan of the upper abdomen which shows an irregular margin (arrowhead) of the lateral border of the inferior vena cava. This could represent a thrombus or tumor. However, it is secondary to beam width artifact and must be recognized as such. By slightly angling the transducer and examining the region more closely, the sonographer will realize it is a transient finding secondary to an artifact. If it were secondary to a pathologic condition, the finding would be there on multiple views. Figure 1–78 demonstrates a clear, sharp border to the IVC of the same patient as in Figure 1–77. There is no evidence of any irregular echoes on the lateral wall of the inferior vena cava.

Evaluation of the walls of cystic masses becomes important on ultrasound. Cystic masses of the kidney, liver, ovary, and other organs are often studied on ultrasound examination. If they are diagnosed as simple cysts, very little further study is needed. if they are thought to be complex cysts, the differential diagnosis changes dramatically. Beam width artifact causes numerous problems in the evaluation of such masses. In Figure 1–79, a large cystic mass anterior to the uterus is identified. Portions of its wall, however, are imaged with the lateral resolving capabilities of the

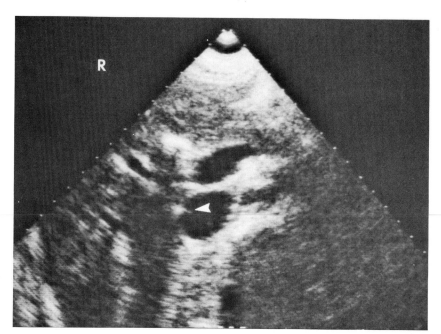

**FIG 1–77.**

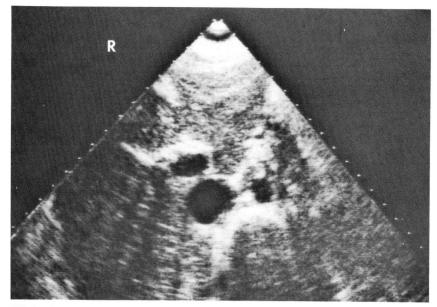

**FIG 1–78.**

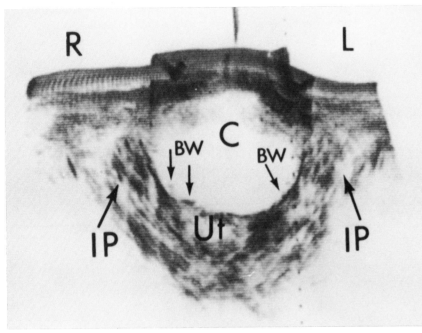

**FIG 1–79.**

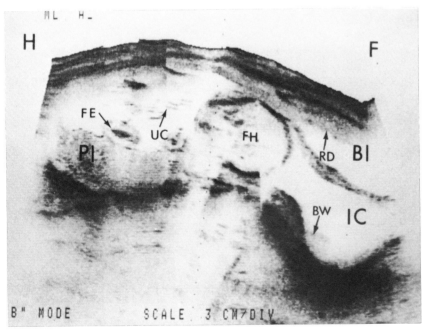

**FIG 1–80.**

beam leading to linear projections into the cyst. This can be mistaken for solid or septated components and thus lead to an incorrect diagnosis. Proper scanning technique helps establish that these findings are not real but secondary to beam width artifact.

Beam width artifact is commonly a problem in association with fluid-containing structures since the artifact is more easily seen in a fluid region rather than a solid region. Figure 1–80 is a longitudinal scan of a gravid uterus in a patient with incompetent cervix. Soft echoes are noted within the fluid in the endocervical canal. The echoes are suggestive of an area of hemorrhage. However, they are secondary to spurious echoes from beam width artifact.

| Arrowhead | = Beam width artifact |
|-----------|----------------------|
| BI | = Urinary bladder |
| BW | = Beam width artifact |
| C | = Ovarian cyst |
| F | = Foot |
| FE | = Fetal extremity |
| FH | = Fetal head |
| H | = Head |
| IC | = Incompetent cervix |
| IP | = Iliopsoas muscle |
| L | = Left |
| PI | = Placenta |
| R | = Right |
| RD | = Ring down |
| UC | = Uterine contraction |
| Ut | = Uterus |

## Total Ultrasound Reflectors

The major complete reflector within the body is air. In addition to the shadowing effect, the very strong reflections lead to a series of reverberation and ring-down artifacts. In Figure 1–81, the typical appearance of artifacts associated with a total reflector is seen. In this case, a linear cap of gas in the stomach overlying the pancreas is illustrated. Each reverberation has regular periodic qualities and is associated with a tail ring-down artifact. Each subsequent reverberation is narrower, thinner, and associated with a smaller ring-down tail.

Figure 1–82 illustrates an additional feature of a reverberation artifact. Since it represents the bouncing back and forth between two surfaces, the configuration of the reverberation is the summation effect of the configuration of the two interfaces. In this case, the configurations of the skin and the linear cap of gas are different; as a result, the configuration of the reverberation is significantly different from that of the total reflector. The source of the reverberation is still easily identified by the associated shadowing and the tail of ring down.

When a gas pocket is spherical in shape, the total reflection is inclined and never returns to the transducer, leading to a clean type of shadowing (Fig 1–83). This most frequently occurs in the small bubble of gas in the duodenal bulb and can mimic the clean shadowing resulting from velocity changes in an abnormal gallbladder. Therefore, when the diagnosis of an abnormal gallbladder, based on shadowing related to velocity changes, is entertained, the duodenum must be specifically identified.

In general, artifacts related to total reflectors are easily identified, but they still may cause problems in scan interpretation. In Figure 1–84, artifacts associated with the total reflectors make determination of the extent of the aneurysm difficult. If the gas pockets were more generalized, the aneurysm could be entirely obscured.

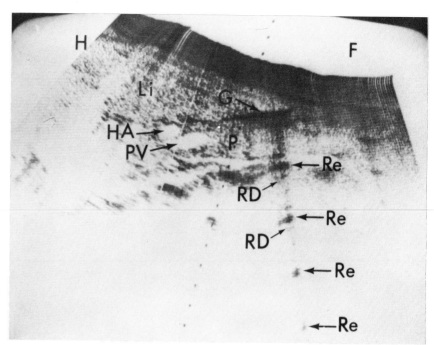

**FIG 1–81.**

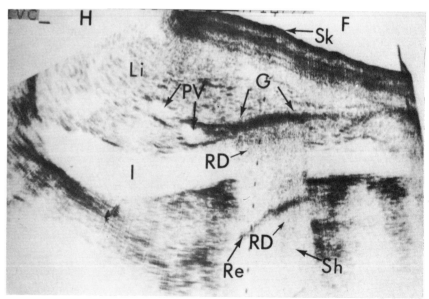

**FIG 1–82.**

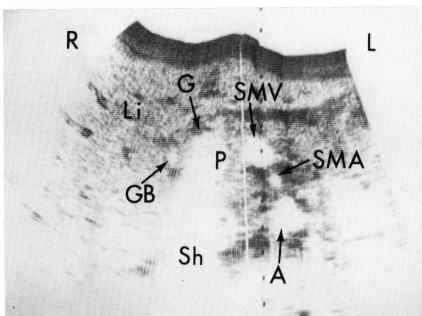

FIG 1–83.

| A | = | Aorta |
|---|---|---|
| An | = | Aneurysm |
| Co | = | Colon |
| F | = | Foot |
| G | = | Gas |
| GB | = | Gallbladder |
| H | = | Head |
| HA | = | Hepatic artery |
| I | = | Inferior vena cava |
| L | = | Left |
| Li | = | Liver |
| P | = | Pancreas |
| PV | = | Portal vein |
| R | = | Right |
| RD | = | Ring down |
| Re | = | Reverberation |
| Sh | = | Shadowing |
| Sk | = | Skin |
| SMA | = | Superior mesenteric artery |
| SMV | = | Superior mesenteric vein |
| St | = | Stomach |

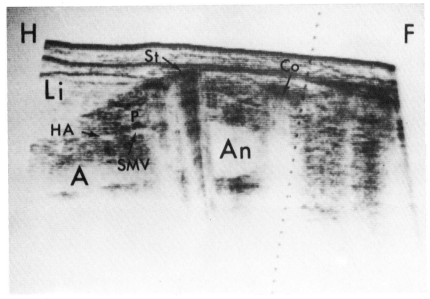

FIG 1–84.

## Total Sound Reflectors

In some cases, the reverberation phenomena created by total reflectors are more difficult to recognize. In Figures 1–85 and 1–86 the transverse and longitudinal scans of a patient being evaluated for pancreatic disease are provided. A flat cap of gas within the duodenal bulb has resulted in a single reverberation artifact that mimics a true, more deeply situated interface. The resulting through-transmission sign is seemingly satisfied, and a mass is misinterpreted in the pancreatic region. The different inclination of the reverberation in Figure 1–86 that results from the differing configurations of the skin and gas pocket further confuses the issue. These types of reverberative phenomena usually can be recognized if multiple scanning approaches are directed at the same interface. Different types of reverberative phenomena usually can be elicited and will allow proper recognition.

Another place where phenomena reverberating off total reflectors frequently occur is in the pelvis. The fluid-filled bladder allows a path of decreased attenuation for such a reverberation even if the total reflecting surface is deep within the pelvis. The apparent mass effect created by reverberation off the gas in the rectal sigmoid portion of the colon passing beneath the adnexa is shown in Figure 1–87. Since the reverberation was associated with very little ring-down noise, a cystic-appearing mass with apparent through-transmission was simulated. The apparent through-transmission, however, represents the reverberation plus its accompanying ring-down noise.

If the reverberation artifact from gas beneath the bladder is associated with a large amount of noise, a solid-appearing mass within the pelvis can be simulated, as demonstrated in Figure 1–88. The mass in this case mimics an enlarged uterus adjacent to an adnexal fluid collection. Careful questioning of the patient, however, revealed that the uterus had been removed some years ago and led to alternative scanning approaches that

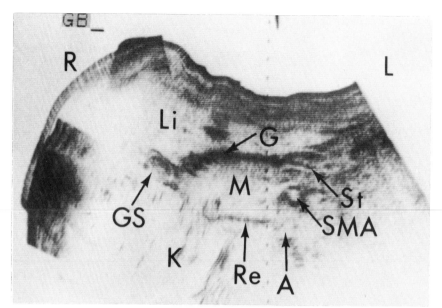

FIG 1–85.

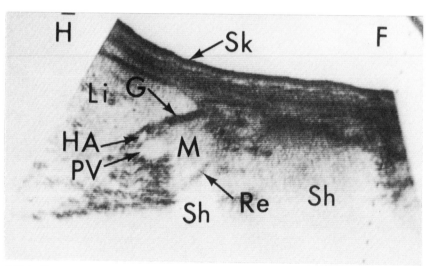

FIG 1–86.

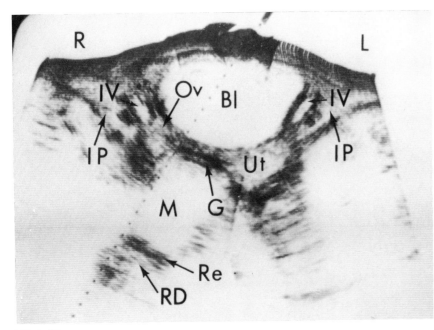

**FIG 1–87.**

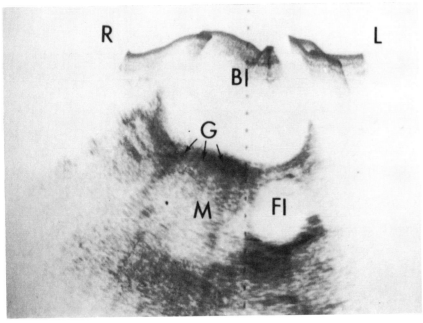

**FIG 1–88.**

demonstrated the artifactual nature of the mass.

SOURCE: Figure 1–87 is reproduced with permission from Sample WF: Normal Anatomy of the female pelvis: Computed tomography and ultrasonography, in Rosenfield AT: *Genitourinary Ultrasonography* (Clinics in Diagnostic Ultrasound Series, vol 2). New York, Churchill Livingstone, Inc., 1979.

| **A**   | = | Aorta |
|---------|---|-------|
| **Bl**  | = | Bladder |
| **F**   | = | Foot |
| **Fl**  | = | Fluid |
| **G**   | = | Gas |
| **GS**  | = | Gallstone |
| **H**   | = | Head |
| **HA**  | = | Hepatic artery |
| **IP**  | = | Iliopsoas muscle |
| **IV**  | = | Iliac vessels |
| **K**   | = | Kidney |
| **L**   | = | Left |
| **Li**  | = | Liver |
| **M**   | = | False mass |
| **Ov**  | = | Ovary |
| **PV**  | = | Portal vein |
| **R**   | = | Right |
| **RD**  | = | Ring down |
| **Re**  | = | Reverberation |
| **Sh**  | = | Shadowing |
| **Sk**  | = | Skin |
| **SMA** | = | Superior mesenteric artery |
| **St**  | = | Stomach |
| **Ut**  | = | Uterus |

## Artifacts Associated With Regions of Low Attenuation

Interposed regions of low attenuation are associated with a number of artifacts. The acoustic impedance differences at the junction of an average and a low-attenuating tissue usually are substantial and generate relatively strong reflections. Therefore, when the region of low attenuation is close to the transducer, a series of reverberation and ring-down artifacts can be generated within the low-attenuating area. These regions have been recognized on ultrasound as the echoes in the near side of the fluid region (Fig 1–89) and usually are easily identified. However, when the region of low attenuation occurs very superficially, the noise and ring-down phenomena, particularly if the gain settings are somewhat high, can totally obscure the region unless careful attention is paid to underlying enhancement. A typical clinical example is illustrated in Figure 1–90, in which a very superficial renal cyst easily could be missed.

More deeply situated regions of diminished attenuation also can lead to artifacts if there is a nearby strong reflecting surface. A common place for such an artifact to occur is in a cystic or fluid mass within the liver adjacent to the diaphragm. Reverberation artifacts result and give the apparent appearance of a similar mass on the other side of the diaphragm, as indicated in Figure 1–91.

An experimental situation simulating this phenomenon is demonstrated in Figure 1–92. A water bath containing a balloon filled with water is placed midway along the ultrasound beam but adjacent to the highly reflective water-bath wall. While the sound beam is insonating the water-bath wall at an inclination, reflections are set up which reverberate off the balloon and simulate a similarly configured mass in the air outside of the container. This experiment was conducted by Fred Gardner.

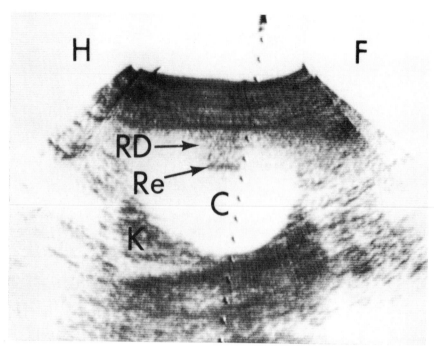

FIG 1–89.

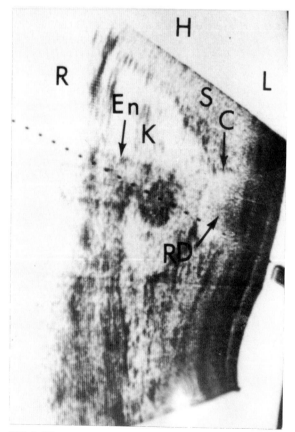

FIG 1–90.

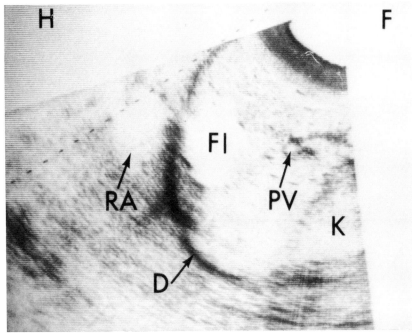

| B | = Balloon |
| C | = Cyst |
| D | = Diaphragm |
| En | = Enhancement |
| F | = Foot |
| FI | = Fluid |
| H | = Head |
| K | = Kidney |
| L | = Left |
| PV | = Portal vein |
| R | = Right |
| RA | = Reduplication artifact |
| RD | = Ring down |
| Re | = Reverberation |
| S | = Spleen |

FIG 1–91.

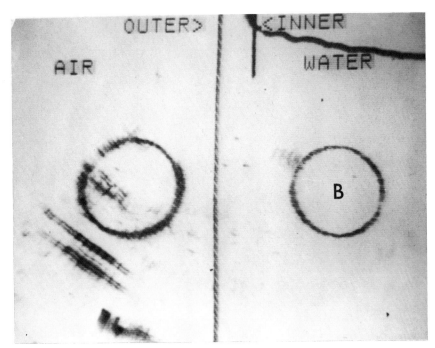

FIG 1–92.

## Duplication Artifact

Duplication artifact can occur secondary to reflection and refraction phenomena. Duplication artifact secondary to reflection is also called a mirror
image artifact. Air is a nearly complete
reflector of ultrasound. Because of
this, it acts as an acoustic mirror. Any
large air interface can act as a potential source of diagnostic problems because of duplication artifact. In the
previous case (see Fig 1–92), the
acoustic mirror was the straight border
of the glass tank. The following images (Figs 1–93 through 1–96) involved a curved acoustic mirror, the
right hemidiaphragm.

Figure 1–93 is a longitudinal scan
of the right upper quadrant in a patient
who has a large echogenic mass (M)
in the midportion of the liver. Since
the diaphragm is in contact with air-
containing lung, this interface acts as
a nearly complete reflector of sound.
After the sound beam hits the diaphragm, it is nearly completely reflected back to the transducer and encounters the echogenic mass on the
return trip. The echogenic mass reflects sound back to the diaphragm,
which then returns the echo for its
final trip to the transducer. Since we
are only measuring time on ultrasound
and then converting it to distance, a
second echogenic mass is created
(DA) in what appears to be the base
of the lung. There are no true echoes
in the base of the lung. The duplication artifact is surrounded by false
liver parenchymal echoes which arise
from the liver beneath the diaphragm.
These are also secondary to duplication artifacts.

Figure 1–95 is another example of
duplication artifact of the diaphragm. A
subdiaphragmatic fluid collection has
been reproduced above the diaphragm (D). There are no true echoes
present above the diaphragm in this
image. The sonolucent area above the
diaphragm is a duplication artifact
(DA) reproducing the subdiaphragmatic fluid (Fl), and the curved line is
a duplication artifact reproducing the
liver capsule.

Occasionally, a mass may be noted
in what appears to be the base of the

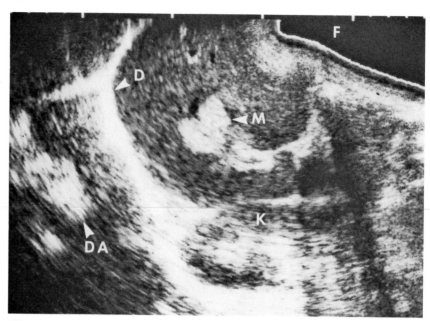

**FIG 1–93.**

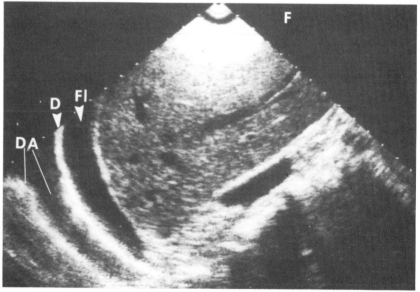

**FIG 1–94.**

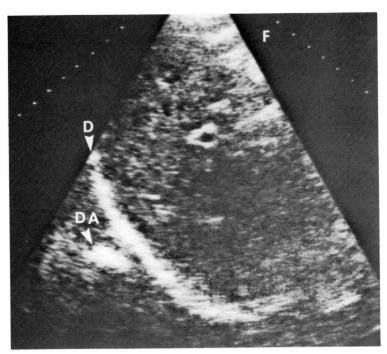

**FIG 1–95.**

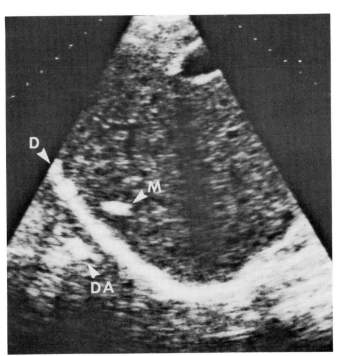

**FIG 1–96.**

lung; that is a clue to liver pathology. By being aware of the mirror image duplication artifact of the diaphragm, the sonographer may detect liver masses that were initially missed. Since the diaphragm is a curved surface, it is not a perfect reflector. Rather, it causes distortion of the ultrasound image above the diaphragm. When the beam path is just to the side of a liver mass, it may miss the mass on the initial trip but encounter the mass on the reflected trip off the diaphragm. Such is the case in Figure 1–95, where the duplication artifact (DA) is noted above the diaphragm but not in the liver. Once this is recognized as a duplication artifact, the liver can more closely be examined. Figure 1–96 is a scan of the same patient as in Figure 1–95, but scanning was carried out in a slightly different plane. Both the liver mass (M) and the duplication artifact (DA) can be seen.

| | | |
|---|---|---|
| **D** | = | Diaphragm |
| **DA** | = | Duplication artifact |
| **F** | = | Foot |
| **FI** | = | Subdiaphragmatic fluid |
| **K** | = | Kidney |
| **M** | = | Liver mass |

## Duplication Artifact

Duplication artifact can occur secondary to refraction. This is most common over the abdominal wall in the region of the rectus muscle. The muscle-fat interface causes a bending of the ultrasound beam, which in turn can create a duplicated image of various anatomic structures. This duplication artifact is secondary to refraction, whereas the duplication artifact associated with the diaphragm in previous cases was secondary to reflection.

Figure 1–97 is a transverse scan of the pelvis which shows a duplication artifact of an intrauterine device (I). The anterior portion of the uterine wall is also duplicated. Figure 1–98 is a scan of the same patient as in Figure 1–97, with the transducer position changed slightly. Now, a truer anatomic representation is present. A single intrauterine device and single contour to the uterine wall are visualized.

Figure 1–99 is a scan showing a duplication artifact of the superior mesenteric artery (arrowheads). Note that the aorta is single in appearance. Duplication of the superior mesenteric artery is secondary to refraction in this case. The transducer position was moved slightly in Figure 1–100. The superior mesenteric artery (arrowhead) is now single in appearance. However, because of the slight change in position of the transducer, the aorta is now duplicated by the same artifact.

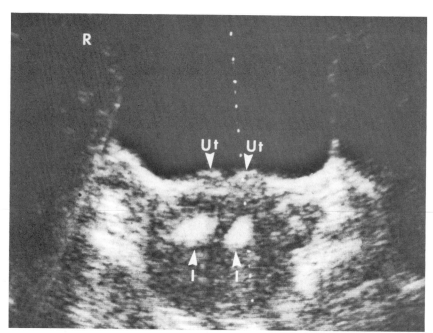

FIG 1–97.

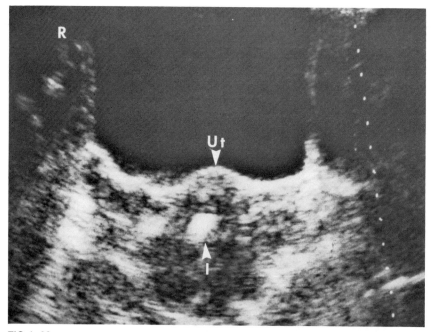

FIG 1–98.

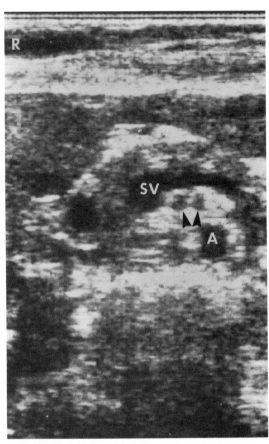

**FIG 1–99.**

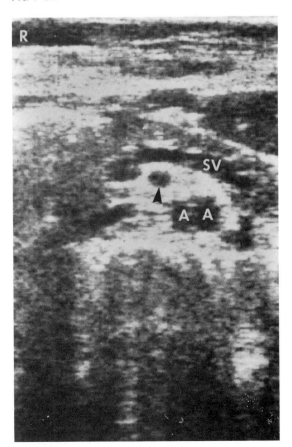

**FIG 1–100.**

| A | = Aorta |
|---|---|
| **Arrowhead** | = Superior mesenteric artery |
| I | = Intrauterine device |
| R | = Right |
| SV | = Splenic vein |
| Ut | = Anterior uterine wall |

## Duplication Artifact Causing a Double Gestational Sac

Because of refraction associated with the abdominal rectus muscles, duplication artifacts in the pelvis can be a common occurrence. When they are present during early gestation, a mistaken diagnosis of a twin pregnancy may be made secondary to the refracted duplication artifact. Figures 1–101 and 1–102 are scans of two different patients; the scans show duplication artifacts of the gestational sac secondary to the refracted phenomenon. This can lead to an embarrassing misdiagnosis of twins, as a single pregnancy will be present later in pregnancy. This error can be avoided by scanning a gestational sac from several directions. If a twin gestation is truly present, a double sac will always be identified in various views. However, if this is only secondary to a refracted phenomenon, a double gestational sac will only be visualized in one position. By slightly altering the transducer position, the sonographer can avoid this diagnostic error.

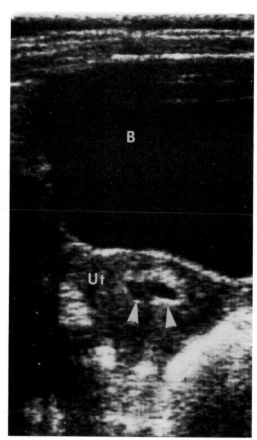

**FIG 1–101.**

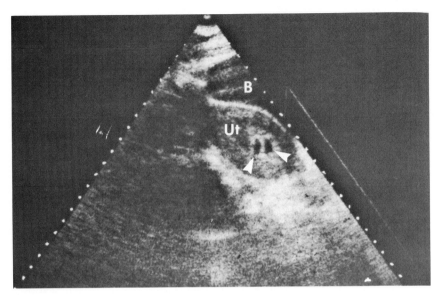

**FIG 1–102.**

| | | |
|---|---|---|
| **Arrowheads** | = | Double gestational sac |
| **DA** | = | Duplication artifact |
| **B** | = | Urinary bladder |
| **Ut** | = | Uterus |

# 2.
# Hepatic Section

Philip W. Ralls, M.D.

## Normal Sonographic Anatomy of the Liver

The liver, the largest parenchymal organ in the body, plays a vital role in abdominal sonography. The liver fills the right upper abdomen, displacing gas-filled structures. This provides an acoustic window through which not only the liver itself, but also the upper abdomen and retroperitoneum may be imaged. Consequently, an understanding of hepatic and perihepatic anatomy is crucial in state-of-the-art abdominal sonography.

The liver is a sonographically complex organ. There is a relatively homogeneous "parenchymal background" of medium-level echogenicity in which many other structures are seen. Within this background are various-sized, fluid-filled tubular structures and many linear and rounded echogenic areas. Basic to understanding this anatomy is an appreciation of the microscopic structure of the liver.

The hepatic parenchyma consists of hepatocytes interspersed with reticuloendothelial cells (Kupffer cells) organized into lobules. Each lobule measures approximately 1 × 2 mm. Within the lobule, the hepatocytes are arranged radially in cords about a central hepatic venule (Fig 2–1). There are approximately one million of these lobules in a typical liver.[1] Peripherally, around each lobule, are several portal triads. The portal triads consist of portal venules, bile ductules, and hepatic arterioles, surrounded by fibrofatty areolar tissue.

The medium-level-echogenic sonographic "parenchymal background" is due primarily to nonspecular reflectors, most of which are probably lobules and their surrounding stroma. Interspersed throughout the parenchyma are numerous small rounded echogenic areas. These areas represent portal regions in which the hepatic artery, bile duct, and portal vein lumina are too small to be imaged. All that one sees is the echogenic periportal fibrofatty tissue.

Many fluid-filled tubular structures are seen in the liver. Most of these are hepatic or portal veins. Generally, only the larger hepatic arteries are imaged, usually near the porta hepatis ventral to the portal veins.[2] Intrahepatic bile ducts usually are not imaged unless they are dilated.

The last important group of intrahepatic anatomic structures consists of the echogenic linear fissures and ligaments. These structures are imaged primarily

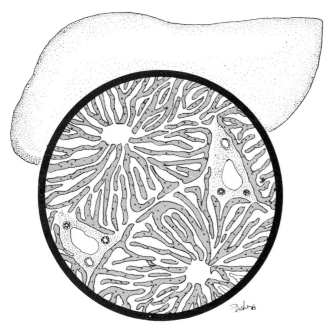

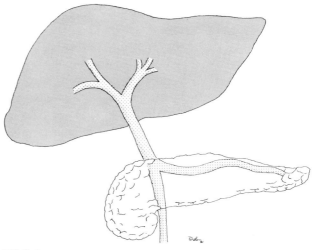

**FIG 2–2.**
*The horizontal splenic vein and vertical superior mesenteric vein are shown to join behind the isthmus of the pancreas, forming the portal vein.*

**FIG 2–1.**
*The inset shows hepatic lobules formed by cords of hepatocytes with sinusoids between them, situated around a central hepatic venule. Portal triads, located between the lobules, contain the larger portal venules and smaller bile ductules and hepatic arterioles.*

because of the fat contained within and about them. One can segregate the liver into lobes and segments using the hepatic ligaments and venous structures as landmarks.

*Portal Veins*

Portal venous structures bring blood from the splenic and mesenteric circulations to the liver. The portal venous system provides about two thirds of the blood reaching the liver, twice as much as the hepatic arteries. The main portal vein is formed behind or dorsal to the cephalad isthmus of the pancreas by the confluence of the splenic and superior mesenteric veins (Fig 2–2). The portal vein then courses cranially, usually following a somewhat lateral and ventral path, through the hepatoduodenal ligament (the free right edge of the lesser omentum) to enter the liver at the porta hepatis (Fig 2–3). At the porta, the portal vein or its major branches, the right and left portal veins, plunge intrahepatically to supply all portions of the liver. Portal veins are primarily intersegmental structures, in contrast to hepatic veins, which are intersegmental or interlobar. Portal veins are easily recog-

nized as they are larger closer to the porta hepatis, and because of the dense peripheral echoes typically seen about them. This prominent peripheral echogenicity is not caused by the venous walls per se, but rather by the surrounding fibrofatty tissue. As noted, this fibrofatty tissue acounts for most of the multiple small echo-dense areas seen throughout the hepatic parenchyma. These areas represent small portal regions whose tubular structures are insufficiently large to be imaged sonographically, but are imaged nonetheless because of the surrounding echogenic fibrofatty tissue.

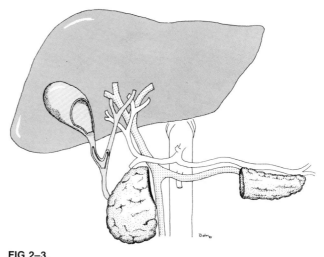

**FIG 2–3.**
*The portal triad contains the portal vein posterior to the hepatic artery and biliary system.*

## Hepatic Arteries and Bile Ducts

Accompanying the portal venous system are the other two components of the portal triad, the hepatic arterial system and the bile ducts. Generally, the bile ducts and the hepatic arterial structures lie ventral to the larger portal venous structures (see Fig 2–3). The relationship of the larger portal vein to the smaller arteries and bile ducts can be seen macroscopically in the hepatoduodenal ligament (main portal vein, common duct, and proper hepatic artery). This relationship is maintained down to the microscopic portal triads. Only the larger hepatic arteries are normally seen ventral to the major portal veins. Intrahepatic bile ducts are rarely imaged unless dilated.

## Hepatic Veins

Hepatic veins drain blood from the hepatic lobules and transport it to the systemic circulation, emptying into the inferior vena cava. Hepatic veins are easily recognized sonographically by their location in the cephalad portion of the liver, becoming larger as they approach the inferior vena cava. Additionally, hepatic veins have much less prominent peripheral echogenicity than portal veins, frequently appearing to have no "walls" at all. Occasionally, major hepatic veins will have some increased peripheral echogenicity, but this is never as prominent as with comparably sized portal veins. Hepatic veins are intersegmental and interlobar and thus may be used to define hepatic lobar and segmental anatomy.

## Lobar and Segmental Anatomy of the Liver

The lobar anatomy of the liver is defined most meaningfully by biliary drainage and vasculature. On this basis, the liver is separable into three lobes—right, left, and caudate. The "quadrate lobe" is the medial segment of the left lobe, rather than an anatomically distinct lobe. Fortunately, hepatic veins and hepatic fissues, both of which run between the lobes and their segments, can be used to define the lobar and segmental anatomy.[3–7]

Ligamentous structures can be identified sonographically because of surrounding echogenic fat. Important fissures and ligaments include the main lobar fissure, the right and left intersegmental fissures, the fissure for the ligamentum venosum, and the falciform ligament, whose dorsal free edge is the ligamentum teres, which is the fissure for the umbilical vein (Table 2–1).

### RIGHT LOBE

The right lobe comprises the bulk of hepatic tissue. It is separated from the left lobe by the main lobar fissure caudally and by the middle hepatic vein cranially (Figs 2–4 through 2–7). The main lobar fissure runs obliquely from the region of the right portal vein down to the gallbladder fossa. On transverse views the main lobar fissure is seen as a comet-tailed echogenic structure extending anteriorly and to the right, just cephalad to the gallbladder fossa. On sagittal views it appears as a linear echogenic structure of variable length extending from the right portal vein down to the gallbladder fossa. Thus, the main lobar

**TABLE 2–1.**

**Important Hepatic Fissures**

| FISSURE | BETWEEN | CONTAINS | COMMENTS |
|---|---|---|---|
| Main lobar fissure | R and L lobes | Gallbladder | Comet-tailed appearance on transverse scans; helps locate gallbladder |
| Ligamentum venosum | L and caudate lobes | . . . | Continuous with the extrahepatic gastrohepatic ligament |
| Ligamentum teres | Medial and lateral segments of L lobe | Obliterated umbilical vein | Runs in free edge of the falciform ligament |
| R intersegmental fissure | Anterior and posterior segments of R lobe | R portal vein, R hepatic duct, R hepatic artery | Usually very short; may not be seen separate from porta hepatis |
| L intersegmental fissure | Medial and lateral segments of L lobe | L portal vein | May be hard to see; location is defined by the distal left portal vein |

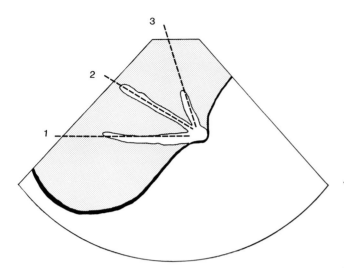

**FIG 2–4.**
*Orientation of a high transverse scan through the three hepatic veins. Line 1 separates the anterior and posterior segments of the right lobe and passes through the right hepatic vein. Line 2 separates the right and left lobes and passes through the middle hepatic vein. Line 3 separates the medial and lateral segments of the left lobe and passes through the left hepatic vein.*

fissure may be used to localize the gallbladder in difficult cases.[8]

The gallbladder, the inferior vena cava, and the middle hepatic vein can also be used as landmarks to define the plane between the right and left lobes. On transverse images, a line connecting the inferior vena

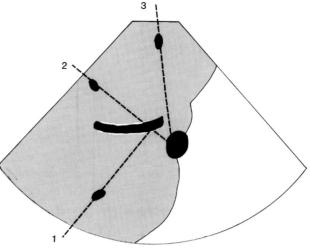

**FIG 2–6.**
*Orientation of a transverse scan lower than that in Figure 2–5, at the level of the right portal vein. Lines 1, 2, and 3 separate the same segmental anatomy as in Figure 2–4. Line 3 extends through the echogenic ligamentum teres.*

cava with the gallbladder in the caudal portion of the liver, or with the middle hepatic vein more cranially, defines this plane. Thus, even when the main lobar fissure is not seen well, the plane delineating right from the left hepatic lobes can be closely approximated.

### LEFT LOBE

The left lobe is separated from the right lobe by the main lobar fissure and the middle hepatic vein (see

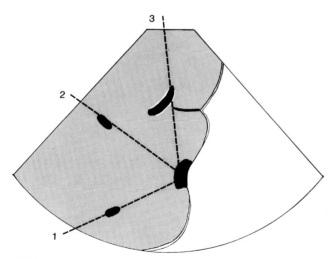

**FIG 2–5.**
*Orientation of a transverse scan slightly inferior to that shown in Figure 2–4. Lines 1, 2, and 3 separate the same segmental anatomy as in Figure 2–4. Lines 1 and 2 pass through the right and middle hepatic veins, respectively. Line 3 passes through the left portal vein. The horizontal line extending to the right from line 3 represents the fissure for the ligamentum venosum and separates the left lobe from the caudate lobe.*

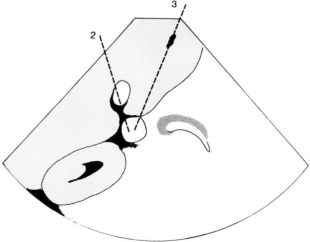

**FIG 2–7.**
*Orientation of a transverse scan lower than that in Figure 2–6. Lines 2 and 3 separate the same segmental anatomy as Figure 2–4. Line 3 extends through the echogenic ligamentum teres. Line 2 extends from the inferior vena cava through the gallbladder fossa.*

Figs 2–4 through 2–7). On its dorsal surface, it is separated from the caudate lobe by the fissure for the ligamentum venosum and by the proximal portion of the left portal vein (see Fig 2–5).

## CAUDATE LOBE

The caudate lobe is the smallest lobe of the liver.[9] It lies dorsal to the left lobe near the cephalad portion of the liver. The caudate lobe is separated from the left lobe by the fissure for the ligamentum venosum and the proximal portion of the left portal vein. The right lateral border of the caudate lobe is formed by the inferior vena cava cephalad. Caudally, the caudate process of the caudate lobe extends down between the inferior vena cava and the portal vein. The caudate process merges with the right lobe of the liver, generally without a sonographically definable border. The length of the caudate process defines the relationship of the inferior vena cava to the main portal vein. The smaller the caudate process, the longer the contiguity between the inferior vena cava and the main portal vein.

## SEGMENTAL ANATOMY

The large right lobe is divided into anterior and posterior segments by the short right intersegmental fissure, which is frequently not separably identifiable from the porta hepatis structures. The plane between the segments is best defined by a line drawn from the porta hepatis to the right hepatic vein (see Figs 2–4 through 2–7). The right hepatic vein runs between the anterior and posterior branches of the right portal vein, which run within their respective segments.

The medial and lateral segments of the left lobe are delineated, cranially to caudally, by the left hepatic vein, the left intersegmental fissure, and ligamentum teres (fissure for the umbilical vein). Cranially, the left hepatic vein segregates the medial and lateral segments, but is somewhat inconsistently imageable. The left intersegmental fissure is defined by the distal portion of the left portal vein. This portion of the left portal vein runs almost vertically dorsally to ventrally (see Fig 2–5), sending branches right and left to the segments of the left lobe. Caudad to the left portal vein, the medial and lateral segments are best defined by the round, echogenic ligamentum teres (see Figs 2–6 and 2–7). The ligamentum teres is the free (dorsal) edge of the falciform ligament and is always easily

seen sonographically because of the fat within it. The falciform ligament itself is generally not seen because of a paucity of fat.

## Perihepatic Relationships

The diaphragm is seen as a dense echogenic line adjacent to the right lateral and cephalad aspect of the liver. The liver capsule itself is very thin and is rarely imaged sonographically.

The liver is tethered in the upper abdomen to the diaphragm and retroperitoneum by ligaments. Additional support is provided by intra-abdominal pressure. The coronary ligament of the liver is the primary support structure. It is formed by the peritoneal reflections, which encompass a nonperitonealized region extending over a variable amount of the right and left lobes. The right-sided portion of the area encompassed by the coronary ligament is called the bare area. The bare area is between the recesses of the anterior and posterior subphrenic spaces, bounded laterally by the right triangular ligament (the right free edge of the coronary ligament) and medially by the inferior vena cava. The nonperitonealized area continues to the left of the inferior vena cava. Its leftmost extent is defined by the left free edge of the coronary ligament, the left triangular ligament.

The falciform ligament originates from the midportion of the coronary ligament, extending from the anterior abdominal wall to the liver. The falciform ligament inserts between the medial and lateral segments of the left lobe. The posterior (dorsal) free edge of the falciform ligament is the round ligamentum teres. The ligamentum teres is virtually always imaged sonographically because of the fat it contains. The remainder of the falciform ligament usually contains insufficient fat to be imaged sonographically. The falciform ligament separates the left and right subphrenic spaces.

The ligamentum teres extends caudally from the most ventral portion of the distal or vertical portion of the left portal vein. It becomes progressively more superficial and ventral, finally emerging from the liver near the anterior abdominal wall peritoneum on its course to the umbilicus.

The gastrohepatic ligament, also known as the lesser omentum, is an important perihepatic structure.

It originates on the undersurface of the liver continuous with the ligamentum venosum. It sweeps caudally to attach to the lesser curvature of the stomach and the first portion of the duodenum. Gastrohepatic ligament pathology is often overlooked. Varices and enlarged nodes may be imaged in this region.

The right free edge of the gastrohepatic ligament is called the hepatoduodenal ligament. The hepatoduodenal ligament is important sonographically because it surrounds the portal vein, proper hepatic artery, and common duct on their way to the porta hepatis. The size of the caudate process of the caudate lobe determines, in part, the length of the hepatoduodenal ligament and its relationship to the inferior vena cava posteriorly (Fig 2–8). The portal vein within the hepatoduodenal ligament and the inferior vena cava are contiguous immediately caudad to the caudate process. This is the location of the foramen of Winslow, a potential space that represents the only communication of the lesser peritoneal sac with the rest of the peritoneal cavity. The ventral portion of the lesser sac is formed in part by the gastrohepatic ligament.

To the right of the hepatoduodenal ligament is the subhepatic space. In this area, the gallbladder is the only structure that has a fossa on the medial under surface of the liver (see Fig 2–8). This fossa is at the caudal extent of the main lobar fissure, indenting a portion of both the medial segment of the left lobe and the anterior segment of the right lobe (see Fig 2–8). The gallbladder can be localized by identifying the main lobar fissure sagittally as it courses down from the right portal vein between the left and right lobes. Laterally, an indentation for the right kidney is seen on the posterior segment of the right hepatic lobe. The subhepatic space is continuous with the anterior and posterior subphrenic spaces as well as with the right paracolic gutter.

## Variants of Normal and Pseudolesions

The normal liver is shaped like a three-sided pyramid with its base formed by the large right lobe and its apex by the tapered tip of the left lobe. Generally, the sagittal area of the liver is largest through the right lateral portions of the right lobe, where it essentially fills the entire depth of the abdomen. The sagittal area then decreases progressively to the left until the tapered tip of the left lobe terminates, usually slightly left

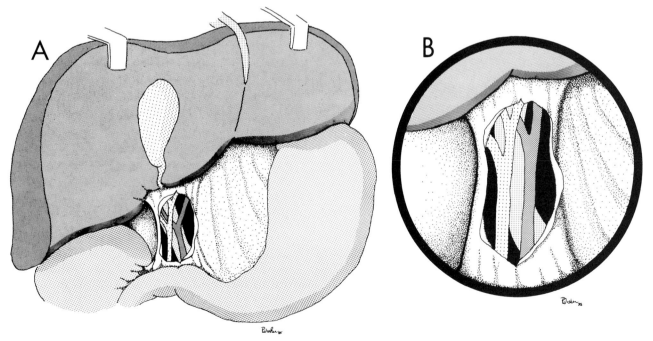

**FIG 2–8.**
*A, hepatoduodenal ligament forming the right free edge of the lesser omentum as it courses from the undersurface of the liver to the lesser curvature of the stomach and the first portion of the duodenum. B, enlarged view of the hepatoduodenal ligament and its contents. The portal vein is the larger posterior structure. The hepatic artery and its branches are the smaller anterior tubular medial structures, and the common bile duct and branches are anterior and lateral. These three structures make up the portal triad.*

of midline. The left lobe is primarily an anterior structure.

Commonly, the left lobe is somewhat smaller and truncated, terminating to the right of midline. These patients are more difficult to examine sonographically because of the decreased acoustic window. Another fairly common variation is an elongated left lobe whose tip extends far left of midline, occasionally extending lateral to the spleen. Rarer hepatic variations include situs inversus, in which the liver is on the left side, and the polysplenia/asplenia complex, in which the liver may be symmetric or midline. Riedel's lobe is a caudal extension of the right lobe. In this entity, the tip of the liver may extend below the right iliac crest. Normal variations in hepatic shape may occasionally prompt sonography for a palpable mass. Sonographers should understand these variants in hepatic shape so that they are not misdiagnosed as hepatic mass lesions.

Diffuse liver disease may cause atrophy and compensatory hypertrophic changes. Usually there is a relative decrease in the size of the right lobe, with enlargement of the left and/or caudate lobes. This situation may be differentiated from normal variants by the presence of altered hepatic echogenicity and the presence of other signs of diffuse liver disease such as splenomegaly and portosystemic collaterals.

Occasionally, indentations of the diaphragm subdivide the hepatic parenchyma, causing "pseudofissures." Pseudofissures are most commonly seen along the cephalad border of the right lobe and occasionally mimic hepatic fissures or lesions.[10] Indentations along the right lateral lobe caused by ribs may also be seen occasionally.

Hepatic pseudolesions may be caused by fat collections within the liver. These usually occur in or near major fissures.[11] The ligamentum teres, which is always seen as a rounded echogenic structure between the medial and lateral segments of the left lobe, is the most frequently encountered pseudolesion of this type. The ligamentum teres frequently exhibits some degree of acoustic shadowing.[9] Acoustic shadowing may be seen from other normal echogenic intrahepatic structures, especially the fibrofatty tissue around portal veins. The presence of acoustic shadowing from these normal structures should not prompt their misdiagnosis as lesions.

Another occasional pseudolesion occurs when transverse scans through the caudal portion of the right lobe intersect the upper pole of the right kidney and perirenal fat. This can result in either an echogenic or a "bull's-eye" pseudolesion in the right hepatic lobe. This pseudolesion, as well as the others mentioned above, is easily recognized with real-time techniques which allow rapid scanning in multiple planes. This, coupled with an understanding of normal hepatic anatomy, will prevent misdiagnosis.

## Hepatic Ultrasound Technique

Although many of the scans reproduced in this chapter were obtained using conventional scanning equipment, real-time imaging is the principal mode used in modern sonography. Real-time scanning not only allows assessment of structures in motion, it also facilitates rapid delineation of pathology, quickly displaying the anatomic relationships and internal characteristics of any lesion. Real-time imaging allows confident and easy identification of normal anatomic structures as well as complete, careful surveys of the liver.

Controversy exists as to whether ultrasound images should be displayed as white echoes against a black background or as gray echoes against a clear background. Although many authors prefer one or the other display technique, no carefully controlled study has proved either superior. This writer finds that echo-free structures are more apparent when viewed against black backgrounds, while subtle gray-scale alterations are more apparent when viewed against clear backgrounds. The "white-on-black" displays looked prettier than "gray-on-clear" displays when early real-time instruments were used, probably because these systems lacked sufficient gray-scale capabilities. Thus, many sonographers have "grown up" with black background real-time imaging, leading to a growing preference for this type of display. However, background preference is extremely varied, especially among experienced ultrasonographers. The important factor is understanding the basic concepts of ultrasound imaging. These include echo amplitude, attenuation, transmission, and parenchymal texture, features evident with both modalities. Choice of display modality is subjective, in the absence of evidence from appropriately conducted experiments in perceptual psychology.

The most useful information derived from any real-time hepatic sonogram can be obtained by observing the study as it is performed. During the examination, hard copy images are made to document pathology and to substantiate that a complete examination was performed. This is analogous to a fluoroscopic radiographic examination. The dynamic relationships are seen during the real-time part of the examination and the hard copy "spot film," are taken to document the findings.

One must ensure that the entire liver is imaged during the examination. One must always ask, "Have I seen the whole liver?" Problem areas include the ventral liver, especially beneath the ribs at the costal margin, the left lateral tip of the left lobe, and the most cephalad and lateral aspects of the right lobe. Generally, a sector real-time device is best since it can scan between ribs to image problem areas. Changing the patient's position, particularly to various degrees of right anterior obliquity, is helpful. Both focal lesions and diffuse changes in echogenicity should be sought. Displacement of normal structures, such as fissures and vessels, is a useful indicator of disease.

Hard copy images should be obtained systematically. The internal architecture of any lesion should be characterized. Each lesion should be precisely localized by demonstrating its relationship to intrahepatic and perihepatic structures in several scan planes. Implicit clinical questions that arise during the examination should be answered. For example, if one sees hepatic metastasis, potential primary lesions in the pancreas and elsewhere should be sought.

If no abnormalities are detected, images of various anatomic landmarks should be recorded to prove that a complete examination was performed. We routinely obtain the following images: (1) transverse images showing the right and left portal veins, the left lobe (including the ligamentum teres), and the gallbladder fossa; (2) several sagittal images of the left and right lobes, including the region of the left portal vein and the region of the right portal vein and gallbladder fossa; (3) transverse subcostal scans angled cephalad showing the hepatic parenchyma and the diaphragm; and (4) oblique images of the long axis of the hepatoduodenal ligament.

Real-time ultrasonography allows expeditious survey examinations of the abdomen to be undertaken. For this reason, each hepatic sonogram should include an examination of the biliary tree, both kidneys, spleen, pancreas, and upper retroperitoneum. Images need not be obtained unless pathology is noted.

## Hepatic Pathology

Recently, computed tomography (CT) and real-time sonography have challenged the role of technetium sulfur colloid liver-spleen scanning as the screening test of choice in cases of suspected hepatic pathology.[12] CT and ultrasound appear to be more sensitive than nuclear medicine scanning.[13] More important, they can better characterize lesions that have been detected. Distinguishing simple cysts from noncystic lesions and diagnosing anatomic variants are more easily performed with CT and ultrasound than with nuclear medicine scanning. This writer believes that real-time sonography should be used to screen patients for suspected hepatic pathology, with CT serving as a backup. Ultrasonography is noninvasive, can be performed rapidly, and provides excellent results. Additionally, ultrasonography is the least expensive of available imaging tests, an important consideration in these times of heightened awareness of cost-effectiveness. High-resolution CT scanning, which has the advantage of being less technically dependent than sonography, is several times more expensive and exposes the patient to the risks attendant on intravenous contrast agent use and irradiation. Innovations may change which test is preferred for screening. The advent of new ultrasound and CT hepatic contrast agents, as well as the promise of magnetic resonance imaging, may alter the situation over the next few years.[14–17]

Few hepatic lesions have specific sonographic features. For this reason, knowledge of the patient's clinical history as well as the usual sonographic patterns of various lesions is important. In the following section sonographic patterns of disease are reviewed as an aid to limiting the differential diagnosis in patients with hepatic abnormalities.

### Benign Localized Lesions

#### HEPATIC CYSTIC LESIONS

Hepatic cystic disease includes simple, nonparasitic cysts, polycystic liver disease, hepatic pseudocysts, and cystadenomas. Simple cysts are usually solitary and may vary in size from millimeters to 20 cm. Sonographically, cysts have thin, well-defined walls, are echo free, and show distal sonic enhancement. Complications such as hemorrhage may occur, causing some changes in the sonographic pattern, and calcification may occur in cyst walls. There is a 4:1 female/male predominance of simple cysts.[18] The typical patient is a middle-aged woman. Most patients are asymptomatic. Large cysts may evoke symptoms, usually pain or mass effect. Symptomatic cysts may be treated surgically. Percutaneous aspiration and drainage is usually not efficacious in the long-term management of these patients.[19] However, we have treated one such patient by simple aspiration alone.

Polycystic liver disease usually consists of innumerable contiguous cysts, seldom over 2–3 cm in diameter.[18] These are histologically identical to simple cysts and have the same watery contents. Polycystic liver disease is less common than adult polycystic kidney disease, which may have associated simple hepatic cysts.[20–23] Polycystic liver disease is one part of a disease spectrum that includes adult polycystic kidney disease. Unlike patients with adult polycystic kidney disease, patients with polycystic liver disease do not have a diminished life expectancy. Rarely, polycystic liver disease may cause biliary obstruction. Malignant degeneration is very rare.

Residua from previous focal hepatic disease may produce lesions indistinguishable from simple cysts. This probably occurs most often after abscess.[24] These lesions are clinically insignificant and differ from simple cysts only in lacking an epithelial lining.

Hepatic cystadenoma is a rare neoplasm that most often occurs in middle-aged women.[25] Patients usually present with palpable abdominal masses. The lesions may be multilocular and as large as 15–20 cm. Cystadenomas contain mucinous fluid, rather than the watery fluid found in the cystic lesions described above. Treatment is surgical. Malignant degeneration is rare.

### INFLAMMATORY LESIONS

Modern antibiotics have changed the clinical spectrum of pyogenic hepatic abscess but have not lessened the incidence of hepatic abscess, which appears to be increasing slightly.[26] Patients currently developing hepatic abscess are older than pre-antibiotic era patients. In the past, appendicitis and gastrointestinal infections with portal venous sepsis were the major causes of hepatic abscess. More recently, hepatic abscesses have occurred most often as complications of biliary tract disease or trauma.[26]

Sonographically, most pyogenic abscesses are round or oval with relatively poorly defined walls. They tend to be centrally located, with only a minority touching the hepatic capsule. Internal echogenicity is usually less than that of the surrounding normal parenchyma, although clumps of increased echogenicity may be interspersed within the abscesses.[27] Gas-containing abscesses may be diffusely hyperechoic, a pattern that is also sometimes seen in non-gas-containing lesions.[28, 29] Diagnosis depends on correlation with the clinical history (usually right upper quadrant pain, fever, and a predisposing condition) and diagnostic percutaneous aspiration. Intrahepatic abscesses traditionally have been treated by surgical drainage. Percutaneous drainage is efficacious and is gaining wider acceptance.[30, 31] Many intrahepatic abscesses can be cured conservatively without either percutaneous or surgical drainage, merely by appropriate antibiotics alone.[32] Enthusiasm for interventional techniques must be tempered by this fact. Appropriate patient selection for surgical or percutaneous drainage is advised.

Hepatic amebic abscess, the most common nonenteric manifestation of amebiasis, is fairly common in patient populations where sanitation is suboptimal. Amebiasis is endemic throughout the United States. Hepatic amebic abscesses usually occur sometime after gastrointestinal infestation with *Entamoeba histolytica*, but hepatic amebiasis can occur coincident with the colonic disease. Many patients with hepatic amebic abscess report no gastrointestinal symptoms. Clinically, these patients present with right upper quadrant pain, relatively low-grade fever, and a mild leukocytosis. Patients with amebic abscesses usually appear less ill than patients with comparably sized pyogenic abscesses.

Sonographically, most amebic abscesses are peripheral, touching the liver capsule. In that respect they differ from pyogenic abscesses, which are primarily central. Amebic abscesses are usually round or oval with well-defined margins but without prominent wall echoes. Internally, the lesions are primarily hypoechoic, but may have areas of clumped echogenicity similar to pyogenic abscesses. Amebic abscesses tend to "fill in" with relatively homogeneous, low-level echogenicity at higher gain settings. Almost all amebic abscesses show some distal sonic enhancement, a finding that is much less consistent in pyogenic abscess.[33] Detection of a lesion with the above characteristics in a patient from a population at risk for amebiasis should prompt the sonographer to suggest hepatic amebic abscess.

Hydatid disease of the liver, caused by infestation with various species of *Echinococcus,* presents an interesting spectrum of sonographic findings. Lesions may be purely cystic, mixed, or solid.[34] Occasionally, daughter cysts or prominent septations may be seen. Patient motion may allow visualization of plumes of "hydatid sand" in an otherwise purely cystic lesion. Calcifications are frequently present but are less sensitively detected by sonography than by plain radiography or CT. Diagnosis depends on appreciation of the sonographic findings and correlation with clinical findings. Most patients with echinococcal disease have a history of contact with rural dogs. Percutaneous aspiration of echinococcal lesions should be avoided, since rupture may cause diffuse peritoneal spread and anaphylaxis. Treatment is surgical.

## TRAUMATIC LESIONS

Trauma is an important public health problem in the United States, representing one of the commonest causes of death in young adults. Although ultrasound plays little role in the imaging of acute hepatic trauma, it is important for sonographers to recognize traumatic lesions and complications of hepatic trauma.

Hepatic hematoma occurs frequently in both blunt and penetrating trauma. The sonographic appearance of blood varies with time. Acute hepatic hemorrhage is generally echogenic.[35] This echogenic appearance will usually persist for one to several days, during which time various changes may occur. A small hematoma may resolve completely, leading to a normal hepatic sonogram. Larger persistent hematomas retract. At this stage, there are usually anechoic areas with internal clumps of highly echogenic material. The echogenic material is primarily composed of fibrin. Over a period of weeks, clots may either disappear or lyse completely, leading to an almost totally echo-free collection.[36] Some dependent sludge-like material is frequently seen. Aspiration of hematomas may prove difficult with little or no return despite a predominantly anechoic "fluid" appearance. The reasons for this are unclear, but may relate to replacement by a gelatinous material or to clot organization.[36]

Seromas are almost always echo-free collections, frequently containing sludge-like debris. Occasionally, serum collections will have higher amplitude internal echoes, but this is uncommon.

Posttraumatic bilomas are interesting fluid collections that develop slowly over a period of several weeks and are due to gradual bile leakage from small duct injuries. Typically, the patients have done well after incurring acute hepatic injury and are discharged from the hospital. Three to four weeks later, they return with mild right upper quadrant pain and occasionally a low-grade fever or palpable mass. Bilomas have characteristics that should lead sonographers to suggest the diagnosis. These lesions are generally totally echo free, although they occasionally contain some sludge-like material. Bilomas are usually distinguishable from other fluid collections, since they exhibit striking distal sonic enhancement.[37] While hematomas and seromas may occasionally have distal sonic enhancement, it is rarely as pronounced as that seen with bilomas. Not infrequently, a biloma will arise in the same region as a hematoma, resulting in fibrinous areas of increased echogenicity adjacent to the bile collection. Pronounced distal sonic enhancement should allow the sonographer to suggest the diagnosis, leading to confirmation by either cholescintigraphy with delayed films or percutaneous aspiration.[37] Percutaneous drainage of these lesions is generally not indicated since most resolve spontaneously.

## BENIGN TUMORS OF THE LIVER

Cavenous hemangiomas are the most benign neoplasm of the liver. They occur at any age and are slightly more common in women. Most lesions are small and single, but they may be multiple (10%) and large.[38] Small hemangiomas tend to be well-defined, highly echogenic lesions. Unfortunately, a spectrum of findings may be present.[38, 39] Hemangiomas may have anechoic peripheral areas, presumably representing larger vessels. Areas of differing echogenicity may be present. Occasionally, hemangiomas may be primarily or entirely less echogenic than the surrounding hepatic parenchyma, or they may be anechoic with echogenic septa.

When a small echogenic lesion is discovered in an asymptomatic patient, hemangioma is likely. Confirmation of the sonographic diagnosis in such patients is probably best done by dynamic CT scanning.[40] Rapid sequential scanning of the lesion after bolus injection of a contrast agent is recommended. Classically, hemangiomas display peripheral contrast enhancement with sequential centripetal "filling in" with time.[40] Such lesions may be observed sonographically at long intervals or ignored. If CT is not diagnostic or if the patient has a known malignancy, angiography should be performed. Despite reports of uncontrollable hemorrhage after large needle biopsy, some believe that thin needle biopsy of hemangiomas is indicated and safe.[40] Biopsies with needles larger than 22-gauge should be discouraged.

Hepatic adenomas were rare prior to the widespread use of birth control pills.[18] Among long-term birth control pill users, there is an estimated annual incidence of three to four per hundred thousand. Adenomas may also occur in patients with glycogen storage disease (von Gierke disease) and in men taking androgens.[18, 41] Most patients are asymptomatic, but rupture with catastrophic hemorrhage may occur. Sonographically, liver cell adenomas are usually well-defined lesions that exhibit slightly increased echogenicity compared to surrounding hepatic parenchyma. Unfortunately, other sonographic patterns are also common. Adenomas may be hypoechoic or may have internal hyperechoic or hypoechoic areas, perhaps related to hemorrhage.[42]

Focal nodular hyperplasia is a nonencapsulated, solid lesion whose blood supply runs through a fibrotic stellate center. Focal nodular hyperplasia is most common in women of menstrual age. No proof exists to suggest that focal nodular hyperplasia is caused by birth control pills. The entity is occasionally seen in males.[18] Focal nodular hyperplasia has a variable ultrasound appearance. It is usually seen as a focal mass of varying echogenicity.

Adenomas and focal nodular hyperplasia can usually be distinguished by [99m]Tc sulfur colloid liver-spleen scanning. Adenomas consist of hepatocytes alone, while focal nodular hyperplasia consists of both hepatocytes and Kupffer cells. Adenomas, therefore, should appear as photopenic areas on liver spleen scans, while focal nodular hyperplasia either is not detectable or is slightly "hot" compared to normal liver.[42]

## SMALL ECHOGENIC FOCI

Intrahepatic stones, intrabiliary and intravascular gas, and dystrophic calcifications may all cause shadowing echogenic foci within the liver.[43] The differential diagnosis can usually be made by correlating the clinical diagnosis with the sonographic findings. A plain film of the abdomen is also frequently helpful. Biliary duc-

tal gas occurs most often in patients who have undergone biliary surgery. Gas usually changes position within the ducts as the patient is moved. Intravascular gas is most often seen with bowel infarction. Generally, suggestive plain film and clinical findings are present in these patients. Intrahepatic biliary calculi, occurring in gallstone disease, Caroli's disease, Oriental cholangiohepatitis, and various other entities, are usually associated with biliary dilatation. Dystrophic calcifications, which are most often associated with granulomatous infections such as tuberculosis, are usually parenchymal and unassociated with bile ducts.

### Focal Malignant Disease

Hepatocellular carcinoma (HCC) is the most common primary malignant tumor of the liver. In the United States, metastatic carcinoma is approximately 20 times more frequent. In parts of Asia and Africa, HCC is the most common hepatic neoplasm, primary or metastatic. Approximately 85% of HCCs arise in patients with cirrhosis or precirrhotic livers. Hepatitis B–related cirrhosis has the highest incidence of HCC, but the more prevalent alcoholic cirrhosis is responsible for more cases in the United States. Cirrhosis-associated HCC occurs five times more often in males than females. HCC arising in a normal liver occurs equally in males and females.[18] Tumors arising in cirrhotic livers tend to be irregular and have a greater propensity to be multifocal. Tumors arising in normal livers tend to be discrete single lesions. Sonographically, HCC has no specific appearance. It is difficult to differentiate from metastatic disease as both are frequently multifocal, occurring in all lobes of the liver.

Tanaka et al. have correlated sonographic findings with histology.[44] Hypoechoic lesions correspond to solid tumors without necrosis, while complex masses are seen in tumors with some necrotic areas. Hyperechoic lesions were seen in two types of tumor, those with fatty metamorphosis and those with marked sinusoidal dilatation. When small (<3 cm), HCCs are usually well-defined, hypoechoic, relatively homogeneous masses. Although angiography remains the most sensitive means of detecting small HCCs, sonography is probably the most cost-effective imaging technique for screening high-risk patients. Initial screening for α-fetoprotein and hepatitis B surface antigen, followed by sonography in positive patients, is probably the most appropriate approach.[45, 46]

METASTATIC TUMORS

Metastatic malignancy is easily the commonest neoplasm involving the liver in the United States. In a large autopsy series, approximately 40% of patients with carcinoma had liver metastasis. Hepatic metastases most often occur with gastrointestinal malignancy, breast carcinoma, and lung carcinoma, but they may arise from virtually any primary tumor. Clinically, metastasis is frequently silent, causing symptoms in only one half of affected patients. Symptoms may include hepatomegaly, jaundice, and pain. Results of liver function tests are frequently abnormal in patients with liver metastasis. Elevated alkaline phosphatase levels in a patient with cancer should prompt evaluation for hepatic metastasis.[18]

Hepatic metastasis is protean in its sonographic manifestations.[47] Metastases are almost always multifocal, although occasionally a large single metastasis may be found. Metastases run the sonographic gamut from purely cystic to diffusely hyperechoic. Usually metastases are multiple, rounded lesions with areas of decreased and increased echogenicity compared to normal hepatic parenchyma. Hypoechoic "halos" are frequently seen, resulting in a bull's-eye pattern. A diffuse parenchymal pattern may also occur with metastatic disease.

Unfortunately, the sonographic appearance does not correlate well with the cell type of origin in hepatic metastases.[48–50] Certain tendencies can be noted but are insufficiently consistent to be used in an individual case. For example, colonic metastases tend to have a significant hyperechoic component, and leiomyosarcomas tend to undergo cystic necrosis.[51, 52]

OTHER MALIGNANT TUMORS

Cholangiocarcinoma usually involves the confluence of hepatic ducts in the porta hepatis. An early manifestation is jaundice. Generally, these infiltrative tumors are not imaged, though proximal intrahepatic biliary dilatation is noted. Cholangiocarcinoma may cause increased peribiliary echogenicity or, rarely, peribiliary mass.[53] We have seen one case in which a well-circumscribed, hypoechoic, peribiliary mass was detected in a patient with cholangiocarcinoma. Peripheral cholangiocarcinoma is a rare tumor that may grow larger than the more central lesions.[18] To our knowledge, sonographic findings in such cases have not been described.

Hepatic involvement by lymphoma is common in later stages of the disease. In autopsy series, hepatic involvement is found in more than half of patients with either Hodgkin's or non-Hodgkin's lymphoma.[54] Nevertheless, detection remains difficult and has been reported at 5%.[54] This low detection rate is probably due to the fact that lymphoma usually involves the liver in a diffuse infiltrative fashion which is difficult to detect sonographically. When focal lesions occur, they tend to be hypoechoic or even anechoic, but other patterns, including mixed and echogenic patterns, are seen.[55] Distinguishing between metastasis and multifocal lymphoma may be difficult, although multiple anechoic lesions should suggest lymphoma. Once again, clinical correlation is useful.

Calcification in hepatic neoplasms is commonest in mucinous adenocarcinoma, most often arising from the colon.[18] Other metastases that may calcify include those from thyroid, lung, stomach, ovary, kidney, and matrix-producing tumors. Metastases from virtually any other primary may calcify occasionally. HCC and cavernous hemangioma may calcify.

Venous invasion by hepatic malignancy is most often seen in HCC. HCC may invade both portal and hepatic venous systems. Metastatic disease or even lymphoma may involve hepatic vascular structures. Vascular invasion may be detected by sonography or CT, but the sensitivity of these modalities for detecting vascular invasion is not known.

Biliary obstruction by malignant disease is usually caused by extrinsic compression. On occasion, intrabiliary invasion with obstruction may occur.

## Diffuse Hepatic Disease

Unfortunately, the sonographic findings in diffuse hepatic disease are not specific. Diffuse diseases are harder to detect than focal processes because they cause less distortion of normal hepatic architectural landmarks, as was mentioned in the discussion of hepatic lymphoma. Once again, correlation with clinical findings is important in establishing the best sonographic diagnosis.

## BENIGN DIFFUSE DISEASE

Acute hepatitis has been described as causing an increased overall echogenicity diffusely dispersed throughout the liver.[56] In this writer's experience, this pattern is only seen occasionally, and most patients with acute hepatitis have no sonographic abnormality. Changes of chronic hepatitis are similar to those seen in cirrhosis.

Hepatic cirrhosis results from the fibrotic reparative processes caused by a diffuse hepatic insult. Many agents may provoke cirrhosis. Common causes include alcohol abuse, chronic active hepatitis, prolonged biliary obstruction, and toxic drugs.[57] Cirrhosis results not only in laying down of fibrotic tissue, but also in alterations in hepatic shape. For reasons not totally understood, but possibly related to differences in blood supply, cirrhosis relatively spares the caudate and left lobes.[58] Some workers have proposed that the size ratio of the caudate and right hepatic lobes might be useful in the diagnosis of cirrhosis.[59] This writer has found the ratio unreliable.

Cirrhosis usually causes diffuse increased echogenicity as well as alterations in shape due to atrophy and hypertrophy.[60] Regenerating nodules, which are usually very small (2–3 mm), often cannot be imaged sonographically. Sometimes micronodular change may be detected in cirrhotic patients with ascites by imaging the nodular anterior hepatic surface with a high-frequency transducer via the ascites.[61] Rarely, large regenerating nodules may simulate a neoplasm sonographically. These cases can generally be sorted out with nuclear medicine imaging.[62] Splenomegaly and portosystemic collaterals that result from portal hypertension may be seen and are useful ancillary signs in severe hepatic cirrhosis.[63]

Fatty infiltration of the liver may cause increased echogenicity indistinguishable from cirrhosis.[60] Patchy geographic fatty infiltration may cause focal rather than diffuse abnormalities. In these instances, focal fatty change may simulate neoplasm.[64] Fatty infiltration has many causes, including diabetes, obesity, chemotherapy, and other diseases.

## OTHER DIFFUSE HEPATIC DISEASES

Inflammatory conditions of the liver can cause diffuse disease. Rarely, diffuse pyogenic abscess will cause heterogeneity and disruption of the normal hepatic parenchyma. Diffuse tuberculosis may cause a "bright liver." Diffuse metastases and other infiltrating processes may also cause sonographic alteration.

## The Future of Hepatic Ultrasonography

Currently, ultrasound plays an important role in the evaluation of hepatic disease. The noninvasiveness and cost-effectiveness of the method are critical advantages. Nevertheless, rapid technological change in imaging means that ultrasound must also progress if it is to maintain its importance in hepatic imaging in competition with magnetic resonance imaging and high-resolution CT scanning. Sonographic contrast agents need extensive further evaluation and hold much promise for assessing hepatic disease.[14]

Other areas of potential improvement include quantitative ultrasound tissue characterization and signal processing based on parameters other than amplitude.[66–68] Frequency-based (phase data) FM imaging hold some promise for the future. Clinical evaluation of these technological developments in sonography as well as the evolving technology of high-resolution CT, magnetic resonance imaging, and the possible development of new modalities will continue to have a major impact on hepatic imaging.

## References

1. Arey LB: *Human Histology,* ed 3. Philadelphia, WB Saunders Co, 1968.
2. Ralls PW, Quinn MF, Rogers W, et al: Sonographic anatomy of the hepatic artery. *AJR* 1981; 136:1059–1063.
3. Kane RA: Sonographic anatomy of the liver. *Semin Ultrasound* 1981; 2(3):190–197.
4. Sexton CC, Zeman RK: Correlation of computed tomography, sonography, and gross anatomy of the liver. *AJR* 1983; 141:711–718.
5. Pagani JJ: Intrahepatic vascular territories shown by computed tomography (CT). *Radiology* 1983; 147:173–178.
6. Parulekar SG: Ligaments and fissures of the liver: Sonographic anatomy. *Radiology* 1979; 130:409–411.
7. Marks WM, Filly RA, Callen PW: Ultrasonic anat-

omy of the liver: A review with new applications. *JCU* 1979; 7:137–146.

8. Callen PW, Filly RA: Ultrasonographic localization of the gallbladder. *Radiology* 1979; 133:687–691.

9. Brown BM, Filly RA, Callen PW: Ultrasonographic anatomy of the caudate lobe. *J Ultrasound Med* 1982; 1:189–192.

10. Auh YH, Rubenstein WA, Zirinsky K, et al: Accessory fissures of the liver: CT and sonographic appearance. *AJR* 1984; 143:565–572.

11. Prando A, Goldstein HM, Bernardino ME, et al: Ultrasonic pseudolesions of the liver. *Radiology* 1979; 130:403–407.

12. Scheible W: A diagnostic algorithm for liver masses. *Semin Roentgenol* 1983; 18:84–86.

13. Bernardino ME, Thomas JL, Makland N: Hepatic sonography: Technical considerations, present applications, and possible future. *Radiology* 1982; 142:249–251.

14. Mattrey RF, Scheible FW, Gosink BB, et al: Perfluoroctylbromide: A liver/spleen-specific and tumor-imaging ultrasound contrast material. *Radiology* 1982; 145:759–762.

15. Miller DL, Rosenbaum RC, Sugarbaker PH, et al: Detection of hepatic metastases: Comparison of EOE-13 computed tomography and scintigraphy. *AJR* 1983; 141:931–935.

16. Doyle FH, Pennock JM, Banks LM, et al: Nuclear magnetic resonance imaging of the liver: Initial experience. *AJR* 1982; 138:193–200.

17. Margulis AR, Moss AA, Crooks LE, et al: Nuclear magnetic resonance in the diagnosis of tumors of the liver. *Semin Roentgenol* 1983; 18(2):123–126.

18. Edmondson HA, Peters RL: Tumors of the liver: Pathologic features. *Semin Roentgenol* 1983; 18(2):75–83.

19. Saini S, Mueller PR, Ferrucci JT Jr, et al: Percutaneous aspiration of hepatic cysts does not provide definitive therapy. *AJR* 1983; 141:559–560.

20. Weaver RM, Goldstein HM, Green B, et al: Gray-scale ultrasonographic evaluation of hepatic cystic disease. *AJR* 1978; 130:849–852.

21. Feldman M: Polycystic disease of the liver. *Am J Gastroenterol* 1958; 29:83–86.

22. Sanfelippo PM, Beahrs OH, Weiland LH: Cystic disease of the liver. *Ann Surg* 1974; 179:922–925.

23. Henson SW Jr, Gray HK, Dockerty MB: Benign tumors of the liver. IV. Polycystic disease of surgical significance. *Surg Gynecol Obstet* 1957; 104(1):63–67.

24. Ralls PW, Quinn MF, Boswell WD Jr, et al: Patterns of resolution in successfully treated hepatic amebic abscess: Sonographic evaluation. *Radiology* 1983; 149:541–543.

25. Henson SW Jr, Gray HK, Dockerty MB: Benign tumors of the liver: VI. Multilocular cystadenomas. *Surg Gynecol Obstet* 1957; 104(5):551–554.

26. Ranson JHC, Madayag MA, Localio SA, et al: New diagnostic and therapeutic techniques in the management of pyogenic liver abscess. *Ann Surg* 1975; 181:508–518.

27. Newlin N, Silver TM, Stuck KJ, et al: Ultrasonic features of pyogenic liver abscesses. *Radiology* 1981; 139:155–159.

28. Kressel HY, Filly RA: Ultrasonographic appearance of gas-containing abscesses in the abdomen. *AJR* 1978; 130:71–73.

29. Powers TA, Jones TB, Karl JH: Echogenic hepatic abscess without radiographic evidence of gas. *AJR* 1981; 137:159–160.

30. Kuligowska E, Connors SK, Shapiro JH: Liver abscess: Sonography in diagnosis and treatment. *AJR* 1982; 138:253–257.

31. vanSonnenberg E, Ferrucci JT Jr, Mueller PR, et al: Percutaneous drainage of abscesses and fluid collections: Technique, results, and applications. *Radiology* 1982; 142:1–10.

32. Maher JA Jr, Reynolds RB, Yellin AE: Successful medical treatment of pyogenic liver abscess. *Gastroenterology* 1979; 77:618–622.

33. Ralls PW, Colletti PM, Quinn MF, et al: Sonographic findings in hepatic amebic abscess. *Radiology* 1982; 145:123–126.

34. Gharbi HA, Hassine W, Brauner MW, et al: Ultrasound examination of the hydatic liver. *Radiology* 1981; 139:459–463.

35. vanSonnenberg E, Simeone JF, Mueller PR, et al: Sonographic appearance of hematoma in liver, spleen, and kidney: A clinical, pathologic, and animal study. *Radiology* 1983; 147:507–510.

36. Wicks JD, Silver TM, Bree RL: Gray scale features of hematomas: An ultrasonic spectrum. *AJR* 1978; 131:977–980.

37. Esensten M, Ralls PW, Colletti P, et al: Posttraumatic intrahepatic biloma: Sonographic diagnosis. *AJR* 1983; 140:303–305.

38. Ishak KG, Radin L: Benign tumors of the liver. *Med Clin North Am* 1975; 59:995–1013.

39. Itai Y, Ohtomo K, Araki T, et al: Computed tomography and sonography of cavernous hemangioma of the liver. *AJR* 1983; 141:315–320.

40. Bree RL, Schwab RE, Neiman HL: Solitary echogenic spot in the liver: Is it diagnostic of a hemangioma? *AJR* 1983; 140:41–45.

41. Grossman H, Ram PC, Coleman RA, et al: Hepatic ultrasonography in type I glycogen storage disease (von Gierke disease). *Radiology* 1981; 141:753–756.

42. Sandler MA, Petrocelli RD, Marks DS, et al: Ultrasonic features and radionuclide correlation in liver cell adenoma and focal nodular hyperplasia. *Radiology* 1980; 135:393–397.

43. Gosink BB: Intrahepatic gas: Differential diagnosis. *AJR* 1981; 137:763–767.

44. Tanaka S, Kitamura T, Imaoka S, et al: Hepatocellular carcinoma: Sonographic and histologic correlation. *AJR* 1983; 140:701–707.

45. Chen DS, Sheu JC, Sung JL, et al: Small hepatocellular carcinoma: A clinicopathological study in thirteen patients. *Gastroenterology* 1982; 83:1109–1119.

46. Takashima T, Matsui O, Suzuki M, et al: Diagnosis and screening of small hepatocellular carcinomas. *Radiology* 1982; 145:635–638.

47. Scheible W, Gosink BB, Leopold GR: Gray scale echographic patterns of hepatic metastatic disease. *AJR* 1977; 129:983–987.

48. Hillman BJ, Smith EH, Gammelgaard J, et al: Ultrasonographic pathologic correlation of malignant hepatic masses. *Gastrointest Radiol* 1979; 4:361–365.

49. Schwerk WB, Schmitz-Moormann PS: Ultrasonically guided fine-needle biopsies in neoplastic liver disease. *Cancer* 1981; 48:1469–1477.

50. Lamb G, Taylor I: An assessment of ultrasound scanning in the recognition of colorectal liver metastases. *Ann R Coll Surg Engl* 1982; 64:391–393.

51. Taylor KJW, Richman TS: Diseases of the liver. *Semin Roentgenol* 1983; 18(2):94–101.

52. Wooten WB, Green B, Goldstein HM: Ultrasonography of necrotic hepatic metastases. *Radiology* 1978; 128:447–450.

53. Meyer DG, Weinstein BJ: Klatskin tumors of the bile ducts: Sonographic appearance. *Radiology* 1983; 148:803–804.

54. Ginaldi S, Bernardino ME, Jing BS, et al: Ultrasonographic patterns of hepatic lymphoma. *Radiology* 1980; 136:427–431.

55. Carroll BA, Ta HN: The ultrasonic appearance of extranodal abdominal lymphoma. *Radiology* 1980; 136:419–425.

56. Kurtz AB, Rubin CS, Cooper HS, et al: Ultrasound findings in hepatitis. *Radiology* 1980; 136:717–723.

57. Schiff ER, Schiff R: Cirrhosis. Fatty infiltration, in Schiff ER, Schiff R (eds): *Diseases of the Liver.* Philadelphia, JB Lippincott, 1982, pp 813, 859.

58. Scott WW, Donovan PJ, Sanders RC: The sonography of diffuse liver disease. *Semin Ultrasound* 1981; 2(3):219–225.

59. Harbin WP, Robert NJ, Ferrucci JT: Diagnosis of cirrhosis based on regional changes in hepatic morphology. *Radiology* 1980; 135:273–282.

60. Gosink BB, Lemon SK, Scheible W, et al: Accuracy of ultrasonography in diagnosis of hepatocellular disease. *AJR* 1979; 133:19–23.

61. Filly RA: Personal communication.

62. Laing FC, Jeffrey RB, Federle MP, et al: Noninvasive imaging of unusual regenerating nodules in the cirrhotic liver. *Gastrointest Radiol* 1982; 7:245–249.

63. Juttner HU, Jenney JM, Ralls PW, et al: Ultrasound demonstration of portosystemic collaterals in cirrhosis and portal hypertension. *Radiology* 1982; 142:459–463.

64. Scott WW Jr, Sanders RC, Siegelman SS: Irregular fatty infiltration of the liver: Diagnostic dilemmas. *AJR* 1980; 135:67–71.

65. Andrew WK, Thomas RG, Gollach BL: Military tuberculosis of the liver: Another cause of the "bright liver" on ultrasound examination. *S Afr Med J* 1982; 62:808–809.

66. Maklad NF, Ophir J, Balsara V: Attenuation of ultrasound in normal liver and diffuse liver disease in vivo. *Ultrasonic Imaging* 1984; 2(4):117–125.

67. Ferrari L, Gopinathan G, Ranalli R: The charac-

teristics of an ultrasound image procured from frequency signal processing of the RF waveform. Presented at the 29th Annual AIUM Meeting, Kansas City, Mo, Sept 16–19, 1984.

68. Trier HG, Reuter R, Epple E, et al: Frequency modulated portions of the time-amplitude ultrasonogram of models. Presented at the Second European Congress on Ultrasound in Medicine, Munich, West Germany, May 12–16, 1975.

## CASES

Dennis A. Sarti

### Normal Hepatic Transverse Scans

Transverse sections of the liver are best obtained with the patient in deep inspiration. This drives the liver caudal so that it can be visualized beneath the right costal margin. In some individuals with very high diaphragms, adequate liver studies are not possible unless we scan laterally through the intercostal spaces.

Figure 2–9 is a transverse scan with cephalad angulation of the transducer. The inferior vena cava is seen anterior to the spine. Hepatic veins are noted draining into the inferior vena cava. The echo pattern of the liver is fairly homogeneous. This even echo pattern is interrupted by tubular structures throughout the liver. Some of the tubular structures have high-amplitude echoes surrounding them. These arise from the fibrous tissue surrounding the portal triad. The tubular structures with the strong surrounding echoes represent branches of the portal venous system. The hepatic veins are also tubular structures coursing through the liver, but they do not have this high-amplitude surrounding echo. Therefore, they can be distinguished from the portal venous system.

Figure 2–10 demonstrates some portal veins with the strong surrounding echoes and a hepatic vein without the strong surrounding echoes. The crus of the diaphragm is seen anterior to the aorta as a thick lucent band.

Figures 2–11 and 2–12 are transverse scans of the liver made using some sector scanning through the intercostal spaces over the right lateral aspect of the abdomen. The major portion of the scan is done in a single-sector sweep anteriorly over the epigastrium. The lateral aspects of the liver, however, are filled in with small sector scans through the intercostal spaces. The left portal vein is seen in both Figures 2–11 and 2–12 in the midportion of the left lobe of the liver.

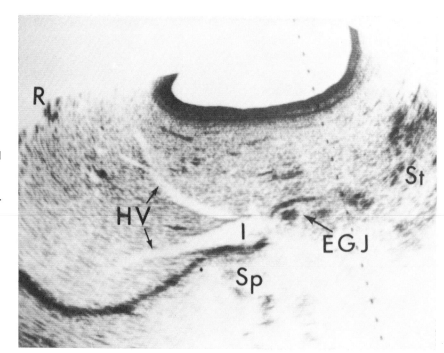

FIG 2–9.

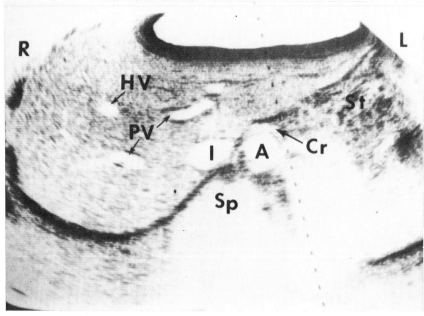

FIG 2–10.

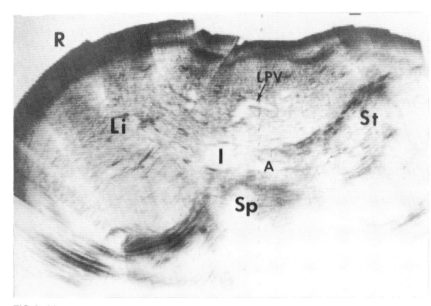

**FIG 2–11.**

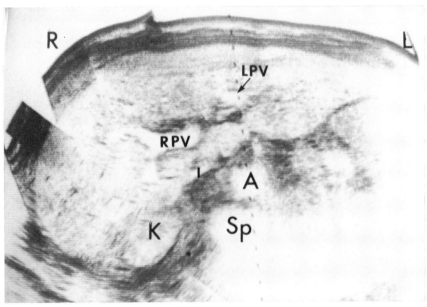

**FIG 2–12.**

This can usually be identified in most studies. Figure 2–12 demonstrates the right portal vein in the midportion of the right lobe of the liver, separating the anterior and posterior portions of this lobe.

| | | |
|---|---|---|
| **A** | = | Aorta |
| **Cr** | = | Crus of the diaphragm |
| **EGJ** | = | Esophagogastric junction |
| **HV** | = | Hepatic vein |
| **I** | = | Inferior vena cava |
| **K** | = | Kidney |
| **L** | = | Left |
| **Li** | = | Liver |
| **LPV** | = | Left portal vein |
| **PV** | = | Portal vein |
| **R** | = | Right |
| **RPV** | = | Right portal vein |
| **Sp** | = | Spine |
| **St** | = | Stomach |

## Normal Hepatic Transverse Sections

Occasionally, the portal vein can be seen in its entirety, as in Figure 2–13. This occurs when it has a horizontal orientation. It can be seen situated anterior to the inferior vena cava. High-level echoes surround the portal vein, secondary to fibrous tissue. This is well seen in Figure 2–14 as dark echoes surrounding the portal vein and separating the caudate lobe from the anterior portion of the left lobe of the liver. It is important to recognize the caudate lobe as arising from the liver. It can occasionally be mistaken for a mass in the head of the pancreas. The echogenicity arising from the caudate lobe, however, is similar to that of the liver.

Figures 2–15 and 2–16 demonstrate an increased echo amplitude arising from the liver when compared to the kidney. The echoes arising from the renal parenchyma are usually several shades of gray lighter than the liver parenchyma. The pancreas seen in Figure 2–16 has a darker echo appearance than the liver. The normal echo amplitude relationship of the three organs is: pancreas > liver > kidney. The gallbladder can be seen within the liver parenchyma; it is usually lateral to the inferior vena cava, as seen in Figures 2–15 and 2–16. The left lateral border of the liver is often demarcated by a strong C-shaped echo arising from the medial wall of the stomach.

A strong circular echo, seen in the left lobe of the liver, arises from the falciform ligament as is present in Figure 2–16. Shadowing behind the falciform ligament is also seen in many instances.

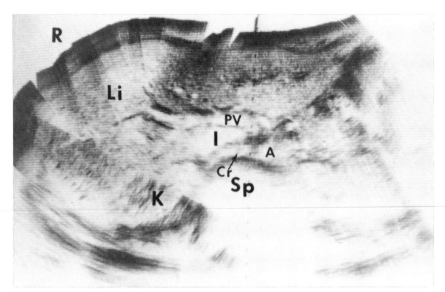

**FIG 2–13.**

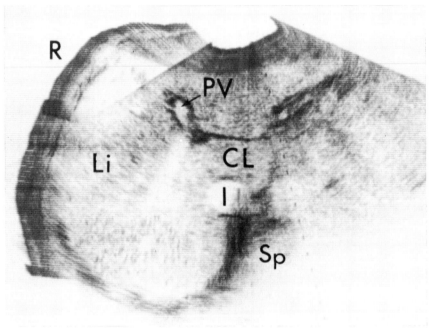

**FIG 2–14.**

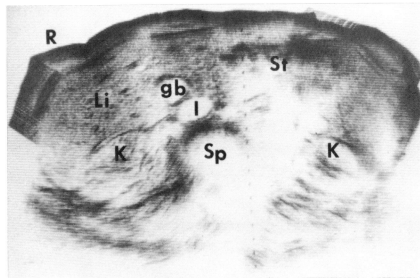

| A | = | Aorta |
|---|---|---|
| CL | = | Caudate lobe of liver |
| Cr | = | Crus of the diaphragm |
| FL | = | Falciform ligament |
| gb | = | gallbladder |
| I | = | Inferior vena cava |
| K | = | Kidney |
| L | = | Left |
| Li | = | Liver |
| P | = | Pancreas |
| PV | = | Portal vein |
| R | = | Right |
| Sh | = | Shadowing |
| SMA | = | Superior mesenteric artery |
| Sp | = | Spine |
| St | = | Stomach |
| SV | = | Splenic vein |

FIG 2–15.

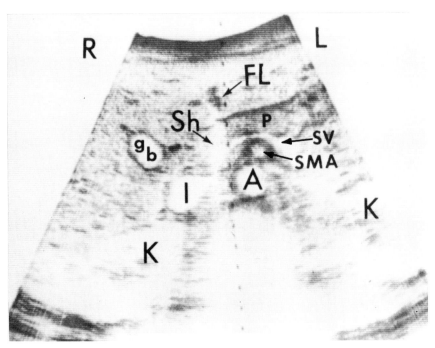

FIG 2–16.

## Normal Hepatic Longitudinal Scans

Evaluation of liver echogenicity and texture is best performed by longitudinal scans. A single sweep of the liver can be made approximately parallel to the diaphragm and continuing down over the abdominal surface. This yields an even texture to the liver parenchyma except for the tubular structures coursing through it. Figure 2–17 is an example of a longitudinal scan obtained quite laterally, over the right abdomen. The diaphragm is a strong curvilinear echo which provides the superior border to the liver echo pattern. As we continue to scan more medially, the right kidney comes into view (Fig 2–18). Numerous tubular structures secondary to the hepatic and portal veins are present within the liver.

Figures 2–18 and 2–19 demonstrate the normal echo relationship of the renal to the liver parenchyma. The echoes arising from the renal cortex and medulla are of a lower amplitude than those arising from the liver. Furthermore, the hepatic veins do not contain the strong high-level surrounding echoes that are present around the portal venous system. As we continue more medially, the gallbladder will come into view, as seen in Figures 2–19 and 2–20.

The inferior vena cava is a large tubular structure present on the posterior aspect of the liver. Figure 2–20 demonstrates the hepatic vein draining into the inferior vena cava. Around the porta hepatis are seen several circular lucencies which represent the right portal vein, the hepatic artery, and the common bile duct. As we scan longitudinally on the right side, the gallbladder also is visible as a lucent structure just posterior to the right lobe of the liver.

Occasionally, some echoes can be seen above the diaphragm, as are present in Figure 2–17. These are reverberations off the diaphragm and also represent liver parenchyma duplication artifacts that are placed in the lower lung field (see chapter 1). It is important to note that the posterior

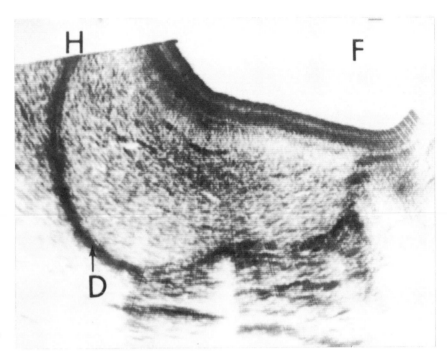

FIG 2–17.

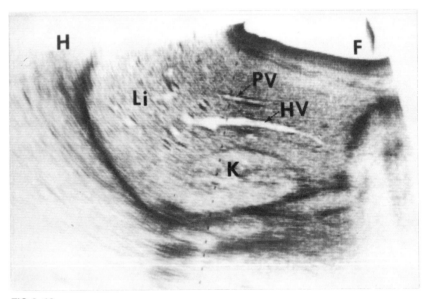

FIG 2–18.

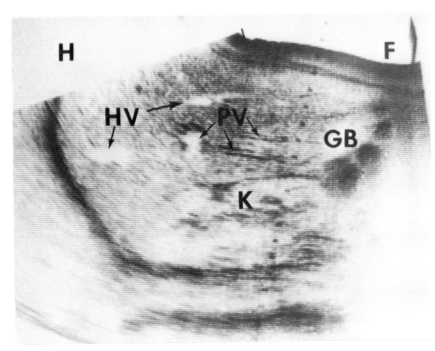

**FIG 2–19.**

thoracic wall is not seen above the diaphragm in any of these cases. The posterior thoracic wall will be seen secondary to the presence of right pleural effusions.

The longitudinal scans provide excellent visualization not only of the liver parenchyma but also of the subdiaphragmatic, subhepatic, and hepatorenal spaces.

| | | |
|---|---|---|
| **CBD** | = | Common bile duct |
| **D** | = | Diaphragm |
| **F** | = | Foot |
| **GB** | = | Gallbladder |
| **H** | = | Head |
| **HA** | = | Hepatic artery |
| **HV** | = | Hepatic vein |
| **I** | = | Inferior vena cava |
| **K** | = | Kidney |
| **Li** | = | Liver |
| **PV** | = | Portal vein |
| **RPV** | = | Right portal vein |

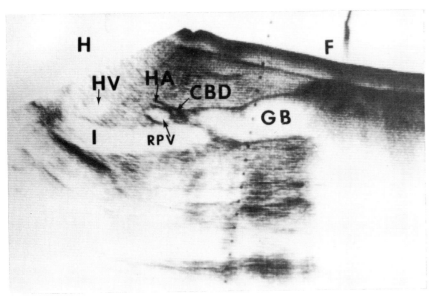

**FIG 2–20.**

## Normal Hepatic Longitudinal Scans

As we scan to the right, the inferior vena cava is seen as a posterior tubular structure with the liver situated anteriorly. We can visualize a small circular structure indenting the posterior aspect of the inferior vena cava. This is the right renal artery (Figs 2–21 through 2–23). The liver maintains its fairly even echo pattern except in the region of the porta hepatis, where numerous tubular structures are identified. The largest of these are secondary to various branches of the portal venous system. Figure 2–21 demonstrates the caudate lobe as seen on longitudinal scans. It is situated anterior to the inferior vena cava. There is also a strong echogenic region just posterior to the liver which arises from the mucosa of the duodenum. We can notice a small lucent area surrounding the mucosa of the duodenum which represents its muscular wall. Some posterior shadowing is noted. The pancreas is evident slightly caudal to the portal vein.

Figure 2–22 demonstrates a small tubular structure coming out of the porta hepatis and situated posterior to the head of the pancreas. This represents the common bile duct. The pancreas often is seen just posterior to the left lobe of the liver. Caudal to this is the strong echo of the air-filled stomach. Figure 2–24 is a longitudinal scan further to the left, in which we see a fairly homogeneous left lobe of the liver. There, a few highly echogenic circular structures represent the portal venous system. Just posterior to the liver we can see the echoes of the pancreas, situated anterior to the splenic vein and splenic artery.

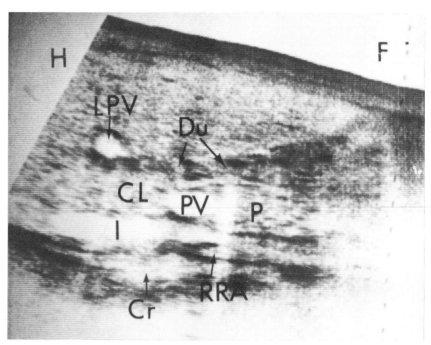

FIG 2–21.

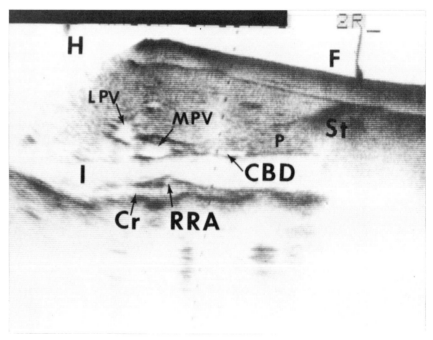

FIG 2–22.

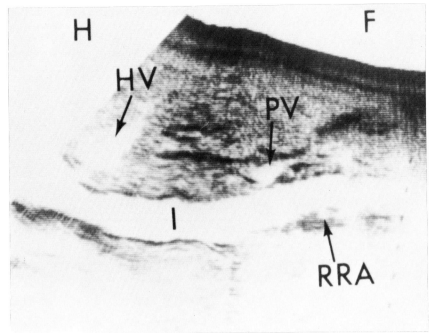

FIG 2–23.

| | |
|---|---|
| **CBD** = | Common bile duct |
| **CL** = | Caudate lobe |
| **Cr** = | Crus of the diaphragm |
| **Du** = | Duodenum |
| **F** = | Foot |
| **H** = | Head |
| **HV** = | Hepatic vein |
| **I** = | Inferior vena cava |
| **Li** = | Liver |
| **LPV** = | Left portal vein |
| **MPV** = | Main portal vein |
| **P** = | Pancreas |
| **PV** = | Portal vein |
| **RRA** = | Right renal artery |
| **SA** = | Splenic artery |
| **St** = | Stomach |
| **SV** = | Splenic vein |

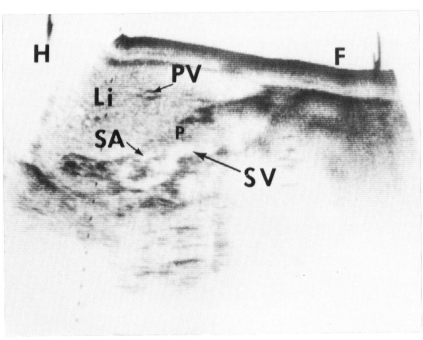

FIG 2–24.

## Segmental Liver Anatomy

Figures 2–25 through 2–28 are transverse scans corresponding to the diagrams shown in Figures 2–4 through 2–7. These transverse scans show the liver anatomy, which will assist the examiner in separating the liver into various segments. Line 1 separates the right lobe of the liver into anterior and posterior segments. Line 2 separates the right from the left lobe of the liver. Line 3 separates the lateral and medial segments of the left lobe of the liver. Figure 2–25 is the most cephalic of the four transverse images and Figure 2–28 being the most caudal of the transverse images. The right lobe of the liver comprises the bulk of hepatic tissue. It is separated into an anterior segment and a posterior segment by line 1 on the various images. In the cephalic portion of the liver, this corresponds to the right hepatic vein seen in Figure 2–25. Figure 2–26 is slightly more caudal, and line 1 represents the line connecting the right hepatic vein with the inferior vena cava. In Figure 2–27 line 1 connects the right portal vein with the right hepatic vein.

Separation of the right from the left lobe of the liver is demonstrated by line 2 in the four images. In Figures 2–25, 2–26, and 2–27, line 2 connects the middle hepatic vein with the inferior vena cava at different levels within the liver. In the most caudal scan obtained, shown in Figure 2–28, line 2 connects the inferior vena cava with the gallbladder. This represents the main lobar fissure.

Line 3 separates the medial from the lateral aspect of the left lobe of the liver. In the more cephalic portion in Figure 2–25, this line is drawn through the left hepatic vein and inferior vena cava. Slightly more caudal in the Figure 2–26, line 3 is drawn through the left portal vein and inferior vena cava. In the most caudad scans, shown in Figures 2–27 and 2–28, line 3 is drawn through the ligamentum teres and the inferior vena cava. These various landmarks will assist the ultrasonographer in determining the segmental anatomy of the liver.

The caudate lobe is the third major lobe of the liver. This is best seen in Figure 2–26. The high echogenic line

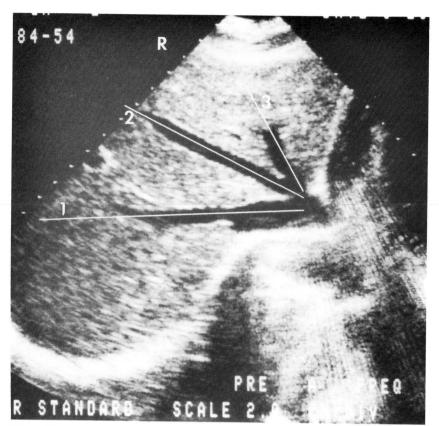

**FIG 2–25.**

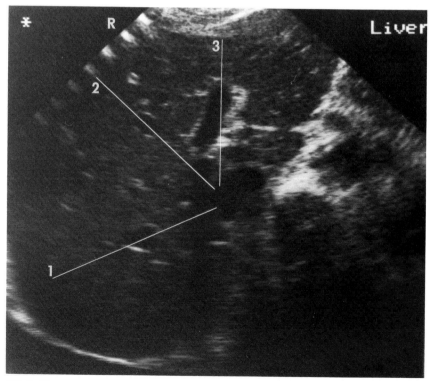

**FIG 2–26.**

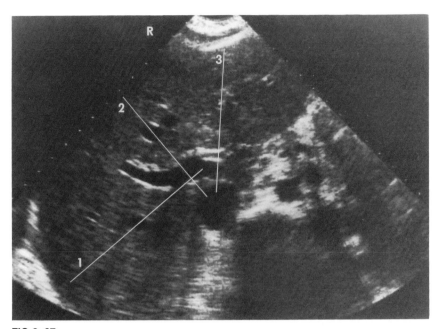

**FIG 2–27.**

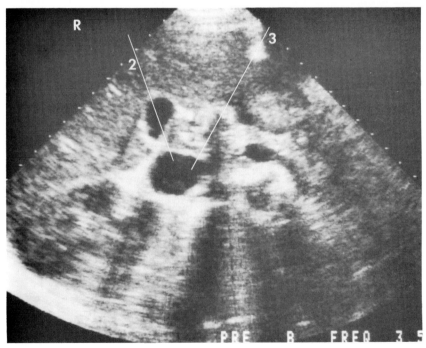

**FIG 2–28.**

situated horizontally and to the left of the left portal vein indicates the separation between the left lobe of the liver and the caudate lobe. The caudate lobe is situated posterior to the horizontal echogenic line and anterior to the inferior vena cava.

**R** = Right
**1** = Line separating the anterior and posterior segments of the right lobe
**2** = Line separating the right from the left lobe
**3** = Line separating the medial from the lateral segments of the left lobe

## Segmental Liver Anatomy

The right and left lobes of the liver are separated by the main lobar fissure caudally and the middle hepatic vein cranially. The main lobar fissure runs obliquely from the portal vein to the gallbladder fossa. Figures 2–29 and 2–30 are longitudinal scans demonstrating the main lobar fissure as it runs from the right portal vein to the gallbladder. The main lobar fissure is identified by the arrows in Figures 2–29 and 2–30. It is an easy structure to identify because of the high echogenicity from the surrounding echogenic fat. The main lobar fissure is a linear echogenic region of variable length that extends from the right portal vein to the gallbladder fossa. When the gallbladder is difficult to identify, the main lobar fissure may assist the examiner in locating the gallbladder fossa. The main lobar fissure contains the gallbladder and separates the right from the left lobe.

The caudate lobe is the smallest lobe of the liver and is separated from the left lobe of the liver by the fissure for the ligamentum venosum. Figures 2–31 and 2–32 are transverse and longitudinal scans demonstrating the fissure for the ligamentum venosum (arrowheads). The caudate lobe is posterior to this echogenic structure. On transverse scans, the fissure for the ligamentum venosum extends medially from the left portal vein, as is seen in Figure 2–31. This structure is continuous with the extrahepatic gastrohepatic ligament. On longitudinal scans, the caudate lobe is situated posterior to the fissure for the ligamentum venosum and anterior to the inferior vena cava. The caudate lobe merges medially with the right lobe of the liver without any discernible anatomic landmark identifying this border. What are structures 1 and 2 in Figure 2–32?

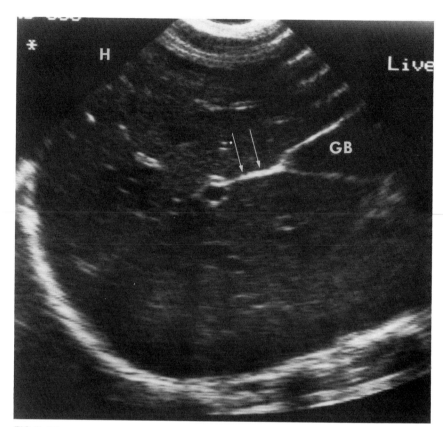

**FIG 2–29.**

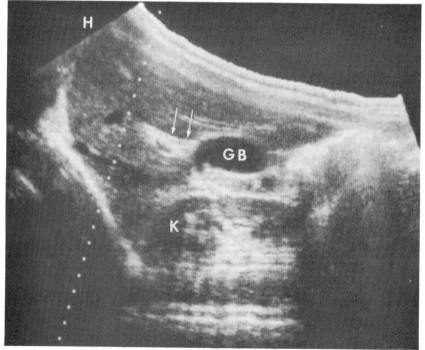

**FIG 2–30.**

| Arrows | = | Main lobar fissure |
| Arrowheads | = | Fissure for the ligamentum venosum |
| CL | = | Caudate lobe |
| GB | = | Gallbladder |
| H | = | Head |
| K | = | Kidney |
| R | = | Right |
| 1 | = | Hepatic vein |
| 2 | = | Superior mesenteric vein |

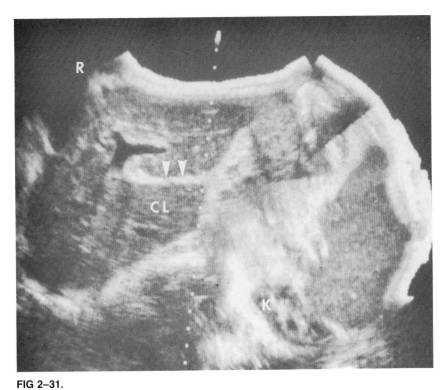

FIG 2–31.

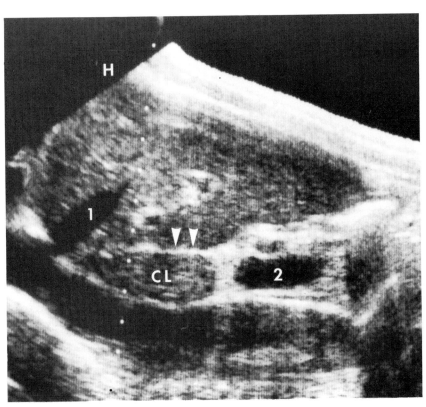

FIG 2–32.

## Normal Variants and Pseudolesions

Occasionally a right-sided abdominal mass is detected on ultrasound as being secondary to enlargement of the liver. In reality, it is secondary to an anatomic variant known as Riedel's lobe. The texture of the liver is within normal limits. There is no evidence of any intrahepatic masses. A Riedel's lobe can be so large that it extends inferior to the iliac crest. In Figure 2–33, we see liver texture anterior to the right kidney. In this instance, the right kidney has an unusual appearance. The central echoes of the collecting system are not seen because of scanning through the renal cortex and medulla.

An interesting finding in this scan is the appearance of a mass on the inferior aspect of the Riedel's lobe (arrowheads). This is a common occurrence of a pseudolesion adjacent to the liver. In reality, the mass is secondary to the transverse colon abutting the inferior aspect of the lobe of the liver. This gives a bull's-eye appearance typical to many collapsed GI structures within the abdomen. The transverse colon cannot be differentiated from the inferior aspect of the liver because the scan plane is not perpendicular to these interfaces. Therefore, a continuity appears between the pseudomass and the liver. This is often seen with the duodenum and stomach adjacent to the liver.

Hepatic pseudolesions are also often caused by normal fatty collections within the liver. These usually occur near major fissures. Figures 2–34 and 2–35 are ultrasound and CT images of the liver. In Figure 2–34, a highly echogenic oval mass is noted in the right anterior aspect of the liver. It could be mistaken for a metastatic lesion. However, the CT scan shown in Figure 2–35 indicates a collection of fat in the major fissure separating the right from the small left lobe. These fatty collections appear quite echogenic on ultrasound and can often be mistaken for pathologic lesions. Visualization of the ligamentum teres in the left lobe of the liver is common.

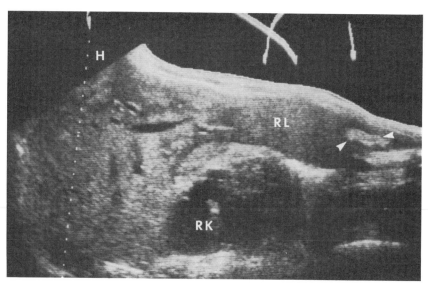

FIG 2–33.

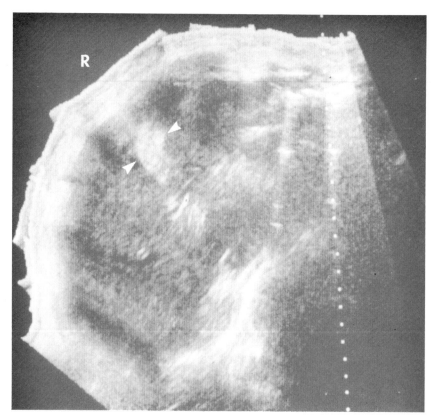

FIG 2–34.

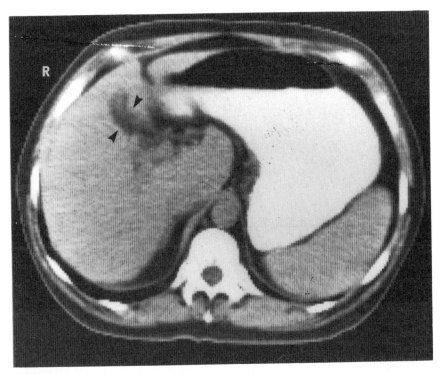

**FIG 2–35.**

However, fatty collections can occur in areas other than the ligamentum teres. In this instance, it is secondary to fat collection in the major fissure.

Figure 2–36 is a transverse scan through the liver in which another echogenic mass appears to be present in the deep portion of the right lobe. This echogenic collection is secondary to fat in the perirenal space. The transverse scan through the liver will sometimes indicate an echogenic region posteriorly. The scan plane has actually passed through the liver, and the scan displays perirenal fat cephalad to the upper pole of the right kidney. Since the scan is not perpendicular to the liver surface, its interface is not seen. Therefore, the appearance of a lesion within the liver parenchyma can be visualized, as in Figure 2–36.

| **Arrowheads** | = | Hepatic pseudolesions |
|---|---|---|
| **H** | = | Head |
| **R** | = | Right |
| **RK** | = | Right kidney |
| **RL** | = | Riedel's lobe |

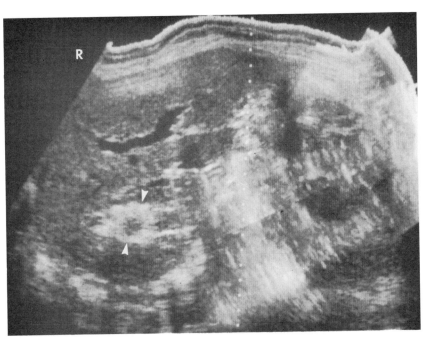

**FIG 2–36.**

# Liver Cysts: Polycystic Liver Disease

Patients with liver cysts are usually referred for ultrasound examination because of an area of decreased uptake on an isotope scan. Ultrasound is an excellent means for detecting a cyst within the liver. Liver cysts stand out as echo-free areas with sharp borders and prominent through-transmission, as they would in any other section of the body. Because of this characteristic finding, the workup of a patient with a liver cyst may end with the ultrasound examination. There is usually a 4:1 female/male predominance of simple liver cysts. Occasionally, the wall of the cyst may be calcified. This will pose diagnostic difficulty on ultrasound since reverberation artifacts off the calcific wall will be present.

Figure 2–37 shows an area of decreased echogenicity in a patient with a filling defect on isotope study. The longitudinal scan over the left lobe of the liver indicates a fluid-filled mass, representing a liver cyst. Posterior to the cyst is an area of increased through-transmission indicating the fluid-filled nature of the mass. Liver cysts are usually smooth walled with fairly sharp borders and excellent through-transmission.

Figures 2–38 and 2–39 are transverse and longitudinal scans of a patient in whom a large filling defect was detected on isotope study. The scans indicate a large sonolucent mass with sharp borders. Prominent through-transmission is noted deep to the mass. The patient had a huge liver cyst involving most of the anterior aspect of the liver. What are structures 1 and 2 in Figure 2–38? What is structure 3 in Figure 2–39?

Frequently, an isotope liver scan will show multiple filling defects within the liver that arouse suspicion of diffuse metastatic disease. Ultrasound may demonstrate numerous anechoic masses spread diffusely throughout the liver. These masses will have prominent through-transmission, indicating their cystic nature. When such a sonographic appearance is encountered, the possibility of metastatic dis-

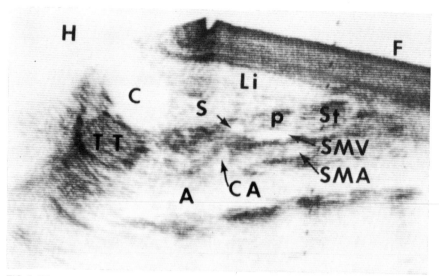

**FIG 2–37.**

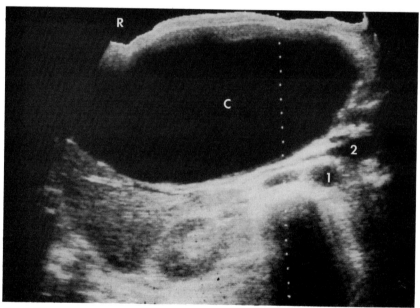

**FIG 2–38.**

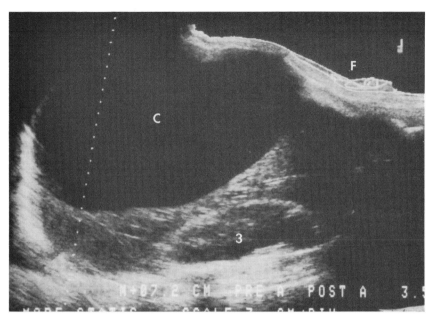

**FIG 2–39.**

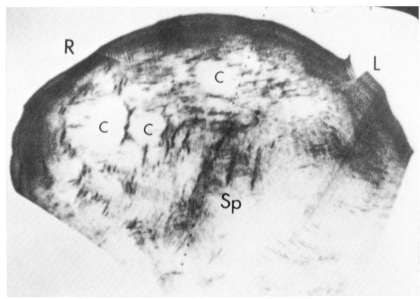

**FIG 2–40.**

ease is ruled out. Figure 2–40 is a transverse scan of the liver showing multiple cystic areas. This characteristic echo pattern is fairly easy to diagnose by ultrasound because of the prominent anechoic areas caused by the liver cysts. When examining a patient with such a finding, the sonographer must also examine the kidneys and pancreas to see if these organs are involved by cystic disease.

| | | |
|---|---|---|
| **A** | = | Aorta |
| **C** | = | Cysts |
| **CA** | = | Celiac axis |
| **F** | = | Foot |
| **H** | = | Head |
| **L** | = | Left |
| **Li** | = | Liver |
| **P** | = | Pancreas |
| **R** | = | Right |
| **S** | = | Splenic artery |
| **SMA** | = | Superior mesenteric artery |
| **SMV** | = | Superior mesenteric vein |
| **Sp** | = | Spine |
| **St** | = | Stomach |
| **TT** | = | Through-transmission |
| **1** | = | Aorta |
| **2** | = | Splenic vein; note how this vessel is compressed posterior to the large cyst |
| **3** | = | Right kidney; scan passes through the renal cortex and medulla and not through the collecting system |

## Amebic and Sterile Abscesses

The ultrasonic findings in amebic abscesses can present as a spectrum. Very often the abscesses are relatively sonolucent with good through-transmission. When debris is present, however, they can yield large masses with numerous soft internal echoes. Figure 2–41 is a scan obtained on a 52-year-old Mexican-American man who had a 3-week history of sore throat and steadily increasing right upper quadrant pain. About 1 day prior to admission, the patient experienced the onset of diarrhea with some blood-tinged stools. A liver-spleen scan demonstrated two large filling defects in the right lobe of the liver. Ultrasound examination demonstrated two large abscesses within the right lobe of the liver. Echoes are noted within the abscesses, especially the more anterior and medial one.

The patient was treated with metronidazole (Flagyl) and his symptoms improved rapidly. Amebic serologies revealed an amebic fluorescent antibody that was markedly positive. This case demonstrates two amebic abscesses in the liver with slightly different echo appearances. The anterior abscess had more echoes within it, indicating debris.

The patient whose scan is shown in Figure 2–42 was a 36-year-old man working in Saudi Arabia. He had a 3-month history of weight loss, right upper quadrant and pleuritic pain. Fever and leukocytosis, along with pleural effusion, developed while the patient was in Saudi Arabia, and treatment was with a course of antibiotics in that country. Further workup in the United States revealed a mass in the right lobe of the liver that was seen on ultrasound. The mass was relatively sonolucent with an echogenic center highly suggestive of an abscess. The patient was treated for a period of time with antibiotics. He eventually underwent surgery for drainage of the abscess. The abscess was found to be sterile, with all cultures remaining negative. Biopsy of the abscess wall also was negative. This is an example

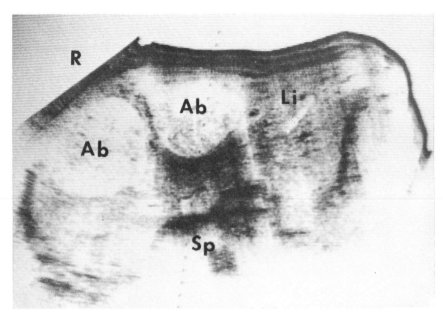

FIG 2–41.

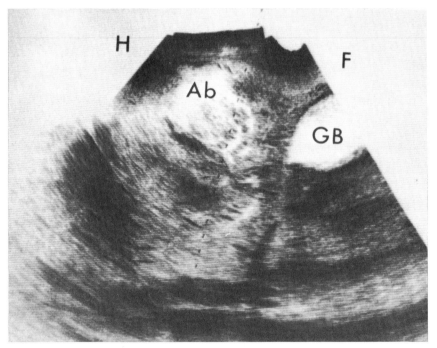

FIG 2–42.

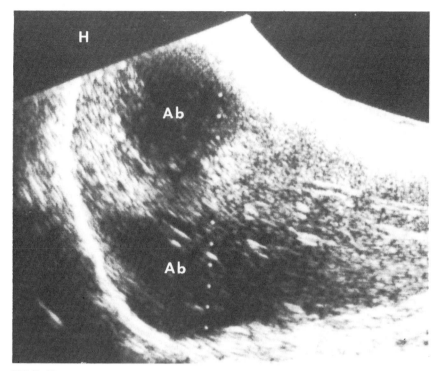

**FIG 2–43.**

of a sterile abscess in which a large amount of debris was found.

Figure 2–43 is a longitudinal scan of the liver. Two large relatively sonolucent masses are present within the liver. Soft echoes are noted within these masses. These findings are compatible with two amebic abscesses. Figure 2–44 is a longitudinal scan of the same patient made several years later. One of the abscesses has resolved into a smooth-walled, cystic-appearing lesion near the dome of the diaphragm. Through-transmission is present deep to this area. Some amebic abscesses will resolve into cystic structures and will appear as liver cysts on later examinations. What is structure 1 in Figure 2–44?

| | | |
|---|---|---|
| **Ab** | = | Abscess |
| **C** | = | Cystic mass several years later |
| **F** | = | Foot |
| **GB** | = | Gallbladder |
| **H** | = | Head |
| **R** | = | Right |
| **Sp** | = | Spine |
| **1** | = | Gallbladder |

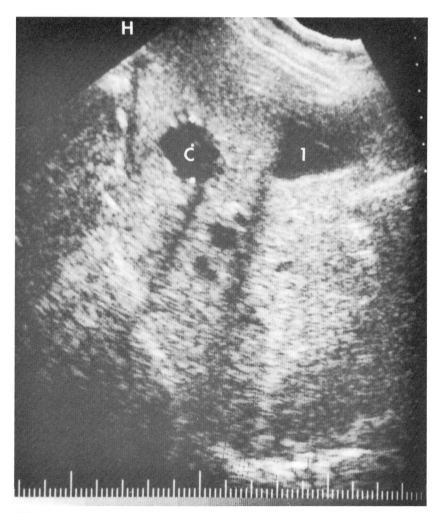

**FIG 2–44.**

## Liver Abscess

Figures 2–45 and 2–46 are the scans of a 72-year-old woman in whom fever of undetermined etiology developed. At hospitalization, a liver scan demonstrated a defect in the superior dome of the right lobe of the liver. Figure 2–45 is a longitudinal scan of the area corresponding to the defect on the liver scan. The scan shows a relatively sonolucent mass near the dome of the liver on the right side. Soft echoes are present within the mass, but it is mainly sonolucent. A pleural effusion is noted in the right pleural space. The patient had a history of chronic congestive heart failure. A portion of the base of the right lung (arrows) is also seen on the scan. The patient was treated with IV antibiotics over a 3-week period, with marked clinical improvement and no further fever. An ultrasound scan obtained at that time is shown in Figure 2–46. The abscess has markedly decreased in size; soft echoes, however, are still present within the central portion. Fluid is still noted in the right pleural space.

Figure 2–47 is a scan obtained from a 65-year-old woman with multiple medical problems, including previous pulmonary emboli and cerebral vascular accident. She reported the acute onset of midepigastric pain that was knifelike and radiated toward the right flank. Fever and signs of peritonitis developed. At operation a perforated jejunum in the proximal portion was found. On the seventh postoperative day, the patient had a persistent right pleural effusion along with fever spikes. The possibility of an abscess was considered. Because of this, an ultrasound examination was performed. Figure 2–47 is a longitudinal scan of the right lobe of the liver. There is evidence of a relatively sonolucent mass in the liver. The borders are slightly irregular, and soft echoes are noted within. A pleural effusion is also seen above the right hemidiaphragm. The patient underwent a repeat operation, and a subdiaphragmatic and intrahepatic abscess was confirmed.

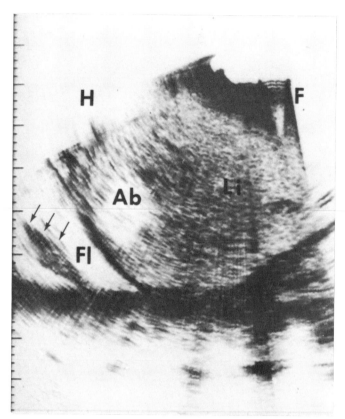

FIG 2–45.

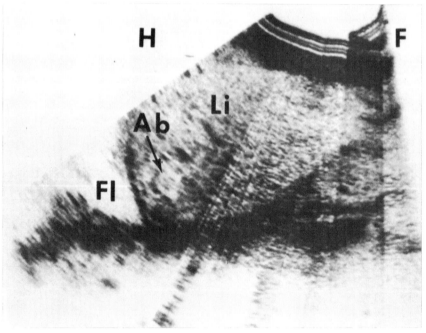

FIG 2–46.

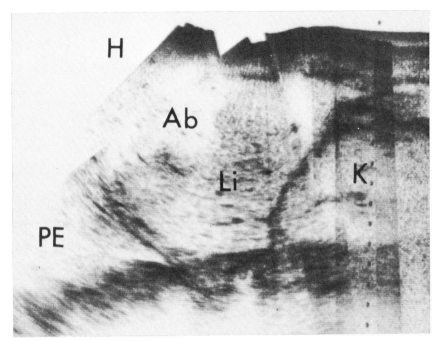

FIG 2–47.

Figure 2–48 is a longitudinal scan through the right lobe of the liver. A large echogenic mass is evident within the right lobe. The initial impression on ultrasound examination was that of a metastatic lesion. However, the clinical history included right upper quadrant pain and fever. Although not common, a liver abscess may have a hyperechoic appearance. This is such an example. The liver abscess is hyperechoic secondary to air. Small pockets of air will manifest as areas of increased echogenicity on ultrasound examination. These cannot be distinguished from solid lesions of the liver. Correlation of sonographic findings with the clinical picture is necessary to come to the correct diagnosis.

| | | |
|---|---|---|
| **Ab** | = | Abscess |
| **Arrows** | = | Inferior portion of collapsed right lung |
| **F** | = | Foot |
| **Fl** | = | Pleural fluid |
| **H** | = | Head |
| **K** | = | Kidney |
| **Li** | = | Liver |
| **PE** | = | Pleural effusion |

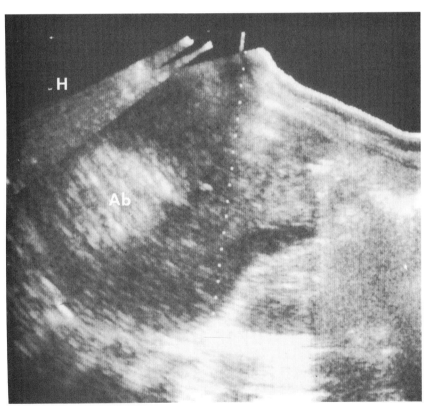

FIG 2–48.

## Echinococcal Cysts

The following case is an excellent example of the different manifestations of an echinococcal cyst. Figures 2–49 and 2–50 are scans of the same patient, a 3-year-old boy. An echinococcal cyst was diagnosed 1 year previously, and a cyst was removed from the right lung. Three weeks before admission, the patient had a high temperature associated with abdominal pain. There was no vomiting or diarrhea. Ultrasound examination revealed a fluid-filled mass in the anterior portion of the left lobe of the liver. Through-transmission is present posterior to the fluid on the images. Also noted during the course of examination was a highly echogenic region in the posterior aspect of the right lobe of the liver. This was secondary to a calcified inactive echinococcal cyst from the previous episode.

Chest x-ray studies revealed a lesion in the right lobe of the lung that was well circumscribed, circular, and consistent with an echinococcal cyst of the lung. A right lobectomy of the lung was performed, along with removal of the left lobe of the liver. The surgical findings were consistent with echinococcal cysts of both lung and liver.

This case illustrates the ultrasonic findings of an echinococcal cyst in different stages of activity. The left lobe cyst appears as a fluid-filled mass with through-transmission and fairly sharp borders. This would be difficult to distinguish from a simple liver cyst. The lesion in the posterior aspect of the right lobe represented calcification within an inactive echinococcal cyst from a previous infection. Abdominal films obtained at admission showed calcification in the right upper quadrant that corresponded to the lesion in the liver.

The patient whose scans are shown in Figures 2–51 and 2–52 underwent surgical removal of a left lower lung echinococcal cyst 17 years before the present admission. She had done well until approximately 1 month prior to admission, when she began experiencing right shoulder and back pain

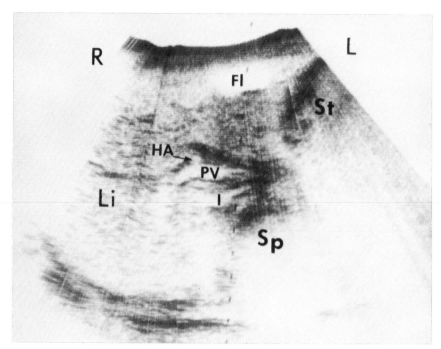

**FIG 2–49.**

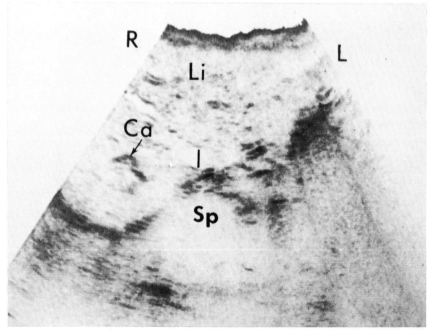

**FIG 2–50.**

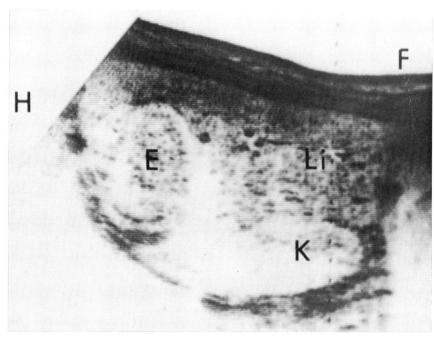

**FIG 2–51.**

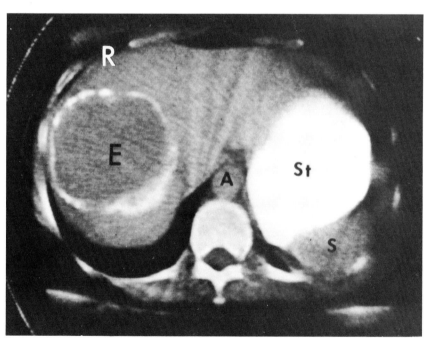

**FIG 2–52.**

that radiated to the right flank. Ultrasound examination and CT studies were performed. Figure 2–51 is an ultrasound scan of the liver in a longitudinal plane. A large calcified echinococcal cyst can be seen in the superior aspect of the liver just beneath the diaphragm. The mass is strongly echogenic, which indicates its solid nature. It also has decreased through transmission because of the calcified walls.

The CT scan shown in Figure 2–52 reveals the calcified wall of the echinococcal cyst. The mass is present in the superior portion of the right lobe of the liver. At operation an echinococcal cyst of the right lobe of the liver was removed.

| | | |
|---|---|---|
| **A** | = | Aorta |
| **Ca** | = | Calcified echinococcal cyst |
| **E** | = | Echinococcal cyst |
| **F** | = | Foot |
| **Fl** | = | Echinococcal cyst with fluid |
| **H** | = | Head |
| **HA** | = | Hepatic artery |
| **I** | = | Inferior vena cava |
| **K** | = | Kidney |
| **L** | = | Left |
| **Li** | = | Liver |
| **PV** | = | Portal vein |
| **R** | = | Right |
| **S** | = | Spleen |
| **Sp** | = | Spine |
| **St** | = | Stomach |

## Hepatic Hematomas

The ultrasound appearance of hepatic hematomas is quite varied and depends to some degree on the time elapsed between trauma and ultrasound evaluation. Very early, hematomas are highly echogenic. Later, some clot formation may be identified within a lucent mass. Even later, the hematoma may completely lyse and appear sonolucent. Correlation with clinical history is necessary to evaluate a hepatic hematoma. Figures 2–53, 2–54, and 2–55 are scans of a patient who sustained a gunshot wound to the right upper quadrant. Figure 2–53 is a transverse scan obtained 2 weeks after the incident. A large sonolucent hematoma is seen within the liver. The echogenic area present posteriorly and medially within the hematoma is secondary to clot formation. Figures 2–54 and 2–55 are transverse and longitudinal scans of the same patient obtained 4 weeks after the incident. The appearance of the hematoma has changed. Instead of the clot noted in Figure 2–53, low-amplitude echoes layer posteriorly (arrowheads). Continued lysis of the hematoma has occurred, along with the accumulation of dependent sludge-like material, seen on the later scans. This is an excellent example of the evolving ultrasonographic appearance of a hematoma.

Figure 2–56 is a longitudinal scan made through the right hepatic lobe of a patient who had recently been stabbed. The scan was made shortly after the incident. The hematoma has an echogenic appearance (arrows). This is the acute phase of a traumatic episode in which a hematoma will appear as an echogenic mass.

What is structure 1 in Figure 2–53? What is structure 2 in Figure 2–56?

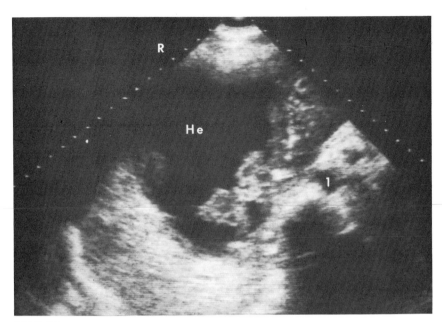

**FIG 2–53.**

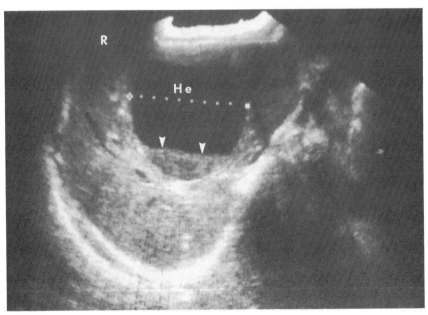

**FIG 2–54.**

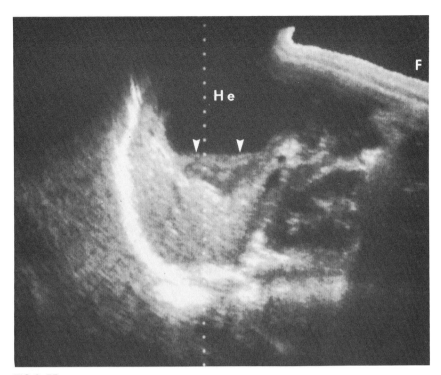

**FIG 2–55.**

| | | |
|---|---|---|
| **Arrows** | = | Hematoma |
| **Arrowheads** | = | Layering of debris posteriorly in a hematoma |
| **F** | = | Foot |
| **He** | = | Hematoma |
| **R** | = | Right |
| **1** | = | Aorta |
| **2** | = | Small right pleural effusion |

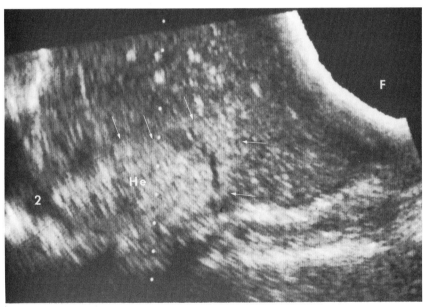

**FIG 2–56.**

## Hepatic Hematoma and Biloma

Figures 2–57 and 2–58 are transverse scans of a patient with sickle cell anemia and multiple complications. He was admitted to the hospital because of a progressive rise in serum bilirubin. An ultrasound study was initially performed to rule out an obstructive cause of the jaundice. Figure 2–57 is a transverse scan obtained at that time which did not show any evidence of a dilated biliary tree within the liver, although prominent portal venous structures were seen. The patient underwent transhepatic cholangiography, which was followed by a drop in hematocrit. He was thought to have sustained a liver laceration, and a repeat ultrasound examination was performed.

Figure 2–58 is a transverse scan from the follow-up study. A relatively sonolucent mass on the lateral aspect of the right lobe of the liver, representing a liver hematoma, is clearly visible. Soft echoes are noted within the hematoma. There is also peritoneal fluid, indicative of an extrahepatic bleed. The liver echoes posterior to the hematoma are increased, indicating some through-transmission. These findings are an example of an intrahepatic and extrahepatic bleed diagnosed by ultrasound.

Trauma to the liver may result in a collection of bile within the liver parenchymal. These bilomas will appear as sonolucent masses on ultrasound with prominent through-transmission. The through-transmission is even more pronounced in the presence of bilomas than in the presence of hematomas. Figures 2–59 and 2–60 are scans from a patient who had recently sustained a gunshot wound to the liver. Figure 2–59 is a cholescintigram which shows a defect 25 minutes after injection of isotope. A later 4-hour scintigram showed an area of increased uptake in the previously noted area of decreased uptake. This finding is compatible with a biloma. Figure 2–60 is a longitudinal ultrasound scan through the right lobe of the liver, corresponding to the area of

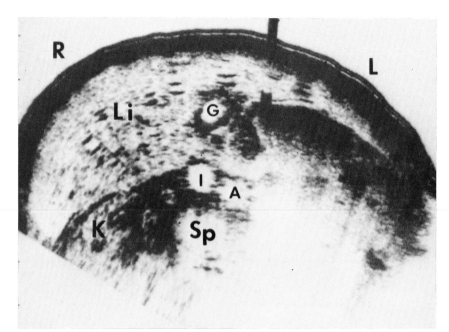

FIG 2–57.

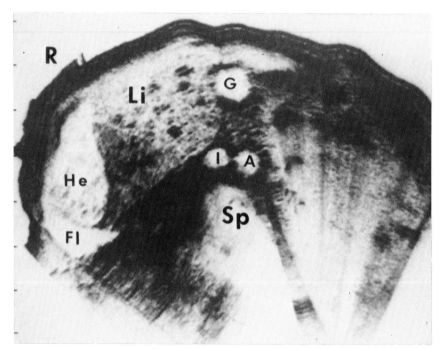

FIG 2–58.

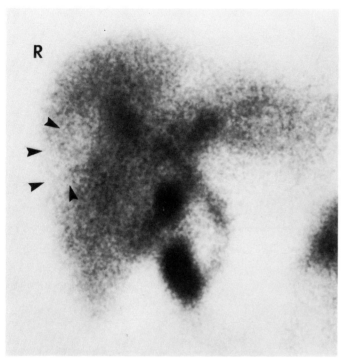

**FIG 2–59.**

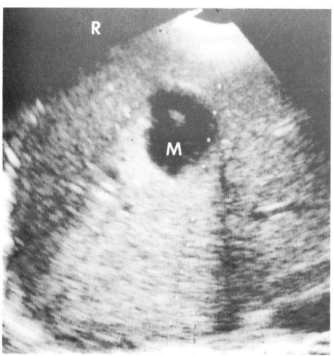

**FIG 2–60.**

decreased uptake in Figure 2–59. A sonolucent mass with prominent through-transmission, indicating a cystic structure, is visible. The findings are compatible with a hepatic biloma. The biloma shown here is somewhat characteristic in appearance, as it is relatively echo free and has prominent through-transmission.

| | | |
|---|---|---|
| **A** | = | Aorta |
| **Arrowheads** | = | Filling defects secondary to biloma |
| **Fl** | = | Fluid |
| **G** | = | Gallbladder |
| **He** | = | Hematoma |
| **I** | = | Inferior vena cava |
| **K** | = | Kidney |
| **L** | = | Left |
| **Li** | = | Liver |
| **M** | = | Biloma |
| **R** | = | Right |
| **Sp** | = | Spine |

## False Liver Masses; Hemangioma

Occasionally, ultrasound examination of the liver will yield an area of decreased echogenicity because of technical factors. Figure 2–61 is an example of a false liver mass in the anterolateral aspect of the right lobe of the liver. Such a false mass is seen quite commonly over the right costal margin. Since the ultrasound beam does not penetrate bone well, the area deep to the right costal margin will not have normal echoes. The anterior portion of the liver over the epigastric region can be filled in quite well since no ribs are present. The technologist can sector scan through the costal spaces laterally. This will often leave an area of decreased echogenicity just beneath the right costal margin that may simulate a hypoechoic liver mass. The sharpness of the borders, however, is an important indication that this is a technical artifact. We can also scan underneath the costal margin with the patient in deep inspiration to rule out such a mass.

Figure 2–62 shows an area of decreased echogenicity within the liver secondary to attenuation of the sound beam from a midline scar from previous surgery. Since scar tissue has a large amount of fibrous tissue present, this will lead to marked attenuation of the sound beam. Therefore, the echoes arising deep to the scar tissue will appear less echogenic than those of the surrounding liver parenchyma. Figure 2–62 is an excellent example of a false liver mass in the left lobe of the liver that actually is a technical problem arising from attenuation posterior to scar tissue.

Figures 2–63 and 2–64 are transverse and longitudinal scans of the liver in which small, well-circumscribed echogenic regions can be seen. The echogenic area in the anterior portion of the left lobe in Figure 2–63 is secondary to the falciform ligament. This is commonly seen and usually does not pose any diagnostic difficulty. However, a second well-circumscribed echogenic region is noted in the mid-

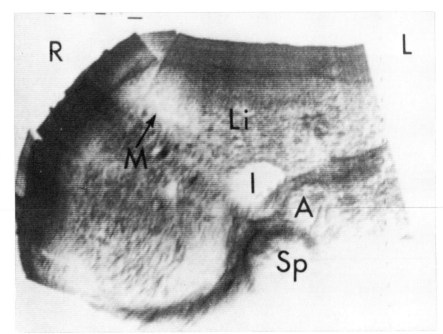

**FIG 2–61.**

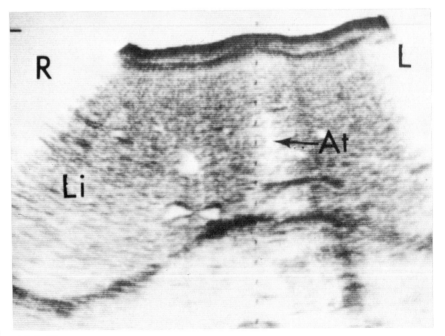

**FIG 2–62.**

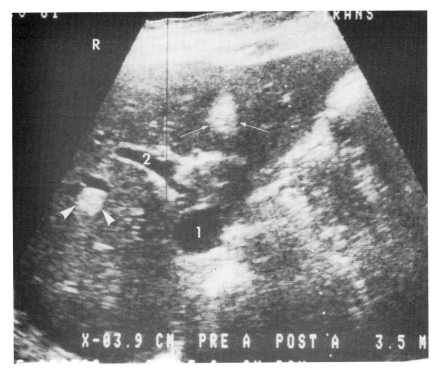

FIG 2–63.

portion of the right lobe (arrowheads) and directly posterior to a hepatic vein. This lesion has the typical appearance of a hemangioma. Hemangiomas are the most common benign hepatic neoplasms. They can occur at any age and are slightly more common in women than in men. Most lesions are small, highly echogenic, and well circumscribed. They are usually single and do not pose diagnostic difficulties. However, a spectrum of findings may be present that can produce diagnostic dilemmas. In these instances a single, well-circumscribed, highly echogenic mass is secondary to a benign hemangioma. If confirmation is necessary, CT can be performed. Rapid sequential CT scans after a bolus injection will usually show peripheral contrast enhancement with later central filling. Because of the highly vascular nature to these lesions, needle biopsies are discouraged.

What are structures 1 and 2 in Figure 2–63?

| A | = Aorta |
| Arrows | = Falciform ligament |
| Arrowheads | = Echogenic hemangioma |
| At | = Attenuation posterior to a scar from previous surgery |
| H | = Head |
| I | = Inferior vena cava |
| L | = Left |
| Li | = Liver |
| M | = False mass secondary to scanning around ribs |
| R | = Right |
| Sp | = Spine |
| 1 | = Inferior vena cava |
| 2 | = Right portal vein |

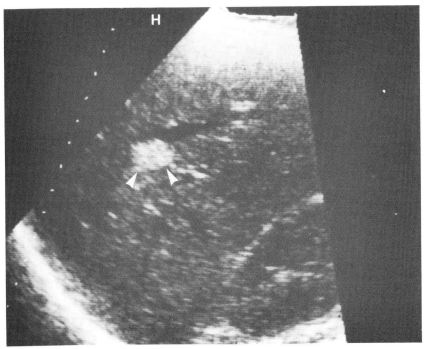

FIG 2–64.

## Hemangiomas; Focal Nodular Hyperplasia

Hemangiomas most commonly occur as very small, well-circumscribed, single echogenic masses in the liver. However, hemangiomas can present as a spectrum and give varying ultrasound appearances. They may be quite large and multiple, and may be sonolucent, echogenic, or mixed. Figure 2–65 is a longitudinal scan through the right lobe of the liver showing a large echogenic mass with a relatively lucent periphery. The ultrasound appearance is highly suspicious for a malignancy. The mass turned out to be a large hepatic hemangioma, discovered incidentally in an asymptomatic female. The patient has remained asymptomatic for 4 years and without change in the size or appearance of the mass. As mentioned previously, dynamic CT can be used to document the presence of a hemangioma with its characteristic presentation.

Figure 2–66 is a longitudinal scan through the right lateral aspect of the liver. In this case the mass is relatively sonolucent with small areas of increased echogenicity. Again, the appearance is highly suspicious for a malignant lesion. The mass turned out to be a hypoechoic hepatic hemangioma.

Hepatic hemangiomas may have a confusing appearance on ultrasound. When they are highly echogenic, small, and well circumscribed, they are usually easy to diagnose. However, if they have an unusual appearance, as in the two cases just mentioned, they do present diagnostic dilemmas. In these instances, dynamic CT scanning is most helpful in making the correct diagnosis.

Figure 2–67 is a longitudinal scan through the left lobe of the liver. An echogenic mass is noted on the posterior aspect. The patient had focal nodular hyperplasia. Focal nodular hyperplasia is a solid lesion of the liver which is not encapsulated. It is seen most often in women of menstrual age, and has a varying ultrasound appearance. Adenomas and focal nodu-

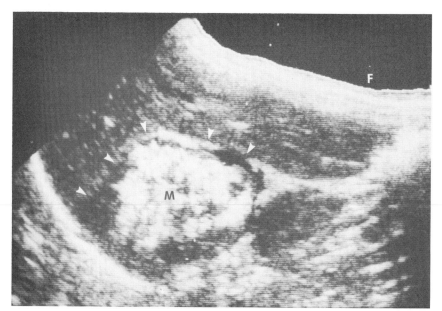

**FIG 2–65.**

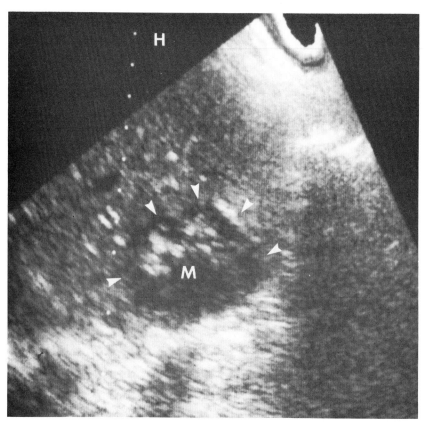

**FIG 2–66.**

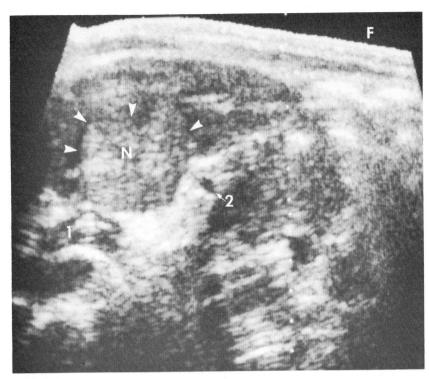

FIG 2–67.

lar hyperplasia can usually be distinguished by technetium sulfur colloid scanning. Adenomas are usually seen as areas of low uptake, while focal nodular hyperplasia either is not detectable or is slightly hot compared to normal liver. What are structures 1 and 2 in Figure 2–67?

Figure 2–68 is a longitudinal scan through the right lobe of the liver. An echogenic mass is present, secondary to focal nodular hyperplasia. Such a mass cannot be distinguished from other lesions of the liver. Isotope studies are necessary to make the correct diagnosis.

**F** = Foot
**H** = Head
**M** = Hemangioma
**N** = Focal nodular hyperplasia
**1** = Gastroesophageal junction
**2** = Splenic artery

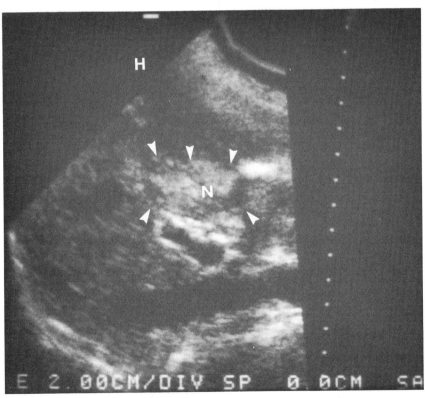

FIG 2–68.

## Hepatoma

Figures 2–69 and 2–70 are scans of a 36-year-old man with a long history of heavy alcohol abuse. Approximately 3 months before admission, he noted the onset of nausea, vomiting, and sharp abdominal pain. A liver isotope study carried out during hospitalization demonstrated a large filling defect in the right lobe of the liver. Figure 2–69 is a transverse scan of the upper abdomen in which we see a large echogenic mass (arrows) in the posterior aspect of the right lobe of the liver. The portal vein is displaced anteriorly. Figure 2–70 is a longitudinal scan of the entire abdomen. The echogenic mass is seen in the superior aspect of the right lobe of the liver. Also noted on this scan is fluid in the pelvis secondary to ascites. The high echogenicity of this mass suggested a vascular lesion, which was confirmed on angiography. The patient had a hepatoma.

Hepatoma or hepatocellular carcinoma is often associated with cirrhosis. The ultrasound appearance of hepatomas is varied. In the previous case the hepatoma was echogenic. In Figure 2–71, a transverse scan of the liver, a large sonolucent mass (arrowheads) is seen in the left lobe of the liver. The mass was a hepatoma, which was primarily hypoechoic in appearance. There is no way to distinguish this hepatoma from other lesions of the liver, such as metastasis.

Figure 2–72 is a longitudinal scan through the right lobe of the liver of another patient with hepatoma. The hepatoma is multifocal. There are three separate lesions in the right lobe of the liver which have a varying ultrasound appearance. An echogenic mass is seen in the inferior border of the right lobe of the liver. Cephalad to the right kidney is a hypoechoic mass. Anterior and just beneath the diaphragm is a target lesion with a central lucency, surrounding echogenicity, and concentric outer sonolucency. This case is an excellent example of the varying appearance of a hepatoma within an individual patient.

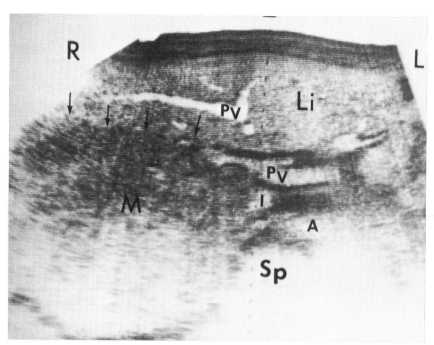

**FIG 2–69.**

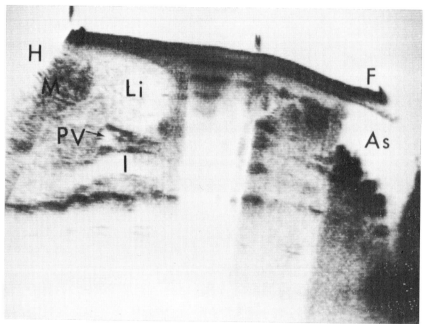

**FIG 2–70.**

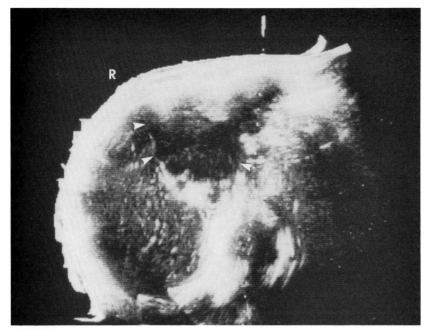

FIG 2–71.

| A | = Aorta |
|---|---|
| **Arrows** | = Hepatoma |
| **Arrowheads** | = Hepatoma |
| As | = Ascites |
| F | = Foot |
| H | = Head |
| I | = Inferior vena cava |
| L | = Left |
| Li | = Liver |
| M | = Hepatoma |
| PV | = Portal vein |
| R | = Right |
| Sp | = Spine |

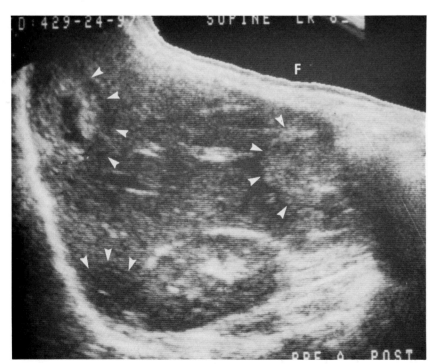

FIG 2–72.

## Hepatoma

The scans shown here illustrate an unusual presentation of hepatomas. Figure 2–73 is a transverse scan through the liver; Figure 2–74 is an accompanying CT scan made at approximately the same level. A highly echogenic structure is noted in the right lobe of the liver (arrowheads), secondary to a hepatoma. An acoustic shadow is noted near the medial posterior aspect of this tumor. The shadow reflects calcification within the hepatoma. The accompanying CT scan shows a low-density (small arrowheads) lesion in the right lobe of the liver. A calcific density can be seen in the posterior medial aspect of this lesion, corresponding to the ultrasound findings. Ascites is present on the CT scan.

Figure 2–75 is an oblique longitudinal scan through the region of the hepatoduodenal ligament. Ascites is seen as an echo-free region inferior to the liver. This is an unusual case in which hepatoma has caused tumor invasion within the common bile duct. The tumor (T) is seen to markedly enlarge the common bile duct, with a soft tissue echogenic appearance. Figure 2–76 illustrates another unusual case of hepatoma in which there is tumor invasion of the portal vein. Figure 2–76 is an oblique longitudinal scan parallel to the course of the portal vein. The soft echoes within the portal vein indicate tumor invasion.

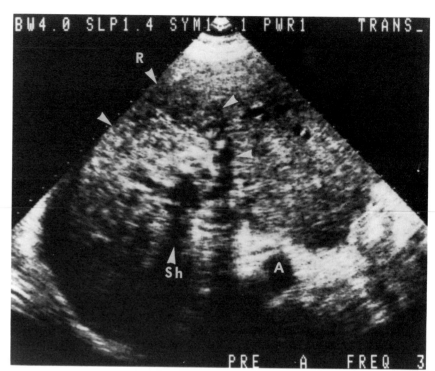

FIG 2–73.

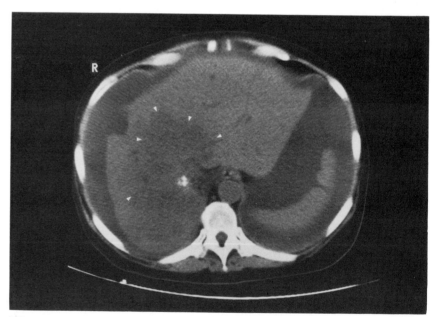

FIG 2–74.

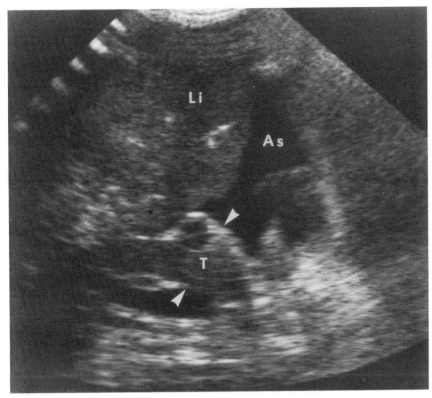

| | |
|---|---|
| **A** | = Aorta |
| **Arrowheads** | = Hepatoma |
| **As** | = Ascites |
| **Li** | = Liver |
| **PV** | = Portal vein |
| **R** | = Right |
| **Sh** | = Shadow from calcification |
| **T** | = Tumor invasion from hepatoma |

FIG 2–75.

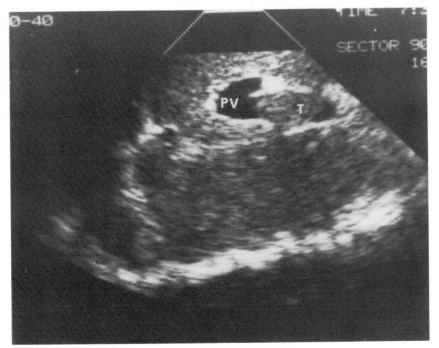

FIG 2–76.

# Hypoechotic Liver Metastases

Metastatic lesions of the liver can present with a variety of ultrasonographic patterns. The following examples demonstrate liver metastases that are decreased in echo amplitude compared to the rest of the liver. Figure 2–77 is a longitudinal scan of the lateral right lobe of the liver in a middle-aged woman with a known gastric carcinoma. A relatively sonolucent mass is seen within the liver. The borders are slightly irregular with no evidence of enhanced through-transmission. Soft echoes are noted within the mass, indicating a solid rather than a fluid nature. The patient was placed on several months of chemotherapy; the liver metastasis, however, continued to enlarge. Figure 2–78 is a scan of the same patient made approximately 3 months later. The liver metastasis has markedly enlarged. The borders have become more irregular, and numerous echoes are noted within. This is an example of a solitary hypoechotic liver metastasis that did not respond to chemotherapy.

Figure 2–79 is a longitudinal scan of a 70-year-old woman with carcinoma of the breast. This scan demonstrates a large metastatic lesion (arrows) of the inferior aspect of the right lobe of the liver. The echo amplitude of the metastatic lesion is not greatly different from the remainder of the liver. A slight hypoechotic rim, however, indicates a separation between the metastatic lesion and the liver. If it were not for this hypoechotic rim, the mass would be quite difficult to distinguish from the surrounding liver parenchyma. To identify liver metastasis, it is necessary to detect either a difference in echogenicity from the surrounding liver parenchyma or a capsular echo which will separate it from the remainder of the liver.

Figure 2–80 is a longitudinal scan of a 53-year-old man with poorly differentiated carcinoma of the left superior pulmonary sulcus. A large liver metastasis is present involving only the caudate lobe (arrows). Again, the echo amplitude of the metastatic le-

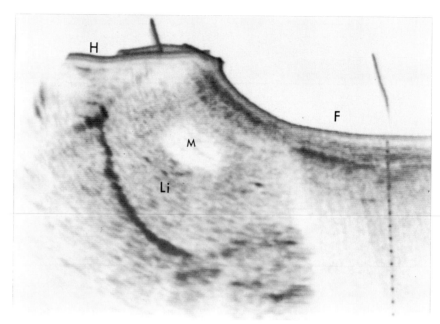

FIG 2–77.

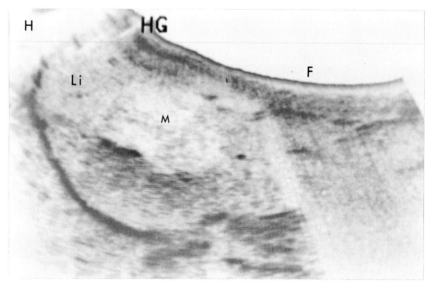

FIG 2–78.

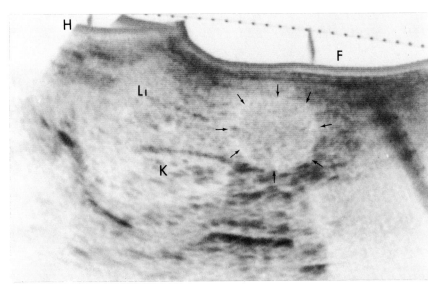

**FIG 2–79.**

sions is approximately the same as the normal liver situated anteriorly. The echoes arising from the metastatic lesion are somewhat coarser than those from the normal liver and are markedly enlarging the caudate lobe, which led to the diagnosis.

SOURCE: Figures 2–77 through 2–80 are provided through the courtesy of Barry Green, M.D.

| Arrows | = | Metastatic lesions |
|--------|---|--------------------|
| CL | = | Caudate lobe tumor |
| F | = | Foot |
| H | = | Head |
| HA | = | Hepatic artery |
| K | = | Kidney |
| Li | = | Liver |
| M | = | Metastases |
| PV | = | Portal vein |
| St | = | Stomach |

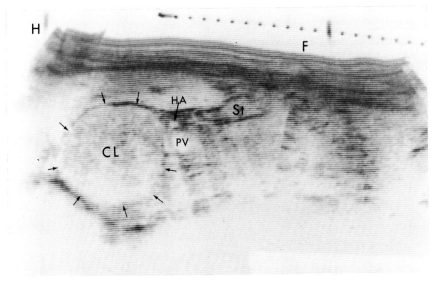

**FIG 2–80.**

## Echogenic Liver Metastasis

Figure 2–81 is a longitudinal scan of the right lobe of the liver in a 58-year-old woman with colonic carcinoma. The scan demonstrates a highly echogenic area in the posterior aspect of the right lobe (arrows), which indicates a single metastatic lesion from the colon. Colonic metastases are often highly echogenic lesions, perhaps because of their increased vascularity or mucinous nature. Tumors usually do not yield a characteristic echo pattern within the liver. However, colonic tumors often are highly echogenic. The patient was placed on combined chemotherapy; the metastatic disease, however, progressed. Figure 2–82 is a longitudinal scan of the right lobe of the liver made 4 months later. Multiple echogenic masses are present throughout the liver (arrows). They are quite varied in size and echogenicity.

Figure 2–83 is a transverse scan of the liver in a different patient. The scan shows a large, well-circumscribed echogenic mass lateral to the portal vein. This patient also had a carcinoma of the transverse colon. The echo amplitude of the metastatic lesion is much greater than that of the surrounding normal liver parenchyma.

Figure 2–84 is a longitudinal scan of the right lobe of the liver of a 72-year-old woman with known carcinoma of the cecum. Liver function studies were abnormal; a liver-spleen scan was markedly abnormal. Liver biopsy confirmed metastatic adenocarcinoma. The scan demonstrates multiple highly echogenic lesions (arrows) within the normal, less echogenic, liver parenchyma. We can see the different sizes of the liver tumors. They are of a much higher echo amplitude than the surrounding liver parenchyma.

All of these cases are examples of echogenic liver metastases arising from the colon.

SOURCE: Figures 2–81 and 2–82 are provided through the courtesy of Barry Green, M.D.

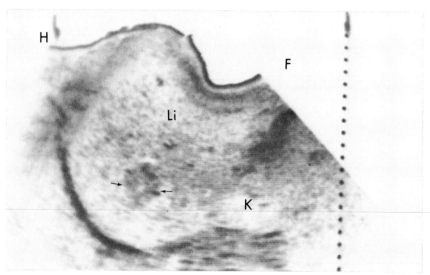

**FIG 2–81.**

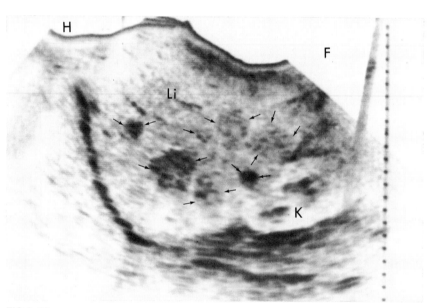

**FIG 2–82.**

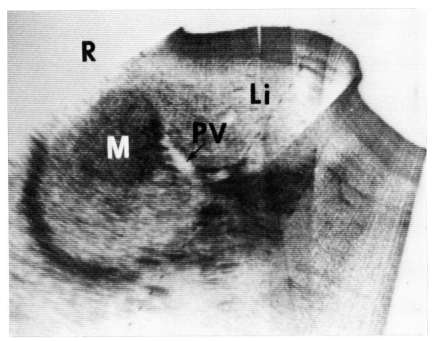

FIG 2–83.

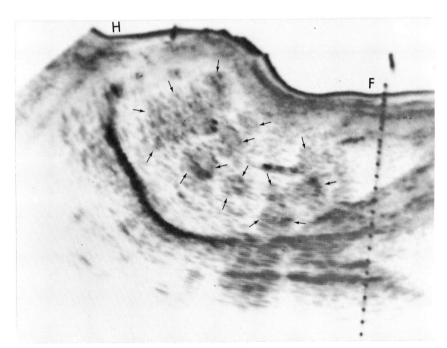

FIG 2–84.

## Necrotic Liver Metastases

Figures 2–85 and 2–86 are scans of a 66-year-old man with proven rectal carcinoid tumor metastatic to the lungs and liver. The initial ultrasound study was performed after several courses of combination chemotherapy. The metastatic lesions of the liver are in various stages of necrosis. Figure 2–85 is a transverse scan over the upper liver demonstrating a highly echogenic metastasis (arrows) in the posterior aspect of the left lobe. Fluid-filled necrotic metastases are noted in the right lobe.

Figure 2–86 is a longitudinal scan through the lateral aspect of the right lobe demonstrating numerous fluid-filled masses which are secondary to necrosis within the tumors. The two larger sonolucent masses have markedly irregular and ratty-appearing borders. Necrotic areas are also seen within the echogenic metastases.

This case illustrates an unusual manifestation of liver metastases in which marked necrotic changes are present. Necrosis has brought about liquefaction of the tumor in which fluid is noted in the central portion of many of these metastatic lesions. The irregular borders rule out a simple cyst. The fluid structures could possibly indicate abscess or hematomas. In light of the echogenic metastatic lesions, however, they are consistent with necrosis of the central portion of the tumor.

Figure 2–87 is a scan of a 24-year-old man with embryonal cell carcinoma of the testes. The scan shows a large necrotic metastasis involving most of the right lobe of the liver. The borders are irregular and ratty in appearance. The mass involves most of the right lobe.

Figure 2–88 is a transverse scan of the liver in a 53-year-old woman with leiomyosarcoma resected from the small intestine 8 years previously. An isotopic scan of the liver was positive, and biopsy confirmed metastatic disease. This scan demonstrates a fluid-filled mass in the left lobe of the liver. A horizontal line indicates a fluid-filled layer within the mass. This layer most

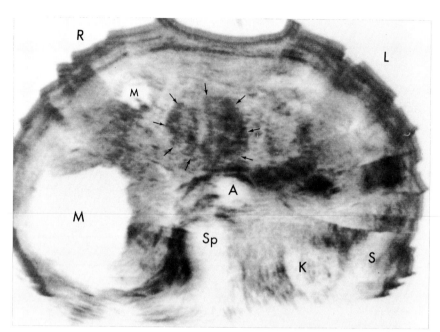

**FIG 2–85.**

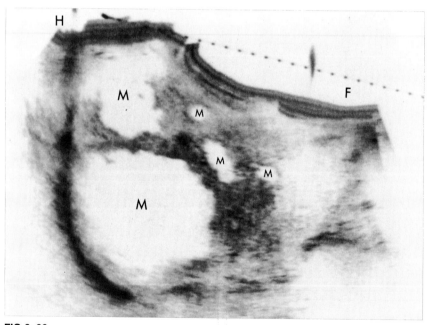

**FIG 2–86.**

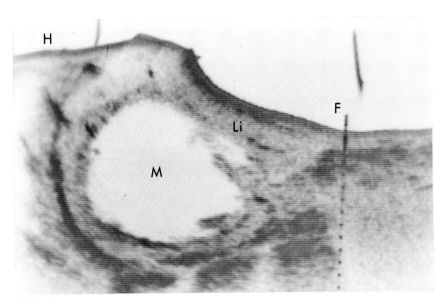

**FIG 2–87.**

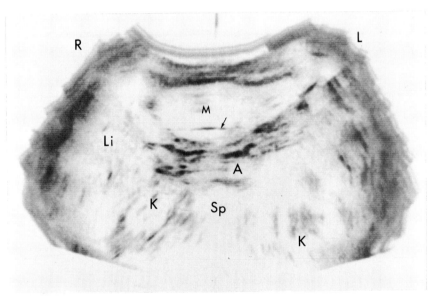

**FIG 2–88.**

likely represents debris within the tumor which is layering out in the fluid.

Source: Figures 2–85 through 2–88 are provided through the courtesy of Barry Green, M.D.

| | | |
|---|---|---|
| **A** | = | Aorta |
| **Arrow** | = | Fluid layer |
| **Arrows** | = | Echogenic metastasis |
| **F** | = | Foot |
| **H** | = | Head |
| **K** | = | Kidney |
| **L** | = | Left |
| **Li** | = | Liver |
| **M** | = | Necrotic metastases |
| **R** | = | Right |
| **S** | = | Spleen |
| **Sp** | = | Spine |

## Metastatic Disease of the Liver With Diffuse Abnormality

Often liver involvement is difficult to detect ultrasonographically because of the diffuse nature of metastatic disease. The liver parenchymagram does not show its even texture. Instead, disruption and disorganization of the liver parenchyma are apparent on ultrasound, and although no discrete lesion can be detected, this disorganization is reflected in the liver echoes.

Figure 2–89 is a longitudinal scan of the right lobe of the liver obtained from a 65-year-old woman with metastatic melanoma. The right lobe of the liver is markedly enlarged. The echo pattern arising from the liver demonstrates diffuse distortion of the usual normal architecture. Although no discrete lesions are easily visualized, destruction of the normal parenchymal echo pattern is evident.

Figure 2–90 is a longitudinal scan of the right lobe of the liver in a 56-year-old woman with metastatic colonic carcinoma. Ultrasound demonstrates a lack of normal homogeneous hepatic pattern, indicating diffuse metastatic disease. Increased echoes are noted posteriorly within the liver and are disorganized in nature. However, the anterior, less echogenic half of the liver also appears disrupted.

Figure 2–91 is a longitudinal scan of the liver in a 65-year-old woman with metastatic sigmoid colon carcinoma. Again, diffuse extensive disruption of the parenchymal pattern is present, with no discrete lesions noted.

Figure 2–92 is a longitudinal scan of the right lobe of the liver in a 66-year-old man with metastatic melanoma. The posterior half of the liver has a subtle inhomogeneous echo architecture. The anterior half of the liver appears to have a fairly even echo pattern that is characteristic of normal liver. The area in the posterior half of the liver (arrows), however, is less echogenic and much coarser in appearance, an indication of diffuse involvement of the liver on this scan. This is a good example of a compari-

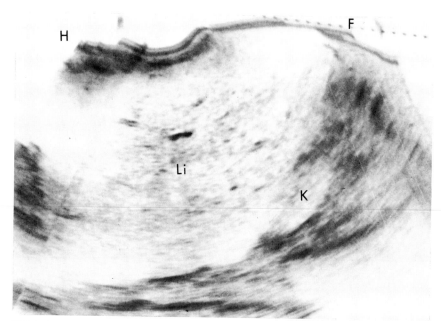

**FIG 2–89.**

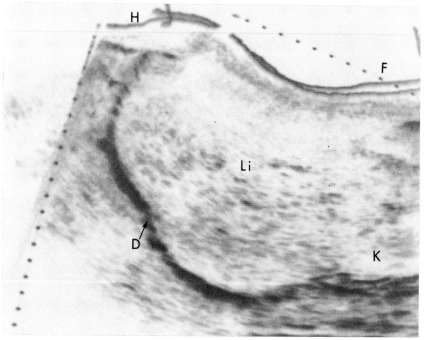

**FIG 2–90.**

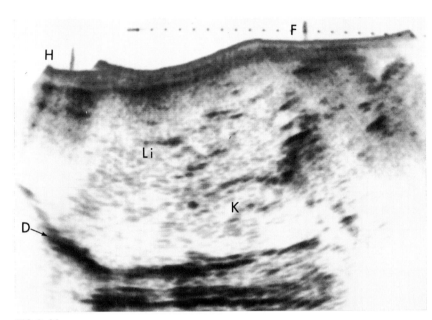

**FIG 2–91.**

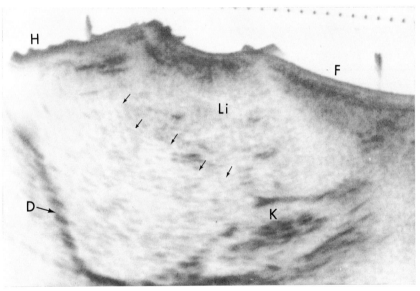

**FIG 2–92.**

son of the normal, soft, even echo pattern of the liver with the diffuse, irregular echogenicity of metastatic disease.

SOURCE: Figures 2–89 through 2–92 are provided through the courtesy of Barry Green, M.D.

| **Arrows** | = | Demarcation between normal and abnormal liver |
|---|---|---|
| **D** | = | Diaphragm |
| **F** | = | Foot |
| **H** | = | Head |
| **K** | = | Kidney |
| **Li** | = | Liver |

## Calcification of Liver Metastasis

Liver metastasis can occasionally calcify and lead to characteristic ultrasound findings. Figure 2–93 is a longitudinal scan in a 56-year-old woman with metastatic colonic carcinoma. Two highly echogenic areas are noted within the inferoposterior portion of the liver. Shadows are noted behind the strong echoes. Figure 2–94 is an x-ray film of the right upper quadrant demonstrating the calcifications within the liver arising from the metastatic colonic lesions.

Figure 2–95 is a transverse scan of a 60-year-old woman with colon carcinoma metastatic to the liver. The scan shows a highly echogenic region (arrows) in the lateral posterior aspect of the right lobe of the liver. The left lobe of the liver has a fairly even echo pattern. Figure 2–96 is a longitudinal scan of the same patient. Again, a high-amplitude echogenic region (arrows) is noted in the anterior aspect of the right lobe of the liver. Quite evident behind these strong echoes is an acoustic shadow arising from the calcified metastatic lesions.

SOURCE: Figures 2–93 through 2–96 are provided through the courtesy of Barry Green, M.D.

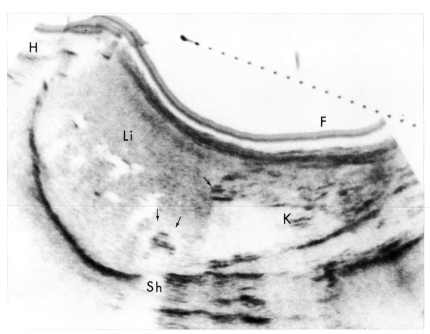

FIG 2–93.

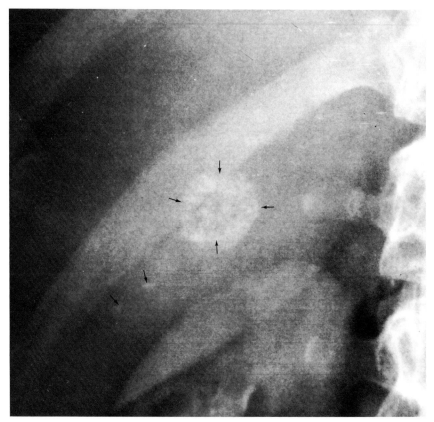

FIG 2–94.

A        = Aorta
Arrows   = Highly echogenic metastatic
           regions and calcified regions
F        = Foot
GB       = Gallbladder
H        = Head
K        = Kidney
L        = Left
Li       = Liver
R        = Right
Sh       = Shadowing
Sp       = Spine

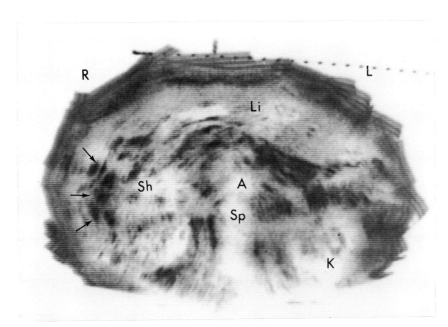

FIG 2–95.

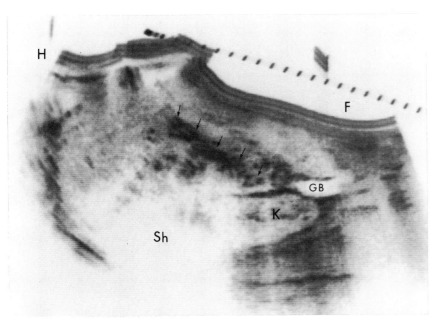

FIG 2–96.

## Lymphoma of the Liver

Lymphoma of the liver usually presents on ultrasound as relatively hypoechoic masses. Although echogenic lesions secondary to lymphoma have been reported, they are extremely rare. There is no way to distinguish lymphoma of the liver from other hypoechoic metastatic lesions.

Figures 2–97 and 2–98 are scans of a 40-year-old man with a long history of lymphocytic lymphoma that had spread to the neck, oral pharynx, lungs, and liver. Figure 2–97 is a transverse scan of the liver in which a relatively sonolucent mass is noted within the left lobe. There is evidence of adenopathy in the region of the porta hepatis. A second smaller mass is seen anterior to the portal vein. The CT scan (Fig 2–98) reveals a decreased density (arrows) corresponding to the site of lymphomatous involvement noted on the ultrasound scan.

Figures 2–99 and 2–100 are transverse and longitudinal scans of a different patient with hepatic lymphoma. A single isolated hypoechoic lesion is present in the liver. There is no way to distinguish this mass from other entities mentioned previously. The only suggestive finding is that lymphoma tends to be hypoechoic.

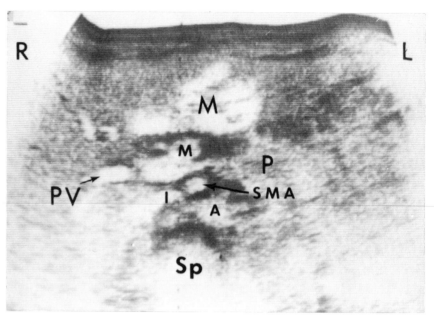

FIG 2–97.

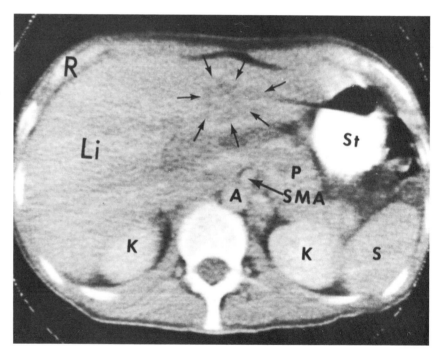

FIG 2–98.

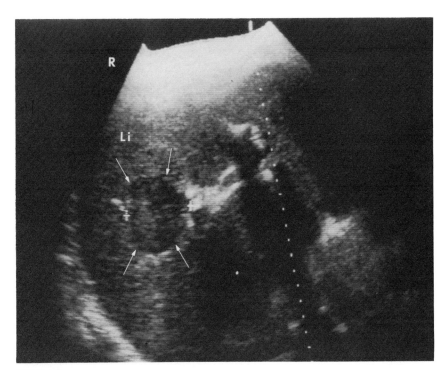

A       = Aorta
**Arrows** = Lymphoma
H       = Head
I       = Inferior vena cava
K       = Kidney
L       = Left
Li      = Liver
M       = Lymphoma
P       = Pancreas
PV      = Portal vein
R       = Right
S       = Spleen
SMA     = Superior mesenteric artery
Sp      = Spine
St      = Stomach

FIG 2–99.

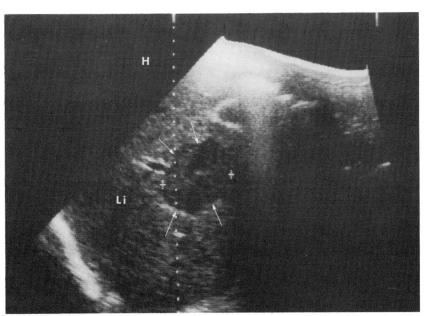

FIG 2–100.

## Cholangiocarcinoma: Ultrasound Contrast Agents

Cholangiocarcinoma often involves the confluence of the hepatic ducts in the region of the porta hepatis. Usually the only ultrasound manifestation will be dilatation of the biliary tree. Most often the carcinomas are quite small and not visualized on ultrasound. As the lesions increase in size, they become evident as a mass proximal to the dilated ducts. Figures 2–101 and 2–102 are transverse and longitudinal oblique scans of a patient with cholangiocarcinoma. The lesion (M) presents as a relatively sonolucent mass in the region of the porta hepatis. Dilated bile ducts (arrowheads) are evident proximal to the mass. This hypoechoic lesion could be secondary to metastatic disease, lymphoma, or primary liver tumor. There is no characteristic ultrasound feature that would suggest the diagnosis of cholangiocarcinoma.

Ultrasound contrast agents show promise of increasing the diagnosis of liver masses. Figures 2–103 and 2–104 are longitudinal scans of the same patient obtained 24 hours apart. The patient has a diagnosis of gastric carcinoma. The initial scan in Figure 2–103 was obtained without the injection of a contrast agent. Note the power and gain settings, and compare them with settings in Figure 2–104. Twenty-four hours after the administration of Fluosol-DA 20% scanning was again performed with the same transducer and at the same power and gain settings. A highly echogenic mass (arrows) can be seen slightly cephalad to the portal vein. There is a dramatic difference in the ultrasound appearance of this lesion between the two scans. The lesion would not have been detected on the non-contrast-enhanced scan. The future of ultrasound contrast agents is quite promising, and further investigation is underway.

SOURCE: Figures 2–103 and 2–104 are provided through the courtesy of Robert F. Mattrey, M.D. From Mattrey RF, Strich G, Shelton RE, et al: Perfluorochemicals as ultrasound contrast agents for tumor imaging and hepatosplenography: Preliminary clinical results. *Radiology*.

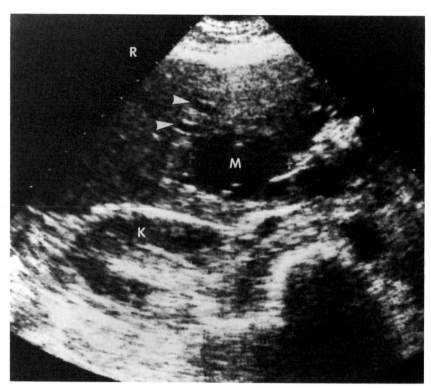

**FIG 2–101.**

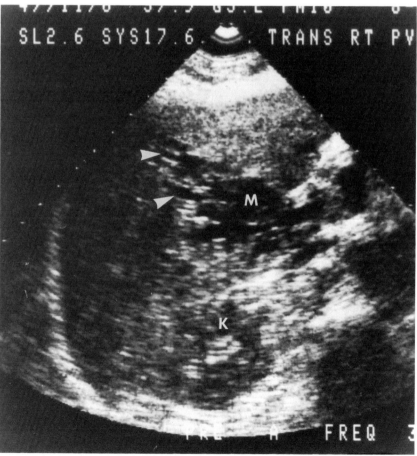

**FIG 2–102.**

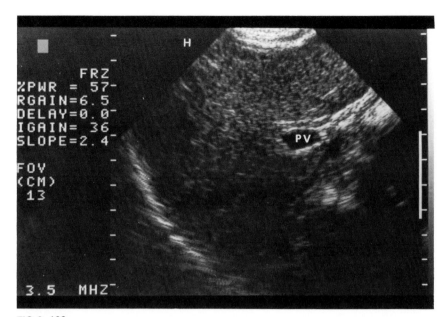

| Arrows | = Metastatic lesion |
| Arrowheads | = Dilated bowel ducts |
| H | = Head |
| K | = Kidney |
| M | = Cholangiocarcinoma |
| PV | = Portal vein |

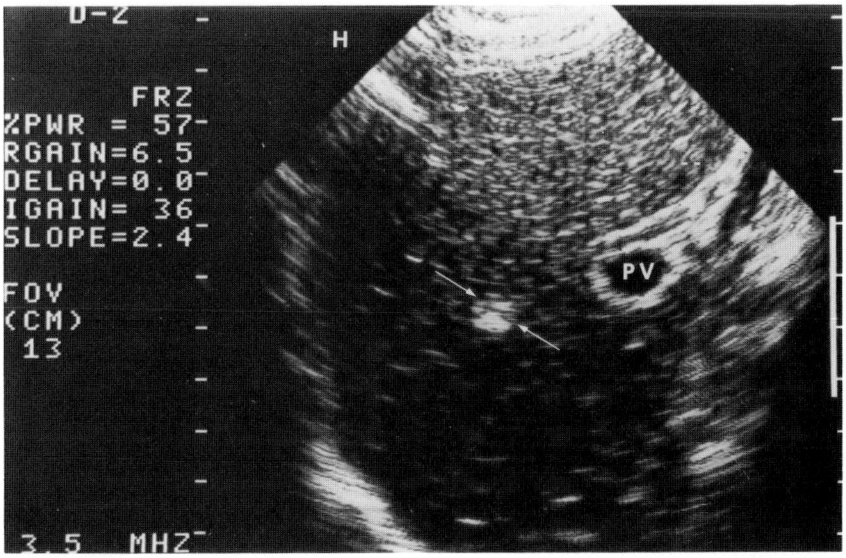

**FIG 2–103.**

**FIG 2–104.**

## Small Echogenic Liver Foci

The fibrofatty tissue surrounding the portal triad consistenly gives high-amplitude echoes within the liver. However, these echoes have a characteristic appearance that is usually not confusing. Occasionally one may encounter a liver ultrasound scan in which numerous highly echogenic foci are dispersed throughout the liver. Depending on their character and location, the correct diagnosis can often be determined. After biliary surgery, such as a choledochojejunostomy, air can be introduced into the biliary tree. Figures 2–105 and 2–106 are transverse scans of a patient who had previously undergone choledochojejunostomy. Reflux of intestinal gas is evident in the biliary tree on these scans. Numerous linear highly echogenic regions are dispersed throughout the liver, paralleling the course of the portal vein. These loculations of gas stand out as high-amplitude echoes within the liver. What is structure number 1 in Figure 2–106?

Stones within the biliary tree have an ultrasound appearance similar to that of stones within the gallbladder. They present as high-amplitude echoes casting acoustic shadows. This is not true when small amounts of air are present. Usually small amounts of air will not cast a shadow unless they are large enough to obstruct a good portion of the ultrasound beam. In the presence of intrabiliary stones, they will give acoustic shadowing similar to that seen with stones in the gallbladder. Figure 2–107 is a longitudinal scan of the right lobe of the liver in a patient with Caroli's disease. The biliary tree was dilated and nearly entirely filled with stones. Note the acoustic shadowing deep to the intrahepatic stones.

Figure 2–108 is a transverse scan of an elderly Vietnamese patient who had previously experienced multiple episodes of cholangitis. The scan illustrates Oriental cholangiohepatis. These patients have massively dilated intrahepatic and common bile ducts with stricturing and intrahepatic

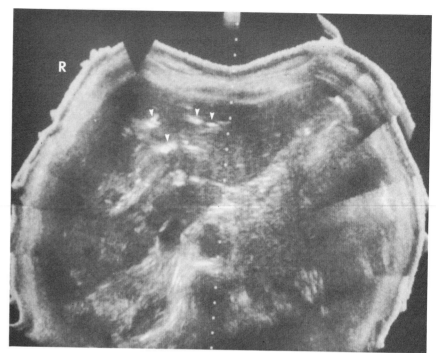

**FIG 2–105.**

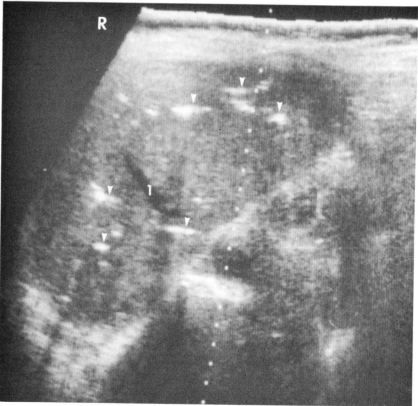

**FIG 2–106.**

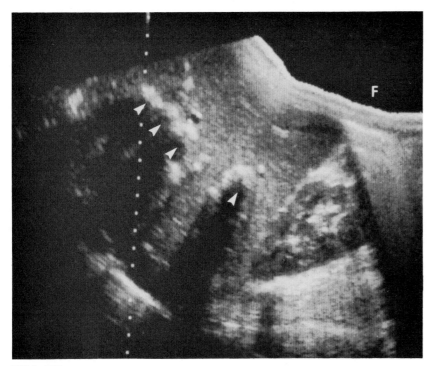

**FIG 2–107.**

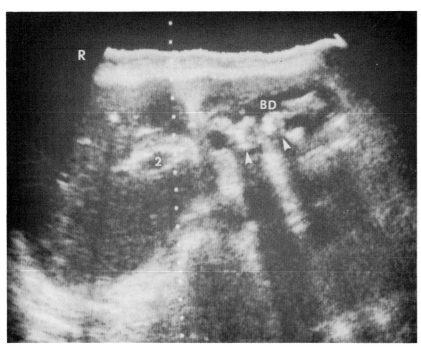

**FIG 2–108.**

stones. In Figure 2–108 one can see highly echogenic stones, with shadowing deep to them. Note the dilated bile ducts proximal to stones. What is structure 2 in Figure 2–108?

| | | |
|---|---|---|
| **Arrowheads (small)** | = | Air in the biliary tree |
| **Arrowheads (large)** | = | Stones in the biliary tree |
| **BD** | = | Dilated left hepatic duct |
| **F** | = | Foot |
| **R** | = | Right |
| **1** | = | Hepatic vein |
| **2** | = | Portal vein |

## Dilated Portal Vein, Hepatomegaly, and Cirrhosis

Figures 2–109 and 2–110 are scans of a patient with a dilated portal vein. The portal vein can be extremely variable in size. Its size is affected by Valsalva maneuvers and respiratory changes. The most dramatic dilatations, however, are found in cases of portal venous hypertension. The portal vein in Figure 2–110 is markedly dilated when compared to the inferior vena cava. Very often a filling defect on the liver spleen scan will be noted in the porta hepatis. Ultrasound examination of this region can be extremely helpful if a large portal vein is diagnosed. This will explain the defect in the porta hepatis. Furthermore, dilated hepatic veins can appear as defects on the nuclear medicine study near the medial portion of the dome of the right hemidiaphragm. Figure 2–109 demonstrates a rather prominent left lobe of the liver, indicating hepatomegaly.

Hepatomegaly is best evaluated on a liver-spleen scan. Unless volume determinations are done, hepatomegaly can be difficult to evaluate on ultrasound, but massively enlarged livers such as is present in Figure 2–111 are easily demonstrated. Figure 2–111 is a longitudinal scan of the right lobe of the liver which extends caudal to the lower pole of the right kidney. There is even evidence of abdominal distention, as is demonstrated by the protuberance of the anterior abdominal wall (arrows).

The ultrasound findings in cirrhotic changes of the liver are mainly those of severe attenuation to the sound. Figure 2–112 is an example of cirrhosis in which strong echoes are noted in the near field, with marked attenuation present more distally. The echoes arising from the liver are fairly even and small, but of high amplitude in the near field. The ultrasound beam is barely able to penetrate the liver to allow visualization of the lateral aspects of the spine and aorta. The marked attenuation of sound is secondary to fibrotic changes within the liver. Other

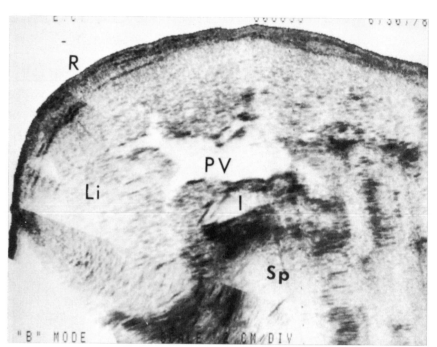

**FIG 2–109.**

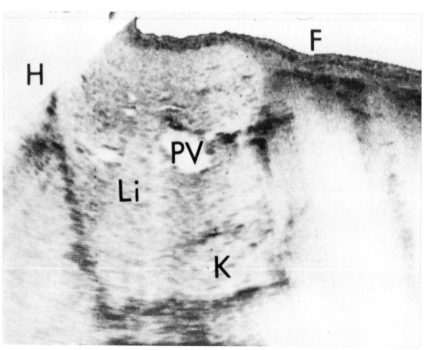

**FIG 2–110.**

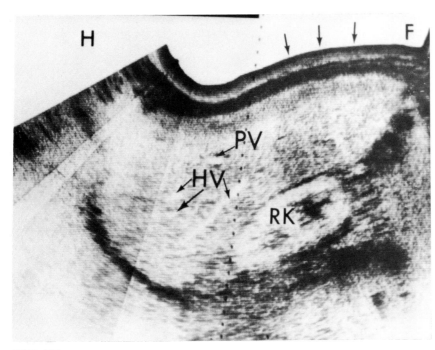

**FIG 2–111.**

causes of attenuation, such as fatty infiltration, may give an ultrasound picture somewhat similar to cirrhosis.

| | | |
|---|---|---|
| **A** | = | Aorta |
| **Arrows** | = | Protuberance of the anterior abdominal wall |
| **F** | = | Foot |
| **H** | = | Head |
| **HV** | = | Hepatic veins |
| **I** | = | Inferior vena cava |
| **K** | = | Kidney |
| **L** | = | Left |
| **Li** | = | Liver |
| **PV** | = | Portal vein |
| **R** | = | Right |
| **RK** | = | Right kidney |
| **Sp** | = | Spine |

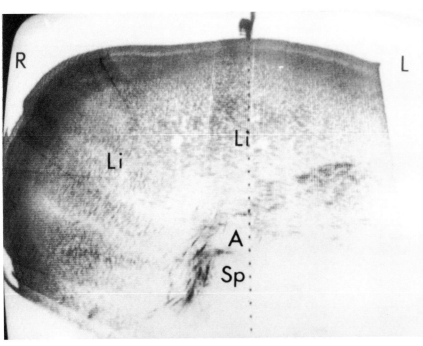

**FIG 2–112.**

## Cirrhosis and Fatty Infiltration

Figure 2–113 is a longitudinal scan of a patient with ascites and marked cirrhotic changes of the liver. The capsule of the liver is seen adjacent to the ascites. The near echoes of the liver are quite dark. Penetration of sound through the liver, however, is extremely poor, as is indicated by the dramatic drop-off of echoes. This finding is compatible with marked fibrotic changes in a liver involved with cirrhosis. The severe attenuation of sound is evident in this case.

Fatty infiltration of the liver can have an ultrasound appearance quite similar to cirrhotic changes. Figures 2–114 through 2–116 are of a patient who had fatty involvement of the liver. Figure 2–116 is a CT scan of the liver in which we see that the density of the liver is much less than the spleen secondary to fatty infiltration. The portal vein is seen within the liver as a much denser structure. Figures 2–114 and 2–115 are transverse and longitudinal ultrasound scans of the same patient. There is marked attenuation of sound by the liver due to the fatty infiltration. The transverse scan in Figure 2–114 shows poor visualization of the spine. The echoes arising from the spine are much weaker than we would usually expect. The longitudinal scan of the liver in Figure 2–115 again demonstrates marked attenuation of sound by fatty infiltration of the liver. The diaphragm (arrows) is barely seen because of this marked attenuation.

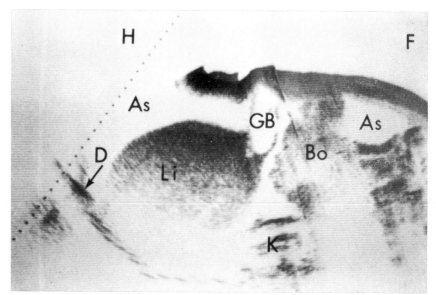

FIG 2–113.

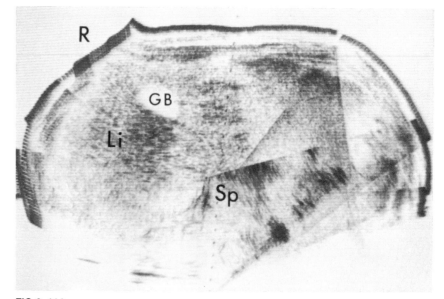

FIG 2–114.

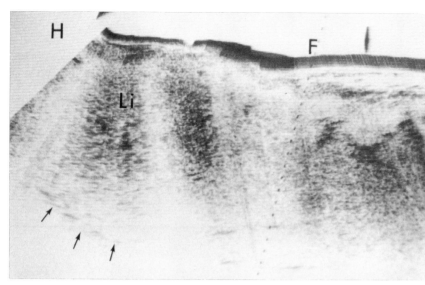

**FIG 2–115.**

| | | |
|---|---|---|
| **A** | = | Aorta |
| **Arrows** | = | Diaphragm |
| **As** | = | Ascites |
| **Bo** | = | Bowel |
| **D** | = | Diaphragm |
| **F** | = | Foot |
| **GB** | = | Gallbladder |
| **H** | = | Head |
| **I** | = | Inferior vena cava |
| **K** | = | Kidney |
| **Li** | = | Liver |
| **PV** | = | Portal vein |
| **R** | = | Right |
| **S** | = | Spleen |
| **Sp** | = | Spine |
| **St** | = | Stomach |

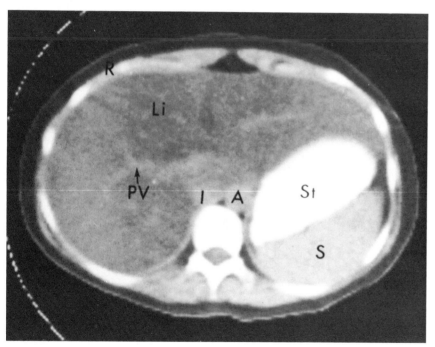

**FIG 2–116.**

## Cirrhosis; Focal Fatty Infiltration

Figures 2–117 and 2–118 are transverse scans through the liver in a patient with cirrhosis. The liver is surrounded by a lucent region that is secondary to ascites. Figure 2–117 is an amplitude-modulation (AM) scan. Figure 2–118 is a frequency-modulation (FM) scan. FM imaging is a recent development which tends to give a slightly different ultrasound appearance. On FM images more liver structure is apparent. There is also suggestive evidence of better lateral resolution on FM images, compared to AM images. In this patient with cirrhosis, the low-amplitude areas within the liver most likely represent micronodular cirrhosis.

Figure 2–119 is a transverse scan through the liver; the ultrasound appearance is confusing. There is a hypoechoic region that appears to be the abnormal area. However, the hypoechoic area (arrowheads) in fact is normal liver. It is the echogenic region laterally that is abnormal secondary to fatty infiltration. Occasionally, focal fatty infiltration may have an extremely confusing ultrasound appearance. Confirmation with CT scanning is suggested in such cases.

Figure 2–120 shows another case of focal fatty infiltration. There is an echogenic region (arrows) in the medial segment of the left lobe. This transverse scan gives the impression of a metastatic lesion or hemangioma in the region. However, the echogenic region is secondary to focal fatty infiltration. What are structures 1, 2, and 3 in Figure 2–120?

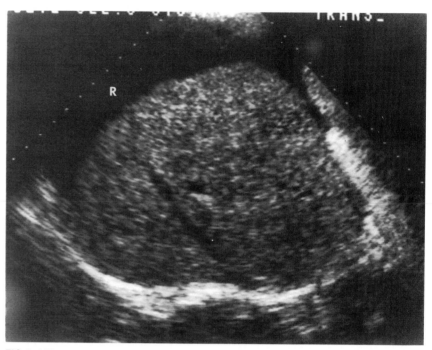

FIG 2–117.

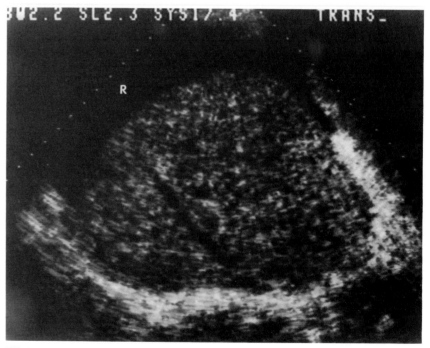

FIG 2–118.

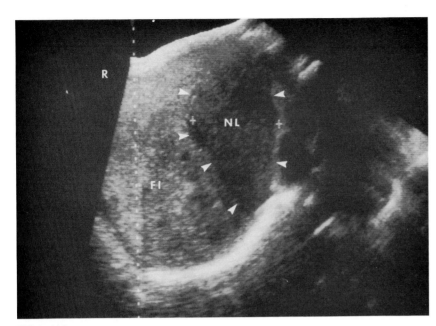

| Arrows | = Focal fatty infiltration |
| Arrowheads | = Normal liver |
| FI | = Focal fatty infiltration |
| NL | = Normal liver |
| R | = Right |
| 1 | = Inferior vena cava |
| 2 | = Right portal vein |
| 3 | = Caudate lobe |

FIG 2–119.

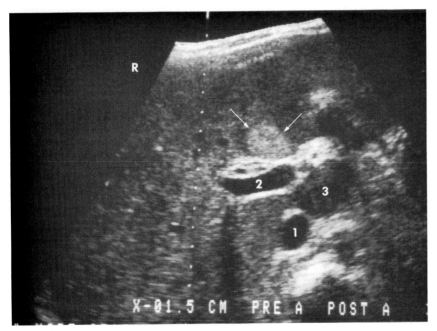

FIG 2–120.

# 3.
# Ultrasonography of the Gallbladder and Biliary Tree

Faye C. Laing, M.D.

The impact of ultrasound on assessment of the hepatobiliary system has been dramatic. Few would disagree that despite the introduction and refinements of other imaging modalities, especially computed tomography (CT) and more recently magnetic resonance imaging ultrasound remains the initial screening modality for evaluating the gallbladder and bile ducts. Because of its high sensitivity and accuracy in detecting gallstones and for determining whether or not biliary dilatation is present, and because it is a rapid, noninvasive, and flexible examination that is independent of organ function, ultrasound is likely to remain the examination of choice for evaluating both jaundiced patients and those suspected of having cholelithiasis.

This chapter is divided into three sections, the gallbladder, the intrahepatic bile ducts, and extrahepatic bile ducts. In each section the anatomy, pathology, and imaging pitfalls are discussed.

## Gallbladder

### Gallbladder Anatomy

A normal gallbladder should be visible in virtually all patients if it is physiologically distended after an 8- to 12-hour fast. The anatomic position of the gallbladder fundus can vary dramatically from one patient to another. It may even vary quite markedly in a single patient, depending on the patient's position. The neck of the gallbladder, however, bears a fixed anatomic relationship to the main lobar fissure and the right portal vein.[1] In approximately 70% of patients a linear echo, thought to represent a portion of the main lobar fissure, can be identified connecting the gallbladder to the right or main portal vein. This anatomic consideration becomes important for conclusively identifying the gallbladder in patients with pathologic conditions such as a small contracted gallbladder, or one filled with calculi.

Because the size and shape of the normal gallbladder vary widely in individual patients, it is difficult to formulate precise size criteria. In general, if the transverse diameter of the gallbladder exceeds 5 cm and if the gallbladder is no longer ovoid but round, it is likely to be hydropic.[2] Conversely, if the diameter is less than 2 cm despite adequate fasting, the gallbladder is likely to be abnormally contracted.

The shape of a typical gallbladder is oval or gourd-like, but frequently it varies from this configuration and contains apparent folds or kinks. Although true septations are rare, in approximately 4% of patients a "phrygian cap" deformity is present in which the gallbladder fundus appears to be folded upon the body. A more frequent variation is the presence of a fold between the body and infundibulum of the gallbladder, known as a junctional fold.[3] Any fold in the gallbladder can produce high-amplitude echoes that may occasionally be associated with posterior acoustic shadowing (due to refractive effects). This appearance can cause folds to be mistaken for polyps and/or calculi. An awareness of these variations as well as meticulous scanning technique should minimize diagnostic errors.

The normal gallbladder wall is visible as a pencil-thin echogenic line less than 3 mm thick. Although the gallbladder may be normally indented by adjacent bowel loops, focal impressions on it from the liver suggest the presence of a hepatic mass. Because bile does not contain particulate material, the gallbladder lumen is normally echo free.

## Scanning Techniques

To ensure adequate gallbladder distention, the examination should be performed after an overnight fast. Adequate fasting is important to avoid diagnostic errors. Physiologic contraction of the gallbladder yields a small, thick-walled gallbladder on ultrasound. These findings will be misinterpreted as pathology. Thorough questioning of the patient about eating or drinking over the previous 12–16 hours is a necessity.

Real-time equipment is preferred to articulated arm machines because it is less operator dependent, and because it allows rapid and complete display of the entire gallbladder. For most patients, a sector transducer is better than a linear array format. The smaller-sized sector transducer can be more optimally positioned subcostally or within rib interspaces. The highest frequency transducer that yields satisfactory images of the gallbladder should be used. For most patients, a 3.5-MHz transducer is adequate. In thin patients or in those with an anteriorly positioned gallbladder, a 5-MHz transducer provides superior resolution. As the gallbladder fossa is scanned, gentle pressure should be applied to the patients abdomen

with the transducer. This is done in an attempt to elicit gallbladder tenderness in patients suspected of having acute cholecystitis.

A thorough examination of the gallbladder can usually be accomplished in 5–10 minutes. The scans are performed with the patient supine or in a left posterior oblique (LPO) position. Occasionally, however, scans should be obtained with the patient in an erect or prone position to convincingly demonstrate calculi mobility. Cholecystosonography requires meticulous scanning technique to avoid overlooking small calculi. Special attention should be directed to the most dependent region of the gallbladder, where most calculi are found. In most patients this is the region of the gallbladder neck and the cystic duct area.

## Gallbladder Pathology

### CHOLELITHIASIS

Detection of cholelithiasis is the primary role of cholecystosonography. Since Hublitz et al. first reported the ultrasonographic detection of gallstones in four of eight patients,[4] cholecystosonographic visualization of calculi has improved dramatically. Recent studies have reported sensitivities and accuracies of greater than 95%.[5–7] As a result of these statistics, ultrasonography has essentially replaced oral cholecystography as the examination of choice for detecting cholelithiasis. It is apparent that ultrasound can even detect gallstones that are not visualized or technically adequate oral cholecystograms.[5, 8] Other advantages of ultrasonography over radiographic cholecystography are that irradiation and contrast material are eliminated, the study can be performed on acutely ill patients, and the examination is independent of gastrointestinal, hepatic, and biliary function.

Because gallstones both absorb and reflect the ultrasound beam, the net sonographic effect is a highly reflective echo originating from the anterior surface of the calculus with a prominent posterior acoustic shadow. The demonstration of a posterior acoustic shadow is important. Shadowing echo densities that originate from within the gallbladder correlate with cholelithiasis in virtually all cases, whereas nonshadowing echo densities correlate with calculi in only 50% of cases.[6] To optimally visualize a posterior acoustic shadow, it is important to use the highest frequency transducer, which is focused maximally at the depth of the stone. Because very small calculi may fail to demonstrate acoustic shadowing, it is sometimes advantageous to reposition the patient in an attempt to pile small stones on one another. The effect of this maneuver is to form an aggregate of small stones that acoustically behaves as a larger stone with respect to casting a posterior acoustic shadow. The patient can also be repositioned so that the stone is within the focal zone.

The diagnosis of calculus disease can be made confidently when gravity-dependent movement of a stone is demonstrated. Except when a stone is impacted in the gallbladder neck or is adherent to the gallbladder wall, calculi should be mobile. On very rare occasions, "sludge balls"[9] or "tumefactive biliary sludge"[10] can appear as mobile masses within the gallbladder lumen. The nature of this material varies from case to case and may include parasites, blood clots, aggregated pus, sludge, or contrast material. In contrast to calculi, this material is evanescent and is not associated with posterior acoustic shadowing.

As the gallbladder becomes filled with stones, its ultrasound appearance changes dramatically. The outline of the gallbladder is no longer seen. Instead, a high-amplitude reflection with a prominent acoustic shadow emanates from the gallbladder fossa. This echo-shadow complex originates from the most superficial layer of stones. The deeper calculi, as well as the intraluminal bile and outline of the gallbladder, are rendered invisible. Close scrutiny of these images usually allows one to identify the anterior gallbladder wall as well as the superficial calculi.[11] These findings lead to a definitive diagnosis of cholethiasis.[12] The sonographic differential diagnosis for this appearance includes calcification in the gallbladder wall (porcelain gallbladder)[13] or air in the gallbladder wall.[14, 15] In patients with emphysematous cholecystitis, reverberation echoes from the air suggest the correct diagnosis.

## WALL CHANGES

The most frequent gallbladder wall abnormality detected by sonography is diffuse thickening, which is diagnosed when the wall is more than 3 mm thick. Wall thickening typically appears as a hypoechoic region between two echogenic lines. Although initially described as highly specific for cholecystitis, diffuse wall thickening is now recognized as neither sensitive nor specific for an inflammatory process. Approximately 50%–75% of patients with acute cholecystitis, have diffusely thickened gallbladder walls, while fewer than 25% of patients with chronic cholecystitis have this finding.[2, 16, 17]

Other conditions associated with diffuse gallbladder wall thickening include hepatic dysfunction (associated with alcoholism, hypoalbuminemia, ascites, and hepatitis), congestive heart failure, renal disease, neoplasm, and sepsis.[18, 19] Although a unifying pathophysiologic mechanism may not explain these diverse disease processes, many of the patients have decreased intravascular osmotic pressure and elevated portal venous pressure. Another cause of generalized gallbladder wall thickening is partial contraction due to eating. If the maximum diameter of the gallbladder is less than 2 cm and if diffuse wall thickening is present, the sonographer should inquire as to whether or not the patient fasted appropriately before the ultrasound examination.

In contrast to diffuse gallbladder wall thickening, focal gallbladder wall thickening strongly suggests primary gallbladder pathology. Gallbladder carcinoma is most often visualized as a mass that fills or replaces the gallbladder lumen. In approximately 40% of cases, it is seen either as a focal mass that protrudes into the gallbladder lumen or as an asymmetrically thickened wall.[20] Additional findings include liver metastases, evidence of direct hepatic invasion, adenopathy, bile duct dilatation, and cholelithiasis (80%–90% of cases). Other causes of focal gallbladder wall thickening are polyps (adenomatous, cholesterol), papillary adenomas, metastatic nodules, adenomyomatosis, and occasionally tumefactive sludge. In patients with adenomyomatosis, anechoic or echogenic foci may sometimes be visible within the thickened gallbladder wall. Intraluminal diverticula (Rokitansky-Aschoff sinuses) that contain bile are most likely responsible for the anechoic areas, while biliary sludge or gallstones within the diverticula are most likely responsible for echogenic foci.[21] Focal gallbladder wall irregularities are also sonographically visible in approximately 50% of patients with gangrenous cholecystitis. These irregularities correspond to areas of mucosal ulceration, hemorrhage, necrosis, and/or microabscess formation.[22]

## SLUDGE

Echogenic bile or "sludge" refers to particulate material (specifically calcium bilirubinate and/or cholesterol crystals) within bile.[23] Unlike gallstones, which generate strong echoes, sludge characteristically displays low to mid-level echoes. It is never accompanied by posterior acoustic shadowing. Because of its viscous nature, sludge moves sluggishly after the patient has been repositioned. This is easily documented with real-time scanning.

The most frequent predisposing factor associated with sludge is bile stasis. This can occur in patients who undergo prolonged fasting or hyperalimentation, as well as in patients with biliary obstruction at the level of the gallbladder, cystic duct, or common bile duct. Occasionally, other types of particulate material are found in bile, such as pus or hemorrhagic clot. Their appearance may be sonographically indistinguishable from sludge.

Although gallbladder sludge suggests an underlying abnormality, its presence does not necessarily imply primary gallbladder pathology. The clinical significance of sludge is uncertain. Further investigations are required to assess whether or not sludge can irritate the gallbladder or mucosa and act as a precursor to stone formation.

## PERICHOLECYSTIC FLUID

Localized pericholecystic fluid is most often due to acute cholecystitis, complicated by gallbladder perforation and abscess formation. Ultrasound can aid in the diagnosis of this condition by displaying an anechoic or complex fluid collection adjacent to or surrounding the gallbladder.

Rarely, an isolated pericholecystic fluid collection can be seen in patients with pancreatitis, peptic ulcer disease, or both.[24] This fluid presumably results from extension of the primary inflammatory process along the hepatoduodenal ligament into the main lobar fissure, where it comes to rest adjacent to the gallbladder neck.

## ACUTE CHOLECYSTITIS

The primary role of ultrasound is in the detection of gallstones. Recent evidence, however, suggests that ultrasonography can also be successfully used in diagnosing acute cholecystitis.[2, 16, 25] Tests using technetium-tagged IDA and IDA-like compounds are extremely sensitive and accurate for determining whether or not acute cholecystitis is present.[26] It is still important to first evaluate the patient with ultrasound, because acute cholecystitis will be present in only one third of patients with acute right upper quadrant

pain.[16] In addition to detecting gallstones with an accuracy of 95%–99%,[5–7] ultrasound can distinguish acute from chronic cholecystitis with an accuracy of 88%.[16] The most sensitive sonographic criteria for diagnosing acute cholecystitis are the presence of gallstones and focal gallbladder tenderness. Other findings that corroborate the diagnosis include gallbladder dilatation, sludge, and wall thickening. Chronic cholecystitis is diagnosed if the gallbladder contains stones but the secondary criteria listed above are missing. An advantage of ultrasound over radionuclide imaging is that the former examination also permits evaluation of the liver, right kidney, pancreas, and pelvic structures. Pathologic processes affecting each of these organs frequently result in symptoms that mimic those of acute cholecystitis. Patients whose ultrasonograms are equivocal for the diagnosis of acute cholecystitis should undergo a nuclear scan with an IDA-like compound.

### Pitfalls in Imaging of the Gallbladder

Real-time ultrasound equipment has not only made the detection of gallbladder calculi faster and easier, it has also eliminated some of the problems associated with static articulated-arm machines. If a static unit is used, it is important to perform single sector scans to eliminate spurious intraluminal echoes that can result from compound scanning. For similar reasons, with static equipment, scans should be performed during suspended respiration. Reverberation artifacts from gas or overlying ribs can be minimized if acoustic windows are chosen that avoid these anatomic areas.

Regardless of the kind of equipment used, shadows that appear to arise from the gallbladder neck can be a source of diagnostic confusion. Because refraction from the edge of the gallbladder is associated with shadowing, it is mandatory to visualize the stone—not merely the acoustic shadow—before diagnosing cholelithiasis. Similarly, shadowing posterior to the gallbladder that originates from within the bowel should not be misinterpreted as suggesting primary gallbladder pathology.

A false positive diagnosis of cholelithiasis can be made if the gallbladder is physiologically contracted and the gastric antrum/duodenum contains material that mimics the appearance of a gallbladder filled with stones. Real-time equipment and if necessary the ingestion of water should be used to further evaluate these problems. Air and water will be seen moving through the antrum and duodenum on real-time studies. Very rarely, particulate material may enter the gallbladder through a spontaneous or surgically created gastrointestinal fistula and may be responsible for a false positive diagnosis of cholelithiasis.[27, 28]

Although the great majority of gallstones appear sonographically "classic," sometimes atypical calculi are encounterd. An example is a stone either adherent to or within the gallbladder wall. Its appearance can mimic the appearance of focal air or calcification within the gallbladder wall. These entities can sometimes be distinguished from one another by plain film radiographs, although in special circumstances CT may be required.

Normally, calculi are positioned dependently in the gallbladder lumen. Rarely they may float in bile. The nondependent position of calculi was initially attributed to the presence of oral cholecystographic contrast material within bile.[29] Recently, however, cholesterol stones and those containing gas fissures have also been observed to "float."[30]

Echoes produced by gallstones are usually high in amplitude. Occasionally, however, they are less echogenic than expected. This appearance occurs most often in patients with soft pigment stones which have a mud-like consistency. Although these calculi are unusual in the gallbladder, they are common in the intrahepatic and extrahepatic biliary tree and are seen in patients with Oriental cholangiohepatitis.[31]

In a small percentage of patients, and despite the use of optimal equipment and scanning techniques, neither the gallbladder nor shadowing from its fossa is seen. In most cases the gallbladders are abnormal, with an obliterated lumen. Rarely, the gallbladder may be difficult to detect because it is filled with sludge that is isoechoic with liver parenchyma.[32] Other causes of gallbladder nonvisualization include physiologic contraction, congenital absence of the gallbladder, an unusual position, or technical error. In these situations, oral cholecystography or technetium-IDA imaging should be done as a confirmatory examination because despite nonvisualization on sonography, the gallbladder will sometimes prove normal.[15]

Sludge-like intraluminal echoes can also be a source of confusion. Occasionally, artifacts may be responsible for intraluminal, dependent low-level echoes. Most often, these are due to either section thickness or side lobe artifacts.[33, 34]

Section thickness artifacts result from partial voluming and occur when a portion of the ultrasound beam interacts with the fluid-filled gallbladder lumen while an adjacent portion of the beam interacts with a true echo reflector. These artifactual echoes can be minimized by using a narrow sound beam focused at the level of the gallbladder and by scanning through the gallbladder's central portion.[33]

Side lobe artifacts are caused by transducer side lobes interacting with highly reflective acoustic surfaces, such as duodenal gas located adjacent to the gallbladder. These echoes, which appear to originate within the main ultrasound beam, can be minimized by repositioning the patient so the gallbladder falls away from adjacent gas-filled structures, by changing the angulation of the transducer, or by decreasing machine intensity.[34] Because section thickness and side lobe artifacts are independent of gravity, "pseudosludge" that is secondary to artifacts will not layer with changes in patient position, unlike true sludge.

## Intrahepatic Bile Ducts

### Normal Anatomy

Because ultrasound can be used to identify and trace tubular fluid-filled structures, it is an ideal modality for evaluating dilated intrahepatic bile ducts. Under normal circumstances, only portal veins are visible within the portal triads of the hepatic parenchyma. Although normal-sized right and left bile ducts can be seen, it is important to realize that they are extrahepatic in location and course with the undivided portion of the right portal vein and the initial portion of the left portal vein, respectively. When intrahepatic bile ducts dilate, they cross the threshold of visibility and accompany the normally visible branches of the intrahepatic portal venous system. Four criteria have been described that allow a distinction to be made between dilated intrahepatic bile ducts and portal veins.[35] These are described below.

### Dilated Intrahepatic Bile Ducts

The first and most reliable differentiating feature is an alteration in the anatomic pattern of the portal veins.

Normally, intrahepatic veins appear as solitary tubular structures because the accompanying hepatic arteries and bile ducts are too small to be resolved by ultrasound. When intrahepatic bile ducts dilate, two or more tubular structures can be identified in the expected location of the solitary portal veins. This alteration of anatomy, which occurs in virtually all patients with generalized intrahepatic bile duct dilatation, is best seen within the right hepatic lobe, where the dilated intrahepatic bile ducts accompany the divisions of the right portal vein.

The second sonographic feature of intrahepatic bile duct dilatation is irregularity of the walls of dilated bile ducts. Similar to changes seen on cholangiograms, progressive biliary dilatation is accompanied by an alteration in the course and caliber of bile ducts such that they become increasingly tortuous and irregular. In contrast, the walls of portal veins, even when dilated, remain smooth and gradually tapering.

In patients with moderate to marked intrahepatic biliary dilatation, a "stellate confluence" of tubular structures may be seen that has been likened to the spokes of a wheel. This finding, which is evident in approximately two thirds of patients, occurs at points of conversion of several large ducts.

The final distinguishing feature of dilated intrahepatic bile ducts is acoustic enhancement behind dilated ducts. This occurs in approximately 55%–60% of cases and is usually not seen behind portal veins. Acoustic enhancement is visible in association with biliary structures because bile does not attenuate the sound beam. Blood, in contrast, because of its high protein content, dramatically attenuates the acoustic beam.[36]

### Pitfalls in Imaging of the Intrahepatic Bile Ducts

Although the finding of dilated intrahepatic bile ducts is specific for active biliary obstruction, it is not highly sensitive because up to 23% of patients with biliary obstruction have normal-sized intrahepatic bile ducts.[37] In a study by Sample et al.,[37] neither the degree of hyperbilirubinemia nor the duration of jaundice bore any relation to the presence or absence of intrahepatic biliary dilatation. Although false negative diagnoses are common, false positive diagnoses are distinctly unusual. They may be made, however, in patients with abnormally large hepatic arteries, in which case the dilated intrahepatic arteries mimic di-

lated intrahepatic bile ducts.[38] This situation occurs most often in patients with severe cirrhosis and portal hypertension. Pseudodilated intrahepatic bile ducts can usually be distinguished from truly dilated bile ducts because in the former, the extrahepatic hepatic artery is large (while the common bile duct is normal in size). The changes are manifest primarily in the left hepatic lobe, and there is evidence of portal hypertension (recanalized umbilical vein, varices, splenomegaly, ascites).

### Extrahepatic Bile Ducts

#### Normal Anatomy

The most easily visualized portion of the extrahepatic ductal system is the common hepatic duct, which results from the union of the right and left hepatic bile ducts. This structure, which is present in the porta hepatis, is visible in virtually all patients regardless of body size or habitus. The anatomic position of the common hepatic duct is constant, and it can be readily detected as it crosses anterior to the undivided right portal vein. At this level, the right hepatic artery is usually visible in cross section between the posterior portal vein and anterior bile ducts. As the common hepatic duct leaves the porta hepatis, it joins the cystic duct (the specific point of union is not usually visible on ultrasound) and forms the common bile duct (CBD). The CBD descends within the hepatoduodenal ligament in a fixed but somewhat confusing anatomic relationship with two other tubular structures, the main portal vein and the proper hepatic artery. Critical for recognizing and distinguishing these three tubular structures is understanding that there is a fixed and reproducible anatomic relationship between them. Proximally within the hepatoduodenal ligament, the portal vein is posterior, while the bile duct is anterior and somewhat laterally positioned (on the same side as the gallbladder). The proper hepatic artery is anteriorly and medially positioned (on the same side as the aorta) relative to the portal vein.

As these three structures descend within the hepatoduodenal ligament, their anatomic relationship changes in accordance with their sites of termination. Because the CBD terminates in the retroperitoneally located second duodenum, as it descends it courses posteriorly. The portal vein descends in a relatively anterior direction to form the splenic and superior mesenteric veins. The third component of this tubular triad, the proper hepatic artery, remains anterior as it gives off the gastroduodenal artery which enters the anterior aspect of the pancreatic head. Proper identification of these similar-appearing but very differently functioning anatomic structures is crucial for correctly analyzing the extrahepatic biliary tree.

The size of the extrahepatic bile duct is the most sensitive means of distinguishing medical from surgical jaundice. Normally, the diameter of the common hepatic duct or CBD is 5 mm or less, with 6–7 mm considered equivocal, and 8 mm or greater considered dilated.[37] These values are somewhat smaller than corresponding ductal measurements made during radiographic procedures such as transhepatic cholangiography, intravenous cholangiography, or endoscopic retrograde cholangiopancreatography, because the ultrasonograms do not include the effects of radiographic magnification or contrast agents.

The size of the common hepatic duct or CBD may be somewhat larger in patients who have undergone previous biliary surgery. Postoperatively, the common hepatic duct may measure up to 10 mm in diameter.[39] Unless baseline postoperative scans are obtained, however, a single measurement of 10 mm should be followed with sequential scans and liver function tests in order to evaluate the possibility of early obstruction. If a symptomatic postoperative patient has a large or equivocal duct measurement (by nonoperated size criteria), further evaluation should also be undertaken.

*Scanning Techniques*

The CBD is most commonly examined by means of parasagittal scans obtained with the patient in a supine left posterior oblique (LPO) position. This approach is based on the widely cited 1978 article by Behan and Kazam.[40] Although scans obtained by this method are acceptable for evaluating the common hepatic duct or proximal CBD, they are frequently suboptimal for visualizing the distal CBD, the most common site of biliary obstruction. Because the duodenum often contains gas when the patient is supine or in an LPO position, the distal bile duct is usually obscured as it passes behind this gas-filled bowel loop. A superior scanning method is to examine the proximal and distal portions of the CBD separately.

Initially, the distal duct should be examined. This is most satisfactorily accomplished by performing scans with the patient in an erect RPO position and by relying on transverse rather than parasagittal scans.[41] The erect RPO position minimizes gas in the antrum and duodenum, while the transverse scan plane maximizes one's ability to trace the course of the intrapancreatic distal bile duct. If overlying bowel gas obscures this region, the patient should be given 16 ounces of water to drink, placed into a right lateral decubitus position for 2–3 minutes, and rescanned in the erect (RPO) position.

Although the proximal CBD can also be evaluated in this position, it is usually seen to better advantage after the patient has been repositioned in the conventional supine LPO position, and on parasagittal scans.[40] In most patients examination of the proximal and distal bile ducts can be completed in 5–10 minutes. In difficult cases, the study may take as long as 15–30 minutes.

*Extrahepatic Bile Duct Pathology*

As a screening modality, the primary function of ultrasound is to determine whether or not biliary obstruction is present. A secondary function is to determine the level and cause of obstruction.

### DIAGNOSING OBSTRUCTION

Because bile ducts expand centrifugally from the point of obstruction, extrahepatic dilatation occurs before intrahepatic dilatation.[42] It is not unusual, therefore, to see isolated or disparate dilatation of the extrahepatic duct in patients with obstructive jaundice. There are two possible explanations for this phenomenon. The first invokes La Place's law, according to which expansion of a fluid-containing structure is proportional to its diameter. Since the gallbladder and CBD have the largest diameters in the biliary system, they preferentially dilate after an obstruction.[42] The second explanation for disparate dilatation is that in patients with fibrosed or infiltrated livers, intrahepatic dilatation cannot readily occur due to lack of compliance of the hepatic parenchyma. Because intrahepatic bile ducts may not always dilate in patients with surgical jaundice, most authorities consider the diameter of the common hepatic duct as the most sensitive indicator for diagnosing biliary obstruction.

Although the reported upper limit of size for the diameter of the common hepatic duct varies from 4 mm[43] to 8 mm,[40] our laboratory accepts as normal a diameter of 5 mm or less, with 6–7 mm considered equivocal and 8 mm or greater considered dilated, based on nosologic probabilities reported by Sample et al.[37]

**Level and Cause of Obstruction.**—Localizing the anatomic site and cause of biliary obstruction is important for determining what other examinations, if any, should be performed for further diagnostic evaluation. This information may also be useful for determining whether further procedures are necessary, such as surgery, endoscopy, or percutaneous drainage. In cases of biliary obstruction, the ultrasonographer should attempt to place the level of obstruction at one of three sites: the intrapancreatic common duct, the suprapancreatic common duct, or the porta hepatis.

Published figures on the ability of ultrasound to display the level and suggest the cause of obstruction vary dramatically. At one extreme are the reports of Haubek et al.[44] and Koenigsberg et al.,[45] who reported the correct level of obstruction in 94% and 95% of cases, respectively, and diagnosed the precise cause of obstruction in 68% and 81% of cases, respectively. At the opposite extreme is the recent report of Honickman et al.,[46] who predicted the correct level of obstruction in only 27% of cases and the correct cause in only 25% of cases. Although one can only speculate as to the reasons for these discrepancies, they most likely relate to variations in equipment, scanning technique, and interpretation of the terms "level" and "cause" of obstruction. If high-resolution sector equipment is used for examining the gallbladder and biliary tree, and if newer scanning techniques are used for evaluating the distal CBD, the sensitivity and accuracy for assessing the level and cause of obstruction will be maximized.

**Intrapancreatic Obstruction.**—The most common site of biliary obstruction is distal, at the level of the pancreatic head. In these patients the extrahepatic bile duct should be dilated throughout its course. Depending on the severity and duration of the obstruction, the intrahepatic bile ducts may or may not be dilated. Tumor, calculi, and inflammatory strictures commonly cause distal CBD obstruction.

In a technically adequate examination, solid masses larger than 2½ cm in diameter should be visible. Because of their anatomic location within the head and/or uncinate process, the pancreatic duct is frequently obstructed and dilated. Although masses smaller than 2.5 cm in diameter are often not visible,

their presence may be inferred if a double duct sign is present. Neoplasm and focal pancreatitis may be indistinguishable unless secondary findings such as adenopathy or distant metastases are visible.

When optimal scanning techniques are used, distal CBD calculi can now be visualized in approximately 70% of patients.[41] They are most often located at the level of the ampulla and are best seen on transverse, RPO erect scans performed over this region. As with gallstones, acoustic shadowing is almost always present. Although choledocholithiasis may be detected in a normal-sized bile duct, calculi are more readily identified in a dilated system. Not surprisingly, ultrasound's sensitivity for diagnosing choledocholithiasis diminishes dramatically if the region over the head of the pancreas is obscured by overlying bowel gas or obesity.

Strictures, the third most common cause of distal obstruction, are a problem for sonography in that the precise etiology for obstruction is not apparent. Nonetheless, after ultrasound indicates a distal site of obstruction, endoscopic retrograde cholangiopancreatography can be performed for precise diagnosis.

**Suprapancreatic Obstruction.**—Suprapancreatic obstruction is defined as obstruction that originates between the pancreas and porta hepatis. Sonographically, the head of the pancreas is normal, as are the diameters of the intrapancreatic bile duct and pancreatic duct. Malignancy (both primary and secondary) is the most common cause of these obstructions. Ultrasound may reveal a mass or adenopathy at this level. Rarely, a mass may be visible within the intraluminal portion of the duct. Although calculi and inflammatory strictures can also cause suprapancreatic obstruction, they do not commonly do so.

**Porta Hepatis Obstruction.**—Obstruction at the level of the porta hepatis is also usually due to neoplasm, either primary or secondary. In these cases, sonography discloses intrahepatic ductal dilatation and a normal-sized CBD. The gallbladder may or may not be obstructed, depending on the level of the lesion relative to the position of the cystic duct. In patients with secondary neoplasms, adenopathy is often present in the region of the porta hepatis. In patients with cholangiocarcinoma, the neoplastic portion of the bile duct can be visualized in approximately 75% of cases.[47] These ducts may be narrowed, normal-sized, or enlarged and may contain intraluminal soft tissue echoes or echogenic bands across their lumens. Occasionally, pathology may involve the right or left ductal systems separately. In these instances only one side of the biliary system will be dilated, while the other side and CBD will be normal. The level of obstruction will be easy to localize when the above ultrasound findings are present.

### Pitfalls in Imaging of the Extrahepatic Bile Ducts

To maximize the use of ultrasound in evaluating the extrahepatic duct, sonographers must have a clear understanding of the problems and pitfalls pertaining to examining the CBD.

#### ANATOMIC PROBLEMS

Variations in the course of the extrahepatic bile duct can occasionally occur. In approximately 20% of patients with CBD dilatation, the course of the duct is more transverse than vertical.[48] In these cases the sonogram can be confusing with respect to distinguishing the bile duct from the oblique to horizontal courses of the portal and splenic veins. Variations in the course of the CBD can also occur in the presence of a pancreatic mass, particularly within the uncinate process. This may result in anterior elevation of the distal duct, such that it mimics the course of the gastroduodenal artery. In addition, patients who have undergone biliary surgery may have anatomic deviations in the position of the extrahepatic bile ducts.

In approximately 8% of patients, redundancy, elongation, or folding of the gallbladder neck on itself can each cause a pattern that mimics dilatation of either the common hepatic duct or proximal CBD.[49] To avoid misinterpreting a redundant or elongated gallbladder neck for a dilated CBD, real-time equipment is essential. Emphasis should be placed on scanning the region of the gallbladder neck in an effort to note redundancy. The CBD can usually be located by angling the transducer along its expected course, just medial to the gallbladder neck.

Variations in the anatomic position of the hepatic artery, which occur in approximately 30% of patients, can also cause diagnostic problems.[50] Because the diameters of both the aberrant artery and duct are usually small, in most circumstances it is not necessary to determine which structure is the duct and which is the artery. A problem may develop, however, if the hepatic artery (aberrant or normally positioned) dilates and becomes larger in diameter than the CBD.

This has been reported to occur in 59% of cases and may result in the hepatic artery being mistaken for an enlarged CBD.[50]

Sonographic signs that may be helpful in definitively recognizing the hepatic artery include arterial pulsations, an arterial indentation or displacement of adjacent structures, and tortuosity, which frequently accompanies hepatic artery enlargement. Although tracing their respective anatomic courses is an obvious way to distinguish the CBD from the hepatic artery, this is not always technically possible. The combined use of pulsed Doppler and real-time sonography has also been suggested as a method for discriminating the artery from the duct.[50] Deep Doppler examination is not widely available, however, nor is it technically easy to position this equipment over relatively small structures which rapidly change position with respiration.

#### SIZE PROBLEMS

Although enlargement of the extrahepatic duct is the most sensitive indicator of biliary obstruction, there are discrepant reports in the literature as to the maximal diameter of the normal-sized CBD. Measurements as small as 4 mm[43] and as large as 8 mm[40] have been reported. The literature is similarly unclear as to whether or not the CBD dilates after cholecystectomy. Articles can be found which both support[43, 51] and refute[39, 52] the claim that CBD dilatation occurs after cholecystectomy.

It is generally accepted that the diameter of the CBD is normally slightly greater in its distal than proximal portion. In most patients this size discrepancy is barely perceptible, although occasionally the duct becomes funneled and the distal diameter is several millimeters wider than the proximal diameter. In this situation, if the duct is measured solely in the porta hepatis, it may be of normal caliber. When measured more distally, it may be borderline or even frankly enlarged. The significance of the funneled appearance is that it may indicate early extrahepatic bile duct obstruction. This finding is nonspecific, however, because a similar appearance may be seen in patients whose obstruction has been relieved.

Recently, it has been suggested that biliary dynamics can be assessed in patients with borderline or mild dilatation by repeating the scan after administering a fatty meal.[53] In normal cases, the common hepatic duct remains the same or decreases in caliber, while in abnormal cases an initially normal duct increases in size, and a slightly dilated duct remains the same or increases in size. Although this provocative test can be useful, the authors considered a 1-mm change in duct caliber significant. Because it may be difficult to measure the duct at precisely the same point before and after fat administration, the significance of a small change becomes difficult to interpret. Furthermore, in our laboratory, many critically ill patients fail to show any biliary response following the administration of either oral fat (Lipomul) or intravenous cholecystokinin (sincalide). Because gallbladder contraction fails to occur, the test loses its validity in these patients.

Although ultrasound can distinguish medical from surgical jaundice in more than 90% of cases, occasionally atypical cases will be encountered. Infrequently, dilatation of the biliary tree can occur without jaundice.[54, 55] In these patients, partial or incomplete biliary obstruction may be present, or only one hepatic duct may be dilated. Rarely, complete obstruction can occur with a significant time delay from the onset of obstruction to the development of clinical signs. In patients with anicteric dilatation, the ultrasound findings and the serum alkaline phosphatase level appear to be more sensitive than the serum bilirubin level for suggesting obstruction. Occasionally, anicteric dilatation of the extrahepatic bile duct may be seen in postcholecystectomy patients or in patients with prior obstruction who exhibit dilatation without obstruction.

The converse situation can also occur. A patient with obstructive jaundice may fail to exhibit dilatation of either the intrahepatic or extrahepatic bile ducts.[37, 56] Cholangitis, partial obstruction, or intermittent obstruction from choledocholithiasis are usually responsible for these cases. Finally, an occasional patient may be encountered whose extrahepatic duct changes rapidly in size (over a period of several minutes to several days).[57, 58] These prominent fluctuations most likely relate to the elasticity and associated distensibility of the duct. Because of these dynamic changes, a patient with significant biliary symptomatology and a normal ultrasound study should have a repeat examination before one excludes obstruction.

Fortunately these cases are unusual. Nonetheless they serve to remind sonographers that although this imaging technique is highly sensitive and accurate, it is not perfect. Both false positive and false negative studies will occasionally be encountered.

DETECTING CHOLEDOCHOLITHIASIS

Until recently, the sonographic detection rate for choledocholithiasis was unacceptably low, in the range of 13%–55%.[59, 60] Improved equipment and scanning techniques currently allow approximately 75% of CBD stones to be visualized.[41] Although experienced sonographers can usually diagnose choledocholithiasis with confidence, there are several possible sources of confusion. Distally, a CBD stone may be mimicked by gas or particulate material in the adjacent duodenum. Transverse scanning with fluid in the duodenum can minimize this problem. Pancreatic calcification can also be confused with a distal calculus. Although careful transverse scanning over the distal duct can usually differentiate these two entities, CT or a radiographic contrast examination of the bile duct may be required for definitive diagnosis.

The sensitivity of ultrasound for detecting calculi in the proximal CBD approximates 90%.[41] Despite this high sensitivity, there are multiple pitfalls which can cause problems for the unwary. Sources of confusion include the right hepatic artery, postcholecystectomy surgical clips, the cystic duct, tortuosity of the duct, reverberation echoes, and air within the bile duct. Although these are potential sources of confusion, it must be emphasized that appropriate equipment and scanning technique, as well as familiarity with these causes of echogenic foci within the common duct, should minimize false positive diagnoses of choledocholithiasis.

*Acknowledgment*

The author wishes to express her appreciation to Mrs. Shirley Soucie for her outstanding assistance in preparation of this manuscript.

**References**

1. Callen PW, Filly RA: Ultrasonographic localization of the gallbladder. *Radiology* 1979; 133:687–691.

2. Worthen NJ, Uszler JM, Funamura JL: Cholecystitis: Prospective evaluation of sonography and $^{99m}$Tc-HIDA cholescintigraphy. *AJR* 1981; 137:973–978.

3. Sukov RJ, Sample WF, Sarti DA, et al: Cholecystosonography: The junctional fold. *Radiology* 1979; 133:435–436.

4. Hublitz UF, Kahn PC, Sell LA: Cholecysto-sonography: An approach to the nonvisual-ized gallbladder. *Radiology* 1972; 103: 645–649.

5. Cooperberg PL, Burhenne HJ: Real time ultraso-nography: Diagnostic technique of choice in cal-culus gallbladder disease. *N Engl J Med* 1980; 302:1277–1279.

6. Crade M, Taylor KJW, Rosenfield AT, et al: Sur-gical and pathologic correlation of cholecysto-sonography and cholecystography. *AJR* 1978; 131:227–229.

7. McIntosh DMF, Penney HF: Gray scale ultraso-nography as a screening procedure in the detec-tion of gallbladder disease. *Radiology* 1980; 136:725–727.

8. deGraaff CS, Dembner AG, Taylor KJW: Ultra-sound and false normal oral cholecystogram. *Arch Surg* 1978; 113:877–879.

9. Jeanty P, Ammann W, Cooperberg P, et al: Mo-bile intraluminal masses of the gallbladder. *J Ul-trasound Med* 1983; 2:65–71.

10. Fakhry J: Sonography of tumefactive biliary sludge. *AJR* 1982; 139:717–719.

11. Laing FC, Gooding GAW, Herzog KA: Gallstones preventing ultrasonographic visualization of the gallbladder. *Gastrointest Radiol* 1977; 1:301–303.

12. Raptopoulos V, D'Orsi C, Smith E, et al: Dy-namic cholecystosonography of the contracted gallbladder: The double-arc-shadow sign. *AJR* 1982; 138:275–278.

13. Kane RA, Jacobs R, Katz J, et al: Porcelain gall-bladder: Ultrasound and CT appearance. *Radiol-ogy* 1984; 152:137–141.

14. Hunter ND, Macintosh PK: Acute emphysema-tous cholecystitis: An ultrasonic diagnosis. *AJR* 1980; 134:592–593.

15. Parulekar SG: Sonographic findings in acute em-physematous cholecystitis. *Radiology* 1982; 145:117–119.

16. Laing FC, Federle MP, Jeffrey RB, et al: Ultra-sonic evaluation of patients with acute right up-per quadrant pain. *Radiology* 1981; 140:449–455.

17. Sanders RC: The significance of sonographic gallbladder wall thickening. *JCU* 1980; 8:143–146.

18. Shlaer WJ, Leopold GR, Scheible FW: Sonogra-phy of the thickened gallbladder wall: A nonspe-cific finding. *AJR* 1981; 136:337–339.

19. Ralls PW, Quinn MF, Juttner HU, et al: Gall-bladder wall thickening: Patients without intrin-sic gallbladder disease. *AJR* 1981; 137: 65–68.

20. Weiner SN, Koenigsberg M, Morehouse H, et al: Sonography and computed tomography in the di-agnosis of carcinoma of the gallbladder. *AJR* 1984; 142:735–739.

21. Raghavendra BN, Subramanyam BR, Balthazar EJ, et al: Sonography of adenomyomatosis of the gallbladder: Radiologic-pathologic correlation. *Radiology* 1983; 146:747–752.

22. Jeffrey RB, Laing FC, Wong W, et al: Gangre-nous cholecystitis: Diagnosis by ultrasound. *Ra-diology* 1983; 148:219–221.

23. Filly RA, Allen B, Minton MJ, et al: In vitro inves-tigation of the origin of echoes within biliary sludge. *JCU* 1980; 8:193–200.

24. Nyberg DA, Laing FC: Ultrasonographic findings in peptic ulcer disease and pancreatitis that sim-ulate primary gallbladder disease. *J Ultrasound Med* 1983; 2:303–307.

25. Shuman WP, Mack LA, Rudd TG, et al: Evalua-tion of acute right upper quadrant pain: Sonogra-phy and $^{99m}$Tc-PIPIDA cholescintigraphy. *AJR* 1982; 139:61–64.

26. Weissmann HS, Frank MS, Bernstein LH, et al: Rapid and accurate diagnosis of acute cholecys-titis with $^{99m}$Tc-HIDA cholescintigraphy. *AJR* 1979; 132:523–528.

27. White M, Simeone JF, Muller PR: Imaging of cholecystocolic fistulas. *J Ultrasound Med* 1983; 2:181–185.

28. Gooding GAW: Food particles in the gallbladder mimic cholelithiasis in a patient with a cholecys-tojejunostomy. *JCU* 1981; 9:346–347.

29. Scheske GA, Cooperberg PL, Cohen MM, et al: Floating gallstones: The role of contrast material. *JCU* 1980; 8:227–231.

30. Rubaltelli L, Talenti E, Rizzatto G, et al: Gas-containing gallstones: Their influence on ultra-sound images. *JCU* 1984; 12:279–282.

31. Federle MP, Cello JP, Laing FC, et al: Recurrent pyogenic cholangitis in Asian immigrants. *Ra-diology* 1982; 143:151–156.

32. Reinig JW, Stanley JH: Sonographic hepatization of the gallbladder: A cause of nonvisualization of

the gallbladder by cholecystosonography. *JCU* 1984; 12:234–236.

33. Fiske CE, Filly RA: Pseudo-sludge: A spurious ultrasound appearance within the gallbladder. *Radiology* 1982; 144:631–632.

34. Laing FC, Kurtz AB: The importance of ultrasonic side-lobe artifacts. *Radiology* 1982; 145:763–768.

35. Laing FC, London LA, Filly RA: Ultrasonographic identification of dilated intrahepatic bile ducts and their differentiation from portal venous structures. *JCU* 1978; 6:90–94.

36. Filly RA, Sommer FG, Minton MJ: Characterization of biological fluids by ultrasound and computed tomography. *Radiology* 1980; 134:167–171.

37. Sample WF, Sarti DA, Goldstein LI, et al: Gray-scale ultrasonography of the jaundiced patient. *Radiology* 1978; 128:719–725.

38. Wing VW, Laing FC, Jeffrey RB, et al: Sonographic differentiation of enlarged hepatic arteries from dilated intrahepatic bile ducts. *AJR* (in press).

39. Graham MF, Cooperberg PL, Cohen MM, et al: The size of the normal common hepatic duct following cholecystectomy: An ultrasonographic study. *Radiology* 1980; 135:137–139.

40. Behan M, Kazam E: Sonography of the common bile duct: Value of the right anterior oblique view. *AJR* 1978; 130:701–709.

41. Laing FC, Jeffrey RB, Wing VW: Improved visualization of choledocholithiasis by sonography. *AJR* 1984; 143:949–952.

42. Shawker TH, Jones BL, Girton ME: Distal common bile duct obstruction: An experimental study in monkeys. *JCU* 1981; 9:77–82.

43. Niederau C, Muller J, Sonnenberg A, et al: Extrahepatic bile ducts in healthy subjects, in patients with cholelithiasis, and in postcholecystectomy patients: A prospective ultrasonic study. *JCU* 1983; 11:23–27.

44. Haubek A, Pedersen JH, Burcharth F, et al: Dynamic sonography in the evaluation of jaundice. *AJR* 1981; 136:1071–1074.

45. Koenigsberg M, Wiener SN, Walzer A: The accuracy of sonography in the differential diagnosis of obstructive jaundice: A comparison with cholangiography. *Radiology* 1979; 133:157–165.

46. Honickman SP, Mueller PR, Wittenberg J, et al: Ultrasound in obstructive jaundice: Prospective evaluation of site and cause. *Radiology* 1983; 147:511–515.

47. Subramanyam BR, Raghavendra BN, Balthazar EJ, et al: Ultrasonic features of cholangiocarcinoma. *J Ultrasound Med* 1984; 3:405–408.

48. Jacobson JB, Brodey PA: The transverse common duct. *AJR* 1981; 136:91–95.

49. Laing FC, Jeffrey RB: The pseudo-dilated common bile duct: Ultrasonographic appearance created by the gallbladder neck. *Radiology* 1980; 135:405–407.

50. Berland LL, Lawson TL, Foley WD: Porta hepatis: Sonographic discrimination of bile ducts from arteries with pulsed Doppler with new anatomic criteria. *AJR* 1982; 138:833–840.

51. Parulekar SG: Ultrasound evaluation of common bile duct size. *Radiology* 1979; 133:703–707.

52. Mueller PR, Ferrucci JT Jr, Simeone JF, et al: Postcholecystectomy bile duct dilatation: Myth or reality? *AJR* 1981; 136:355–358.

53. Simeone JF, Mueller PR, Ferrucci JT Jr, et al: Sonography of the bile ducts after a fatty meal: An aid in detection of obstruction. *Radiology* 1982; 143:211–215.

54. Weinstein BJ, Weinstein DP: Biliary tract dilatation in the nonjaundiced patient. *AJR* 1980; 134:899–906.

55. Zeman R, Taylor KJW, Burrell MI, et al: Ultrasound demonstration of anicteric dilatation of the biliary tree. *Radiology* 1980; 134:689–692.

56. Muhletaler CA, Gerlock AJ Jr, Fleischer AC, et al: Diagnosis of obstructive jaundice with nondilated bile ducts. *AJR* 1980; 134:1149–1152.

57. Glazer GM, Filly RA, Laing FC: Rapid change in caliber of the nonobstructed common duct. *Radiology* 1981; 140:161–162.

58. Mueller PR, Ferrucci JT Jr, Simeone JF, et al: Observations on the distensibility of the common bile duct. *Radiology* 1982; 142:467–472.

59. Cronan JJ, Mueller PR, Simeone JF, et al: Prospective diagnosis of choledocholithiasis. *Radiology* 1983; 146:467–469.

60. Laing FC, Jeffrey RB Jr: Choledocholithiasis and cystic duct obstruction: Difficult ultrasonographic diagnosis. *Radiology* 1983; 146:475–479.

## CASES

Dennis A. Sarti

### Normal Gallbladder

Ultrasound examination of the gall-bladder is performed following over-night fasting or fasting greater than 12 hours. Fasting allows normal disten-tion of the gallbladder with bile. This enhances ultrasonic visualization of the gallbladder. If the patient has re-cently eaten, the gallbladder will con-tract and often will not be seen on ul-trasound examinations. Inability to visualize it with ultrasound is indicative of gallbladder disease if the patient has been fasting. Therefore it is ex-tremely important to determine when the patient has last eaten before start-ing a gallbladder examination. It is common to find that a patient has re-cently eaten after he has initially indi-cated otherwise. It is most helpful to ask the patient if he swallowed some water when he brushed his teeth in the morning. If he answers no to this question, one can be fairly confident that he has not had anything to eat.

Examination of the gallbladder usu-ally begins with the patient in the su-pine position. With current real-time equipment, a gallbladder examination can be performed quickly and easily. Initially, supine transverse scans in the subcostal region on the right side are obtained. After the long axis of the gallbladder has been determined, oblique longitudinal scans following the long axis are obtained. It is ex-tremely important to scan more medi-ally than anticipated because this is where the cystic duct is positioned. Occasionally it is difficult to see a gall-bladder in the right subcostal region secondary to a high position of the liver. In these instances, right coronal intercostal scans are helpful in visual-izing a high gallbladder.

After the patient has been scanned in the supine position, he should be placed in a decubitus position with the right side up. When the patient is in a supine position, cystic duct stones will be dependent posteriorly. However, if the patient is turned to the decubitus position with the left side down, these stones will be displaced into the body

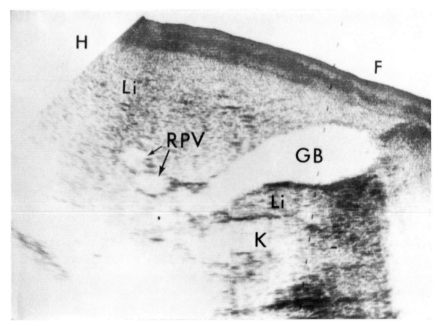

FIG 3–1.

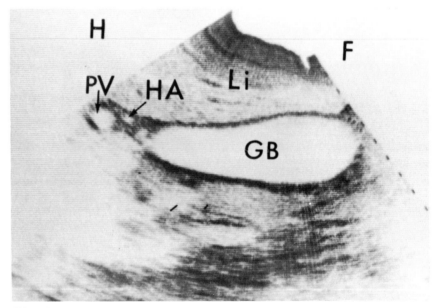

FIG 3–2.

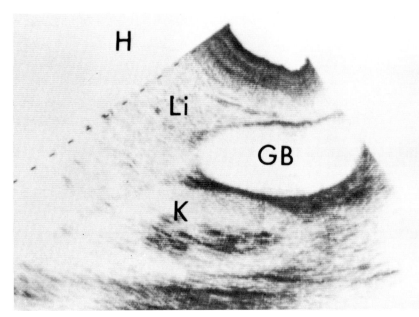

**FIG 3–3.**

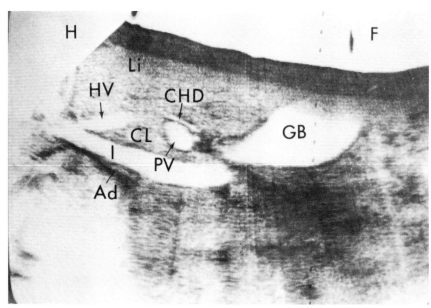

**FIG 3–4.**

and fundus of the gallbladder. Very often the gallbladder will be difficult to visualize when the patient is in the decubitus position. Difficulty of visualization is consequent on movement of the gallbladder across the midline anterior to the aorta and the inferior vena cava. One will often keep scanning in the right upper quadrant when the patient is in the decubitus position. The gallbladder is highly mobile and will often be seen in the midline and even in the left side of the abdomen.

Figures 3–1 through 3–4 are examples of longitudinal scans of the normal gallbladder. The gallbladder walls are fairly smooth, sharp, and not markedly thickened. Figure 3–1 demonstrates the gallbladder with liver parenchyma noted both anterior and posterior to the gallbladder. The characteristic pear shape of the gallbladder is seen anterior to the right kidney.

The gallbladder is easily recognizable in the right upper quadrant because of the sonolucent bile. Figure 3–2 is a longitudinal scan of the gallbladder with liver parenchyma again noted posteriorly. Very often, the right kidney can be seen through the gallbladder (Fig 3–3). This can facilitate examination of the right kidney. Figure 3–4 demonstrates a tubular structure anterior to the portal vein and representing the common hepatic duct. This structure often is visualized coursing over the portal vein before it joins with the cystic duct to form the common bile duct. Figure 3–4 also demonstrates echoes on the anterior wall of the fundal region of the gallbladder; they are secondary to the reverberation artifacts commonly seen in sonolucent masses on the anterior wall (see chapter 1).

| | | |
|---|---|---|
| **Ad** | = | Adrenal gland |
| **CHD** | = | Common hepatic duct |
| **CL** | = | Caudate lobe |
| **F** | = | Foot |
| **GB** | = | Gallbladder |
| **H** | = | Head |
| **HA** | = | Hepatic artery |
| **HV** | = | Hepatic vein |
| **I** | = | Inferior vena cava |
| **K** | = | Kidney |
| **Li** | = | Liver |
| **PV** | = | Portal vein |
| **RPV** | = | Right portal vein |

## Normal Gallbladder

Since the gallbladder is a fluid-filled structure, through-transmission is seen posterior to the gallbladder when liver parenchyma or kidney is visualized. This is present in Figure 3–5, in which the gallbladder is seen as the characteristic pear structure in the right upper quadrant with increased echogenicity present in the liver posterior to the gallbladder. On transverse scans the gallbladder appears as a circular or oval structure in the right upper quadrant. It is most often seen anterior to the right kidney, as in Figures 3–6 and 3–7. Figure 3–6 demonstrates the characteristic circular echo of the gallbladder in the right upper quadrant. The borders are sharp and distinct. The gallbladder can be used as an ultrasonic window for visualization of the right kidney.

Figure 3–7 demonstrates slight decreased visualization of the medial wall of the gallbladder secondary to overlying bowel gas. Since the duodenum is adjacent to the medial aspect of the gallbladder, this border may be indistinct or not seen, because it has become obscured by bowel air. Occasionally, the gallbladder may be in a slightly unusual position (Fig 3–8). Here the gallbladder is situated more laterally than usual. This scan may be misinterpreted as showing ascitic fluid in the hepatorenal angle.

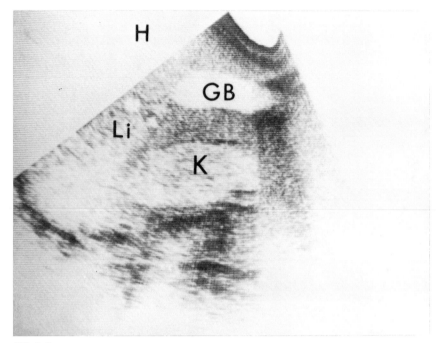

FIG 3–5

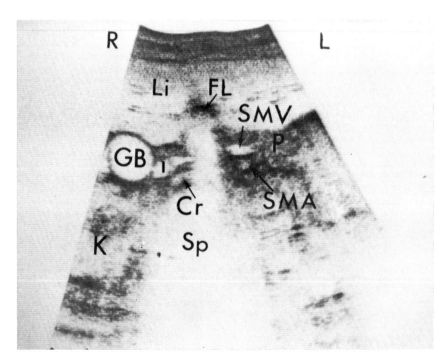

FIG 3–6.

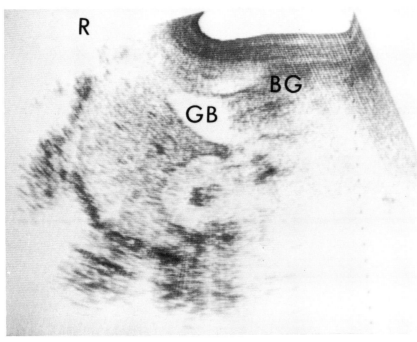

A   = Aorta
BG  = Bowel gas
Cr  = Crus of the diaphragm
FL  = Falciform ligament
GB  = Gallbladder
H   = Head
I   = Inferior vena cava
K   = Kidney
L   = Left
Li  = Liver
P   = Pancreas
PV  = Portal vein
R   = Right
SMA = Superior mesenteric artery
SMV = Superior mesenteric vein
Sp  = Spine

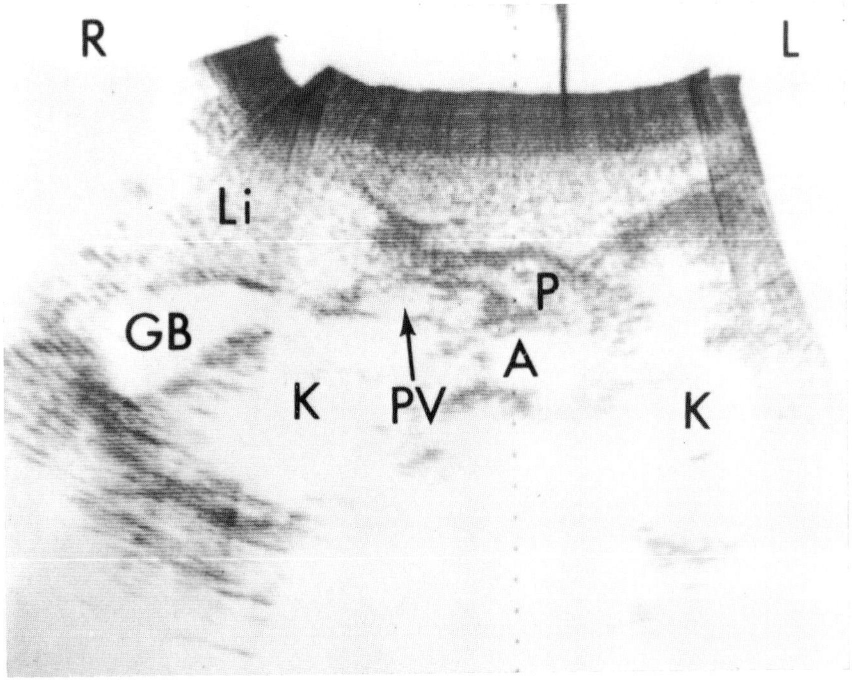

FIG 3–7.

FIG 3–8.

## Normal Variants

Occasionally the gallbladder can assume a rather unusual configuration that may be initially confusing. One anatomic variant that can give an unusual picture is a gallbladder that has a phrygian cap. Because of the unusual folding of the phrygian cap, it can be confused with several other entities, including a liver cyst, fluid around the gallbladder, abscess or hematoma, or perforation of the gallbladder. Occasionally fluid in the duodenum can give a similar appearance.

Figure 3–9 is a longitudinal scan of a gallbladder with a strongly anteroposterior orientation. The phrygian cap is situated quite superficially, near the skin. It is folded in a cephalad direction and could be mistaken for a liver cyst. However, its location and appearance will usually lead to the correct diagnosis.

Figure 3–10 is a longitudinal scan of a different patient. The gallbladder has a more normal orientation. Narrowing of the gallbladder near the fundus indicates the presence of a phrygian cap. The sharp echo of the phrygian cap is not as well seen in this scan as in the scan shown in Figure 3–9. The reason is that the phrygian cap is perpendicular to the ultrasonic beam in Figure 3–9, and since it is a specular reflector, it will be well seen. In Figure 3–10, however, the phrygian cap is markedly off the perpendicular and is not well seen. There is only a faint suggestion of an echo caused by the septum of the phrygian cap.

Figures 3–11 and 3–12 are longitudinal and transverse scans of the same patient. In Figure 3–12, a confusing ultrasound picture is present. Anterior to the gallbladder is a small sonolucent area that could be an abscess, a hematoma, or a liver cyst. The longitudinal scan in Figure 3–11 clarifies the image in Figure 3–12. One should always scan in two different planes before attempting a diagnosis. In this instance, Figure 3–11 reveals the anatomy correctly. The phrygian cap is well seen relative to the remainder of the gallbladder.

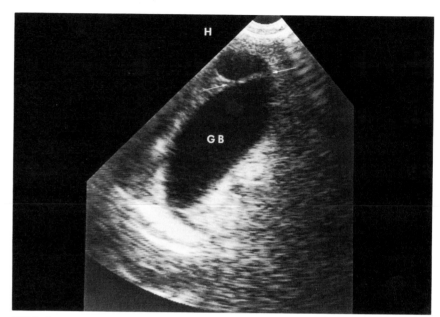

FIG 3–9.

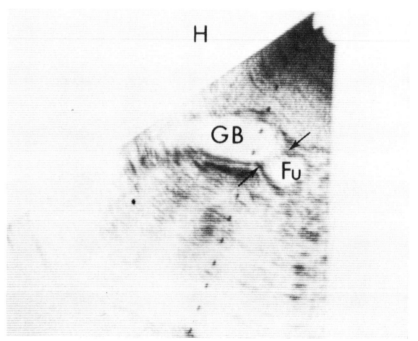

FIG 3–10.

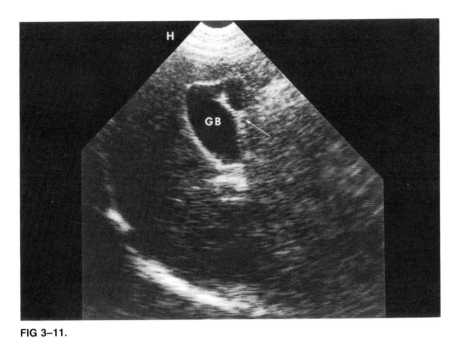

| **Arrows** | = | Phrygian cap |
| **Fu** | = | Fundus of the gallbladder |
| **GB** | = | Gallbladder |
| **H** | = | Toward head of patient |
| **R** | = | Right |

**FIG 3–11.**

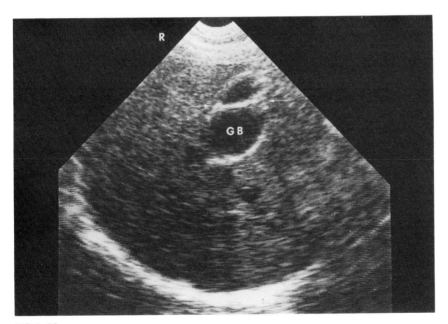

**FIG 3–12.**

## Normal Variants

Often the gallbladder is folded over on itself in an unusual position. The resulting ultrasonic picture can be confusing. Such a dilemma is usually clarified by scanning through the long axis of the gallbladder.

Figure 3–13 is a longitudinal oblique scan made through the long axis of the gallbladder. A common anatomic variant of the gallbladder, a junctional fold (arrowhead), is seen. The junctional fold usually represents folding of the gallbladder in its proximal portion. If the long axis of the gallbladder is not scanned correctly, the junctional fold may have the appearance of a liver cyst or dilated bile duct. Occasionally, shadowing will be associated with the junctional fold because of the critical angle phenomenon. In such instances, a stone will be mistakenly diagnosed. A junctional fold may also be mistaken for a gallbladder polyp. If the patient is turned into the decubitus position with the left side down, the gallbladder will unfold itself and lead to the correct diagnosis. Figure 3–14 is the scan of another patient with a smaller junctional fold (arrowhead). This is a longitudinal oblique scan made through the long axis of the gallbladder. The small linear echo in the proximal portion of the gallbladder is secondary to a junctional fold. It could be confused with a small calculus, especially if shadowing from critical angle were present. Having the patient take a deep inspiration or turn into the decubitus position will usually eliminate the junctional fold.

Figures 3–15 and 3–16 are oblique longitudinal scans of a different patient. In Figure 3–15, there is the suggestion of a dilated common bile duct, as indicated by the question mark. The dilated tubular structure is in the correct position for a dilated common bile duct. The circular region of the portal vein is seen slightly cephalad to this area. Inferior to the tubular structure is the gallbladder, folded on itself. However, meticulous scanning in Figure 3–16 shows the dilated tubular structure in continuity with the proximal portion of the gallbladder. The ar-

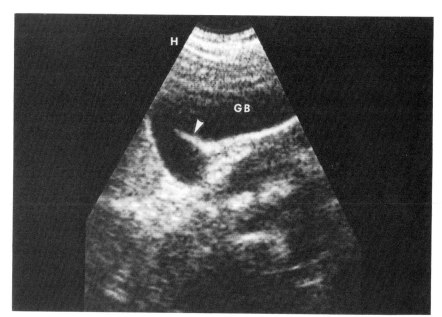

FIG 3–13.

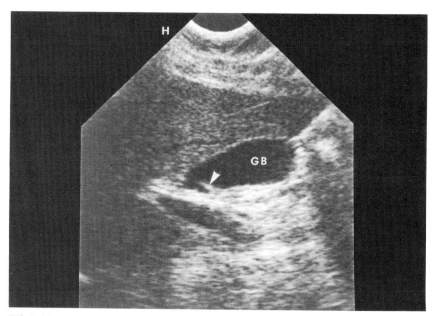

FIG 3–14.

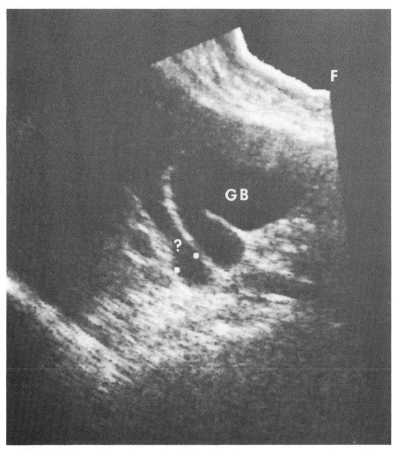

**FIG 3–15.**

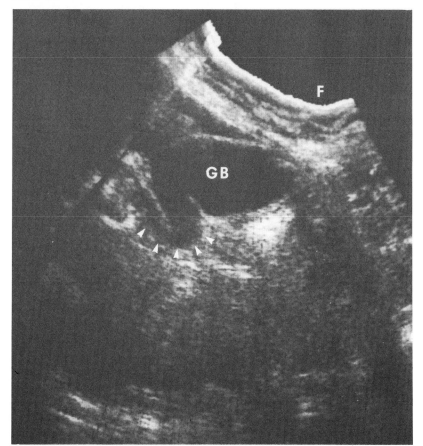

**FIG 3–16.**

rowheads indicate continuity of the proximal portion of the gallbladder with this tubular region. In reality, we are seeing not the common bile duct but rather a fold within the gallbladder. Often scanning along the long axis of the gallbladder will yield the correct anatomic relationship of such structures.

**Arrowhead** (Figs 3–13, 3–14)
    = Junctional fold
**Arrowheads** (Fig 3–16)
    = Continuity of the proximal portion
      of the gallbladder
**F**   = Foot
**GB**  = Gallbladder
**H**  = Toward head of patient
**?**  = Proximal portion of the gallbladder,
      not a dilated common bile duct

## Normal Variants

Junctional folds of the gallbladder are usually present with the fundus of the gallbladder reflected posteriorly and inferiorly. Figure 3–17 shows an unusual presentation of the gallbladder: the fundus is displaced anteriorly and superiorly. This would be a difficult examination unless a scan through the long axis of the gallbladder was obtained. Such a scan, shown in Figure 3–17, displays the anatomy of the gallbladder quite well, including the fundus, the body, and the proximal portion of the gallbladder.

Occasionally a mass is noted adjacent to the gallbladder. Such a mass could be secondary to numerous pathologic entities. However, several normal findings can also be present adjacent to the gallbladder. Fluid around the gallbladder may represent abscess, hematoma, or loculated fluid such as ascites or a pancreatic pseudocyst. However, whenever fluid is identified in the abdomen, a loop of fluid-filled bowel must be considered. Figure 3–18 is a longitudinal scan through the region of the gallbladder in which a fluid area is situated posterior to the gallbladder lumen. In this instance, fluid was present in the duodenum. Real-time studies demonstrate peristaltic activity, which confirms the diagnosis.

Figure 3–19 is a longitudinal scan made through the right upper quadrant in a patient who was supposedly fasting before the examination. The gallbladder cannot be identified. There is a region of acoustic shadowing (arrowhead) that is highly suggestive of a gallbladder filled with stones. The patient eventually admitted that he did have something to eat just before the examination. It is extremely important that the patient be thoroughly questioned when the gallbladder is not visualized on ultrasound. If the patient truly has not eaten for 16 hours and the gallbladder is not visualized, then gallbladder pathology can be diagnosed. However, an accurate history must be obtained. Because of the questionable history, another gallbladder examination with overnight fasting

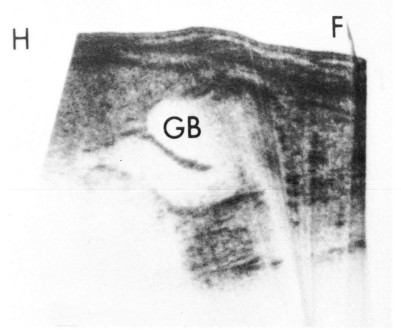

**FIG 3–17.**

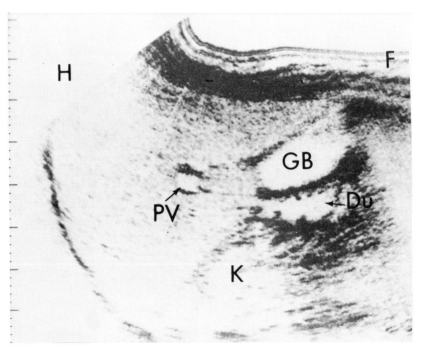

**FIG 3–18.**

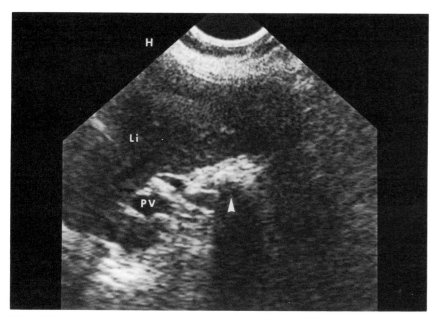

**FIG 3–19.**

was ordered. On this scan, shown in Figure 3–20, the gallbladder is now seen. It is long and narrow, but within normal range. No stones are evident within the gallbladder lumen. This is an excellent example of the difficulty that can arise when a gallbladder is not visualized because of a recently ingested meal. Careful clinical history of food intake is mandatory in such instances.

| | | |
|---|---|---|
| **Arrowhead** | = | Shadowing secondary to air in duodenum |
| **Du** | = | Fluid in the duodenum |
| **F** | = | Foot |
| **GB** | = | Gallbladder |
| **H** | = | Head |
| **K** | = | Kidney |
| **Li** | = | Liver |
| **PV** | = | Portal vein |

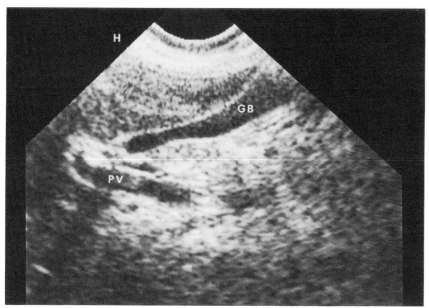

**FIG 3–20.**

## Cholelithiasis

The most common pathology of the gallbladder to be diagnosed by ultrasound is cholelithiasis. It characteristically presents as a strong echo within the sonolucent lumen of the gallbladder (Figs 3–21 and 3–22). The strong echogenicity of a gallstone is due to the marked acoustic mismatch between the stone and the bile. Posterior to the majority of the stones will be acoustic shadowing. This often aids in distinguishing between a gallstone and a polyp. Figures 3–21 and 3–22 are scans of a patient with multiple stones. Figure 3–21 demonstrates the numerous strong echoes consistent with cholelithiasis in the posterior aspect of the gallbladder.

When the gallbladder is well distended, visualization of the gallstones is quite easy. Often the gallbladder is not markedly distended in the presence of cholelithiasis, and so the diagnosis becomes more difficult. Figure 3–23 is an example of cholelithiasis with a somewhat smaller gallbladder. Because fluid is still present in the gallbladder, however, the gallstones stand out quite easily. Two gallstones are seen in Figure 3–23.

One of the more difficult areas for detection of a gallstone is near the cystic duct region of the gallbladder. Figure 3–24 shows a gallstone that casts a shadow in the cystic duct area. In all of the examples in this section (Figs 3–21 through 3–24), the gallbladder wall remains fairly sharp. Therefore, we cannot make a diagnosis of coincident cholecystitis based on these examinations.

Since the gallbladder is adjacent to the duodenum and hepatic flexure, we may have difficulty in visualizing a gallstone in the fundal region adjacent to the bowel gas. Fairly characteristic findings from bowel gas, however, may be present. Figure 3–21 is an example of bowel gas adjacent to the fundal region of the gallbladder. Behind the bowel gas echo are reverberation artifacts, along with ring down of the transducer (see chapter 1).

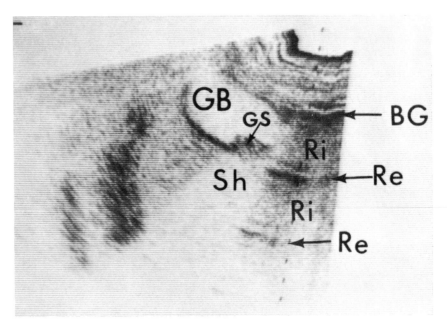

**FIG 3–21.**

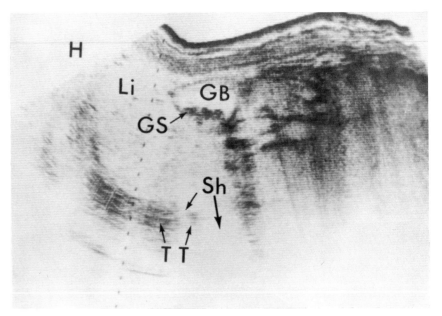

**FIG 3–22.**

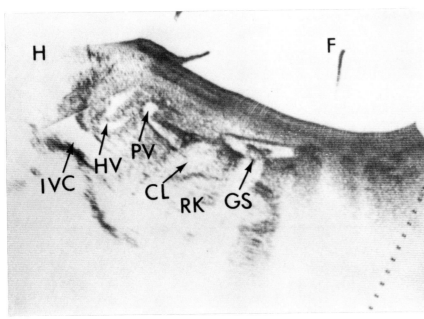

| BG | = | Bowel gas |
| CL | = | Caudate lobe |
| F | = | Foot |
| GB | = | Gallbladder |
| H | = | Head |
| HV | = | Hepatic vein |
| IVC | = | Inferior vena cava |
| Li | = | Liver |
| PV | = | Portal vein |
| Re | = | Reverberation |
| Ri | = | Ring down |
| RK | = | Right kidney |
| Sh | = | Shadowing |
| TT | = | Through-transmission |

FIG 3–23.

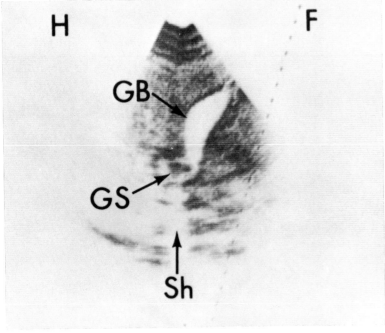

FIG 3–24.

## Cholelithiasis

An intraluminal echo within the gall-bladder is suggestive evidence of cholelithiasis. If acoustic shadowing is present, it confirms the diagnosis. However, acoustic shadowing cannot always be demonstrated when a gallstone is present. The diagnosis might also be suggested on the basis of a change in the internal echoes within the gallbladder lumen when the patient is scanned in a different position. Figures 3–25 and 3–26 are two scans of the same patient. Figure 3–25 is a longitudinal scan of the right upper quadrant made with the patient supine. The gallbladder is well visualized. A high-amplitude echo (arrowhead) on the back wall of the proximal portion of the gallbladder does not cast an acoustic shadow. Figure 3–26 is a scan made of the same patient in the erect position immediately after the scan in Figure 3–25. The gallbladder is again well visualized. The high-amplitude echo is now positioned near the inferior aspect of the gallbladder. The internal echo has moved with a change in the patient's position. Even though acoustic shadowing is not definitely seen on these scans, the diagnosis of a stone can usually be made with such a change in position. Real-time imaging is extremely helpful in this diagnosis. Stones change position quite rapidly. Occasionally very thick sludge balls up into a rounded echo. However, sludge changes position fairly slowly. This can be documented with real-time imaging.

Whether or not gallstones cast an acoustic shadow depends on several factors. The size of the stone is critical. If the stone is quite small, there can be no evidence of shadowing. In Figure 3–27, a longitudinal scan of the gallbladder, there is a small echogenic mass (arrow) on the posterior wall, suggestive of a gallstone. However, there is no evidence of acoustic shadowing. Since the stone is quite small, it may not be obstructing enough of the sound beam to yield an acoustic shadow. Most likely the transducer beam was slightly off center in relation to the gallstone. By min-

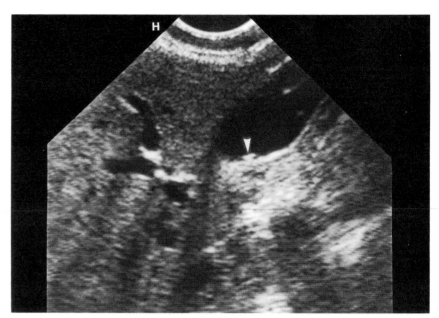

FIG 3–25.

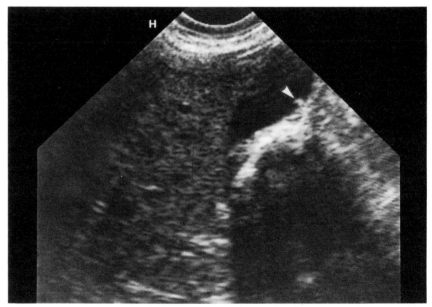

FIG 3–26.

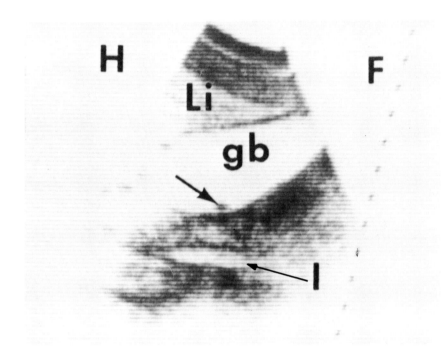

**FIG 3–27.**

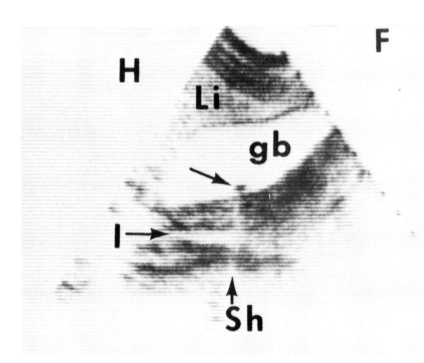

**FIG 3–28.**

utely altering the transducer path on longitudinal scans, the sonographer was able to demonstrate acoustic shadowing, as shown in Figure 3–28. Only a slight change in the position of the transducer was required to place the gallstone within the central portion of the beam.

Acoustic shadowing may also be absent if the gallstone is not in the focal zone. If the gallstone is close to the transducer or deep in the far field, acoustic shadowing may not be seen. If the stone is placed in the focal zone, acoustic shadowing can then be identified. Because of these factors, correct choice of the transducer is important in assisting in the diagnosis of gallstones.

SOURCE: Figure 3–25 is reproduced with permission from Sample WF: Diagnostic value and limitations in digestive disorders, in Berk JE (ed): *Developments in Digestive Diseases: Clinical Relevance.* Philadelphia, Lea & Febiger, 1977.

| **Arrow** | = Gallstone |
|---|---|
| **Arrowhead** | = Gallstone |
| **F** | = Foot |
| **gb** | = Gallbladder |
| **H** | = Head |
| **I** | = Inferior vena cava |
| **Li** | = Liver |
| **Sh** | = Shadowing |

## Cholelithiasis

Often gallstones are embedded in the proximal portion of the gallbladder adjacent to the cystic duct. This area is usually difficult to image with ultrasound. It is important to establish a habit of scanning the patient in a decubitus view with the left side down so that any stones will dislodge from the region of the cystic duct. When the patient's position is changed, the stones will go into a dependent portion near the fundus of the gallbladder where they will be more readily visible.

Figure 3–29 is a transverse scan of the gallbladder in which no definite stones are seen. There is a region of very high amplitude echoes (arrowhead) on the posterior wall of the gallbladder. No definite shadowing is seen deep to this area of increased echogenicity. Scanning was repeated with the patient almost prone (Fig 3–30). With the change in position, the high-amplitude echoes noted posteriorly have now been displaced into the gallbladder lumen. The multiple stones (arrowhead) are demonstrated within the gallbladder lumen as high-amplitude echoes. At surgery, multiple small stones were found. No acoustic shadowing is present because of the small size of the stones. This case is an excellent example of how the gallbladder wall may be lined with stones that are not visible when the patient is supine. With a change in the patient's position, these stones are displaced into the gallbladder lumen.

The scans shown in Figures 3–31 and 3–32 are from a 27-year-old woman with a 1-month history of right upper quadrant pain. This pain lasted for up to 2 hours and usually followed meals. There was no evidence of obstruction of the biliary tract and no chemical evidence of jaundice. Figure 3–31 is a longitudinal scan made with the patient supine. The gallbladder is well distended and is within normal limits for size. Any gallbladder diameter less than 5 cm is considered within normal limits. High-amplitude echoes are noted in the posterosuperior aspect of the gallbladder. The gallstones

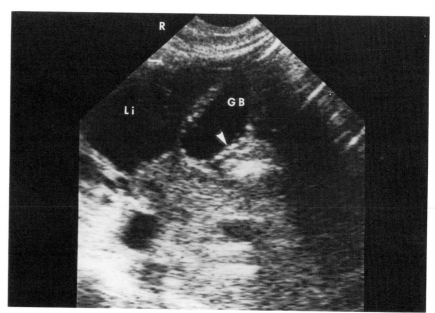

**FIG 3–29.**

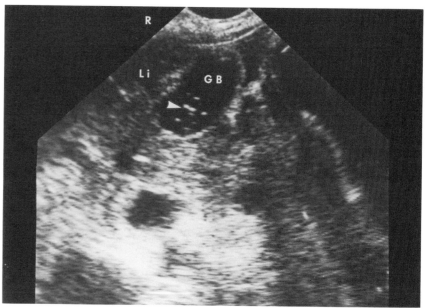

**FIG 3–30.**

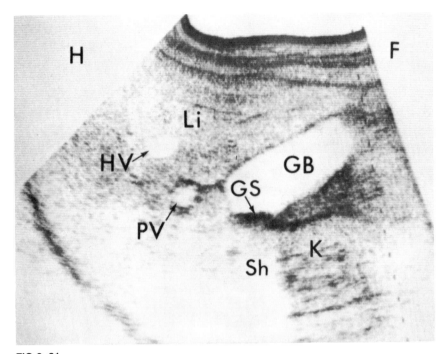

**FIG 3–31.**

are prominent enough to cause acoustic shadowing. When the patient was turned into a left-side-down decubitus position (Fig 3–32), the stones were displaced from the region of the cystic duct. They are now in the gallbladder lumen rather than lying posteriorly against the gallbladder wall, as in Figure 3–31.

If the sonographer routinely examines the gallbladder with the patient in the decubitus, prone, or upright position, cases such as the ones described above will always be correctly diagnosed. Small gallstones can layer posteriorly against the gallbladder wall and may be easily missed unless there is a change in the patient's position.

| | | |
|---|---|---|
| **Arrowhead** | = | Gallstones |
| **F** | = | Foot |
| **GB** | = | Gallbladder |
| **GS** | = | Gallstones |
| **H** | = | Head |
| **HV** | = | Hepatic vein |
| **K** | = | Kidney |
| **Li** | = | Liver |
| **PV** | = | Portal vein |
| **R** | = | Right |
| **Sh** | = | Shadowing |

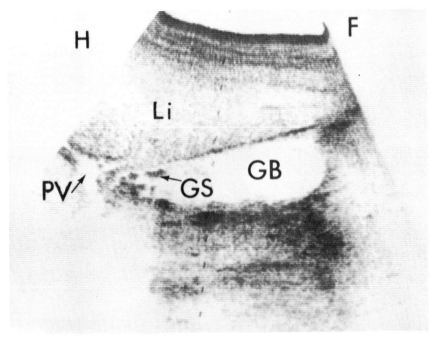

**FIG 3–32.**

## Cholelithiasis

Figure 3–33 is a transverse scan of a woman who was seen with acute right upper quadrant pain. Onset of pain occurred 2 hours after dinner on the evening before admission. She had no previous history of abdominal pathology. Figure 3–33 is a transverse oblique scan displaying the gallbladder and its proximal portion. A high-amplitude curvilinear echo is seen in the proximal portion of the gallbladder near the cystic duct. This echo represented a cystic duct stone lodged in the region. The patient was turned into a decubitus position, but the stone could not be displaced. The sharply curved surface of the gallstone led to the correct diagnosis.

Figure 3–34 is the scan of a different patient who reported acute right upper quadrant pain. Again, a high-amplitude echo accompanied by acoustic shadowing is seen in the proximal portion of the gallbladder near the cystic duct region. This scan is different in that the gallbladder wall is thickened. The diagnosis of cystic duct stone with accompanying acute cholecystitis was made because of the ultrasound findings.

Figures 3–35 and 3–36 are two scans of the same patient. Figure 3–35 was obtained with the patient supine. As in the previous two cases, a high-amplitude echo near the cystic duct area casts an acoustic shadow. A second high-amplitude echo is seen that does not cast an acoustic shadow. The patient was turned slightly into a decubitus position. Both stones were displaced into the body of the gallbladder (Fig 3–36), and both stones then had shadows. The reason for the lack of shadowing in Figure 3–35 is that the second stone was slightly off center with respect to the transducer beam. In Figure 3–36, both stones were within the central portion of the beam and therefore cast acoustic shadows. These cases demonstrate cystic duct stones that may be impacted in the cystic duct region. Turning the patient into the decubitus position will displace the stone in some instances but not in others.

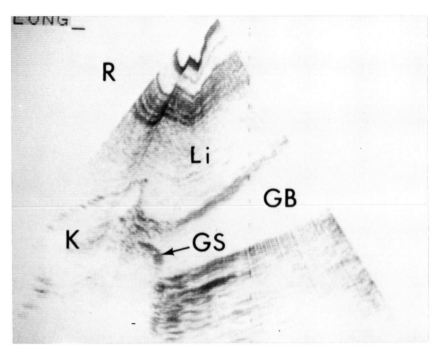

**FIG 3–33.**

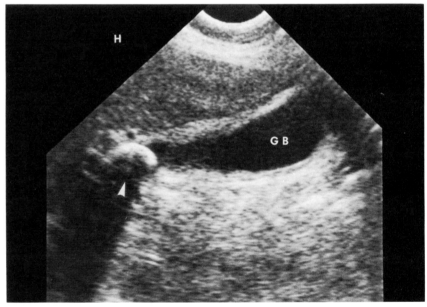

**FIG 3–34.**

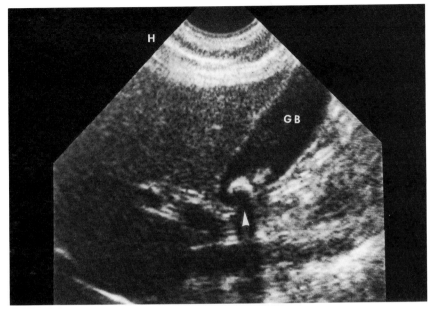

**FIG 3–35.**

| Arrowhead | = Shadowing |
|---|---|
| GB | = Gallbladder |
| GS | = Gallstone |
| H | = Head |
| K | = Kidney |
| Li | = Liver |
| R | = Right |

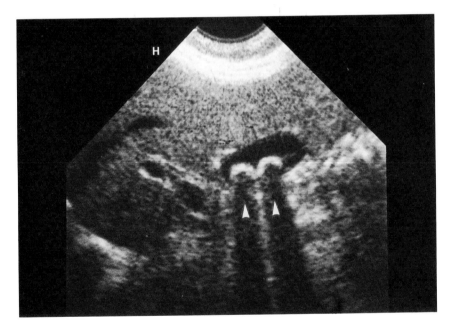

**FIG 3–36.**

## Cholelithiasis

Frequently, cholelithiasis will be present when there is no evidence of bile within the gallbladder. This is secondary to chronic inflammation of a gallbladder completely filled with stones. The case illustrated in Figures 3–37 and 3–38 is of a 64-year-old woman with chronic right upper quadrant pain. Ultrasound examination demonstrated a strong shadow in both the longitudinal and transverse sections. Figure 3–37 is a longitudinal scan in which the superficial border of the gallstones is seen as very highly reflective echoes. Behind the stones is a clear shadow. Figure 3–38 is a transverse scan of the gallbladder adjacent to the duodenum. Here we see a "dirty" appearance to the shadowing noted by the duodenum, whereas there is a "clean" shadow behind the gallstone. The superficial border of the gallstone is easily visible.

Figures 3–39 and 3–40 similarly show a gallbladder completely filled with gallstones. No fluid is evident within the gallbladder. The superficial borders of the gallstones are more clearly evident as a strong curvilinear echo. Again posterior to the gallstones is a clean shadowing area. It is important to recognize that a gallbladder filled with stones is not easily visualized and that the diagnosis of cholelithiasis can be easily misinterpreted as bowel gas in the area.

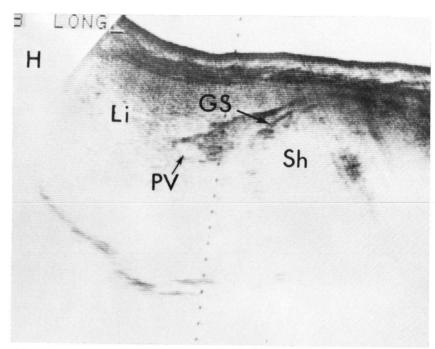

**FIG 3–37.**

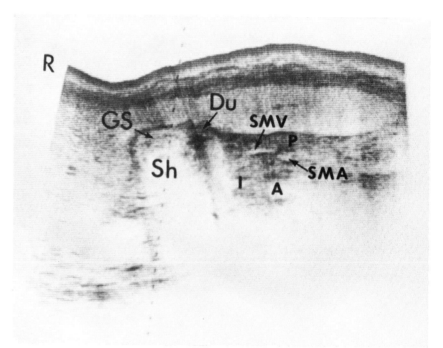

**FIG 3–38.**

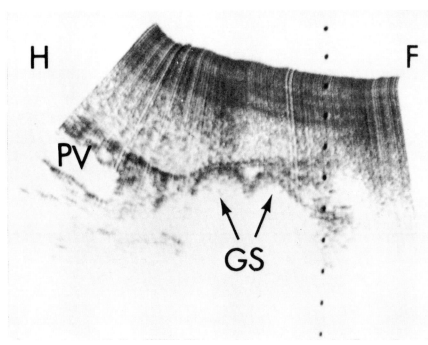

A = Aorta
Du = Duodenum
F = Foot
GS = Gallstones
H = Head
I = Inferior vena cava
K = Kidney
L = Left
Li = Liver
P = Pancreas
PV = Portal vein
R = Right
Sh = Shadowing
SMA = Superior mesenteric artery
SMV = Superior mesenteric vein

FIG 3–39.

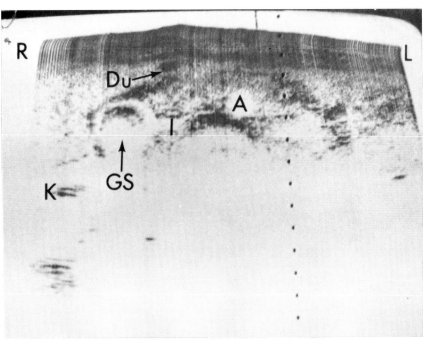

FIG 3–40.

## Cholelithiasis

The diagnosis of cholelithiasis often is extremely difficult to make, because it frequently is impossible to visualize the gallbladder, or even a large stone. Often, a gallstone will be present with a border that cannot be seen, and only the shadow from the stone itself will be visible. This usually will appear as a "clean" shadow, as opposed to the "dirty" shadow noted by the reflection from bowel air. Figures 3–41 and 3–42 are scans of a patient with a large shadow present in the right upper quadrant on ultrasound examination. The longitudinal scan in Figure 3–41 demonstrates the clear shadowing behind the gallstone, as opposed to the bowel air, which has a dirty shadow posteriorly. The border of the gallstone is very difficult to see because of its irregular surface. The transverse scan in Figure 3–42 again demonstrates the clean shadowing, obscuring visualization of the medial portion of the right kidney, as compared with the dirty shadowing present behind the duodenum.

Figure 3–43 illustrates another case in which clean shadowing appears behind a gallstone. This time there is a suggestion of visualization of the anterior border of the gallstone, but the important information here is the contrast between the echoes behind the duodenum, which are caused by ring down and reverberation, and the extremely clean shadow behind the gallstone.

Figure 3–44 is another example of clean shadowing seen behind a right upper quadrant gallstone. There is only slight suggestion of a curvilinear echo at the superficial border of the gallstone. Without this clean shadowing, the diagnosis easily would be missed. This right upper quadrant finding cannot be overemphasized since many gallbladders completely filled with gallstones will present in this manner.

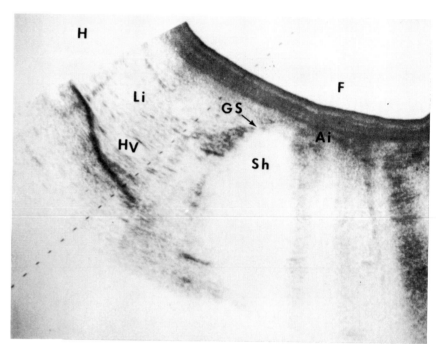

FIG 3–41.

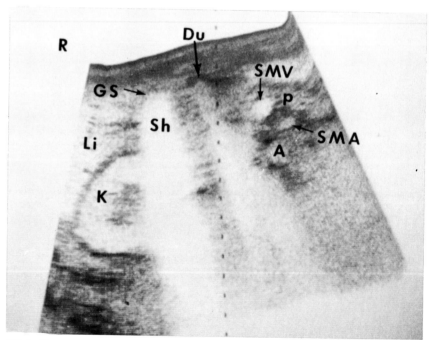

FIG 3–42.

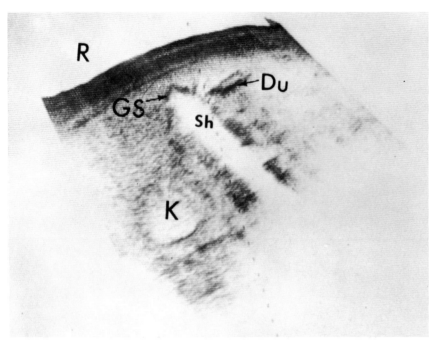

| A | = Aorta |
| Ai | = Air |
| Du | = Duodenum |
| F | = Foot |
| GS | = Gallstone |
| H | = Head |
| HV | = Hepatic vein |
| K | = Kidney |
| Li | = Liver |
| P | = Pancreas |
| R | = Right |
| Sh | = Shadowing |
| SMA | = Superior mesenteric artery |
| SMV | = Superior mesenteric vein |

FIG 3–43.

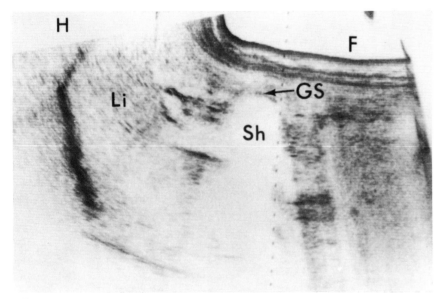

FIG 3–44.

## Biliary Sludge

Biliary sludge is a term that has come into the medical literature since the development of diagnostic ultrasound. Prior to diagnostic ultrasound, this entity was not visualized. Biliary sludge denotes the presence of particulate material suspended within bile. This particulate material is made up usually of either calcium bilirubinate or cholesterol crystals. The gallbladder is usually echo free, with evidence of internal echoes. However, in some instances a soft level of echoes can be detected on the posterior aspect of the gallbladder. This is not accompanied by acoustic shadowing. Usually biliary sludge is quite viscous and moves slowly when the patient is repositioned. This is easily documented with real-time equipment. The factor most frequently associated with biliary sludge is bile stasis. This occurs in patients who have undergone prolonged fasting, such as the postoperative patient. However, biliary sludge can occur in a normal individual and need not be of clinical significance.

Figure 3–45 is a transverse scan of the right upper quadrant of a patient. The gallbladder is seen as an oval sonolucent area with soft midlevel echoes on its dependent portion. The gallbladder is half-filled with biliary sludge. Note the fluid level present on the superficial surface of the sludge. This is common when the patient has been recumbent for a short period of time. There is no acoustic shadowing deep to the sludge. In some instances a small amount of sludge may be present; in other instances the entire gallbladder may be filled with sludge.

Figure 3–46 is a transverse scan of the same patient, who has been turned into a left-side-down decubitus position. The scan was obtained almost immediately after the patient was turned. The softly echogenic sludge remains on the posterior portion of the gallbladder. Approximately 20 seconds later, the sludge layered out into the dependent half of the gallbladder. This is a very typical appearance. The sludge moved slowly into the dependent portion once the patient's position was changed.

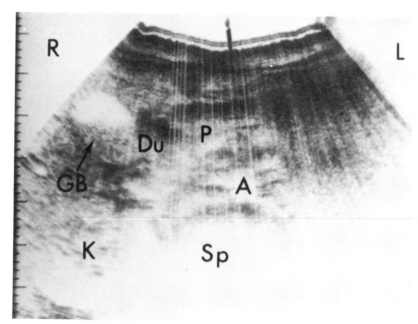

FIG 3–45.

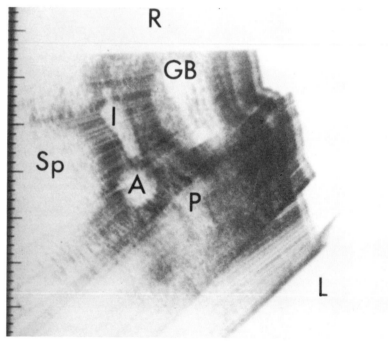

FIG 3–46.

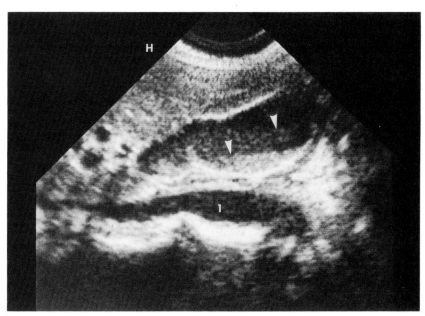

**FIG 3–47.**

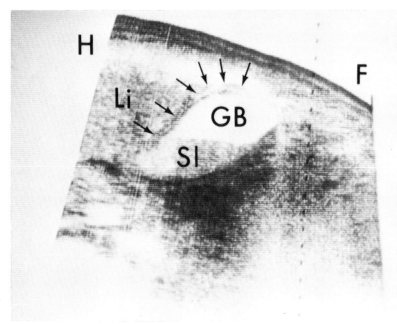

**FIG 3–48.**

Figure 3–47 is a longitudinal scan of the right upper quadrant, examining the gallbladder. Biliary sludge is seen in the dependent portion of the gall-bladder but has a rather unusual appearance. There are two fluid levels present (arrowheads). The most dependent fluid level has relatively highly echogenic sludge situated posteriorly. Superficial to this level is a second layer of slightly less echogenic sludge. Finally, on top of this layer is echo-free bilious material. Therefore, there are really three layers of fluid within this gallbladder. The most dependent layer has the highest concentration of crystalline material. As mentioned previously, biliary sludge is not necessarily indicative of a pathologic process. It is just a sign that stasis has occurred. Usually complete emptying of the gallbladder clears the patient of any biliary sludge. In this instance, the patient has biliary stasis secondary to metastatic disease causing obstruction of the biliary tree.

Figure 3–48 is a longitudinal scan of the right upper quadrant. Biliary sludge is noted on the dependent portion of the gallbladder. In this instance there is a pathologic entity present, as indicated by the lucent rim (arrows) around the gallbladder. The pathology is secondary to cholecystitis. If a pathologic condition is accompanied by bile stasis, biliary sludge will be identified on the posterior aspect of the gallbladder.

What is structure 1 in Figure 3–47?

| | | |
|---|---|---|
| **Arrows** | = | Thick gallbladder wall secondary to cholecystitis |
| **Arrowheads** | = | Biliary sludge layering |
| **A** | = | Aorta |
| **Du** | = | Duodenum |
| **F** | = | Foot |
| **GB** | = | Gallbladder |
| **H** | = | Head |
| **I** | = | Inferior vena cava |
| **K** | = | Kidney |
| **L** | = | Left |
| **Li** | = | Liver |
| **P** | = | Pancreas |
| **R** | = | Right |
| **Sl** | = | Sludge |
| **Sp** | = | Spine |
| **1** | = | Inferior vena cava |

## Biliary Sludge

Although biliary sludge is often visualized in normal patients, it may also be
associated with pathologic entities.
Very often biliary sludge will be present in the presence of cholelithiasis.
Figure 3–49 is a longitudinal scan of
the right upper quadrant in which a
single gallstone is identified as a high-
amplitude echo with acoustic shadowing deep to it. Some soft echoes are
present slightly inferior to the gallstone. These soft echoes do not have
any acoustic shadowing deep to them.
The findings indicate biliary sludge in
association with gallstone. Figure 3–
50 is a longitudinal scan of the right
upper quadrant of the same patient. In
Figure 3–50 the patient is upright, and
the scan was made almost immediately on change of position. The gallstone is now in an inferior position
and the biliary sludge is cephalad to it.
This is a common finding. The gallstones move quickly with a change in
position but sludge moves slowly.

Figure 3–51 is another example of
cholelithiasis accompanied by biliary
sludge. The soft echoes on the posterior aspect of the gallbladder are secondary to sludge, and the stronger
echo is secondary to a gallstone.
There is acoustic shadowing deep to
the gallstone but not behind the region
of biliary sludge.

Figure 3–52 is a transverse scan of
the right upper quadrant with visualization of the gallbladder partially filled
with echo-free fluid. Within the lateral
aspect of the gallbladder are numerous soft echoes in midrange. There is
a slightly irregular border between the
soft echoes and the fluid within the
gallbladder. Within the soft echoes,
which represent thickened sludge,
there is a high-amplitude echo casting
an acoustic shadow. This represents a
small gallstone, which is in an unusual
position within the biliary sludge. In
this instance the sludge is quite thick
and is not layering out, as usually
happens. The gallbladder wall is also
slightly thickened, compatible with the
diagnosis of cholecystitis. The patient
has cholecystitis, cholelithiasis, and
markedly thickened biliary sludge.

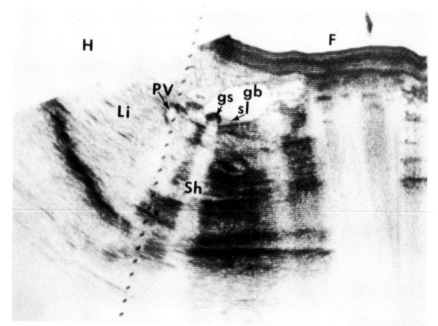

FIG 3–49.

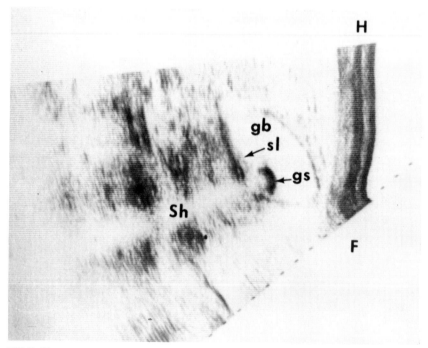

FIG 3–50.

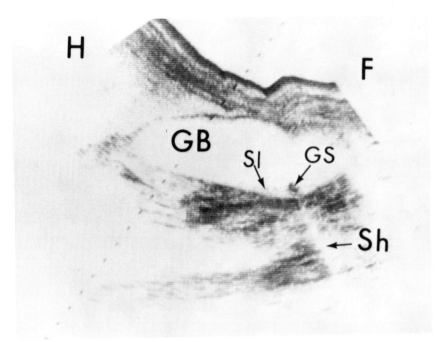

**FIG 3–51.**

| | | |
|---|---|---|
| **F** | = | Foot |
| **GB** | = | Gallbladder |
| **gb** | = | Gallbladder |
| **GS** | = | Gallstone |
| **gs** | = | Gallstone |
| **H** | = | Head |
| **Li** | = | Liver |
| **PV** | = | Portal vein |
| **R** | = | Right |
| **Sh** | = | Shadow to gallstone |
| **Sl** | = | Biliary sludge |
| **sl** | = | Biliary sludge |

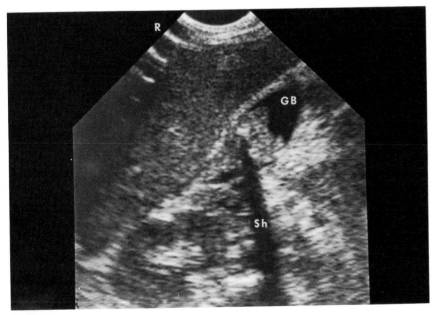

**FIG 3–52.**

## Gallbladder Polyps; Cholecystitis

Often, internal echoes not secondary to gallstones are noted within the gallbladder. Figure 3–53 is a scan of a patient who had a gallbladder polyp on OCG. There is an internal echo within the gallbladder. Several important features are present that help distinguish the polyp from a stone. First, the size of the polyp is approximately 8 mm. Most gallstones of this size will shadow. There is no shadow distal to the gallbladder polyp. This indicates that the polyp is composed of soft tissue. Furthermore, the polyp is notably adherent to the lateral gallbladder wall. If this were a stone, it would most likely be in the dependent portion of the gallbladder adjacent to the posterior wall. Most polyps will present as soft internal echoes within the gallbladder and without evidence of shadowing. By changing the patient's position, in an effort to cause the stone to drop into a dependent position in the gallbladder, the diagnosis of a gallstone can be made. If the internal echo does not fall into a posterior position, the diagnosis of a polyp is quite likely. If there also is a lack of shadowing, we are fairly safe in diagnosing a gallbladder polyp.

Also of interest is the manner in which the scan in Figure 3–53 was performed. We can see a small sector scan through an intercostal space, yielding a great deal of information. When we attempted to scan this patient anteriorly we were unable to visualize the gallbladder, because of overlying bowel air in the hepatic flexure.

Figure 3–54 is a longitudinal scan of the right upper quadrant in a 24-year-old patient who had intermittent right upper quadrant pain. The gallbladder is well visualized as a sonolucent oval region deep to liver parenchyma. Within the gallbladder lumen attached to the anterior wall is a circular soft tissue echogenic region. Acoustic shadowing is not present deep to the mass. This mass is large enough that acoustic shadowing would be expected if it represented a

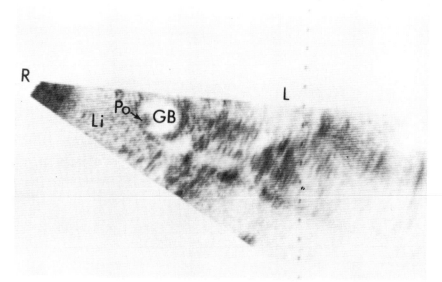

FIG 3–53.

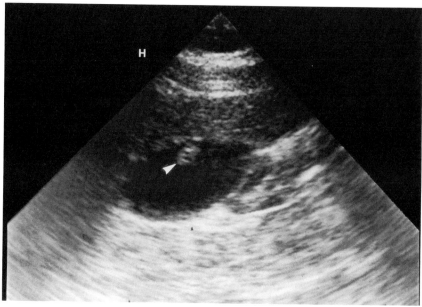

FIG 3–54.

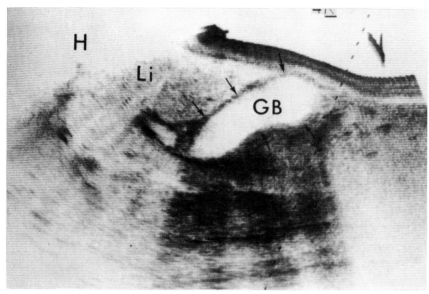

**FIG 3–55.**

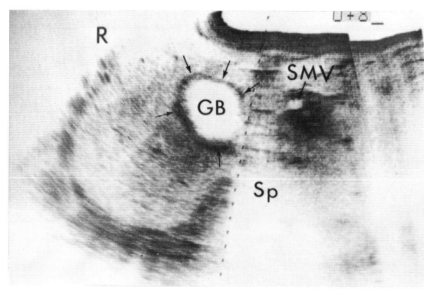

**FIG 3–56.**

gallstone. Therefore, the findings were most consistent with a gallbladder polyp. The soft tissue echogenic appearance, along with lack of acoustic shadowing, would be most consistent with a soft tissue lesion. Also, the mass adheres to the anterior wall. Because of continued pain, the patient was operated on and the diagnosis of cholesterolosis was made.

A gallbladder wall thickness up to 3 mm has been considered normal for ultrasound criteria. When the gallbladder wall is thicker than 3 mm, the possibility of pathology should be considered. It is imperative that the patient be fasting for more than 12 hours. If the patient has recently eaten, the gallbladder wall may appear thickened as a result of normal contraction. However, if the patient has fasted, gallbladder wall thickening is consistent with pathologic entities.

The most common pathologic entity is cholecystitis. In acute cholecystitis, an early finding is slight gallbladder thickening without evidence of a lucent rim. Figures 3–55 and 3–56 are longitudinal and transverse scans of a patient who had right upper quadrant pain. These scans demonstrate a fuzzy, thickened gallbladder wall (arrows). There is no lucent rim as is often seen in cholecystitis. However, the irregular gallbladder wall thickening is an early sign of cholecystitis. The examiner should gently press on the patient's abdomen over the region of the gallbladder. This will often elicit some pain and tenderness, which confirm the diagnosis.

| | |
|---|---|
| **Arrows** | = Thickened gallbladder wall consistent with cholecystitis |
| **Arrowheads** | = Gallbladder polyp |
| **GB** | = Gallbladder |
| **H** | = Head |
| **L** | = Left |
| **Li** | = Liver |
| **Po** | = Gallbladder polyp |
| **R** | = Right |
| **Sp** | = Spine |
| **SMV** | = Superior mesenteric vein |

## Cholecystitis

Figures 3–57 through 3–59 are scans obtained from the same patient but several weeks apart. The patient was a 20-year-old woman who had recently had a cesarean operation. One day after the operation, she experienced an episode of epigastric pain that shifted to the right upper quadrant. An ultrasound examination of the right upper quadrant was performed on the third postoperative day. Figure 3–57 is a transverse scan of the right upper quadrant. A high-amplitude echo with acoustic shadowing is seen in the proximal portion of the gallbladder. A diagnosis of cholelithiasis was made. At the time of this examination, the gallbladder wall is not thickened or lucent. The patient's right upper quadrant pain subsided and she was discharged from the hospital.

Approximately 3 weeks after the initial scan, the patient returned to the emergency room with an episode of acute right upper quadrant abdominal pain. Longitudinal and transverse scans were obtained, as shown in Figures 3–58 and 3–59. The appearance of the gallbladder wall has dramatically changed from the earlier scan shown in Figure 3–57. The gallbladder wall is now thickened (approximately 5 mm) and lucent (arrows). The changes are best seen on the anterior surface of the gallbladder, which is in contact with the liver. The dramatic change in wall thickness is compatible with acute cholecystitis. In Figure 3–59 there is a high-amplitude echogenic region medial to the gallbladder which is compatible with a cystic duct stone. The cystic duct stone was causing obstruction of the gallbladder.

At surgery the diagnosis of severe acute cholecystitis was made. The gallbladder wall measured approximately 4–5 mm in thickness. A 1.5-cm gallstone was found impacted in the cystic duct.

Figure 3–60 is a transverse scan of the right upper quadrant in a patient with chronic right upper quadrant pain. Although the patient had been fasting, the gallbladder was difficult to visual-

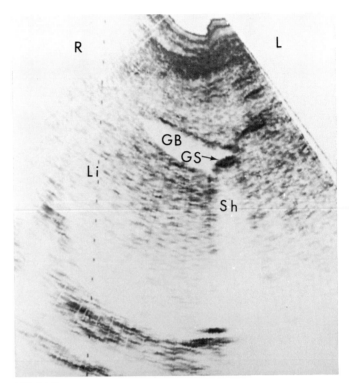

**FIG 3–57.**

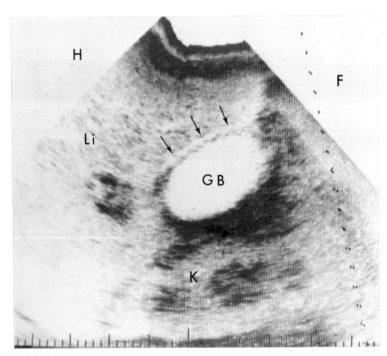

**FIG 3–58.**

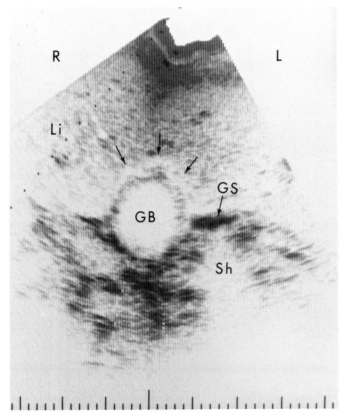

**FIG 3–59.**

ize on ultrasound. This often happens when the gallbladder is small and shrunken as a result of pathology. The scan shows the fairly characteristic appearance of a gallstone surrounded by a small shrunken gallbladder. The high-amplitude echo indicates a gallstone with acoustic shadowing deep to it. A lucent rim compatible with the gallbladder wall (arrows) completely surrounds the gallstone. This rim is often easy to miss during ultrasound examination. However, once the characteristic echo pattern has been identified, a diagnosis of cholelithiasis and cholecystitis can be made. Occasionally, the duodenum may have a similar appearance. An incorrect diagnosis can be avoided by having the patient drink water during the examination. The stomach and duodenum will show movement of water and air.

| Arrows | = Thickened gallbladder wall |
|--------|------------------------------|
| F | = Foot |
| GB | = Gallbladder |
| GS | = Gallstone |
| H | = Head |
| K | = Kidney |
| L | = Left |
| Li | = Liver |
| R | = Right |
| Sh | = Shadowing |

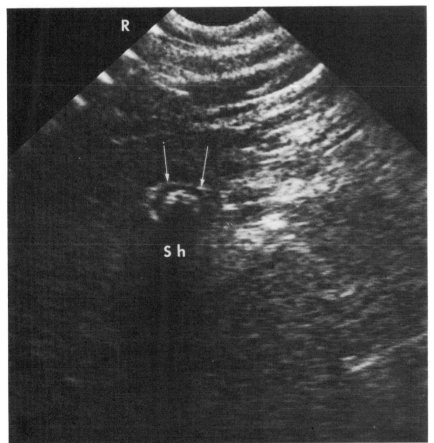

**FIG 3–60.**

## Cholecystitis

More severe forms of cholecystitis are illustrated in the two cases reviewed here. Figures 3–61 and 3–62 are scans obtained from a 34-year-old alcoholic with cirrhosis and right upper quadrant pain. Figure 3–61 is a longitudinal scan obtained on the initial ultrasound examination. Gallbladder wall thickening (arrowheads) is identified on the posterior aspect of the gallbladder. The anterior half of the gallbladder lumen is relatively sonolucent. In the posterior half of the gallbladder lumen are soft level echoes in which the surface has a cauliflower appearance. This is most likely secondary to sludge and hemorrhage. Although the patient had some pain, he was not acutely ill, and surgery was deferred.

Figure 3–62 is a transverse scan obtained on the same patient 3½ weeks later. The patient was ill and had dramatic right upper quadrant tenderness. The gallbladder is shrunken and the gallbladder wall is thickened (arrowhead). Surrounding the gallbladder is a large sonolucent rim representing fluid. There is an echogenic region present posterior and medial to the gallbladder that is secondary to adherent omentum. At surgery the gallbladder was noted to have a thick wall secondary to hemorrhagic cholecystitis along with necrosis. A large fluid collection was present around the gallbladder which was serosanguineous in appearance. Omentum was adherent to the posterior aspect of the gallbladder. These findings indicate changes secondary to severe cholecystitis with associated hemorrhage and necrosis.

Figures 3–63 and 3–64 are longitudinal and transverse scans of a different patient who also had severe right upper quadrant pain. Figure 3–63 is a longitudinal scan that shows the dramatic changes of gangrenous cholecystitis. The gallbladder wall is enlarged and thickened posteriorly (arrowheads). Soft amplitude echoes are present in the posterior aspect of the gallbladder secondary to biliary sludge. A high-amplitude echo is pres-

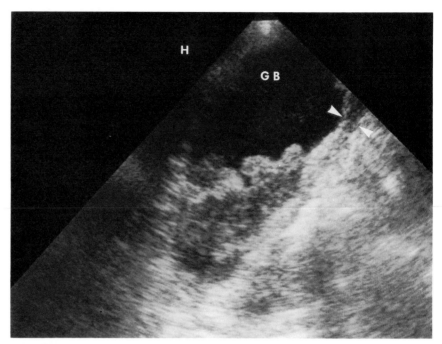

**FIG 3–61.**

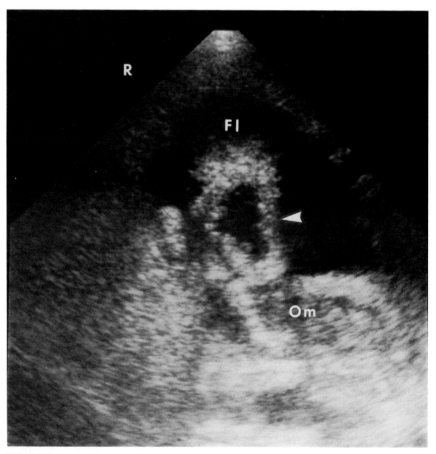

**FIG 3–62.**

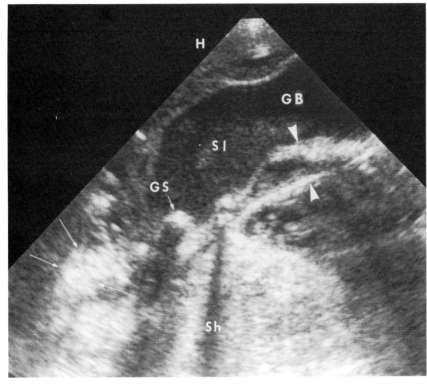

FIG 3–63.

ent in the region of the cystic duct secondary to a gallstone which is casting an acoustic shadow. There is evidence of a shadow arising from a high-amplitude echo within the gall-bladder wall. This is separate from the gallstone. This was found to be secondary to air within the gallbladder wall. Also noted on this scan is a high-amplitude region (arrows) cephalad to the gallbladder and gallstone. Figure 3–64 is a transverse scan through the high-amplitude region. The high-amplitude echoes (arrows) have slight shadowing. The high-amplitude region is secondary to an abscess near the gallbladder neck, confirmed at surgery. The patient had gangrenous cholecystitis with gallbladder wall thickening along with air in the gallbladder wall. The region of increased echogenicity cephalad to the gallbladder was secondary to an abscess.

| | |
|---|---|
| **Arrows** | = Abscess |
| **Arrowheads** | = Gallbladder wall thickening |
| **FI** | = Pericholecystic fluid |
| **GB** | = Gallbladder |
| **GS** | = Gallstone |
| **H** | = Head |
| **Om** | = Inflamed omentum |
| **R** | = Right |
| **Sh** | = Shadow |
| **SI** | = Biliary sludge |

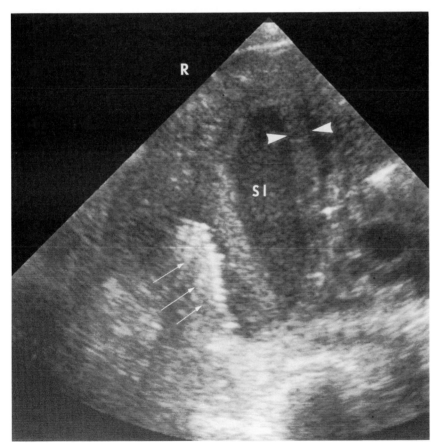

FIG 3–64.

## Gangrenous Cholecystitis With Gallbladder Hematoma

The case illustrated in Figures 3–65 through 3–68 is a 44-year-old man with carcinoma of the cecum. An ultrasound examination performed near the time of diagnosis (Figs 3–65 and 3–66) revealed a gallbladder in the right upper quadrant. The walls are fairly sharp, and there is no evidence of any internal echoes indicating stones. This was thought to be a normal study. The longitudinal scan in Figure 3–65 also demonstrates an interesting finding of pleural fluid in the right lower pleural space. The posterior thoracic wall can be seen due to the fluid in the pleural space. It should not be seen under normal circumstances. The patient underwent a hemicolectomy for carcinoma of the cecum a few days after the initial ultrasound study.

Approximately 6 weeks later, the patient experienced the sudden onset of abdominal pain, and his white blood cell count became elevated. Because of the possibility of a postoperative abscess, an ultrasound study was performed. The scans (Figs 3–67 and 3–68) show a dramatic change in the gallbladder, as compared to the study performed 6 weeks earlier. The gallbladder is completely filled with echoes, and there is hardly any evidence of sonolucent bile. The walls are minimally thickened, as compared to the previous study. Because of the elevated white blood cell count and the findings on ultrasound, the patient was taken to the operating room. At operation, a gangrenous gallbladder was found, and when the gallbladder was opened, the lumen was entirely filled with a hematoma. This case is an excellent example of the rapid development of cholecystitis followed by hemorrhage into the gallbladder lumen. Figures 3–67 and 3–68 show the soft internal echoes nearly completely filling the gallbladder lumen, secondary to a hematoma.

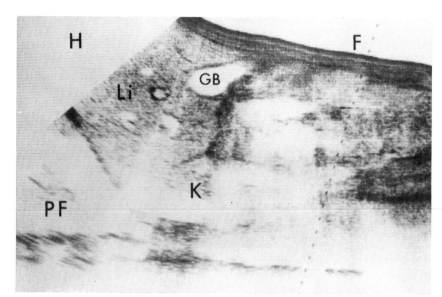

FIG 3–65.

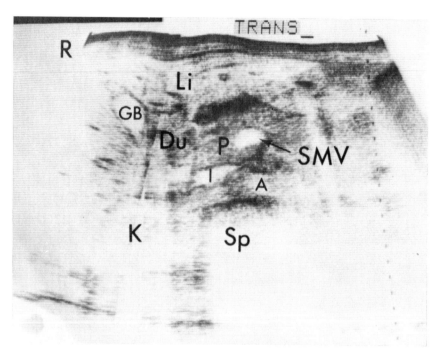

FIG 3–66.

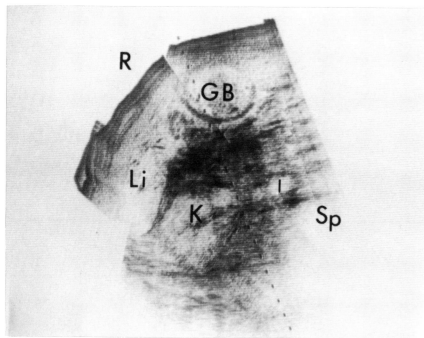

**FIG 3–67.**

| | | |
|---|---|---|
| **A** | = | Aorta |
| **Du** | = | Duodenum |
| **F** | = | Foot |
| **GB** | = | Gallbladder |
| **H** | = | Head |
| **I** | = | Inferior vena cava |
| **K** | = | Kidney |
| **Li** | = | Liver |
| **P** | = | Pancreas |
| **PF** | = | Pleural fluid |
| **R** | = | Right |
| **SMV** | = | Superior mesenteric vein |
| **Sp** | = | Spine |

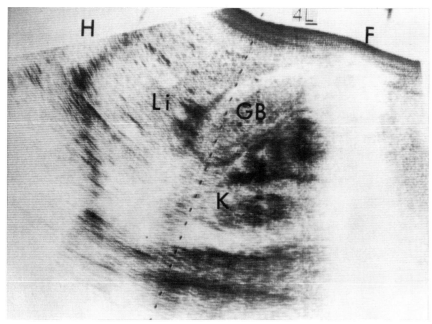

**FIG 3–68.**

## Cholecystitis

The gallbladder wall is not always thickened on ultrasound examination in the presence of cholecystitis. It is reported to be enlarged in only about 50%–75% of cases. The patient whose scan is shown in Figure 3–69 was admitted for ultrasound examination because of acute right upper quadrant pain. During examination, localized tenderness was detected in the right upper quadrant. The gallbladder was difficult to visualize. Figure 3–69 is a longitudinal scan of the right upper quadrant in which the gallbladder is barely detectable. The gallbladder wall is not thickened (arrowheads), as may happen in acute cholecystitis. The gallbladder itself is completely filled with biliary sludge and has a parenchymal appearance similar to that of the liver. This has been termed hepatization of the gallbladder and is characterized by biliary sludge that is nearly isoechoic with the hepatic parenchyma. The gallbladder wall is not thickened but is detected only as a slight area of decreased echogenicity, compared to liver parenchyma and the sludge. Localized tenderness was elicited over the region of the gallbladder, which confirmed the diagnosis of acute cholecystitis.

Figure 3–70 is a transverse scan of another patient in whom localized tenderness of the gallbladder bed was elicited on palpation during an ultrasound examination. In this instance, the gallbladder wall is thickened (arrowheads), which confirms the diagnosis of acute cholecystitis. There is a multiloculated fluid collection medial to the gallbladder that demonstrated peristalsis during real-time examination. On a static scan, this could be confused with a pericholecystic fluid collection. Because of real-time examination, the area was determined to be the duodenum. However, there is a smaller fluid collection present in the posterior lateral aspect of the gallbladder bed. This fluid collection persisted and did not manifest any peristaltic activity. Therefore, a diagnosis of fluid in the gallbladder bed was made. At

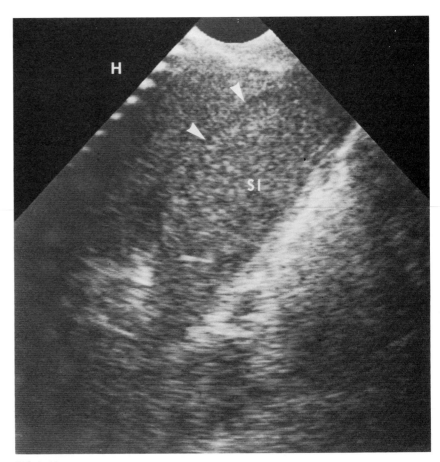

FIG 3–69.

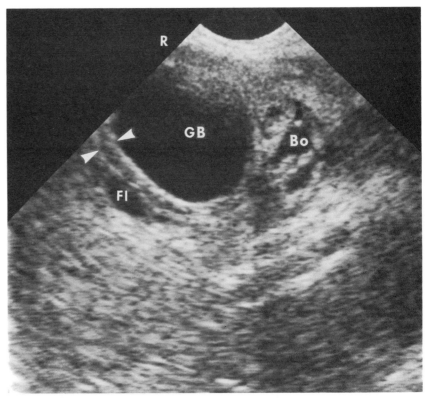

FIG 3–70.

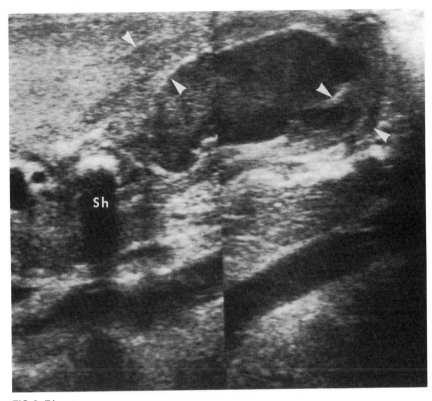

**FIG 3–71.**

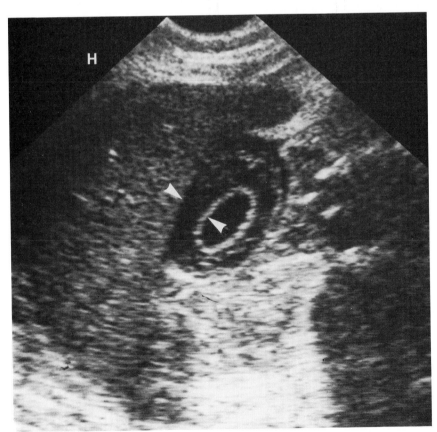

**FIG 3–72.**

operation acute cholecystitis was diagnosed along with a perforated gallbladder and small fluid collection. Real-time ultrasound is important in evaluating patients with right upper quadrant pain as it allows visualization of bowel loops. When there is any doubt, the patient may be given water, and further determination of bowel loops can be made.

Figure 3–71 is two side-by-side linear array scans of the gallbladder bed. This patient also had right upper quadrant pain and localized tenderness. The gallbladder wall is markedly thickened and irregular (arrowheads). The gallbladder is nearly entirely filled with sludge. In the region of the neck of the gallbladder is a high-amplitude echo with acoustic shadowing, secondary to an impacted cystic duct stone. When the gallbladder wall is markedly thickened and irregular, hemorrhage and gangrenous cholecystitis is quite likely. At operation the diagnosis of gangrenous cholecystitis was confirmed.

Gallbladder wall thickening visualized on ultrasound is not always secondary to cholecystitis. Other causes of diffuse gallbladder wall thickening include alcoholism, hypoalbuminemia, ascites, hepatitis, congestive heart failure, renal disease, neoplasm, and sepsis. Figure 3–72 is a longitudinal scan of a patient with abnormal liver function tests. The gallbladder wall is markedly thickened (arrowheads). The patient had severe hypoalbuminemia, which accounted for the gallbladder wall thickening. No gallstones were present. There was no clinical evidence of acute cholecystitis.

| **Arrowheads** | = | Gallbladder wall |
| **Bo** | = | Bowel |
| **Fl** | = | Pericholecystic fluid |
| **GB** | = | Gallbladder |
| **H** | = | Head |
| **R** | = | Right |
| **Sh** | = | Shadow |
| **Sl** | = | Biliary sludge |

## Gallbladder Carcinoma

When the gallbladder wall is irregularly thickened or there is a soft tissue mass in the gallbladder bed, the possibility of gallbladder carcinoma should be considered. Often the gallbladder will be difficult to visualize. Instead, a soft tissue mass with irregular echogenicity will be present in the region and may be mistaken for a liver metastasis. The possibility of gallbladder carcinoma should always be considered.

Figure 3–73 is a longitudinal scan of a 79-year-old woman who had a 3-week history of right-sided abdominal pain, nausea, and vomiting, and recent weight loss. Ultrasound examination demonstrates a large mass in the region of the gallbladder bed. The mass is solid in appearance with numerous low-level echoes. Shadowing is noted in the inferior aspect secondary to calcification. Often gallstones are present in association with gallbladder carcinoma. At operation a gallbladder carcinoma with necrosis was found.

Figure 3–74 is a transverse scan of the right upper quadrant of a different patient who presented with right upper quadrant pain of 2–3 weeks' duration. Ultrasound examination demonstrates a solid mass in the region of the gallbladder bed (arrows). At surgery, adenocarcinoma of the gallbladder was found.

Figure 3–75 is a longitudinal scan of another patient with acute right upper quadrant pain. The gallbladder wall is thickened and irregular (arrowheads). There is evidence of a gallstone near the cystic duct region that is casting an acoustic shadow. These findings are highly suggestive of acute cholecystitis with possible hemorrhage and necrosis. However, a soft tissue mass cannot be distinguished from edema, and the possibility of gallbladder carcinoma should always be considered. At operation gallbladder carcinoma was diagnosed. There was also evidence of a cystic duct stone obstructing the common bile duct. There is a high association of cholelithiasis with gallbladder carcinoma.

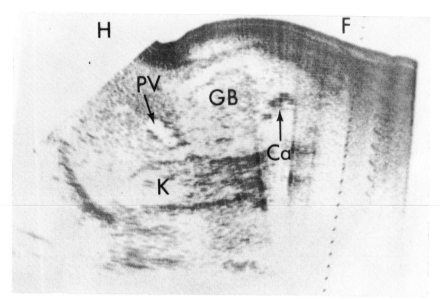

**FIG 3–73.**

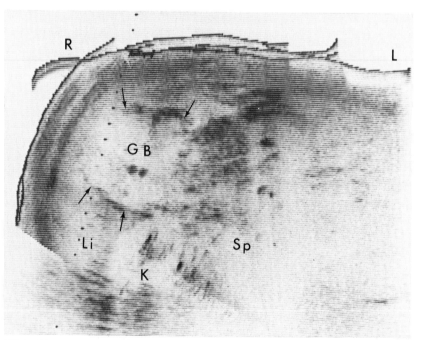

**FIG 3–74.**

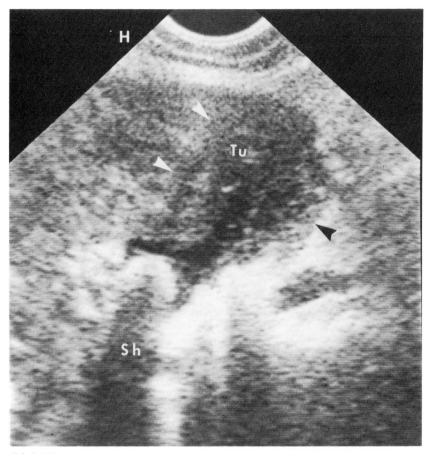

**FIG 3–75.**

Figure 3–76 is the scan of another patient with acute right upper quadrant pain. There is localized thickening of the anterior gallbladder wall. The posterior aspect of the gallbladder is filled with sludge. Numerous high-amplitude stones are present on the posterior wall, casting acoustic shadows. The gallbladder carcinoma was localized to the anterior wall of the gallbladder. It was already metastatic to the liver.

SOURCE: Figure 3–73 is reproduced with permission from Sample WF: Diagnostic value and limitations in digestive disorders, in Berk JE (ed): *Developments in Digestive Diseases: Clinical Relevance.* Philadelphia, Lea & Febiger, 1977.

| | | |
|---|---|---|
| **Arrowheads** | = | Gallbladder carcinoma |
| **Ca** | = | Calcification |
| **F** | = | Foot |
| **GB** | = | Gallbladder bed with tumor |
| **GB and arrows** | = | Gallbladder carcinoma |
| **H** | = | Head |
| **K** | = | Kidney |
| **L** | = | Left |
| **Li** | = | Liver |
| **PV** | = | Portal vein |
| **R** | = | Right |
| **Sh** | = | Shadow |
| **Sl** | = | Sludge |
| **Sp** | = | Spine |
| **Tu** | = | Gallbladder tumor |

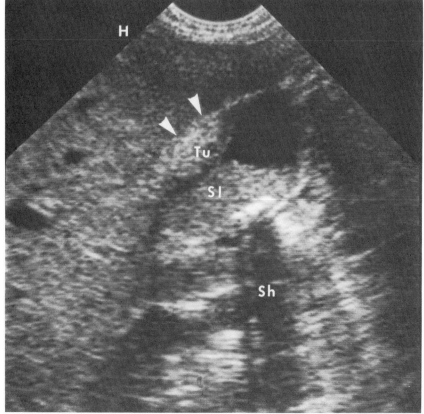

**FIG 3–76.**

## Normal Biliary System

In an examination of the biliary system, it is important to understand the anatomy of the portal venous system. Normally, the portal venous system yields the largest tubular structures within the parenchyma of the liver. These vessels are surrounded by strong echoes arising from the fibrous tissue. The hepatic veins are the second tubular structures seen within the liver. They have less of an echogenic surrounding because there is less fibrous tissue. We do not usually see the biliary system within the parenchyma of the liver. When, on occasion, it is visualized within the parenchyma of the liver, it presents as a second tubular structure adjacent to the portal venous system, yielding the "parallel channel" sign.

Figures 3–77 and 3–78 are transverse scans of the same patient and demonstrate the normal anatomy of the portal venous system. The vertical lines, numbered 1–4, correspond to the longitudinal scans in Figures 3–79 through 3–82.

The main portal vein branches into the left portal vein and the right portal vein. Figure 3–77 shows bifurcation of the right portal vein in the lateral aspect of the right lobe of the liver. Figure 3–79 is a longitudinal scan corresponding to vertical line 1 in Figure 3–77. In Figure 3–79 we see bifurcation of the right portal vein. This is important to recognize so as not to misdiagnose biliary dilatation. The longitudinal scans should demonstrate a second tubular structure, parallel to the portal vein, which will aid in the diagnosis of biliary obstruction. We do, however, see bifurcation of the portal venous system at certain anatomic sites. Peripheral bifurcation at one of these sites is seen at the right portal vein. If we follow the right portal vein medially, we will see only one circular structure in the porta hepatis. Figure 3–80 is a longitudinal scan corresponding to line 2 in Figure 3–77. Here we see the juncture of the right portal vein as it approaches a single circular structure.

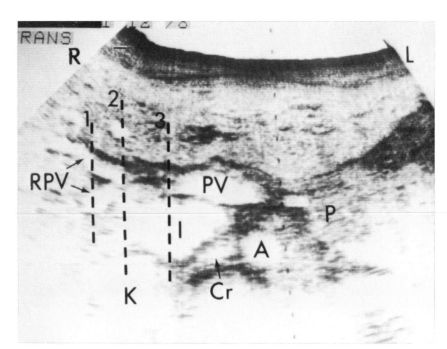

**FIG 3–77.**

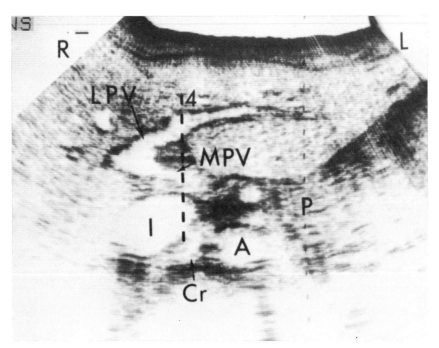

**FIG 3–78.**

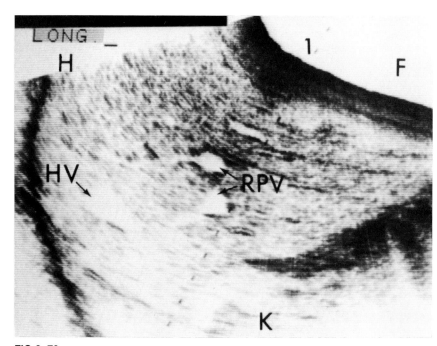

FIG 3–79.

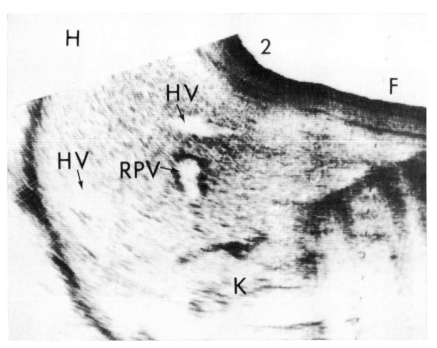

FIG 3–80.

## Normal Biliary System

Figure 3–81 is a longitudinal scan through the liver corresponding to line 3 in Figure 3–77. Here we are scanning through the main portion of the right portal vein, which appears as a single circular sonolucency. This is the important part of an examination to rule out biliary obstruction. At this point, we should see only one circular sonolucency on longitudinal scans within the porta hepatis. This corresponds to that segment of the right portal vein before bifurcation and before the left portal vein can be seen. If we do not see a single circular sonoluency but instead see two or three, we have evidence consistent with biliary obstruction. As we move medially, we will see two circular sonolucencies once we encounter the left portal vein (Fig 3–82). Figure 3–82 is a longitudinal scan corresponding to line 4 in Figure 3–78. The left portal vein is situated anterior to the main portal vein. Again, there are two circular sonolucencies. This is a normal finding and not to be mistaken for biliary obstruction.

This conception of the portal venous system is extremely important in order not to misdiagnose biliary obstruction. There are certain anatomic positions where two large circular sonolucencies on longitudinal scans, corresponding to bifurcations in the portal venous system, can be seen. The segment of the right portal vein where we should see only a single sonolucency on longitudinal scan corresponds to Figure 3–81. It is important to look for this site in order to rule out biliary obstruction. If two circular sonolucencies of approximately the same size are seen consistently, biliary obstruction is most likely present.

Transverse scans in the region of the porta hepatis often show several circular sonolucencies anterior to the portal vein. Figures 3–83 and 3–84 exemplify this finding. Usually the hepatic artery is the medial sonolucency and the common bile duct or common hepatic duct is the lateral sonolucency. Ordinarily, these are only 3–4 mm in diameter. If they are larger, ob-

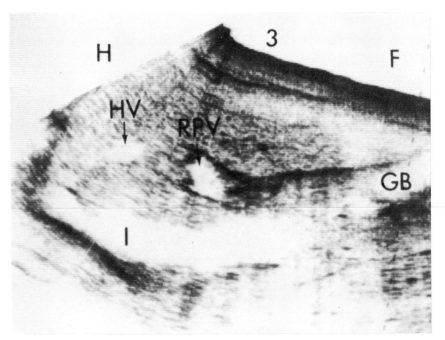

**FIG 3–81.**

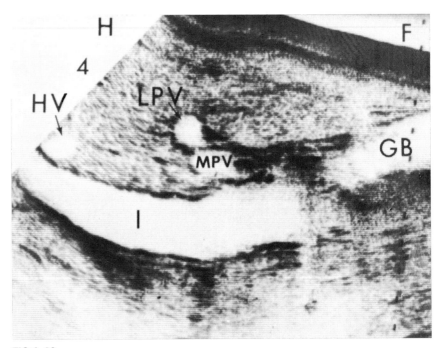

**FIG 3–82.**

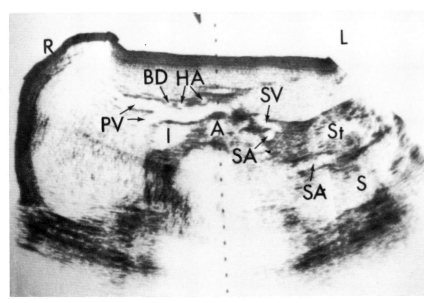

**FIG 3–83.**

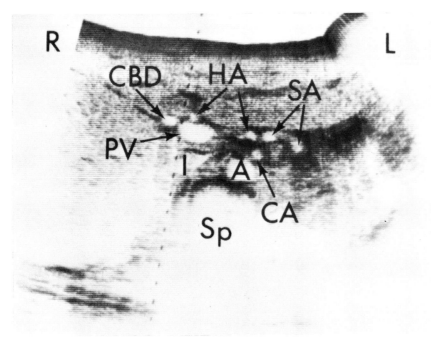

**FIG 3–84.**

struction should be suspected. The portal vein is the larger sonolucency noted posteriorly. This is best evident in Figure 3–84, which demonstrates the portal triad of the common bile duct, hepatic artery, and portal vein.

SOURCE: Figure 3–83 is reproduced with permission from Sample WF: Normal abdominal anatomy defined by gray scale ultrasound. *Radiol Clin North Am* 1979; 17:3-11.

| | | |
|---|---|---|
| **A** | = | Aorta |
| **BD** | = | Bile duct |
| **CA** | = | Celiac axis |
| **CBD** | = | Common bile duct |
| **F** | = | Foot |
| **GB** | = | Gallbladder |
| **H** | = | Head |
| **HA** | = | Hepatic artery |
| **HV** | = | Hepatic vein |
| **I** | = | Inferior vena cava |
| **L** | = | Left |
| **LPV** | = | Left portal vein |
| **MPV** | = | Main portal vein |
| **PV** | = | Portal vein |
| **RPV** | = | Right portal vein |
| **S** | = | Spleen |
| **SA** | = | Splenic artery |
| **Sp** | = | Spine |
| **St** | = | Stomach |
| **SV** | = | Splenic vein |
| **3** | = | Longitudinal scan corresponding to the vertical line Figure 3–77 |
| **4** | = | Longitudinal scan corresponding to the vertical line in Figure 3–78 |

## Normal Biliary System

Transverse scans of the porta hepatis are continued in a caudal direction until the head of the pancreas is visualized. Occasionally, a circular sonolucency corresponding to the common bile duct can be seen just lateral to the head of the pancreas. Often, however, visualization of the common bile duct is obscured by air in the duodenum. The upper normal limits for the common bile duct in a patient who has not had a previous cholecystectomy is in the range of 6–7 mm. Figure 3–85 is a transverse scan showing the common bile duct and gastroduodenal artery situated between the duodenum and head of the pancreas. The lumen of this common bile duct (sonolucent portion) measures approximately 3–4 mm. This is within normal limits. In a patient who has had a cholecystectomy, the common bile duct can be larger without obstruction present. Obstruction of the common bile duct often can be seen in this area and will appear as a large circular sonolucency just lateral to the head of the pancreas.

It is important to attempt to visualize the common bile duct on longitudinal scans. Figure 3–86 is a longitudinal scan in the region of the porta hepatis in which the common hepatic duct is seen anterior to the portal vein. The common hepatic duct is draped over the portal vein and begins its course posteriorly, so that it may end up posterior and lateral to the head of the pancreas. Figure 3–87 is a longitudinal scan showing the common bile duct coursing more posteriorly and situated behind the head of the pancreas. A tubular sonolucent area anterior to the head of the pancreas is caused by the gastroduodenal artery. These two tubular structures surround the head of the pancreas on longitudinal scans and provide excellent anatomic landmarks. The common bile duct in this case (Fig 3–87) is approximately 2–3 mm in diameter. Figure 3–88 is another example of the common bile duct and gastroduodenal artery surrounding the head of the pancreas. The common bile duct here is

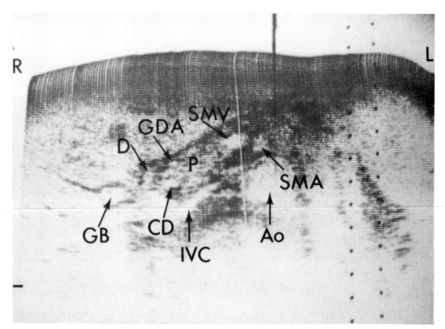

FIG 3–85.

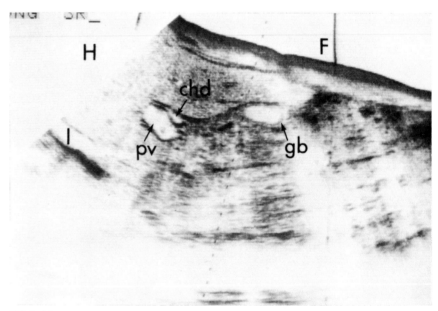

FIG 3–86.

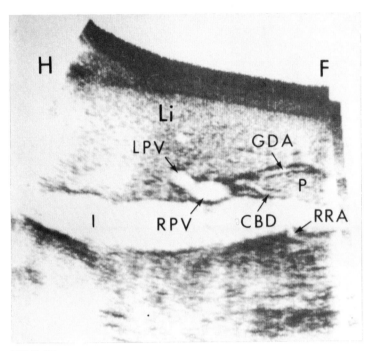

FIG 3–87.

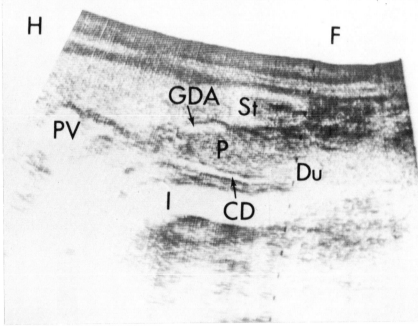

FIG 3–88.

approximately 2–3 mm in diameter, within the normal range. The common bile duct courses anterior to the portal vein and dips posteriorly behind the head of the pancreas, frequently just anterior to the inferior vena cava. To confirm the diagnosis of biliary obstruction, it is necessary to visualize on longitudinal scans the common bile duct draping over the portal vein and posterior to the pancreas. The technologist must be certain he or she is not visualizing the superior mesenteric vein.

SOURCE: Figure 3–88 is reproduced with permission from Sample WF: Normal abdominal anatomy defined by gray scale ultrasound. *Radiol Clin North Am* 1979; 17:3-11.

| | | |
|---|---|---|
| **A** | = | Aorta |
| **CBD** | = | Common bile duct |
| **CD** | = | Common bile duct |
| **chd** | = | Common hepatic duct |
| **D** | = | Duodenum |
| **Du** | = | Duodenum |
| **F** | = | Foot |
| **GB** | = | Gallbladder |
| **gb** | = | Gallbladder |
| **GDA** | = | Gastroduodenal artery |
| **H** | = | Head |
| **I** | = | Inferior vena cava |
| **L** | = | Left |
| **Li** | = | Liver |
| **LPV** | = | Left portal vein |
| **P** | = | Pancreas |
| **PV** | = | Portal vein |
| **pv** | = | Portal vein |
| **R** | = | Right |
| **RPV** | = | Right portal vein |
| **RRA** | = | Right renal artery |
| **SMA** | = | Superior mesenteric artery |
| **SMV** | = | Superior mesenteric vein |
| **St** | = | Stomach |

## Biliary Obstruction

When biliary obstruction is present, a second tubular structure adjacent to the portal vein will be identified. This has been described as the "parallel channel" sign. Figure 3–89 is an example of this sign seen in a patient with extrahepatic jaundice secondary to choledocholithiasis. The portal vein is seen posterior to a second tubular structure that represents a dilated intrahepatic biliary duct.

Very often, the dilated biliary ducts appear as knobby, irregularly branching tubular patterns within the liver. Usually the portal venous system has a fairly even, smooth, branching pattern. Figure 3–90 is an example of a dilated biliary tree secondary to carcinoma of the pancreas in a 53-year-old man. The tubular structures within the liver have a "knotty" appearance, rather than the even branching noted in the normal portal venous system.

Figure 3–91 is the scan of a 64-year-old woman who also had carcinoma of the head of the pancreas. Again, an irregular "knotty" appearance to the dilated bile ducts is noted in the anterior half of the liver on this longitudinal scan. The common bile duct is also markedly dilated, to approximately 2 cm in diameter.

Figure 3–92 is a transverse scan near the region of the head of the pancreas. The portal triad is seen with the portal vein, noted posteriorly. Anterior and medial to the portal vein is the hepatic artery. Lateral and anterior to the portal vein is the dilated common bile duct. The portal triad is easily recognized within the porta hepatis of the liver. The common bile duct should be approximately the size of the hepatic artery or slightly smaller. Here it is approximately 2–3 times the size of the hepatic artery. The pancreas is less echogenic than the liver. This is consistent with pancreatitis, which was the cause of the biliary obstruction.

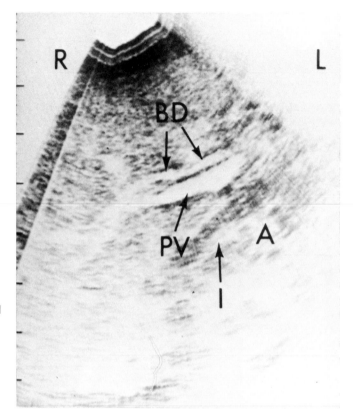

FIG 3–89.

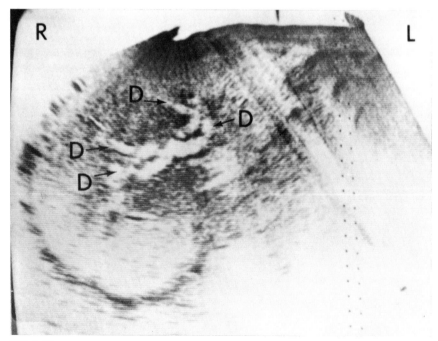

FIG 3–90.

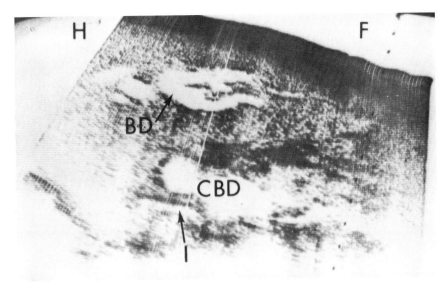

**FIG 3–91.**

SOURCE: Figures 3–90, 3–91, and 3–92 are reproduced with permission from Sample WF: Diagnostic value and limitations in digestive disorders, in Berk JE (ed): *Developments in Digestive Diseases: Clinical Relevance.* Philadelphia, Lea & Febiger, 1977.

| | | |
|---|---|---|
| **A** | = | Aorta |
| **BD** | = | Dilated bile ducts |
| **CBD** | = | Common bile duct |
| **D** | = | Dilated bile ducts |
| **F** | = | Foot |
| **H** | = | Head |
| **HA** | = | Hepatic artery |
| **I** | = | Inferior vena cava |
| **K** | = | Kidney |
| **L** | = | Left |
| **P** | = | Pancreas |
| **PV** | = | Portal vein |
| **R** | = | Right |
| **SMA** | = | Superior mesenteric artery |

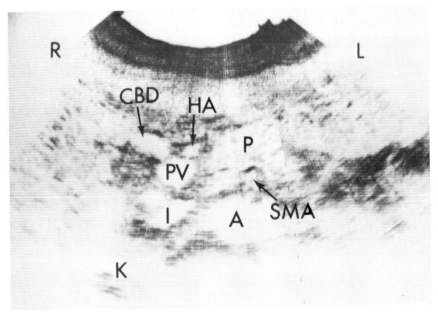

**FIG 3–92.**

## Biliary Obstruction

The portal vein is usually smooth and gradually tapering. When biliary obstruction is present and causes intrahepatic bile duct dilatation, there is a fairly characteristic appearance to the tubular structures within the liver. These structures become increasingly tortuous and irregular in their course and caliber. They have what has been termed a stellate configuration with an irregular tortuous branching pattern.

Figure 3–93 is a transverse scan of the right upper quadrant in a patient with jaundice. It is difficult to determine which of the tubular structures in the midportion of the liver are secondary to bile ducts or portal venous structures. However, the irregular tortuous appearance of the tubular structures indicates that most are secondary to obstructed bile ducts. Enhanced through-transmission is noted deep to these tubular structures, further evidence that they are secondary to biliary dilatation. Usually through-transmission is identified deep to dilated bile ducts but is not present behind portal venous structures. Therefore the combination of tortuous, dilated tubular structures with enhanced through-transmission is confirmatory ultrasound evidence of biliary obstruction. One is structure 1 in Figure 3–93?

In an evaluation of biliary obstruction it is important to visualize the right hepatic duct. This is usually seen anterior to the right portal vein. The right portal vein is the portion of the portal vein after the takeoff of the left portal vein and before the bifurcation of the right portal vein into anterior and posterior branches. If a tubular structure is noted anterior to the right portal vein, it may represent the right hepatic artery or right bile duct. As long as the lumen of this tubular structure is 4 mm or less in diameter, it is considered normal. If the diameter is larger, one must determine whether the tubular structure is arising from the arterial system or the biliary system. By following its course medially, one can see whether or not it arises from the celiac axis. If the structure from the celiac axis, it is the hepatic artery. If it does not arise from the celiac axis, it is secondary to dilatation of the right hepatic duct.

Figure 3–94 is an oblique scan made parallel to the long axis of the

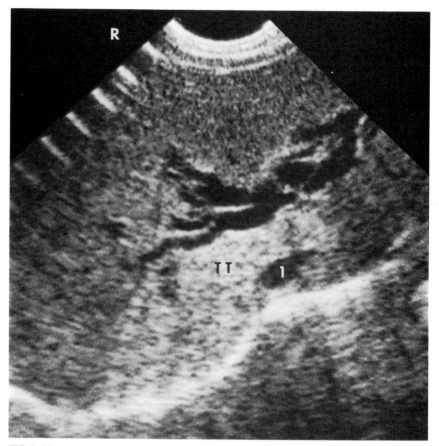

FIG 3–93.

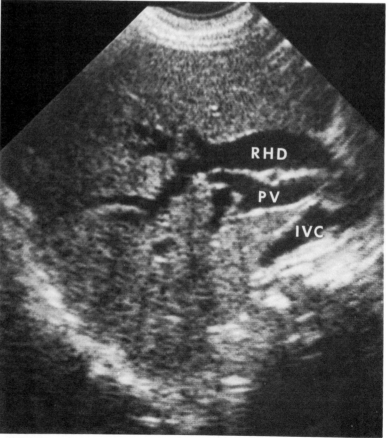

FIG 3–94.

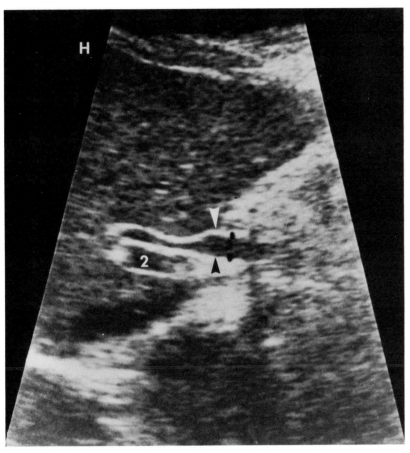

**FIG 3–95.**

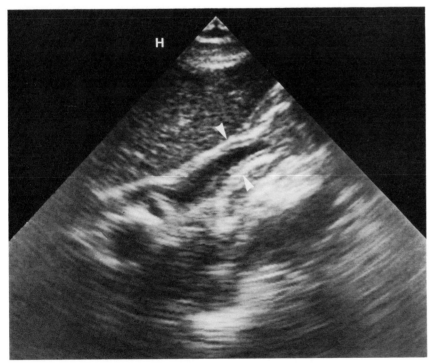

**FIG 3–96.**

right portal vein. Anterior to the right portal vein is a large tubular structure that is secondary to a dilated right hepatic duct. Between the right hepatic duct and portal vein is a small circular lucency that is secondary to the right hepatic artery. The area of the right hepatic duct is the most easily identifiable region of the biliary tree on ultrasound examination. Very often the common bile duct and common hepatic duct are obscured by bowel air. However, the region of the right hepatic duct can be seen in almost-all cases because of the surrounding liver. Therefore, one should regularly look in the area of the right hepatic duct.

Although the finding of dilated intrahepatic bile ducts is very helpful in the diagnosis of biliary jaundice, it is not highly specific. There is evidence that up to 23% of patients with biliary obstruction have normal-sized intrahepatic bile ducts. The dilatation will only be visualized in the extrahepatic biliary system. Therefore, evaluation of the extrahepatic biliary system is necessary. Figure 3–95 is a longitudinal scan made through the common hepatic and common bile duct region. The common bile duct is markedly larger than the region of the common hepatic and right hepatic duct. This appearance has been termed funneling. The common bile duct has a larger diameter because it tends to be the part of the biliary system that dilates first. Therefore, the intrahepatic biliary system may have a normal appearance while the distal common bile duct is dilated. What is structure 2 in Figure 3–95?

Figure 3–96 is a longitudinal scan in a patient who has jaundice and a markedly elevated alkaline phosphatase level. The common bile duct (arrowheads) is slightly dilated. A striking feature of this scan is evidence of wall thickening in the common bile duct, an unusual finding. In this case, wall thickening was secondary to sclerosing cholangitis, which explains the ultrasound findings.

| | |
|---|---|
| **Arrowheads** | = Dilated common bile duct |
| **H** | = Head |
| **IVC** | = Inferior vena cava |
| **PV** | = Portal vein |
| **R** | = Right |
| **RHD** | = Dilated right hepatic duct |
| **TT** | = Through-transmission |
| **1** | = Inferior vena cava |
| **2** | = Portal vein |

## Biliary Obstruction

The extrahepatic biliary tree may often be dilated without evidence of the cause of dilatation. This is because the distal portion of the common bile duct is not visualized because of overlying bowel air. However, the finding of biliary dilatation will lead to further tests.

Figure 3–97 is a longitudinal oblique scan through the region of the porta hepatis. The diameters of the common hepatic and common bile ducts are at the upper limits of normal. There is a suggestion of mild biliary dilatation. Figure 3–98 is a scan of the same patient made a few seconds later. The common bile duct is now definitely dilated, indicating biliary obstruction. The only difference between the two scans is that increased pressure was applied during the scan shown in Figure 3–97. Scanning with increased abdominal pressure causes the common bile duct to appear less dilated than when scanning is done without pressure. This is a technical artifact that could lead to an incorrect diagnosis. Proper scanning techniques must be used to avoid a false negative diagnosis. In this instance, too much abdominal pressure during imaging led to the appearance of a minimally dilated common bile duct. When proper pressure techniques were used (Fig 3–98), the common bile duct was easily identified as dilated.

Figures 3–99 and 3–100 are transverse and longitudinal scans of the right upper quadrant in a 28-year-old woman with an 8-day history of right upper quadrant pain. She also reported the recent onset of nausea and vomiting. The transverse scan in Figure 3–99 shows a dilated common bile duct lateral and posterior to the head of the pancreas. The common bile duct measured 12 × 14 mm at this level. A longitudinal scan through the dilated common bile duct is shown in Figure 3–100. The large tubular structure seen in the scan represents a dilated common bile duct posterior to the head of the pancreas. The distal end of the common bile duct is not well seen. The biliary dilatation was

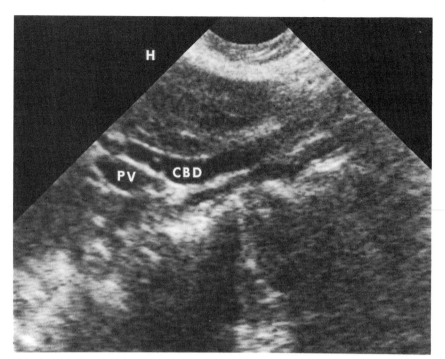

**FIG 3–97.**

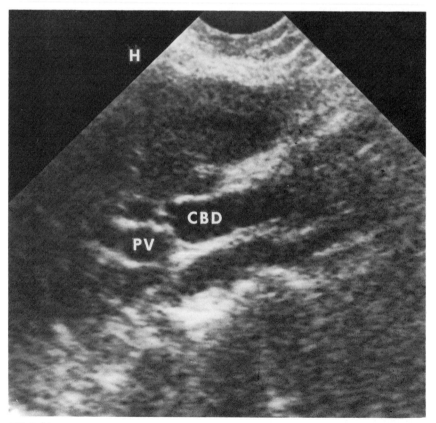

**FIG 3–98.**

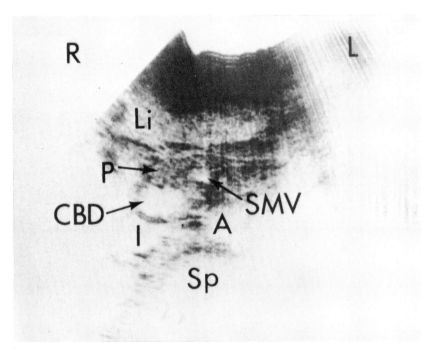

FIG 3–99.

the result of choledocholithiasis. The stone in the common bile duct cannot be seen. This is not unusual. However, biliary dilatation is easily identified. The cause of biliary dilatation cannot always be determined from ultrasound imaging. Numerous attempts should be made to see the distal end of the common bile duct in an effort to diagnose the cause of obstruction.

| | | |
|---|---|---|
| **A** | = | Aorta |
| **Arrows** | = | Dilated intrahepatic bile ducts |
| **CBD** | = | Dilated common bile duct |
| **F** | = | Foot |
| **H** | = | Head |
| **I** | = | Inferior vena cava |
| **L** | = | Left |
| **Li** | = | Liver |
| **P** | = | Pancreas |
| **PV** | = | Portal vein |
| **R** | = | Right |
| **SMV** | = | Superior mesenteric vein |
| **Sp** | = | Spine |

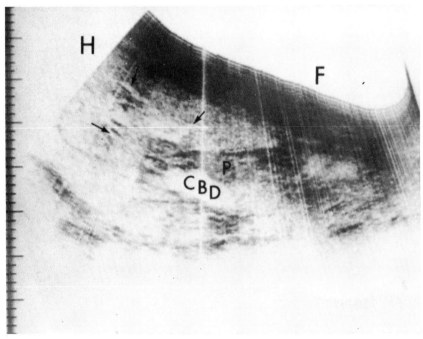

FIG 3–100.

## Biliary Obstruction With Choledocholithiasis

The scans shown here were obtained in a 20-year-old woman who was 10 weeks pregnant. She had experienced colicky right upper guadrant pain for 4 weeks. The pain was episodic in nature and usually came after eating. Ultrasound examination demonstrated a dilated biliary tree, which is seen in a transverse section of the liver in Figure 3–101. The portal vein is seen on transverse section with a dilated biliary duct situated anterior to it. A transverse scan more caudal and near the region of the head of the pancreas (Fig 3–102) showed a circular sonolucency lateral to the head of the pancreas, measuring approximately 15 mm, and representing a dilated common bile duct. A longitudinal scan following this circular structure is seen in Figure 3–103. The common bile duct is seen nearly in its entirety, with a circular echo noted in its distal portion. This circular echo was found at surgery to be a common bile duct stone.

During the early part of the ultrasound examination, Figure 3–102 was obtained while the patient was in a great deal of pain. During the latter half of the ultrasound examination, the patient reported that the pain had disappeared.

Figure 3–104 is the transverse scan near the head of the pancreas obtained a few minutes after the scan shown in Figure 3–102. The only difference was the cessation of the patient's pain. The common bile duct is still visible adjacent to the head of the pancreas. However, its size has decreased dramatically. Figure 3–104 shows a common bile duct approximately 9 mm in diameter. The patient had most likely decompressed herself during the course of the examination and thereby relieved her pain temporarily. This surely is a therapeutic triumph for ultrasound.

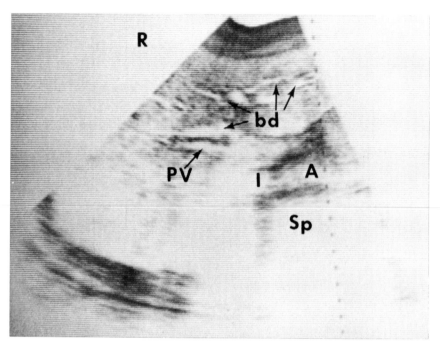

FIG 3–101.

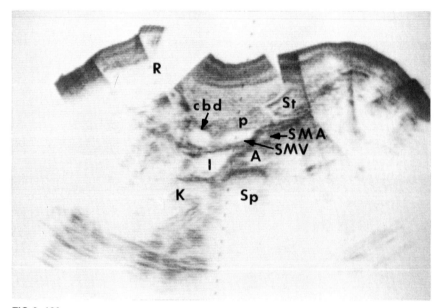

FIG 3–102.

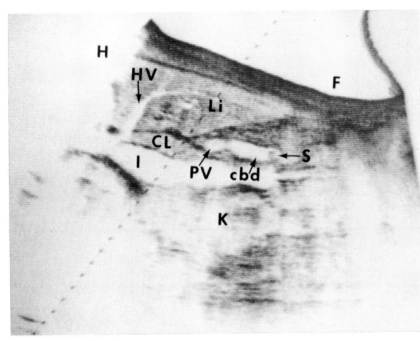

| A | = | Aorta |
|---|---|---|
| **BD** | = | Dilated bile duct |
| **cbd** | = | Common bile duct |
| **CL** | = | Caudate lobe |
| **Cr** | = | Crus of the diaphragm |
| **F** | = | Foot |
| **H** | = | Head |
| **HV** | = | Hepatic vein |
| **I** | = | Inferior vena cava |
| **K** | = | Kidney |
| **Li** | = | Liver |
| **LRV** | = | Left renal vein |
| **P** | = | Pancreas |
| **PV** | = | Portal vein |
| **R** | = | Right |
| **S** | = | Stone |
| **SC** | = | Spinal canal |
| **SMA** | = | Superior mesenteric artery |
| **SMV** | = | Superior mesenteric vein |
| **Sp** | = | Spine |
| **St** | = | Stomach |

**FIG 3–103.**

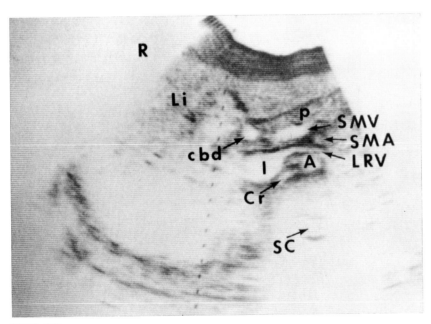

**FIG 3–104.**

## Biliary Obstruction With Choledocholithiasis

When biliary obstruction is visualized, attempts should be made to see the distal portion of the common bile duct. Very often the anatomic cause of obstruction can be identified. The duodenum often obscures the region because of bowel air. However, if the patient is initially scanned in the upright position, bowel air is often not present in the duodenum. This technique allows better visualization of the region of the distal common bile duct. It is best to examine the jaundiced patient initially in the upright position. This will improve visualization of the distal common bile duct and of pathology in the area.

Figure 3–105 is a longitudinal oblique scan of a patient with acute right upper quadrant pain. A markedly dilated common bile duct is present anterior to the portal vein. Note the small circular structure between the portal vein and the common bile duct. This is secondary to the hepatic artery. The distal end of the common bile duct is not well seen because of overlying air in the duodenum. Figure 3–106 is a transverse scan of the same patient that was obtained earlier in the upright position. A stone (arrowhead) is now visible in the distal common bile duct that was not seen on a later scan made with the patient supine. High-amplitude echoes were noted in the gallbladder, confirming the diagnosis of cholelithiasis. A fluid-filled structure (1) is seen lateral to the stone in the common bile duct. It may represent the inferior vena cava, pseudocysts, fluid in the duodenum, abscess, or some other entity. What are structures 1, 2, and 3?

Figure 3–107 is a longitudinal scan of another patient with acute right upper quadrant pain. The common bile duct is only minimally dilated, with a 7-mm diameter. In the distal portion of the common bile duct, a high-amplitude echo with acoustic shadowing is present (arrowhead). This represents a stone in the distal portion of the common bile duct causing partial obstruction. Notice the funnel appear-

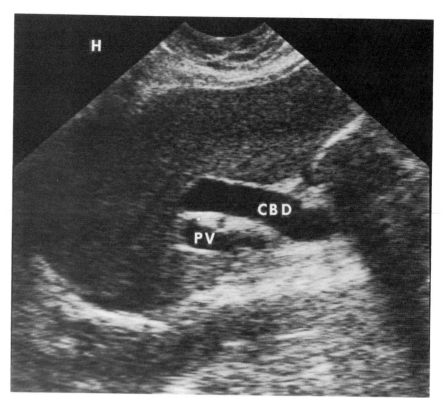

FIG 3–105.

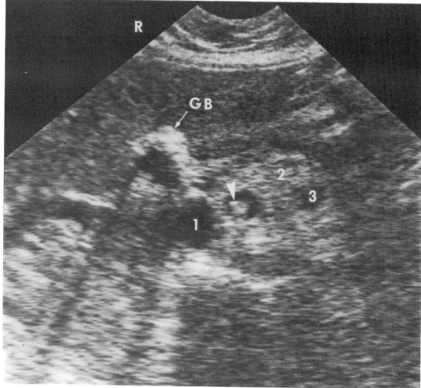

FIG 3–106.

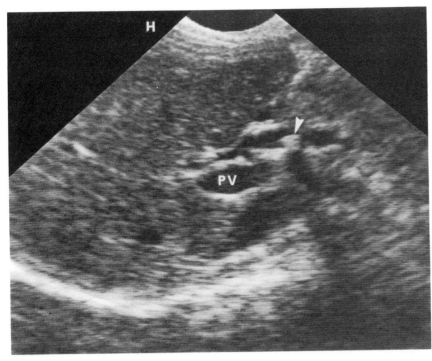

**FIG 3–107.**

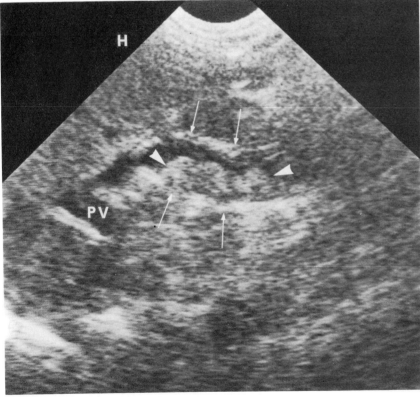

**FIG 3–108.**

ance of the common hepatic duct compared to the common bile duct. This appearance is common in early dilatation, as the distal portion of the common bile duct dilates first.

Figure 3–108 is a longitudinal scan of a patient who has had several previous episodes of cholangitis. The common bile duct is markedly dilated (arrows). Within the common bile duct are numerous pigmented stones (arrowheads) that have a soft echo consistency and may be suggestive of sludge. Pigmented stones do not always shadow. To the unwary, this common bile duct may seem of normal caliber. The border of the pigmented stones could be confused with the border of the common bile duct. Close examination reveals that the common bile duct is markedly dilated (arrows).

| | | |
|---|---|---|
| **Arrowhead** | = | Choledocholithiasis |
| **Arrows** | = | Dilated common bile duct |
| **CBD** | = | Dilated common bile duct |
| **GB** | = | Stones in gallbladder |
| **H** | = | Head |
| **PV** | = | Portal vein |
| **1** | = | Fluid in the duodenum, documented on real-time examination |
| **2** | = | Head of the pancreas |
| **3** | = | Superior mesenteric vein |

## Biliary Obstruction

One should always attempt to visualize the distal end of the common bile duct. Very often a soft tissue density will be present near the distal duct, indicating a tumor as the cause of obstruction. Figure 3–109 is a longitudinal scan through a dilated common bile duct in which only soft tissue echoes are noted distal to it. Note the irregular border to the distal end of the common bile duct. This scan was obtained in a patient with jaundice secondary to gastric carcinoma. The gastric carcinoma was invading the region of the porta hepatis and obstructing the common bile duct. The soft echoes in the common bile duct are secondary to biliary sludge. In this case, biliary sludge cannot be differentiated from tumor in the common bile duct. If sludge is layering out and a fluid level can be seen, biliary sludge can be diagnosed. However, if sludge is filling the entire lumen, it can be difficult to distinguish from a soft tissue tumor. What is structure 1 in Figure 3–109.

Figure 3–110 is a scan of a patient with an elevated bilirubin level. The common bile duct is dilated and ends abruptly in its distal portion. The common bile duct contains numerous soft amplitude echoes, as in the previous case. However, the soft echoes in Figure 3–110 are secondary to tumor growing within the common bile duct. This patient also had gastric carcinoma. Ultrasound cannot usually differentiate tumor, pigmented stones, sludge, and blood clot. After surgery in which a bypass stint was placed in the common bile duct, another scan was obtained (Fig 3–111). The stint is visualized (small arrowheads) as high-amplitude parallel echoes arising from the tube walls.

Figure 3–112 is a longitudinal oblique scan of another patient with right upper quadrant pain and abnormal liver function tests. The common bile duct is markedly dilated (large arrowheads). Within the common bile duct is an echogenic tubular structure. The appearance is similar to the appearance in the previously described

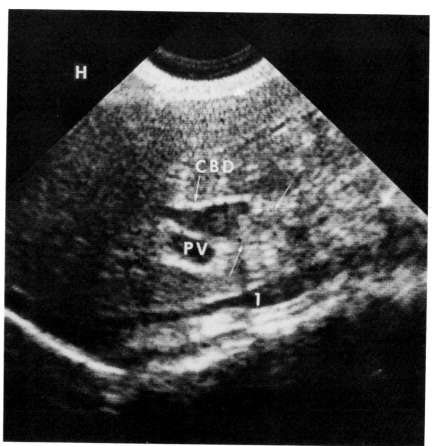

FIG 3–109.

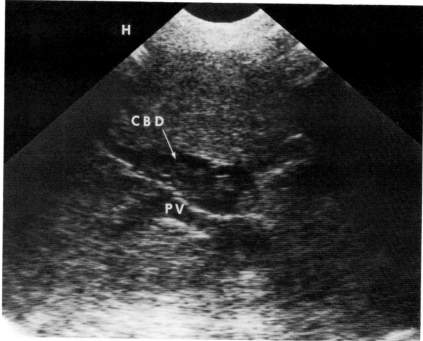

FIG 3–110.

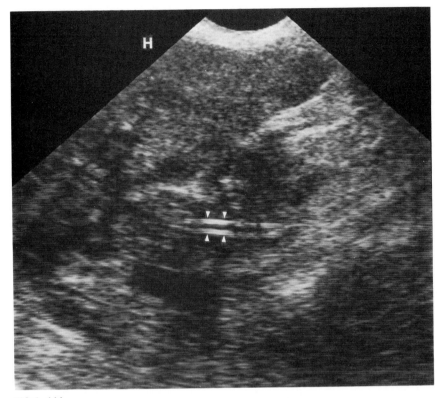

**FIG 3–111.**

patient. However, the walls of this tube are not as prominent or as high in echogenicity. The tubular structure is secondary to a long ascaris that is present within the common bile duct and causing biliary dilatation. The ascaris does not have as high amplitude echoes as the stint.

| | |
|---|---|
| **Arrows** | = Gastric carcinoma obstructing common bile duct |
| **Arrowheads (large)** | = Dilated common bile duct |
| **Arrowheads (small)** | = Stint |
| **CBD** | = Dilated common bile duct |
| **H** | = Head |
| **PV** | = Portal vein |
| **1** | = Inferior vena cava |

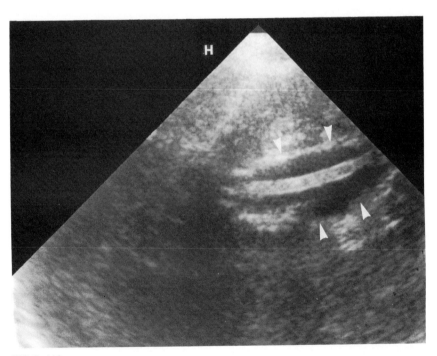

**FIG 3–112.**

## Echogenic Foci

Numerous echogenic foci in the liver may be secondary to metastatic disease. However, multiple echogenic foci can also be identified in the biliary system. These echogenic foci are usually from intrabiliary stones or intrabiliary air. Figure 3–113 is a transverse scan of a 14-year-old patient who had undergone multiple abdominal surgeries. High-amplitude echoes are noted within the liver, casting acoustic shadows. These are secondary to intrabiliary stones, which represent the echogenic foci within the liver.

Figure 3–114 is a longitudinal scan of an Oriental patient who had previously undergone surgery. The patient presented with right upper quadrant pain and signs of sepsis. Numerous high-amplitude echoes are seen within the liver. Other scans confirmed that these echoes are within the biliary system because of their anatomic distribution. The high-amplitude echoes are casting acoustic shadows and are consistent with biliary calculi. The patient had Oriental cholangiohepatitis, and the findings are consistent with intrabiliary calculi.

Figure 3–115 is a transverse scan of an 83-year-old man with a history of cholelithiasis. Three years before the scan shown here was made, the patient underwent cholecystectomy and choledochojejunostomy. After operation there were repeated episodes of ascending cholangitis. The patient was found to have reflux of intestinal contents into the biliary tree, which resulted in the cholangitis. In numerous instances, air was noted in the biliary tree. Figure 3–115 is a transverse scan of the liver showing numerous highly echogenic circular regions. These regions followed the distribution of the biliary system. X-ray findings indicated air within the biliary tree.

Figure 3–116 is a longitudinal scan of another patient, made 6 days after a small bowel anastomosis to the biliary system was performed. The patient developed increasing abdominal pain and fever. The ultrasound scan shows a high-amplitude echo in the

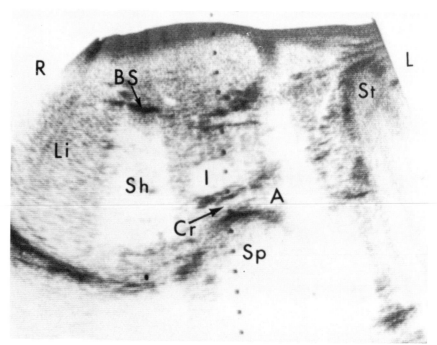

FIG 3–113.

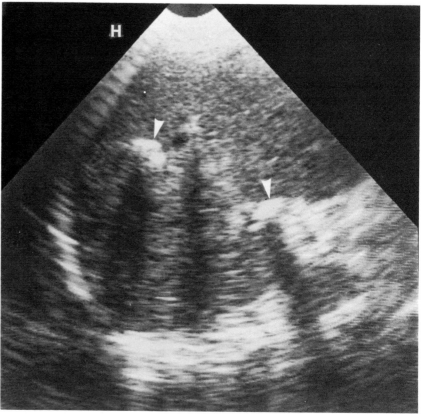

FIG 3–114.

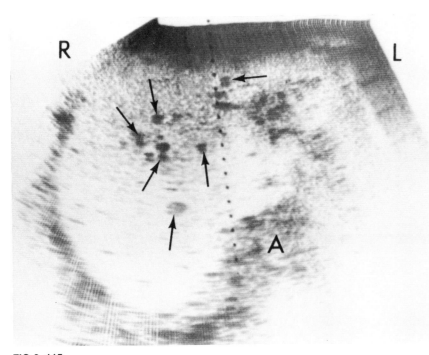

**FIG 3–115.**

region of the porta hepatis. This has a tapering artifact, consistent with air. Real-time ultrasound revealed that air was present along the course of the portal vein rather than in the biliary system. An anastomatic leak accounted for the portal vein gas. Separation of portal from biliary anatomy is extremely important in all cases.

| | | |
|---|---|---|
| **A** | = | Aorta |
| **Arrow** | = | Air in the portal vein (Fig 3–116) |
| **Arrows** | = | Air in the biliary tree (Fig 3–115) |
| **Arrowheads** | = | Intrabiliary stones |
| **BS** | = | Intrabiliary stones |
| **Cr** | = | Crus of the diaphragm |
| **H** | = | Head |
| **I** | = | Inferior vena cava |
| **L** | = | Left |
| **Li** | = | Liver |
| **R** | = | Right |
| **Sh** | = | Shadowing behind biliary stone |
| **Sp** | = | Spine |
| **St** | = | Stomach |

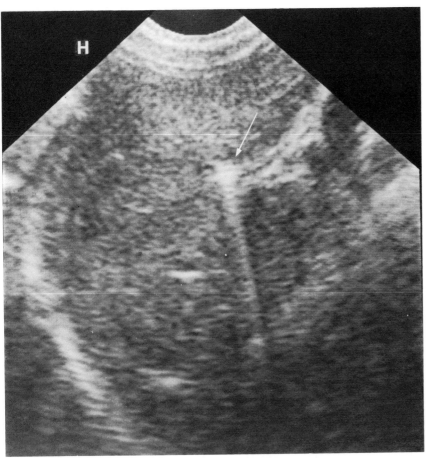

**FIG 3–116.**

## Choledochal Cyst; Congenital Stenosis of the Common Hepatic Duct

Figures 3–117 and 3–118 are ultrasound scans of a 2-month-old girl who had had jaundice since birth. A rose-bengal study suggested obstruction of the bile ducts. Ultrasound examination showed a sonolucency near the region of the common bile duct. This sonolucent area was situated just lateral to the pancreas, as is best seen in the transverse scan (Fig 3–117). There was no evidence of marked biliary dilatation. At operation a 1-cm choledochal cyst contiguous with the cystic duct was found. The gallbladder at the time of surgery was notably atretic and contracted.

Figures 3–119 and 3–120 are ultrasound scans of a 22-year-old woman with pruritus and jaundice of recent onset. She was initially thought to have jaundice secondary to hepatitis. An ultrasound examination, however, demonstrated two large fluid-filled masses in the porta hepatis. Figure 3–119 is a transverse scan in which we see two large dilated ducts situated anterior to the portal vein. Figure 3–120 is a longitudinal scan that again shows the dilated ducts anterior to the left portal vein. At operation congenital stenosis of the common hepatic duct was found. This stenotic lesion led to massive dilatation of the right and left intrahepatic ducts, which yielded the sonolucencies on ultrasound. Note the through-transmission behind these ducts on both the transverse and longitudinal scans.

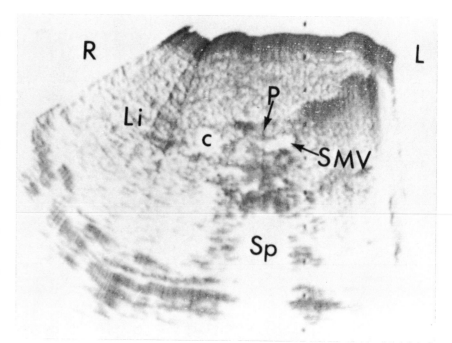

FIG 3–117.

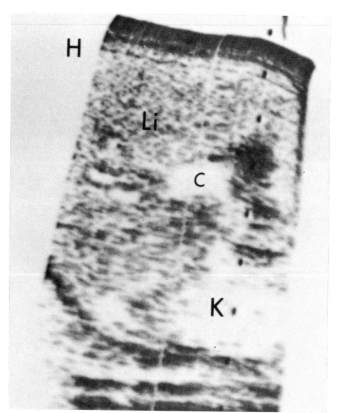

FIG 3–118.

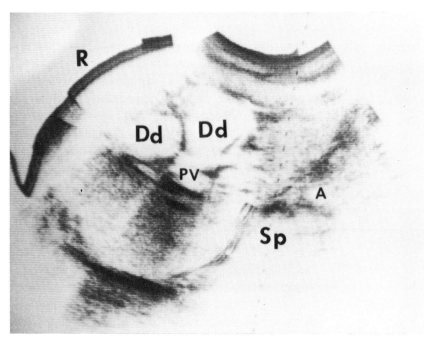

A   = Aorta
c   = Choledochal cyst
Dd  = Dilated intrahepatic ducts
F   = Foot
H   = Head
I   = Inferior vena cava
K   = Kidney
L   = Left
Li  = Liver
LPV = Left portal vein
MPV = Main portal vein
P   = Pancreas
PV  = Portal vein
R   = Right
SMV = Superior mesenteric vein
Sp  = Spine
St  = Stomach

FIG 3–119.

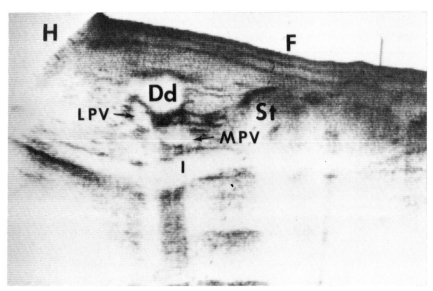

FIG 3–120.

# 4.
# Ultrasonography of the Pancreas

Dennis A. Sarti, M.D.

## Introduction

Before ultrasound, computed tomography (CT), and nuclear magnetic resonance (MR) imaging were developed the pancreas was not directly visualized except by means of selective angiography. With the development of these recent imaging modalities, the pancreas has come under closer scrutiny.

Diagnostic ultrasound permits direct visualization of the pancreas. The pancreas can be seen in its normal and abnormal state. Ultrasound gives information different from x-ray studies, since it has to do with acoustic properties. Tissue echogenicity is an important aid in differentiating various masses. Unlike CT scanning the highest quality scans are obtained in thinner patients. The major disadvantage of ultrasound imaging relates to the high reflectivity at bone and air interfaces. Adequate visualization of the pancreas is often obscured by ribs, stomach, and colon. Nevertheless, even with its inherent drawbacks, diagnostic ultrasound has found an important role in the workup of a patient with suspected pancreatic pathology. Because ultrasound is noninvasive, serial examinations are possible and allow the examiner to follow the progress of pathologic states. The tissue character information obtained from ultrasound scans can also narrow the differential possibilities.

## Normal Anatomy

In a discussion of pancreatic ultrasound examination technique, a review of the anatomic structures adjacent to the pancreas is important. Increased resolution allows visualization of small (1–2 mm) structures and reveals the characteristic echo pattern of the normal pancreas.

Numerous vascular structures are situated in close proximity to the pancreas, and their identification is necessary for adequate localization of the pancreas. Important branches of the aorta to be identified are the celiac axis, hepatic artery, splenic artery, gastroduodenal artery, superior mesenteric artery, and bilateral renal arteries. The celiac axis arises slightly cephalad to the superior portion of the body of the pancreas and then divides into three major branches: the left gastric, the common hepatic, and the splenic arteries. The first branch of the common hepatic artery is the gastroduodenal artery, which courses anterior to the common bile duct and gives off the pancreaticoduodenal artery on the medial aspect of the second portion of the duodenum, adjacent to the head of the pancreas. The splenic artery courses from the celiac axis to the spleen, usually on the dorsal cephalic surface of the pancreas, to which it gives off numerous branches. The pancreas is often 1–2 cm caudal to the splenic artery and need not be situated directly anterior to this vessel. The superior mesenteric artery originates at the aorta, approximately 1–2 cm below the celiac axis. It courses inferiorly on the posterior aspect of the junction of the head and body of the pancreas and passes anterior to the uncinate process and third portion of the duodenum. Except for the uncinate process, the pancreas lies anterior to the proximal portion and origin of the superior mesenteric artery. The renal arteries arise from the lateral aspect of the aorta, below the origin of the superior mesenteric artery and posterior to the head and body of the pancreas.

The portal venous system includes several easily identifiable vessels adjacent to the pancreas that run parallel to smaller arterial structures. The splenic vein arises from the hilum of the spleen and courses from left to right, indenting the superoposterior aspect of the pancreas. It is situated posteriorly from the midportion to the superior aspect of the pancreas, but seldom on its inferior portion. In these situations the pancreas is directly anterior to the splenic vein. The splenic vein, however, is often found cephalad to the pancreas, and transverse scans must be obtained slightly inferior to the splenic vein in order to detect pancreatic tissue.

The superior mesenteric vein drains the intestines and courses superiorly just to the right of the superior mesenteric artery. Parallel to the artery, it travels anterior to the third portion of the duodenum and uncinate process and posterior to the junction of the head and body of the pancreas. Near the origin of the superior mesenteric artery, the superior mesenteric vein joins the splenic vein, and this confluence of vessels forms the portal vein. The portal vein is approximately 8 cm long and courses superiorly and to the right, after its formation by the splenic and superior mesenteric veins. It travels upward behind the superior part of the duodenum and enters the porta hepatis posterior to the common bile duct and hepatic artery. As it enters the liver, it divides into right and left with the corresponding branches of the hepatic artery and biliary tree.

The inferior vena cava is situated anterior to the right side of the vertebral bodies and to the right of the aorta. It courses posterior to the duodenum, head of the pancreas, portal vein, and common bile duct. The left renal vein drains the left kidney and courses directly anterior to the aorta just beneath the origin of the superior mesenteric artery. This vessel has a curvilinear shape similar to the splenic vein, with which it may be confused. The left renal vein, however, is in close proximity to the anterior surface of the aorta beneath the superior mesenteric artery, whereas the splenic vein is situated anterior to the superior mesenteric artery. These vessels also can be distinguished by the vessels into which they drain: the left renal vein empties into the inferior vena cava and the splenic vein empties into the portal vein.

Other structures demonstrated by ultrasound can delineate the region of the pancreas. The antrum of the stomach appears as a "bull's-eye" when it is airless, and the pancreas is often seen directly posterior to this or slightly cephalad and posterior. The C-loop of the duodenum nestles around the head of the pancreas and often obscures visualization when it is filled with air. The pancreatic tail is difficult to visualize when the patient is supine. This is secondary to the fundus of the stomach and splenic flexure, which are often air filled. The tail of the pancreas is situated directly anterior to the left kidney and continues on into the hilum of the spleen. This anatomic relation allows visualization of the tail of the pancreas through the left kidney with the patient prone.

A thorough understanding of this anatomy is necessary for an adequate ultrasound examination. It is also very helpful in interpreting CT and MR images. Without an understanding of the above-mentioned anatomic structures, numerous diagnostic errors in interpretation of pancreatic studies will occur.

**Technique for Pancreatic Ultrasound Examination**

Numerous ultrasound studies have been undertaken to determine the most valuable technique for pancreatic examination. There is no superior method of patient preparation for pancreatic examination, although various procedures have been attempted. Adequate patient hydration is helpful in yielding high-quality studies.[1] The difficulty in visualizing the pancreas arises because of bowel air in the midabdomen. Patients with a transverse stomach are difficult to scan because this air-filled viscus is directly anterior to the pancreas. A small truncated left lobe of the liver is another important anatomic variant that yields nondiagnostic studies. The left lobe of the liver is used as an ultrasonic window for visualization of the pancreas. Since air is the major culprit, the patient is often scheduled for examination early in the morning and kept without oral intake overnight. Some limited imaging success has been reported using simethicone and other drugs.[2] Other investigators have studied the pancreas after the patient has ingested large quantities of water. These different techniques have been undertaken in an attempt to visualize the pancreas through a fluid-filled stomach or duodenum.[3-5] Some investigators have also used glucagon to decrease peristaltic activity.[3, 6] Although the patient is usually scanned in a supine position, some have attempted imaging with the patient upright or in a sitting position for better visualization of the pancreas.[3, 4] No single technical procedure is universally accepted at this time. A successful study is most dependent on individual patient anatomy. Ultrasound is usually performed before barium examinations because of the high reflectivity of barium.[7] Some penetration is possible if the barium study was performed several days earlier.[8]

The patient is initially scanned in the supine position with adequate oil or gel applied to the upper abdomen for acoustic coupling. Before the examiner searches for the pancreas, the output and sensitivity settings must be adjusted to yield maximum information from the reflected pancreatic echoes.[9] The pancreas is usually as or slightly more echogenic than the liver.[10] The increased echogenicity of the pancreas compared to the liver is thought to be due to the presence of fat and fibrotic tissue. Ultrasound echogenicity has been correlated with CT findings of fatty infiltration in the pancreas.[11] Fatty deposition within the pancreas and the patient's age are major factors contributing to increased echogenicity of the pancreas.[12] If the output and sensitivity are set at too high a level, the pancreatic echoes will be lost in the highly reflective echoes of the fatty retroperitoneum. Therefore it is necessary to adjust the liver echoes in the midranges of gray. The pancreas will then register one to two shades higher than the liver but will not be placed in the highest level of the retroperitoneal fat.

The correct transducer choice is extremely important for obtaining the highest quality pancreatic scans. A transducer must be chosen that is focused at the depth of the pancreas in the patient. Recent studies have showed that the average depth of the pancreas in most patients is approximately 5–6 cm.[13] Therefore, the choice of a transducer that places the pancreas in the focal zone will yield the highest quality scans. B-scanning and real-time imaging of the pancreas are done today. It is important that compound scanning be avoided when examining the patient with a B-mode scan unit. Single-sector scans are best for recorded images.[14] When real-time studies are performed, it is important to remember that the pancreas is a retroperitoneal organ which can undergo respiratory movements.[15] Respiratory movement of the pancreas should not be a difficulty during real-time studies but may be a problem on B-scan examinations.

On both longitudinal and transverse scans, identification of the portal vein is the first and easiest method for finding the pancreas.[16, 17] On transverse scans the left lobe of the liver is used as an ultrasonic window. The portal vein is easily identified as a large tubular structure in the right upper quadrant. The patient should take a deep breath to drive down the diaphragm and cause the left lobe of the liver to displace the lesser curvature of the stomach as inferiorly as possible. Transverse scans are continued caudally following the course of the portal vein.[18, 19] Anterior to the portal vein, the hepatic artery and common bile duct will be visualized. More inferiorly the celiac axis arising from the aorta will come into view, along with its major branches, the splenic and hepatic arteries. The portal vein joins the curvilinear sonolucency of the splenic vein, which is situated anterior to the aorta and inferior vena cava. It is at this point that the pancreatic echo pattern may come into view. The "cobblestone" echo pattern is often but not always seen anterior to the splenic vein.[1]

The portal and splenic veins are joined by the superior mesenteric vein, which is just to the right of the superior mesenteric artery. The pancreas should be seen at this level, and the head of the pancreas will be seen on the right if the duodenum is not markedly air filled. The uncinate process of the pancreas is situated posterior to the superior mesenteric vein and anterior to the inferior vena cava. Near the origin of the superior mesenteric artery, a curvilinear lucency similar in shape to the splenic vein is seen coursing directly over the aorta behind the superior mesenteric artery and joining the inferior vena cava. This is the left renal vein.[20, 21] It is closer to the aorta than the splenic vein and will not be seen until the superior mesenteric artery comes into view. The origin of the left renal vein is recognizable, because the inferior vena cava loses its oval shape and becomes pointed on its left side.

As all of these vessels come into view, the echo pattern of the pancreas will be seen anterior to them.[22] Within the confines of the pancreatic parenchymal pattern, the pancreatic duct may be visualized. The pancreatic duct may appear as a single linear echo or as a small tubular structure.[23, 24] The upper limit of the pancreatic duct in the body of the pancreas has been reported as 2 mm.[25, 26] The size of the pancreatic duct in the region of the head of the pancreas has been given the upper limit of 3 mm.[27] On the right side of the head of the pancreas at its juncture with the duodenum, a small circular sonolucency that represents the common bile duct is occasionally seen. Anterior to it is a second circular sonolucency, representing the gastroduodenal artery or one of its branches.[12]

With a small left lobe of the liver only a portion of the portal vein may be seen before it joins the splenic vein. In these instances the pancreas is often obscured by overlying bowel air. Occasionally we can visualize the pancreas by angling the transducer 15° to 20° in a caudad direction. This often will enable visualization of the pancreas in a study that would ordinarily have been aborted. Another potential ultrasonic window is the gallbladder, which can be used for visualizing the pancreatic head. Air, food, or fluid in the duodenal bulb often creates the impression of a false mass.[5, 28]

Longitudinal scans should also start with identification of the portal vein. On longitudinal scans to the right of midline, the portal vein is a circular sonolucency situated anterior to the inferior vena cava. As scanning proceeds toward the midline, the pancreatic head will come into view inferior to the portal vein and anterior to the inferior vena cava. The common bile duct occasionally can be seen as a tubular sonolucency coursing posterior to the pancreatic head.

As scans progress toward the midline, the portal vein is joined by the superior mesenteric vein, which is seen as a longitudinal sonolucent tubular structure posterior to the neck of the pancreas. If the stomach is collapsed and airless, a "bull's-eye" is often seen anterior to the body of the pancreas. If the stomach is fluid filled, this will appear as a sonolucent mass. Fur-

ther scans to the left show the splenic vein as a circular sonolucency posterior to the cephalad portion of the pancreas. The portal and splenic veins can be differentiated on longitudinal scans only if the examiner knows the location of the superior mesenteric vein. As we progress past the midline to the left, a long posterior tubular structure representing the aorta will be easily recognized. The origins of the celiac axis and superior mesenteric artery can be seen off the anterior aortic wall with the pancreas situated directly anterior to the superior mesenteric artery.[1, 21, 29] The left renal vein appears as a slit-like sonolucency between the aorta and superior mesenteric artery just caudal to the origin of the superior mesenteric artery.

The pancreatic head and body are fairly consistent in location, but there is variability in the location of the tail. The tail is most often situated cephalad in the splenic hilum; but it may also course straight laterally, anterior to the left kidney, or, less commonly, turn inferiorly. Because of this axis, scans along the length of the pancreas are not possible unless the transducer plane is aligned parallel to the long axis of the pancreas.[30]

Because of air in the left upper quadrant, the pancreatic tail is difficult to visualize. As mentioned earlier, a fluid-filled stomach may act as an ultrasonic window.[14] The tail of the pancreas can also be visualized when the patient is examined in the prone position. Either posterior or coronal scans often will show the tail of the pancreas anterior to the left kidney and medial to the hilum of the spleen. When the left kidney is absent, the tail of the pancreas may be displaced into the left renal fossa.[31]

The size of the pancreas has been determined from several studies. The anteroposterior diameter of the head of the pancreas is approximately 2.2–2.7 cm, while the body is approximately 1.8–2.2 cm.[32, 33] The head and body of the pancreas are seen in a higher percentage of cases than is the tail of the pancreas. The head and body of the pancreas are seen in approximately 70%–80% of cases, while the tail is seen in approximately 30%–40%.[34]

## Ultrasound and CT Evaluation of the Pancreas

Early comparison studies of ultrasound and CT of the pancreas tended to yield fairly similar results.[35–38] Early reports stated that ultrasound and CT were comparable in evaluation of the pancreas but that further study was needed. It was usually thought that CT did better in the fat patient whereas ultrasound was more useful in the thin patient. The obvious advantage CT had over ultrasound was in the region of air and bone. CT was found to be of greater value in the tail of the pancreas because of the inherent difficulties of sonographic imaging of the left upper quadrant.

More recent comparative studies have indicated that CT has a higher sensitivity and diagnostic accuracy in detecting pancreatic pathology.[39-43] These studies indicate that a certain percentage of ultrasound examinations are nondiagnostic because of air in the upper abdomen. In these instances CT can be used to evaluate such patients because air is not a problem with that modality. In a comparison of diagnostic examinations with both modalities, CT has been reported to have higher accuracy.[40, 41] In the next section, the usefulness of CT and ultrasound in diagnosing several pathologic entities will be discussed and compared.

Different opinions have been expressed as to where ultrasound fits into the workup of a patient with suspected pancreatic disease. In many institutions ultrasound is still the initial imaging modality. If an ultrasound study is positive, the diagnosis, such as pseudocyst, carcinoma or pancreatitis, can be made. However, if the ultrasound study is negative, some suggest that CT be performed. The sequential use of these imaging modalities has been proposed because of the number of false negative ultrasound studies. Some groups suggest performing CT first in nonjaundiced patients and ultrasound first in jaundiced patients.[38] Since ultrasound permits good visualization of vessels and tubular structures, the workup of the jaundiced patient is the ideal setting for ultrasonographic evaluation of the upper abdomen. CT is better able to display the complete size and extent of a disease process such as pancreatitis. In patients with pancreatitis, bowel air will often inhibit visualization of the entire extent of the disease on ultrasound.

Both CT and ultrasound have had a dramatic effect on the role of angiography in the workup of pancreatic patients.[44-46] Angiography is no longer used as a screening tool for evaluating patients. CT and ultrasound are used to screen patients suspected of having pancreatic pathology. Depending on the results of these two modalities, a pancreatic angiogram may be scheduled or bypassed. Angiography has been sug-

gested in patients who have a potentially resectable pancreatic carcinoma, or in a patient with a normal or equivocal ultrasound or CT examination.[45] Other groups think that pancreatic angiography is unnecessary in most cases because CT, ultrasound, endoscopic retrograde cholangiopancreatography, and transhepatic cholangiography can answer most clinical questions.[44] It has become apparent in recent years that both ultrasound and CT have dramatically changed the workup of a patient with suspected pancreatic disease.

## Pancreatitis

Acute and chronic pancreatitis may be caused by numerous conditions and disease processes. Among the most common causes are alcoholism, gallstones, trauma, and peptic ulcer disease. Less common causes are complications of pregnancy, mumps, diffuse vascular diseases such as periarteritis nodosa, essential hyperlipemia, hereditary pancreatitis, and hyperparathyoidism. Elevated amylase levels and white blood cell counts are the pertinent laboratory findings. X-ray films show a "sentinel" loop or, in chronic pancreatitis, calcification in the pancreatic bed. Another finding on plain film x-ray studies of pancreatic patients is the renal "halo" sign.[47] This is a lucent rim around the left kidney, which is caused by enhancement of the perirenal fat secondary to edema from pancreatitis. The retroperitoneal exudate in the left anterior perirenal space is seen as a soft tissue density on x-ray studies. This allows the fat between the kidney and the perirenal space to stand out on plain films.

Acute pancreatitis can be diffuse or localized. Alcoholism most often results in the generalized form. The ultrasound changes in pancreatitis involve increased size and decreased echogenicity.[48] Diffuse edematous involvement changes the echogenicity of the pancreas, which appears more sonolucent than in the uninvolved state.[49-51] The normal liver-pancreas echo relationship is reversed. Because of increased pancreatic sonolucency, the liver is more echogenic than the pancreas. Since a cirrhotic liver manifests increased echogenicity, this echo relationship can be difficult to assess in the alcoholic patient. A normal pancreas will appear less echogenic when the liver is cirrhotic.

Pancreatic size may be increased in acute pancreatitis. This has been documented on both ultrasound and CT.[52, 53] However, the possibility of pancreatic carcinoma must also be considered when localized pancreatic enlargement is seen. In these instances, the clinical history is usually helpful in separating the two entities.

Comparison studies of CT and ultrasound in the diagnosis of pancreatitis have indicated that CT has a higher diagnostic accuracy. The discrimination usually arises because of the number of nondiagnostic ultrasound studies due to bowel air. CT is thought to yield a better view of the entire pancreas.[52] Very often the tail of the pancreas is not seen on ultrasound, and the tail is where much of the edema of pancreatitis occurs. The left anterior perirenal space can be a site of edema and fluid collection. This is well documented on CT.[53, 54] Acute pancreatitis is often associated with fluid collections.[55] These can be diagnosed from both CT and ultrasound studies. Well-circumscribed fluid collections often are secondary to pseudocysts, which will be discussed later. However, early fluid collections in pancreatitis are most likely due to pancreatic secretions which enter the lesser sac, left anterior perirenal space, or adjacent to the surface of the pancreas.[55] Acute pancreatitis can lead to aneurysms of the adjacent arteries.[56] Examination of the vascular structures in the pancreatic bed is important. Gallbladder wall thickening has also been reported in cases of acute pancreatitis[57] and is attributable to the adjacent inflammatory edema of the pancreas and the surrounding organs.

Pancreatitis in children has a similar ultrasound appearance as in the adult. Pediatric ultrasound examination usually yields high-quality scans because of the lack of retroperitoneal fat in most children compared to adults. Ultrasound is very helpful, especially when the study is positive in a child with abdominal discomfort.[58] As in the adult, the size of the pancreas will be increased and the echogenicity decreased.[59]

Chronic pancreatitis may be diffuse or localized. The diffuse variety is usually associated with alcohol abuse, whereas localized pancreatitis is usually secondary to obstruction of the pancreatic duct. The normal cobblestone pancreatic appearance and echogenicity are lost. The pancreas will have an irregular, echogenic appearance due to fibrosis and early calcification.[49, 60] The borders are often irregular, and distinction from neoplasm is extremely difficult. When

the pancreas is calcified, it is difficult if not impossible to localize on ultrasound. Plain film x-ray studies and CT are much more advantageous since calcification is not a problem with these two modalities. The increased echogenicity seen in chronic pancreatitis is thought to be secondary to fibrotic and calcific changes.

Similar ultrasound findings are seen in children with cystic fibrosis where increased fibrous tissue occurs. It has been shown that the longer a patient has cystic fibrosis, the more fibrotic changes occur in the pancreas. Ultrasound examination of children of different ages reveals that as patient age increases, pancreatic echogenicity also increases, because of the long-standing cystic fibrosis.[61, 62] The ultrasound findings in children with cystic fibrosis and in patients with chronic pancreatitis are similar. The size of the pancreas is decreased, but the echo amplitude is markedly increased. In acute episodes of pancreatitis in patients with cystic fibrosis, the pancreas is more edematous and increases slightly in size.[63] In the later stages of cystic fibrosis, the pancreas is of markedly increased echogenicity. CT studies will often reveal complete fatty replacement of the entire pancreas.[46] In an evaluation of the severity of pancreatic involvement in cystic fibrosis, increased echogenicity is the most important ultrasound parameter. Size measurements are of no value in determining the severity of the disease. A hyperechoic pancreas is dramatically prominent in patients with severe cystic fibrosis.[65]

## Pancreatic Pseudocysts

Pseudocysts occur in 11%–18% of patients with acute pancreatitis. Before ultrasound became available, the diagnosis of a pancreatic pseudocyst was made by palpation or an upper gastrointestinal (GI) tract series. Although these methods show the position of a mass, they do not necessarily confirm its nature. Carcinoma, edema, abscess, or other mass should be ruled out. By revealing whether a mass is fluid or solid, ultrasound can indicate whether or not the mass is secondary to a pseudocyst.[66–69] Successful surgical drainage of a pancreatic pseudocyst is dependent on cyst wall maturation for anastomosis to the GI tract. A 4–6-week period is necessary for adequate cyst wall maturity. In the past, however, cyst-wall maturity was verified by a palpating hand or the

GI radiologist's eye. With ultrasound we can follow serially the development and evolution of pancreatic pseudocysts.

Pancreatic pseudocysts are mainly sonolucent masses with enhanced through-transmission. Their borders are highly echogenic and somewhat thicker and more irregular than the borders of simple cysts of the kidney or ovary. They may be unilocular or multilocular, a distinction which is important to determine for surgical drainage.[70] Debris secondary to necrosis and enzymatic action on surrounding tissue presents as echogenic regions within a pseudocyst. In these instances, a solid lesion of the pancreas is suspected. Such unusual locations as the neck and anterior thigh have been reported as sites for pseudocyst migration along tissue planes.[71] Most pseudocysts, however, will be found in close proximity to the pancreatic bed and in contact with the stomach, duodenum, liver, kidneys, and spleen.

When a sonolucent structure is noted in the upper abdomen, it is important to rule out a fluid-filled loop of bowel before prematurely diagnosing a pseudocyst.[72] There are several ways to rule out a fluid-filled loop of bowel. If only B-scan equipment is available, the examination is repeated 24 hours later. However, with real-time imaging bowel loops can easily be ruled out by documenting peristaltic activity. Fluid in the stomach, duodenum, proximal jejunum, and colon is easily diagnosed with modern real-time ultrasound equipment. Bowel loops will pose a problem only in the case of an ileus. This can often be ruled out by evaluating the mucosal lining of the bowel loops. Other fluid-filled masses in the upper abdomen must be considered, including vascular aneurysms.[56, 73] Usually cardiac pulsations can be visualized on real-time ultrasound. Lesions such as bile leaks, gallbladder rupture, hepatic and echinococcal cysts, cystadenomas of the pancreas, and splenic and renal cysts should be considered.[74, 75] The entity of liquefactive necrosis of the pancreas has been described. In this entity the pancreatic bed itself is necrotic and can appear quite sonolucent. It will give a confusing picture. On ultrasound and CT this may be misinterpreted as a pseudocyst of the pancreas.[76]

Occasionally pancreatic cysts in the pancreatic bed and surrounding region will have an unusual appearance. They can arise within the wall of adjacent intestine.[77] An elongated tubular pseudocyst of the pancreas has been reported that mimicked a dilated pancreatic duct.[78] Pseudocysts in the region of the kidney may be misinterpreted as renal cysts rather than pancreatic pseudocysts.[79] Correlation with the clinical history and amylase level determinations will avoid this mistaken diagnosis. Fluid in the region of the pancreatic bed should not automatically lead to the diagnosis of a pseudocyst. Fluid, such as ascites, can collect in areas around the pancreas without having a thickened wall typical of a pseudocyst.[55]

The diagnosis of pancreatic pseudocysts has increased dramatically since the development of ultrasound and CT scanning. Both modalities are thought to be quite useful in this disease entity. A recent study indicated that CT is more accurate than ultrasound in detecting pancreatic pseudocysts, although ultrasound is quite useful.[80] CT is thought to be more accurate in the diagnosis of pseudocysts because it allows the entire abdomen to be imaged without concern for bowel air. However, pseudocysts are quite easily diagnosed on ultrasound and can be followed serially because of the noninvasive and relatively inexpensive nature of ultrasound.

We have encountered several cases of spontaneous regression of pseudocysts without the expected morbidity and mortality. Approximately 50% of ruptured pseudocysts drain into the peritoneal cavity and 50% drain into the GI tract.[67, 81] A 50% mortality is associated with spontaneous regression into the GI tract and a 70% mortality is associated with decompression into the peritoneal cavity.[82, 83] These figures were reported before ultrasound became available as a routine diagnostic tool. Serial ultrasound examinations have shown that in many more cases than was originally estimated, pseudocysts drain spontaneously without adverse effect. Serial examinations have also demonstrated the rapid development of pseudocysts in patients with acute pancreatitis. An acute episode of pain in a patient with pancreatitis may signal imminent pseudocyst development, and serial ultrasound examinations are indicated. We followed up a patient in whom a pseudocyst developed within 6 days after the last negative ultrasound examination.[84] The pseudocyst wall was mature enough to anastomose to a loop of jejunum 21 days after the pseudocyst began to develop. A period of 4–6 weeks is thought to be necessary for adequate wall maturation. Other reports have since documented the spontaneous regression of pancreatic pseudocysts on both CT and ultrasound in adults and children.[85, 86] These reports have resulted in a more conservative approach to the management of pancreatic pseudocysts. Although uncommon, pancreatic pseudocysts also occur in children, most often after blunt trauma. Ultrasound has proved effective in the management of these cases.[87]

Congenital pancreatic cysts range in size from microscopic to 3–5 cm and are secondary to the anomalous development of pancreatic cysts. Low cuboidal epithelial cells line these cysts, which are found in conjunction with polycystic disease of the liver, kidney, or ovary. When ultrasound detects multiple cysts in the liver or kidneys, the pancreatic bed should be examined. Often it will be normal. Occasionally, numerous cystic lesions also will be evident in the pancreas.

Retention cysts are smaller than congenital cysts, rarely exceeding several centimeters in diameter. They are usually secondary to obstruction of the pancreatic ducts and are rarely of clinical significance.

## Pancreatic Abscess

Pancreatic abscesses may arise as a direct extension of a neighboring infection such as perforated peptic ulcer, acute appendicitis, or acute cholecystitis. Bacteria may reach the pancreas through the lymph system. The ultrasonographic appearance depends on the amount of suppurative material and debris. If abundant suppuration is present, the mass will appear sonolucent. The walls of an abscess are usually thick, irregular, and highly echogenic. If air bubbles are present, they yield a highly echogenic region and occasional shadows, depending on their size. CT has been found to be superior to ultrasound in the diagnosis of pancreatic abscess. In abscess formation, air may be present that will obscure visualization on ultrasound scans. However, on CT, gas collection in the region of the pancreas may be a definitive feature of infection in the area. This was seen in only approximately 29% of patients studied with CT.[88] It was not possible to distinguish infected from noninfected pseudocysts or pancreatic abscesses by using other CT criteria. The only finding suggestive of a pancreatic abscess was air in the pancreatic region. Percutaneous needle aspiration is helpful in the diagnosis. This will be discussed in a later section.

## Pancreatic Neoplasms

Carcinoma of the pancreas has been increasing in frequency and now is the fourth most common malignancy. This neoplasm is usually detected late, and medical intervention has not markedly improved survival. Earliest detection occurs in the head of the pancreas where the common bile duct is obstructed. Carcinomas occur twice as often in the head of the pancreas as in the body and tail. The gross specimen is a gray-white scirrhous homogeneous mass that silently grows to a large size. The normal cobblestone appearance of the pancreas is lost and replaced by a less echogenic, coarser mass.[60, 89] There is enlargement of the pancreas and often an irregular, nodular border.[51]

CT and ultrasound have both been used in the detection of pancreatic neoplasm. When sonographic visualization of the pancreas is adequate, both CT and ultrasound are similar in diagnostic accuracy, although CT is slightly better. The diagnostic accuracy of CT has been reported at 96% versus 84% for ultrasound.[90] When the ultrasound examination is technically good, it is quite accurate. However, if the ultrasound examination is not satisfactory, then CT is recommended since imaging will not be obscured by bone or air.

Ultrasound demonstrates not only a mass but also distortion of parenchymal texture. CT findings of pancreatic carcinoma include a pancreatic mass, lucent areas within the mass, dilatation of the pancreatic and common bile ducts, hepatic metastasis, atrophy of the tail of the pancreas, and periaortic lymphadenopathy.[91, 92] Small lesions of the pancreas are difficult to detect with CT. One is usually looking for a mass or contour deformity of the pancreas. Ultrasound can reveal a parenchymal change even before there are any changes in size or contour of the pancreas.[93] Therefore, ultrasound has been found to be more informative in the diagnosis of small and resectable lesions. In fact, ultrasound, ERCP, and cytology have been found to be most reliable for detecting small resectable pancreatic carcinoma, while CT has a higher sensitivity for unresectable lesions, especially in the region of the tail of the pancreas.[94] Newer CT technology may improve the diagnosis of small lesions. If a bolus injection of contrast agent is given and dynamic CT scanning is performed, the tumor vascularity can be evaluated, which allows the boundary between the tumor and the normal pancreas to be visualized. This technique has increased the CT detection of small tumors in the pancreas.[95, 96] Other masses in the pancreatic region and upper abdomen may be mistaken for pancreatic carcinoma on both ultrasound and CT.[97–99] These masses include primary tumors of other organs, metastasis, intussusception, bowel infarction, ileus, abscess, pancreatitis, and pseudocyst.

Ultrasonographic detection of neoplasm is easiest in the pancreatic head, where displacement of numerous surrounding vessels is often noted. Tumors as small as 2 cm have been detected.[100] The smallest lesions are usually found in the region of the uncinate process, and lesions may be detected earliest in that region because of the prominent anatomy in the area. Ultrasound can reveal parenchymal changes in this region before contour deformity is identified. This is not the case for CT.

A dilated common bile duct signals the immediate need for meticulous scanning of the head of the pancreas to determine the cause of obstruction. A dilated pancreatic duct may also be associated with tumors of the head of the pancreas. It appears as a tubular sonolucency within the pancreas anterior to the splenic vein, with which it may be confused. By demonstrating that it does not join the portal vein and that it is contained within the pancreatic echoes, ultrasound can confirm pancreatic duct dilatation.[101] As was discussed in the section on normal anatomy, the pancreatic duct has a fairly characteristic appearance on ultrasound. It appears as a linear echo throughout the length of the pancreas up to a small 2-mm tube.[23–27] Ultrasound is an excellent means of visualization of the numerous tubular structures in the upper abdomen. Dilatation of the biliary tree is quite easily documented by ultrasound. In both jaundiced and nonjaundiced patients, ultrasound will image a dilated biliary tree if it is secondary to pancreatic tumor. In fact, early detection of pancreatic carcinoma is first suggested from visualization of the dilated biliary tree in the anicteric patient.[102] Once a dilated biliary tree is identified, visualization of a dilated pancreatic duct will yield confirmatory evidence. A dilated pancreatic duct will also appear as a tubular lucent structure in the soft tissue of the pancreas on CT scans.[103, 104] A dilated pancreatic duct may appear as a large tubular structure within the echoes of the pancreas on ultrasound. However, it will occasionally have a cystic appearance and may be mistaken for a pseudocyst on

ultrasound.[105] The important point to be made is that any time an unusual tubular structure is visualized in the region of the pancreatic bed, the possibility of pancreatic carcinoma should immediately come to mind. Close scrutiny of the pancreatic head will often disclose a small lesion that would otherwise be missed.

Tumors of the tail are more difficult to detect because of air in the stomach and splenic flexure. They are best seen through the left kidney or the spleen. An increased size of the pancreatic tail alone is not sufficient evidence. Angiography performed on several patients with increased pancreative tail size but normal echogenicity has been negative. This is most likely due to an anteroposterior orientation to the tail as it drapes over the aorta and courses straight back toward the left kidney. Peripancreatic adenopathy can often be confused for pancreatic masses. Lymphadenopathy on ultrasound usually presents as a relatively lucent mass similar in appearance to pancreatic carcinoma.[106, 107] Such a mass may be difficult to distinguish from pancreatic carcinoma. CT may play a helpful role in separating the pancreas from the surrounding adenopathy.

Percutaneous aspiration biopsy under ultrasonographic guidance has been found to be useful in the diagnosis and may render laparotomy unnecessary.[50, 108–110] Percutaneous aspiration biopsy and percutaneous drainage of the pancreas duct and biliary tree will be discussed in more detail in the next section. Ultrasound also may be of assistance in planning radiation therapy and in following tumor response.[111]

Islet cell tumors are difficult to detect because of their small size. However, ultrasound has been effective in evaluating islet cell tumors because of the parenchymal change compared to normal pancreatic texture.[112, 113] Lesions as small as 7 mm have been detected on ultrasound scans.[114] There is differing opinion as to whether islet cell tumors are better detected on CT, arteriography, or sonography.[115–117] A case can be made for any of the three modalities. The most prudent course of action in patients suspected of having islet cell lesions would be to start with ultrasound, since it is the least expensive examination. If the ultrasound examination is positive, the workup can stop here. If the ultrasound examination is negative, CT followed by angiography would be suggested. In some cases in which all three studies have been negative but there was still a high clinical suspicion, intraoperative real-time ultrasound has localized small pancreatic lesions.[118]

Cystadenomas and cystadenocarcinomas have an ultrasound appearance similar to that of a multiloculated pseudocyst. The mass is mainly sonolucent with numerous curvilinear echoes arising from septa coursing through it.[119] A higher echogenicity may be present about these septa, secondary to the mucous secretions. Although cystadenomas cannot be distinguished from cystadenocarcinomas with certainty, there are suggestive findings on ultrasound and CT which may indicate malignancy. Macrocystic adenomas are usually premalignant. If the cysts are larger than 2 cm on ultrasound and CT, the possibility of malignancy should be entertained. Microcystic adenomas are usually without malignant potential. When cysts 2 cm or less are detected on ultrasound and CT, this often represents a benign lesion.[120–122]

## Percutaneous and Intraoperative Procedures

Ultrasound has been used with increasing frequency in percutaneous biopsy and intraoperative detection of pancreatic lesions. Both CT and ultrasound can be used for guidance of fine-needle biopsy of pancreatic masses.[123–126] When mass lesions are easily visualized on ultrasound, the mass may be located for needle placement. Thin-needle aspiration biopsies have decreased the number of operations required for definitive diagnosis of pancreatic carcinoma. With real-time transducers, one can follow the needle as it moves into the center of the lesion. If bowel gas is present, CT can be used for needle placement.

Thin-needle placement into dilated bile ducts or the pancreatic duct is also possible with ultrasound guidance.[127–130] When a dilated tubular structure is identified in the upper abdomen, real-time ultrasound can be used to guide the placement of a thin needle into the tubular structure. Drainage of the structure is possible along with placement of an indwelling catheter for therapeutic purposes.

Cystic masses are easily identifiable on ultrasound scans. Therapeutic percutaneous aspiration of cystic masses such as pseudocysts and pancreatic abscesses is possible with ultrasound guidance.[131–134] Many times surgery can be avoided with percutaneous aspiration of the cystic masses. Occasionally pancreatic pseudocysts may have to be drained several times before complete resolution occurs. A recent report discussed the ultrasonographically guided percutaneous implantation of I-125 for therapeutic reasons in cancer therapy.[135] The radioactive material is placed in the center of the lesion under ultrasonographic guidance. Complications of percutaneous thin-needle placement have been rare. However, malignant seeding of tumor along the track after thin-needle aspiration biopsy has been reported.[136, 137] A fatal necrotizing pancreatitis has also been reported after thin-needle aspiration biopsy of the pancreas.[138]

The intraoperative use of ultrasound has also increased in recent years. Many lesions of the pancreas are too small to be detected before operation. Even at operation, the surgeon may not be able to palpate a small lesion in the pancreas. The surface of the pancreas can look quite normal. With intraoperative ultrasound, small lesions such as insulinomas or pseudocysts can be located by their texture change.[134, 139, 140] Biliary or renal stones and the degree of tumor spread can be more readily detected on intraoperative ultrasound than by the palpating hand.[141, 142]

## Pitfalls in Ultrasonographic Examination of the Pancreas

Numerous problems can arise during the course of an ultrasonographic pancreatic examination that may lead to erroneous diagnoses and interpretations. A common error arises from the false appearance of a mass in the region of the pancreatic bed. The false mass is often seen around the head of the pancreas and is caused by air or food in the duodenum. It is important to analyze the orientation of the echoes to determine where the transducer was at the time of scanning. The criterion of through-transmission is also extremely important in ruling out a mass lesion.[128]

Another common error that deserves mention is the misinterpretation of a fluid-filled loop of bowel as a pseudocyst. This is most likely if the stomach is filled with fluid or food. Since the stomach is in close proximity to the pancreatic bed, any sonolucency caused by this structure can easily be misinterpreted as pancreatic pseudocyst. Real-time examination allows one to detect peristaltic activity.

Many patients will have had surgery before an ultrasound examination. Since there is a preponderance of fibrous tissue within scars, high attenuation occurs. When scanning a patient over the region of a scar, we must be aware that the scan deep to the scar will be less echogenic because of the marked attenuation of the ultrasound beam through the scar tissue. This can often give the appearance of a more lucent mass. Pancreatic tissue will appear less echogenic than the remaining, normal-appearing pancreas and often is confused for edema and neoplasm. This mistake can be avoided by scanning on either side of the scar with angulation over the area of interest.

Pancreatic echogenicity is affected by the structures situated directly anterior to the pancreas. On ultrasound a normal-appearing pancreas will have normal structures situated anteriorly. Whenever the liver is cirrhotic, it has increased fibrous tissue which attenuates sound. This will give a higher amplitude echo to the liver but will also yield lower amplitude echoes to the pancreas because of the attenuation prior to the sound waves reaching the pancreatic tissue and returning to the transducer. Therefore, a mistaken diagnosis of pancreatitis may be made if the left lobe of the liver is cirrhotic. Furthermore, a fluid-filled mass anterior to the pancreas, such as a pseudocyst, loculated ascites, or fluid-filled stomach, will cause the pancreas to appear more echogenic than usual. This appearance is secondary to the lack of attenuation by a fluid-filled mass. The decreased attenuation will result in a higher amplitude echo returning from the pancreas than is seen in the normal situation. Therefore, a possible erroneous diagnosis of increased echogenicity suggesting chronic pancreatitis may be made. An awareness of the structures anterior to the pancreatic tissue will help avoid these mistakes.

These numerous pitfalls can be very disturbing, especially in the early attempts at pancreatic evaluation. With experience, however, they become less troublesome. By paying attention to technique and some basic concepts of physics, the examiner can avoid most of these pitfalls.

## References

1. Leopold G: Echographic study of the pancreas. *JAMA* 1975; 232:287.
2. Sommer G, Filly R: Patient preparation to decrease bowel gas: Evaluation by ultrasonic measurement. *JCU* 1977; 5:87.
3. Bowie JD, MacMahon H: Improved techniques in pancreatic sonography. *Semin Ultrasound* 1980; 1:170.
4. MacMahon H, Bowie JD, Beezhold C: Erect scanning of pancreas using a gastric window. *AJR* 1979; 132:587.
5. Oliva L, Biggi E, Derchi L, et al: Ultrasonic anatomy of the fluid-filled duodenum. *JCU* 1981; 9:245.
6. Weighall SL, Wolfman NT, Watson NE: The fluid-filled stomach: A new sonic window. *JCU* 1979; 7:353.
7. Leopold G, Asher WN: Deleterious effects of gastrointestinal contrast material on abdominal echography. *Radiology* 1972; 104:365.
8. Sarti DA, Lazere A: Re-examination of the deleterious effects of gastrointestinal contrast material on abdominal echography. *Radiology* 1978; 126:231.
9. Filly RA, Carlsen E: Newer ultrasonic anatomy in the upper abdomen: II. The major systemic veins and arteries with a special note on localization of the pancreas. *JCU* 1976; 4:91.
10. Filly RA, London SS: The normal pancreas: Acoustic characteristics and frequency of imaging. *JCU* 1979; 7:121.
11. Marks WM, Filly RA, Callen PW: Ultrasonic evaluation of normal pancreatic echogenicity and its relationship to fat deposition. *Radiology* 1980; 137:475.
12. Worthen NJ, Beabeau D: Normal pancreatic echogenicity: Relation to age and body fat. *AJR* 1982; 139:1095.
13. Kwa A, Bowie JD: Transducer selection for pancreatic ultrasound based on skin to pancreas distance in the supine and upright position. *Radiology* 1980; 134:541.
14. Sample WF, Po JB, Gray RK, et al: Gray scale ultrasonography: Techniques in pancreatic scanning. *Appl Radiol* 1975; 4:63.
15. Bryan PJ, Custar S, Haaga JR, et al: Respiratory movement of the pancreas: An ultrasonic study. *J Ultrasound Med* 1984; 3:317.
16. Burger J, Blauenstein VW: Current aspects of ultrasonic scanning of the pancreas. *AJR* 1974; 122:406.
17. Sarti DA, Lindstrom JR, Tabrisky J: Correlation of the ultrasonic appearance of the portal vein with abdominal arteriography. *JCU* 1975; 3:263.
18. Carlsen E, Filly RA: Newer ultrasonographic anatomy in the upper abdomen: I. The portal hepatic venous anatomy. *JCU* 1976; 4:85.
19. Sanders RC, Conrad MR, White RI: Normal

and abnormal upper abdominal venous structures as seen by ultrasound. *AJR* 1977; 128:657.

20. Leopold G: Gray scale ultrasonic angiography of the upper abdomen. *Radiology* 1975; 117:665.

21. Sample WF: Techniques for improved delineation of normal anatomy of the upper abdomen and high retroperitoneum with gray scale ultrasound. *Radiology* 1977; 124:197.

22. Weinstein BJ, Weinstein DP: Sonographic anatomy of the pancreas. *Semin Ultrasound* 1980; 1:156.

23. Weinstein DP, Weinstein BJ: Ultrasonic demonstration of the pancreatic duct: An analysis of 41 cases. *Radiology* 1979; 130:729.

24. Parulekar SG: Ultrasonic evaluation of the pancreatic duct. *JCU* 1980; 8:457.

25. Bryan PJ: Appearance of the normal pancreatic duct: A study using real time ultrasound. *JCU* 1982; 10:63.

26. Lawson TL, Berland LL, Foley WD, et al: Ultrasonic visualization of the pancreatic duct. *Radiology* 1982; 144:865.

27. Hadidi A: Pancreatic duct diameter: Sonographic measurement in normal subjects. *JCU* 1983; 11:17.

28. Freimanis AK, Asher WM: Development of diagnostic criteria in echographic study of abdominal lesions. *AJR* 1970; 108:747.

29. Skolnick ML, Royal DR: Normal upper abdominal vasculature: A study correlating contact B-scanning with arteriography and gross anatomy. *JCU* 1976; 4:399.

30. Ghorashi B, Rector WR: Gray scale sonographic anatomy of the pancreas. *JCU* 1977; 5:25.

31. Charnsangavej C, Elkin M: Displacement of the tail of the pancreas in the absence of the left kidney. *Radiology* 1980; 137:156.

32. Haber K, Freimanis AK, Asher WM: Demonstration and dimensional analysis of the normal pancreas with gray scale echography. *AJR* 1976; 126:624.

33. Niederau C, Sonnenberg A, Miller J, et al: Sonographic measurements of the normal liver, spleen, pancreas, and portal vein. *Radiology* 1983; 149:537.

34. Arger PH, Mulhern CB, Bonavita JA, et al: Analysis of pancreatic sonography in suspected pancreatic diseases. *JCU* 1979; 7:91.

35. Lee JKT, Stanley RJ, Melson GL, et al: Pancreatic imaging by ultrasound and computed tomography. *Radiol Clin North Am* 1979; 17:105.

36. Simeone JF, Simonds BD: Normal anatomy of the pancreas by computed tomography and diagnostic ultrasound. *Clin Diagn Ultrasound* 1979; 1:73.

37. Sample WF, Sarti DA: Diagnosis of pancreatic disease by ultrasound and computed tomography. *Clin Diagn Ultrasound* 1979; 1:85.

38. Katz RJ, Behan M, Herbstman C, et al: Sonography and CT of the pancreas. *Semin Ultrasound* 1980; 1:209.

39. Ferrucci JT, Wittenberg J: A comprehensive approach for diagnosing pancreatic disease. *Radiology* 1980; 136:255.

40. Kamin PD, Bernardino ME, Wallace S, et al: Comparison of ultrasound and computed tomography in the detection of pancreatic malignancy. *Cancer* 1980; 46:2410.

41. McCain AH, Berkman WA, Bernardino ME: Pancreatic sonography: Past and present. *JCU* 1984; 12:325.

42. Hessel SJ, Siegelman SS, McNeil BJ, et al: A prospective evaluation of computed tomography and ultrasound of the pancreas. *Radiology* 1982; 143:129.

43. Foley WD, Stewart ET, Lawson TL, et al: Computed tomography, ultrasonography, and endoscopic retrograde cholangiopancreatography in the diagnosis of pancreatic disease: A comparative study. *Gastrointest Radiol* 1980; 5:29.

44. Stanley RJ, Sagel SS, Evens RG: The impact of new imaging methods on pancreatic arteriography. *Radiology* 1980; 136:251.

45. Freeney PC, Ball TJ, Ryan J: Impact on new diagnostic imaging methods on pancreatic angiography. *AJR* 1979; 133:619.

46. Levin DC, Wilson R, Abrams HL: The changing role of pancreatic arteriography in the era of computed tomography. *Radiology* 1980; 136:245.

47. Susman N, Hammerman AM, Cohen E: The renal halo sign in pancreatitis. *Radiology* 1982; 142:323.

48. Sarti DA, King W: The ultrasonic findings in inflammatory pancreatic disease. *Semin Ultrasound* 1980; 1:178.

49. Doust BD: Ultrasonic examination of the pancreas. *Radiol Clin North Am* 1975; 13:467.

50. Hancke S: Ultrasonic scanning of the pancreas. *JCU* 1976; 4:223.

51. Stuber JL, Templeton AW, Bishop K: Sonographic diagnosis of pancreatic lesions. *AJR* 1972; 116:406.

52. Silverstein W, Isikoff MB, Hill MC, et al: Diagnostic imaging of acute pancreatitis: Prospective study using CT and sonography. *AJR* 1981; 137:497.

53. Hill MC, Barkin J, Isikoff MB, et al: Acute pancreatitis: Clinical vs CT findings. *AJR* 1982; 139:263.

54. Nicholson RL: Abnormalities of the perinephric fascia and fat in pancreatitis. *Radiology* 1981; 139:125.

55. Donovan PJ, Sanders RC, Siegelman SS: Collections of fluid after pancreatitis: Evaluation by computed tomography and ultrasonography. *Radiol Clin North Am* 1982; 20:653.

56. Gooding GAW: Ultrasound of a superior mesenteric artery aneurysm secondary to pancreatitis: A plea for real time ultrasound of sonolucent masses in pancreatitis. *JCU* 1981; 9:255.

57. Nyberg DA, Laing FC: Ultrasonic findings in peptic ulcer disease and pancreatitis that simulate primary gallbladder disease. *J Ultrasound Med* 1983; 2:303.

58. Fleischer AC, Parker P, Kirchner SG: Sonographic findings of pancreatitis in children. *Radiology* 1983; 146:151.

59. Coleman BG, Arger PH, Rosenberg HK, et al: Gray scale sonographic assessment of pancreatitis in children. *Radiology* 1983; 146:145.

60. Weill F, Bourgoin A, Aucant D, et al: Pancreatite chronique cancer du pancreas: Differenciation par ultrasons. *Nouv Presse Med* 1975; 4:567.

61. Phillips HE, Cox KL, Reid MH, et al: Pancreatic sonography in cystic fibrosis. *AJR* 1981; 137:69.

62. Spehl-Robberecht M, Baran D, Dab I, et al: Ultrasonic study of pancreas in cystic fibrosis. *Ann Radiol* 1981; 24:49.

63. Cox KL, Ament ME, Sample WF, et al: The ultrasonic and biochemical diagnosis of pancreatitis in children. *J Pediatr* 1980; 96:407.

64. Daneman A, Gaskin K, Martin DJ, et al: Pancreatic changes in cystic fibrosis: CT and sonographic appearances. *AJR* 1983; 141:653.

65. Shawker TH, Linzer M, Hubbard VS: Chronic pancreatitis: The diagnostic significance of pancreatic size and echo amplitude. *U Ultrasound Med* 1984; 3:267.

66. Holmes JH, Findley L, Frank B: Diagnosis of pancreatic pathology utilizing ultrasound. *Trans Am Clin Climatol Assoc* 1973; 85:224.

67. Leopold GR, Berk RN, Reinke RT: Echographic radiological documentation of spontaneous rupture of a pancreatic pseudocyst into the duodenum. *Radiology* 1972; 120:699.

68. Sokoloff J: Pitfalls in the echographic evaluation of pancreatic disease. *JCU* 1974; 2:321.

69. Walls WJ, Gonzales G, Martin NL, et al: B-scan ultrasound evaluation of the pancreas. *Radiology* 1975; 114:127.

70. Duncan JG, Imrie CW, Blumgart LH: Ultrasound in the management of acute pancreatitis. *Br J Radiol* 1976; 49:858.

71. Gooding GAW: Pseudocyst of the pancreas with mediastinal extension: An ultrasonographic demonstration. *JCU* 1977; 5:121.

72. Holm HH, Rasmussen SN, Kristensen JK: Errors and pitfalls in ultrasonic scanning of the abdomen. *Br J Radiol* 1972; 45:835.

73. Shultz S, Druy EM, Friedman AC: Common hepatic artery aneurysm: pseudopseudocyst of the pancreas. *AJR* 1985; 144:1287.

74. Miller CE, Cooperberg PL, Cohen MM: Pitfalls in the ultrasonographic diagnosis of the pancreatic pseudocyst. *J Can Assoc Radiol* 1978; 29:239.

75. Andrew WK, Thomas RG: Hydatid cyst of the pancreatic tail. *S Afr Med J* 1981; 59:235.

76. Burrell M, Gold JA, Simeone J, et al: Liquefactive necrosis of the pancreas. *Radiology* 1980; 135:157.

77. McCowin MJ, Federle MP: Computed tomography of pancreatic pseudocysts of the duodenum. *AJR* 1985; 145:1003.

78. Semogas P, Cooperberg PL, Li D: A typical pseudocyst of pancreas mimicking a dilated pancreatic duct. *J Can Assoc Radiol* 1980; 31:258.

79. Baker MK, Kopecky KK, Wass JL: Perirenal pancreatic pseudocysts: Diagnostic management. *AJR* 1983; 140:729.

80. Williford ME, Foster WL, Halvorsen RA: Pancreatic pseudocyst: Comparative evaluation by

sonography and computed tomography. *AJR* 1983; 140:53.

81. Clements JL, Bradley EL, Eaton SB: Spontaneous internal drainage of pancreatic pseudocysts. *AJR* 1976; 126:985.

82. Hanna WA: Rupture of pancreatic cysts: Report of a case and review of the literature. *Br J Surg* 1960; 47:495.

83. Littmann R, Pichaczevsky R, Richter R: Spontaneous rupture of a pancreatic pseudocyst into the duodenum. *Radiology* 1972; 120:699.

84. Sarti DA: Rapid development and spontaneous regression of pancreatic pseudocysts documented by ultrasound. *Radiology* 1977; 125:789.

85. Petruschak MJ, Haaga JR, Padres J: CT demonstration of spontaneous internal drainage of a pancreatic pseudocyst. *CT* 1981; 5:534.

86. Bloom RA, Abu-Dalu K, Pollak C: Spontaneous resolution of a large pancreatic pseudocyst in a child. *JCU* 1983; 11:37.

87. Slovis TL, Von Berg VJ, Milkelic V: Sonography in the diagnosis and management of pancreatic pseudocysts and effusions in childhood. *Radiology* 1980; 135:153.

88. Federle MP, Jeffrey RB, Crass RA: Computed tomography of pancreatic abscesses. *AJR* 1981; 136:879.

89. Engelhart G, Blauenstein VW: Ultrasound in the diagnosis of malignant pancreatic tumours. *Gut* 1970; 11:443.

90. Kamin PD, Bernardino ME, Wallace S: Comparison of ultrasound and computed tomography in the detection of pancreatic malignancy. *Cancer* 1980; 46:2410.

91. Itai Y, Araki T, Tasaka A: Computed tomographic appearance of resectable pancreatic carcinoma. *Radiology* 1982; 143:719.

92. Ward EM, Stephens DH, Sheedy PF: Computed tomographic characteristics of pancreatic carcinoma: An analysis of 100 cases. *Radiographics* 1983; 3:547.

93. Taylor KJW, Buchin PJ, Viscomi GM, et al: Ultrasonographic scanning of the pancreas. *Radiology* 1981; 138:211.

94. Moosa AR, Levin B: The diagnosis of early pancreatic cancer: The University of Chicago experience. *Cancer* 1981; 47:1688.

95. Rossi P, Baert A, Passariello R: CT of functioning tumors of the pancreas. *AJR* 1985; 144:57.

96. Hosoki T: Dynamic CT of pancreatic tumors. *AJR* 1983; 140:959.

97. Zeman RK, Schiebler M, Clark LR: The clinical and imaging spectrum of pancreaticoduodenal lymph node enlargement. *AJR* 1985; 144:1223.

98. Lee TG, Forsberg FG, Koehler PR: Post-splenectomy: True mass and pseudomass ultrasound diagnosis. *Radiology* 1980; 134:707.

99. Morgan CL, Trought WS, Oddson TA, et al: Ultrasound patterns of disorders affecting the gastrointestinal tract. *Radiology* 1980; 135:129.

100. Otto P, Lucke C, Mitzkat HJ: Sonographische Darstellung eines Inselzelladenomas. *Dtsch Med Wochenschr* 1974; 99:2344.

101. Gosink BB, Leopold GR: The dilated pancreatic duct: Ultrasonic evaluation. *Radiology* 1978; 126:475.

102. Zeman R, Taylor KJW, Burrell MI, et al: Ultrasound demonstration of anicteric dilatation of the biliary tree. *Radiology* 1980; 134:689.

103. Berland LL, Lawson TL, Foley WD, et al: Computed tomography of the normal and abnormal pancreatic duct: Correlation with pancreatic ductography. *Radiology* 1981; 141:715.

104. Fishman A, Isikoff MD, Farkin JS, et al: Significance of a dilated pancreatic duct on CT examination. *AJR* 1979; 133:225.

105. Kuligowska E, Miller K, Birkett D, et al: Cystic dilatation of the pancreatic duct simulating pseudocysts on sonography. *AJR* 1981; 136:409.

106. Bradley WG, Brown TW, Jacobs RP: Mobile mesenteric adenopathy: Sonographic distinction from pancreatic mass. *AJR* 1980; 135:849.

107. Schnur MJ, Hoffman JC, Koenigsberg M: Gray-scale ultrasonic demonstration of peripancreatic adenopathy. *J Ultrasound Med* 1982; 1:139.

108. Hancke S, Holm HH, Koch F: Ultrasonically guided percutaneous fine needle biopsy of the pancreas. *Surg Gynecol Obstet* 1975; 140:361.

109. Smith EH, Bartrum RJ, Chang YC: Ultrasonically guided percutaneous aspiration biopsy of the pancreas. *Radiology* 1974; 112:737.

110. Smith EH, Bartrum RJ, Chang YC, et al: Percutaneous aspiration biopsy of the pancreas under ultrasonic guidance. *N Engl J Med* 1975; 292:825.

111. Brascho DJ: Computerized radiation treatment planning with ultrasound. *AJR* 1974; 120:213.

112. Shawker TH, Doppman JL, Dunnick NR, et al: Ultrasonic investigation of pancreatic islet cell tumors. *J Ultrasound Med* 1982; 1:193.

113. Raghavendra BN, Glickstein ML: Sonography of islet cell tumor of the pancreas: Report of two cases. *JCU* 1981; 9:331.

114. Kuhn FP, Gunther R, Ruckert K, et al: Ultrasonic demonstration of small pancreatic islet cell tumors. *JCU* 1982; 10:173.

115. Dunnick NR, Long JA, Krudy A, et al: Localizing insulinomas with combined radiographic methods. *AJR* 1980; 135:747.

116. Gunther RW, Klose KJ, Ruckert K, et al: Islet-cell tumors: Detection of small lesions with computed tomography and ultrasound. *Radiology* 1983; 148:485.

117. Krudy AG, Doppman JL, Jensen RT, et al: Localization of islet cell tumors by dynamic CT: Comparison with plain CT, arteriography, sonography, and venous sampling. *AJR* 1984; 143:585.

118. Charboneau JW, James M, Heerden JA, et al: Intraoperative real time ultrasonographic localization of pancreatic insulinoma: Initial experience. *J Ultrasound Med* 1983; 2:251.

119. Wolson AH, Walls WJ: Ultrasonic characteristics of cystadenoma of the pancreas. *Radiology* 1976; 119:203.

120. Wolfman NT, Ramquist NA, Karstaedt N, et al: Cystic neoplasms of the pancreas: CT and sonography. *AJR* 1982; 138:37.

121. Friedman AC, Lichtenstein JE, Dachman AH: Cystic neoplasms of the pancreas: Radiological-pathological correlation. *Radiology* 1983; 149:45.

122. Itai Y, Moss AA, Ohtomo K: Computed tomography of cystadenoma and cystadenomacarcinoma of the pancreas. *Radiology* 1982; 145:419.

123. Harter LP, Moss AA, Goldberg HI, et al: CT guided fine needle aspirations for diagnosis of benign and malignant disease. *AJR* 1983; 140:363.

124. Mitty HA, Efremids SC, Yeh HC: Impact of fine needle biopsy on management of patients with carcinoma of the pancreas. *AJR* 1981; 137:1119.

125. Yamanaka T, Kimura K: Differential diagnosis of pancreatic mass lesion with percutaneous fine needle aspiration biopsy under ultrasonic guidance. *Dig Dis Sci* 1979; 24:694.

126. Ohto M, Karasawa E, Tsuchiya Y, et al: Ultrasonically guided percutaneous contrast medium injection and aspiration biopsy using a real time puncture transducer. *Radiology* 1980; 136:171.

127. Ohto M, Saotome N, Saisho H, et al: Real time sonography of the pancreatic duct: Application to percutaneous pancreatic ductography. *AJR* 1980; 134:647.

128. Cooperberg PL, Cohen MM, Graham M: Ultrasonographically guided percutaneous pancreatography: Report of two cases. *AJR* 1979; 132:662.

129. Gobien RP, Stanley JH, Anderson MC, et al: Percutaneous drainage of pancreatic duct for treating acute pancreatitis. *AJR* 1983; 141:795.

130. Makuuchi M, Bandai Y, Ito T, et al: Ultrasonically guided percutaneous transhepatic cholangiography and percutaneous pancreatography. *Radiology* 1980; 134:767.

131. MacErlean DP, Bryan PJ, Murphy JJ: Pancreatic pseudocyst: Management by ultrasonically guided aspiration. *Gastrointest Radiol* 1980; 5:255.

132. Barkin JS, Smith FR, Pereiras R, et al: Therapeutic percutaneous aspiration of pancreatic pseudocysts. *Dig Dis Sci* 1981; 26:585.

133. Karlson KB, Martin EC, Fankuchen EI, et al: Percutaneous drainage of pancreatic pseudocysts and abscesses. *Radiology* 1982; 142:619.

134. Smith SJ, Vogelzang RL, Donovan J, et al: Intraoperative sonography of the pancreas. *AJR* 1985; 144:557.

135. Holm HH, Stroyer I, Hansen H, et al: Ultrasonically guided percutaneous interstitial implantation of iodine 125 seeds in cancer therapy. *Br J Radiol* 1981; 54:665.

136. Ferrucci JT, Wittenberg J, Margolies MN, et al: Malignant seeding of the tract after thin needle aspiration biopsy. *Radiology* 1979; 130:345.

137. Kim WS, Barth KH, Zinner M: Seeding of pancreatic carcinoma along the transhepatic catheter tract. *Radiology* 1982; 143:427.

138. Evans WK, Ho CS, McLoughlin MJ, et al: Fatal necrotizing pancreatitis following fine needle

aspiration biopsy of the pancreas. *Radiology* 1981; 141:61.

139. Gooding GAW, Linkowski GD, Deveney C, et al: Intraoperative sonography of perisplenic pseudocysts. *AJR* 1985; 145:1013.

140. Sigel B, Duarte B, Coelho JCU, et al: Localization of insulinomas of the pancreas at operation by real time ultrasound scanning. *Surg Gynecol Obstet* 1983; 156:145.

141. Plainfosse MC, Merran S: Work in progress: Intraoperative abdominal ultrasound. *Radiology* 1983; 147:829.

142. Rifkin MD, Weiss SM: Intraoperative sonographic identification of nonpalpable pancreatic masses. *J Ultrasound Med* 1984; 3:409.

## CASES

Dennis A. Sarti, M.D.

### Transverse Scans of the Normal Pancreas

Transverse scans are obtained above the level of the pancreas. We usually start transversely within the liver, progressing caudally until certain vascular structures come into view. Figure 4–1 shows some of the vascular structures seen cephalad to the pancreas. The celiac axis can be seen arising from the anterior surface of the aorta and dividing into the hepatic and splenic arteries. Figure 4–1 also shows the portal vein situated posterior to the hepatic artery. Frequently, air in the stomach will obscure visualization of the pancreas. If the patient takes in a deep breath, the left lobe of the liver can caudally displace the lesser curvature of the stomach. This maneuver often increases visualization of the pancreas.

Near the origin of the hepatic artery, a small vessel will occasionally be noted. This is the left gastric artery (Fig 4–2). Also seen in Figure 4–2 is the origin of the superior mesenteric artery. This scan was made with caudal angulation. The hepatic artery can be seen anterior to the superior mesenteric artery. This is due to the fact that the transducer is aimed toward the foot of the patient.

Figure 4–3 illustrates a situation in which too many tubes appear in the region of the head of the pancreas. This occasionally happens when a replaced right hepatic artery is present. The anterior structure represents the portal vein and splenic vein. Posterior to this structure is the circular superior mesenteric artery. Coming off the superior mesenteric artery and heading toward the right of the patient is the replaced right hepatic artery. A small circular structure posterior to this artery represents the common bile duct, which is only approximately 3 mm in diameter. Just to the right is the gallbladder. The left renal vein can be seen coursing anterior to the aorta and emptying into the inferior vena

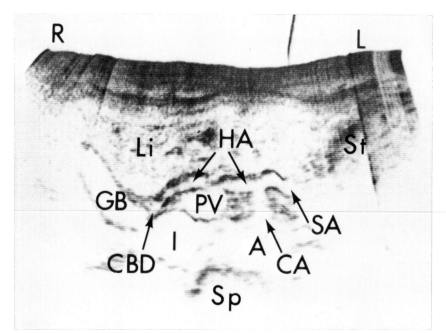

FIG 4–1.

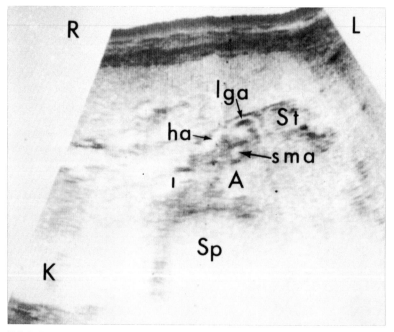

FIG 4–2.

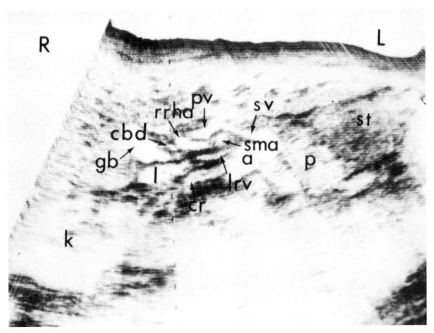

**FIG 4–3.**

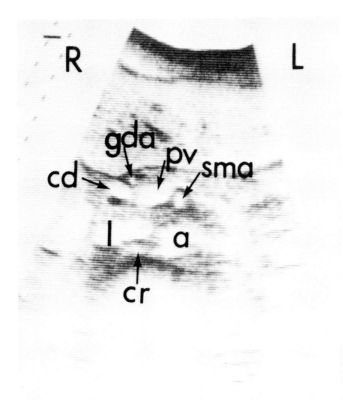

**FIG 4–4.**

cava. A relatively lucent structure, posterior to the left renal vein and adjacent to the aorta, represents the crus of the diaphragm. Figure 4–3 is our first visualization of echoes arising from the pancreas. A portion of the body and tail of the pancreas can be seen here. The tail of the pancreas usually comes into view first, since it is often situated more cephalad than is the head of the pancreas. The head of the pancreas will come into view on more caudal sections.

Figure 4–4 shows the gastroduodenal artery and common bile duct. Just to the left of these vessels a portion of the pancreas situated anterior to the superior mesenteric artery and portal vein can be seen. The pancreatic echoes in Figures 4–3 and 4–4 are equal to or slightly greater in amplitude than the echoes arising from the liver.

SOURCE: Figure 4–3 is reproduced with permission from Sample WF: Normal abdominal anatomy defined by gray scale ultrasound. *Radiol Clin North Am* 1979;17:3-11.

| | | |
|---|---|---|
| **A** | = | Aorta |
| **a** | = | Aorta |
| **CA** | = | Celiac axis |
| **CBD** | = | Common bile duct |
| **cbd** | = | Common bile duct |
| **cd** | = | Common bile duct |
| **Cr** | = | Crus of the diaphragm |
| **GB** | = | Gallbladder |
| **gb** | = | Gallbladder |
| **gda** | = | Gastroduodenal artery |
| **HA** | = | Hepatic artery |
| **ha** | = | Hepatic artery |
| **I** | = | Inferior vena cava |
| **K** | = | Kidney |
| **k** | = | Kidney |
| **L** | = | Left |
| **lga** | = | Left gastric artery |
| **Li** | = | Liver |
| **LRV** | = | Left renal vein |
| **p** | = | Pancreas |
| **PV** | = | Portal vein |
| **pv** | = | Portal vein |
| **R** | = | Right |
| **rrha** | = | Replaced right hepatic artery |
| **SA** | = | Splenic artery |
| **sma** | = | Superior mesenteric artery |
| **Sp** | = | Spine |
| **St** | = | Stomach |
| **SV** | = | Splenic vein |

## Transverse Scans of the Normal Pancreas

Figures 4–5 through 4–8 illustrate the normal increased echogenicity of the pancreas compared to the liver. Usually the pancreatic echoes are equal to or greater in amplitude than the liver. The duodenum is usually situated just lateral to the head of the pancreas. It may be air filled, fluid filled or collapsed. Figure 4–5 shows an air-filled duodenum with posterior shadowing. A portion of the head of the pancreas, just medial to air-filled duodenum, can still be seen. The level of the pancreas is determined by visualization of the superior mesenteric vein. A small portion of the pancreas is obscured by the air shadowing of the duodenum (Fig 4–5). The gallbladder, duodenum, and pancreas are in their normal relationships in this figure. This relationship is fairly consistent on most ultrasound examinations.

Figure 4–6 is a transverse scan at the confluence of the portal vein and splenic vein. A portion of the head of the pancreas is seen lateral to the portal vein. The echo amplitude of the pancreas is greater than that of the liver. The small sonolucency anterior to the inferior vena cava represents the common bile duct. This anatomic landmark is helpful in locating the lateral border of the head of the pancreas. The superior mesenteric artery is seen as a circular lucency posterior to the splenic vein.

Figure 4–7 is a transverse scan at the level of the splenic vein. A small portion of pancreatic tissue is seen anterior to the splenic vein. The echo amplitude of the pancreas is between that of the liver and that of the highly echogenic surrounding retroperitoneal fat. If the sensitivity and output of the ultrasound unit are set too high, the pancreatic texture will be lost in the surrounding highly echogenic fat. This is why understanding the vascular anatomy is so important in a pancreatic examination. Once the correct vascular anatomy has been identified, the output and sensitivity of the unit must be adjusted to bring out the tex-

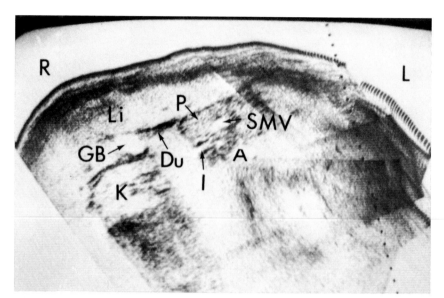

FIG 4–5.

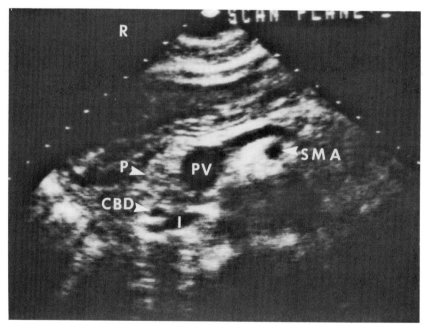

FIG 4–6.

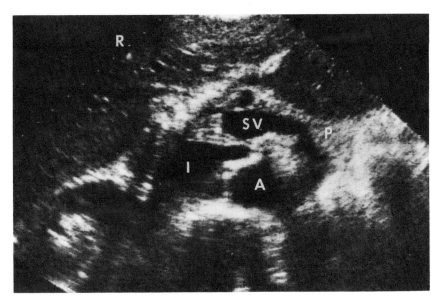

**FIG 4–7.**

ture of the pancreatic echoes separate from the highly echogenic fat. Also of interest in this scan are the aorta and inferior vena cava. The vessel arising from the anterior aspect of the aorta represents the origin of the superior mesenteric artery. The vessel arising from the left side of the inferior vena cava is the left renal vein.

The common bile duct and the gastroduodenal artery are important landmarks that define the limits of the head of the pancreas. They help the examiner identify the lateral borders of the pancreatic head and allow pancreatic echoes to be distinguished from duodenal echoes. Figure 4–8 shows the duodenum in a collapsed state. The duodenal bulb and second portion of the duodenum are collapsed. This could suggest a pancreatic mass. However, Figure 4–8 also shows the gastroduodenal artery and the common bile duct. These two structures separate the head of the pancreas from the collapsed duodenum. Some fluid is noted in the stomach in Figure 4–8. The stomach in this view is partially air filled and fluid filled. The important part of these images is the echogenicity of the pancreas relative to the liver. A good portion of the head, body, and tail of the pancreas can be seen on these scans. The pancreas is slightly more echogenic than the liver.

SOURCE: Figure 4–5 is reproduced with permission from Sample WF: Normal abdominal anatomy defined by gray scale ultrasound. *Radiol Clin North Am* 1979; 17:3-11.

| | | |
|---|---|---|
| **A** | = | Aorta |
| **CBD** | = | Common bile duct |
| **DB** | = | Duodenal bulb |
| **DS** | = | Second portion of the duodenum |
| **Du** | = | Duodenum |
| **GB** | = | Gallbladder |
| **GDA** | = | Gastric duodenal artery |
| **I** | = | Inferior vena cava |
| **IVC** | = | Inferior vena cava |
| **K** | = | Kidney |
| **L** | = | Left |
| **Li** | = | Liver |
| **P** | = | Pancreas |
| **PV** | = | Portal vein |
| **R** | = | Right |
| **SMA** | = | Superior mesenteric artery |
| **SMV** | = | Superior mesenteric vein |
| **St** | = | Stomach |

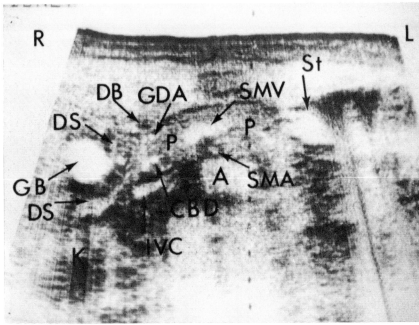

**FIG 4–8.**

## Transverse Scans of the Normal Pancreas

The superior mesenteric artery and superior mesenteric vein are important landmarks that aid the examiner in visualizing the pancreas. They are in the region of the juncture of the head and body of the pancreas. A strong linear echo, representing the pancreatic duct (Fig 4–9), can be seen within the pancreas. The examiner must be certain not to conclude that the wall of the stomach is the pancreatic duct. Therefore, it is important to identify pancreatic echoes on each side of this linear echo. To see the pancreatic duct, a careful study must be performed at small scan intervals over the midportion of the pancreas. With present-day equipment, the pancreatic duct is usually visualized.

In Figure 4–10 the pancreatic head is well displayed to the right of the superior mesenteric artery and vein. The gallbladder, partially filled duodenum, head of the pancreas, and superior mesenteric vein are in normal relationship. Some air is noted in the third portion of the duodenum to the left of the aorta. The head of the pancreas is more caudally situated than the body of the pancreas.

A technique was discussed in the chapter on biliary imaging that improved visualization of the distal common bile duct. If the patient is scanned upright before lying down, the distal common bile duct is better seen. Improved imaging results from air remaining the fundus of the stomach but relatively airless duodenal and antral regions when the patient is upright. The upright position also places the liver more inferiorly, permitting its use as an ultrasonic window. Since this technique has led to increased visualization of the common bile duct, it can be used in visualization of the head of the pancreas. Figure 4–11 is a transverse scan of the abdomen in an upright patient. The head of the pancreas is well visualized. The patient was then placed supine and a routine pancreatic examination was performed. The pancreatic region could not be visualized because of air.

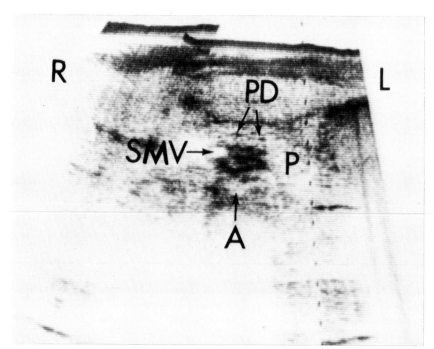

**FIG 4–9.**

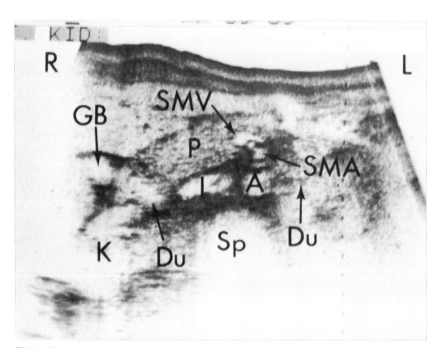

**FIG 4–10.**

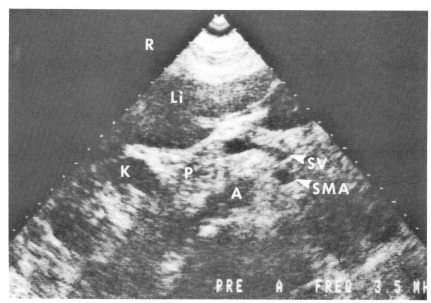

**FIG 4–11.**

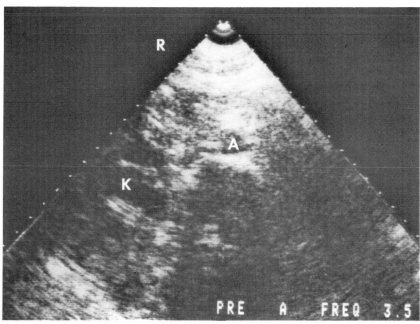

**FIG 4–12.**

Figure 4–12 is a transverse scan of the same patient supine and shows the only area in the upper abdomen that ultrasound can penetrate. The pancreas is not seen. It is suggested that pancreatic and biliary ultrasound studies should be initiated with the patient upright. The distal common bile duct and pancreatic head region are examined, then the rest of the study is performed with the patient supine.

SOURCE: Figures 4–9 and 4–10 are reproduced with permission from Sample WF, Sarti DA: Computed tomography and gray scale ultrasonography of the adrenal gland: A comparative study. *Radiology* 1978; 128: 377–383.

| | | |
|---|---|---|
| **A** | = | Aorta |
| **Du** | = | Duodenum |
| **GB** | = | Gallbladder |
| **I** | = | Inferior vena cava |
| **K** | = | Kidney |
| **L** | = | Left |
| **Li** | = | Liver |
| **P** | = | Pancreas |
| **PD** | = | Pancreatic duct |
| **R** | = | Right |
| **SMA** | = | Superior mesenteric artery |
| **SMV** | = | Superior mesenteric vein |
| **Sp** | = | Spine |
| **SV** | = | Splenic vein |

## Longitudinal Scans of the Normal Pancreas

Longitudinal scans are usually started to the right of midline and within the liver progress toward the left until the head of the pancreas comes into view. The best way to find the pancreas is to identify the portal vein within the liver and follow it medially. Figure 4–13 is a longitudinal scan to the right of midline in which the head of the pancreas is beginning to appear. The left portal vein and main portal vein can also be seen. Just anterior to the main portal vein is the hepatic artery. The common bile duct is situated anterior to the main portal vein in the porta hepatis. It then courses over the portal vein and continues posteriorly behind the head of the pancreas (Figs 4–13 and 4–14).

The gastroduodenal artery is the first branch of the hepatic artery. It courses anterior to the head of the pancreas. The head of the pancreas is located between the posterior common bile duct and the anterior gastroduodenal artery on many longitudinal scans. The position of these structures is well seen in Figure 4–14. The common bile duct is seen as a tubular structure coursing caudally and situated inferior to the main portal vein (Fig 4–15). The common bile duct is posterior and the gastroduodenal artery is anterior. For visualization of the head of the pancreas, either the liver must be anterior to it, or the stomach and duodenum must be airless (Fig 4–16). If air is present in the duodenum and stomach, the pancreas may not be visualized unless there is a prominent left lobe of the liver. Air in the duodenum bulb usually obscures at least a portion of the head of the pancreas.

Occasionally, a small circular structure can be seen posterior to the inferior vena cava and displacing it anteriorly. This is due to the right renal artery coursing behind the inferior vena cava. Figure 4–16 shows the relationship of the pancreas to the stomach and third portion of the duodenum. The third portion of the duodenum is situated caudal to the

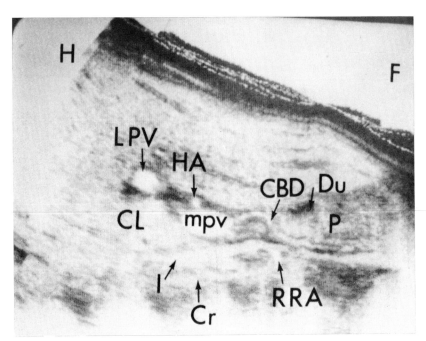

**FIG 4–13.**

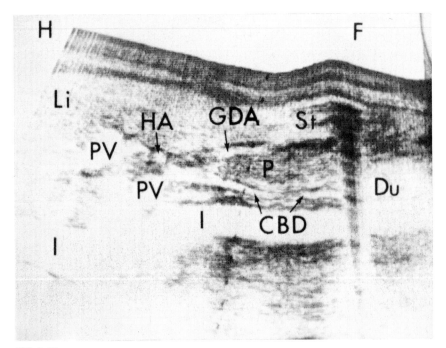

**FIG 4–14.**

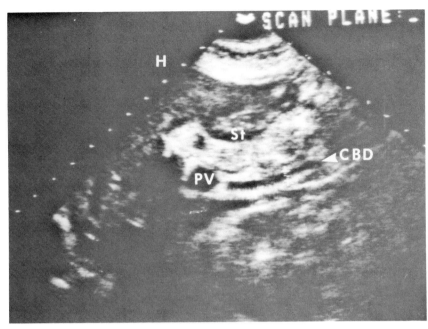

**FIG 4–15.**

head of the pancreas. The stomach is often situated anterior to the pancreas. If the stomach were air filled in Figure 4–16, the head of the pancreas would not be imaged.

SOURCE: Figure 4–13 is reproduced with permission from Sample WF: Normal abdominal anatomy defined by gray scale ultrasound. *Radiol Clin North Am* 1979; 17:3-11.

| | | |
|---|---|---|
| **CBD** | = | Common bile duct |
| **CL** | = | Caudate lobe |
| **Cr** | = | Crus of the diaphragm |
| **Du** | = | Duodenum |
| **F** | = | Foot |
| **GDA** | = | Gastroduodenal artery |
| **H** | = | Head |
| **HA** | = | Hepatic artery |
| **HV** | = | Hepatic vein |
| **I** | = | Inferior vena cava |
| **Li** | = | Liver |
| **LPV** | = | Left portal vein |
| **mpv** | = | Main portal vein |
| **P** | = | Pancreas |
| **PV** | = | Portal vein |
| **RRA** | = | Right renal artery |
| **SC** | = | Spinal canal |
| **St** | = | Stomach |
| **VB** | = | Vertebral body |

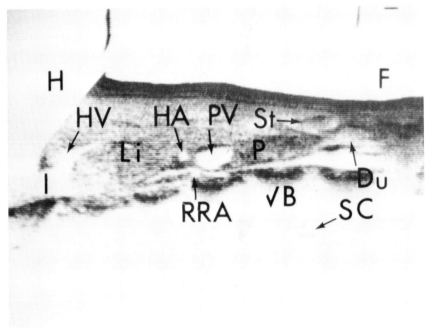

**FIG 4–16.**

## Longitudinal Scans of the Normal Pancreas

As scans progress toward the left, we see the pancreas anterior to the inferior vena cava, the aorta, and the superior mesenteric vein. In Figure 4–17 a linear lucency posterior to the inferior vena cava represents the crus of the diaphragm. This should not be confused with a vascular structure. Figure 4–17 also demonstrates the pancreas caudal to the portal vein. Again, the duodenum is seen caudal to the head of the pancreas. The pancreas does not indent the inferior vena cava in Figures 4–17 and 4–18. Figure 4–18 shows the hepatic artery and the portal vein cephalad to the head of the pancreas. As we continue to the left, the pancreas is seen anterior to the aorta (Fig 4–19). In an unusual finding, the inferior mesenteric artery (Fig 4–19) is seen caudal to the head of the pancreas and posterior to the stomach. We also visualize the right renal artery toward us, as it is on the right side of the aorta. The head of the pancreas is again situated between the portal vein and the stomach.

The most important longitudinal structure for the identification of the pancreas is the superior mesenteric vein (Fig 4–20). This identifies the juncture of the head and body of the pancreas. The pancreas is usually seen anterior to the superior mesenteric vein, as in Figure 4–20. However, there is also some pancreatic tissue posterior to the superior mesenteric vein (Fig 4–20). This tissue is the uncinate process of the pancreas. The prominent left lobe of the liver allows excellent visualization of the body of the pancreas. The stomach is somewhat airless and caudal to the body of the pancreas. The duodenum is posterior to the stomach and contains air. The transverse colon can be seen even more caudally to the duodenum.

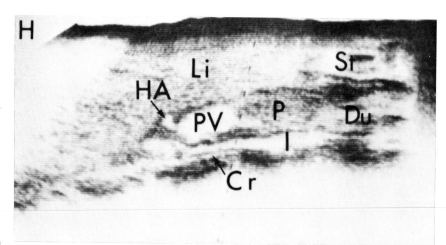

**FIG 4–17.**

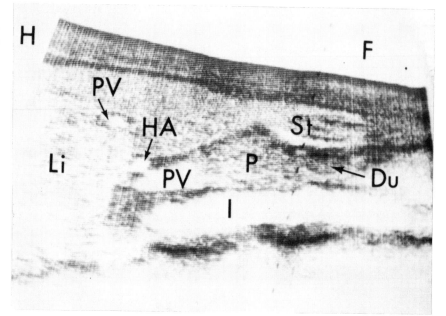

**FIG 4–18.**

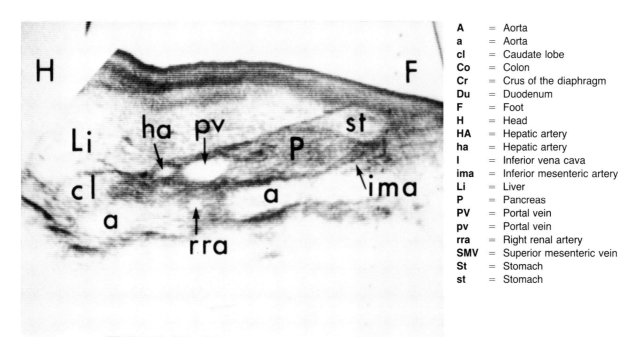

**A** = Aorta
**a** = Aorta
**cl** = Caudate lobe
**Co** = Colon
**Cr** = Crus of the diaphragm
**Du** = Duodenum
**F** = Foot
**H** = Head
**HA** = Hepatic artery
**ha** = Hepatic artery
**I** = Inferior vena cava
**ima** = Inferior mesenteric artery
**Li** = Liver
**P** = Pancreas
**PV** = Portal vein
**pv** = Portal vein
**rra** = Right renal artery
**SMV** = Superior mesenteric vein
**St** = Stomach
**st** = Stomach

**FIG 4–19.**

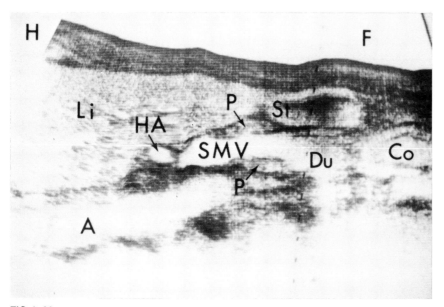

**FIG 4–20.**

## Longitudinal Supine and Prone Scans of the Normal Pancreas

As scanning continues toward the left, the vessels arising from the aorta come into view. Figure 4–21 shows the celiac axis and the superior mesenteric artery as they arise from the aorta. A vessel is seen coming off the celiac axis somewhat anteriorly; it most likely represents the left gastric artery. The splenic vein is seen as a circular lucency situated on the posterior aspect of the cephalic portion of the pancreas. The splenic vein is usually situated posterior to the upper third of the pancreas. Occasionally it is located completely cephalad to the pancreas. When trying to identify the pancreas, the examiner should find the splenic vein and look directly anterior to it for the characteristic pancreatic echoes. If these are not seen anteriorly, the examiner should look somewhat caudally, since the pancreas may be situated slightly caudal to the splenic vein.

It is also important to set the ultrasound unit so that the pancreatic echoes are not in the highest shade. If the unit is set up with too high an output or sensitivity, the pancreatic echoes will blend in with the echoes of the fibrofatty retroperitoneum. Therefore, in an effort to bring out the echoes of the pancreas, it is important to adjust the unit so that the shades of the liver are somewhat light.

Occasionally a "bull's-eye" mass appears just beneath the diaphragm on the left side. This mass represents the esophageal gastric junction (Figs 4–21 and 4–23). Another "bulls-eye" mass is seen in Figures 4–22 and 4–23, representing the stomach. A slit-like lucency anterior to the aorta and inferior to the origin of superior mesenteric artery represents the renal vein (Fig 4–22). The renal vein is an important vessel to identify since the body of the pancreas is often situated anterior to it. Progressing toward the left, the pancreas can be seen anterior to the splenic vein as it approaches the hilum of the spleen. In Figure 4–23 a large left lobe of the

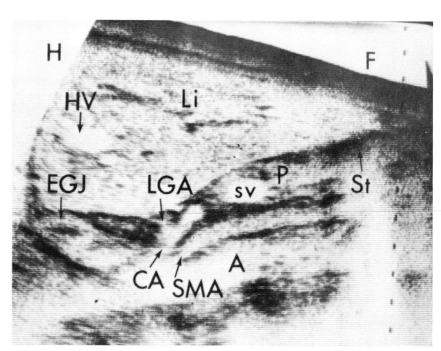

**FIG 4–21.**

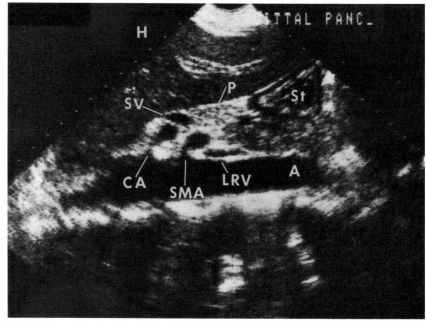

**FIG 4–22.**

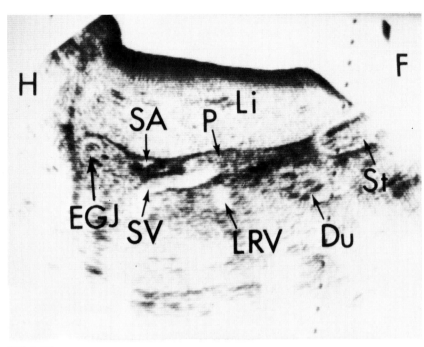

**FIG 4–23.**

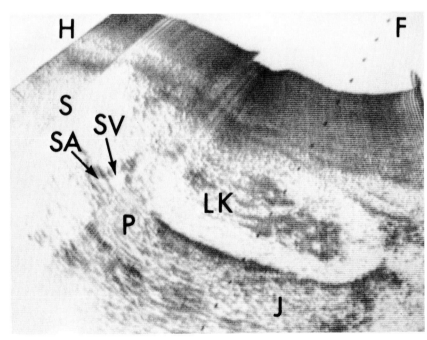

**FIG 4–24.**

liver allows visualization of the tail of the pancreas, which is situated anterior to the splenic vein and the splenic artery. The tail of the pancreas is visualized anteriorly only when there is a large left lobe of the liver or a left upper quadrant mass.

When attempting to visualize the tail of the pancreas, it is often necessary to turn the patient to the prone or decubitus position. Because of air in the stomach and splenic flexure, the tail of the pancreas rarely can be seen when the patient is supine. Figure 4–23 is an unusual case because of the large left lobe of the liver. When the patient is prone, the left kidney (Fig 4–24) is used as an ultrasonic window. The pancreas is seen just caudal to the splenic artery and splenic vein. We must be careful not to diagnose a mass anterior to the left kidney when it is actually secondary to the proximal jejunum. The jejunum often will give an ill-defined echogenic region anterior to the left kidney. The sonographer should attempt to identify the splenic artery and vein with the patient prone to be certain of the location of the tail of the pancreas. If this is not done, bowel loops may be called masses in the tail of the pancreas. By scanning the patient coronally, both the kidney and spleen can be used as ultrasonic windows for visualizing the tail of the pancreas.

SOURCE: Figure 4–21 is reproduced with permission from Sample WF: Normal abdominal anatomy defined by gray scale ultrasound. *Radiol Clin North Am* 1979; 17:3-11/

| | | |
|---|---|---|
| **A** | = | Aorta |
| **CA** | = | Celiac axis |
| **Du** | = | Duodenum |
| **EGJ** | = | Esophagogastric junction |
| **F** | = | Foot |
| **H** | = | Head |
| **HV** | = | Hepatic vein |
| **J** | = | Jejunum |
| **LGA** | = | Left gastric artery |
| **Li** | = | Liver |
| **LK** | = | Left kidney |
| **LRV** | = | Left renal vein |
| **P** | = | Pancreas |
| **S** | = | Spleen |
| **SA** | = | Splenic artery |
| **SMA** | = | Superior mesenteric artery |
| **St** | = | Stomach |
| **SV** | = | Splenic vein |

## Acute Pancreatitis

Pancreatitis is difficult to diagnose from ultrasound studies. Whenever the echoes arising from the pancreas are of less amplitude than those arising from the liver, the diagnosis of acute pancreatitis is suggested. Figure 4–25 is a scan of a 39-year-old man who entered the hospital for a head trauma and was noted to have an elevated amylase level. His history suggested alcohol abuse. During his hospital stay, the diagnosis of acute pancreatitis was determined by clinical and laboratory findings. The scan shown in Figure 4–25 demonstrates a pancreas less echogenic than the liver. The major drawback to this diagnostic technique is that liver echogenicity is used as the standard for comparison. If the liver is of increased echogenicity, as happens in cirrhosis or fatty infiltration, then the pancreas will appear much more lucent than usual, but may in fact be normal. Also, the patient may have clinical and laboratory evidence of pancreatitis but the ultrasound findings may appear to be normal.

Figure 4–26 is a transverse scan of the upper abdomen of a young female with abdominal pain and an elevated amylase level. The pancreas has decreased echogenicity compared to the liver. The high-amplitude echoes (arrowheads) with posterior acoustic shadowing are secondary to gallstones. This scan is typical of a patient with gallstone pancreatitis.

Figure 4–27 illustrates another case of acute pancreatitis. The pancreas is less echogenic than the liver. It is important to compare the echogenicity in the liver at approximately the same depth as the pancreas. Normal body attenuation in the liver can give rise to varying echo amplitude if the anterior to posterior echoes are compared. This is especially true if the time gain compensation is incorrectly set. With correct time gain compensation settings, a normal pancreas should have higher amplitude echoes than a normal liver at the same depth.

Figure 4–28 is a longitudinal scan made over the midabdomen of a 35-

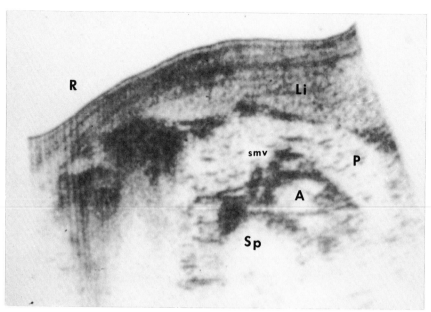

FIG 4–25.

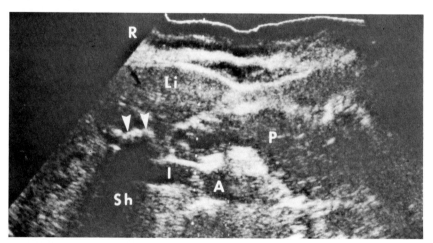

FIG 4–26.

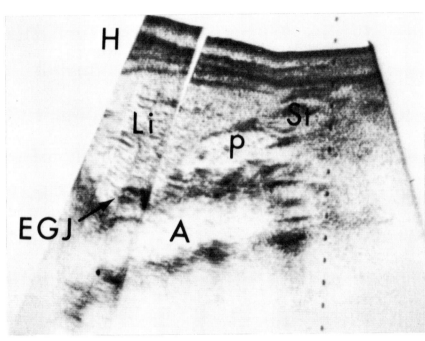

FIG 4–27.

year-old man with a history of alcohol abuse. The pancreas is diffusely enlarged and sonolucent relative to the liver. A patient with an alcoholic history may also have cirrhotic liver changes which make evaluation of the pancreas relative to liver quite difficult. Pancreatitis is present in this case not only because of the increased sonolucency of the pancreas, but also because of pancreatic enlargement. What are structures 1, 2, and 3 in Figure 4–28?

| **A** | = Aorta |
| **Arrowheads** | = Gallstone |
| **EGJ** | = Esophagogastric junction |
| **H** | = Head |
| **I** | = Inferior vena cava |
| **Li** | = Liver |
| **P** | = Pancreas |
| **R** | = Right |
| **Sh** | = Acoustic shadowing |
| **smv** | = Superior mesenteric vein |
| **St** | = Stomach |
| **1** | = Splenic vein |
| **2** | = Celiac axis |
| **3** | = Superior mesenteric artery |

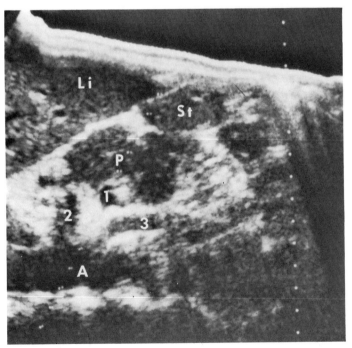

FIG 4–28.

## Chronic Pancreatitis; Cystic Fibrosis

With increasing fibrosis, the pancreas manifests increased echogenicity. Patients with chronic pancreatitis have an even higher amplitude echo arising from the pancreas. This can be so high that the pancreas will be lost in the highly echogenic fibrofatty retroperitoneum. Figures 4–29 and 4–30 are examples of chronic pancreatitis in which the pancreas is extremely echogenic. Identification of the pancreas is confirmed by the surrounding anatomy. In Figure 4–29 the pancreas is seen lateral to the superior mesenteric vein. The liver is much less echogenic than the pancreatic head. On the longitudinal scan (Fig 4–30), the head of the pancreas is markedly increased in echogenicity compared to the liver. The fluid-filled mass anterior to the pancreatic head represents fluid in the stomach. Increased pancreatic echogenicity may also be seen in elderly patients, probably as part of the aging process; the increased fibrosis causes increased echogenicity to the pancreatic parenchyma.

Increased pancreatic echogenicity also has been noted in patients with cystic fibrosis. Figures 4–31 and 4–32 are scans obtained from a 19-year-old patient with severe cystic fibrosis. Figure 4–31 is a longitudinal scan through the head of the pancreas; the pancreas is of markedly increased echogenicity compared to the adjacent liver parenchyma. Figure 4–32 is a longitudinal scan through the body of the pancreas anterior to the superior mesenteric vein and the superior mesenteric artery. The pancreas is extremely echogenic compared to the liver parenchyma. It can be lost, however, in the highly echogenic fibrofatty retroperitoneal echoes.

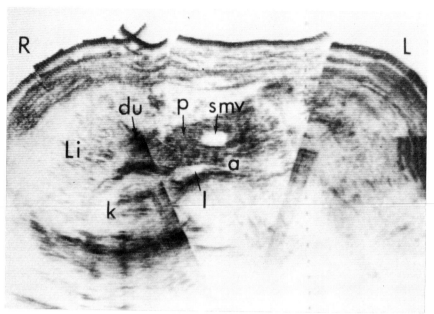

**FIG 4–29.**

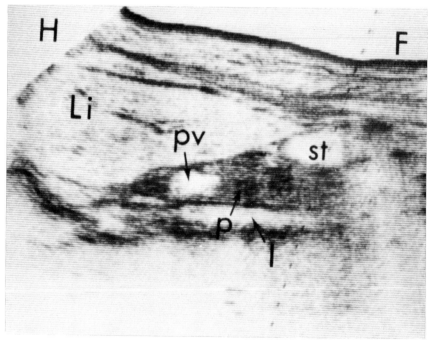

**FIG 4–30.**

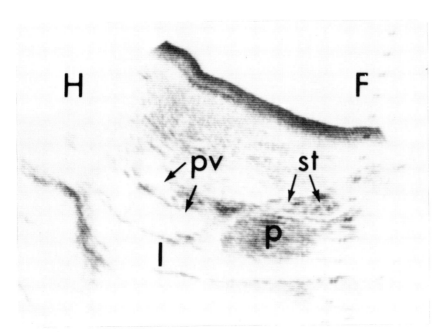

A   = Aorta
a   = Aorta
CA  = Celiac axis
du  = Duodenum
F   = Foot
H   = Head
I   = Inferior vena cava
K   = Kidney
L   = Left
Li  = Liver
P   = Pancreas
p   = Pancreas
pv  = Portal vein
R   = Right
SMA = Superior mesenteric artery
SMV = Superior mesenteric vein
smv = Superior mesenteric vein
St  = Stomach

FIG 4–31.

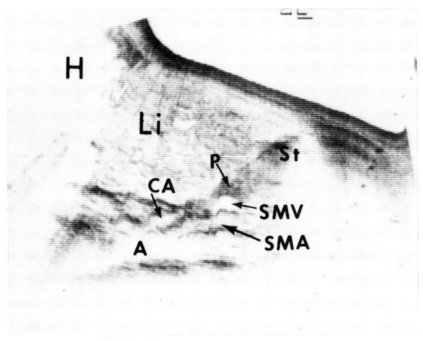

FIG 4–32.

## Chronic Pancreatitis With Calcification

When chronic pancreatitis progresses, calcification will eventually involve the region of the pancreatic bed. The ultrasonographic indication of a calcified pancreas is an extremely high-amplitude echo to the surrounding pancreatic bed. Often the calcification will be large enough to cause shadowing. A markedly calcified pancreas may be extremely difficult to diagnose because it can be confused with bowel air. Figures 4–33 through 4–35 are scans of a 40-year-old man with a long history of alcohol abuse. The patient had previously had alcoholic hepatitis. He was admitted with a 2-month history of nausea and abdominal pain. The scans in Figures 4–33 and 4–34 show a markedly enlarged pancreas (arrows). The central portion of the pancreatic bed is highly echogenic, consistent with calcification. The periphery is less echogenic, indicating the surrounding pancreatic tissue. Figure 4–35 is an x-ray film of the same patient. The calcifications are best seen to the right of midline.

Figure 4–36 is a transverse scan of a 45-year-old man whose first episode of alcholic pancreatitis was noted 11 years earlier. The present examination demonstrates a highly echogenic pancreatic bed. We are unable to see the area posterior to the pancreatic bed because of shadowing arising from the calcification within the pancreas. It is evident, however, that the pancreas can easily be confused with bowel air. It is the nodular irregular appearance of the high-level echoes that gives the clue that calcification is present within the pancreatic bed.

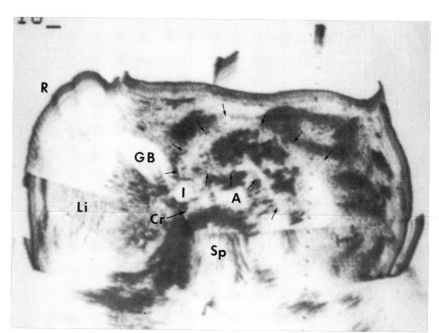

**FIG 4–33.**

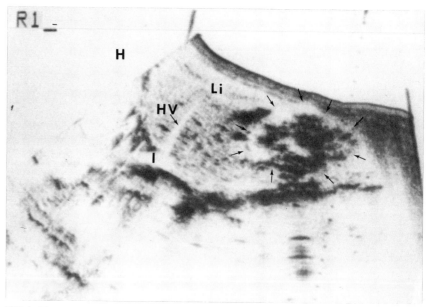

**FIG 4–34.**

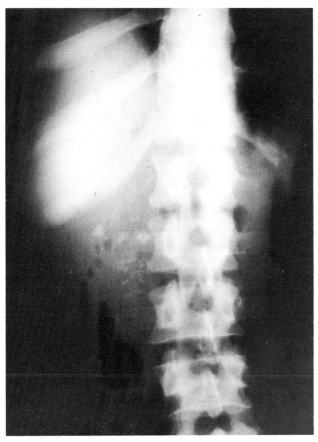

| | | |
|---|---|---|
| **A** | = | Aorta |
| **Arrows** | = | Outline the pancreatic bed |
| **Cr** | = | Crus of the diaphragm |
| **GB** | = | Gallbladder |
| **H** | = | Head |
| **HV** | = | Hepatic vein |
| **I** | = | Inferior vena cava |
| **K** | = | Kidney |
| **Li** | = | Liver |
| **P** | = | Pancreatic bed |
| **R** | = | Right |
| **Sh** | = | Shadow from the calcified pancreas |
| **Sp** | = | Spine |

FIG 4–35.

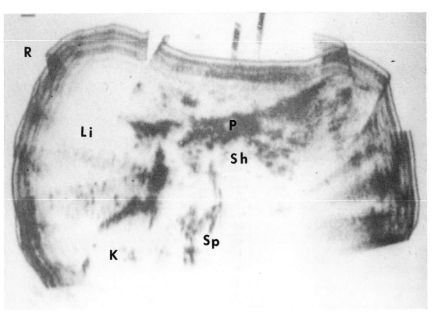

FIG 4–36.

## Pancreatic Calcification

Calcification in the pancreatic bed gives a confusing picture on ultrasound. Unless the ultrasonographer has seen this entity before or is considering the possibility while scanning, it will easily be overlooked. The coarse, high-amplitude echoes arising from the calcific areas are often thought to be secondary to air or retroperitoneal fat when they are first seen. As with an echogenic dermoid in the pelvis, these characteristic findings are easily missed unless one considers their possibility while scanning. Figure 4–37 is an oblique scan of the right upper quadrant of a middle-aged man. The common bile duct was dilated. As the sonographer scanned the distal common bile duct in an effort to determine the cause of dilatation, several high-amplitude echoes were noted in the region. The echoes did not appear to be within the lumen of the common bile duct but rather were surrounding the common bile duct and were situated more caudally. The findings were thought to be secondary to calcification within the pancreatic head. A CT scan was ordered for confirmation (Fig 4–38). Calcification is noted within the pancreatic head (arrowheads), along with dilatation of the distal common bile duct (arrow). The patient had had a pancreatic abscess that was surgically drained 5 years earlier. On the present examination, the calcifications in the pancreatic head were causing strictures of the distal common bile duct. The patient underwent a choledochojejunostomy.

Figures 4–39 and 4–40 are transverse and longitudinal scans of a young man with numerous previous episodes of pancreatitis. These scans show typical calcification in the region of the pancreatic head. Acoustic shadowing is present deep to the high-amplitude echoes, which suggests that the echoes are calcific. The biliary tree is not dilated. These findings are typical of chronic calcific pancreatitis. What are structures 1, 2, and 3 in Figure 4–39?

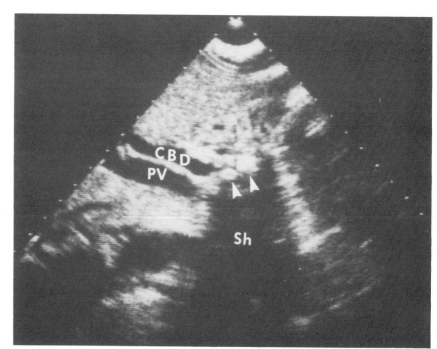

**FIG 4–37.**

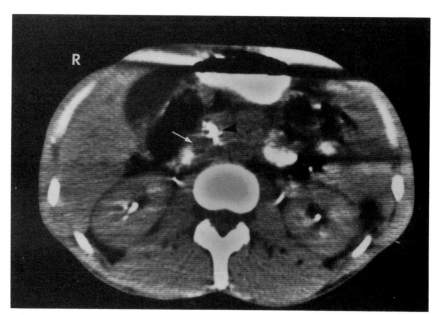

**FIG 4–38.**

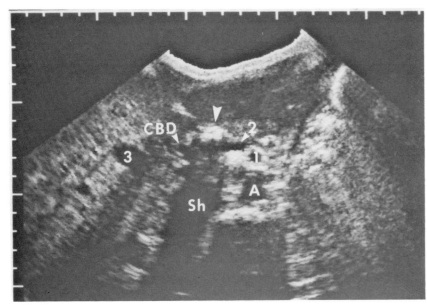

A          = Aorta
**Arrow**      = Common bile duct
**Arrowheads** = Pancreatic calcification
**CBD**        = Common bile duct
I          = Inferior vena cava
P          = Portal vein
R          = Right
**Sh**         = Acoustic shadowing
1          = Superior mesenteric artery
2          = Superior mesenteric vein
3          = Gallbladder

**FIG 4–39.**

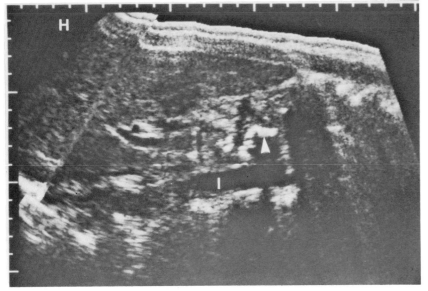

**FIG 4–40.**

## Chronic Pancreatitis Versus Neoplasm

Often, chronic pancreatitis leads to a pancreatic mass that is difficult to distinguish from carcinoma of the pancreas. Figures 4–41 through 4–44 illustrate such a case. A 25-year-old woman had complaints suggestive of jaundice of approximately 2–3 months' duration. Viral hepatitis was suspected, and she underwent ultrasound examination. Figure 4–41 is a transverse scan through the liver showing both a dilated biliary tree (arrows) and a dilated common bile duct. Transverse scans through the head of the pancreas (Fig 4–42) reveal a pancreatic mass. The borders are somewhat irregular, and the mass is less echogenic than the liver. A longitudinal scan through the head of the pancreas (Fig 4–43) again reveals the dilated biliary tree (arrows) and the dilated common bile duct. Some indentation is noted on the inferior vena cava due to this pancreatic mass. The findings are highly suggestive of a pancreatic tumor within the head. An upper gastrointestinal series demonstrated enlargement of the C-loop with effacement of the second portion of the duodenum. A transhepatic cholangiogram (Fig 4–44) shows dilatation of the biliary tree and narrowing of the distal common bile duct.

The patient underwent laparotomy, and biopsy revealed chronic pancreatitis. There was no evidence of neoplasm. The common bile duct was obstructed, and choledochojejunostomy was performed. This ultrasound study illustrates that severe chronic pancreatitis can present as a mass that cannot be distinguished from a neoplasm.

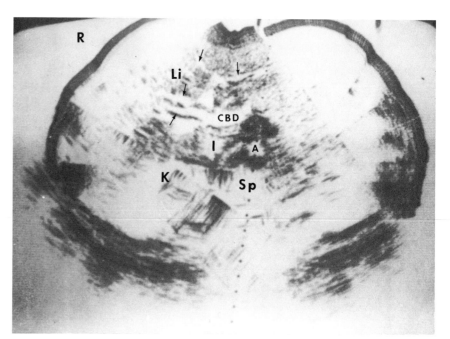

**FIG 4–41.**

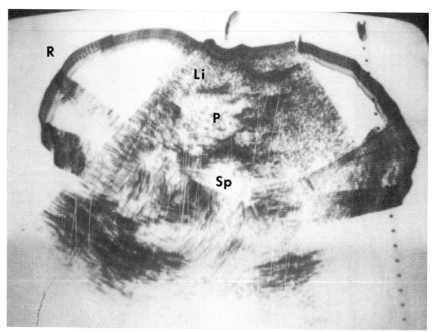

**FIG 4–42.**

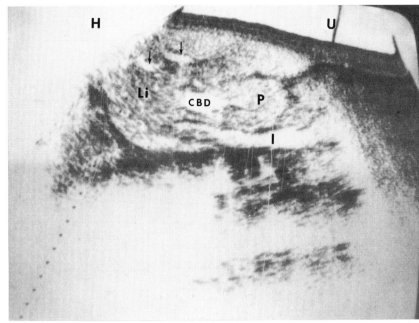

A = Aorta
Arrows = Dilated biliary tree
CBD = Common bile duct
H = Head
I = Inferior vena cava
K = Kidney
Li = Liver
P = Pancreas
R = Right
Sp = Spine
U = Umbilical level

**FIG 4–43.**

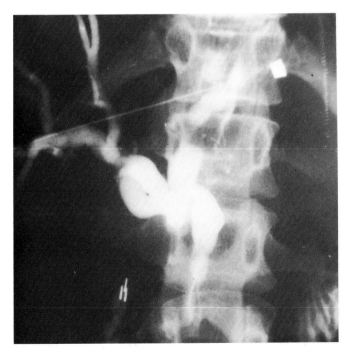

**FIG 4–44.**

## Pancreatic Abscess

A 31-year-old man experienced the sudden onset of a sharp midepigastric pain. He had a long history of chronic alcohol abuse. His white blood cell count and amylase level were elevated. Figures 4–45 and 4–46 are ultrasound scans of the patient. Figure 4–45 is a transverse scan of the midepigastric region. Two large sonolucent masses with fairly thick walls are present. These masses represent pancreatic abscesses. A longitudinal scan (Fig 4–46) shows a sonolucent mass in the pancreatic bed anterior to the aorta and crus of the diaphragm. The pancreatic abscess would be difficult to distinguish from a pseudocyst or from severe edema of the pancreas, as it is present in a pancreatic phlegmon. Figure 4–47 is an x-ray film of the upper abdomen obtained several days later. Air is noted in the pancreatic abscess just to the left of T-12.

Pancreatic abscesses usually appear as a large sonolucent mass in the pancreatic bed on ultrasound examination. Abscesses cannot be differentiated from other lucent masses in the pancreatic region. However, when combined with clinical history, the ultrasound findings usually lead to the correct diagnosis. Figure 4–48 is a transverse scan of the upper abdomen in a 65-year-old male with abdominal pain, fever, and elevated white blood cell count. He was admitted to the hospital and an ultrasound examination was ordered because of the abdominal pain. A large 9 × 12 cm sonolucent mass with thick borders was found in the pancreatic bed. The ultrasound findings and clinical history indicated that the most likely diagnosis was pancreatic abscess. At operation a large pancreatic abscess was drained.

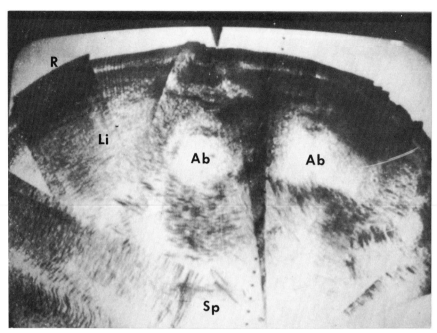

FIG 4–45.

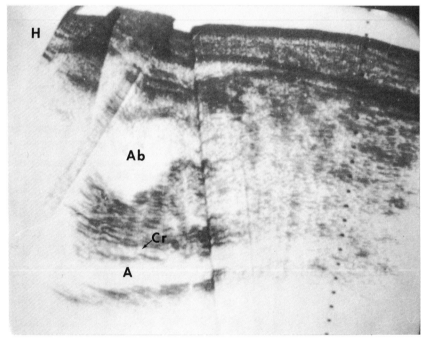

FIG 4–46.

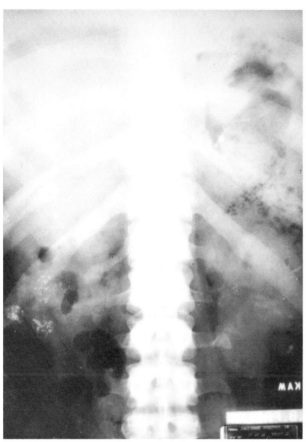

**FIG 4–47.**

A   = Aorta
**Ab** = Pancreatic abscess
**Cr** = Crus of the diagphragm
**H**  = Head
**Li** = Liver
**R**  = Right
**Sp** = Spine

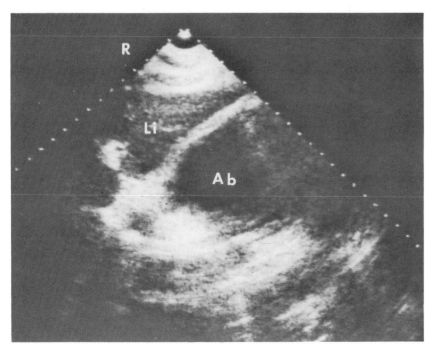

**FIG 4–48.**

## Pancreatic Pseudocyst

Ultrasound is an excellent means of diagnosing a pancreatic pseudocyst. Pancreatic pseudocysts are usually large sonolucent masses that stand out on ultrasound examination. Although they have been reported to dissect along tissue planes to distant sites, such as the thorax and lower abdomen, most pancreatic pseudocysts are located in the region of the pancreatic bed. Pseudocysts can be single, multiple, unilocular, multilocular, and filled with debris. Their internal structure determines their ultrasonographic appearance. Figures 4–49 and 4–50 are transverse and longitudinal scans of a young adult man with abdominal pain, abnormal results on liver function tests, and a history of alcoholism. The scans show the typical appearance of a unilocular pancreatic pseudocyst. The walls are fairly sharp and there are no internal echoes. Prominent through-transmission is present deep to the mass, indicating its fluid-filled structure. This is typical of a cystic mass anywhere in the body. In Figure 4–50 biliary dilatation cephalad to the pseudocyst can be seen. Biliary dilatation is not uncommon when the pseudocyst is located in the head of the pancreas. The pancreatic duct is dilated (Fig 4–49). The small sonolucency lateral to the pseudocyst in Figure 4–49 is the gallbladder.

Figure 4–51 is a transverse intercostal scan of the left upper quadrant of a 26-year-old woman with vague upper abdominal pain. A 5-cm sonolucent mass is seen in the left upper quadrant, representing a pancreatic pseudocyst of the tail. At operation the pseudocyst was drained and a distal pancreatectomy was performed. The ultrasound examination revealed a unilocular mass with increased through-transmission and slightly irregular borders.

Figure 4–52 is a longitudinal scan of the right upper quadrant of a middle-aged man. A sonolucent mass with increased through-transmission is present in the region of the head of the pancreas. Close examination of

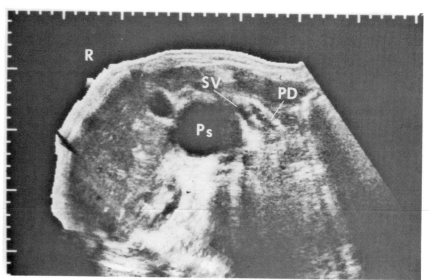

**FIG 4–49.**

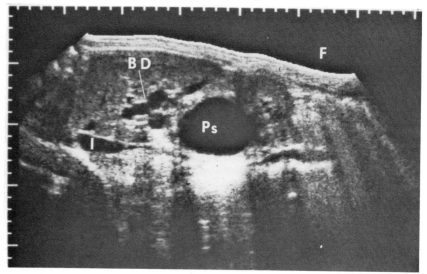

**FIG 4–50.**

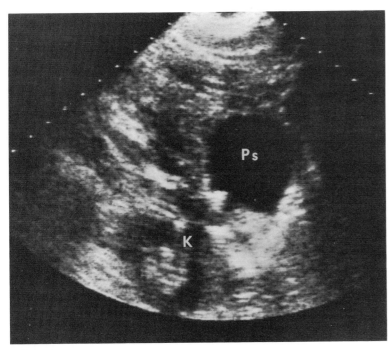

**FIG 4–51.**

the wall of this mass reveals a slightly increased lucency and thickening, especially in the superior region of the mass. This appearance is not uncommon in a pancreatic pseudocyst because of the adjacent surrounding edema. It must be remembered that a pancreatic pseudocyst is not a true cyst but a false cystic mass created by enzymatic action of the pancreatic juices. Very often tissue surrounding a pancreatic pseudocyst will be edematous and thickened, as in this case. No biliary dilatation is present. What are structures 1 and 2 in Figure 4–52?

| | | |
|---|---|---|
| **BD** | = | Biliary dilatation |
| **F** | = | Foot |
| **H** | = | Head |
| **I** | = | Inferior vena cava |
| **K** | = | Kidney |
| **PD** | = | Dilated pancreatic duct |
| **Ps** | = | Pancreatic pseudocyst |
| **R** | = | Right |
| **1** | = | Hepatic vein |
| **2** | = | Portal vein |

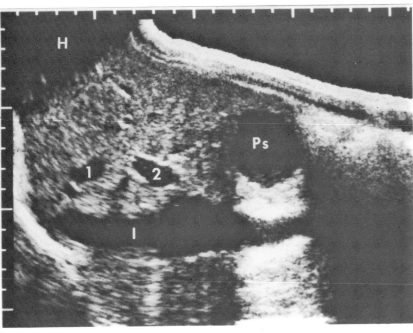

**FIG 4–52.**

## Multilocular Pseudocysts

Pseudocysts may be unilocular, multi-locular, completely fluid filled, or contain debris. This information about the internal structure of a pseudocyst can be extremely helpful before surgery. Severely multiloculated pseudocysts are often difficult to drain completely. Recurrence after surgery is common. Figures 4–53 and 4–54 are transverse and longitudinal scans of the upper abdomen of a patient with a pancreatic pseudocyst that is mainly fluid filled. Some curvilinear echoes are present within the pseudocyst (arrows) and represent septations. The walls are somewhat irregular.

Figure 4–55 is a transverse scan of the upper abdomen of a 56-year-old woman with severe epigastric pain 3 weeks before admission. Ultrasound examination demonstrates a 10 × 8 cm mass in the middle to upper abdomen compatible with a pancreatic pseudocyst. A few echoes representing septations are present on the posterior wall (arrows). The patient was observed for several weeks before surgery while the pseudocyst wall matured. She became febrile and an ultrasound-guided diagnostic aspiration was performed; the aspirate yielded *Staphylococcus*. At operation a pancreatic pseudocyst and a lesser sac abscess were drained.

Figure 4–56 shows a multiloculated pseudocyst with many more septations than in the previous cases. The patient was a 19-year-old woman who was referred because of recurrence of a pancreatic pseudocyst. The pseudocyst was supposedly drained at an earlier operation, but the mass did not disappear. It is not unusual for a multiloculated pseudocyst not to disappear completely after surgery. Not all of the chambers may have been drained. It is important to notify the surgeon specifically that a multiloculated pseudocyst is present. Figure 4–56 shows a multiloculated pseudocyst in the right abdomen. It has numerous small circular sonolucencies, which explains the difficulty of adequate surgical drainage.

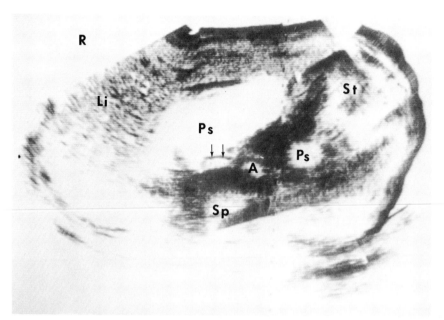

FIG 4–53.

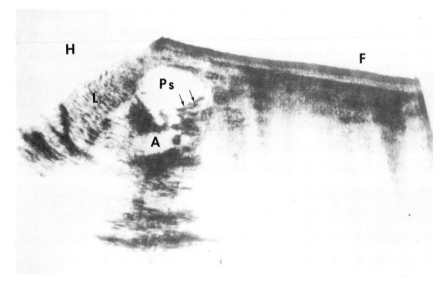

FIG 4–54.

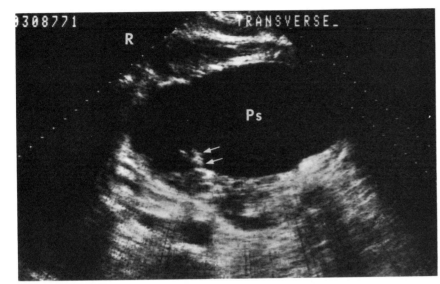

| | | |
|---|---|---|
| **A** | = | Aorta |
| **Arrows** | = | Septations |
| **F** | = | Foot |
| **H** | = | Head |
| **K** | = | Kidney |
| **L** | = | Left |
| **Li** | = | Liver |
| **M** | = | Multiloculated pseudocyst |
| **Ps** | = | Pseudocyst |
| **R** | = | Right |
| **Sp** | = | Spine |
| **St** | = | Stomach |

FIG 4–55.

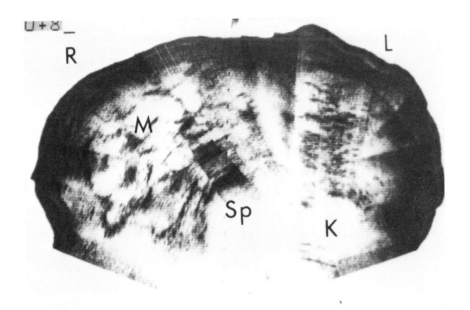

FIG 4–56.

## Pancreatic Pseudocysts With Debris

Pancreatic pseudocysts arise from an inflammatory process caused by escape of pancreatic juices. A false wall or capsule builds up around the pancreatic juices. This false wall is the source of the term "pseudocyst." Very often the central portion of the pseudocyst is fluid filled. Since the pancreatic enzymes digest adjacent tissue, some pseudocysts may be filled with necrotic debris. The debris will appear as internal echoes on ultrasound, especially in the dependent portion. Figures 4–57 and 4–58 are transverse and longitudinal scans of a man with a long history of alcoholism and a 4-day history of nausea, vomiting, epigastric pain, and hematemesis. Ultrasound examination reveals a large fluid-filled mass in the left upper abdomen. Soft echoes are present in the posterior region, compatible with debris. At operation, a pancreatic pseudocyst with necrosis and hemorrhagic tissue was removed from the posterior region of the pancreas.

Figure 4–59 is a transverse scan of the upper abdomen of a 38-year-old woman with a history of scleroderma. Pancreatitis had recently developed and the woman was thought to have a pancreatic pseudocyst. An ultrasound examination was ordered because of abdominal pain and an increased amylase level. A 5-cm fluid-filled mass with posterior internal echoes was visualized near the head of the pancreas. This was secondary to a pancreatic pseudocyst with debris (arrowheads). The pancreatic duct was also noted to be dilated. Detecting pancreatic duct dilatation can be difficult unless the vascular anatomy of the upper abdomen is well understood.

Figure 4–60 is a transverse scan of the upper abdomen of a 51-year-old man with a long history of episodic upper abdominal pain. In the immediately preceding 3–4 months, this pain had become constant. Ultrasound reveals a 7-cm pseudocyst in the upper abdomen. Internal echoes are present on the medial border. At operation a

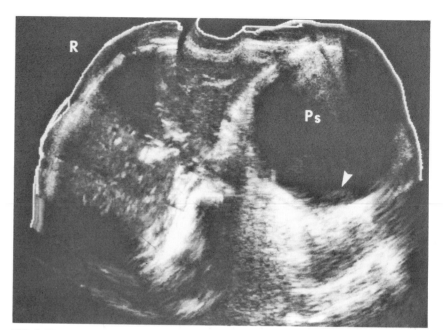

FIG 4–57.

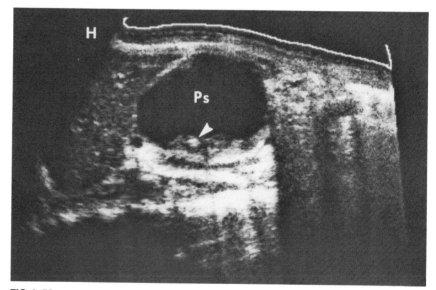

FIG 4–58.

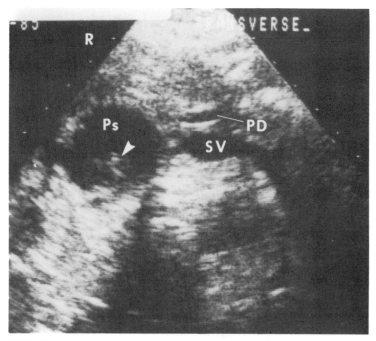

FIG 4–59.

necrotic, fibrotic pseudocyst was found.

| **Arrowheads** | = Internal debris |
| --- | --- |
| **H** | = Head |
| **PD** | = Dilated pancreatic duct |
| **Ps** | = Pseudocyst |
| **SV** | = Splenic vein |
| **R** | = Right |

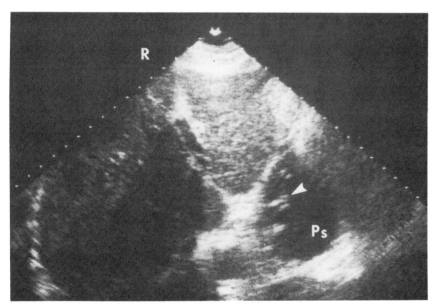

FIG 4–60.

## Unilocular Pancreatic Pseudocyst With Spontaneous Resolution

Ultrasound plays an important role in the diagnosis of pancreatic pseudocysts. Since fluid can easily be detected by ultrasound, it is the imaging modality of choice in the differential diagnosis of pseudocysts. Pseudocysts may be unilocular or multiloculated. Figures 4–61 through 4–64 are scans of a unilocular pseudocyst. The patient was a 52-year-old woman who had a long history of alcoholic pancreatitis. She was admitted with epigastric pain. A sonolucent mass posterior to the left lobe of the liver was noted and was thought to be a pseudocyst (Figs 4–61, 4–62). The patient was scheduled for surgery and followed serially by ultrasound. Just prior to surgery the pseudocyst began to decrease in size (Fig 4–63). Surgery was postponed, and follow-up examination demonstrated complete disappearance of the pseudocyst (Fig 4–64).

This case illustrates the dynamic nature of pancreatic pseudocysts. Many cysts do drain spontaneously without any marked side effects. Ultrasound should be used to serially follow all patients with pseudocysts who do not go on to surgery.

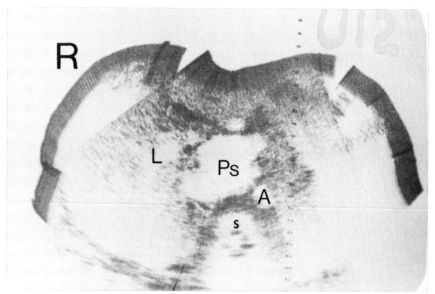

FIG 4–61.

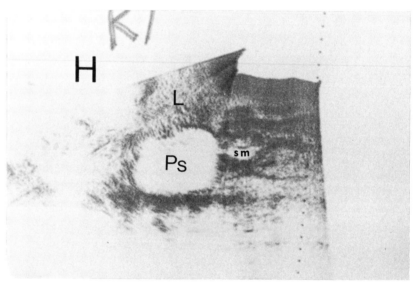

FIG 4–62.

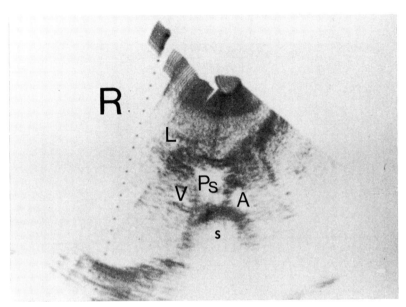

**FIG 4–63.**

SOURCE: Figures 4–61, 4–62, 4–63, and 4–64 are reproduced with permission from Sarti DA: Rapid development and spontaneous regression of pancreatic pseudocysts documented by ultrasound. *Radiology* 1977; 125:789-793.

**A** = Aorta
**H** = Head
**L** = Liver
**Ps** = Pseudocyst
**R** = Right
**S** = Spine
**sm** = Superior mesenteric vein
**V** = Inferior vena cava

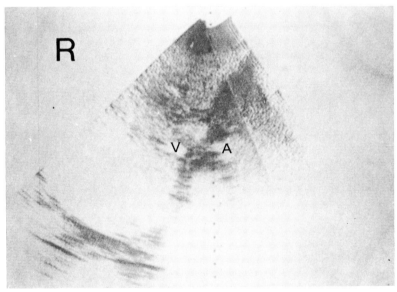

**FIG 4–64.**

## Rapid Development of a Pancreatic Pseudocyst

Pancreatic pseudocysts may arise quite rapidly. Ultrasound is an excellent means of following a patient with acute pancreatitis. A change in the clinical symptoms such as acute pain indicates that ultrasound should be ordered to detect whether or not a pseudocyst has developed. The case illustrated in Figures 4–65 and 4–66 is an excellent example of the rapid development of a pancreatic pseudocyst. A 33-year-old man with a long history of alcohol abuse was in the hospital for several months and underwent serial ultrasound examinations. The patient had somehow managed to continue drinking during his hospitalization and while on hyperalimentation. Figures 4–65 and 4–66 show a relatively normal pancreas (arrows), with no mass noted anteriorly. Figures 4–67 and 4–68 are scans made approximately 1 week later, followed an episode of acute abdominal pain. A large sonolucent mass secondary to a pancreatic pseudocyst is now visible. At operation a pancreatic pseudocyst was found anterior to the body of the pancreas.

This case illustrates the rapid development of a pancreatic pseudocyst, which can be followed best by ultrasound examination.

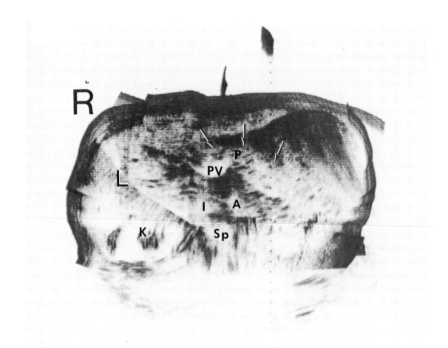

**FIG 4–65.**

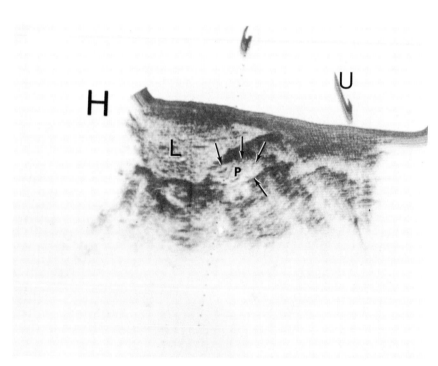

**FIG 4–66.**

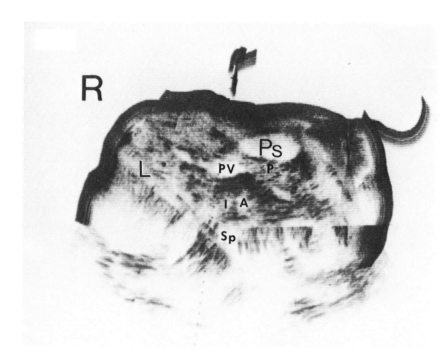

**FIG 4–67.**

SOURCE: Figures 4–65, 4–66, 4–67, and 4–68 are reproduced with permission from Sarti DA: Rapid development and spontaneous regression of pancreatic pseudocysts documented by ultrasound. *Radiology* 1977; 125:789-793.

| | | |
|---|---|---|
| **A** | = | Aorta |
| **H** | = | Head |
| **I** | = | Inferior vena cava |
| **K** | = | Kidney |
| **L** | = | Liver |
| **P** | = | Pancreas |
| **Ps** | = | Pseudocyst |
| **PV** | = | Portal vein |
| **R** | = | Right |
| **SA** | = | Splenic artery |
| **Sp** | = | Spine |
| **SV** | = | Splenic vein |
| **U** | = | Umbilical level |

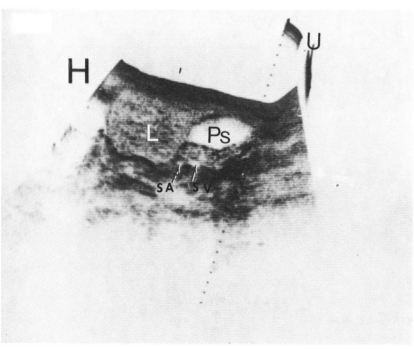

**FIG 4–68.**

## Pseudocyst of the Uncinate Process

The smallest pathologic entity of the pancreas can best be diagnosed in the area of the uncinate process. This is due to excellent vascular anatomy, which can delineate small masses. Figure 4–69 and 4–70 are ultrasound scans of a patient with chronic alcoholism and continual abdominal pain. The head of the pancreas is slightly enlarged, but no masses are noted in Figure 4–69. Figure 4–70 shows the superior mesenteric vein to have a straight course.

On follow-up examination 2 months later, a small pseudocyst was seen in the uncinate process of the pancreas (Fig 4–71). Figure 4–72 is a longitudinal scan showing an altered course to the superior mesenteric vein, which is now draped over the small pseudocyst in the uncinate process of the pancreas.

This case illustrates the excellent visualization of anatomy about the head of the pancreas, especially the uncinate process, that can be achieved with ultrasound. It also illustrates the development of a pancreatic pseudocyst over a short period of time.

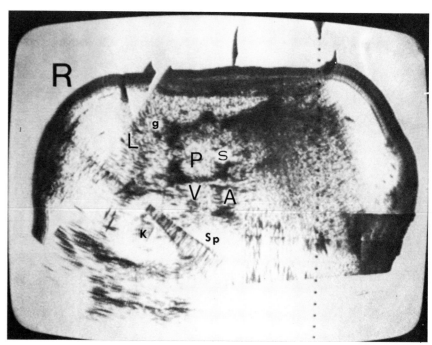

FIG 4–69.

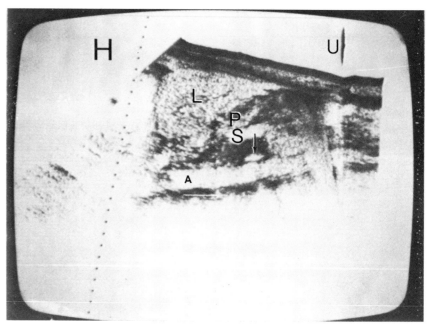

FIG 4–70.

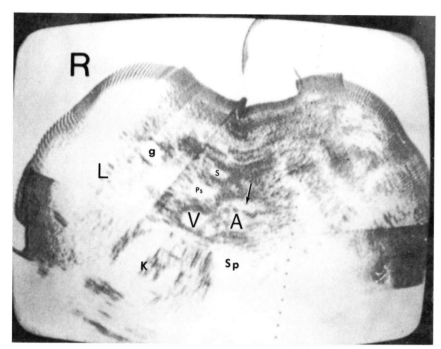

FIG 4–71.

SOURCE: Figures 4–69, 4–70, 4–71, and 4–72 are reproduced with permission from Sarti DA: Rapid development and spontaneous regression of pancreatic pseudocysts documented by ultrasound. *Radiology* 1977; 125:789-793.

| | | |
|---|---|---|
| **A** | = | Aorta |
| **Arrow** | = | Left renal vein |
| **G** | = | Gallbladder |
| **H** | = | Head |
| **K** | = | Kidney |
| **L** | = | Liver |
| **P** | = | Pancreas |
| **Ps** | = | Pseudocyst |
| **R** | = | Right |
| **S** | = | Superior mesenteric vein |
| **Sp** | = | Spine |
| **U** | = | Umbilical level |
| **V** | = | Inferior vena cava |

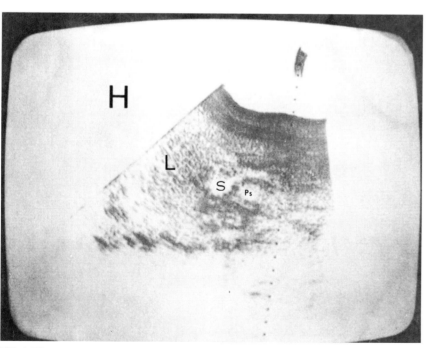

FIG 4–72.

## Other Sonolucent Masses Near the Pancreas

Any time a fluid-filled mass is seen in the upper abdomen, a pseudocyst is usually considered in the differential diagnosis. Other entities must, however, be ruled out before the diagnosis can be made. The most common error in the diagnostic interpretation is visualization of a fluid-filled loop of bowel. Figure 4–73 is an example of a fluid-filled stomach with echoes noted posteriorly due to food in the posterior aspect of the stomach. It is important to repeat the examination the next day with the patient having had no oral intake. If a similarly shaped sonolucency is present in the same location, the diagnosis of a pancreatic pseudocyst is quite likely.

The scans in Figures 4–74 through 4–76 are from serial ultrasound examinations of a fluid-filled loop of bowel. In Figure 4–74 the duodenum is air filled as it lies between the gallbladder and the pancreas. The patient was given a small amount of water, and the duodenum became partially fluid filled (Fig 4–75). There is now some enhanced through-transmission posterior to the duodenum and adjacent to the head of the pancreas. A portion of fluid-filled stomach is also seen to the left of the body of the pancreas. The patient was given more water, and the duodenum enlarged (Fig 4–76). The duodenum now presents as a larger sonolucent mass with through-transmission between the gallbladder and the pancreas. If this fluid-filled mass had been present initially, the diagnosis of a pseudocyst would most likely have been made. It is always necessary to reexamine the patient the following day. We have used nasogastric suction on inpatients to rule out a fluid-filled loop of bowel. An outpatient should be requested to remain without oral intake after midnight prior to the day of examination. Real-time examination may be used to detect peristalsis.

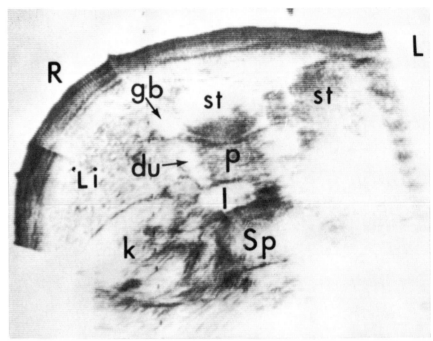

**FIG 4–73.**

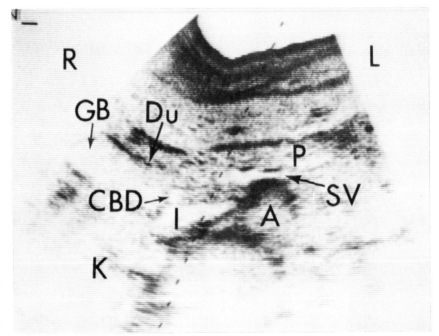

**FIG 4–74.**

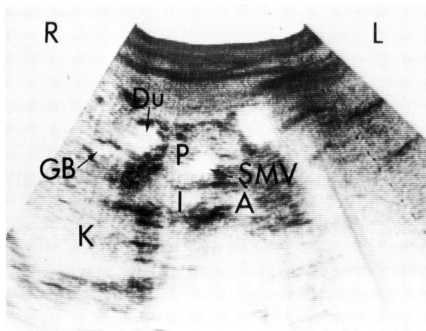

| A | = | Aorta |
| CBD | = | Common bile duct |
| Du | = | Duodenum |
| du | = | Duodenum |
| GB | = | Gallbladder |
| gb | = | Gallbladder |
| I | = | Inferior vena cava |
| K | = | Kidney |
| k | = | Kidney |
| L | = | Left |
| Li | = | Liver |
| P | = | Pancreas |
| p | = | Pancreas |
| R | = | Right |
| SMV | = | Superior mesenteric vein |
| Sp | = | Spine |
| St | = | Stomach |
| SV | = | Splenic vein |

**FIG 4–75.**

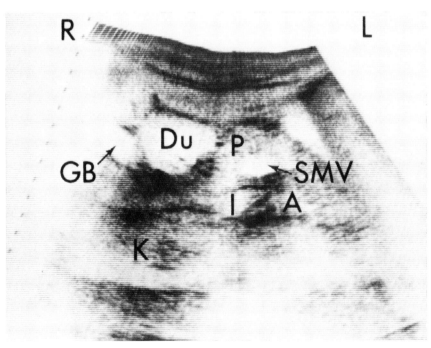

**FIG 4–76.**

## Other Sonolucent Masses Near the Pancreas

Another cause of a fluid-filled mass in the upper abdomen can be loculated ascites. The lesser sac is a common spot for a pancreatic pseudocyst to occur. However, ascites can be present in unusual loculations and shapes, and the lesser sac can be the site of loculated ascites. Figures 4–77 and 4–78 are scans of a 40-year-old woman with a diagnosis of ovarian carcinoma. A fluid-filled area was noted in the region of the lesser sac anterior to the pancreas. Figure 4–77 demonstrates a large sonolucency anterior to the pancreas and secondary to loculated ascites. A longitudinal scan shows the ascites anterior to the body of the pancreas (Fig 4–78). The patient underwent laparotomy, and poorly differentiated diffuse carcinoma of the pelvis was noted along with loculated ascites.

Occasionally, large dilated vessels may present as fluid-filled masses in the upper abdomen. Very prominent portal and splenic veins are quite commonly seen. Figures 4–79 and 4–80 demonstrate an unusual aneurysm of the celiac axis. Figure 4–79 is a transverse section of the upper abdomen in which the celiac axis appears as a sonolucency anterior to the aorta. On longitudinal scans the communication between the celiac artery aneurysm and the celiac artery can be identified as it takes off from the aorta. Any time we see a sonolucent mass in the upper abdomen, it is important to attempt to determine whether or not it communicates with any of the vessels in the area. If this communication can be demonstrated, the diagnosis of an aneurysm or a dilated venous structure can be made. If it cannot be shown, the possibility of a small pseudocyst must be considered.

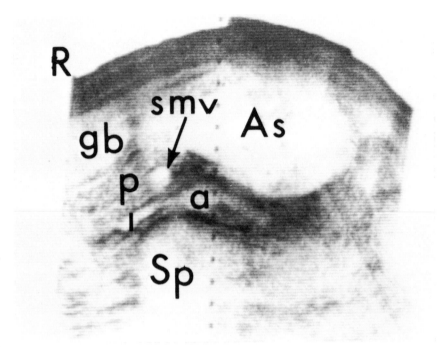

FIG 4–77.

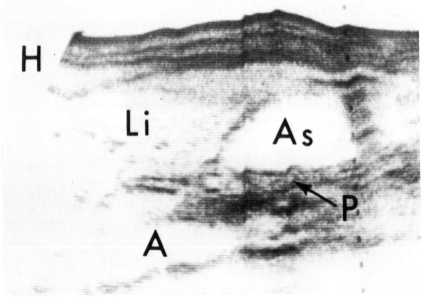

FIG 4–78.

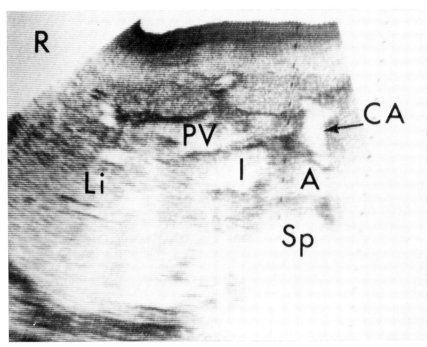

A   = Aorta
a   = Aorta
As  = Ascites
CA  = Celiac artery aneurysm
F   = Foot
gb  = Gallbladder
H   = Head
I   = Inferior vena cava
Li  = Liver
P   = Pancreas
p   = Pancreas
PV  = Portal vein
R   = Right
SA  = Splenic artery
smv = Superior mesenteric vein
Sp  = Spine
SV  = Splenic vein

FIG 4–79.

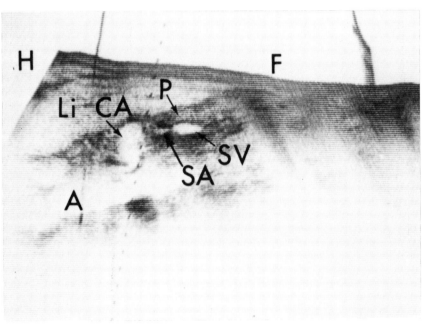

FIG 4–80.

## Pancreatic Carcinoma

Tumors of the pancreas usually appear on ultrasound scans as masses that are less echogenic than the normal pancreas and have irregular borders. They appear solid with diffuse echoes throughout. Often, they are less echogenic than the normal liver. The borders are somewhat irregular or ill-defined. The even echo pattern seen in the normal pancreas is not present in pancreatic carcinoma. Figures 4–81 and 4–82 are scans of a 47-year-old man with progressive weight loss. An upper GI tract examination revealed anterior displacement of the stomach. Ultrasound examination showed a large hypoechoic mass in the head of the pancreas. The borders of the mass are irregular and the splenic vein is displaced anteriorly along with the superior mesenteric vein. In Figure 4–81, the superior mesenteric artery is in a normal position, but the superior mesenteric vein is displaced anteriorly. The longitudinal scan (Fig 4–82) shows the mass anterior to the aorta, displacing the superior mesenteric vein anteriorly. The mass is in the head and uncinate process of the pancreas and is displacing the superior mesenteric vein. The biliary tree is obstructed, as numerous tubular structures are noted in the liver (arrows in Fig 4–82).

Figures 4–83 and 4–84 are transverse and longitudinal scans of a 76-year-old woman who entered the hospital with a history of guaiac-positive stools and progressive weight loss. Ultrasound examination revealed a mass in the pancreatic head. The transverse scan (Fig 4–83) shows a pancreatic carcinoma (arrows) in the region of the head of the pancreas. Figure 4–84, a longitudinal scan through the carcinoma of the head of the pancreas, shows a markedly dilated common bile duct ending abruptly at the site of the tumor. This represents a solid mass of the head of the pancreas obstructing the biliary tree. When the common bile duct is dilated, attempts should be made to determine the reason for obstruction. By scanning along the long axis of the

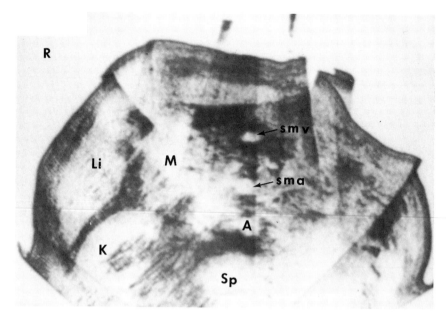

FIG 4–81.

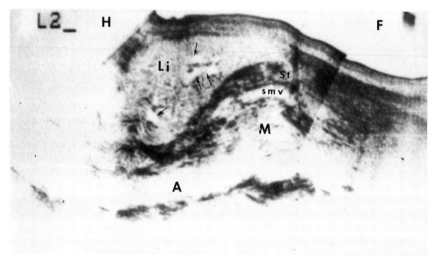

FIG 4–82.

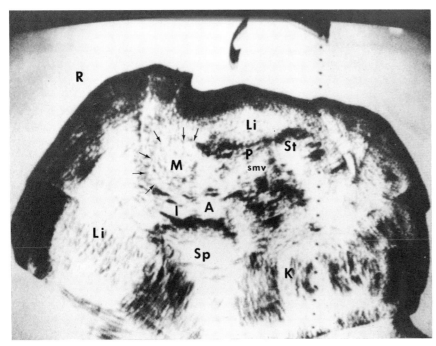

**FIG 4–83.**

common bile duct, the region of the distal common bile duct can be visualized. It may often be obscured by air. However, the reason for biliary obstruction can often be determined. The dilated common bile duct ends abruptly in a soft tissue tumor, consistent with pancreatic carcinoma.

| | | |
|---|---|---|
| **A** | = | Aorta |
| **Arrows** | = | Biliary dilatation |
| **cbd** | = | Dilated common bile duct |
| **F** | = | Foot |
| **H** | = | Head |
| **I** | = | Inferior vena cava |
| **K** | = | Kidney |
| **Li** | = | Liver |
| **M** | = | Pancreatic carcinoma |
| **M + arrows** | = | Pancreatic carcinoma |
| **P** | = | Pancreas |
| **PV** | = | Portal vein |
| **R** | = | Right |
| **sma** | = | Superior mesenteric artery |
| **smv** | = | Superior mesenteric vein |
| **Sp** | = | Spine |
| **St** | = | Stomach |

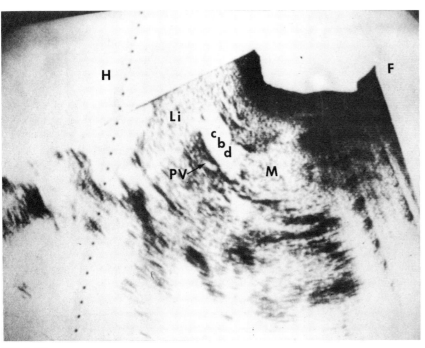

**FIG 4–84.**

## Pancreatic Carcinoma

Hypoechoic, solid masses in the pancreatic bed must always be regarded as possible pancreatic carcinoma. Ultrasound can be used in the diagnosis by assisting in the percutaneous needle biopsy. Figures 4–85 and 4–86 are transverse and longitudinal scans of a 58-year-old man with recent weight loss. Ultrasound and CT examination demonstrated a mass in the head of the pancreas (M). Ultrasound was used to obtain a percutaneous biopsy specimen, which was positive for pancreatic adenocarcinoma. Note the irregular texture pattern to the liver in Figure 4–85. This is secondary to diffuse liver metastases.

Figures 4–87 and 4–88 are scans of a 45-year-old woman with vague abdominal discomfort. An upper GI series, abdominal CT, and ERCP all were negative. Figure 4–87 is a transverse scan from the earlier abdominal study. A mass was noted near the uncinate process of the pancreas. It did not appear to be the inferior vena cava because of the soft internal echoes. The possibility that the mass represented the duodenum was considered. However, the common bile duct (arrowheads) in Figure 4–87 was identified, and the mass was medial to it. The duodenum is usually lateral to the common bile in this location. For better localization of the duodenum, the patient was given water. Figure 4–88 is a transverse scan made after the patient had ingested several glasses of water. The duodenum is well distended and separate from the mass. The duodenum is now fluid filled. The mass measured 2.5 cm and was located in the head and uncinate process of the pancreas. Operation was performed on the basis of the ultrasound findings alone, since all other studies were negative. A small adenocarcinoma of the head of the pancreas was removed at surgery.

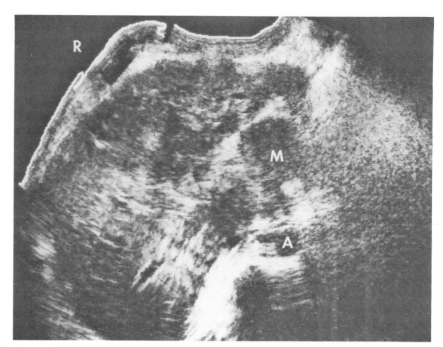

**FIG 4–85.**

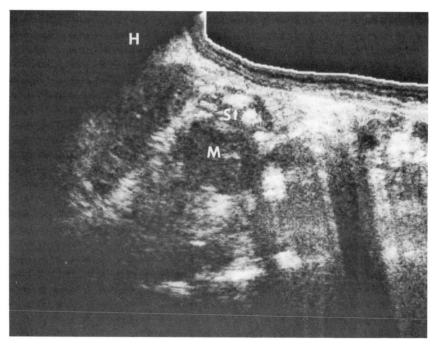

**FIG 4–86.**

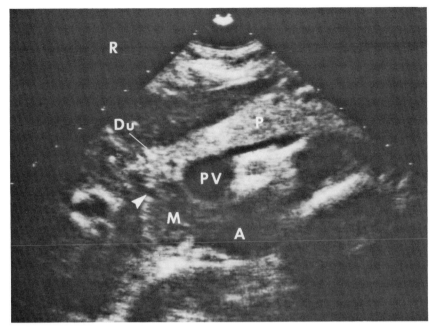

FIG 4–87.

| A | = Aorta |
| **Arrowhead** | = Common bile duct |
| **Du** | = Duodenum |
| **H** | = Head |
| **M** | = Pancreatic carcinoma |
| **P** | = Pancreas |
| **PV** | = Portal vein |
| **R** | = Right |
| **St** | = Stomach |

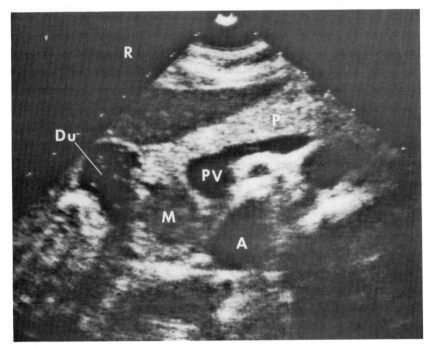

FIG 4–88.

## Pancreatic Tumors

Solid lesions in the pancreatic bed which are demonstrated by ultrasound are usually secondary to neoplasm. The type of neoplasm cannot be determined from any characteristic echo appearance. The only information that can be derived is that a solid lesion in the pancreatic bed is present.

Figure 4–89 is a longitudinal scan of the upper abdomen of a 34-year-old woman who had recently had a cesarean section. A diagnosis of cervical carcinoma was made at the time of the operation, and an ultrasound examination of the abdomen was ordered after surgery. In Figure 4–89, a mass can be seen in the region of the head of the pancreas. This was solid in appearance. There is evidence of dilatation of the proximal pancreatic duct (PD). The patient died approximately 4 weeks after the ultrasound examination. Cervical carcinoma with diffuse abdominal metastasis was found. The solid lesion in the pancreas was secondary to cervical carcinoma metastasis. There is no sonographic feature that would discriminate such a lesion from pancreatic carcinoma or any other solid tumor.

Tumors in the tail of the pancreas are more difficult to detect on ultrasound if the patient is imaged in a supine position. The left upper quadrant is often obscured by air in the stomach and splenic flexure. Therefore, other orientations must be used to visualize the tail of the pancreas. The patient may be examined prone. The left kidney is used as an ultrasonic window to visualize the pancreatic tail. Coronal scans through an intercostal space can also be performed, with the spleen and kidney acting as ultrasonic windows. Figure 4–90 is an intravenous pyelogram of a patient with marked distortion and deformity of the upper pole collecting system of the left kidney. A mass is present and was suspected of being a hypernephroma. Ultrasound examination of the patient was performed with the patient in a prone position. Figure 4–91 is a longitudinal scan through the long axis of the left kidney. The mass is markedly

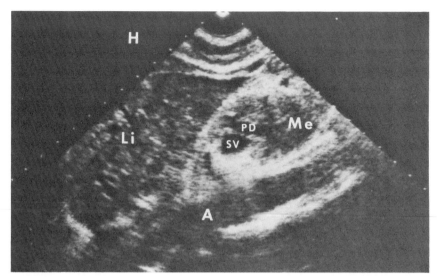

FIG 4–89.

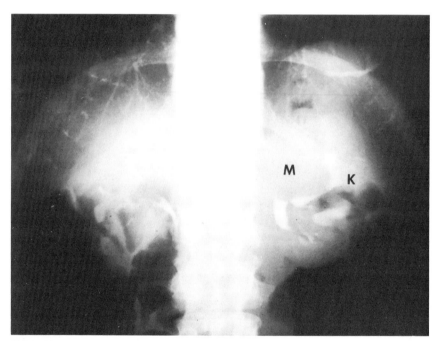

FIG 4–90.

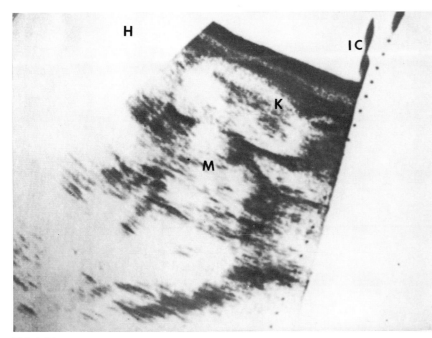

**FIG 4–91.**

anterior to the kidney, more in the region of the tail of the pancreas. There is loss of the renal contour adjacent to the mass, indicating invasion. This turned out to be a carcinoma of the tail of the pancreas that invaded the kidney.

Figure 4–92 is a coronal scan through an intercostal space. The patient was a 24-year-old woman with vague abdominal discomfort. A large solid mass is seen in the left upper quadrant, displacing the spleen and kidney posteriorly and medially. The mass was thought to be in the tail of the pancreas on ultrasound examination, and distal pancreatectomy for islet cell tumor of the pancreas was performed.

| | | |
|---|---|---|
| **A** | = | Aorta |
| **H** | = | Head |
| **IC** | = | Iliac crest |
| **K** | = | Kidney |
| **Li** | = | Liver |
| **M** | = | Pancreatic carcinoma |
| **Me** | = | Cervical carcinoma metastasis |
| **PD** | = | Dilated pancreatic duct |
| **S** | = | Spleen |
| **SV** | = | Splenic vein |
| **T** | = | Islet cell tumor |

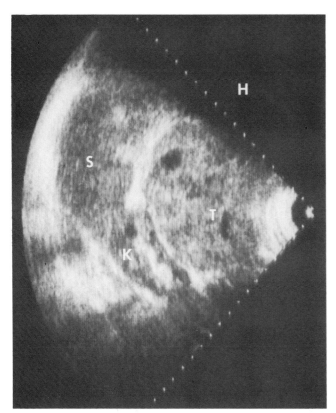

**FIG 4–92.**

## Insulinoma and Cystadenocarcinoma

As mentioned earlier, detection of a small mass is easiest in the uncinate process of the pancreas, because of the surrounding vascular anatomy. Figures 4–93 and 4–94 show a 1.5-cm insulinoma of the uncinate process of the pancreas. The transverse section in Figure 4–93 shows a relatively sonolucent solid mass in the uncinate process of the pancreas, just posterior to the superior mesenteric vein. The mass is medial to the common bile duct. On a longitudinal scan (Fig 4–94) the insulinoma appears as a relatively less echogenic region in the posterior aspect of the pancreas.

A cystadenocarcinoma usually presents as a sonolucent mass with multiple septations (Figs 4–95, 4–96). The mass is often confused with a multiloculated pseudocyst of the pancreas. Figure 4–95 is a transverse scan showing a mass in the region of the body and tail of the pancreas. There are some linear echoes and some wall thickening to the lateral aspect of the mass. Figure 4–96, a CT scan of approximately the same area, shows a large mass anterior to the left kidney and medial to the spleen. The mass is less dense centrally with some increased density representing the septations (arrow).

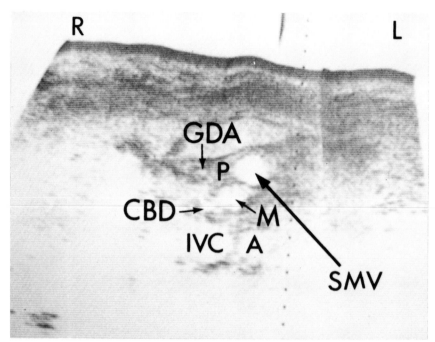

FIG 4–93.

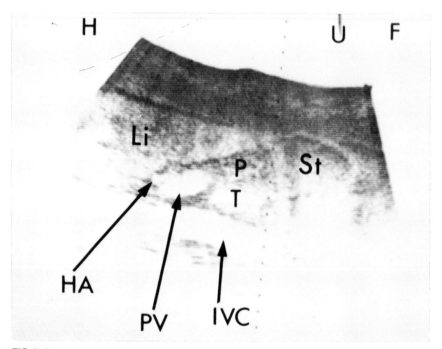

FIG 4–94.

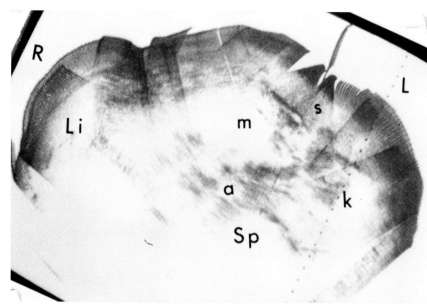

**FIG 4–95.**

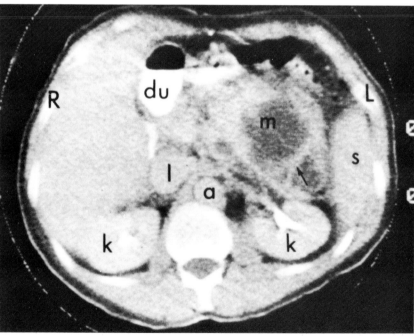

**FIG 4–96.**

SOURCE: Figures 4–95 and 4–96 are reproduced with permission from Carroll B, Sample WF: Pancreatic cystadenocarcinoma: CT body scan and gray scale ultrasound appearance. *AJR* 1978; 131:339–341.

| A | = | Aorta |
|---|---|---|
| a | = | Aorta |
| **Arrows** | = | Septations within cystadeno-carcinoma |
| **CBD** | = | Common bile duct |
| **Du** | = | Duodenum |
| **F** | = | Foot |
| **GDA** | = | Gastroduodenal artery |
| **H** | = | Head |
| **HA** | = | Hepatic artery |
| **I** | = | Inferior vena cava |
| **IVC** | = | Inferior vena cava |
| **k** | = | Kidney |
| **L** | = | Left |
| **Li** | = | Liver |
| **M** | = | Insulinoma |
| **m** | = | Cystadenocarcinoma |
| **P** | = | Pancreas |
| **PV** | = | Portal vein |
| **R** | = | Right |
| **s** | = | Spleen |
| **SMV** | = | Superior mesenteric vein |
| **Sp** | = | Spine |
| **St** | = | Stomach |
| **T** | = | Insulinoma tumor |
| **U** | = | Umbilical level |

## Dilated Pancreatic Duct

The patient whose scans are shown here had ampullary carcinoma, with dilatation of the common bile duct and the pancreatic duct. Figures 4–97 and 4–98 are transverse scans made at different levels through the pancreas. Figure 4–97 is close to the level of the splenic vein. Anterior to the splenic vein is another tubular structure representing a dilated pancreatic duct. We can also see a dilated common bile duct. The transverse scan in Figure 4–98 was made slightly lower, at the level of the superior mesenteric vein. It shows the uncinate process of the pancreas posterior to the superior mesenteric vein. The dilated pancreatic duct is seen to approach the common bile duct.

Figures 4–99 and 4–100 are longitudinal scans showing the dilated common bile duct of the same patient. The dilated pancreatic duct (Fig 4–99) is seen coursing caudally, just anterior to the dilated common bile duct. Finally, Figure 4–100 shows the region close to the ampulla where the dilated common bile duct and proximal portion of the pancreatic duct near the ampulla can be seen. The head of the pancreas, anterior to the common bile duct and cephalad to the stomach, is also visible. Dilated bile ducts are noted also within the liver. These scans illustrate the finding of dilatation of the pancreatic duct, normally seen as a strong linear echo, not as a tubular structure within the pancreas.

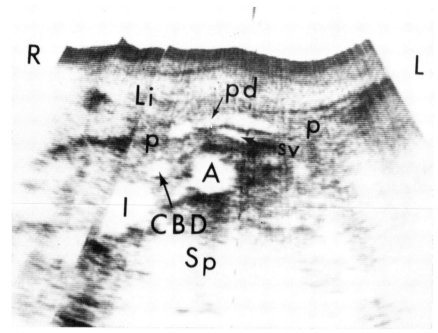

FIG 4–97.

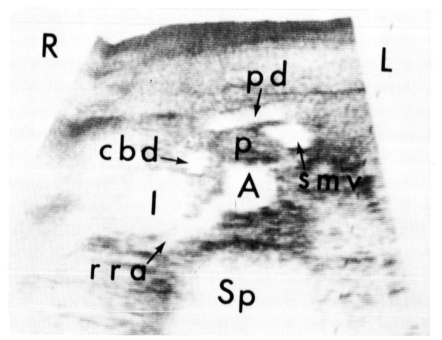

FIG 4–98.

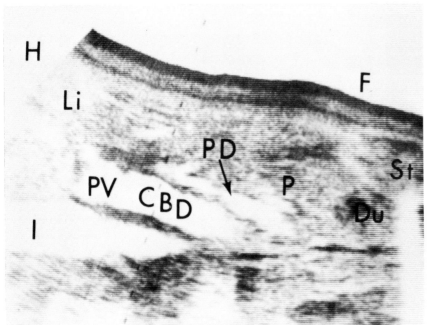

A = Aorta
BD = Dilated bile duct
CBD = Common bile duct
cbd = Common bile duct
Du = Duodenum
F = Foot
H = Head
ha = Hepatic artery
hv = Hepatic vein
I = Inferior vena cava
L = Left
Li = Liver
P = Pancreas
p = Pancreas
PD = Pancreatic duct
pd = Pancreatic duct
PV = Portal vein
pv = Portal vein
R = Right
rra = Right renal artery
smv = Superior mesenteric vein
Sp = Spine
St = Stomach
sv = Splenic vein

FIG 4–99.

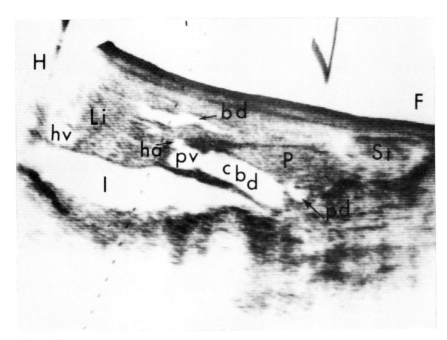

FIG 4–100.

## Dilated Pancreatic Duct

Figures 4–101 and 4–102 illustrate another case of a dilated pancreatic duct. The patient was a 28-year-old woman who had a perforated duodenal ulcer. The perforation and surgery in the area caused stricture around the ampulla of Vater. This in turn led to dilatation of the pancreatic duct. A transverse scan (Fig 4–101) shows the dilated pancreatic duct anterior to the splenic vein. It is important to identify the splenic vein so as not to confuse it with a dilated pancreatic duct. A longitudinal scan (Fig 4–102) shows the pancreatic duct again anterior to the splenic vein. The celiac axis and the superior mesenteric artery arising from the aorta are also seen.

Figures 4–103 and 4–104 again illustrate dilatation of the pancreatic duct, in this case secondary to ampullary carcinoma. On a transverse scan through the pancreas (Fig 4–103), pancreatic tissue is well seen on both sides of the slightly dilated pancreatic duct. Figure 4–104 is a longitudinal scan through the body of the pancreas at the region of the superior mesenteric vein. A small circular sonolucency is seen, representing the pancreatic duct in the central portion of the body of the pancreas.

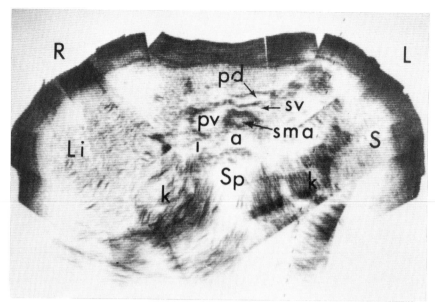

FIG 4–101.

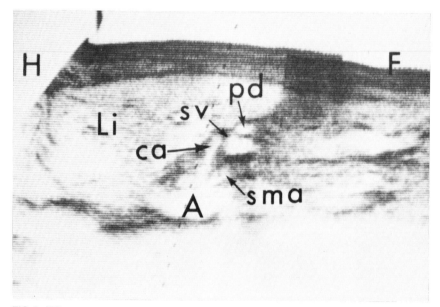

FIG 4–102.

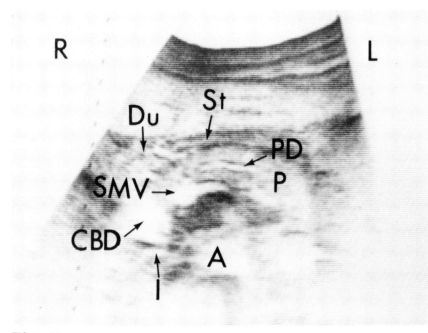

A   =  Aorta
a   =  Aorta
bd  =  Dilated intrahepatic bile ducts
ca  =  Celiac axis
CBD =  Common bile duct
Du  =  Duodenum
F   =  Foot
H   =  Head
I   =  Inferior vena cava
k   =  Kidney
L   =  Left
Li  =  Liver
P   =  Pancreas
PD  =  Pancreatic duct
pd  =  Pancreatic duct
pv  =  Portal vein
R   =  Right
S   =  Spleen
sma =  Superior mesenteric artery
SMV =  Superior mesenteric vein
smv =  Superior mesenteric vein
Sp  =  Spine
St  =  Stomach
sv  =  Splenic vein

FIG 4–103.

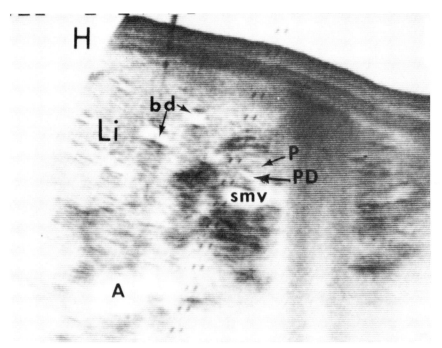

FIG 4–104.

## Dilated Pancreatic Duct

A dilated pancreatic duct is another tubular structure in the upper abdomen that poses diagnostic difficulties. The splenic vein, splenic artery, left renal vein, wall of the stomach, and fluid in the stomach may all be confused with a dilated pancreatic duct. If the ultrasonographer has never seen a dilated pancreatic duct before, he or she will confuse it with a normal structure and not recognize its importance. By identifying the above-mentioned normal anatomic structures and recognizing that an extra tubular lucency is present, the ultrasonographer may then consider the possibility of a dilated pancreatic duct.

Figure 4–105 is a transverse scan of the upper abdomen of a 60-year-old man with carcinoma of the head of the pancreas. The posterior tubular structure represents the splenic vein; a dilated pancreatic duct is anterior to it. The wall of the dilated pancreatic duct has an irregular contour. Figure 4–106 is a CT scan at the same level. The splenic vein is again seen posterior to a dilated pancreatic duct (arrow).

Figures 4–107 and 4–108 are scans of a 58-year-old man who also had pancreatic carcinoma of the head. Figure 4–107 is an oblique scan following the long axis of the common bile duct, which is massively dilated. Figure 4–108 is a transverse scan that shows the massively dilated common bile duct and a slightly dilated pancreatic duct (arrow). When these findings are demonstrated, the level of the lesion is near the ampulla of Vater. When no mass is seen, the differential diagnosis would include ampullary carcinoma, common bile duct stone, common bile duct stricture or edema, postsurgical stenosis, and small pancreatic head tumor. In this case, the dilatation of the common bile duct and pancreatic duct was secondary to a small pancreatic head tumor.

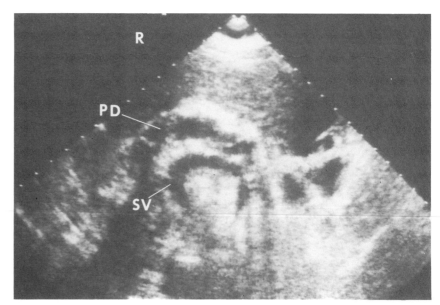

**FIG 4–105.**

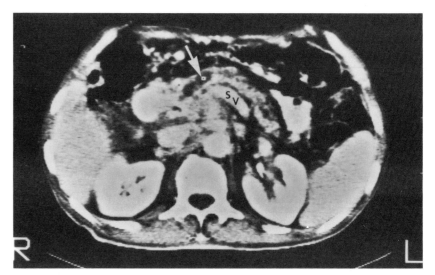

**FIG 4–106.**

| A | = | Aorta |
|---|---|---|
| **Arrow** | = | Dilated pancreatic duct |
| **CBD** | = | Dilated common bile duct |
| **GB** | = | Gallbladder |
| **H** | = | Head |
| **PD** | = | Dilated pancreatic duct |
| **R** | = | Right |
| **SV** | = | Splenic vein |

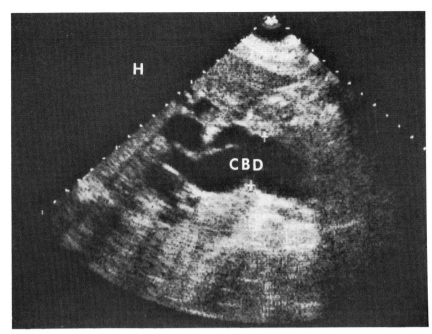

**FIG 4–107.**

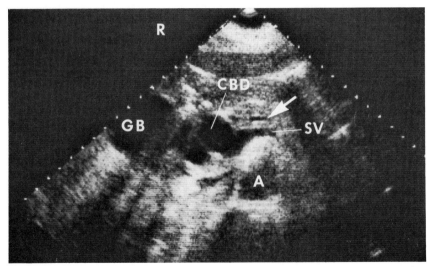

**FIG 4–108.**

# 5.
# Ultrasonography of the Aorta

Nancy J. Worthen, M.D.

## Anatomy of the Aorta

The aorta is the main arterial trunk of the systemic circulation. The abdominal aorta is the last segment of the aorta and enters the abdomen at the level of the 12th thoracic vertebral body, behind the diaphragm and through the aortic hiatus. It descends in the abdomen to the left of the midline and anterior to the lumbar vertebral bodies. The aorta tapers in caliber and approximately at the level of the fourth lumbar vertebral body bifurcates and becomes the common iliac arteries. The average diameter of the aorta varies with age and anatomic level. The aorta dilates with advancing age. Mean aortic diameters in females vary from 12.3 mm in the second decade to 16.9 mm in the sixth decade. In males, the diameter increases from 12.2 mm to 22.8 mm in the corresponding time interval.[1] Aortic diameters greater than 30 mm on ultrasound are considered abnormal.

The diameter of the aorta tapers as branches arise from it. Branches of the aorta are considered in three groups: visceral, parietal, and terminal. The visceral branches in the abdomen are the celiac, middle suprarenal, superior mesenteric, renal, gonadal, and inferior mesenteric arteries. The celiac axis and the superior mesenteric artery are the only visceral branches commonly seen on routine abdominal sonography. The renal arteries are less frequently seen. The right renal artery is more frequently observed than the left. The celiac axis arises perpendicular to the anterior surface of the aorta and just caudad to the abdominal entrance of the aorta. The superior mesenteric artery also arises from the ventral surface of the aorta about 1.25 cm below the celiac axis. Its origin forms an obtuse angle with the aorta. The renal arteries are paired arteries that arise caudad to the superior mesenteric artery off the lateral aspect of the aorta. The parietal branches of the aorta are not seen sonographically. The terminal branches of the aorta are the common iliac arteries.

The abdominal aorta comes in contact with several structures within the abdominal cavity. To the right lies the inferior vena cava. Anteriorly, the aorta comes in contact with the pancreas, splenic vein, left renal vein, third portion of the duodenum, and many loops of small bowel. Several nerve ganglia, the celiac plexus, and the intermesenteric portion of the aortic plexus lie anterior to the aorta. The left ureter lies to the left of the aorta. These anatomic relationships should be kept in mind when evaluating a patient for aortic disease.

## Ultrasound Technique

No special patient preparation is necessary except that sonograms must be scheduled before barium studies. The patient is examined in a supine position. If the aorta is obscured by bowel gas, or for demonstration of the aortic bifurcation, the patient may be positioned in a left lateral decubitus position. In this position the liver is used as an acoustic window.[2] The left lateral decubitus position is also helpful for delineating the origin of the renal arteries.[3] Scans should be made with the patient in deep inspiration so the full effect of the liver as an acoustic window can be realized.

The typical evaluation should include both static and real-time examinations. Transducer selection is based on body habitus and aortic position. The most routinely used transducers include the 3.5-MHz medium or long focus transducers or the 5.0-MHz medium focus transducer.

Static scans are begun in the transverse plane at the xyphoid and proceed in 1- to 2-cm steps to an area 3 cm below the umbilicus. The aorta may be easily mapped out during transverse scanning, thus allowing easier alignment of longitudinal scans. Longitudinal scans are performed at 0.5-cm intervals over the mapped-out course of the aorta. If an aneurysm is identified in the distal aorta, if iliac artery enlargement is suspected, or if the patient has had an aortoiliac or aortofemoral bypass graft implanted, the examination should be extended to include the common iliac, external iliac, and femoral arteries bilaterally.[4] These scans are made in an oblique plane from the umbilicus to the inguinal canal. Doppler evaluation of the aorta and its branches is under investigation and may prove to be a new tool for aortic examinations.

On transverse scans the normal aorta appears as an anechoic circular structure anterior and to the left of the vertebral body. On longitudinal scans the aorta is seen as an anechoic tapering tubular structure to the left of the midline and anterior to the vertebral bodies. Aortic pulsations are seen on real-time studies of the aorta. Ease of the transducer manipulation fa-

cilitates real-time studies, often making them easier to perform than static scans, because the transducer head may be used to manually dislodge or move bowel gas masking the aorta.

## Normal Aging Changes of the Aorta

The aorta consists of elastic fibers, collagen fibers, smooth muscle, and mucoid ground substance. All of these components change with age.[5] The end result is a weakening of the aorta leading to enlargement. These ectatic changes have long been noted at autopsy and confirmed by in vivo computed tomographic (CT) appearances.[1] Dixon et al. reported normal sizes of the aorta for men and women from the second to the eighth decade. Dilation of the aorta is more often seen in men than in women.[1] The median diameter in the eighth decade is 22.8 mm ± 2.8 mm for men and 16.9 mm ± 2.5 mm for women. Sonographically, these aging changes correspond to an increasing caliber and decreasing taper of the aorta.

## Pathology of the Aorta

### Atherosclerosis

The most common disease of the aorta is atherosclerosis. It is prevalent in all societies in which the mean serum cholesterol level in adults is above 200 mg/dl. After approximately 20 years, the disease manifests with plaques in the abdominal portion of the aorta. The major consequences of severe atherosclerosis of the aorta are luminal dilatation (aneurysms) and luminal obstruction. Aneurysms are more common. Aortic plaque secondary to atherosclerosis can be recognized sonographically by irregularities in the typically smooth lumen/wall interface. Calcifications of the plaques can be recognized as areas of irregularity that cast an acoustic shadow.

### Obstruction

Aortic obstruction most commonly affects the abdominal aorta. It may be missed on static sonography.[6, 7] The aorta is of normal diameter in this condition and on static scans appears as a typical anechoic vascular channel, rather than having a hyperechogenic center (as in thrombosis). Real-time sonography will demonstrate prominent pulsations in the patent proximal aorta and an absence of pulsations in the occluded aorta.[7]

*Aneurysm*

The abdominal aorta is the most frequent site of atherosclerotic aneurysm formation. Occasionally aneurysms of the abdominal aorta may be secondary to other conditions such as trauma, infection, dissection, syphilitic aortitis, degenerative conditions (e.g., Ehlers-Danlos syndrome, Marfan's syndrome), or, less frequently, surgery. More than 96% of abdominal aortic aneurysms are atherosclerotic in nature.[8] Atherosclerotic aneurysms occur in as many as 2% of the elderly population.[9] They are more common in men and occur in increasing frequency directly related to age. As the longevity of the American population increases, the incidence of aneurysmal disease is also expected to increase.

Aortic aneurysms tend to occur as multifocal disease. A recent review found that 12.6% of patients treated for aortic aneurysms had multiple aneurysms, 72% of which occurred simultaneously.[10] In 28% of the patients, another aneurysm developed within 10 years. The most frequent combination found was thoracic aortic and infrarenal abdominal aneurysms. Multiplicity tended to be associated with causes other than atherosclerosis, such as Marfan's syndrome, dissection, infection, and previous operation.

True aneurysms involve all three layers of the abdominal aorta wall—the intima, media, and adventitia. There are two types of aneurysms, fusiform and saccular. The fusiform type is more common and is so named because the entire circumference of the aortic wall is involved. Fusiform aneurysms tend to arise distal to the renal arteries. Saccular aneurysms involve only a portion of the aortic wall. They tend to occur more frequently in the thorax. Abdominal saccular aneurysms generally are confined to the region proximal to the renal arteries. Most aneurysms are located to the left of midline since the expansion of the aneurysm is limited on the right and posteriorly by the spine. This anterior expansion usually pushes aside the bowel gas, thus creating a good sonographic window for examination. The common iliac arteries are frequently involved—in more than 65% of aortic aneurysms. Less often, peripheral arterial aneurysms are concomitantly present.

Most abdominal aortic aneurysms are asymptomatic. An aneurysm is usually suspected on a routine physical examination in an older person when a pulsatile abdominal mass is found. The role of ultrasound is to document the presence or absence of aneurysm and to exclude other etiologies for the pulsatile mass.

Sonographically, aneurysms appear as focal areas of aortic enlargement (>3 cm) or as a bulge in the normally tapering distal aorta.[11] The thrombus within the aneurysm usually appears as low level echogenic material surrounding the aneurysm. Not all thrombi are detected sonographically. Recent thrombi or thrombi that are homogeneous or of similar age will appear anechoic.[6]

Ultrasound has been reported to be 94%–100% accurate in detecting abdominal aortic aneurysms.[12–16] Failure to detect an aneurysm has been attributed to overlying bowel gas[13, 16] and confusion of para-aortic masses with aneurysms when bistable equipment was used.[12, 14] Confusion of para-aortic lymph nodes or other para-aortic lesions for aneurysm has become far less common with the advent of gray-scale equipment.

In recent reports, ultrasound has been helpful in defining normal aortas in patients with pulsatile masses and in delineating other possible etiologies of the suspected aneurysms.[17, 18] Tortuous aortas, pancreatic pseudocysts, pancreatic carcinoma, metastatic disease, lymphomatosis, para-aortic lymph nodes, and low-lying livers all have been described as pulsatile masses clinically mimicking abdominal aneurysms.

The aneurysm should be measured at the time of sonographic examination. The most accurate indicator of aneurysmal size is the anteroposterior (AP) diameter of the aneurysm. The AP diameter should be measured on both longitudinal and transverse scans. AP diameter measurement is most accurate in the axial plane. The transverse diameter is less accurate because of dependence on lateral resolution and because the transverse dimension may be elongated due to an accidental tangential scan through a tortuous aorta. Graeve et al. have shown that the best correlation between aneurysmal size and sonographic measurement occurs when measurements are taken from the leading echo of the anterior aortic wall to the anterior echo of the spine.[19] Discrepancies between sonographic aneurysmal size and operative aneurysmal measurements do exist. Leopold et al. reported a measured accuracy of ±3 mm.[11] Maloney et al. reported an average difference between measured and actual diameters of ±4 mm.[15] Brewster et al. found ultrasound to underestimate aneurysm size by as much as 20%, with an inaccuracy of slightly more than 1 cm.[20] In another report, the mean aortic measurement on ultrasound in 58 patients was 6.1 cm and the intraoperative mean was 6.3 cm. The measurements were identical in 34% of patients and were within 0.5 to 1 cm in 75% and 92% of patients, respectively.[21] Gomes et al. found ultrasound to underestimate aneurysm size, with variations from −2 to 16 mm.[22–24] Comparisons, however, were made with transverse diameter measurements. Graeve et al. found ultrasound to underestimate aneurysm size from 0 to −9 mm when AP diameter measurements were used.[19] They also found that the best correlation occurred using aorta to spine measurements. Ultrasound is accurate in the diagnosis of abdominal aortic aneurysms when the aorta is visualized. Slight discrepancies in size are not of concern.

The current surgical management of an aortic aneurysm is controversial. Some authors believe that resection is indicated in all cases, while others have suggested that close observation is the best choice for aneurysms less than 5 cm in size. In patients who are poor surgical risks, the course of the aortic aneurysm may be followed by sonography. Bernstein et al. examined the growth rates of aneurysms less than 6 cm in size.[25] The mean growth rate was 0.26 cm/year in aneurysms ranging from 3 to 5.9 cm. The growth rate was higher in aneurysms larger than 6 cm. If patients are being studied by serial ultrasound examinations, it is important that comparable images with good points of reference be obtained for accurate measurements. Any rapid change in the size of an abdominal aortic aneurysm may indicate impending rupture.

If an aneurysm is detected on a sonographic examination, it is important to determine whether or not the aneurysm extends into the iliac arteries.[4] Sonography may be requested to delineate the relationship of the aortic aneurysm to the renal arteries. Ericksson et al. reported poor results when they attempted to identify the renal arteries and measure their distance from the aneurysmal borders.[16] This information, however, may be derived from knowledge that the renal arteries arise at approximately the same level as the superior mesenteric artery (SMA), which is a constant landmark. If the aneurysm extends to the SMA, it will involve the renal arteries. It is also possible to estimate the relationship of the aneurysm and the renal arteries by marking the skin at the level where the aneurysm extends cranially and at the midpoint of the kidneys. The renal arteries are almost never involved if the midpoint of the lowest kidney is cranial to the aneurysm.[26] Most experienced surgeons can readily anticipate suprarenal extension by the aortic aneurysm, so the information is interesting but not critical to successful surgical repair of the lesion.[27, 28]

The most common major complication of an aortic aneurysm is rupture. Aneurysms may rupture into the retroperitoneum, the free peritoneum, or an adjoining viscus such as the duodenum, left renal vein, inferior vena cava, or urinary tract. The rate of rupture depends on the site of the aneurysm. In an autopsy series of 473 patients with aneurysms, Darling et al. found that 24% of the aneurysms had ruptured and were the cause of death.[29] Aneurysms 4–7 cm in diameter had a rupture rate of 25%. Aneurysms 7–10 cm had a 45% rupture rate. Aneurysms larger than 10 cm had a 60% rupture rate.

Because of patient instability, ultrasound plays no role in the diagnosis of abdominal aortic aneurysm rupture. However, ultrasound has been useful in detecting a contained aortic aneurysmal rupture.[30] The findings are those of an aneurysm with an adjacent complex mass, or an aneurysm with a complex mass anterior to the left psoas muscle. These patients survived because the aneurysm ruptured into a confined anatomic space. A series of five patients with aortic aneurysm rupture were examined postoperatively.[31] Significant hematomas were found persisting for several months in the retroperitoneal and periaortic areas.

In summary, sonography serves the following functions in patients with clinically suspected abdominal aortic aneurysm:

1. To document the aneurysm.
2. To delineate anatomic causes of pulsatile masses.
3. To measure the aneurysm.
4. To document aneurysmal extension (iliac, renal arteries).
5. To document changing size of the aneurysm.

## Dissection

Aortic dissection is unusual. It usually begins in the thoracic aorta and is characterized by the development of a hematoma within the middle to outer third of the aortic media. The dissecting hematoma may extend for a variable distance around the circumference of the vessel, but the major force of the dissection is longitudinal, paralleling the blood flow. Aortic dissections are classified on the basis of duration and anatomic location. Acute dissection is defined as having occurred within 2 weeks before the institution of therapy. Chronic dissection is defined as having existed for more than 2 weeks before the institution of therapy. Debakey et al. have formulated the most widely used classification of dissection.[32] This classification is based on the anatomic site of the initial tear and on the extent of the hematoma. Types I and III, although arising in different areas of the thoracic aorta, both tend to extend beyond the thoracic aorta.

Hypertension is the most consistent factor that predisposes to aortic dissection. Aneurysms may develop in an aorta that has a preexisting chronic dissection.

Sonography plays little role in the diagnosis of acute aortic dissection. The major imaging examinations ordered in cases of suspected aortic dissection are CT and aortography.[33] On sonography, dissection appears as an extralinear echo in the aortic lumen.[34] If the intimal flap at the site of the original tear is free and pulsating, it sometimes may be demonstrated by slow static B-mode scanning, and it is easily seen using real-time modality. The site of reentry may be visualized as the area where the aorta regains its normal appearance.

## Postoperative Ultrasonography of the Aorta

Both aneurysms and aortic occlusive disease are treated by placement of bypass grafts. An uncomplicated infrarenal aortic aneurysm is repaired by placement of a prosthetic tube graft from the area of disease-free aorta above the aneurysm to a disease-free section of vessel below the aneurysm. The distal section of vessel may be the aorta, the common iliac artery, or the femoral artery, depending on the size of the intervening aneurysm. The graft is inserted end-to-end into the aorta and the aneurysm is closed directly over the graft. The graft is seen sonographically as parallel straight echogenic walls or lines in the distal aorta. They occupy the same position as the replaced aorta and iliofemoral branches. Postoperative complications include hematoma, infection, and false aneurysms. Static sonography delineates these complications as sonolucent masses extrinsic to the grafts.[35]

In bypass surgery for occlusive disease, the diseased segments of the aorta and iliac vessels are left in place and the proximal end of the graft is sewn to the anterior aorta. The iliac limbs of the graft follow the course of the native vessels. On sagittal scans the bypass graft may be seen anterior to the aorta as an anechoic structure with discrete borders. Without a proper patient history this structure could be confused with a para-aortic mass.[35] Complications of aortic graft surgery include hematoma, infections, false aneurysms, and occlusions. As with replacement grafts, the complications on static scans appear as anechoic masses extrinsic to the grafts. False aneurysm fluid collections may be differentiated from the other complications by their pulsations, seen on real-time scanning. In 87 patients with aortofemoral grafts, sonography was able to delineate the proximal anastomoses in 84%, the iliac graft limbs in 88%–91%, and the distal anastomoses in all but one.[36]

Persistent fluid seen around the graft is always abnormal. Hematomas secondary either to surgery or to initial rupture do occur, but they decrease in size over time. A persistent fluid collection around a graft should raise the suspicion of infection.[36] Occluded bypass or replacement grafts will appear as normal vascular grafts on static scans. On real-time examination they are nonpulsatile.[7]

## Comparison of Ultrasound With Other Examination Methods

### Physical Examination

Aortic aneurysms can be diagnosed on physical examination in up to 91% of cases.[20] Measurements on physical examination overestimate the size of the aneurysm. Detection is related to the experience of the examiner and to the size of the lesion.

*Plain Film Radiography*

Lateral lumbar spine films can be diagnostic of abdominal aortic aneurysms if the aneurysms are calcified. Calcifications are seen in up to 70% of patients.[20] Measurements made from lateral x-ray films will also overestimate the aneurysm size. The size of abdominal aortic aneurysms measured on plain films were compared with sonographic measurements.[37] The cross-table lateral measurements were larger than ultrasound measurements by a factor of 1.3 to 1.

*Angiography*

Since only the lumen is opacified, aortography underestimates aneurysmal size, because the aneurysmal area is filled by thrombus, which does not opacify. Aortography may be helpful in providing vascular data on the involvement of other vessels such as the renal, iliac, or femoral arteries. Recent reports have concluded that aortography should not be a routine part of workup for abdominal aortic aneurysm because of low yield to cost ratio, the time delay, and the risk of the procedure.[27, 28] Indications for aortography include thoracic or thoracoabdominal aneurysm suggested by chest x-ray, mesenteric or visceral ischemia, severe hypertension or hypertension in patients under 60 years of age, symptomatic or clinically evident iliofemoral occlusive disease, and horseshoe kidney.

*Computed Tomography*

CT is 100% accurate in diagnosing abdominal aortic aneurysms.[22–24] Some studies have found CT more accurate than ultrasound for delineating aneurysmal size,[22, 23] while others have found little difference between the two techniques.[19] When contrast is used, CT provides better definition of the aortic lumen and thrombus than does ultrasound.[22] CT better delineates the position of the inferior vena cava and ureters in relation to the aneurysm,[24] and CT is also better than ultrasound in demonstrating the cranial extension of an aneurysm, its relation to the renal arteries, and involvement of the iliac arteries.[16, 24, 25]

Both ultrasound and CT can be used to accurately diagnose abdominal aortic aneurysms. Ultrasound should be the primary diagnostic imaging procedure used to evaluate the aorta in nonemergency situations. CT is best used in diagnosing abdominal aortic aneurysms in the acute situation, in extremely obese patients, and when the aorta cannot be visualized on ultrasound.

## References

1. Dixon AK, Lawrence JP, Mitchell JRA: Age-related changes in the abdominal aorta shown by computed tomography. *Clin Radiol* 1984; 35: 33–37.
2. Athey PA, Tamez L: Lateral decubitus position for demonstration of the aortic bifurcation. *JCU* 1979; 7:154–155.
3. Isikoff MB, Hill MC: Sonography of the renal arteries: Left lateral decubitus position. *AJR* 1980; 134:1177–1179.
4. Gooding GAW: Ultrasonography of the iliac arteries. *Radiology* 1980; 135:161–163.
5. Schlatmann TJ, Becker AE: Histologic changes in the normal aging aorta. *Am J Cardiol* 1977; 39:13–16.
6. Anderson JC, Baltaxe HA, Wolf GL: Inability to show clot: One limitation of ultrasonography of the abdominal aorta. *Radiology* 1979; 132: 693–696.
7. Gooding GAW, Effeney DJ: Static and real-time B-mode sonography of arterial occlusions. *AJR* 1982; 139:949–952.
8. Blau SA, Kernstein MD, Deterling RA: Abdominal aortic aneurysms, in Kernstein MD, Mulder PV, Webb WR (eds): *Aneurysms.* Baltimore, Williams & Wilkins Co, 1983, pp 127–196.
9. Carlsson J, Sternby NH: Aortic aneurysm. *Acta Chir Scand* 1964; 127:466–473.
10. Crawford ES, Cohen ES: Aortic aneurysm: A multifocal disease. *Arch Surg* 1982; 117:1393–1400.
11. Leopold GR, Goldberger LE, Bernstein EF: Ultrasonic detection and evaluation of abdominal aortic aneurysms. *Surgery* 1972; 72(6):939–945.
12. Nusbaum JW, Freimanis AK, Thomford NR: Echography in the diagnosis of abdominal aortic aneurysm. *Arch Surg* 1971; 102:385–388.
13. Winsberg F, Cole-Beuglet C, Mulder DS: Contin-

uous ultrasound "B" scanning of abdominal aortic aneurysms. *AJR* 1974; 121(3):626–633.

14. Lee KR, et al: A practical approach to the diagnosis of abdominal aortic aneurysms. *Surgery* 1975; 78(2):195–201.

15. Maloney JD, et al: Ultrasound evaluation of abdominal aortic aneurysms. *Circulation* 1977; 56(suppl 2):80–85.

16. Eriksson I, Hemmingsson A, Lindgren PG: Diagnosis of abdominal aortic aneurysms by aortography, computed tomography and ultrasound. *Acta Radiol Diagn* 1980; 21:209–214.

17. Lee TG, Henderson SC: Ultrasonic and aortography: Unexpected findings. *AJR* 1977; 128:273–276.

18. Shawker TH, Steinfeld AD: Ultrasonic evaluation of pulsitile abdominal masses. *JAMA* 1978; 239(5):419–422.

19. Graeve WH, et al: Discordance in the sizing of abdominal aortic aneurysm and its significance. *Am J Surg* 1982; 144:627–634.

20. Brewster DC, et al: Assessment of abdominal aortic aneurysm size. *Circulation* 1977; 56(11):164–169.

21. Hertzer NR, Beven EG: Ultrasound aortic measurement and elective aneurysmectomy. *JAMA* 1978; 240(18):1966–1968.

22. Gomes MN, Hakkal HG, Schellinger D: Ultrasonography and CT scanning: A comparative study of abdominal aortic aneurysms. *Comput Tomogr* 1978; 2:99–110.

23. Gomes MN, Schellinger D, Hufnagel CA: Abdominal aortic aneurysms: Diagnostic review and new technique. *Ann Thorac Surg* 1979; 27(5):479–488.

24. Gomes MN: Clinical and surgical aspects of abdominal aortic aneurysms. *Semin Ultrasound* 1982; 111(2):156–169.

25. Bernstein EF, Harris RD, Leopold GR: Ultrasound and CT scanning in the noninvasive evaluation of abdominal aortic aneurysms, in Bergen JJ, Yao JS (eds): *Surgery of the Aorta and Its Body Branches.* New York, Grune & Stratton, 1979, pp 43–68.

26. Kristensen JK, Holm HH: Abdominal ultrasound angiography. *Acta Chir Scand* 1980; 502:75–80.

27. Bell DB, Gaspar MR: Routine aortography before abdominal aortic aneurysmectomy. *Am J Surg* 1982; 144(2):191–193.

28. Nuno IN, et al: Should aortography be used routinely in the elective management of abdominal aortic aneurysm? *Am J Surg* 1982; 144:53–57.

29. Darling RC, et al: Autopsy study of unoperated abdominal aortic aneurysms. *Circulation* 1977; 56(11):161–163.

30. Clayton MJ, Walsh JW, Brewer WH: Contained rupture of abdominal aortic aneurysms: Sonographic and CT diagnosis. *AJR* 1982; 138:154–156.

31. Gooding GAW: Ruptured abdominal aorta: Postoperative ultrasound appearance. *Radiology* 1982; 145:781–783.

32. Debakey ME, et al: Surgical management of dissecting aneurysms of the aorta. *J Thorac Cardiovasc Surg* 1965; 49:130.

33. Goodwin JD, Korobkin M: *Radiol Clin North Am* 1983; 21(3):551–574.

34. Mulder DS, et al: Ultrasonic "B" scanning of abdominal aneurysms. *Ann Thorac Surg* 1973; 16(4):361–367.

35. Gooding GAW, et al: B-mode ultrasonography of prosthetic vascular grafts. *Radiology* 1978; 127:763–766.

36. Gooding GAW, Effeney MB, Goldstone J: The aortofemoral graft: Detection and identification of healing complications by ultrasonography. *Surgery* 1981; 89:94–101.

37. Hardy DC, et al: Measurement of the abdominal aortic aneurysm. *Radiology* 1981; 141:821–823.

# CASES

## Dennis A. Sarti, M.D.

### Normal Aorta

Scans of the abdominal aorta are obtained with the patient supine. They may be performed with B-mode or real-time equipment. Initially, transverse scans are obtained to determine the position of the aorta relative to the spine and midline. Longitudinal scans are then obtained that parallel the long axis of the aorta. Sometimes the distal aorta will be difficult to visualize because of overlying bowel air. Gentle pressure with the transducer on the abdomen may displace some of the bowel air. Often transverse scans allow visualization of the aorta only from the lateral aspect. In this case, longitudinal scans that parallel the aorta but angle in through the ultrasonic window, detected on the transverse scans, may have to be obtained.

Figure 5–1 is a transverse scan of the upper abdomen through the major portion of the liver. The large sonolucent structure to the right of the spine is the inferior vena cava. The crus of the diaphragm drapes over the abdominal aorta at this level. The abdominal aorta usually can be visualized high in the abdomen, because the liver acts as an ultrasonic window. As we continue lower in the abdomen, bowel air often obscures visualization of the aorta. Figure 5–2 is a transverse scan in which the aorta can be seen anterior to the spine. The scan was made at the level of the pancreas, which can also act as an ultrasonic window for visualizing the aorta. Anterior to the aorta in this scan are the superior mesenteric artery and the superior mesenteric vein.

Longitudinal scans of the abdominal aorta are usually obtained close to the midline. Figures 5–3 and 5–4 show normal abdominal aortic anatomy in the longitudinal plane. Often the inferior vena cava gives a confusing picture and may be misinterpreted as the aorta. The inferior vena cava, however, courses anteriorly to empty into the right atrium as it goes through the

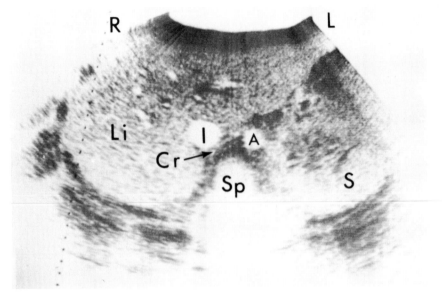

FIG 5–1.

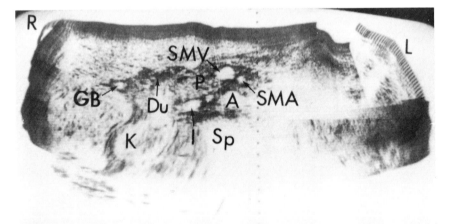

FIG 5–2.

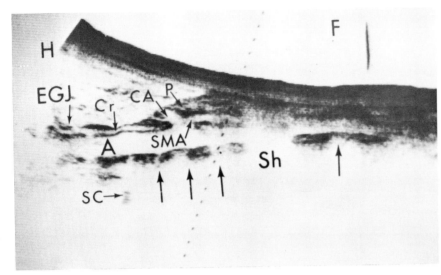

**FIG 5–3.**

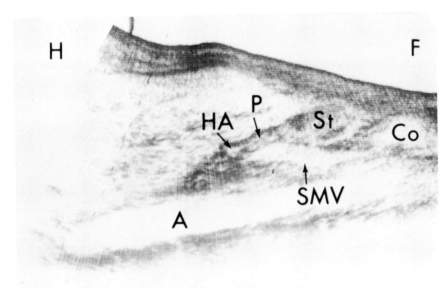

**FIG 5–4.**

hemidiaphragm. The tubular lucency of the aorta continues straight back as it goes through the left hemidiaphragm. Since the aorta is often situated directly anterior to the spine, the examiner may be able to see the vertebral bodies on its posterior aspect. The vertebral bodies appear as strong step-like echoes intermixed with decreased echoes, representing the disk space. The disk spaces (arrows) are well imaged in Figure 5–3. Often the sonographer can penetrate through the disk spaces to view the spinal canal (Fig 5–3). Sound waves are sent through the cartilaginous disk structure to image the canal, but the vertebral bodies cannot be penetrated.

Numerous structures, such as the superior mesenteric artery and the celiac axis, arise from the aorta. If bowel air is present, the aorta cannot be seen because of shadowing. In an airless abdomen the aorta may be seen from the diaphragm to the umbilical level. The normal aortic diameter is approximately 2.5 cm in women and 3.0 in men.

| | | |
|---|---|---|
| **A** | = | Aorta |
| **Arrows** | = | Intervertebral disk spaces |
| **CA** | = | Celiac axis |
| **Co** | = | Colon |
| **Cr** | = | Crus of the diaphragm |
| **Du** | = | Duodenum |
| **EGJ** | = | Esophagogastric junction |
| **F** | = | Foot |
| **GB** | = | Contracted gallbladder following eating |
| **H** | = | Head |
| **HA** | = | Hepatic artery |
| **I** | = | Inferior vena cava |
| **K** | = | Kidney |
| **L** | = | Left |
| **Li** | = | Liver |
| **P** | = | Pancreas |
| **R** | = | Right |
| **S** | = | Spleen |
| **SC** | = | Spinal canal |
| **Sh** | = | Shadowing |
| **SMA** | = | Superior mesenteric artery |
| **SMV** | = | Superior mesenteric vein |
| **Sp** | = | Spine |
| **St** | = | Stomach |

## Abdominal Aortic Aneurysms

Figures 5–5 through 5–7 are scans of a 63-year-old man admitted because of a palpable mass in the midabdomen. Ultrasound examination demonstrated a 4.5–5-cm aneurysm of the distal aorta. A longitudinal scan of the aorta (Fig 5–5) shows the distal half of the aneurysm. The size of the proximal aorta is within normal limits. A transverse scan through the normal proximal portion (Fig 5–6) shows the aorta to be normal in size and just posterior to the superior mesenteric artery and the splenic vein. Figure 5–5 demonstrates elevation of the superior mesenteric artery and the superior mesenteric vein over the aneurysm in the lower abdomen. The origin of the superior mesenteric artery in Figure 5–5 is not, however, involved with dilatation of the abdominal aorta at that site. A transverse section (Fig 5–7), more caudally, over the level of the aneurysm, delineates the enlarged aorta adjacent to the much smaller inferior vena cava. An angiogram confirmed the presence of a 5-cm aneurysm in this region. The ultrasound scans did not show any large thrombus, and no thrombus was evident on angiography.

Figure 5–8 is a longitudinal scan of a 55-year-old man with a large calcified abdominal aortic aneurysm. It demonstrates a normal-sized aorta posterior to the liver. Distal to the take-off of the celiac axis, however, is a large aneurysm measuring 7 cm in diameter and 12 cm in length. This is an excellent example of an extremely large aneurysm originating below the level of the celiac axis. Again, no thrombus is evident with the aneurysm.

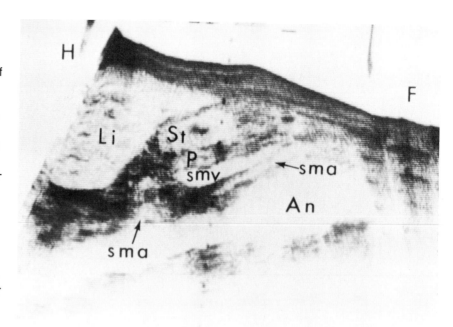

FIG 5–5.

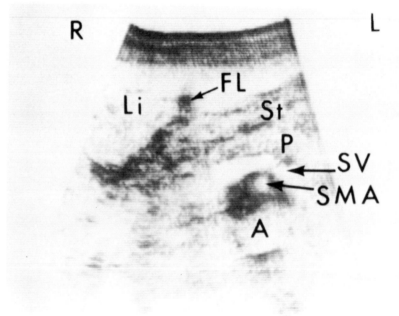

FIG 5–6.

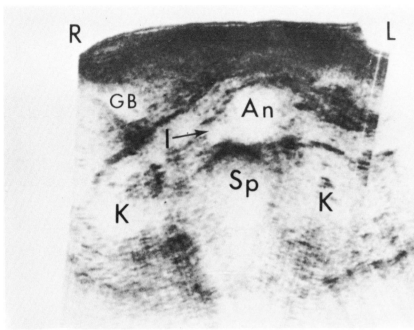

**FIG 5–7.**

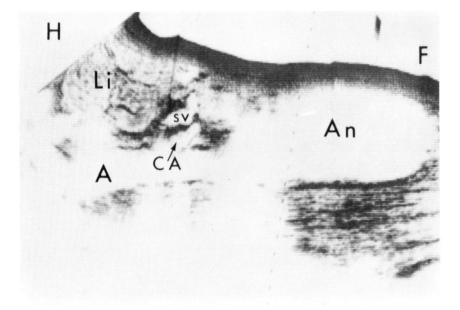

**FIG 5–8.**

| | | |
|---|---|---|
| **A** | = | Normal aorta |
| **An** | = | Aneurysm |
| **CA** | = | Celiac axis |
| **F** | = | Foot |
| **FL** | = | Falciform ligament |
| **GB** | = | Gallbladder |
| **H** | = | Head |
| **I** | = | Inferior vena cava |
| **K** | = | Kidney |
| **L** | = | Left |
| **Li** | = | Liver |
| **P** | = | Pancreas |
| **R** | = | Right |
| **SMA** | = | Superior mesenteric artery |
| **sma** | = | Superior mesenteric artery |
| **SMV** | = | Superior mesenteric vein |
| **Sp** | = | Spine |
| **St** | = | Stomach |
| **SV** | = | Splenic vein |

## Abdominal Aortic Aneurysms

The abdominal aorta tends to become smaller in diameter as it approaches the iliac arteries. Aortic dilatation of greater than 3 cm in men is considered aneurysmal. The main advantage of ultrasound over angiography is that we can see the thrombus along with the lumen of the aorta, as Figures 5–9 and 5–10 illustrate. These two scans were obtained from a 61-year-old man who had a chief complaint of continual aching pain in the abdomen. A palpable mass was noted over the midabdomen. Ultrasound examination just above the umbilical level demonstrated a large aortic aneurysm (Fig 5–9). The aortic lumen is approximately one third the size of the actual diameter of the aorta, including the thrombus.

Figure 5–10 is a longitudinal scan of the same patient; the thrombus is localized to the lower abdominal aorta. The lumen is quite visible and sonolucent, as compared with the echogenicity present within the thrombus. There was protuberance over the anterior abdominal wall (arrows) secondary to the palpable mass.

Figures 5–11 and 5–12 are transverse scans from two different patients who also had abdominal aortic aneurysms of the lower abdominal aorta. In Figure 5–11, the lumen of the aorta is somewhat eccentrically located, as compared with the entire thrombus. Figure 5–12 is an example of a centrally situated lumen. Here the thrombus is fairly even in thickness and completely surrounds the aortic lumen. In these instances an angiogram would only show the size of the abdominal aorta to be that of the lumen. Ultrasound is necessary to determine the exact extent of an abdominal aortic aneurysm. If calcification is present in the wall of the aorta, an angiogram or an abdominal x-ray film will give the accurate dimensions of an abdominal aortic aneurysm.

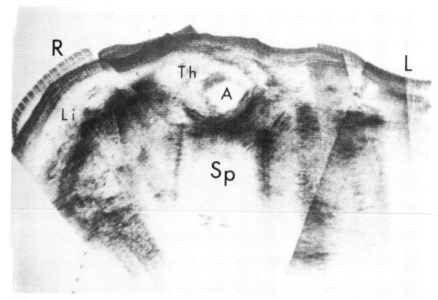

**FIG 5–9.**

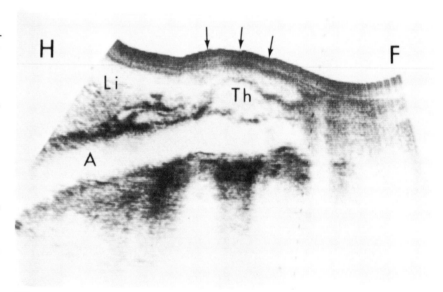

**FIG 5–10.**

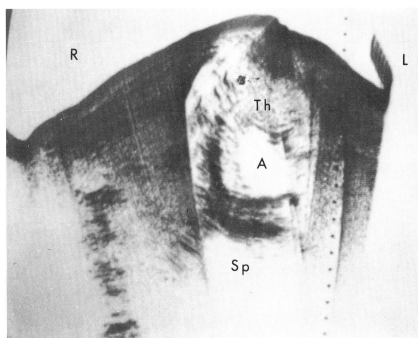

A       = Aortic lumen
Arrows  = Protuberant abdomen second-
          ary to an aortic aneurysm
F       = Foot
H       = Head
I       = Inferior vena cava
L       = Left
Li      = Liver
R       = Right
Sp      = Spine
Th      = Aortic aneurysm thrombus

FIG 5–11.

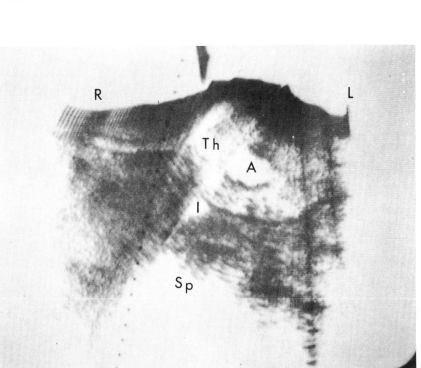

FIG 5–12.

## Abdominal Aortic Aneurysm

Figure 5–13 is a longitudinal scan made in the midline of the abdomen over the abdominal aorta. It shows a large aortic aneurysm, with a thrombus noted peripherally. The aneurysm involves nearly all of the abdominal aorta. It extends from the umbilical level to well under the left lobe of the liver. There is a sharp bend (arrow) in the midportion of the abdominal aorta. The lumen of the aorta is well defined, since it is quite sonolucent. The solid thrombus is echogenic on ultrasound.

Figure 5–14 is a transverse abdominal scan of a 73-year-old man who was experiencing severe abdominal pain. An aortic aneurysm is seen over the midabdomen. A large mass is noted on the right side of the aneurysm and is quite echogenic. At surgery, the mass turned out to be a large hematoma. The aortic aneurysm had ruptured into the right posterior retroperitoneum.

Figures 5–15 and 5–16 are transverse and longitudinal scans of a fusiform aneurysm of the distal abdominal aorta. The abdominal aorta tapers normally and narrows as it reaches the unbilical level. In this case, the distal aorta widens because of aneurysmal dilatation. The distal aorta is elevated off the lumbar spine by a relatively lucent region. Occasionally a tortuous aorta will appear displaced from the lumbar spine. In other instances a mass may be situated posterior to the aorta, elevating it off the spine. These two entities may be difficult to distinguish from one another. Figures 5–15 and 5–16 show metastatic retroaortic nodes (arrowheads) elevating the distal aorta off the spine. The transverse scan in Figure 5–15 demonstrates a discrete oval sonolucent retroaortic mass consistent with adenopathy. The longitudinal scan in Figure 5–16 also shows elevation of the aorta by a mass (arrowheads). However, Figure 5–16 alone could be an example of tortuousity. The transverse view in Figure 5–15 is necessary for the correct diagnosis.

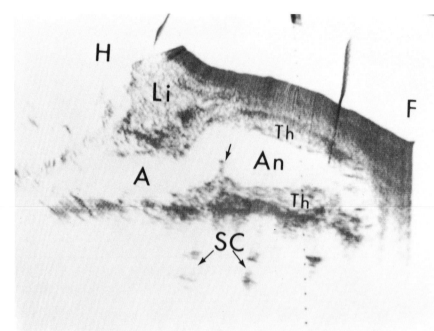

**FIG 5–13.**

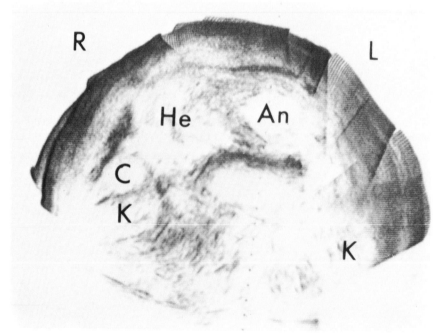

**FIG 5–14.**

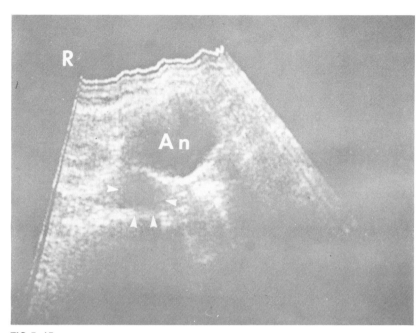

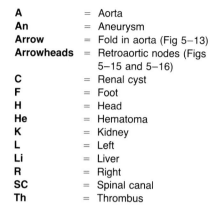

| | | |
|---|---|---|
| **A** | = | Aorta |
| **An** | = | Aneurysm |
| **Arrow** | = | Fold in aorta (Fig 5–13) |
| **Arrowheads** | = | Retroaortic nodes (Figs 5–15 and 5–16) |
| **C** | = | Renal cyst |
| **F** | = | Foot |
| **H** | = | Head |
| **He** | = | Hematoma |
| **K** | = | Kidney |
| **L** | = | Left |
| **Li** | = | Liver |
| **R** | = | Right |
| **SC** | = | Spinal canal |
| **Th** | = | Thrombus |

Source: Figures 5–15 and 5–16 were contributed by Albert Yu, M.D.

FIG 5–15.

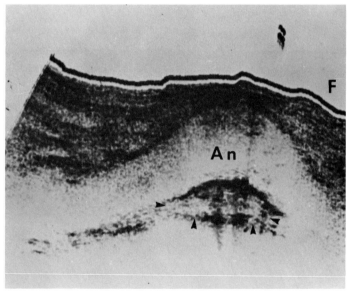

FIG 5–16.

## Aortic Aneurysms; Fistula

Figures 5–17 and 5–18 are transverse ultrasound and CT images of the midabdomen at approximately the same level. The patient was a middle-aged man with a palpable abdominal mass thought to be an abdominal aortic aneurysm. Figures 5–17 and 5–18 indicate excellent correlation between these two modalities in demonstrating this large abdominal aortic aneurysm with thrombus. Intravenous contrast material was given for the CT scan. The aortic lumen is of higher density than the surrounding thrombus. In the ultrasound image (Fig 5–17) the aortic lumen is echo free while the thrombus is filled with moderately high-amplitude echoes.

Figure 5–19 is a longitudinal midline scan of a 30-year-old woman. The impressive finding on this scan is the generalized dilatation of the abdominal aorta throughout its entire length. The normal tapering as the aorta approaches the bifurcation is absent. This patient has Takayasu's disease, or pulseless arteritis. It is most commonly seen in the young female.

Figure 5–20 is the scan of a 54-year-old man with congestive heart failure. Abdominal ultrasound was performed to rule out pancreatic disease secondary to a long history of alcoholism. Figure 5–20 is a longitudinal scan made slightly to the right of midline. A mass was found in the lower abdomen secondary to an abdominal aortic aneurysm **(An).** Inferior and posterior to this mass is a tubular structure which is a dilated right iliac vein. A fistula was found between the aortic aneurysm and the inferior vena cava. The increased size of the right iliac vein is secondary to the shunt.

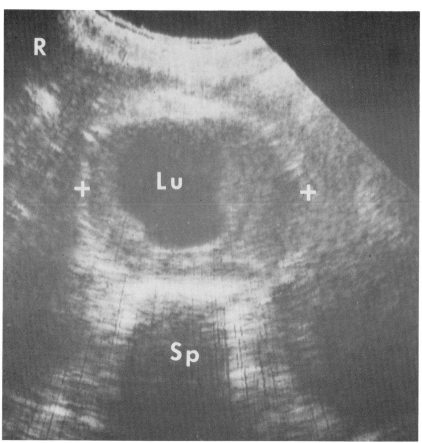

**FIG 5–17.**

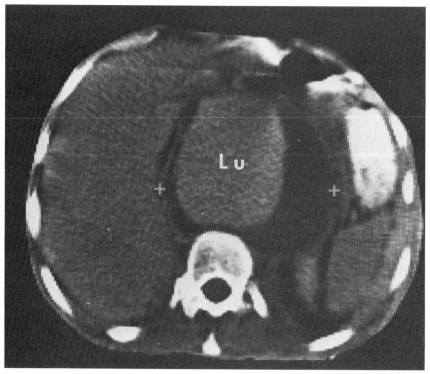

**FIG 5–18.**

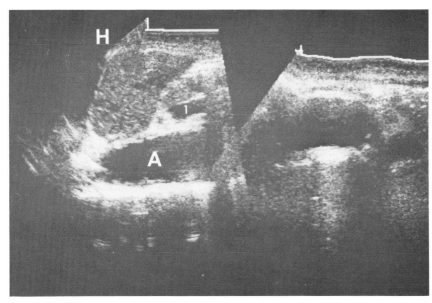

FIG 5–19.

A  = Aorta
An = Aortic aneurysm
H  = Head
IV = Right iliac vein
Lu = Aortic lumen
R  = Right
+  = Lateral margins of aortic aneurysm
     (Figs 5–17 and 5–18)
1  = Superior mesenteric vein with pan-
     creas anterior to it

Source: Figures 5–17 and 5–18 were contributed
by Albert Yu, M.D.

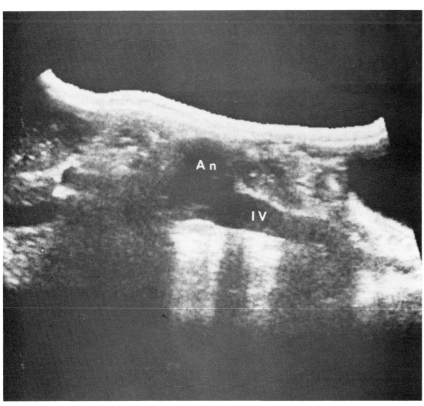

FIG 5–20.

## Infected Aortic Graft

Figures 5–21 through 5–24 are scans of a middle-aged woman who had recently undergone surgery with the placement of an aortic graft. She had had recent onset of abdominal pain with fever and an elevated white blood cell count. Figures 5–21 and 5–22 are transverse and longitudinal scans of the abdomen that demonstrate a mass surrounding the aorta. The mass is quite circumferential. It would be compatible with an aortic aneurysm, but the patient had a graft in place at this site. In fact, the extremely strong echoes of the distal aorta (Fig 5–22, arrows) are fairly characteristic of those echoes arising from the graft. It is evident from Figure 5–22 that the mass is surrounding the site of the graft.

Because of the ultrasonic findings, angiography was performed (Fig 5–23). The distal aorta is narrowed (arrows) in the same area where the mass was noted on ultrasound. The patient was taken to the operating room, and an infected aortic graft was found. An abscess surrounding the distal aorta was over the region of the graft. Figure 5–24 is a contrast examination of the abscess cavity, performed at the time of surgery. The filling defect of the distal aorta is seen in the superior aspect of the abscess cavity. The findings at the time of surgery corresponded to the findings on the previous ultrasound examinations.

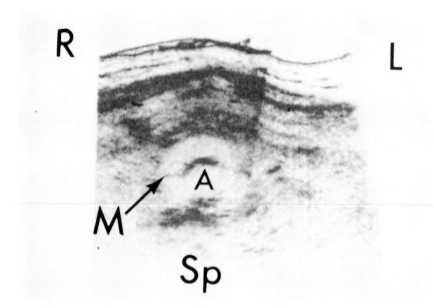

FIG 5–21.

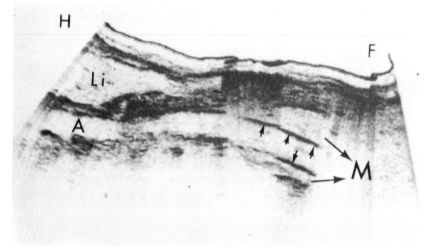

FIG 5–22.

A       = Aorta
**Arrows** = Strong echoes arising from
          the aortic graft (Fig 5–22)
**Arrows** = Indentation from the abscess
          on the aortic lumen (Fig 5–23)
**F**     = Foot
**H**     = Head
**L**     = Left
**Li**    = Liver
**M**     = Abscess surrounding the aor-
          tic graft
**R**     = Right
**Sp**    = Spine

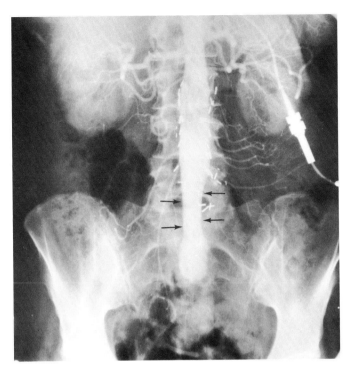

**FIG 5–23.**

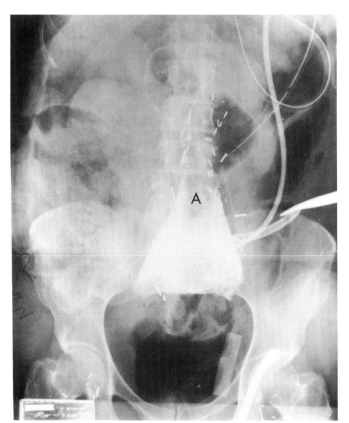

**FIG 5–24.**

## Atherosclerosis

The images in this section are from two different patients with atherosclerotic changes of the abdominal aorta demonstrated by ultrasound. Figures 5–25 and 5–26 are from a 63-year-old woman and Figures 5–27 and 5–28 are from a 65-year-old woman. Although not as thin and sharp as the inferior vena cava, the walls of the aorta are usually fairly smooth. In cases of severe atherosclerosis, however, they can appear quite irregular. The longitudinal scans of both cases (Fig 5–25 and 5–27) show the aortas to have markedly irregular borders, especially in the posterior aspect. Numerous atheromatous plaques (arrows) indent the aortic lumen. Transverse scans of both cases (Figs 5–26 and 5–28) demonstrate marked irregularity and narrowing of the usually smooth and circular aorta.

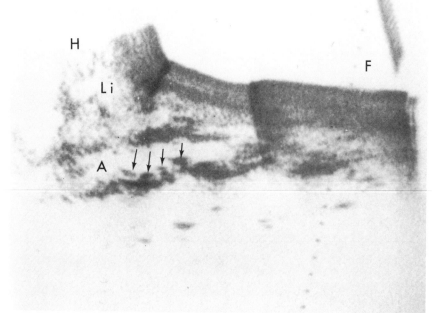

FIG 5–25.

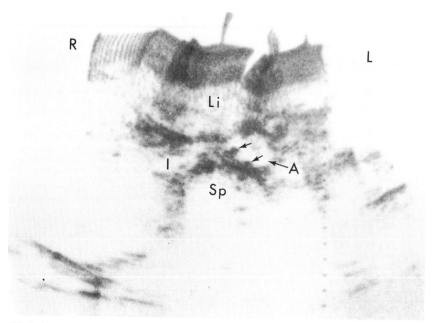

FIG 5–26.

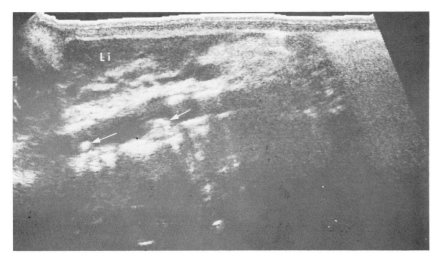

A       = Aorta
**Arrows** = Atherosclerotic plaques
F       = Foot
H       = Head
I       = Inferior vena cava
L       = Left
Li      = Liver
R       = Right
Sp      = Spine
1       = Gallbladder
2       = Inferior vena cava

FIG 5–27.

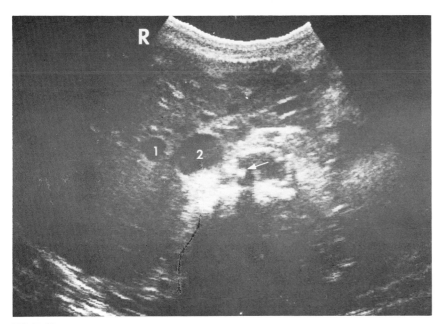

FIG 5–28.

## Dissecting Aneurysm; Recanalization

Figures 5–29 and 5–30 are ultrasound scans of a 45-year-old man with known cystic medial necrosis. Just before his last hospital admission, he noted the sudden onset of back pain which was not relieved by positional changes. He also noted abdominal pain with nausea and vomiting. Abdominal ultrasound was performed to evaluate the abdominal pain. Figure 5–29 is a transverse scan of the initial portion of the study. At first the study appears unremarkable. A close look at the lateral posterior right border of the aorta, however, reveals a strong echo (arrow) within the lumen of the aorta. This unusual finding prompted closer scrutiny of the abdominal aorta.

Figure 5–30 is a longitudinal B-mode scan of the same patient performed at a slow scan speed. The echo within the aortic lumen was noted to have cardiac pulsations, and the diagnosis of dissecting aortic aneurysm was made. This diagnosis is more readily made with real-time equipment. The intraluminal echo can be continuously monitored, and the cardiac pulsations of the intraluminal flap are easily recognizable. The same is not true if only B-mode equipment is available. To make the diagnosis with B-mode equipment, a very slow scan speed over the site of the intraluminal echo is necessary. The cardiac pulsations of the intimal flap will be visualized as the flap moves toward and away from the transducer during slow scanning (Fig 5–30).

Figures 5–31 and 5–32 are transverse and longitudinal scans of a patient with an abdominal aortic aneurysm. The aneurysm has a lucent echogenic then lucent concentric appearance. The central lucency represents the aortic lumen, which is smooth walled and not dilated. Surrounding the lumen is a circular echogenic region representing thrombus and clot. Peripheral to the thrombus is a lucent region that is not usually seen in abdominal aortic aneurysms. This lucent area is secondary to recan-

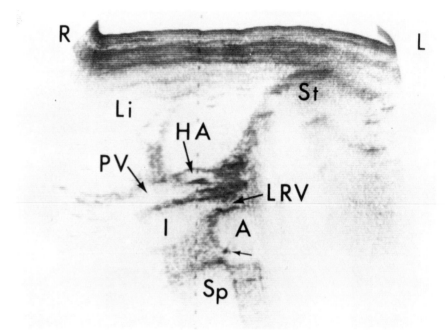

**FIG 5–29.**

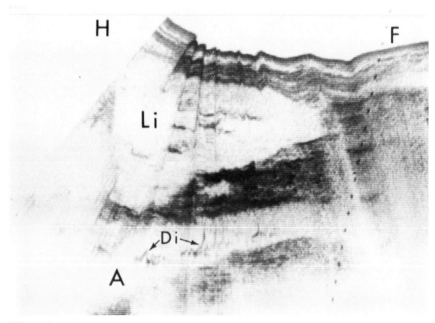

**FIG 5–30.**

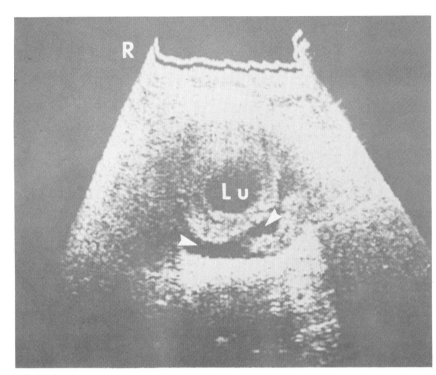

**FIG 5–31.**

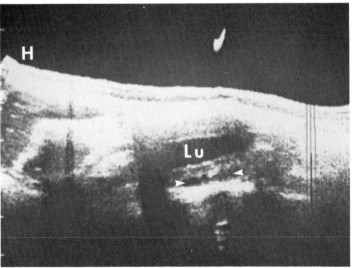

**FIG 5–32.**

alization (arrowheads) through the thrombus. On longitudinal scan (Fig 5–32), the recanalized lumen has slightly irregular borders.

| | | |
|---|---|---|
| **A** | = | Aorta |
| **Arrowheads** | = | Recanalized lumen |
| **Di** | = | Dissection |
| **F** | = | Foot |
| **H** | = | Head |
| **HA** | = | Hepatic artery |
| **I** | = | Inferior vena cava |
| **L** | = | Left |
| **Li** | = | Liver |
| **LRV** | = | Left renal vein |
| **Lu** | = | Lumen of aorta |
| **PV** | = | Portal vein |
| **R** | = | Right |
| **Sp** | = | Spine |
| **St** | = | Stomach |

Source: Figures 5–31 and 5–32 were contributed by Albert Yu, M.D.

# 6.
# Ultrasonography of the Spleen

Peter L. Cooperberg, M.D.

Prior to the widespread availability of real-time sector scan ultrasound, examination of the spleen, and particularly the normal, nonenlarged spleen, was very difficult. It was because of this difficulty, and the pain felt by the patient as a manual transducer was passed over bruised ribs, that ultrasound was relegated to a secondary role in the evaluation of the spleen and left upper quadrant, and nuclear medicine and CT became the primary diagnostic imaging tools. However, with the advent and extensive availability of high-quality real-time sector scan techniques, the spleen can be easily and well visualized, and ultrasound has regained some prominence in the evaluation of possible splenic abnormalities. Certainly real-time ultrasound is easy when the spleen is enlarged and pushes the bowel gas out of the way. If a coronal plane of section from a relatively posterior intercostal window is used, and if the patient is studied supine, even normal and small spleens can be easily visualized.

**Examination Technique**

All routine abdominal sonograms, regardless of the indication, should include at least one view of the spleen and upper pole of the left kidney. Whereas imaging of this area was fraught with difficulties when the older static scan technique was used, real-time ultrasound, and particularly real-time sector scanning, makes visualizing the spleen relatively easy. The most common approach to visualizing the spleen using real-time scanning is to maintain the patient in the supine position and place the transducer in the coronal plane of section posteriorly in one of the lower left intercostal spaces. Different degrees of inspiration should be attempted to maximize the window to the spleen without introducing too much air into the lung in the lateral costophrenic angle to obscure visualization, yet enough inspiration to bring the central portion of the left hemidiaphragm and the spleen inferiorly so that they can be visualized. The plane of section should then be swept posteriorly to anteriorly to view the entire volume of the spleen. We generally find that a thorough examination in the coronal plane of section is highly accurate for ruling out any lesion within or around the spleen and for documenting the approximate size of the spleen. If an abnormality is discovered within or around the spleen, other planes of section can be used. A transverse plane from a lateral, usually intercostal, approach may help define the location of the lesion within the spleen anteriorly and posteriorly. In this regard, especially for beginners, it bears emphasis that the point of a sector image is always placed at the top of the screen or photograph. However, if a left lateral intercostal approach is used, then the top of the screen (apex of the sector) is actually to the patient's left, the right side of the sector on the image is posterior, and the left side of the image is anterior. To look at the image appropriately, one should therefore rotate the image 90° clockwise. If the spleen is not enlarged and if there is no large mass around the spleen, scanning from an anterior position (as one would for imaging the liver) is not helpful because of the interposition of gas within the stomach and splenic flexure of the colon.[1] However, if the patient has a relatively large liver, one may be able to see the spleen through the left lobe of the liver and the collapsed stomach, analogous to the image seen on a transverse CT scan through the upper abdomen. Also, free intraperitoneal fluid around the spleen and a left pleural effusion can help in the visualization of even a normal-sized spleen.

Occasionally it is beneficial to have the patient roll onto his right side, as much as 45° or even 90°, so that an even more posterior approach can be used to visualize the spleen. However, this is rarely necessary since the normal spleen can be seen in most patients when they are supine. We virtually never use the prone position for scanning.

Generally, the same technical settings of gain, time gain compensation, and power are used for examination of the spleen as for examination of other organs in the upper abdomen. Since the spleen is a superficial structure and since there is generally little absorption of sound within the spleen, a frequency of 5 MHz with a medium-length internally focused transducer is recommended. Most commonly mechanical sector scanners, with or without annular-array transducers for beam focusing, are used. Phased-array sector scanners have no particular advantage and frequently have disadvantages in intercostal scanning because of the fairly wide aperture of the transducers. Linear-array transducers are almost completely useless in examination of the spleen, especially if it is not enlarged. The intercostal window is simply too small for larger transducers. It is important to note that sometimes the ribs are broader and flatter than expected. In this case, the width of the ribs encroaches on the intercostal spaces, making them particularly narrow. These instances severely limit the applicability of phased sector and linear arrays. We find no use whatsoever for conventional static-arm scanners in the clinical practice of ultrasonography. Not only are they very difficult and cumbersome to use, they can cause pain as they bump over the left lower ribs, especially in traumatized patients. Occasionally the larger field of view afforded by static scans can be helpful to make a teaching point.

### Examination of the Normal Spleen

The shape of the normal spleen is variable. The spleen consists of two components, joined at the hilum: a superomedial component and an inferolateral component. On transverse scanning, more superiorly the spleen has the typical fat comma shape with a component extending anteriorly and another component extending medially either superior to or adjacent to the upper pole of the kidney. This is the component that can be seen to indent the gastric fundus on plain films of the abdomen and on barium studies. As one moves the scan plane inferiorly, still in the transverse plane, only the inferior component will be noted. This is the component that can be outlined by gas in the splenic flexure or fat on the plain film of the abdomen. It may extend inferior to the costal margin and present as a palpable spleen clinically. Either component can enlarge early without enlargement of the other component. The subjective assessment of mild degrees of splenic enlargement can be exceedingly difficult. The shape of the spleen on coronal views in a posterior scan plane shows a rounded contour of the superior aspect of the spleen with a more pointed configuration to the medial component as well as the inferior component. Between the medial and inferior components is the region of the splenic hilum, which is usually seen slightly more anteriorly.

It is important to recognize the normal structures that are anatomically related to the spleen. The diaphragm cradles the spleen posteriorly, superiorly, and laterally. The normal liver usually does not touch the spleen. If the left lobe is enlarged, it may extend into the left upper quadrant anterior to the spleen. Occasionally, in a thin patient, the normal left lobe of the liver may insinuate itself between the superior aspect of the spleen and the left hemidiaphragm. On the usual coronal view of the spleen, this can mimic the appearance of a subcapsular hematoma or a subphrenic abscess. The fundus of the stomach and lesser sac are medial and anterior to the splenic hilum. It is important to appreciate that the stomach can fill in the concavity near the splenic hilum. It is therefore possible to make a scan showing spleen surrounding or almost surrounding the region of the splenic hilum, with stomach containing air or fluid appearing to be within the middle of the spleen. A transverse scan plane can easily show the true relationship of these structures. Because of this close anatomic relationship, one must be careful not to diagnose a splenic abscess or hematoma. The tail of the pancreas lies posterior to the stomach and lesser sac and also approaches the hilum of the spleen. The left kidney generally lies inferior and medial to the spleen. Rarely, the medial component of the spleen may extend anterior to the upper pole of the left kidney. A useful landmark in identifying the spleen and splenic hilum is the splenic vein, which can generally be demonstrated, especially in splenic enlargement.

The splenic parenchyma is extremely homogeneous, and therefore the textural appearance of the spleen on gray-scale ultrasonography generally shows a diffuse homogeneous low-level echo pattern. In large patients, especially those with broad and flat ribs and therefore with small intercostal spaces, the low-level echoes from the spleen can be difficult to demonstrate. This is especially true unless great care is taken in adjusting the near gain. Older static scans may show the spleen to be completely echo free. This is usually not a problem with real-time scanners in which the time gain compensation and gain adjustments are correctly made. Occasionally, and particularly with static scanning, there may be differential attenuation of the sound passing through the costal margin. This can mimic the appearance of a focal hypoechoic area within the spleen. This type of artifact should not occur with real-time scanning.

It is commonly thought that the liver is more echogenic than the spleen. However, in those cases where we can visualize the liver superior to the spleen, it appears to have decreased echogenicity.[2] The explanation for this is not obvious, but usually the echogenicity of the spleen and liver can be compared only in patients with splenomegaly. It is more difficult to compare the two structures when the spleen is not enlarged. In some cases, one can see the liver close to the spleen, and the spleen does appear to be less echogenic. Attempts have been made in the past to relate the echogenicity of the spleen to the type of pathology. It was said that "reactive" splenomegaly could be differentiated from malignant involvement, such as with Hodgkin's disease, by the degree of echogenicity.[3] These results have not been confirmed.[4]

## Pathologic Conditions of the Spleen

### Splenomegaly

The differential diagnosis of splenomegaly is a lengthy one. Ultrasonography is not generally useful in establishing the etiology of splenomegaly. Several exceptions will be discussed here.

Frequently the question is whether or not there is splenomegaly. This again can be a difficult decision to make on the sonographic study if only mild enlargement is present. With static scanning or CT scanning, one proposed rule of thumb is that if the anterior margin of the spleen extends more anteriorly than the anterior wall of the abdominal aorta on a transverse scan made with the patient supine, splenomegaly is present. This is certainly not a highly accurate rule. It depends on the body habitus of the patient as well as the size of the spleen. Techniques have been described to measure serial sections of the spleen by planimetry and add the product of the areas and the thickness of the sections, but these techniques are cumbersome and not widely popular.[5, 6] Linear measurements can be obtained through the longest axis of the spleen, but since the spleen may enlarge medially more than inferiorly, such measurements also are not particularly useful.[7] We once used the rule that if the entire spleen could not be visualized within the sector image on coronal scans, then splenomegaly was present. However, different sector scanners have wider or narrower sector angles and larger footprints on the surface of the patient, so the rule no longer applies. The most common method applied is still the "eyeball" technique: if it looks big, it is. Unfortunately, this method of assessment requires considerably more experience than is necessary with other imaging techniques. It is relatively inaccurate with lesser degrees of splenic enlargement but is probably the best we have to offer. Needless to say, plain radiography of the abdomen and radionuclide spleen scans with technetium-99m are alternative methods of evaluation of splenic size. These techniques also suffer from the inability to accurately evaluate mild degrees of splenic enlargement.

The spleen is capable of growing to an enormous size. It may extend inferiorly into the left iliac fossa. When the spleen enlarges, it can cross the midline and present as a mass inferior to the left lobe of the liver on a longitudinal section near the midline. This is more obvious on a static image and is not particularly a problem with real-time scanning.

Occasionally a mass is found in the left upper quadrant. The clinical dilemma is whether the mass is an enlarged spleen or an extrinsic mass located against the spleen. It can be helpful if the spleen is demonstrated separately from the mass. Another helpful feature is the demonstration of the splenic vein entering the splenic hilum. This indicates that the mass is, in fact, an enlarged spleen.

If there is splenomegaly, ultrasound can be useful to diagnose focal lesions within the spleen, including lymphomatous involvement, metastatic disease, cysts, or hematomas. Ultrasonography can be helpful to identify other evidence of lymphoma such as lymph node enlargement or liver involvement. Ultrasound may demonstrate recanalization of the umbilical vein or other evidence of portosystemic collaterals and ascites to establish portal hypertension as the cause of splenomegaly. However, in numerous cases, splenomegaly may be the only one or one of several nonspecific findings.

*Focal Abnormalities*

With or without splenic enlargement, old granulomatous disease may cause focal areas of calcification, with deep shadowing if they are large enough. Histoplasmosis and tuberculosis are the most common causes. Gas in an abscess within the spleen may have a similar appearance on ultrasound as a focal echogenic area with deep shadowing. However, gas, especially if it is in small bubbles, frequently causes a "dirty" shadow with numerous ring-down artifacts that differentiate it from calcification. A plain film or CT scan of the abdomen can easily differentiate calcification from the gas of an intrasplenic abscess. An abscess need not contain gas and may present as a cystic structure within the spleen.[8, 9] Generally there

are some low-level debris echoes to differentiate abscess from a simple cyst. Occasionally one may see a characteristic target appearance in a small lesion within the liver or spleen in immunocompromised patients. This may represent a *Candida* or other fungal type of abscess, the echogenic spot in the center supposedly representing the mycelium within the fungal abscess. Simple cysts of the spleen are common. Their etiology is unclear but may be related to trauma. As elsewhere in the body, splenic cysts characteristically appear as echo-free areas with smooth, sharp borders and enhancement of the echoes deep to the lesions. When small, they may be demonstrated to be within the outline of the spleen. Occasionally these cysts attain a very large size. Several years ago we detected large cysts in several patients.[10] However, in the last few years we have only seen smaller cysts in the spleen. Perhaps the cysts are being detected earlier and never reach the large size. Splenic cysts may appear relatively echogenic due to the presence of cholesterol crystals or other debris.[11] Also, hemorrhage into a splenic cyst may occur and therefore may show up on a CT scan as radiodense relative to the splenic parenchyma.[12] Occasionally there the splenic cyst has a calcified rim. This finding should suggest the possibility of an echinococcal cyst.

There may be focal solid lesions within the spleen in a limited number of conditions.[13-16] Primary involvement of the spleen only occurs with the lymphomas, such as lymphosarcoma. Metastasis may present in the spleen, most commonly secondary to malignant melanoma, but other conditions, including pulmonary primaries, can also spread to the spleen.[17] Unfortunately, as in other parts of the body, the sonographic appearance of solid lesions within the spleen is nonspecific. Solid lesions may be echogenic or echo poor and no one type of primary has been associated with a particular appearance of focal splenic lesions.[18] Furthermore, the characteristics of the lesion can change after chemotherapy or radiation therapy. Primary hemangiomas have been described in the spleen and have the same appearance as in the liver.

The sonographic appearance of splenic infarct still has not been clearly defined and depends considerably on the duration of time since the infarct occurred. Early on, there is said to be a wedge-shaped echo-poor region.[19, 20] Subsequently the area may become smaller and more echogenic. Studies from which these findings were reported were performed in patients who had splenic embolization for portal hypertension. However, in most clinical situations, there will be no subsequent pathologic proof of the type of lesion and therefore it is difficult to make sonographic correlations. One must therefore do follow-up examinations to show a decrease in size of the lesion to confirm first that they are benign and second that they are likely to be infarcts.

*Splenic Trauma*

Ultrasound can be very useful and highly accurate in the diagnosis of splenic trauma. This is one area where CT has proved particularly useful since more of the upper abdominal pathology can be identified in one examination.[21, 22] Nonetheless, splenic trauma from blunt nonpenetrating injuries of the left upper quadrant is frequently not an emergency, and ultrasound can be useful. On the other hand, if the patient is in extreme distress, the CT scanner often cannot be freed up quickly enough, so ultrasound can again play an important role.

If the spleen is involved in blunt abdominal trauma, two avenues of pathogenesis are possible. If the capsule remains intact, one may have an intraparenchymal or subcapsular hematoma. Or the capsule may rupture and lead to a focal or free intraperitoneal hematoma. In the latter situation, it might be possible to demonstrate a fluid space separate from the spleen in the left upper quadrant. However, it is important to appreciate the timing of the examination relative to the trauma. Immediately after the traumatic incident, the hematoma is liquid and might be easily differentiated from the splenic tissue. Very soon, and for the next 24–48 hours, the blood is clotted and may closely resemble in echogenicity the normal splenic parenchyma. Subsequently the blood reliquefies and the diagnosis again becomes easy. Usually, by the time the patient has been admitted and settled down, one only sees an irregularly echogenic mass larger than one would expect for a normal spleen. Furthermore, there are usually focal areas of inhomogeneity within the spleen to indicate that there is an abnormality. Since current therapy for stable patients with suspected splenic trauma consists of nonintervention and temporization, we suggest a follow-up sonogram in 2–3 days to demonstrate liquefaction of the hematomas. Although the blood may spread within the intraperitoneal cavity and be found in the flanks or in Morison's

pouch, most commonly it becomes walled off in the left upper quadrant. As time progresses, one may clearly see the subcapsular hematoma differentiated from the pericapsular walled off hematoma by the capsule itself.[23] We have followed up for weeks and even months several patients with fluid collections around the spleen after trauma, even when they were relatively asymptomatic.[24] In one case fine needle aspiration 3 months after the original injury showed dark old blood-stained serous fluid. Evacuation of the fluid collection through a catheter was performed and the fluid did not recur. Although there may actually be a condition of delayed rupture of the spleen, it is at least possible that all ruptures of the spleen occur at the time of injury and are walled off initially. Delayed rupture may only be the extension of a perisplenic hematoma into the peritoneal cavity.

Aside from splenic capsule rupture, there may be internal damage to the spleen with an intact splenic capsule. This can result in an intraparenchymal or a subcapsular hematoma of the spleen which initially appears only as an inhomogeneous area. Subsequently the fluid can clear, and repeat scans characteristically show relatively cystic structures resulting from the splenic hematoma.[23]

A perisplenic hematoma can closely mimic a perisplenic abscess sonographically. A hematoma can easily become infected and thus transform into a left subphrenic abscess.[25] Generally, the clinical situation can help to distinguish these conditions, but if it is not clear, fine needle aspiration can easily differentiate the two. Catheter drainage can then be performed under ultrasound or CT guidance for definitive therapy.

*Congenital Anomalies*

Congenital absence of the spleen is rare and can be ruled out by the demonstration of a splenic structure. Accessory spleens are easier to demonstrate but simulate enlarged lymph nodes and must be differentiated from lymphoma.[26] Isotope studies with agents that tag the reticuloendothelial system are better to confirm the presence or absence of splenic tissue.

### References

1. Hicken P, Sauerbrei EE, Cooperberg PL: Ultrasonic coronal scanning of left upper quadrant. *J Can Assoc Radiol* 1981; 32:107–110.

2. Li DKB, Cooperberg PL, Graham MF, et al: Pseudoperisplenic "fluid collections": A clue to normal liver and spleen echogenic texture. *Ultrasound Med,* to be published.

3. Taylor KJW, Milan J: Differential diagnosis of chronic splenomegaly by gray scale ultrasonography: Clinical observations and digital A-scan analysis. *Br J Radiol* 1976; 49:519–525.

4. Sommer FG, Joynt LF, Carroll BA, et al: Ultrasonic characterization of abdominal tissues via digital analysis of backscattered waveforms. *Radiology* 1981; 141:811–817.

5. Breiman RS, Beck JW, Korobkin M, et al: Volume determinations using computed tomography. *AJR* 1982; 138:329–333.

6. Henderson JM, Heymsfield SB, Horowitz J, et al: Measurement of liver and spleen volume by computed tomography: Assessment of reproducibility and changes found following a selective distal splenorenal shunt. *Radiology* 1981; 141:525–527.

7. Niederau C, Sonnenberg A, Müller JE, et al: Sonographic measurements of the normal liver, spleen, pancreas, and portal vein. *Radiology* 1983; 149:537–540.

8. Kay CJ, Pawar SV, Rosenfield AT: Sonography of splenic abscesses. *Semin Ultrasound, CT MR* 1983; 4:91.

9. Ralls PW, Quinn MF, Colletti P, et al: Sonography of pyogenic splenic abscess. *AJR* 1982; 138:523–525.

10. Bhimji SD, Cooperberg PL, Naiman S: Ultrasound diagnosis of splenic cysts. *Radiology* 1977; 122:787–789.

11. Thurber LA, Cooperberg PL, Clement JG, et al: Echogenic fluid: A pitfall in the ultrasonographic diagnosis of cystic lesions. *JCU* 1979; 7:273–278.

12. Propper RA, Weinstein BJ, Skolnick ML, et al: Ultrasonography of hemorrhagic splenic cysts. *JCU* 1979; 7:18–20.

13. Adler DD, Silver TM, Abrams GD: The sonographic appearance of splenic plasmacytoma. *J Ultrasound Med* 1982; 1:323–324.

14. Anjou A, Cholat L, Bret PM, et al: Computed tomography for focal splenic pathology. *Ann Radiol* 1983; 26:275–283.

15. Costello P, Kane RA, Oster J, et al: Focal splenic pathology demonstrated by ultrasound and computed tomography. *J Can Assoc Radiol* 1985; 36:22–28.

16. Solbiati L, Bossi MC, Bellotti E, et al: Focal lesions in the spleen. *AJR* 1983; 140:59–65.

17. Murphy JF, Bernardino ME: The sonographic findings of splenic metastases. *JCU* 1979; 7:195–197.

18. Mittelstaedt CA, Partin CL: Ultrasonic-pathologic classification of splenic abnormalities: Gray-scale patterns. *Radiology* 1980; 134:697–705.

19. Shirkhoda A, Wallace S, Sokhandan M: Computed tomography and ultrasonography in splenic infarction. *J Can Assoc Radiol* 1985; 36:29–33.

20. Weingarten MJ, Fakhry J, McCarthy J, et al: Sonography after splenic embolization: The wedge-shaped acute infarct. *AJR* 1984; 142:957–959.

21. Jeffrey RB Jr, Laing FC, Federle MP, et al: Computed tomography of splenic trauma. *Radiology* 1981; 141:729–732.

22. Korobkin M, Moss AA, Callen PW, et al: Computed tomography of subcapsular splenic hematoma. *Radiology* 1978; 129:441–445.

23. Lupien C, Sauerbrei EE: Healing in the traumatized spleen: Sonographic investigation. *Radiology* 1984; 151:181–185.

24. Johnson MA, Cooperberg PL, Boisvert J, et al: Spontaneous rupture of the spleen in infectious mononucleosis: Sonographic diagnosis and follow-up. *AJR* 1981; 136:111–114.

25. Epstein MB, Omar GM: Infective complications of splenic trauma. *Clin Radiol* 1983; 34:91–94.

26. Subramanyam BR, Balthazar EJ, Horii SC: Sonography of the accessory spleen. *AJR* 1984; 143:47–49.

## CASES

### Dennis A. Sarti, M.D.

### Normal Spleen

Figures 6–1 and 6–2 are transverse scans of a normal spleen. In Figure 6–1 the spleen is visualized through the intercostal spaces, laterally on the left side. Because of the collapsed and airless stomach, however, the spleen can be seen from an anterior projection. Here we are scanning through the left lobe of the liver and the collapsed stomach to visualize the spleen. Figure 6–2 is a transverse scan of the spleen through the intercostal spaces, laterally on the left. Most of the information comes from scans obtained through the intercostal spaces, rather than from scans obtained from an anterior location. The spleen may be horizontal in orientation and difficult to visualize on ultrasound because of air in the stomach or the splenic flexure. Spleens with a lateral orientation are best seen through intercostal spaces.

Longitudinal scans of the spleen are best obtained with the patient in a decubitus position with the left side up. Scans are then obtained in the midaxillary line beneath the costal margin and in the intercostal spaces.

Figures 6–3 and 6–4 are longitudinal scans of the spleen with the patient in the decubitus position. They demonstrate the splenic parenchyma excellently. The spleen is situated cephalad to the left kidney and caudal to the left hemidiaphragm. By sector scanning through the intercostal space, we can achieve excellent visualization of the splenic parenchyma. The aorta is seen deep to the spleen, because the patient is in a decubitus position. By varying the patient's respiration, the sonographer can move the spleen into an optimal position, with excellent visualization.

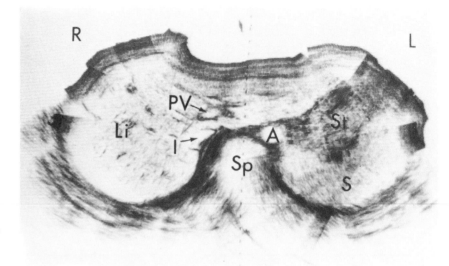

FIG 6–1.

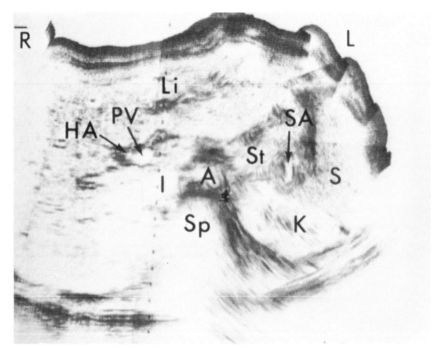

FIG 6–2.

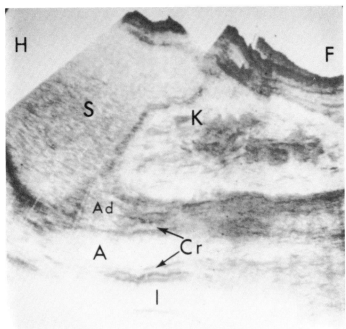

A   = Aorta
Ad  = Left adrenal gland
Cr  = Crus of the diaphragm
D   = Left hemidiaphragm
F   = Foot
H   = Head
HA  = Hepatic artery
I   = Inferior vena cava
K   = Left kidney
L   = Left
Li  = Liver
PV  = Portal vein
R   = Right
S   = Spleen
SA  = Splenic artery
Sp  = Spine
St  = Stomach

FIG 6–3.

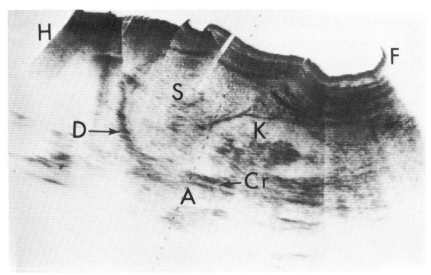

FIG 6–4.

## Normal Spleen

Occasionally the left lobe of the liver is situated anterior to the spleen. The ultrasound picture can be confusing, especially in thin patients. The left lobe of the liver may be confused with entities such as a subcapsular hematoma or left upper quadrant abscess. Figure 6–5 is a longitudinal scan obtained anteriorly over the left upper quadrant. Figure 6–6 is a coronal view of the same patient. The liver is anterior to the spleen. It has an appearance suggestive of subcapsular hematoma. This is an unusual finding but often seen in thin patients. Figure 6–7 is a magnetic resonance image of the same patient as in Figure 6–5 and Figure 6–6. Note that the left lobe of the liver is situated cephalad to the spleen. In examining such patients the sonographer must be aware that a large left lobe of the liver can be situated between the left hemidiaphragm and the spleen.

Figure 6–8 shows a similar finding on a patient with polycystic liver disease. In this instance, the left lobe of the liver is cephalad to the spleen. However, present within the left lobe of the liver are numerous cysts from liver disease. The differential diagnosis includes splenic infarct, splenic cyst, splenic abscess, and subcapsular hematoma. However, the cystic areas (arrows) between the diaphragm and the spleen are secondary to polycystic disease of the liver. This represents cysts in the left lobe of the liver, which are cephalad to the spleen. What is structure 1 in Figure 6–8?

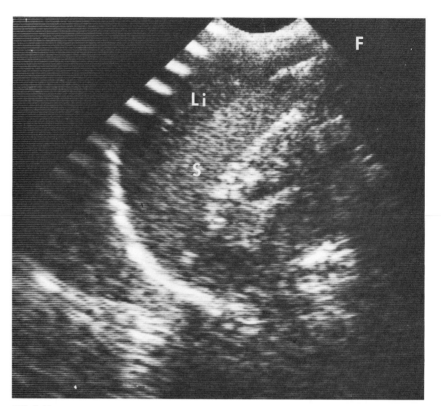

**FIG 6–5.**

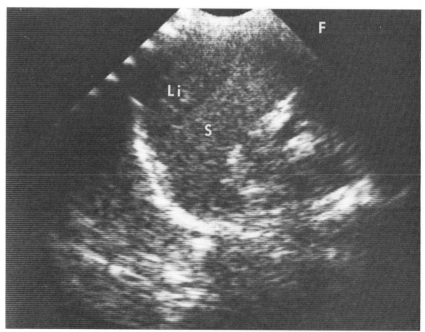

**FIG 6–6.**

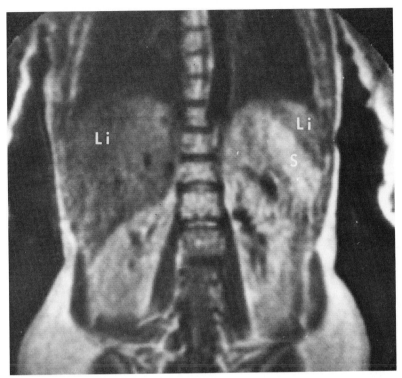

| Arrows | = Polycystic liver |
| --- | --- |
| **F** | = Foot |
| **Li** | = Liver |
| **S** | = Spleen |
| **1** | = Left Kidney |

**FIG 6–7.**

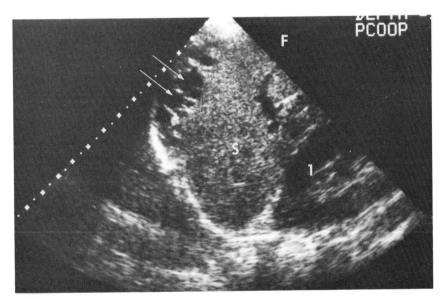

**FIG 6–8.**

## Splenic Visualization

Certain anatomic findings facilitate improved visualization of the spleen. The spleen is situated in the left upper quadrant, often a difficult area for ultrasound examination because of air in the stomach and splenic flexure. However, by utilizing the intercostal spaces, as noted in previous cases, the sonographer can achieve excellent visualization of the spleen. Certain anatomic considerations also improve visualization of the spleen. If the left lobe of the liver is enlarged, one can scan through this ultrasound window and visualize the spleen. When the stomach is airless, it can also function as an ultrasound window. Figure 6–9 is a transverse scan through the subxyphoid region. In this instance, the left lobe of the liver is slightly increased. The important finding is a collapsed stomach between the left lobe of the liver and the spleen. Since the stomach is airless, the sound beam penetrates through the stomach and allows visualization of the spleen deep to the airless stomach. This permits excellent visualization of the splenic parenchyma from an anterior view. Two factors, a large left lobe and a collapsed stomach, are necessary for visualization of the spleen in this case.

When fluid is present in the abdomen or in the left pleural space, the spleen can be visualized to a greater degree, for two reasons. First, the fluid acts as an ultrasound window through which the sound beam can penetrate to the spleen. Second, fluid in the intraperitoneal region will displace the spleen in a caudad direction, permitting better visualization. Figures 6–10 and 6–11 are coronal and transverse scans of the left upper quadrant. Fluid is noted between the diaphragm and spleen and is secondary to ascites (A). There is also evidence of fluid cephalad to the diaphragm that is related to a left pleural effusion (PE). Fluid in the left pleural space and in the subdiaphragmatic region facilitate visualization of the spleen and act as ultrasound windows. The spleen is also noted to be

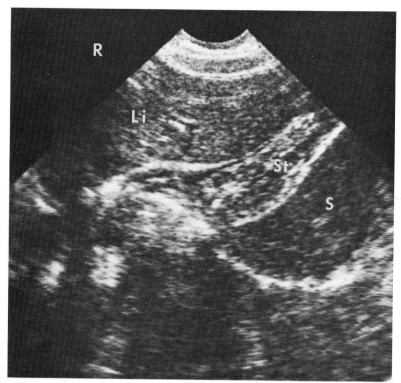

FIG 6–9.

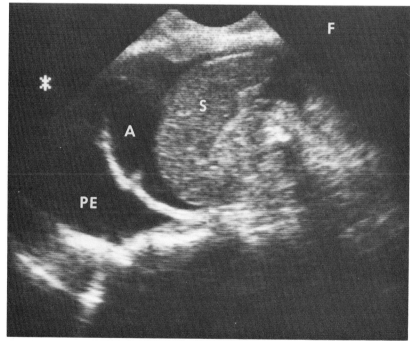

FIG 6–10.

displaced in a caudad direction by the ascitic fluid in Figure 6–10.

Figure 6–12 is a transverse scan through the anterior approach in the subxyphoid region. The left lobe of the liver is again enlarged, facilitating visualization of the spleen. The spleen is seen deep to the left lobe of the liver. Also noted in this scan is ascitic fluid posterior to the spleen. A left pleural effusion is present. The soft tissue echoes situated between the ascitic fluid and pleural effusion are secondary to collapsed lung adherent to the left hemidiaphragm.

**A** = Ascites
**F** = Foot
**Li** = Liver
**Lu** = Collapsed left lung
**PE** = Left pleural effusion
**R** = Right
**S** = Spleen
**St** = Airless stomach

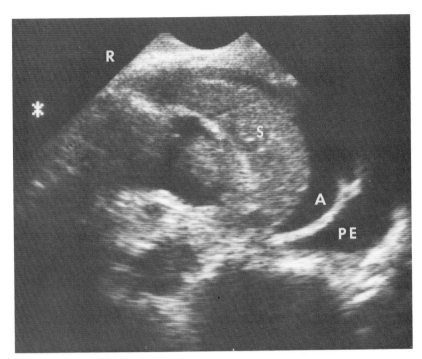

FIG 6–11.

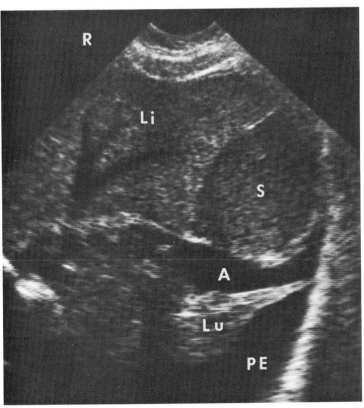

FIG 6–12.

## Mild Splenomegaly

Figures 6–13 and 6–14 are scans of a 76-year-old woman with a history of breast carcinoma. She entered the hospital with a palpable left upper quadrant mass that was thought to be due to splenic enlargement. A transverse ultrasound scan (Fig 6–13) revealed enlargement of the spleen in the left upper quadrant. There is a fairly even parenchymagram to the spleen. A CT scan was also performed (Fig 6–14). This again demonstrated splenomegaly. A rule of thumb in diagnosing splenomegaly is to find the spleen situated anterior to the aorta. In this case, it was situated quite anterior to the abdominal aorta. Also seen in Figure 6–13 is cholelithiasis in the right upper quadrant.

Figure 6–15 is another example of splenomegaly. This is a transverse scan showing marked enlargement of the spleen, which is situated in the anterior abdomen and markedly anterior to the abdominal aorta.

Figure 6–16 is an example of splenomegaly due to chronic alcoholism. Ascites is visualized surrounding the liver and the spleen. When splenomegaly is present, there is usually little difficulty in visualizing the spleen on ultrasound. The reason for this is that the spleen is very often situated below the left costal margin, which gives ready access to the transducer.

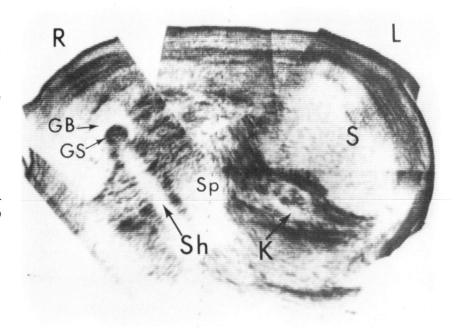

**FIG 6–13.**

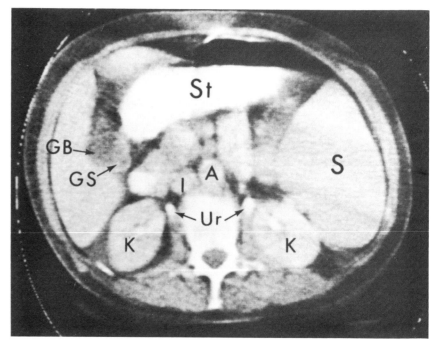

**FIG 6–14.**

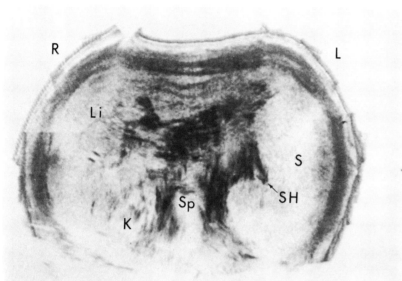

**FIG 6–15.**

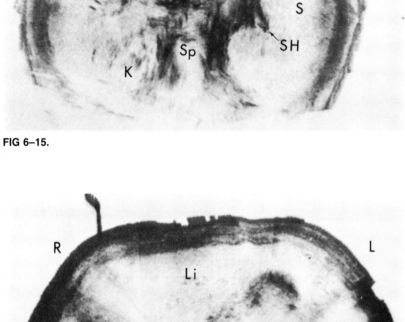

**FIG 6–16.**

| | | |
|---|---|---|
| **A** | = | Aorta |
| **As** | = | Ascites |
| **GB** | = | Gallbladder |
| **Gs** | = | Gallstone |
| **I** | = | Inferior vena cava |
| **K** | = | Kidney |
| **L** | = | Left |
| **Li** | = | Liver |
| **R** | = | Right |
| **S** | = | Spleen |
| **SH** | = | Splenic hilum |
| **Sh** | = | Shadowing from the gallstone |
| **Sp** | = | Spine |
| **St** | = | Stomach |
| **Ur** | = | Ureters |

## Massive Splenomegaly

Figures 6–17 through 6–20 are scans obtained from a patient with chronic myelogenous leukemia. Here we see massive splenomegaly.

Figure 6–17 is a transverse scan high up in the abdomen in which we see the spleen as large as the liver. As we move more caudally in Figure 6–18, we see that the spleen is involving the entire abdomen across the midline and to the right side. At this point, the liver is quite small over its caudal portion.

Figure 6–19 is a longitudinal scan on the left side. The spleen is seen displacing the left kidney somewhat caudally. Another longitudinal scan (Fig 6–20) reveals massive splenomegaly well below the umbilical level. The spleen is seen anterior to the pancreas. It has continued to enlarge to the point that it is visualized below the bifurcation of the aorta.

Figure 6–17 shows an example of a false mass created by sector scanning through the left lateral aspect of the patient. A sonolucent mass appears because of technical factors rather than because of any real mass within the spleen.

The splenic parenchyma is best evaluated on longitudinal scans. Transverse scans obtained through the intercostal spaces very often will have numerous artifacts. This case shows massive splenomegaly in which the spleen is seen across the midline and below the umbilical level.

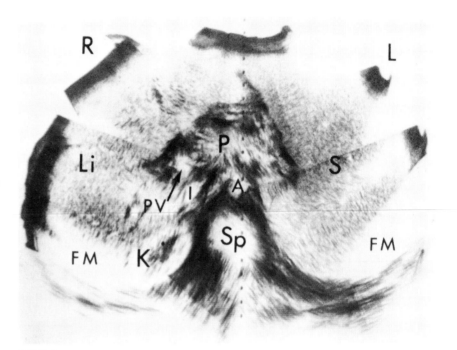

**FIG 6–17.**

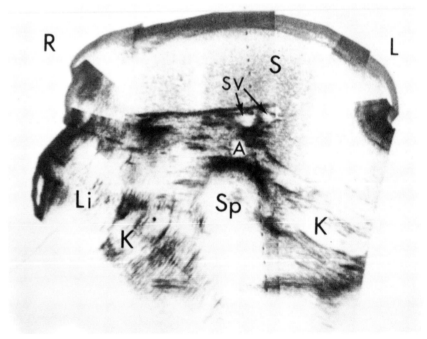

**FIG 6–18.**

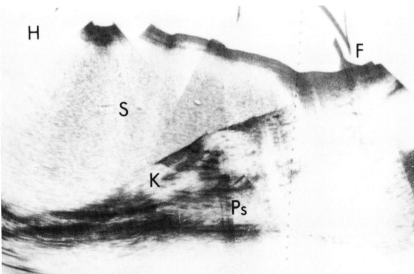

FIG 6–19.

A  = Aorta
B  = Urinary bladder
F  = Foot
FM = False mass
H  = Head
I  = Inferior vena cava
K  = Kidney
L  = Left
Li = Liver
P  = Pancreas
Pu = Level of the symphysis pubis
Ps = Psoas muscle
PV = Portal vein
R  = Right
Re = Reverberations off bowel air
S  = Spleen
Sp = Spine
SV = Splenic vein
U  = Umbilical level

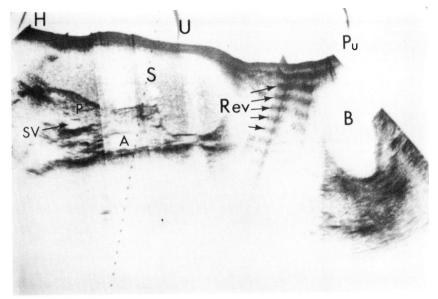

FIG 6–20.

## Splenic Vein Enlargement

Splenomegaly may be secondary to portal hypertension. The splenic vein is variable in size and appearance. When splenomegaly is present, evaluation of the splenic vein becomes helpful in diagnosing the correct etiology. A dilated tortuous splenic vein often indicates portal hypertension.

Figures 6–21 and 6–22 are scans of a 38-year-old man with a long history of alcohol abuse. He had mild splenomegaly. The large circular sonolucencies near the splenic hilum are secondary to a dilated splenic vein. Also noted is some fluid surrounding the spleen in Figure 6–21 due to ascites. The large circular sonolucencies in the splenic hilum are secondary to dilated splenic vein. Although hematomas, abscesses, and other fluid collections may be confused with these sonolucencies, a dilated, tortuous splenic vein has a fairly characteristic tubular appearance.

Figure 6–23 is a coronal scan of a patient with mild splenomegaly. A tortuous and mildly dilated splenic vein is seen in the splenic hilum. The findings are compatible with portal hypertension and splenic enlargement.

Figure 6–24 is an oblique scan of the left upper quadrant in a patient with a history of chronic alcohol abuse. This scan demonstrates increased size and tortuosity to the splenic vein. However, an unusual finding is present adjacent to the spleen. Tubular sonolucent areas are present in the left upper quadrant in close proximity to the spleen. These areas are secondary to large dilated varices. These sonolucencies can be confusing if the sonographer has never seen them before. Other entities such as ascites, hematoma, abscess, or splenic cyst will be considered initially. However, the characteristic tubular, beaded appearance will lead to the correct diagnosis of dilated varices.

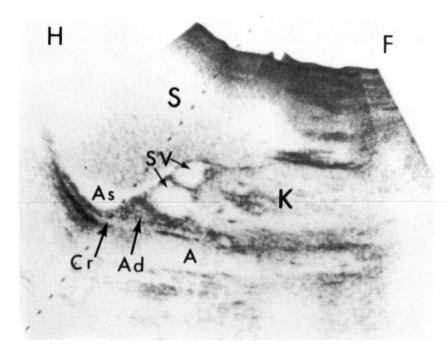

FIG 6–21.

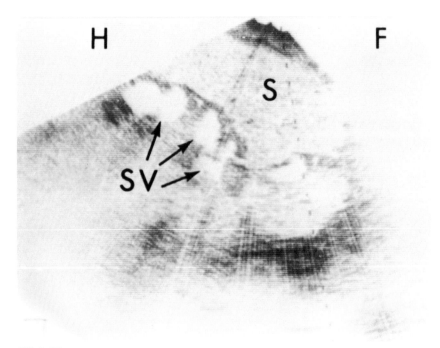

FIG 6–22.

A   = Aorta
**Ad** = Adrenal gland
**As** = Ascites
**Cr** = Crus of the diaphragm
**F**  = Foot
**H**  = Head
**K**  = Kidney
**S**  = Spleen
**SV** = Splenic vein
**V**  = Dilated varices

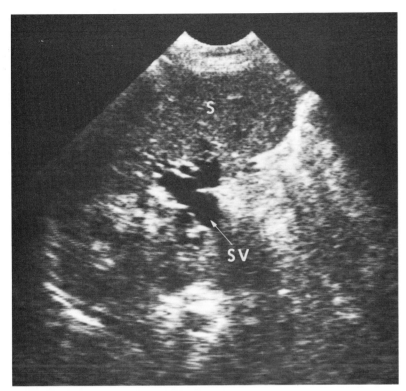

**FIG 6–23.**

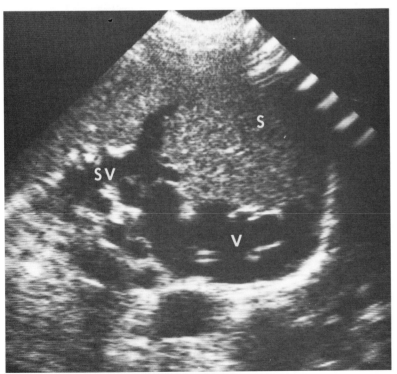

**FIG 6–24.**

## Lymphoma; Lymphosarcoma

Splenic enlargement may be present secondary to an infiltrative process. This is often difficult to distinguish from splenic enlargement secondary to portal hypertension unless a diffusely uneven parenchymal pattern is present. Figure 6–25 is a transverse scan of a patient with lymphoma. A large mass involving the spleen is present in the left upper quadrant. This mass was secondary to lymphomatous involvement within the spleen. The texture pattern of the mass in Figure 6–25 is uneven compared to what is seen in a normal spleen. The mass completely disappeared after radiation therapy and chemotherapy. Usually, splenic enlargement secondary to lymphoma or chronic leukemia gives a fairly even splenic parenchymal texture. It is not easy to distinguish lymphomatous infiltrate from normal splenic echoes. However, this case shows an uneven parenchymal pattern to the left upper quadrant mass.

Figure 6–26 is a longitudinal coronal scan of the left upper quadrant in a patient with lymphosarcoma of the spleen. An isotope study demonstrated numerous filling defects within an enlarged spleen. Figure 6–26 shows numerous highly echogenic regions within the spleen. The appearance is markedly abnormal compared to what is expected on a splenic ultrasound scan. The discrete lesions were secondary to lymphosarcoma (arrows) in this unusual case.

Figures 6–27 and 6–28 are ultrasound and CT scans of a patient who also had lymphosarcoma. Figure 6–27 is a transverse scan of the upper abdomen obtained in the subxyphoid region. The spleen is visualized posterior to the left lobe of the liver. In this instance, the splenic parenchymal pattern has an uneven, irregular texture compared to what one sees in a normal spleen. This uneven texture was secondary to lymphosarcoma. A CT scan (Fig 6–28) confirms the irregular appearance of the spleen. Low-density and high-density regions are noted in the spleen in this patient.

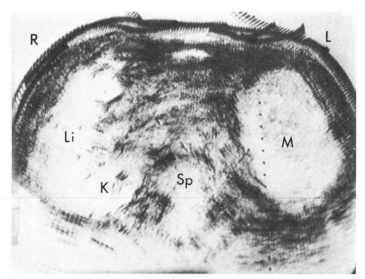

FIG 6–25.

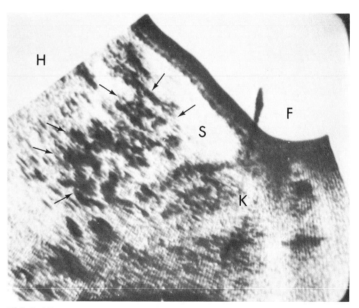

FIG 6–26.

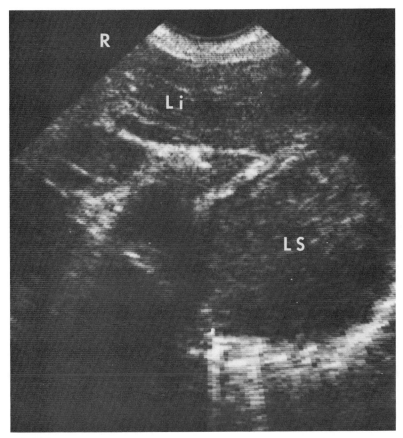

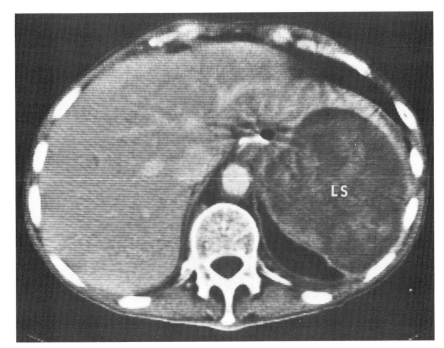

| Arrows | = | Lymphosarcoma |
| --- | --- | --- |
| **F** | = | Foot |
| **H** | = | Head |
| **K** | = | Kidney |
| **L** | = | Left |
| **Li** | = | Liver |
| **LS** | = | Lymphosarcoma |
| **M** | = | Lymphoma |
| **R** | = | Right |
| **Sp** | = | Spine |

**FIG 6–27.**

**FIG 6–28.**

## Splenic Metastasis

Metastatic lesions are not commonly seen in the spleen. They are certainly much less common than in the liver. However, when solid-appearing masses are identified in the spleen, the possibility of splenic metastasis must be considered. Figures 6–29 and 6–30 are transverse and coronal scans in a 31-year-old man who had malignant melanoma. A large mass is noted within the splenic parenchyma. This mass has a solid inhomogeneous appearance. The findings are secondary to malignant melanoma metastatic to the spleen. A rim of normal splenic parenchymal tissue is seen around the mass.

Figures 6–31 and 6–32 are ultrasound and CT scans of the spleen in a patient who had lung carcinoma. A filling defect was noted on an isotope study. The ultrasound scan in Figure 6–31 reveals an uneven parenchymal pattern in the midportion of the spleen. There are numerous internal echoes and the appearance of a capsule. The findings indicate a solid mass within the spleen. The CT scan in Figure 6–32 confirmed the presence of a mass within the central portion of the spleen. The mass appears as a low-density region in the spleen on a postinfusion scan. The findings are secondary to metastatic disease from a lung primary.

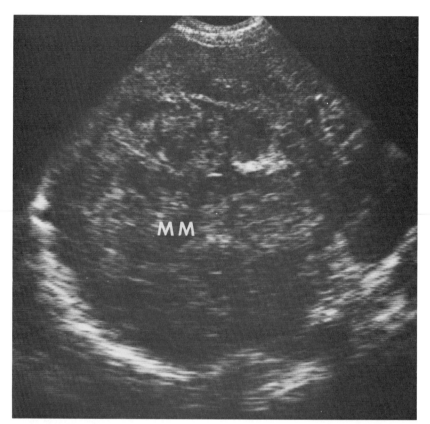

FIG 6–29.

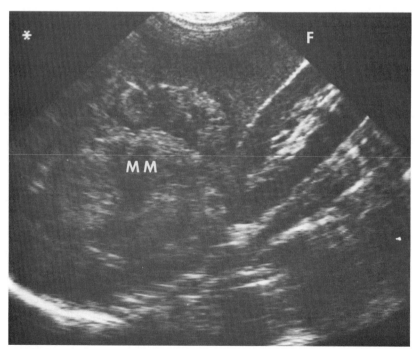

FIG 6–30.

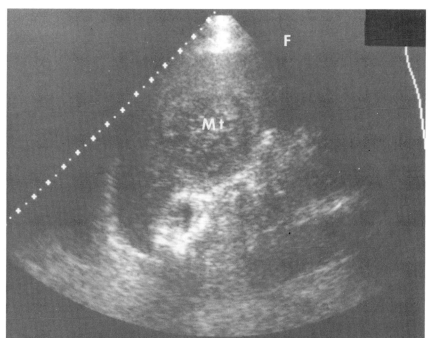

F  = Foot
MM = Metastatic melanoma
Mt = Metastasis from lung primary

FIG 6–31.

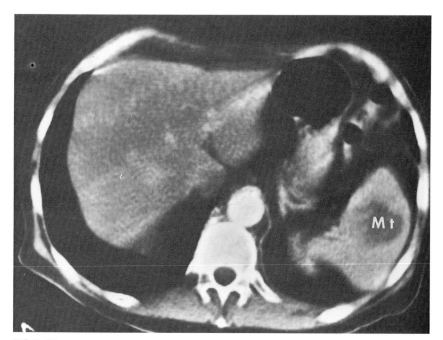

FIG 6–32.

## Small Splenic Cysts

Figure 6–33 is an isotope study of the spleen with a filling defect in the medial aspect of its lower portion. As with a liver examination, ultrasound is an excellent means for detecting the nature of defects noted on isotope study. A transverse scan of the same patient (Fig 6–34) shows a large fluid-filled mass anterior to the spleen. This represents a small splenic cyst.

A longitudinal scan (Fig 6–35) shows the cyst as a sonolucent mass with sharp borders within the spleen. Deep to the cyst are increased splenic echoes due to through-transmission; this confirms the fluid nature of the splenic mass.

Figure 6–36 is an isotope study of a spleen with a large filling defect. Ultrasound is an excellent means for determining the nature of such defects. The case shown in Figure 6–36 follows (Figs 6–37 through 6–40).

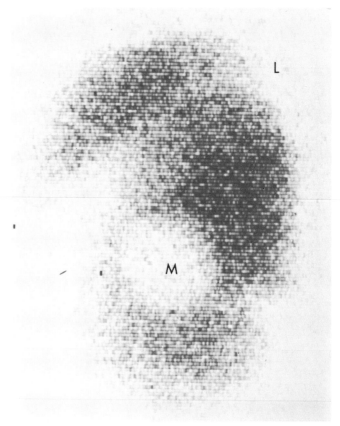

**FIG 6–33.**

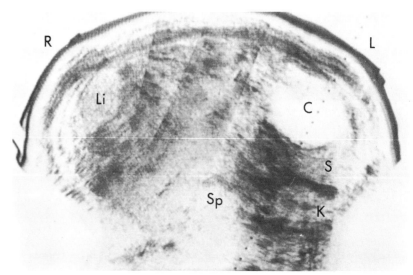

**FIG 6–34.**

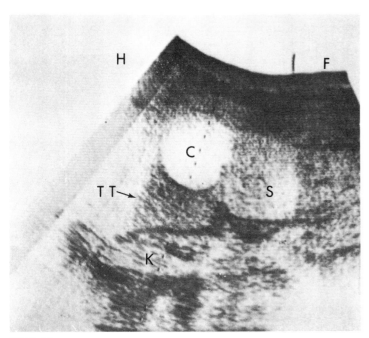

**FIG 6–35.**

| | | |
|---|---|---|
| **C** | = | Small splenic cyst |
| **F** | = | Foot |
| **H** | = | Head |
| **K** | = | Kidney |
| **L** | = | Left |
| **Li** | = | Liver |
| **M** | = | Mass noted on isotope study of the spleen |
| **R** | = | Right |
| **S** | = | Spleen |
| **Sp** | = | Spine |
| **TT** | = | Through-transmission behind the cyst |

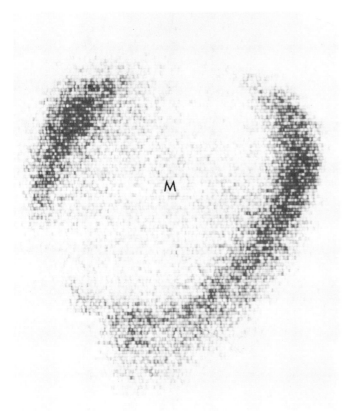

**FIG 6–36.**

## Large Splenic Cyst

Figures 6–37 through 6–39 are ultrasound scans of the spleen showing a large sonolucent mass in the anterior aspect of the left upper quadrant. This mass was found to be a large splenic cyst. The fluid-filled mass is situated anterior to the spleen in Figures 6–37 and 6–38. The excellent through-transmission and fairly sharp borders indicate the fluid-filled nature of the mass.

A prone scan (Fig 6–39) indicates the cyst situated anterior to the left kidney. The upper pole of the left kidney is compressed by this large splenic cyst. Figure 6–40 is an angiogram of the same patient. A large avascular mass is seen in the left upper quadrant with splaying and stretching of the vessels from the splenic artery.

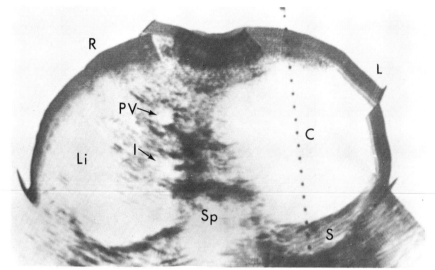

**FIG 6–37.**

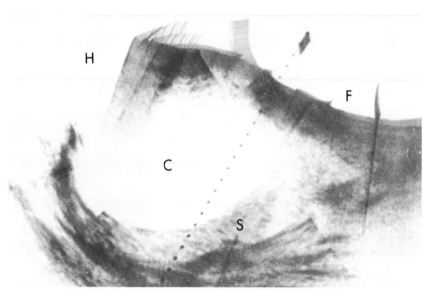

**FIG 6–38.**

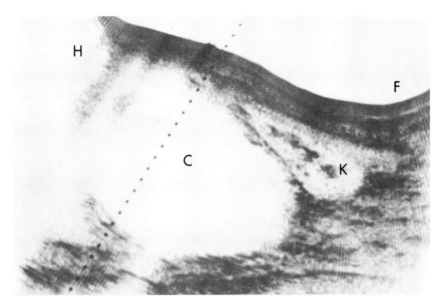

C   = Large splenic cyst
F   = Foot
H   = Head
I   = Inferior vena cava
K   = Left kidney
L   = Left
Li  = Liver
PV  = Portal vein
R   = Right
S   = Spleen
Sp  = Spine

**FIG 6–39.**

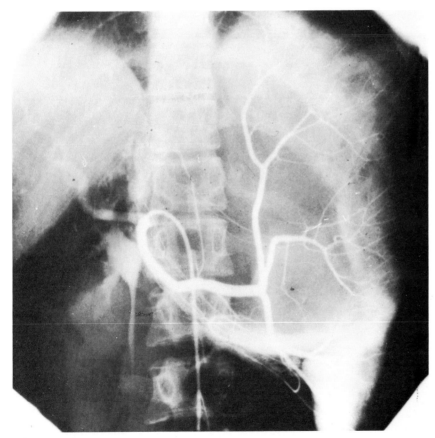

**FIG 6–40.**

## Splenic Cysts

The four images on these pages are from three separate patients who had splenic cysts. Figures 6–41 and 6–42 are scans of the same patient. Figure 6–41 is a longitudinal coronal scan in which we see a sonolucent well-circumscribed mass of the inferior border of the spleen. This mass meets all of the ultrasonographic criteria of a cystic lesion. No internal echoes, and prominent through-transmission, indicate the fluid-filled nature of the structure. Figure 6–42, a scan of the liver through the right upper quadrant, demonstrates two cystic areas near the diaphragm (arrows). The possibility of polycystic disease or simple cysts of the liver would be considered. However, following the sonolucent areas medially, the diagnosis of hepatic veins was made. This is an important example of always making a diagnosis in two planes. On this one scan, the possibility of liver cysts would be quite likely. However, with scanning in a second plane, the cystic areas appeared more tubular. They were found to empty into the inferior vena cava, and represented hepatic veins. Note the pleural effusion above the diaphragm on this scan.

Figures 6–43 and 6–44 are coronal scans from two separate patients. Again, sonolucent masses are seen within the splenic parenchyma. The borders are quite sharp, with prominent through-transmission noted deep to the masses. These findings indicate cysts of the spleen. There is a slight irregularity to the inferior border of the cyst in Figure 6–43. Figure 6–44 demonstrates very sharp borders through the entirety of the cyst. Splenic cysts are usually easily identified. They stand out quite dramatically as sonolucent regions within the splenic parenchyma.

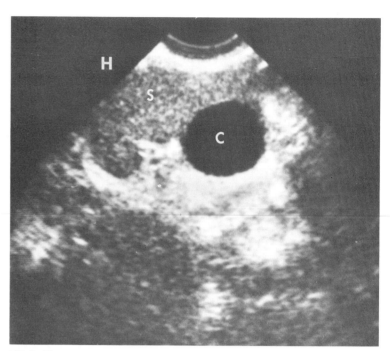

**FIG 6–41.**

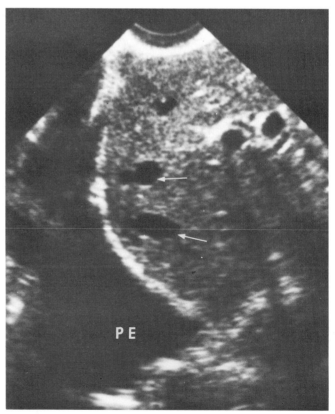

**FIG 6–42.**

| Arrows | = | Hepatic veins |
| C | = | Splenic cyst |
| F | = | Foot |
| H | = | Head |
| K | = | Kidney |
| PE | = | Pleural effusion |
| S | = | Spleen |

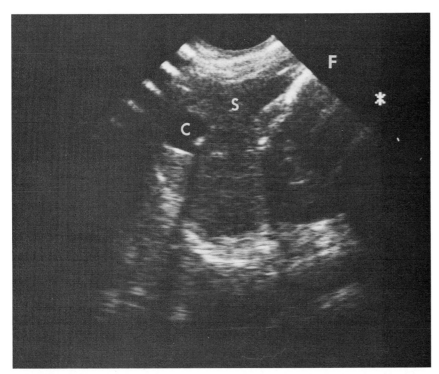

FIG 6–43.

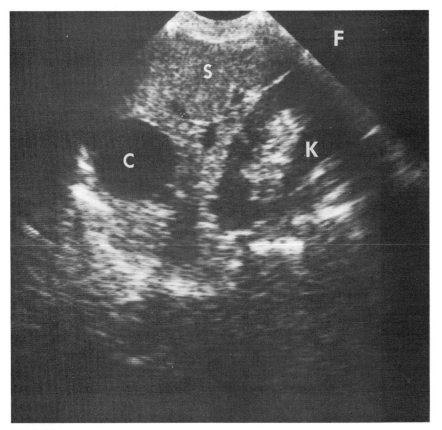

FIG 6–44.

## Splenic Masses

Splenic cysts are often secondary to previous long-standing trauma. However, if trauma has been more recent, hemorrhagic areas in the spleen can have the appearance of splenic cysts. Figure 6–45 is a longitudinal coronal scan in which a sonolucent region is noted in the spleen. Through-transmission is not as pronounced as in the previous cases of splenic cyst. A CT scan in Figure 6–46 demonstrates an area of increased density corresponding to the area on ultrasound. These two findings indicate a splenic hematoma. The relative lucency of the hematoma on ultrasound and the lack of through-transmission are suggestive of hematoma. The CT scan shows an area of increased density which can be seen at various stages of hematoma.

A splenic hematoma or splenic cyst may have a calcified border. Figure 6–47 is a longitudinal scan of a patient with no definite history of trauma. However, a highly echogenic ring with some attenuation is evident in the spleen, compatible with calcification. Patients with previous trauma may have calcification of a hematoma or a calcified wall to a splenic cyst. Figure 6–48 is an x-ray film of the left upper quadrant confirming the presence of a calcified mass within the spleen.

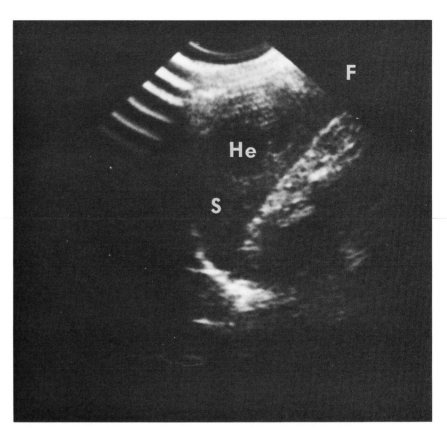

**FIG 6–45.**

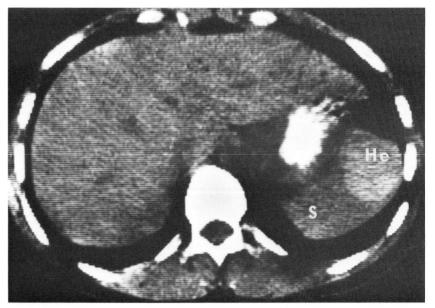

**FIG 6–46.**

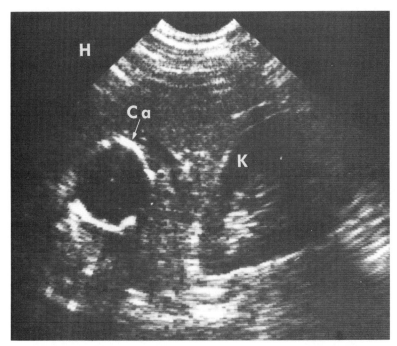

**FIG 6–47.**

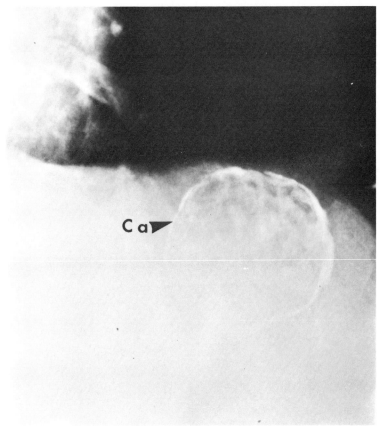

**FIG 6–48.**

Ca = Calcified splenic mass
F = Foot
H = Head
He = Splenic hematoma
K = Kidney
S = Spleen

## Splenic Calcification

Occasionally various high-amplitude echoes can be identified with the splenic parenchyma. Figure 6–49 is a transverse scan in which several high-amplitude echoes are noted in the spleen. Acoustic shadowing is present deep to these echoes. This patient had granulomatous disease of questionable etiology. Some calcifications were noted on an abdominal x-ray film.

Figures 6–50 and 6–51 are splenic ultrasound scans of two different patients with histoplasmosis. In both cases high-amplitude, small echoes are seen within the splenic parenchyma. Some acoustic shadowing is present, especially in Figure 6–50. Note the uneven parenchymal pattern to the spleen. These findings are compatible with small calcifications within the splenic parenchyma, often seen in patients with histoplasmosis.

Figure 6–52 is a transverse scan of the left upper quadrant. A region of high echogenicity is noted near the splenic hilum. Acoustic shadowing is present deep to this region. Also present in the splenic parenchyma are two small oval sonolucent regions. The patient had tuberculosis. Some calcification was noted in the spleen. The patient was thought to have both old and active tuberculosis. The calcific area with shadowing was secondary to old tuberculosis. The sonolucent oval regions in the spleen are most likely secondary to the acute phase of the disease process.

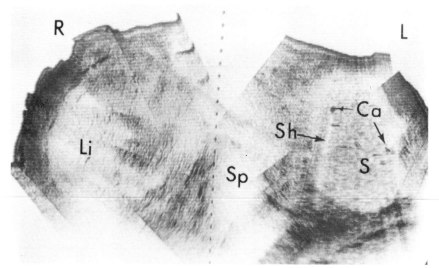

FIG 6–49.

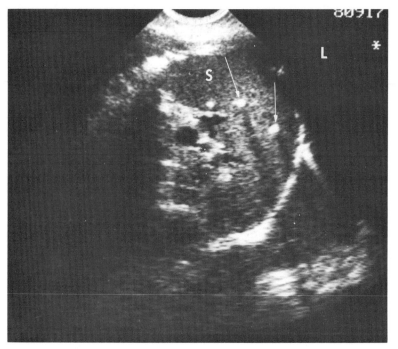

FIG 6–50.

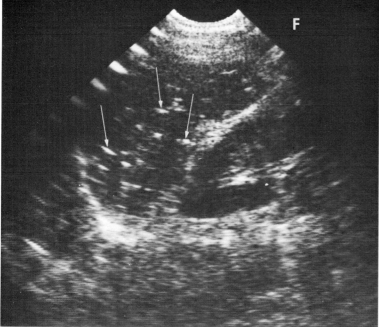

FIG 6–51.

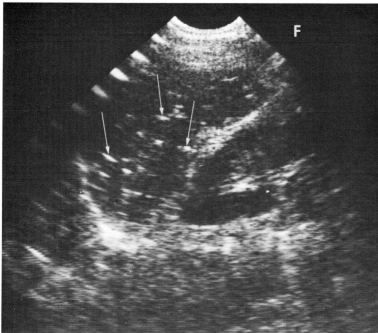

FIG 6–52.

| | | |
|---|---|---|
| **Arrows** | = | Splenic calcification |
| **Ca** | = | Splenic calcification |
| **F** | = | Foot |
| **L** | = | Left |
| **Li** | = | Liver |
| **R** | = | Right |
| **S** | = | Spleen |
| **Sh** | = | Acoustic shadow |
| **Sp** | = | Spine |

## Splenic Hematomas

Figures 6–53 and 6–54 are scans of a patient with a left-sided empyema. Multiple attempts at thoracentesis were made. However, they were unsuccessful because of the loculated nature of the empyema. A few hours after the thoracocentesis attempts, the patient became hypotensive, with a decreased hematocrit. Ultrasound was performed to evaluate the left thorax and left upper quadrant. A sonolucent mass representing a splenic hematoma is seen in the central portion of the spleen. Splenic hematomas may be within the splenic parenchyma or extracapsular, in the peritoneal cavity. At operation performed after the ultrasound examination, a large splenic hematoma was found near the hilum of the spleen, corresponding to the ultrasound findings. The sonolucent mass within the midportion of the spleen is consistent with a hematoma. Very little through-transmission was identified at this time, although some is noted in Figure 6–54.

Figure 6–55 is a longitudinal coronal scan of the left upper quadrant of a middle-aged woman who had recently experienced trauma. The ultrasound findings indicate a relatively sonolucent mass with some soft echoes present. The mass is markedly different from the normal splenic parenchyma. Based on the ultrasound findings alone, the differential diagnosis would include abscess, hematoma, infarct, and metastatic lesion. However, with the history of recent trauma, splenic hematoma was the most likely diagnosis.

Figure 6–56 is a longitudinal coronal scan in a young man with recent acute abdominal trauma. Two sonolucent areas (arrows) are identified within normal splenic parenchyma. They are relatively sonolucent and consistent with splenic hematomas. All of the cases represent intrasplenic hematomas. The relatively lucent masses displace some of the normal splenic parenchymal tissue. There is no free intraperitoneal fluid in any of these cases. These lucent masses in conjunction with a recent traumatic

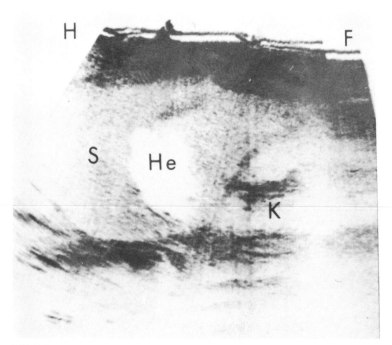

**FIG 6–53.**

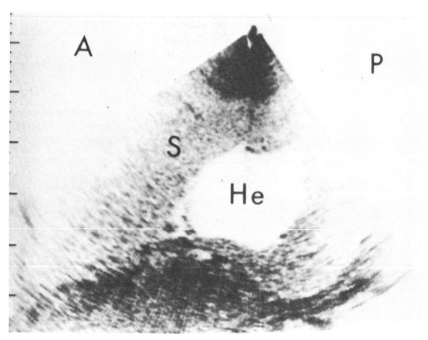

**FIG 6–54.**

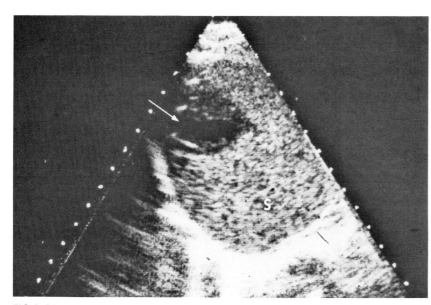

**FIG 6–55.**

history are highly consistent with intrasplenic hematomas.

| | | |
|---|---|---|
| **A** | = | Anterior |
| **Arrow** | = | Splenic hematoma |
| **F** | = | Foot |
| **H** | = | Head |
| **He** | = | Splenic hematoma |
| **K** | = | Kidney |
| **P** | = | Posterior |
| **S** | = | Spleen |

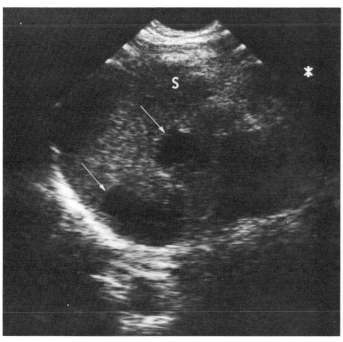

**FIG 6–56.**

## Splenic Hematomas

Figure 6–57 is a longitudinal coronal scan of the left upper quadrant in a patient who had recently sustained upper quadrant trauma. A large sonolucent mass is present displacing the spleen posteriorly and medially. Although the mass is relatively sonolucent, several linear echoes are present within the mass. This ultrasound appearance is often seen in clot formation and fibrotic changes in a hematoma. The splenic hematoma was localized in the left upper quadrant. There was no evidence of any free interperitoneal fluid.

Figure 6–58 is a longitudinal scan of another patient with recent abdominal trauma. A large sonolucent mass is identified cephalad to the spleen. Note the compressed appearance of the remaining splenic parenchymal echoes. This is a common observation when the hematoma remains loculated in the left upper quadrant. The enlarging hematoma and increasing pressure caused compression of the normal splenic parenchymal texture.

Figure 6–59 is a longitudinal scan of another patient with a subcapsular hematoma. The patient was a 50-year-old man who had recently sustained trauma to the left upper quadrant. A large sonolucent mass is present compressing the splenic parenchymal texture posteriorly and medially. The findings are compatible with a splenic hematoma.

In the three preceding cases, the splenic hematoma was localized to the left upper quadrant. In all cases the rest of the abdomen and pelvis was examined to rule out intraperitoneal hemorrhage. Occasionally a patient is scanned and few abnormal findings are seen in the left upper quadrant. However, a thorough search of the abdomen and pelvis may disclose free peritoneal fluid secondary to intraperitoneal hemorrhage. Figure 6–60 is such a case. Frequently, blunt abdominal trauma leads to splenic rupture. The fluid can progress into the peritoneal cavity and may not be loculated in the left upper quadrant. Figure 6–60 shows such a case—

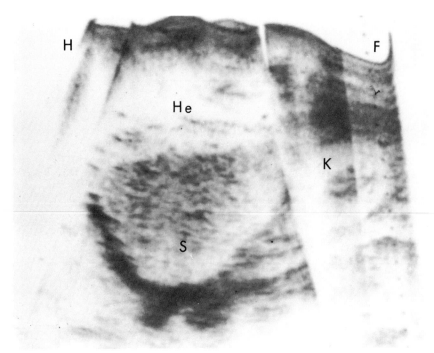

**FIG 6–57.**

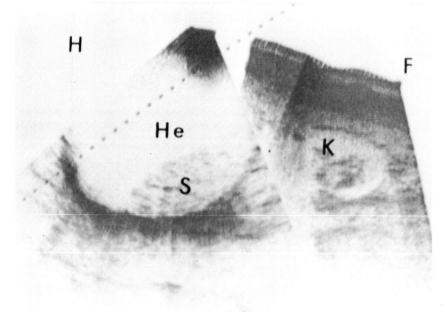

**FIG 6–58.**

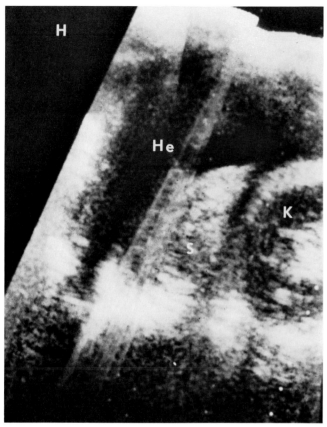

**FIG 6–59.**

fluid is identified in the hepatorenal angle. Note the sonolucent rim of fluid situated between the liver and the kidney. This was secondary to intraperitoneal hemorrhage. It is also most helpful to examine the pelvis. Since the patient is often supine, fluid will collect in the pelvis because it is in the most dependent position in the abdomen.

| | | |
|---|---|---|
| **F** | = | Foot |
| **H** | = | Head |
| **He** | = | Hemorrhage |
| **K** | = | Kidney |
| **Li** | = | Liver |
| **S** | = | Spleen |

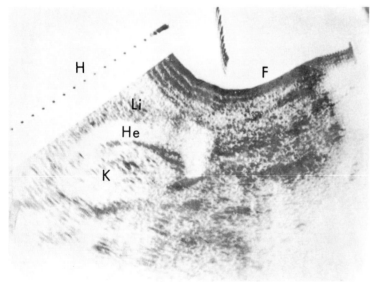

**FIG 6–60.**

## Splenic Hematoma

Figures 6–61 and 6–62 are transverse scans of a 39-year-old man with a history of chronic alcoholism. Approximately 2 weeks earlier, he had been found unconscious with numerous regions of ecchymosis over his abdomen. There was physical evidence of trauma to the left upper quadrant. The ultrasound scans show a large sonolucent collection lateral to the splenic parenchymal echoes. The spleen is enlarged and displaced medially. There is evidence of a large fluid collection lateral to the spleen, consistent with a splenic hematoma. No free fluid was evident in the rest of the abdomen.

Figure 6–63 is a coronal scan of another patient. A large fluid collection is evident lateral and cephalad to the spleen. Most of the fluid collection is echo free. However, there are some curvilinear interfaces present. Sometimes this may represent clot formation or disruption of the splenic parenchymal structure itself.

Figure 6–64 is a coronal scan showing a sonolucent region in the subdiaphragmatic region. The spleen is displaced inferiorly. The splenic parenchymal texture inferior to the region of hematoma is normal. In this instance, a small fluid collection is present cephalad to the left hemidiaphragm, representing a region of pleural effusion secondary to reaction from the hematoma.

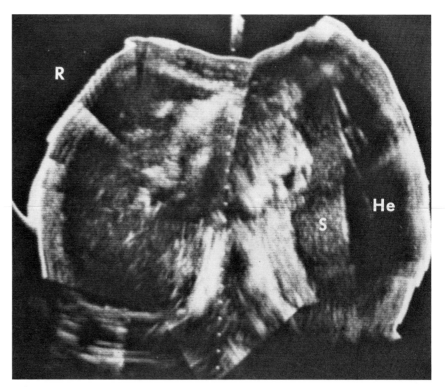

FIG 6–61.

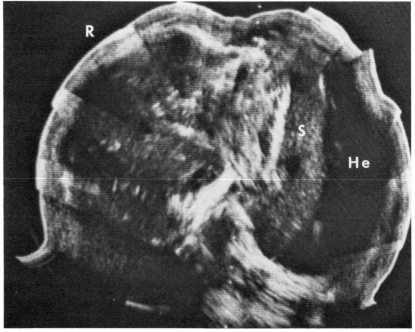

FIG 6–62.

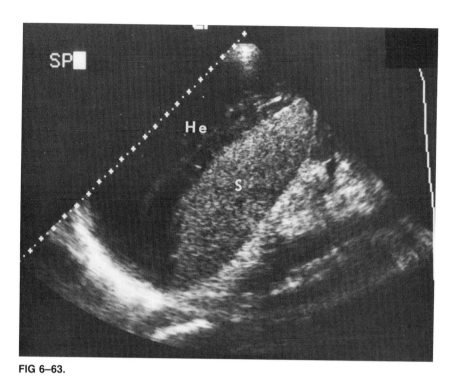

He = Hemorrhage
PE = Pleural effusion
R = Right
S = Spleen

FIG 6–63.

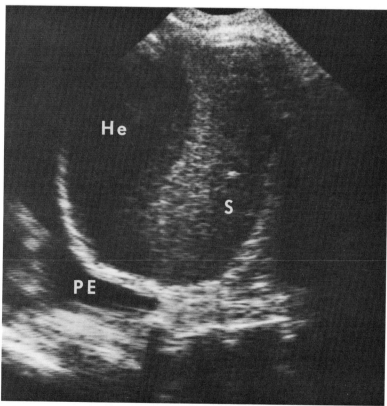

FIG 6–64.

## Splenic Hematoma and Splenic Abscess

Figure 6–65 is a longitudinal coronal scan of the left upper quadrant in a patient with a recent abdominal trauma. An inhomogeneous region is present within the midportion of the spleen (arrows). It does not have the appearance noted in previous cases. Rather, the ultrasound appearance indicates an inhomogeneous structure within the central portion of the splenic parenchyma. The findings are compatible with hematoma, abscess, or a solid metastatic lesion. However, the patient had recently sustained abdominal trauma, and the inhomogeneous structure represented a splenic hematoma. A follow-up scan is shown in Figure 6–66. This scan was obtained 2½ weeks after the scan shown in Figure 6–65. Figure 6–66 shows three relatively lucent areas in the same region that was noted to be inhomogeneous in Figure 6–65. These findings indicate that the hemorrhagic region has undergone lysis. The lysed blood now has a sonolucent appearance. Eventually, the lucent areas of lysis may turn into splenic cysts. Note the difference in the echo pattern of the splenic hematoma in this case. The reason for the difference is the time since the injury. The earlier scan (Fig 6–65) represents clotted blood. The later scan (Fig 6–66) demonstrates an extremely fluid hematoma secondary to lysis of the blood.

Occasionally, relatively lucent masses can be identified in the spleen that are secondary to infection. There is no way to differentiate an abscess from hematoma on ultrasound. Clinical history is necessary to distinguish between the two, along with laboratory data. Figure 6–67 is a longitudinal scan of the left upper quadrant in a 62-year-old woman who had recently undergone aortofemoral graft bypass. Purulent drainage developed in the left groin, and the patient was treated with antibiotics. An abdominal ultrasound examination was performed and revealed a large lucent mass in the midportion of the spleen. A solid component to the mass is present.

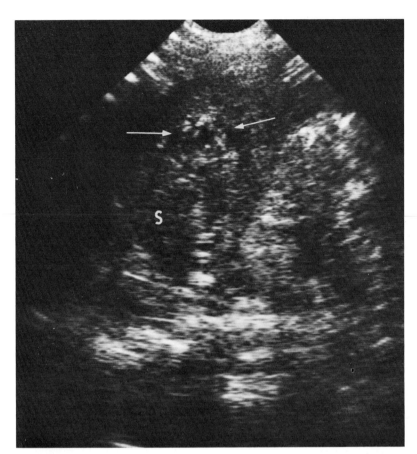

**FIG 6–65.**

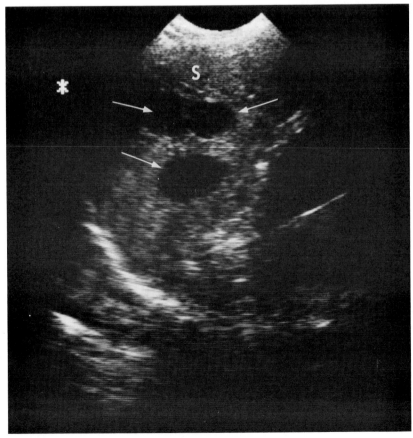

**FIG 6–66.**

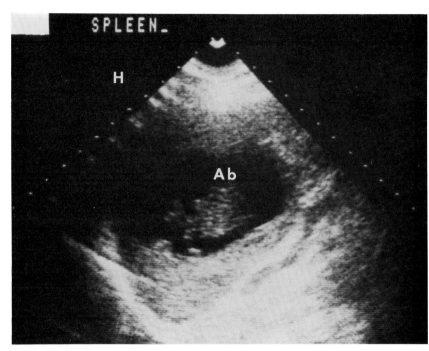

**FIG 6–67.**

The findings indicate a splenic abscess. Blood cultures were positive for *E. coli.* The ultrasound findings cannot distinguish among abscess, hematoma, or necrotic tumor. However, the clinical history usually points to the correct diagnosis.

Figure 6–68 is a longitudinal coronal scan of the spleen in a patient with *Candida* infection and lymphoma. The region developed quite rapidly and is most consistent with a *Candida* abscess. The possibility of a lymphomatous infiltrate cannot be entirely ruled out.

| | | |
|---|---|---|
| **Ab** | = | Splenic abscess |
| **Arrows** | = | Hematoma |
| **F** | = | Foot |
| **H** | = | Head |
| **S** | = | Spleen |

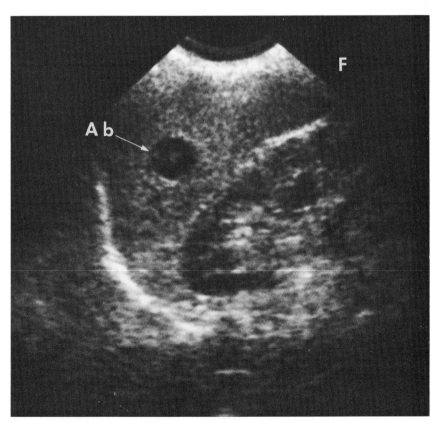

**FIG 6–68.**

## Splenic Abscess

Figure 6–69 is longitudinal coronal scan in which a sonolucent mass is noted cephalad to the spleen. The mass is secondary to a perisplenic abscess. A reactive pleural effusion is evident cephalad to the left hemidiaphragm. Figure 6–70 is the scan of another patient with a left upper mass secondary to a left subphrenic abscess. It is difficult to distinguish an abscess from a hematoma on ultrasound examination. The clinical history will contribute to the correct diagnosis. A pleural effusion is also present in this patient and appears as a sonolucent region cephalad to the left hemidiaphragm. Below the left hemidiaphragm is a sonolucent mass with numerous internal echoes, compatible with a left subphrenic abscess.

Figure 6–71 is a longitudinal scan of a 70-year-old man with longstanding diabetes. A high-amplitude echogenic region (arrows) is noted in the tip of the spleen. There is also evidence of some attenuation deep to the echogenic region. The ultrasound findings were highly suspicious for an air-containing region in the spleen. There was also a slight lucent rim noted around the air-containing region. Therefore, a CT scan was obtained (Fig 6–72) and disclosed air in the central portion of the spleen, along with a low-density region near the splenic hilum. These findings were secondary to a splenic abscess.

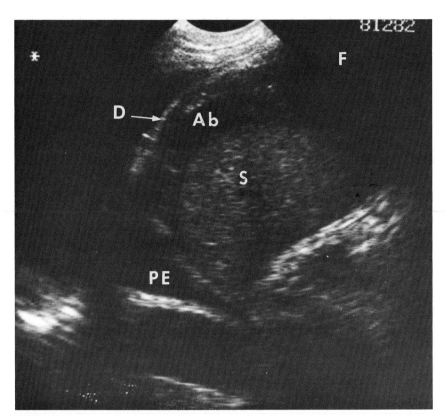

**FIG 6–69.**

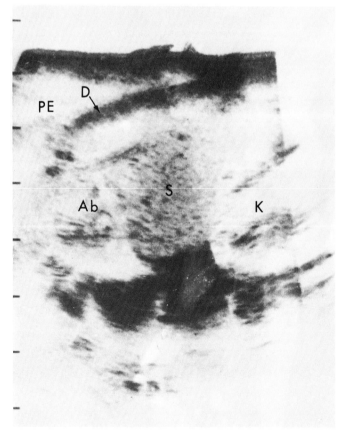

**FIG 6–70.**

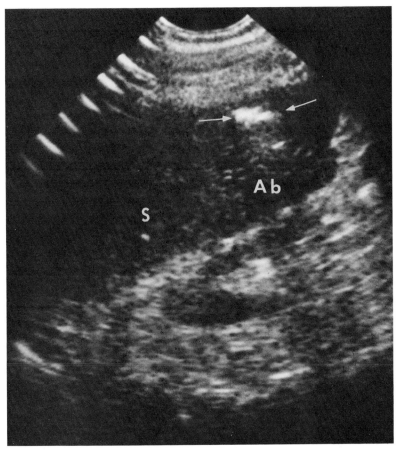

Ab      = Splenic abscess
**Arrows** = Air in abscess
D       = Diaphragm
F       = Foot
K       = Kidney
PE      = Pleural effusion
S       = Spleen

**FIG 6–71.**

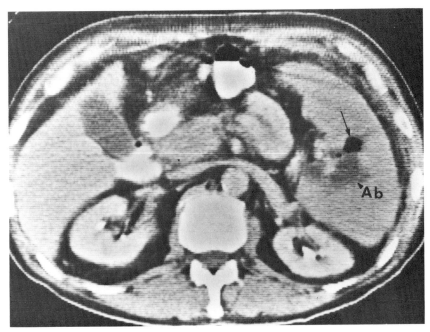

**FIG 6–72.**

# 7.
# Renal Ultrasound

Hedvig Hricak, M.D.

## Introduction

Over the past 15 years ultrasonography has assumed an increasingly important role in the evaluation of various urinary tract abnormalities. The kidneys were among the first organs for which sonography was clinically useful. When bi-stable units were the only equipment available, sonography was limited to the diagnosis of hydronephrosis or of large renal masses deforming the renal contour. Renal anatomy can be well delineated with the superior resolution provided by currently commercially available gray-scale units. The internal architecture of the kidney is now routinely displayed with a clarity approaching that of the cut surface of a gross anatomic specimen. Not only can the kidney be evaluated for anatomic abnormalities, but with the use of Doppler ultrasound and dynamic scanning, renal blood flow alterations can be identified and studied. Furthermore, with ultrasound guidance, biopsy of renal masses or renal parenchyma can be performed and fluids aspirated. Ultrasound has become indispensable in the evaluation of many kidney afflictions.

## Renal Scanning Techniques

The kidneys have been traditionally studied with transverse and longitudinal scans performed with the patient prone.[1] Although the renal size can be assessed and many lesions detected with this approach, the thick paraspinal muscles and bony impingements frequently prevent optimal visualization of the renal architecture, especially of the upper pole. Furthermore, the prevertebral and renal vessels cannot be visualized. As a result, a complete renal study should include transverse and longitudinal scans with the patient in both the decubitus and supine positions. While this may represent a problem when a static scanner is used, examination of the kidney is more flexible and the kidney display is easier with the real-time units.

The right kidney is best imaged through the anterior axillary line, or the intercostal or anterior subcostal ports. As it is important to compare the echo amplitude of the renal parenchyma with that of the liver, anterior or lateral projections should be used that include the liver in the same image as the kidney. Regardless of the approach selected, imaging should always be performed in two projections at right angles to each other. The posterior oblique longitudinal scan, advocated by Bazzocchi and Rizzatto,[2] provides information about renal anatomy, particularly the renal parenchyma and hilus in their vertical axis. This approach is particularly useful in patients with pseudotumors, hydronephrosis, or pelvic lipomatosis.[2] In our experience, as well as that of Thompson et al.[3] and Dana et al.,[4] the optimal image of the renal parenchyma and pelvocalyceal system is obtained in the coronal view. This image is also called the "bivalve" true frontal section.[4] Coronal sections correlate best with the kidney anatomy seen on excretory urograms and are easily understood by physicians and surgeons. A coronal longitudinal sonogram of the kidney presents the renal pelvis to the ureteropelvic junction and proximal ureter in continuity and is useful in the detection of hydronephrosis. Sonograms of the right kidney may be technically inferior in a patient with a short liver and an abundant amount of bowel gas. Rotating the patient into a lateral decubitus position can allow easy visualization of the entire kidney. In addition to the coronal view of the left kidney introduced by Pochhammer,[5] a scoliotic position is useful in allowing better demarcation of the upper pole of the kidney. It is especially helpful in differentiating between the upper pole of the left kidney and the spleen. Another alternative is the display of the left kidney through a fluid-filled stomach which is used as an acoustic window.[6]

A few points are worth mentioning about the technique used in the examination of the patient in acute renal failure (ARF). Such patients are often critically ill and cannot be transported to the ultrasound scanning room. High-resolution portable real-time scanners are therefore mandatory. While supine or prone longitudinal and transverse scans are useful, coronal images that display the renal pelvis and calyces in continuity, allowing optimal evaluation for urinary tract dilatation in patients with ARF, are essential. Posterior oblique longitudinal scanning, producing images between the coronal and sagittal planes, can be used as an alternative.[2] In either case, real-time sector scanning not only provides portability but facilitates identification of the appropriate scanning plane and results in the rapid acquisition of images without any loss of diagnostic accuracy.

## Normal Anatomy

Renal sonography is excellent for imaging all renal and juxtarenal tissue. The position of the kidneys is variable, but they are normally located between the iliac crests and the lower ribs. As many of the surrounding structures as possible should be identified for proper localization. On the right, the liver, gallbladder, second portion of the duodenum, adrenal gland, inferior vena cava (IVC), crus of the diaphragm, psoas muscle, and quadratus lumborum muscle should be identified in the relative scanning planes. On the left, the spleen, pancreas, adrenal, fourth portion of the duodenum, aorta, crus of the diaphragm, psoas muscle, and quadratus lumborum muscle are potentially identifiable structures. Medial to the kidney is a psoas muscle. Psoas muscle hypertrophy, which is often seen in young males, should be recognized and not mistaken for either retroperitoneal fibrosis[7] or abscess. Renal vascular pedicles are easily imaged. The left renal vein extends from the hilum of the left kidney to the IVC. It runs between the aorta and the superior mesenteric artery (SMA). The segment of the left renal vein from the hilus of the left kidney to the point at which it passes between the aorta and SMA may be unusually prominent. This narrowing of the left renal vein between the aorta and the SMA is the "nutcracker" phenomenon and should not be mistaken for pathologic change. The prominence of the left renal vein and the incompletely imaged normal aortic wall adjacent to it may give the false impression of a left renal artery aneurysm.[8] The right renal vein is seen as a linear hypoechoic structure running from the right kidney to the IVC. The alterations in size of the right renal vein with respiration and transmitted pulsations from the IVC can be appreciated. In the workup of a patient with renal cell carcinoma, the display of the renal vein is an important factor in staging the disease.[9–11] Venous tumor thrombus is diagnosed ultrasonically on the basis of diffuse, low-intensity, intraluminal echoes or focal nodules with or without luminal distention.[9, 12] Anechoic enlargement of the renal vein may be due to tumor or arteriovenous shunting, but it is not proof of venous tumor extension.[9] The results of ultrasonic velocimetry performed in the course of resection of renal arteriovenous fistulas have been reported.[13] The anatomic relationship of the renal arteries and veins should be familiar to all using ultrasound. The renal artery passes posterior to the vein. The right renal artery is retrocaval and the left renal vein is preaortic. The sonographic diagnosis of renal artery thrombosis has been reported.[7] The renal arteries are visualized less frequently than the veins, and care must be exercised to distinguish them from the diaphragmatic crura.

The renal parenchyma can be separated into the more echogenic cortex and septum of Bertin from the centrally located hypoechoic medulla.[15, 16] High-amplitude punctate echoes reflected from the arcuate arteries and veins help further to discriminate the cortical medullary junction. A triangular echogenic focus in the upper pole parenchyma on the right or posteriorly in the lower pole on the left can be seen. These defects result from normal extension of the renal sinus[17] and should not be confused with parenchymal atrophy. The renal cortex in the normal adult patient is equal to or less echogenic than the liver.[15, 16] Comparison of hepatic and renal echogenicity should always be performed at the same depth. Scans in which the gallbladder is anterior to the kidney should be avoided to eliminate distal sound enhancement. Comparison of echogenicity of the renal cortex and the liver is valid only if hepatic disease is not present.[15, 16] Normal liver echogenicity can be assessed on scans because the normal liver has an echo amplitude one-third to one-half the height of the diaphragmatic echoes.[18] It was reported that renal cortex and medulla can be clearly differentiated in approximately one half of adults.[15] With new equipment, however, the distinction between the two is much better. The pyramids appear as relatively hypoechoic zones defined by the cortex and renal sinus. The detectability and the sonographic characteristics of the medulla change in response to the diuretic status of the kidney.[19] With increased diuresis, the medulla becomes prominent and anechoic and is readily visible. Normal pyramids should not be mistaken for cysts or other pathologic changes. In the normal adult, the echo amplitude of the parenchymal abdominal organs in ascending order is as follows: renal medulla, spleen, liver, pancreas, diaphragm, and renal sinus. Alterations in this relation are used to define disease. In normal neonates the renal cortex may be equally as echogenic or more echogenic than the liver.[20, 21] Children differ from adults in two additional aspects: the medullary zones are proportionately larger, and there is comparatively less renal

sinus fat.[21] Intense central renal sinus echoes are primarily caused by hilar adipose tissue. Blood vessels and collecting structures are secondary contributors.[22] The renal sinus echoes are compact and homogeneous, and their amplitude is equal to that of the renal capsule. The high-amplitude echoes are due to the inherent scattering properties of fat cells and are not attributable to coexisting fibrous tissue septa.[22, 23]

Regardless of etiology, any infiltrative process, such as edema, mononuclear cell infiltration of fibrosis (as seen during the allograft rejection), infiltration and fibrosis (present in pyelonephrosis), or tumor cell infiltration, will produce changes in the sonographic appearance of the renal sinus. The earliest architectural changes resulting from infiltration are an uneven widening of the interlobar septa.[23] Small blood vessels and collecting structures may be seen coursing through the highly echogenic renal sinus fat. The renal veins may be prominent in normal patients and should not be mistaken for a dilated renal pelvis. Visualization of the intrarenal collecting system on ultrasound was previously equated with dilatation of these structures. With current improved resolution, this sweeping statement is no longer valid.

## Abnormal Anatomy

### Congenital Anomalies

The urinary tract is a common site for congenital anomalies. It has been estimated that 10% of individuals are born with some urinary tract abnormality. Since the kidneys migrate cephalad to the upper abdomen, a variety of malpositions can result if the migration is altered during the gestational period. Malpositions range from simple ptosis to a pelvic kidney.

When the kidneys are not orthotopic, a search for them should be carried out. Sonography can easily display an ectopic pelvic or thoracic kidney and outline the adjacent diaphragmatic deformation.[24–26] The thoracic kidney may be either a true ectopic kidney or the result of a congenital transdiaphragmatic hernia. In either case, no treatment is needed. The diagnosis can be suggested by sonography if the renal artery is well displayed. In a true ectopic kidney the renal artery arises from the thoracic aorta, while in transdiaphragmatic herniation of the kidney a normal vascular pedicle extends through the hernia.[24] Discovering a kidney in the thoracic cage following trauma raises the possibility of traumatic diaphragmatic rupture.

Duplication of the urinary tract is a common congenital abnormality. The upper pole ureter is malpositioned and may be obstructed, leading to an ectopic ureterocele. The lower pole system may also be dilated due to vesical ureteral reflux or obstruction from the upper pole system. If the obstructed upper pole system does not function and if the moiety is small, identification at excretory urography may be difficult.[27] Sonography, which is independent of renal function, permits localization of the upper half of the kidney in such a case and identification of the ureterocele within the bladder. Ultrasound may also be used to guide percutaneous puncture for antegrade pyelography when this is indicated.

Horseshoe kidney is a common congenital abnormality found in 0.25% of the general population. It is generally asymptomatic but can be associated with hydronephrosis, infection, or calculus formation. Multiple arteries to the kidney are typical. Although the isthmus of the horseshoe kidney can be identified sonographically, bowel gas may preclude visualization of these structures.[28] This can be a particular problem in the patient who has an abdominal aortic aneurysm. If the horseshoe kidney is not clearly appreciated, the surgeon may not be alert to the presence of multiple vessels.

Medullary cystic disease is an inherited autosomal recessive trait condition. Patients with this disease are typically young adults with renal failure. Ultrasonography is a safe technique for identifying medullary and corticomedullary cysts in small kidneys, permitting the correct diagnosis. Although nephrotomography can sometimes demonstrate the renal cysts, this study is equivocal due to poor renal function. Sonography should be the method of choice. The findings of medullary or corticomedullary cysts in small kidneys in young adults should raise the suspicion of medullary cystic disease.

Dominant adult polycystic kidney disease (APKD) is characterized by nephromegaly and bilateral renal cystic disease. Hepatic cysts occur in at least one third of patients. Cysts may be seen in other organs as well, particularly in the spleen and pancreas. Ultrasound can be used to identify the cysts in APKD in both kidneys and other organs. In addition, ultrasonography can be used to evaluate patients with known APKD and fever to search for infected cysts.

The infected cysts generally have internal echoes and may have a debris-fluid level. Aspiration of the cyst under ultrasound guidance can be performed to confirm the diagnosis. Ultrasonography is the technique of choice to evaluate patients during renal failure for evidence of APKD.

*Acute Renal Failure*

Once the diagnosis of ARF has been established and a prerenal cause has been excluded, an ultrasound examination should be performed as the primary screening procedure to differentiate between urinary tract outflow obstruction and parenchymal disease. Although obstruction accounts for only 5% of patients with ARF, its distinction from renal medical disorders is crucial. Postrenal ARF is potentially correctable. Furthermore, prompt diagnosis and intervention are necssary to prevent secondary renal parenchymal loss.[29] Obstruction must be bilateral in order to cause ARF. Unilateral obstruction as a cause of ARF should be considered in association with renal agenesis, contralateral nephrectomy, or severe contralateral renal parenchymal diminution. In patients with stable chronic renal failure, unilateral obstruction may tip the balance against the patient resulting in acute biochemical deterioration.

Postrenal ARF most often occurs in patients with malignant neoplasms of the bladder, prostate, uterus, ovaries, or rectum. Retroperitoneal fibrosis, para-aortic lymph node metastases, primary retroperitoneal neoplasms, renal calculi, and sloughed papillae are less common etiologies of postrenal ARF.

Tomography of the kidney before the ultrasonographic examination in patients with renal insufficiency has been advocated by Moreau.[30] In our experience[29] and that of Maklad,[31] this is not necessary.

The presence or absence of urinary tract dilatation is the single most important issue that must be addressed in patients with ARF. With minimal dilatation, calyces and minor infundibula become readily visible and can be demonstrated in continuity. More marked dilatation produces bulbous enlargement of the calyces, infundibula, and renal pelvis. The criteria regarding the severity of dilatation are similar to those employed in excretory urography. While dilatation of the intrarenal and extra-renal collecting system is accurately assessed with ultrasound, it should be emphasized that the degree of dilatation does not necessarily reflect either the presence or the severity of an obstruction.[32, 33] Dilatation of the collecting system is the result of a complex balance between the amount of urine produced, compliance of the collecting system, and the degree of outflow obstruction. Therefore, when urinary obstruction is clinically suspected, even a minimal dilatation of the pelvocalyceal system should be assessed by additional diagnostic procedures such as an antegrade or retrograde pyelography. In the presence of established hydronephrosis, the brightness of the parenchyma of the kidney may be more intense. The etiology of this is currently not fully understood. This increased echogenicity may be due both to compressed parenchyma and reactive renal ischemia.

If bilateral dilatation is detected, the scanning procedure should be continued to determine the level and etiology of the obstructing lesion. A dilated proximal ureter can often be demonstrated. Scanning of the pelvis with the urinary bladder distended (retrograde if necessary) is required to identify obstructing masses of pelvic origin. It is also mandatory to examine the pelvis for an ectopically positioned kidney if none is found in the flank. Ultrasound can distinguish between renal and postrenal causes of ARF with a high degree of accuracy.

The sensitivity of sonography for the diagnosis of urinary dilatation has ranged from 90% to 100%.[34–37] Reported sonographic specificity in the diagnosis of hydronephrosis is 98% and 97%.[36] One early study showed a relatively low specifity of 74%,[38] but subsequent studies have all shown a greater than 90% specificity.[34–37]

A normal ultrasound examination does not totally exclude urinary obstruction. In the clinical setting of acute obstruction secondary to calculi a nondistended collecting system can be present. Urinary dilatation has been missed in patients with large calculi in the renal pelvis. Regardless of their chemical composition, renal calculi cause acoustic shadowing. The ability to detect calculus and produce shadowing is directly related to the size of the stone.[39] Calculi can be recognized by sonography and their presence should forewarn the sonographer of the potential for the stone to mask associated dilatation. Early or partial obstruction may only be identified when the patient is stressed with fluid or diuretics. This has been a partic-

ular pitfall in patients with retroperitoneal fibrosis.[40] Rarely, there will be little or no dilatation even with an established high-grade urinary obstruction, presumably because of reduced glomerular filtration combined with mechanism for urine resorption. For these reasons, nephrotomography or retrograde urography have been recommended for ARF patients with nondilated, normal to large-sized kidneys on ultrasound. While this concept provides the ultimate in safety, it is impractical, as the vast majority of patients with ARF have kidneys of normal size without upper tract dilatation.

Urinary dilatation may also be mistakenly diagnosed on sonography.[29] Patients with polyuric ARF are usually not suspected of having urinary tract obstruction. It is helpful to realize that in these rare individuals, dilatation does not equate with obstruction. However, if dilatation is marked, even in such a patient more invasive evaluation is indicated. Pregnant women with ARF are particularly difficult to evaluate as hydronephrosis is to be normally anticipated.[41–44] Because sonography has a screening role, it is best to err on the false positive side.

Additional false positive diagnoses result from the incorrect identification of renal and pararenal abnormalities. Peripelvic cysts in particular[45, 46] and vascular aneurysms and arteriovenous malformations also have been mistaken for urinary tract dilatation. Peripelvic cysts (i.e., a single cyst in the renal hilus) can be distinguished from a dilated renal pelvis by careful scanning.

Adult polycystic kidney disease (APKD) and the multicystic dysplastic kidney (MCDK) are other entities that have been reported to simulate urinary dilatation. We feel that this problem is overstated. In both APKD and MCDK, the renal cysts are randomly distributed throughout the kidney. The renal contour is distorted in MCDK, whereas a hydronephrotic kidney usually maintains a normal shape with dilated calyces radiating from a larger central fluid collection, the renal pelvis.[47, 48] In APKD, identification of cysts in the liver or pancreas also confirms the correct diagnosis. The presence of renal cystic disease does not preclude the simultaneous recognition of pelvocaliectasis.

There are a variety of nonobstructive causes of urinary dilatation occurring in association with or preceding ARF. These include diabetes insipidus, vesicoureteral reflux, postobstructive atrophy, atony associated with infection, postinflammatory calyceal clubbing, and congenital megacalyces and papillary necrosis. Using ultrasound alone, it is impossible to differentiate between obstruction and nonobstructive urinary dilatation. Furthermore, in patients with obstructive urinary dilatation, it is frequently impossible to define the level of obstruction using sonography. Attempts should be made to evaluate the ureters and bladder in these patients. When urinary dilatation is demonstrated by sonography, further studies (antegrade or retrograde pyelography) should be recommended to determine the existence of obstruction and to define its site and probable etiology. If mechanical drainage is indicated, a percutaneous interventional radiologic procedure should be rapidly instituted to prevent further deterioration of the renal function. Percutaneous stone manipulation can be performed if calculi are the cause of obstruction.[49, 50] In one report, percutaneous stone manipulation by direct ultrasonographic disintegration, extraction, or hemolysis was successfully performed in 34 patients.[49] The primary goal of removing the obstructing pelvic stone was achieved in all cases. Minor complications, reported in three cases, were managed conservatively. Stone manipulation was done either through an established operative nephrostomy (15 of 34 patients) or by percutaneous nephrostomy (19 of 34 patients).[49] In addition to diagnosing primary obstruction, ultrasound can be used for monitoring progress after plastic surgery on the efferent urinary passages.[49, 50] Detecting and monitoring the progression of hydronephrosis in pregnant women is a further use for ultrasound.[41–44]

*Renal medical disease* is a consideration once it has been shown that azotemia is not due to obstruction. Renal medical disease is without question the leading cause of ARF, and usually results from acute tubular necrosis (ATN). The many entities that cause ATN can be divided into two etiologic categories: ischemic and nephrotoxic injury. Uncomplicated ATN is usually reversible, with patients recovering up to 80% of normal renal function, but death occurs in approximately 50% of affected patients.[51]

Other renal medical disorders are less frequently responsible for ARF. These include abnormalities of glomeruli, interstitium, small renal vessels, or less commonly of major renal blood vessels.[15, 16, 52–57] Renal artery occlusion is a rare cause of ARF because it is nearly always unilateral. However, complete traumatic avulsion of a renal pedicle may result in ATN of the contralateral kidney. By contrast, renal vein thrombosis is often bilateral and may be associated with ARF.

For the initial diagnosis of renal parenchymal disease, percutaneous renal biopsy is essential. Renal biopsy has a definite attendant risk, with a complication rate ranging from 0.17% to 0.7%. Among the complications that can be followed by ultrasound are hematomas.[58] In a study on CT, the incidence of hematoma was over 50%.[59] However, significant perirenal hematomas occur in approximately 0.6% of cases.[58] Within the first 3 days, a fresh perirenal hematoma has echo characteristics similar to those of the surrounding soft tissue, and the diagnosis lies in the detection of renal displacement by a mass.[52] In our experience, after 4 days hematomas present as predominantly hypoechoic perirenal collections that are indistinguishable from abscess or urinoma. It is the clinical history that will lead to the correct diagnosis.

After the diagnosis of the renal medical disease has been made, progression of the disease can be monitored by ultrasound, obviating the need for further percutaneous biopsy.[15, 16, 53, 54] The cortical echogenicity can be graded as normal—0—when the echo amplitude of the renal cortex is less than that of the adjacent liver, grade I when the amplitude of the cortical echoes equals the liver, grade II when the amplitude of the cortical echoes is greater than that of the adjacent liver but less than that of the renal sinus, and grade III when the renal parenchyma is markedly echogenic and the amplitude of the echoes approaches that of the renal sinus. There is a statistically significant correlation between cortical echogenicity and the percentage of global sclerosis, focal tubular atrophy, hyaline casts, and leukocytic infiltration, as was shown in an analysis of 109 patients.[16] While there is such a significant correlation between cortical echogenicity and the degree of histopathologic change, no distinct sonographic features are seen that are specific to the individual renal medical disease. While different parenchymal infiltrative processes appear similar sonographically, calcium deposition in either the cortex or medulla has a characteristic appearance.[60–62] Medullary nephrocalcinosis produces characteristic highly echogenic foci within the renal medulla. Acoustic shadowing is mainly not seen because of the very small size of calcium deposit. Vascular calcification should not be mistaken for nephrocalcinosis.[63]

## Involvement of the Solitary Kidney

Although all of the aforementioned renal and post-renal causes of ARF can affect a solitary kidney, their relative frequencies change. Urinary tract obstruction is the most common cause of ARF[37, 64] and the etiologies of unilateral obstruction such as calculi and sloughed papillae assume a more prominent role. Unusual entities, such as obstruction by a polyhydramniotic gravid uterus,[41] can produce ARF in a solitary kidney. A single kidney is also more susceptible to major renal vessel disease, either arterial or venous.[37, 64]

In the setting of ARF of a solitary kidney, additional entities must be considered as well. Acute pyelonephritis is usually unilateral and thus rarely causes ARF when two functioning kidneys are present. Renal sonography is often normal[64] in a patient with acute pyelonephritis, but may reveal renal enlargement with hypoechoic parenchyma and increased through-transmission of sound.[65] ARF of a solitary kidney may also result from an extensive renal neoplasm, particularly when there is invasion of the renal vein. Perirenal abnormalities such as abscess or hematoma may also result in ARF.[37, 64]

## Renal Infection

Diffuse or local renal inflammatory diseases have nonspecific sonographic appearances. In acute pyelonephritis, renal enlargement with hypoechoic appearance of the parenchyma has been reported.[65] Acute focal bacterial nephritis (a focal infection without liquefaction) is seen as a mass which sonographically may be interpreted as either tumor or an abscess.[66] The echogenicity of the mass can vary and can be equal to or less than that of adjacent renal parenchyma. If the echogenicity of a renal mass is greater than that of the normal parenchyma, in a patient with symptoms of renal infection, the lesion is either an abscess or renal tumor.[71, 66–68] However, the combination of clinical presentation, the sonogram which demonstrates focal mass with echogenicity equal to or less than that of the solid lesion, and the findings on excretory urography or CT suggest the diagnosis. Sonography is available as an initial screening technique to evaluate patients with suspected inflammatory disease.

## Pyonephrosis

The value of sonography is not only in the diagnosis of parenchymal involvement. The diagnosis of pyonephrosis is suggested when debris is seen within the dilated collecting system. However, in two situations echoes can be present in the collecting system: when infection is superimposed on hydronephrosis, and when blood is present within the collecting system. The clinical findings generally permit the differentiation between the two entities.[69–74] Aspiration of the collecting system may be needed for a firm diagnosis.[69] In pyonephrosis ill-defined echoes within the dilated collecting system presumably represent cellular debris.

## Vascular Compromise

The sonographic findings in patients with renal disease and hypertension have been reported.[75] In a prospective study of 51 patients with hypertension, characteristic changes made the differentiation of renal vascular and renal parenchymal disease possible.[75] Hypertension caused by perirenal hematoma (Page kidney) is well displayed by sonography.[76] A spectrum of sonographic findings was shown in patients and laboratory animals[77, 78] with acute renal vein thrombosis. Acute renal vein thrombosis led to nephromegaly and decreased cortical echogenicity. Parenchymal anechoic areas representing hemorrhage and hemorrhagic infarctions were also seen. There was an increase in cortical echogenicity between 10 days and 3 weeks, with preservation of the corticomedullary definition. A decrease in renal size, an increase in cortical echogenicity, and a loss of corticomedullary definition were seen at a later phase. Real-time ultrasonography can demonstrate the absence of transmitted pulsations to the affected renal vein and Doppler ultrasound will show the absence of flow. With currently available ultrasound units, a combination of the above-described sonographic findings supplemented with data obtained on excretory urography are sufficient to diagnose clinically suspected renal vein thrombosis.

Renal arterial infarction has been reported in human and animal studies.[79–82] The sonographic pattern of renal infarction is time dependent. Segmental occlusion causes hypoechoic appearance at the beginning and a late infarction can be seen as parenchymal scar. In complete arterial occlusion no sonographic findings were seen in the animal model.[80] Doppler studies are useful in the diagnosis of renal vascular diseases.[81-82]

## Perirenal Collections

Sonography is a sensitive modality in demonstrating perirenal fluid collections. It is difficult to differentiate urinomas from lymphoceles, hematomas, abscesses, or pancreatic pseudocysts with ultrasound alone. Aspiration of fluid under ultrasound guidance, followed by biochemical analysis of the fluid, will help in the differential diagnosis. Extravasation and urinoma formation should be suspected if ancillary findings, such as hydronephrosis, are seen in addition to the perirenal fluid collection. Radionuclide scanning with $^{99m}$Tc-DTPA could then be performed to see if the diagnosis of urinoma can be confirmed.[83] When perinephric abscess is diagnosed, percutaneous drainage under combined ultrasound and fluoroscopy guidance should be considered, eliminating the need for open surgical intervention.[70] In a trauma patient, renal fractures, contusions, intrarenal subcapsular and perirenal hematomas can be detected sonographically with a high degree of accuracy.

## Renal Masses

Ultrasound is often the modality of choice in further evaluating a renal mass found on excretory urography.[84, 85] Ultrasonography is a highly sensitive modality that differentiates cystic from solid renal masses with a reported accuracy as high as 97%.[85-89]

To diagnose a simple renal cyst sonographically, these criteria should be met: (1) no internal echoes are seen (one or two simple thin septa are accepted), (2) all the walls of the cyst are smooth and sharply defined, and (3) the presence of acoustic enhancement beyond the posterior wall is proportional to the fluid content of the cyst. Only when these three major criteria are met can the mass be diagnosed as a benign cyst that does not require further evaluation.

The minor criteria include refraction artifact and reverberation artifact. The artifact from the edges of a renal cyst are due to refraction of the ultrasound beam. Reverberation artifacts are seen as internal echoes in the anterior aspect of the cyst. Changing the scanning plane demonstrates that these echoes are not actually within the cyst but represent the artifact. Another important point is the position of the cyst within the beam and its relation to lesion echogenicity. Due to beam width artifact, small cysts may appear echo free only in the focal zone of the transducer.[90]

Intrarenal masses as small as 1.2 cm can be accurately diagnosed with ultrasound.[91] Livingstone et al. reported, however, that ultrasound is only accurate in evaluating renal lesions of 3 cm or more, while scanning can accurately characterize lesions as small as 1.5 cm in diameter.[85] An atypical renal cyst, such as a multilocular septate cyst, an infected cyst with poorly defined and thickened walls that presents with a complex pattern of internal echoes, should be punctured[86] or studied by CT or magnetic resonance imaging. Six percent of renal cysts will hemorrhage. The blood may clot and appear as a complex echo pattern. When the cyst walls are calcified, there is diminished sound transmission, which makes an accurate diagnosis difficult. Furthermore, because of sound reflection by calcification, the lesions may appear solid. When the ultrasound examination is technically suboptimal or the sonographic appearance of the cyst is equivocal, a CT study should be performed. If, by CT criteria, the lesion is a simple cyst, no further studies are necessary.

Evaluation of renal cysts is especially useful in patients on hemodialysis.[92] Not only can simple cysts be diagnosed by sonography, but the distinction among cystic diseases of the kidney can also be made. The criteria applied include the size of the cysts, their number, their distribution within the kidneys, and their involvement in other organs. Ultrasound is more specific than excretory urography in diagnosing polycystic kidney disease.[93] The presence of numerous small medullary cysts is characteristic for medullary cystic disease.[94]

An accuracy of 94% has been reported[88] in the evaluation of solid renal masses by sonography. A study by O'Reilly et al. showed that, in clarifying the nature of renal space-occupying lesions, ultrasound, radionuclide imaging, and CT scanning had similar results with lesions that were 2 cm or greater in diameter. When lesions were smaller than 2 cm in diameter, ultrasound and radionuclide studies were not useful. In that category, the accuracy of CT and angiography was similar.[88] In the analysis of 100 patients with histologically proved renal cell carcinoma, the accuracy was 84% for excretory urography, 93% for ultrasound, 98% for CT, and 100% for angiography.[95] The sonographic appearance of renal masses is nonspecific, and benign and malignant tumors cannot be differentiated.[96–107]

In another study no direct correlation was found between the sonographic appearance of renal cell carcinoma and the vascularity present on angiograms in 43 patients with histologically proved renal cell carcinoma.[95] There are reports of linear correlation between the echogenicity of the tumor and the degree of renovascularity[96]; Coleman et al. showed that there was considerable overlap between vascular and sonographic classifications of hypernephroma.[97] In the same study, no significant correlation was found between the pathologic and sonographic appearances of the tumor when classified as moderately or markedly echogenic. On the other hand, minimally echogenic tumors were grossly inhomogeneous, suggesting that the sparsity of echoes is most likely due to hemorrhage, necrosis, or cystic degeneration.[97]

In patients with renal cell carcinoma, preoperative staging will determine tumor resectability and influence the surgeon in determining the surgical approach. In tumor staging, CT is superior to ultrasound. However, sonography is usually the first step after the discovery of a renal mass on excretory urography. If a solid renal mass is detected, abdominal scanning should be performed for staging purposes. This procedure may add valuable information and does not significantly prolong the examination; it is therefore routinely recommended.

The appearance of a markedly echogenic intrarenal mass is thought to be pathognomonic for angiomyolipoma.[98–101] Furthermore, when ultrasound is performed in addition to CT, characteristic findings of marked echogenicity on ultrasonography and areas of fat density on CT are seen.[98] These combined findings should resolve the diagnostic dilemma of these benign lesions, and prevent the need for operative intervention in most cases.[98–103] While there are fairly characteristic ultrasound and CT patterns of renal angiomyolipoma, it should be stressed that, in our experience and that of Hartman et al.,[100] the ultrasound findings in angiomyolipoma range from hyperechoic and isoechoic to hypoechoic.[100] The presence of an echo-dense intrarenal mass, while suggestive of an-

giomyolipoma, is not pathognomonic. Renal cell carcinoma may present as a hyperechoic renal mass indistinguishable from angiomyolipoma.[100]

Wilms' tumors tend to be very large, predominantly solid, and well circumscribed. They show variable echogenicity ranging from less than that of a kidney to greater than that of liver.[104] Small anechoic areas may be seen within the masses, representing necrosis. Calcifications may also be present in Wilms' tumors, although they may be less common in neuroblastomas. Another renal mass seen in childhood is nephroblastoma. Nephroblastoma consists of small nodules or sheets of primitive metanephric epithelium which, when present, may be precursors of Wilms' tumors. Although the nodules of nephroblastomas may occasionally be large, most of them are quite small and difficult to identify sonographically.

Lymphomatous involvement of the kidney may be seen on ultrasound as a single or multiple anechoic, or weakly echogenic mass.[105] The sonographic findings are not specific. Lymphomatous involvement of the kidney is usually a secondary process. Most of the patients have a known diagnosis of lymphoma and, at the time of renal sonography, are being examined for nodal mass size, flank pain, or deteriorating renal function. If lymphoma of the kidney is suspected, the ultrasound findings may be confirmed by gallium scanning.[105]

Transitional cell carcinoma is the most common tumor of the renal pelvis. Sonographically it presents as a mass in the renal pelvis containing low-level echoes. The sonographic findings described include a widening of the central sinus echoes, a hypoechoic central area, and inability to detect any abnormalities. The differential diagnosis of such a mass includes other tumors of the renal pelvis, such as squamous cell or adenocarcinoma. Furthermore, blood clot or fungal ball may have a similar appearance.

## Renal Transplantation

The role of sonography in renal transplantation has extended beyond the diagnosis of obstruction and perirenal fluid collections. When dilatation of the collecting system is sonographically present, antegrade pyelography, using both sonographic and radiologic techniques, is advocated.[108] While ultrasound is a sensitive modality in diagnosing perirenal collections,[108-115] the sonographic appearance of fluid collections is nonspecific, and, to reach a correct diagnosis under ultrasound guidance, percutaneous puncture and aspiration of fluid is desirable.[108, 114] Sonography has proved to be more sensitive than either excretory urography or radionuclide studies in detecting perirenal fluid collections.[109] The accuracy in detecting fluid collections is 100% with sonography, 86% with radionuclide studies, and 68% with excretory urography.[109]

Following transplantation, the kidney undergoes normal renal hypertrophy.[110, 116] By the end of the second week, the increase in renal volume in a successful transplant is between 7% and 21%, with a mean value of 16%. By the end of the third week, the increase in renal volume, as compared with the baseline study, is between 14% and 32%, with a mean value of 22%.[118] The remarkable capacity of the human kidney to hypertrophy rapidly was demonstrated in a 16-year-old recipient of a renal transplant from a 16-month-old child.[116] Within 8 weeks, the glomerular filtration rate (GFR) increased more than six times from the estimated pretransplant clearance.

Due to the superficial position of the renal transplant, renal anatomy and pathology can be well delineated.[110-120] Sonographically, during the course of ATN the renal anatomy remains unaltered from the baseline study and the increase in renal volume remains within the range of normal renal hypertrophy.[110] In our experience, an increase in renal volume with enlargement of the renal pyramids is an early and common sonographic (88%) finding[65] in acute rejection. Enlarged medullary pyramids have been seen in moderate, marked, and severe rejection in a similar number of patients (63%).[112] As reported by Fried et al., prominence of the medullary pyramids has limited predictive value in the determination of transplant rejection.[118]

Other sonographic findings indicative of rejection include decreased amplitude of the renal sinus echoes (74%), indistinctness of the corticomedullary boundary (58%), increased echogenicity of the renal cortex (58%), decreased echogenicity of the renal parenchyma (47%), focal anechoic appearance of the renal parenchyma (21%), and sparsely distributed cortical echoes (47%).[110] Also reported was submucosal edema of the collecting system present at the clinical peak of acute rejection.[119] Perirenal fluid collections consisting of either hematomas or lymphoceles were

seen in 4 of 19 patients[110] and 3 of 6 patients.[112] In a report by Meier et al.,[117] the correct diagnosis of rejection was achieved in 84% of the patients. In 7% of patients, the researchers were not able to differentiate between acute and chronic rejection.[117] In histologically proved rejection, false negative sonograms were present in only 8% of the cases reported by Frick et al.[112] Meier et al. sonographically distinguished acute from chronic rejection.[117] They felt that the initial findings in acute rejection consisted of an increase in renal size of at least 20%, with the kidney becoming globular in shape, and enlargement of the medullary pyramids, which become hypoechoic and have indistinct corticomedullary boundaries as a result of decreased contrast between the medulla and cortex. In an advanced stage of acute rejection, there are localized hypoechoic areas within the cortex and medulla. In the end-stage of acute rejection, confluent hypoechoic areas in the medulla and cortex are probably the result of hemorrhagic infarction. In the end-stage of acute rejection there is a change of renal contour.[117]

In chronic rejection, the initial findings consist of renal enlargement with blending of the cortex and medulla and nondifferentiation of the central sinus echoes. There is a diffuse increase in echo density throughout the kidney, with a coarse spatial distribution of the echoes and a smooth kidney contour. In the end-stage of chronic rejection, the kidney is small, very echogenic, and irregularly contoured due to scarring. Differentiation between the parenchymal and central sinus echoes is not possible.[117]

Recently reported is the evaluation of renal transplants with pulsed Doppler duplex sonography.[121] To provide an indicator of renal blood flow pattern, a pulsed Doppler index (PDI) was developed. Interpretation of transplant status based on clinical function studies on PDI yielded the correct diagnosis in 90% of cases.[121] The introduction of duplex sonography will further increase diagnostic accuracy in the evaluation of posttransplantation renal failure.

## References

1. Finberg H: Renal ultrasound: Anatomy and technique. *Semin Ultrasound* 1981; 2(1):7–19.
2. Bazzocchi M, Rizzatto G: The value of the posterior oblique longitudinal scan in renal ultrasonography. *Urol Radiol* 1980; 1:221–225.

3. Thompson IM, Kovac A, Geshner J: Coronal renal ultrasound II. *Urology* 1981; 17(1):210–213.

4. Dana A, Moreau JF: Note de technique. *J Radiol* 1981; 62(1):59–62.

5. Pochhammer KF, Hollstein H, Bohlke E: Modifizierte sonographische Darstellung der Nieren durch Skolioselagerung. *Ultraschall* 1980; 1:57–59.

6. Rosenberg ER, Clair MR, Bowie JD: The fluid-filled stomach as an acoustic window to the left kidney. *AJR* 1982; 138(1):175–176.

7. McCloughlin MJ: Pitfalls to avoid: Psoas hypertrophy mimicking retroperitoneal fibrosis. *J Can Assoc Radiol* 1981; 32(1):56–57.

8. Kurtz AB, Dubbins PA, Zegel HG, et al: Normal left renal vein mimicking left renal artery aneurysm. *JCU* 1981; 9(3):105–108.

9. Levine E, Maklad NF, Rosenthal SJ, et al: Comparison of computed tomography and ultrasound in abdominal staging of renal cancer. *Urology* 1980; 16(3):317–322.

10. Karp W, Ekelund L, Olafsson G, et al: Computed tomography, angiography and ultrasound in staging of renal carcinoma. *Acta Radiol* 1981; 22(6):625–633.

11. Schwerk WB, Schwerk WN, Rodeck G: Venous renal tumor extension: A prospective US evaluation. *Radiology* 1985; 156(2):491–495.

12. Thomas JL, Bernandino ME: Neoplastic-induced renal vein enlargement: Sonographic detection. *AJR* 1981; 136:75–79.

13. Boyce WH: Ultrasonic velocimetry in resection of renal arteriovenous fistulas and other intrarenal surgical procedures. *J Urol* 1981; 125:610–613.

14. Barber-Riley P, Patel AS: Ultrasonic demonstration of renal artery thrombosis. *Br J Radiol* 1981; 54:351–352.

15. Rosenfield AT, Siegel NJ: Renal parenchymal disease: Histopathologic-sonographic correlation. *AJR* 1981; 137(4):793–798.

16. Hricak H, Cruz C, Romanski R, et al: Renal parenchymal disease: Sonographic-histologic correlation. *Radiology* 1982; 144(1):141–147.

17. Carter AR, Horgan JG, Jennings TA, et al: The junctional parenchymal defect: A sonographic variant of renal anatomy. *Radiology* 1985; 154(2):499–502.

18. Taylor KJW, Carpenter DA, Hill CR, et al: Gray-scale ultrasound imaging: The anatomy and pathology of the liver. *Radiology* 1976; 119:415–523.

19. Hricak H, Cruz C, Eyler WR, et al: Acute post-transplantation renal failure: Differential diagnosis by ultrasound. *Radiology* 1981; 139(2):441–449.

20. Haller JO, Berdon WE, Friedman AP: Increased renal cortical echogenicity: A normal finding in neonates and infants. *Radiology* 1982; 142(1):173–174.

21. Hricak H, Slovis TL, Alperd C, et al: Neonatal kidneys: Sonographic anatomic correlation. *Radiology* 1983; 147:699–702.

22. Behan M, Kazam E: The echographic characteristics of fatty tissues and tumors. *Radiology* 1978; 129:143–151.

23. Hricak H, Romanski RN, Eyler WR: The renal sinus during allograft rejection: Sonographic and histopathologic findings. *Radiology* 1982; 142(3):693–699.

24. Darracq-Parries JC, Dombriz M, Coste G, et al: Ectopie thoracique du rein. *J Urol* 1980; 86(9):695–698.

25. Pagliari U: Ectopia alta del rene: Valore diagnostico dell'ecotomografia. *Radiol Med* 1980; 66:387–391.

26. McCarthy S, Rosenfield AT: Ultrasonography in crossed renal ectopia. *J Ultrasound Med* 1984; 3(3):107–112.

27. Jeffrey RB Jr, Laing FC, Wing WW et al: Sonography of the fetal duplex kidney. *Radiology* 1984; 153(1):123–124.

28. Mindell HJ, Kupic EA: Horseshoe kidney: Ultrasonic demonstration. *AJR* 1977; 129:526–527.

29. Hricak H: Ultrasound in the azotemic patient, in Margulis AR, Gooding CA (eds): *Diagnostic Radiology.* San Francisco, Radiology Research and Education Foundation, 1982, pp 385–392.

30. Moreau JF: Urographie intraveineuse vs. echographie ultrasonore ou U.I.V. + ultrasons. *J Urol* 1981; 87:217–218.

31. Maklad NF: Ultrasound in acute renal failure, in Taylor KJW, Viscomi G (eds): *Diagnostic Ultrasound in Emergency Medicine Clin Diagn Ultrasound* 1981; 7:166–181.

32. Curry NS, Gobien RP, Schabel ST: Minimal-dilatation obstructive nephropathy. *Radiology* 1982; 143(2):531–534.

33. Malave SR, Neiman HL: Diagnosis of hydronephrosis: Comparison of radionuclide scanning and sonography. *AJR* 1980; 135(6):1179–1185.

34. Lee JKT, Baron RL, Melson GL, et al: Can real-time ultrasonography replace static B-scanning in the diagnosis of renal obstruction? *Radiology* 1981; 139:161–165.

35. Talner LB, Scheible W, Ellenbogen PH, et al: How accurate is ultrasonography in detecting hydronephrosis in azotemic patients? *Urol Radiol* 1981; 3:1–6.

36. Malave SR, Neiman HL, Spies SM, et al: Diagnosis of hydronephrosis: Comparison of radionuclide scanning and sonography. *AJR* 1980; 135:1179–1185.

37. Behan M, Wixson D, Kazam E: Sonographic evaluation of the nonfunctioning kidney. *JCU* 1979; 7:449–458.

38. Ellenbogen PH, Scheible RW, Talner LB, et al: Sensitivity of gray scale ultrasound in detecting urinary tract obstruction. *AJR* 1978; 130:731–733.

39. King W 3d, Kimme-Smith C, Winter J: Renal stone shadowing: An investigation of contributing factors. *Radiology* 1985; 154(1):191–196.

40. Brown JM: The ultrasound approach to the urographically nonvisualizing kidney. *Semin Ultrasound* 1981; 2(I):44–48.

41. Homons DC, Blake GD, Harrington JT, et al: Acute renal failure caused by ureteral obstruction by a gravid uterus. *JAMA* 1981; 246:1230–1231.

42. Bernaschek G, Kratochwill A: Pregnancy-conditioned dilatation of the calyceal system: Sonographic diagnosis and urologic control. *Geburtshilfe Frauenheilkd* 1981; 41(3): 208–212.

43. Peake SL, Rosburgh HB, Langlois SL: Ultrasonic assessment of hydronephrosis of pregnancy. *Radiology* 1983; 146(1):167–170.

44. Fried AM, Woodring JH, Thompson DJ: Hydronephrosis of pregnancy: A prospective sequential study of the course of dilatation. *J Ultrasound Med* 1983; 2(6):255–259.

45. Hidalgo H, Dunnick NR, Rosenberg ER, et al: Parapelvic cysts: Appearance on CT and sonography. *AJR* 1982; 138(4):667–671.

46. Cronan JJ, Amis ES Jr., Yoder IC, et al: Peripelvic cysts: An imposter of sonographic hydronephrosis. *J Ultrasound Med* 1982; 1(6):229–236.

47. Sanders RC, Hartman DS: The sonographic distinction between neonatal multicystic kidney and hydronephrosis. *Radiology* 1984; 151(3):621–625.

48. Ralls PW, Esensten ML, Boger D, et al: Severe hydronephrosis and severe renal cystic disease: Ultrasonic differentiation. *AJR* 1980; 134(3):473–475.

49. Alken P, Hutschenreiter G, Gunther R, et al: Percutaneous stone manipulation. *J Urol* 1981; 125(4):463–466.

50. Zegel HG, Pollack HM, Banner MC, et al: Percutaneous nephrostomy: Comparison of sonographic and fluoroscopic guidance. *AJR* 1981; 137(5):925–927.

51. Epstein FH: Acute renal failure, in Wintrobe MM, Thorn GW, Adams RD, et al: (eds): *Harrison's Principles of Internal Medicine.* New York, McGraw-Hill, 1974, pp 1383–1388.

52. Hricak H: Sonography of renal parenchymal disease, in Margulis AR, Gooding CA (eds): *Diagnostic Radiology.* San Francisco, Radiology Research and Education Foundation, 1982; pp 355–362.

53. Moccia WA, Kaude JV, Wright PC, et al: Evaluation of chronic renal failure by digital gray-scale ultrasound. *Urol Radiol* 1980; 2:1–7.

54. Rosenfield AT: Ultrasound evaluation of renal parenchymal disease and hydronephrosis. *Urol Radiol* 1982; 4:125–133.

55. Schaffer RM, Schwartz GE, Becker JA, et al: Renal ultrasound in acquired immune deficiency syndrome. *Radiology* 1984; 153(2):511–513.

56. Stanley JH, Cornella R, Loevinger E, et al: Sonography of systemic lupus nephritis. *AJR* 1984; 142(6):1165–1168.

57. Pardes JG, Auh YH, Kazam E: Sonographic findings in myoglobinuric renal failure and their clinical implications. *J Ultrasound Med* 1983; 2(9):391–394.

58. Ralls PW, Colletti P, Boger DC, et al: Ultrasonographic diagnosis of post-percutaneous renal biopsy hematoma. *Urol Radiol* 1980; 2:23–24.

59. Alter AJ, Zimmerman S, Kirachaiwanich C: Computerized tomographic assessment of retroperitoneal hemorrhage after percutaneous renal biopsy. *Arch Intern Med* 1980; 140:1323–1326.

60. Garel LA, Habib R, Pariente D, et al: Juvenile nephrolithiasis: Sonographic appearance in children with severe uremia. *Radiology* 1984; 151(1):93–95.

61. Foley LC, Luisiri A, Graviss ER, et al: Nephro-

calcinosis: Sonographic detection in Cushing syndrome. *AJR* 1982; 139(3):610–620.

62. Glazer GM, Callen PW, Filly RA: Medullary nephrocalcinosis: Sonographic evaluation. *AJR* 1982; 138(1):55–57.

63. Kane RA, Manco LG: Renal arterial calcification simulating nephrolithiasis on sonography. *AJR* 1983; 140(1):101–104.

64. Marangola JP, Bryan PJ, Azimi F: Ultrasonic evaluation of the unilateral nonvisualized kidney. *AJR* 1976; 126:853–862.

65. Edell SL, Bonavita JA: The sonographic appearance of acute pyelonephritis. *Radiology* 1979; 132:683–685.

66. Rosenfield AT, Glickman MG, Taylor KJW: Focal bacterial nephritis (acute lobar nephronia). *Radiology* 1979; 132:553–561.

67. Van Kirk OC, Go RT, Wedel VJ: Sonographic features of xanthogranulomatous pyelonephritis. *AJR* 1980; 134(5):1035–1039.

68. Hartman DS, David CJ Jr., Goldman SM, et al: Xanthogranulomatous pyelonephritis: Sonographic-pathologic correlation of 16 cases. *J Ultrasound Med* 1984; 3(11):481–488.

69. Kuligowska E, Newman B, White SJ, et al: Interventional ultrasound in detection and treatment of renal inflammatory disease. *Radiology* 1983; 147(2):521–526.

70. Elyaderani MK, Subramanian VP, Burgess JE: Diagnosis and percutaneous drainage of a perinephric abscess by ultrasound and fluoroscopy. *J Urol* 1981; 125:405–407.

71. Andrew WK, Thomas RG: Renal amoebic abscess detected on grey-scale ultrasonography: A case report. *S Afr Med J* 1981; 59(16):571–574.

72. Jeffrey RB, Laing FC, Wing VW, et al: Sensitivity of sonography in pyonephrosis: A reevaluation. *AJR* 1985; 144(1):71–73.

73. Coleman BG, Arger PH, Mulhern CB Jr, et al: Pyonephrosis: Sonography in the diagnosis and management. *AJR* 1981; 137(5):939–943.

74. Subramanyan BR, Raghavendra BN, Bosniak MA, et al: Sonography of pyonephrosis: A prospective study. *AJR* 1983; 140(5):991–993.

75. Ergebnisse V: Sonographische Befunde bei Nierenerkrankugen mit Hypertonie. *Dtsch Med Wouhenschr* 1981; 106:539–543.

76. Chamorro HA, Forbes TW, Padkowsky GO: Multi-imaging approach in the diagnosis of

Page kidney. *AJR* 1981; 136:620–621.

77. Rosenfield AT, Zeman RK, Cronan JJ: Ultrasound in experimental and clinical renal vein thrombosis. *Radiology* 1980; 137:735–741.

78. Hricak H, Sandler MA, Madrazo BL: Sonographic manifestations of acute renal vein thrombosis: An experimental study. *Invest Radiol* 1981; 16(1):30–35.

79. Erwin BC, Carroll B, Walter JF, et al: Renal infarction appearing as an echogenic mass. *AJR* 1982; 138(4):759–761.

80. Spies JB, Hricak H, Slemmer TM, et al: Sonographic evaluation of experimental acute renal arterial occlusion in dogs. *AJR* 1984; 142(2):341–346.

81. Avasthi PS, Voyles WF, Greene ER: Noninvasive diagnosis of renal artery stenosis by echo-Doppler velocimetry. *Kidney Int* 1984; 25(5):824–829.

82. Avasthi PS, Green ER, Voyles WF, et al: A comparison of echo-Doppler and electromagnetic renal blood flow measurements. *J Ultrasound Med* 1984; 3(5):213–218.

83. Yeh E, Chiang L, Meade R: Ultrasound and radionuclide studies of urinary extravasation with hydronephrosis. *J Urol* 1981; 125:730.

84. Zimmer WD, Williamson B Jr., Hartman GW, et al: Changing patterns in the evaluation of renal masses: Economic implications. *AJR* 1984; 143(2):285–289.

85. Livingston WD Jr, Collins TL, Novicki DE: Incidental renal mass. *Urology* 1981; 17(3):257–259.

86. Elyaderani MK, Gabriele OF: Ultrasound of renal masses. *Semin Ultrasound* 1981; 5(1):21–43.

87. Appel L, Broos J, Declrecq G: Evaluation of upper urinary tract by CT scan and ultrasonography. *Comput Tomogr* 1981; 5:139–151.

88. O'Reilly PH, Osborn DE, Testa HJ, et al: Renal imaging: A comparison of radionuclide, ultrasound, and computed tomographic scanning in investigation of renal space-occupying lesions. *Br Med J* 1981; 282:943–945.

89. Pollack HM, Banner MP, Arger PH, et al: The accuracy of gray-scale renal ultrasonography in differentiating cystic neoplasms from benign cysts. *Radiology* 1982; 143(3):741–745.

90. Jaffe CC, Rosenfield AT, Sommer G, et al: Technical factors influencing the imaging of

small anechoic cysts by B-scan ultrasound. *Radiology* 1980; 135(2):429–433.

91. Deyesa TM, Castellano FL, Torres JAM: Estudio ultrasonografico de la patologia quistica renal. *Actas Urol Esp* 1980; 5(1):13–18.

92. Andersen BL, Curry NS, Gobien RP: Sonography of evolving renal cystic transformation associated with hemodialysis. *AJR* 1983; 141(5):1003–1004.

93. Shirkhoda A: Gray-scale patterns and ultrasonic spectrum of adult polycystic kidney disease. *Appl Radiol Ultrasound* 1981; 99–102.

94. Rego JD Jr, Laing FC, Jeffrey RB: Ultrasonographic diagnosis of medullary cystic disease. *J Ultrasound Med* 1983; 2(10):433–436.

95. Crone-Munzebrock W, Brassow F: Das hypernephroide Nierendarzinom: Treffsichereit and artdiagnostische Aussagen von i.v. Pyelogram, Sonographie, Computertomographie und Angiographie. *Rontgen Bl* 1981; 34:199–204.

96. Ladwig SH, Jackson D, Older RA, et al: Ultrasonic angiographic and pathologic correlation of noncystic-appearing renal masses. *Urology* 1981; 17(2):204–209.

97. Coleman BG, Arger PH, Mulhern B, et al: Gray-scale sonographic spectrum of hypernephromas. *Radiology* 1980; 137:757–765.

98. Pitts WR Jr, Kazam E, Gray G, et al: Ultrasonography, computerized transaxial tomography and pathology of angiomyolipoma of the kidney: Solution to a diagnostic dilemma. *J Urol* 1980; 124:907–909.

99. Fiegler W: Ultrasonic demonstration of lipomatous tissues and tumors. *ROFO* 1981; 134(2):157–161.

100. Hartman DS, Goldman M, Friedman AC, et al: Angiomyolipoma: Ultrasonic-pathologic correlation. *Radiology* 1981; 139:451–458.

101. Kutcher R, Rosenblatt R, Mitsudo SM, et al: Renal angiomyolioma with sonographic demonstration of extension into the inferior vena cava. *Radiology* 1982; 143(3):755–756.

102. Ragnavendra BN, Bosniak MA, Megibow AJ: Small angiomyolipoma of the kidney: Sonographic-CT evaluation. *AJR* 1983; 141(3):575–578.

103. Bret PM, Bretagnolle M, Gaillard D, et al: Small asymptomatic angiomyolipomas of the kidney. *Radiology* 1985; 154(1):7–10.

104. Jaffe MH, White SJ, Silver TM, et al: Wilms tumor: Ultrasonic features, pathologic correlation, and diagnostic pitfalls. *Radiology* 1981; 140(1):147–152.

105. Shirkhoda A, Staabd EVE, Mittelstaedt CA: Renal lymphoma imaged by ultrasound and gallium-67. *Radiology* 1980; 137:175–180.

106. Goeney RC, Goldenberg L, Cooperberg PL, et al: Renal oncocytoma: Sonographic analysis of 14 cases. *AJR* 1984; 143(5):1001–1004.

107. Press GA, McClennan BL, Melson GL, et al: Papillary renal cell carcinoma: CT and sonographic evaluation. *AJR* 1984; 143(5):1005–1009.

108. Heckemann R, Hartmann HG, Eickenberg HU: Combined ultrasound-radiographic detection of ureteral obstruction in renal transplants. *Urol Radiol* 1980; 1:233–235.

109. Coyne SS, Walsh JW, Tisnado J, et al: Surgically correctable renal transplant complications: An integrated clinical and radiologic approach. *AJR* 1981; 136(6):1113–1119.

110. Hricak H, Cruz C, Eyler WR, et al: Acute post-transplantation renal failure: Differential diagnosis by ultrasound. *Radiology* 1981; 139:441–449.

111. Jafri SZ, Kaude JV, Wright PG: Ultrasound in renal transplant rejection. *Acta Radiol* 1981; 22(3A):245–253.

112. Frick M, Feinberg S, Sibley R, et al: Ultrasound in acute renal transplant rejection. *Radiology* 1981; 138:657–660.

113. Silver TM, Campbell D, Wicks JD, et al: Peritransplant fluid collections: Ultrasound evaluation and clinical significance. *Radiology* 1981; 138(1):145–151.

114. Slovis TL, Babcock DS, Hricak H, et al: Renal transplant rejection: Sonographic evaluation in children. *Radiology* 1984; 153(3):659–665.

115. Hildell J, Aspelin P, Nyman U, et al: Ultrasonography in complications of renal transplantation. *Acta Radiol* 1984; 25(4):299–304.

116. Ingelfinger JR, Teele R, Treves S: Renal growth after transplantation: Infant kidney received by adolescent. *Clin Nephrol* 1981; 15(1):28–32.

117. Meier J, Otto R, Binswanger U: Die Sonographie bei Funktionseinschrankung von Nierentransplantaten. *Fortschr Rontgenstr* 1981; 134(2):142–147.

118. Fried AM, Woodring JH, Loh FJ, et al: The

medullary pyramid index: An objective assessment of prominence in renal transplant rejection. *Radiology* 1983; 149(3):787–791.

119. Birnholz JC, Merkel FK: Submucosal edema of the collecting system: A new ultrasonic sign of severe, acute renal allograft rejection. *Radiology* 1985; 154(1):190.

120. Blumhardt R, Growcock G, Lasher JC: Cortical necrosis in a renal transplant. *AJR* 1983; 141(1):95–96.

121. Berland LL, Lawson TL, Adams MB, et al: Evaluation of renal transplants with pulsed Doppler duplex sonography. *J Ultrasound Med* 1982; 1(6):215–222.

## CASES

Dennis A. Sarti, M.D.

### Normal Renal Scans

A renal examination can be performed with the patient in the prone, supine, or decubitus position. Each kidney can be scanned individually, or both kidneys can be scanned together when the patient is prone. During a transverse scan, it is often very helpful if the patient takes in a deep breath. This will place the kidney more caudally and allow better visualization below the 12th rib. Most scanning is performed through the intercostal spaces. Transverse, longitudinal, and coronal scans can be obtained through these intercostal spaces with small-head real-time transducers.

Figure 7–1 is a transverse scan of both kidneys with the patient prone. The characteristic appearance of the kidneys—strong central echoes surrounded by relatively lucent renal parenchyma—can be seen. The normal kidney borders are usually easily visualized since the strong echoes of Gerota's fascia and the renal capsule stand out against the renal parenchyma. Just medial to the kidneys is the psoas muscle parallel to the sonolucent spine. The muscle bundle posterior to the kidney is the quadratus lumborum. Anterior to the right kidney are echoes arising from the liver. The renal contour and size are usually fairly symmetric. The left kidney usually has a more cephalad position than the right.

It is extremely important to evaluate the renal echogenicity in comparison with other organs. This is best performed using the liver as a standard.

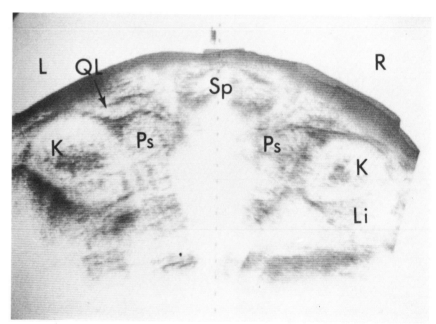

FIG 7–1.

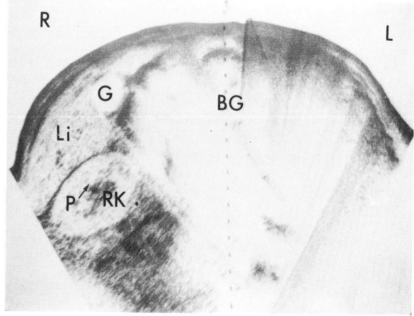

FIG 7–2.

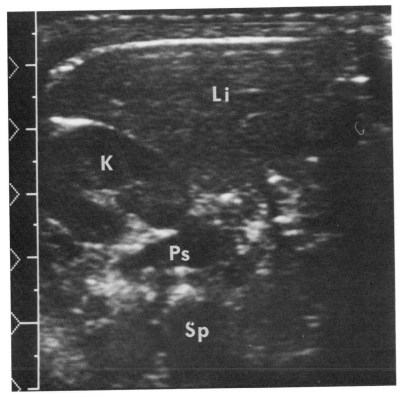

**FIG 7–3.**

The liver and pancreas are routinely compared when one is trying to decide whether or not pancreatic pathology is present. A comparison of the liver and the right kidney is also helpful. Figures 7–2 and 7–3 are transverse scans of the right kidney. Scanning through the liver and right kidney usually shows the kidney to be less echogenic in amplitude than the liver. The parenchyma of the right kidney is slightly less echogenic than the liver. The lucent areas seen in the kidney are secondary to the renal pyramids. Transverse scans of the left kidney (Fig 7–4) are more difficult to obtain because the liver is not present to be used as an acoustic window. Also, comparison of the left renal parenchyma with the liver on the same scan is not possible. The echo amplitude relation of the three organs of the upper abdomen are important and must be remembered. The pancreas usually has a higher amplitude than the liver, which usually has a higher amplitude than the kidney. If this normal relationship is not present, then all three organs must be examined to determine which one is abnormal.

| | | |
|---|---|---|
| **BG** | = | Bowel gas |
| **G** | = | Gallbladder |
| **K** | = | Kidney |
| **Li** | = | Liver |
| **P** | = | Renal pyramid |
| **Ps** | = | Psoas muscle |
| **QL** | = | Quadratus lumborum muscle |
| **R** | = | Right |
| **RK** | = | Right kidney |
| **Sp** | = | Spine |

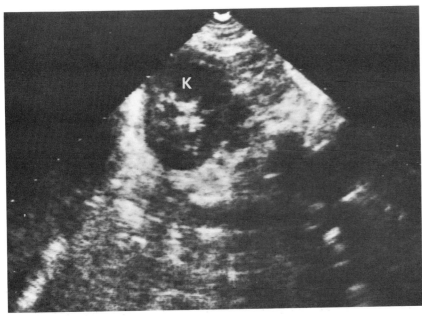

**FIG 7–4.**

## Normal Renal Scans

The right kidney can be examined with the patient supine if the right lobe of the liver is large enough. Figures 7–5 and 7–6 are longitudinal supine scans of the right kidney. The renal outline is seen deep to the right lobe of the liver. Scanning the kidney with the patient supine is usually not possible on the left side unless the left lobe of the liver is dramatically enlarged.

A longitudinal scan through the right lobe of the liver can be very helpful in evaluating the kidney, especially in the upper pole region. Often the upper pole of the kidney is difficult to visualize when the patient is scanned prone because of the overlying ribs. In any attempt to visualize the upper pole of the right kidney, the patient should be scanned supine. Again, the normal echo relationship, in which the liver is more echogenic than the right kidney, is seen.

Usually the left kidney cannot be visualized when the patient is scanned supine because of overlying air in the stomach and splenic flexure. Coronal scans are very helpful in evaluating both kidneys. Evaluation through the intercostal spaces is most helpful, especially with small-head real-time transducers. Coronal scans permit excellent visualization of the lateral border of the kidney for evaluating a mass in that region. Figure 7–7 is a longitudinal coronal scan of a left kidney that is caudal to the spleen. Deep to the left kidney is a tubular structure that represents the aorta. The crus of the diaphragm is also visible. This coronal scan permits excellent visualization of the lateral border of the kidney, and the splenic indentation on this border.

During routine scanning, normal anatomic variants of the kidney may be seen. Figure 7–5 is an example of a bifid renal collecting system. High-amplitude echoes of the renal collecting system are noted centrally and are separated by renal parenchyma (arrow). Figure 7–8 is a coronal scan of the right kidney in a 4-month-old baby. The contour of this kidney is more irregular than in the previous scans of normal kidneys. The contour indenta-

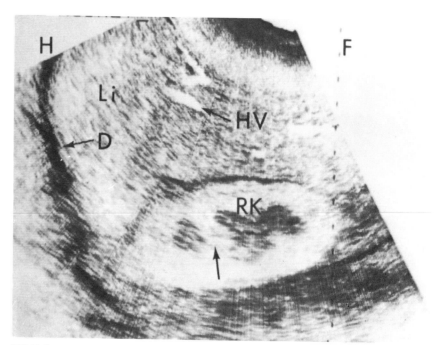

**FIG 7–5.**

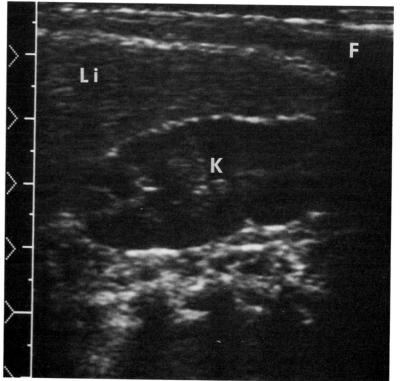

**FIG 7–6.**

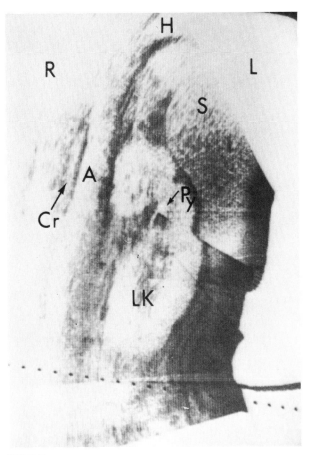

**FIG 7-7.**

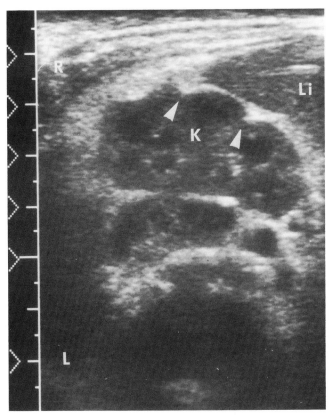

**FIG 7-8.**

tions (arrowheads) are caused by fetal lobulations of the kidney.

| | | |
|---|---|---|
| **A** | = | Aorta |
| **Arrow** | = | Renal parenchyma separating a duplex collecting system (Fig 7-5) |
| **Arrow-heads** | = | Fetal lobulation |
| **Cr** | = | Crus of the diaphragm |
| **D** | = | Diaphragm |
| **F** | = | Foot |
| **H** | = | Head |
| **HV** | = | Hepatic vein |
| **K** | = | Kidney |
| **L** | = | Left |
| **Li** | = | Liver |
| **LK** | = | Left kidney |
| **Py** | = | Renal pyramid |
| **R** | = | Right |
| **S** | = | Spleen |

## Normal Renal Vascular Anatomy

Knowledge of the renal vascular anatomy can be extremely helpful in ruling out certain lesions and in identifying the many tubular structures situated around the retroperitoneal area. Figure 7–9 is a transverse supine scan of a tubular structure arising from the inferior vena cava (IVC) and coursing posteriorly to the right kidney. When communication with the IVC is demonstrated, the right renal vein is visualized.

The right renal vein can be confused for a renal cyst when the right kidney is scanned near its medial aspect. The right renal vein can be seen entering the renal hilum. It is sonolucent and may be quite large on deep inspiration. It can be misdiagnosed as a renal cyst. Figure 7–10 is a supine longitudinal scan in which the right renal vein can be seen as it enters the right hilum.

A longitudinal scan (Fig 7–11) shows the position of the right renal artery in relation to the IVC. The IVC is a tubular structure coursing posterior to the liver. Deep to the IVC are two circular structures that represent right renal arteries. Usually a singular circular structure is seen deep to the IVC. In this case two right renal arteries are supplying the right kidney—not an unusual finding.

When the retroperitoneal area is evaluated, the crus of the diaphragm may be wrongly identified as the right renal artery. The crus of the diaphragm can attain fairly large size, especially on the right side. It is situated adjacent to the aorta and may be difficult to separate completely from the aorta.

Figure 7–12 is a transverse scan of the upper abdomen that shows a soft tissue mass posterior to the IVC. This is the right crus of the diaphragm, which may be misinterpreted as lymphadenopathy if one is not aware of this anatomic variation. Figure 7–12 also shows the left renal artery as it arises from the posterior aspect of the aorta. (The right renal artery is situated more anteriorly.) Anterior to the

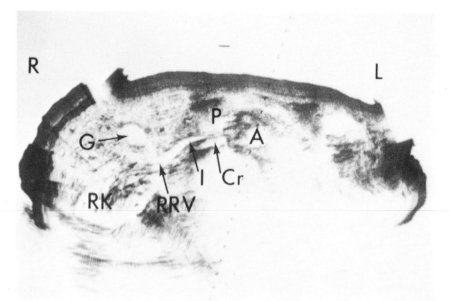

FIG 7–9.

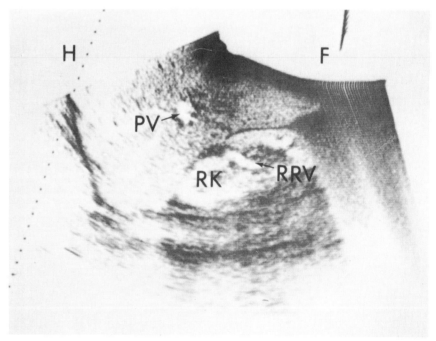

FIG 7–10.

left renal artery on this scan is the left renal vein, which drapes over the aorta and empties into the IVC. Another C-shaped lucency anterior to the left renal vein is the splenic vein. The splenic vein is anterior to the superior mesenteric artery, the structure that best aids the examiner in determining whether the splenic vein or the left renal vein is being seen. The splenic vein courses anterior to the superior mesenteric artery, while the left renal vein is posterior to the superior mesenteric artery.

| | | |
|---|---|---|
| **A** | = | Aorta |
| **Cr** | = | Crus |
| **F** | = | Foot |
| **G** | = | Gallbladder |
| **H** | = | Head |
| **I** | = | Inferior vena cava |
| **L** | = | Left |
| **LPV** | = | Left portal vein |
| **LRA** | = | Left renal artery |
| **LRV** | = | Left renal vein |
| **MPC** | = | Main portal vein |
| **P** | = | Pancreas |
| **PV** | = | Portal vein |
| **R** | = | Right |
| **RK** | = | Kidney |
| **RRA** | = | Right renal artery |
| **RRV** | = | Right renal vein |
| **SMA** | = | Superior mesenteric artery |
| **SV** | = | Splenic vein |

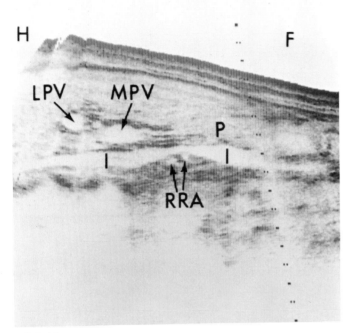

FIG 7–11.

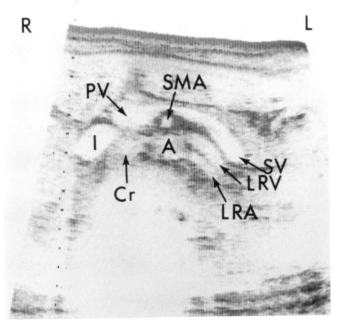

FIG 7–12.

## Low-lying Kidney; Hypoplastic Kidney

Patients are often referred for ultrasound examination because of a palpable right abdominal mass. In many cases the mass turns out to be the lower pole of the right kidney, especially in thinner patients. Figure 7–13 is a longitudinal scan of a patient with a palpable mass in the right abdomen. By simultaneously examining the patient and performing ultrasound, the physician can usually determine the etiology of the palpable mass. In this scan, the right kidney is situated below the right lobe of the liver. The lower pole of the right kidney, approximately 1 cm beneath the patient's skin, could be palpated. This is not an unusual occurrence and can be an extremely helpful diagnosis to the referring clinician.

Figures 7–14 and 7–15 show another example of a low-lying kidney with palpable masses. A transverse scan over the right midabdomen demonstrates the kidney in a longitudinal plane (Fig 7–14). It is not only low in position, but it lies in an unusual orientation.

Figure 7–15 is a longitudinal scan of the same patient. The right kidney is situated below the right lobe of the liver. The inferior vena cava and portal vein can be seen on this scan also. The kidney is not only low in position but has a horizontal orientation.

Frequently we are asked to evaluate the kidneys with ultrasound because one kidney cannot be seen on the intravenous pyelogram. Ultrasound can provide very important information in this instance. First, we can determine whether or not a kidney is present in its normal location. Second, if a kidney is present we can obtain information about its architecture. It may be small or difficult to visualize, it may be obstructed and hydronephrotic, or it may be extremely large and edematous.

Figure 7–16 is a transverse scan in which a normal right kidney is seen in its usual position although there is marked difficulty in visualizing the left kidney. Here we see a hypoplastic

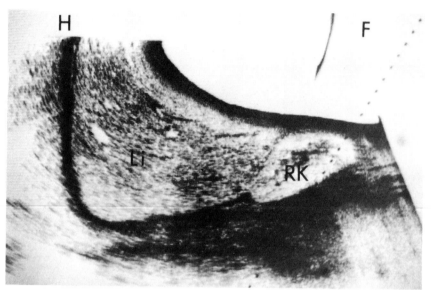

**FIG 7–13.**

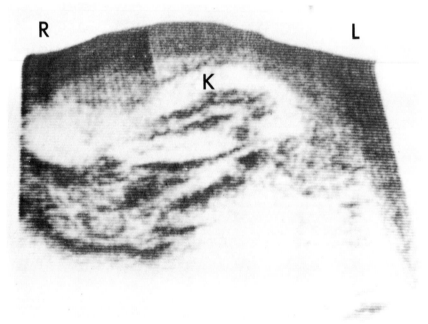

**FIG 7–14.**

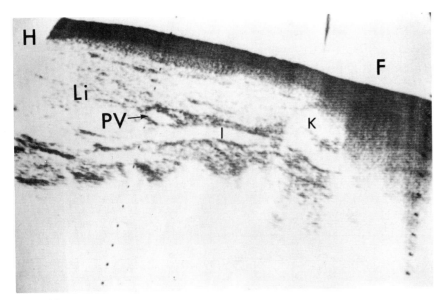

**FIG 7–15.**

kidney that is markedly smaller than the normal right kidney. Another diagnostic possibility in this instance would be severe renal inflammatory disease such as unilateral chronic pyelonephritis.

F  = Foot
H  = Head
HK = Hypoplastic kidney
I  = Inferior vena cava
K  = Right kidney situated below the right lobe of the liver
L  = Left
Li = Liver
LK = Left kidney
PV = Portal vein
R  = Right
RK = Right kidney

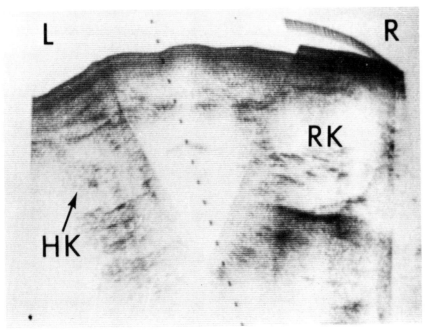

**FIG 7–16.**

## Renal Ectopy

Occasionally, examination of the renal fossae will disclose an unusual appearance or even absence of the kidney. One of the entities to be considered when a kidney is absent on ultrasound examination is renal ectopy. Figure 7–17 is a longitudinal scan of the right abdomen in a supine patient who has crossed fused ectopy. No kidney was identified in the left renal fossa. Figure 7–17 shows an enlarged 15-cm structure on the right side of the abdomen which is secondary to crossed fused ectopy.

Figure 7–18 is a transverse scan over the middle to lower abdomen in a patient with a horseshoe kidney. The central collecting system is visible as high-amplitude echoes surrounded by the lucent renal parenchymal. This appearance can be confused with abnormal bowel loops. In such cases kidneys may not be visualized in the renal bed on ultrasound, or they may have an unusual-appearing axis. A CT scan can be obtained for confirmation.

Ultrasound plays an important role when only a single kidney is seen on the intravenous pyelogram. The retroperitoneal region should be examined to determine whether or not a kidney is present. If no kidney is present, the possibility of agenesis or ectopy should be considered. After routine examination of the renal beds, the pelvis should then be evaluated to rule out a pelvic kidney. Figure 7–19 is a pelvic scan in which a pelvic kidney is seen superior to the uterus and urinary bladder. Since ultrasound studies do not need renal function and are not hindered by the bony structures of the sacrum, visualization of a pelvic kidney is usually easy.

Figure 7–20 shows another pelvic kidney different in appearance from that shown in Figure 7–19. In Figure 7–20 the pelvic kidney is obstructed and the renal pelvis is markedly dilated. The hydronephrotic renal pelvis appears as a cystic mass cephalad to the urinary bladder. In a female patient the kidney could be misinterpreted as the uterus, and the hydronephrosis could be misinterpreted as a cyst. Fortunately, the patient was a

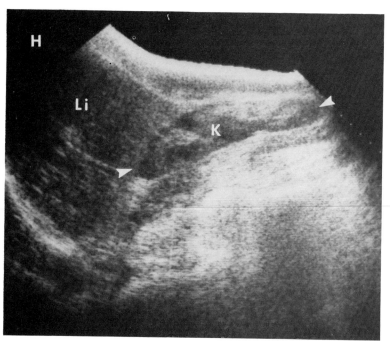

**FIG 7–17.**

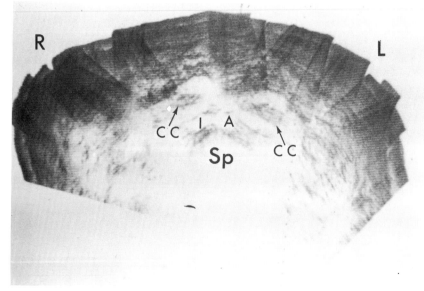

**FIG 7–18.**

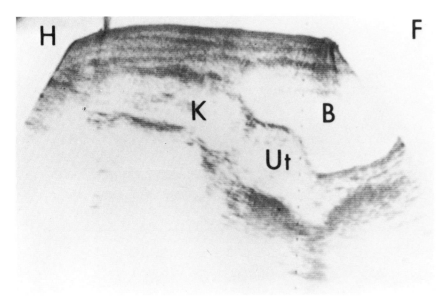

**FIG 7–19.**

male with a recent history of left lower quadrant pain and hematuria. No kidney was present in the right renal fossa. A hydronephrotic, ectopic pelvic kidney was found cephalad to the urinary bladder.

| | | |
|---|---|---|
| **A** | = | Aorta |
| **Arrowheads** | = | Crossed fused ectopy |
| **B** | = | Bladder |
| **CC** | = | Central collecting systems |
| **F** | = | Foot |
| **H** | = | Head |
| **Hy** | = | Hydronephrosis |
| **I** | = | Inferior vena cava |
| **K** | = | Kidney |
| **L** | = | Left |
| **Li** | = | Liver |
| **R** | = | Right |
| **Sp** | = | Spine |
| **Ut** | = | Uterus |

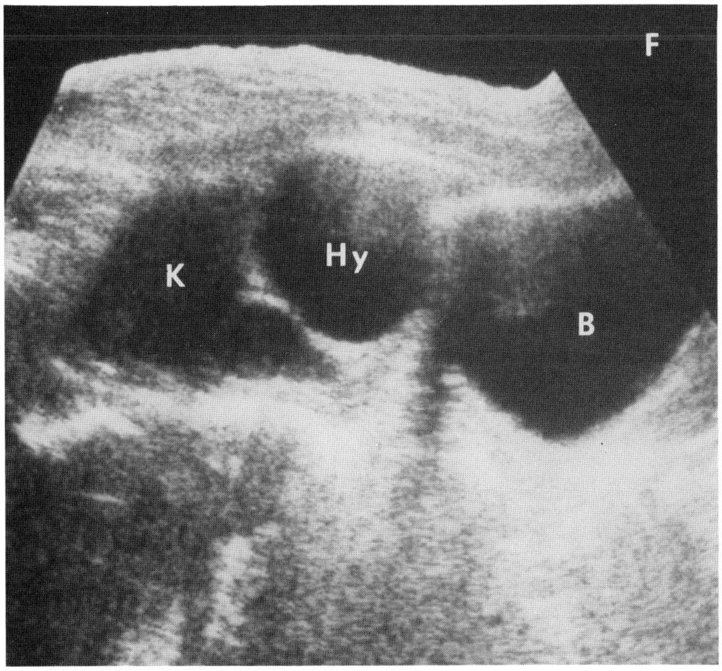

**FIG 7–20.**

## Renal Cyst

One of the most common reasons for performing renal ultrasound examination is to evaluate a renal mass detected on the intravenous pyelogram. If the ultrasonographer can provide information that determines that the mass is a simple cyst, angiography is unnecessary. A cyst puncture can be performed to establish the diagnosis. If the patient is quite elderly and the diagnosis of a simple cyst is confirmed, nothing further need be done.

Some of the problems arising in evaluation of a renal cyst are due to its location. Some problems are caused by artifacts due to overlying ribs. A cyst arising in the lower pole can be evaluated more easily than one arising in the upper pole. Upper pole cysts are more difficult to define because of the overlying 11th and 12th ribs. Figure 7–21 is a longitudinal supine scan demonstrating a lower pole cyst of the right kidney. The walls are quite sharp. Through-transmission is evident and is an important sign in the evaluation of a sonolucent mass. Through-transmission indicates the fluid-filled nature of the mass.

A supine scan through the right kidney (Fig 7–22) shows a sonolucent mass in the anterior renal parenchyma. When examining a cyst in this region, the sonographer must know where the gallbladder is situated. It can be confused with a renal cyst if it is situated adjacent to the kidney.

Figure 7–23 shows a larger cyst of the right lower pole. It has the appearance of a sonolucent mass with through-transmission.

The most difficult cysts to evaluate are those arising from the upper pole of either kidney. A longitudinal prone scan of the left kidney (Fig 7–24) illustrates a cyst in the posterosuperior aspect of the kidney. Through-transmission is present. However, echoes are noted on the near wall of the cyst (arrows). As discussed earlier, these represent reverberation artifacts off a cystic structure in the urinary bladder or in any other fluid-filled masses. If there is any doubt as to whether or not the echoes represents artifact, it is necessary to examine the cyst in dif-

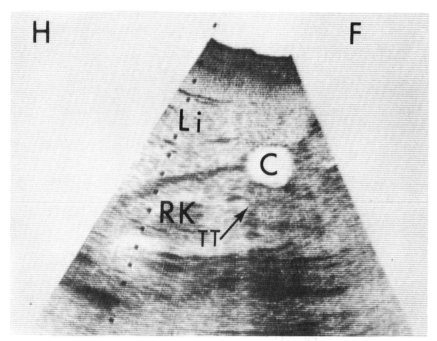

**FIG 7–21.**

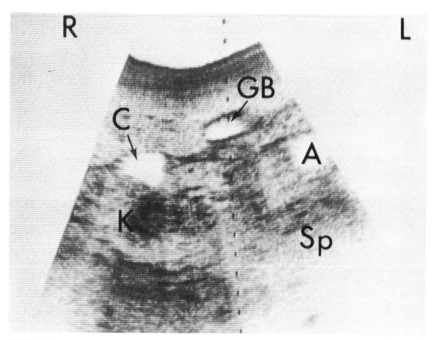

**FIG 7–22.**

ferent positions to rule out the possibility of internal echoes.

| | | |
|---|---|---|
| **A** | = | Aorta |
| **Arrow** | = | Reverberation artifact (Fig 7–24) |
| **C** | = | Renal cyst |
| **F** | = | Foot |
| **GB** | = | Gallbladder |
| **H** | = | Head |
| **K** | = | Kidney |
| **L** | = | Left |
| **Li** | = | Liver |
| **LK** | = | Left kidney |
| **R** | = | Right |
| **RK** | = | Right kidney |
| **S** | = | Spleen |
| **Sp** | = | Spine |
| **TT** | = | Through-transmission |

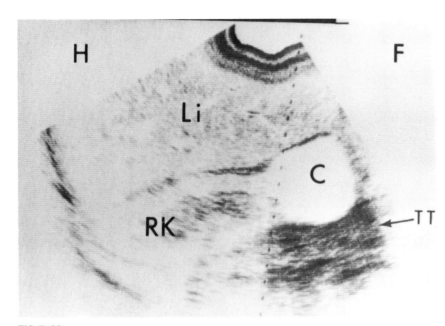

**FIG 7–23.**

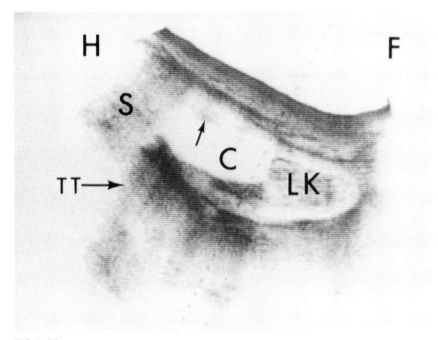

**FIG 7–24.**

## Renal Cyst

As mentioned earlier, evaluation of upper pole masses is quite difficult. The longitudinal scan in Figure 7–25 was obtained with the patient supine. Adequate visualization of the upper pole mass was impossible with the patient prone because of the overlying ribs. In Figure 7–25 we see the right kidney situated deep to the liver. A sonolucent mass is noted in the upper pole; this was thought to be a renal cyst. Although the mass was sonolucent, the borders were not extremely sharp, and there was a suggestion of soft echoes within it. The echoes turned out to be secondary to artifact. The cyst was situated so deep in the abdomen that the output of the ultrasound unit was high enough to cause these artifacts. A simple cyst of the upper pole was found. Ultrasound could not completely clear the borders of the cyst, and a cyst puncture had to be performed.

A longitudinal scan (Fig 7–26) of the right kidney demonstrates a peripelvic cyst splaying the highly echogenic central echoes of the right kidney. Peripelvic cysts may be difficult to distinguish from hydronephrosis. Usually they have circular to oval borders in all dimensions. The lucent portion of a hydronephrosis continues toward the midline as it drains into a proximal dilated ureter.

Figure 7–27 is a transverse scan of an unusual renal cyst which could have been confused for the gallbladder had we not visualized the latter elsewhere during the course of the study. The cyst is situated quite laterally and appears to be completely separate from the right kidney. We were fortunate to visualize the gallbladder more medially. Within the gallbladder is an echogenic region consistent with cholelithiasis.

Figure 7–28 is a longitudinal scan of the right upper quadrant with the patient supine. Acites is present between the liver and the right kidney. The patient was in renal failure secondary to chronic renal disease. The right kidney has increased echogenicity, compared with the liver. This is difficult to evaluate secondary to the

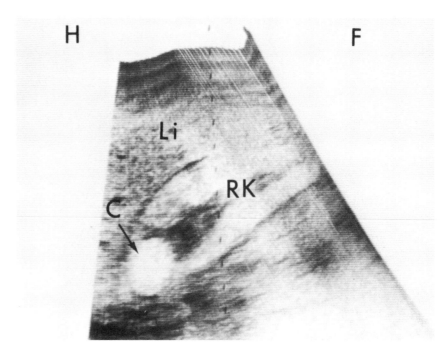

FIG 7–25.

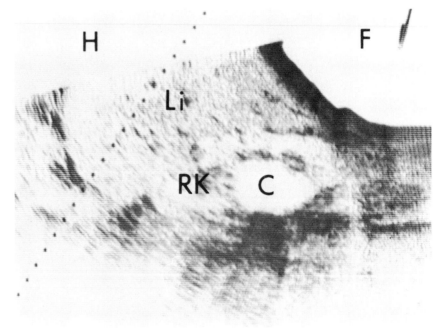

FIG 7–26.

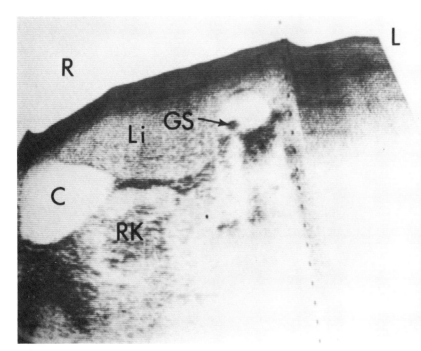

**FIG 7–27.**

through-transmission arising from the ascitic fluid. However, the overall echogenicity of the kidney is increased relative to the liver. There are three circular sonolucent masses in the upper pole of the right kidney. The borders of these masses are fairly sharp. A small amount of through-transmission is noted deep to the masses. These findings indicate three cysts of the right upper pole in this highly echogenic kidney.

| | | |
|---|---|---|
| **As** | = | Ascites |
| **C** | = | Renal cyst |
| **F** | = | Foot |
| **GS** | = | Gallstone |
| **H** | = | Head |
| **K** | = | Kidney |
| **L** | = | Left |
| **Li** | = | Liver |
| **R** | = | Right |
| **RK** | = | Right kidney |

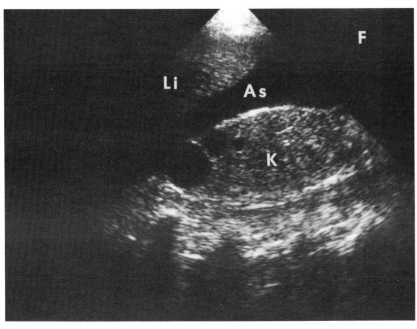

**FIG 7–28.**

## Septated and Bilobed Renal Cysts

It is important to evaluate the walls and lumen of a renal cyst to rule out any internal echoes. Figure 7–29 demonstrates a septated cyst with a linear echo arising from a septum within the renal cyst. There is through-transmission present behind the cyst, but diagnosis of a simple cyst is impossible with the linear echo noted within the cyst. Another example (Fig 7–30) shows a small septum situated within the renal cyst. Cyst puncture with the injection of contrast material confirmed a septated renal cyst in both instances.

The transverse scan in Figure 7–31 shows a renal cyst which is not characteristically oval or circular in shape. We can see what appears to be two compartments to the cyst; these represent a bilobed renal cyst. The renal cyst demonstrates through-transmission and has a smaller compartment (arrows) situated laterally.

Figure 7-32 makes an important diagnostic point in the evaluation of renal cysts. Frequently, the portion of a renal cyst that is in contact with the renal parenchyma will show an irregular border. This scan shows how the entire borders of the renal cyst were cleared except for that portion which was in contact with the renal parenchyma (arrows). This most likely means that the renal cyst is not markedly distended and is somewhat collapsible when it is adjacent to renal parenchyma. Although this represented a simple cyst, we could not completely clear it as such because of the suggestion of indentation on this portion of the kidney. We must be very concerned about the border of a cyst which shows this type of finding. Even though it is secondary to normal parenchymal compression, the diagnosis of an uncomplicated simple cyst cannot be made, a cyst puncture is indicated.

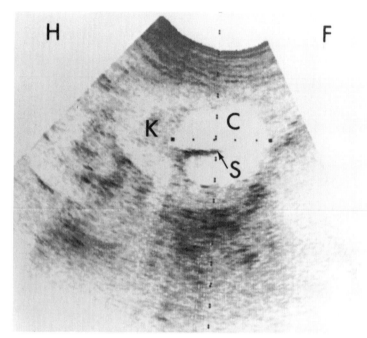

**FIG 7–29.**

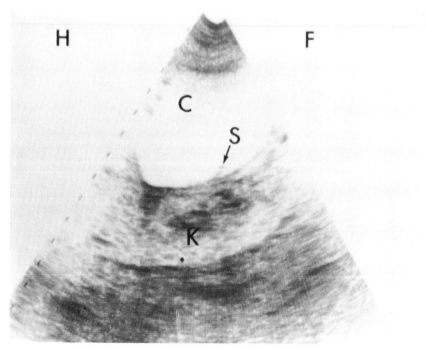

**FIG 7–30.**

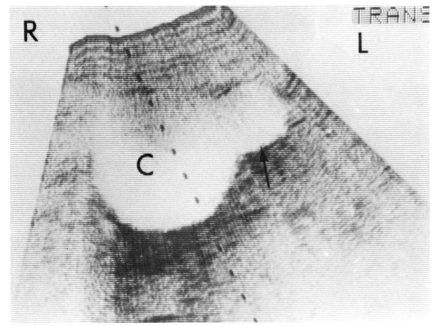

TRANS

**FIG 7–31.**

| **Arrow** | = | Bilobed renal cyst (Fig 7–31) |
|---|---|---|
| **Arrow** | = | Compression of the renal cyst by renal parenchyma (Fig 7–32) |
| **C** | = | Renal cyst |
| **F** | = | Foot |
| **H** | = | Head |
| **K** | = | Kidney |
| **L** | = | Left |
| **R** | = | Right |
| **S** | = | Septum |

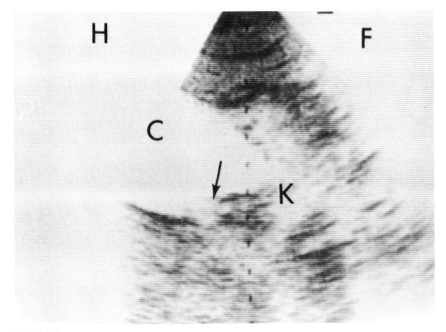

**FIG 7–32.**

## Polycystic Renal Disease

Ultrasound is an excellent means of diagnosing polycystic disease of the kidneys. Usually polycystic disease is not diagnosed on an intravenous pyelogram until the patients are in their 30s or 40s. Ultrasound can, however, demonstrate multiple renal cysts much earlier than intravenous pyelography. Since the cysts themselves, rather than their effects on the collecting system, are visualized on ultrasound, the diagnosis of polycystic disease can be made when patients are in their teens or 20s. Ultrasound evaluation of family members of patients with polycystic kidneys is recommended for earlier diagnosis.

Figure 7–33 is a transverse supine scan of a patient with severe polycystic disease. Numerous sonolucent masses can be seen in both flanks. These masses are separated by multiple curvilinear echoes. The patient initially came to medical attention because of right upper quadrant pain and possible gallbladder disease. The huge bilateral polycystic kidneys, each approximately the size of a football, were completely unexpected findings.

Figure 7–34 is a longitudinal scan of the right upper quadrant of another patient with polycystic kidneys. This patient has the added complication of polycystic liver disease. When polycystic kidneys are visualized on ultrasound, the liver and pancreas are closely examined next. In this patient multiple cystic areas are seen in the liver.

When examining polycystic kidneys, the examiner should not forget the possibility of other diagnoses. In Figure 7–35 we see not only evidence of polycystic kidney, but also a soft tissue echo with a fluid level (arrow) situated in one of the cysts. Such a finding should raise concern, since most polycystic kidneys are mainly fluid filled. The echo eventually was discovered to represent hemorrhage within a polycystic kidney.

Figure 7–36 is a scan of a patient with polycystic kidneys associated with renal cell carcinoma in the right kidney. Figure 7–36, a longitudinal scan of the right kidney, shows multi-

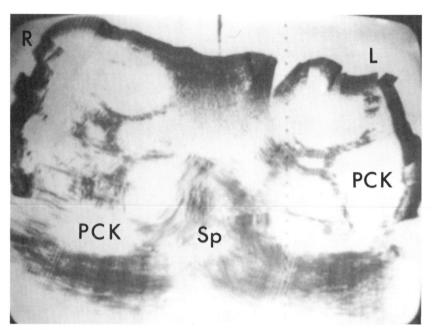

**FIG 7–33.**

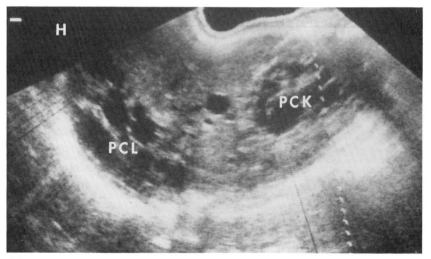

**FIG 7–34.**

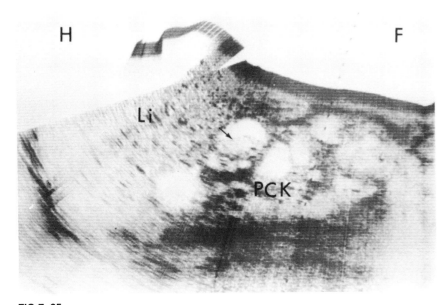

FIG 7–35.

ple sonolucent cysts, indicative of polycystic disease. An area of high echogenicity (arrows) deep to the cyst corresponded to calcification on the abdominal x-ray film. A solid mass is present in this polycystic kidney. The mass was determined to be renal cell carcinoma involving a polycystic kidney.

| **Arrow** | = | Hemorrhage in a cyst (Fig 7–35) |
| **Arrows** | = | Renal carcinoma (Fig 7–36) |
| **F** | = | Foot |
| **H** | = | Head |
| **L** | = | Left |
| **Li** | = | Liver |
| **PCK** | = | Polycystic kidneys |
| **PCL** | = | Polycystic liver |
| **R** | = | Right |
| **Sp** | = | Spine |

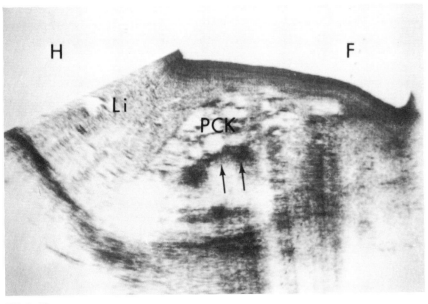

FIG 7–36.

## Multicystic Kidney

Ultrasound examination of the newborn is often requested after an abdominal mass has been palpated. Figures 7–37 and 7–38 are examples of a palpable right abdominal mass which turned out to be a multicystic kidney. This often appears as a highly echogenic region since numerous extremely small cysts are present. However, very large sonolucent masses are also seen on ultrasound in cases of multicystic kidneys. Many of the cysts can attain large size. Figure 7–37 is a transverse scan of a prone patient; the scan shows a normal left kidney and a large fluid-filled multicystic kidney on the right. The multicystic kidney would be difficult to distinguish from hydronephrosis. The cysts in the kidney are so large that hydronephrosis could not be ruled out on this scan alone. Figure 7–38 is a longitudinal scan made with the patient supine. The scan shows a large multicystic mass that does not have the typical appearance of hydronephrosis.

Figures 7–39 and 7–40 are fetal (Fig 7–39) and neonatal (Fig 7–40) scans of the same patient. Figure 7–39, an obstetric sonogram, shows a multicystic mass in the left fetal renal bed. Such masses are often picked up in utero on routine obstetric examinations. The follow-up scan in the neonatal period (Fig 7–40) reveals numerous cystic regions consistent with a multicystic kidney. What is structure 1 in Figure 7–39?

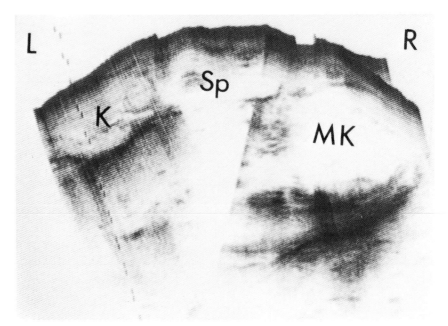

**FIG 7–37.**

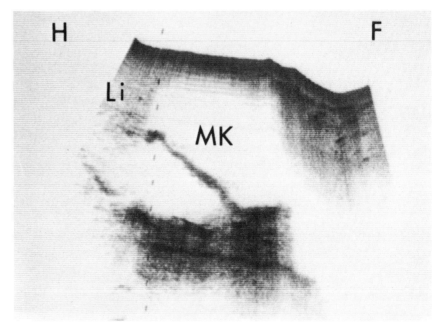

**FIG 7–38.**

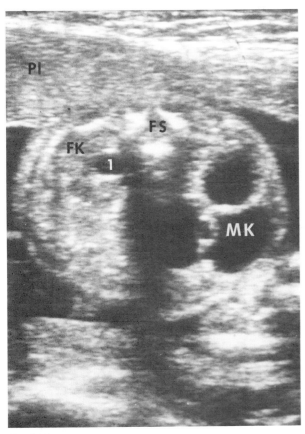

| F | = | Foot |
| FK | = | Fetal kidney |
| FS | = | Fetal spine |
| H | = | Head |
| K | = | Kidney |
| L | = | Left |
| Li | = | Liver |
| MK | = | Multicystic kidney |
| Pl | = | Placenta |
| R | = | Right |
| Sp | = | Spine |
| 1 | = | Collecting system of normal fetal kidney |

**FIG 7–39.**

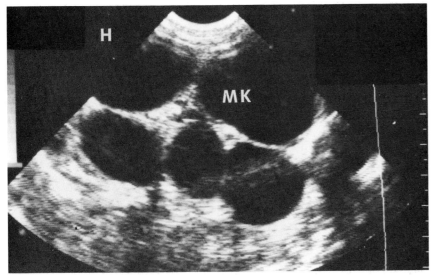

**FIG 7–40.**

## Duplex Collecting System

Various degrees of duplication of the renal collecting system can be visualized on ultrasound. Figure 7–41, a longitudinal coronal scan of the left kidney, demonstrates a sonolucent mass in the upper pole collecting system. A moderate degree of obstruction can be detected. This hydronephrotic duplex system in the upper pole of the left kidney could be confused for an upper pole cyst. An intravenous pyelogram, however, confirmed the suspected ultrasound diagnosis of an obstructed upper pole collecting system.

In Figure 7–42, another longitudinal coronal scan of the left kidney, an extremely large sonolucent mass is seen in its superior portion displacing the lower pole. This also turned out to be a hydronephrotic sac of the upper pole collecting system. The obstruction is much greater than in the previous case. A transverse scan of the pelvis of the same patient (Fig 7–43) suggested a mass within the bladder. This was found to be an ectopic ureterocele.

Figure 7–44 is a transverse scan of another patient. An ectopic ureterocele is located slightly to the left of midline. The scan illustrates the typical appearance of this entity, which presents as a cystic mass arising in the posterior wall of the urinary bladder. When hydronephrosis or suspected hydronephrosis is identified on a renal examination, the sonographer should then scan the pelvis to see if the distal ureter is dilated. Occasionally the cause of distal ureteral obstruction will be identified, as in these cases.

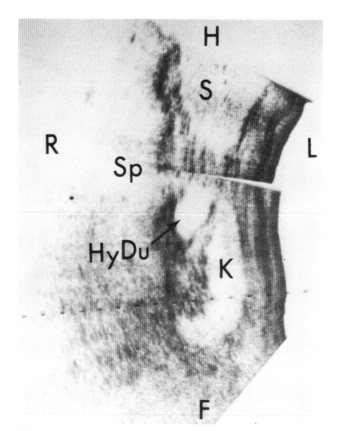

FIG 7–41.

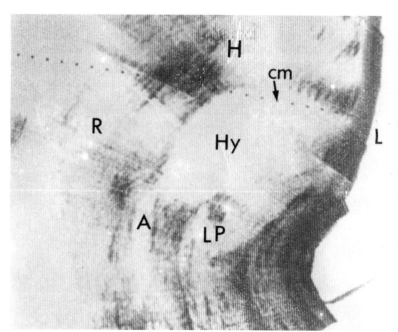

FIG 7–42.

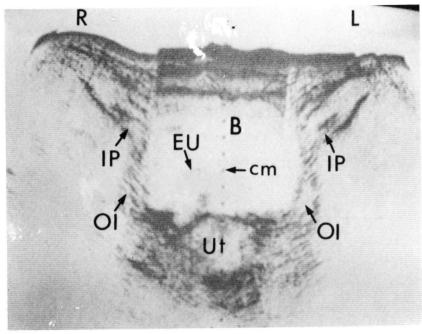

| A | = | Aorta |
| B | = | Urinary bladder |
| cm | = | Centimeter |
| EU | = | Ectopic ureterocele |
| F | = | Foot |
| H | = | Head |
| HyDu | = | Hydronephrosis of a duplex collecting system |
| IP | = | Iliopsoas muscle |
| K | = | Kidney |
| L | = | Left |
| LP | = | Lower pole of left kidney |
| OI | = | Obturator internus muscle |
| R | = | Right |
| S | = | Spleen |
| Sp | = | Spine |
| Ut | = | Uterus |

FIG 7–43.

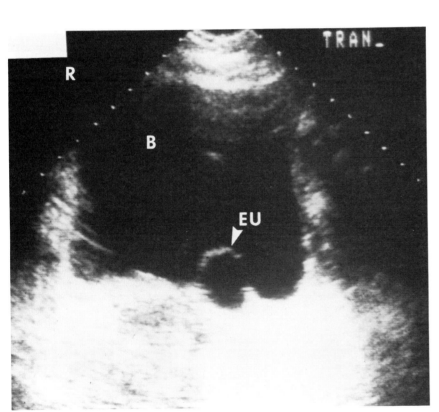

FIG 7–44.

## Hydronephrosis

Ultrasound evaluation can be difficult in the early stages of hydronephrosis. The central echoes of the kidney are usually highly echogenic and present no diagnostic difficulty in the normal state. However, an extrarenal pelvis may be present and may be mistaken for mild hydronephrosis. An extrarenal pelvis will present as a sonolucent fluid collection in the central highly echogenic region. Very early hydronephrosis is best diagnosed on intravenous pyelography since blunting of the calyceal systems can be identified quite early. The difficulty with ultrasound arises secondary to an extrarenal pelvis, which can be quite large in some patients with no hydronephrosis present.

The figures in this section illustrate the ultrasound appearance of hydronephrosis with a large amount of renal parenchyma remaining. Very often a nonfunctioning kidney is found on intravenous pyelography. Since ultrasound is not dependent on renal function, it is an excellent means of examining such nonfunctioning kidneys. Coronal scans are the most useful for evaluating hydronephrosis on ultrasound. Figure 7–45 is a coronal scan of the right kidney showing dilatation of the collecting systems. A dilated renal pelvis is present, along with the finger-like appearance of the infundibulae and calyces.

Figures 7–46 and 7–47 are coronal scans of the left and right kidneys, respectively, of two different patients. The finger-like projections of the dilated infundibulae (arrowheads) are well visualized in Figures 7–46 and 7–47. When such findings are observed on ultrasound, the diagnosis of hydronephrosis can be made with confidence. Note the large amount of renal parenchyma present in these cases, and that the renal pelvis is not markedly dilated. The diagnosis of hydronephrosis was based on visualization of the dilated infundibulae.

Figure 7–48 is a coronal scan of the left kidney. Both the renal pelvis and the infundibulae are quite dilated. In fact, the infundibulae are so dilated as not to be identifiable. The hydrone-

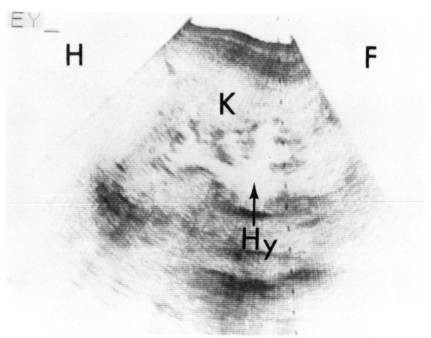

**FIG 7–45.**

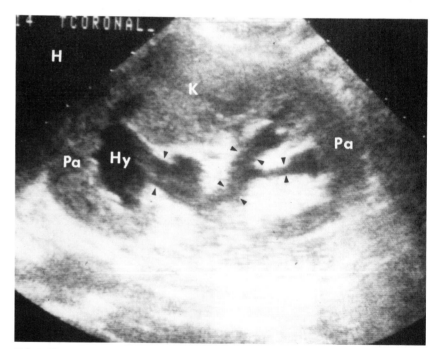

**FIG 7–46.**

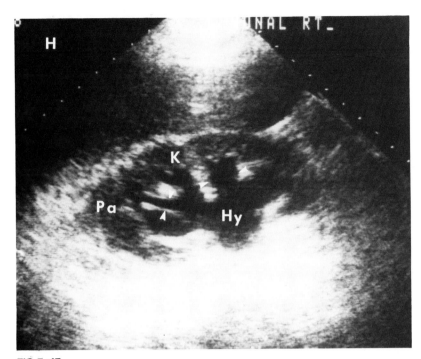

**FIG 7–47.**

phrosis is more severe than in the previous cases. However, a large amount of renal parenchyma still remains.

**Arrowheads** = Dilated infundibulae
**F** = Foot
**H** = Head
**Hy** = Hydronephrosis
**K** = Kidney
**Pa** = Renal parenchyma

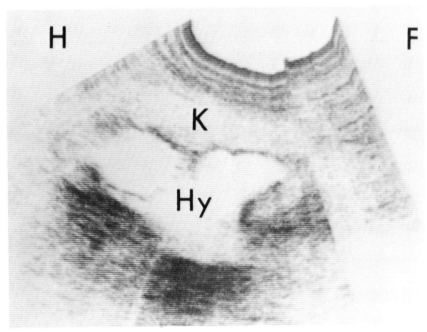

**FIG 7–48.**

## Hydronephrosis

In long-standing cases of hydrone-phrosis, the renal parenchyma decreases in quantity. The decrease can be documented on ultrasound. The cases in this section illustrate the dramatic decrease in renal parenchyma that occurs with long-standing hydronephrosis. A transverse prone scan (Fig 7–49) shows a normal right kidney and a large fluid-filled sac in the region of the left kidney. The hydronephrotic sac extends medially, somewhat anterior to the spine. This finding helps to establish a diagnosis of hydronephrosis as opposed to cystic lesions. When the hydronephrotic sac is present, it tends to be visualized anterior to the spine. A marked paucity of renal parenchyma is also noted. In Figure 7–49, almost no left renal parenchyma is evident. This is consistent with long-standing hydronephrosis. Also note that the renal parenchyma is increased in echogenicity when compared to the spleen. Although the spleen is not usually used as a reference, the increased echogenicity of the left kidney is quite dramatic.

Figure 7–50 is a longitudinal supine scan through the right renal bed. Numerous large cystic areas are visualized and were shown to communicate, an indication of severe hydronephrosis. In the center is a staghorn calculus (arrowhead) with deep acoustic shadowing. Because of the very long-standing hydronephrosis, no recognizable renal parenchyma is present. Some soft echoes are layering out posteriorly in the hydronephrotic sacs. This is secondary to superimposed infection and pyonephrosis.

Figures 7–51 and 7–52 are transverse and longitudinal scans of the right kidney in a patient with long-standing hydronephrosis. The hydronephrotic sacs of fluid nearly fill the entire renal bed. No renal parenchyma is visualized. The patient had a long history of nephrolithiasis and a previous nephrolithotomy. A recent intravenous pyelogram revealed a nonfunctioning right kidney, and ultrasound examination indicated the

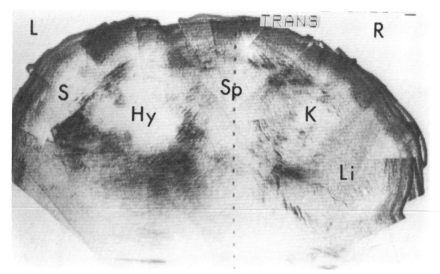

**FIG 7–49.**

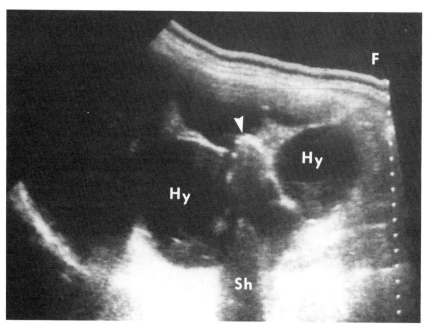

**FIG 7–50.**

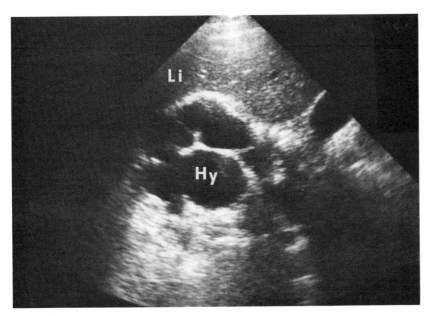

**FIG 7–51.**

reason for the nonfunction: practically no renal parenchymal tissue remains.

| | | |
|---|---|---|
| **Arrowhead** | = | Staghorn calculus |
| **F** | = | Foot |
| **Hy** | = | Hydronephrosis |
| **K** | = | Kidney |
| **L** | = | Left |
| **Li** | = | Liver |
| **R** | = | Right |
| **S** | = | Spleen |
| **Sh** | = | Acoustic shadow |
| **Sp** | = | Spine |

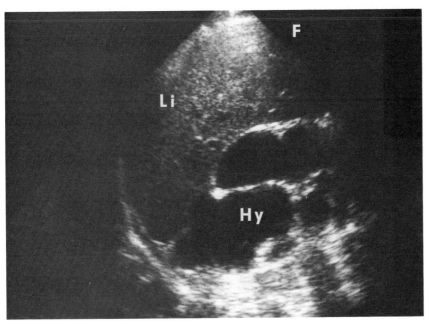

**FIG 7–52.**

## Hydronephrosis and Pyonephrosis

As mentioned previously, long-standing hydronephrosis causes atrophy of the renal parenchyma which can be documented on ultrasound. Figure 7–53 is a real-time transverse scan of the right kidney through an intercostal space. A large hydronephrotic sac is present along with very little renal parenchymal tissue (arrowheads). The small amount of renal parenchymal tissue remaining is increased in echogenicity compared to the liver, indicating underlying chronic renal disease. A CT scan of the same patient (Fig 7–54) reveals bilateral hydronephrosis. Markedly decreased parenchymal tissue is confirmed bilaterally on CT (arrowheads). Frequently long-standing hydronephrosis will yield soft internal echoes in the dependent portion of the hydronephrotic sac. Figure 7–55 is an example of hydronephrosis with layering (arrow) on the dependent portion. With this ultrasound finding, hemorrhage, infection, or debris must be considered and correlated with clinical history. In this case no signs of infection or hemorrhage were present. Most likely the layering represents debris in the collecting system from long-standing hydronephrosis.

Figure 7–56 is an example of pyonephrosis in which we see a dilated hydronephrotic sac in the superior portion of the left kidney. Again, soft echoes (arrow) are noted in the dependent portion. The distinction between pyonephrosis and hydronephrosis with debris cannot be made in these two instances on ultrasound alone. Clinical information is needed in both cases. The patient in Figure 7–56 had pyonephrosis, as was documented by clinical history and follow-up therapy.

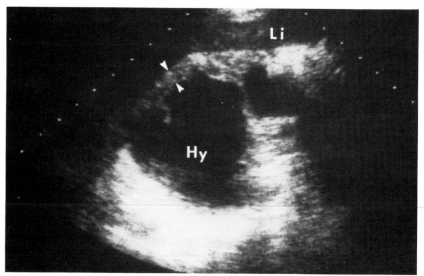

**FIG 7–53.**

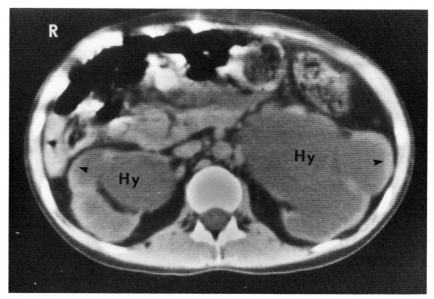

**FIG 7–54.**

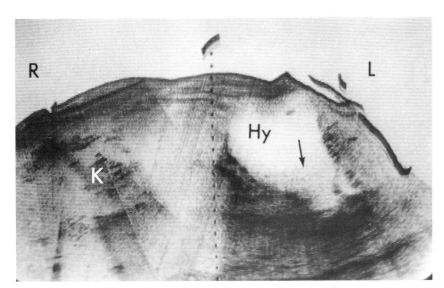

| Arrow | = | Layering of debris in hydronephrotic sac |
| Arrowheads | = | Decreased renal parenchyma |
| F | = | Foot |
| H | = | Head |
| Hy | = | Hydronephrosis |
| K | = | Kidney |
| L | = | Left |
| Li | = | Liver |
| R | = | Right |
| S | = | Spleen |

FIG 7–55.

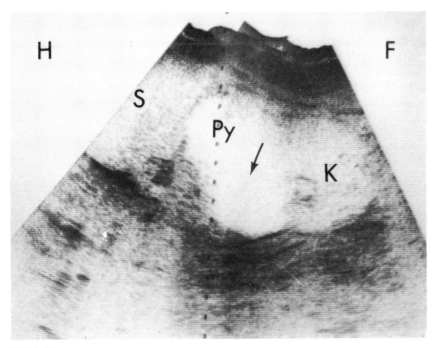

FIG 7–56.

## Hydroureter

It can be extremely helpful to the clinician to localize the level of obstruction when making the ultrasonic diagnosis of hydronephrosis. A dilated ureter over the midabdomen usually cannot be visualized when the patient is imaged supine, because of overlying air. It is extremely important to perform a pelvic ultrasound examination when hydronephrosis is identified. By distending the urinary bladder, a dilated ureter posterior to the urinary bladder may be visualized.

Figures 7–57 and 7–58 are longitudinal scans through the right abdomen and pelvis in a newborn. Figure 7–57 shows the typical ultrasound appearance of hydronephrosis, with dilated infundibulum and calcyes, especially in the upper pole region. When such findings are noted, attempts to visualize the lower collecting system are made in an effort to determine the level of obstruction. Figure 7–58 is a longitudinal scan of the right lower abdomen and pelvis. The long tubular structure is a dilated right ureter. The findings of hydroureter were secondary to an ectopic ureterocele with a right duplex collecting system.

Figures 7–59 and 7–60 are scans of a 14-year-old girl who had ureteral reimplantation approximately 10 years previously. On a recent intravenous pyelogram the left kidney was not visualized. A longitudinal prone scan (Fig 7–59) shows a hydronephrotic sac in the central portion of the left kidney. A decreased amount of renal parenchyma is evident. Because of the hydronephrosis, a pelvic examination was carried out with a distended urinary bladder. Figure 7–60 is a longitudinal scan of the pelvis with the transducer angled to the left side for better visualization of the left ureter. The urinary bladder is situated anteriorly. Posteriorly, a J-shaped tubular structure is seen that represents the dilated distal ureter. The ultrasound findings indicated a hydroureter with ureterovesicular junction obstruction.

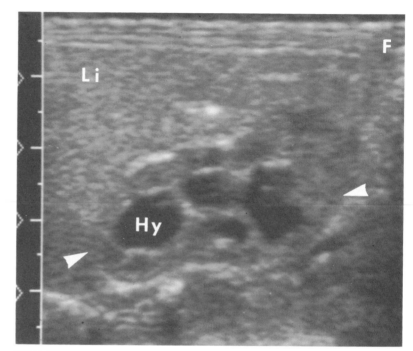

FIG 7–57.

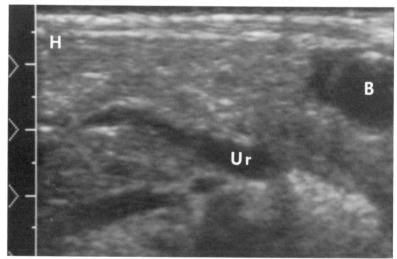

FIG 7–58.

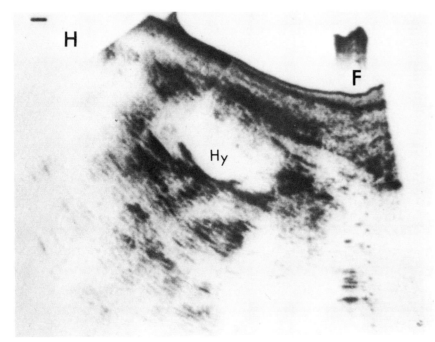

**Arrowheads** = Right kidney
**B** = Bladder
**F** = Foot
**H** = Head
**Hy** = Hydronephrosis
**Li** = Liver
**Ur** = Hydroureter

FIG 7–59.

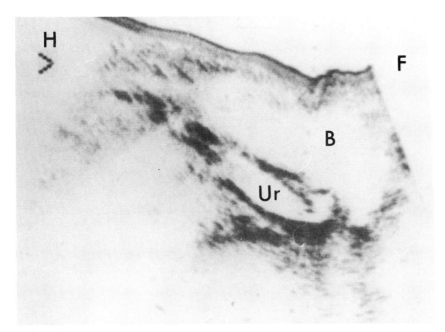

FIG 7–60.

## Renal Calculi

Ultrasound is not the imaging procedure of choice in diagnosing renal calculi, as it is in diagnosing cholelithiasis. The ideal ultrasound parameters are present when a gallstone is identified in a fluid-filled gallbladder. In this situation, highly reflective structures are located in a fluid-filled region. This is an ideal ultrasound picture which leads to a high degree of diagnostic accuracy. The opposite is true in the case of renal calculi. Here, the highly reflective renal stones are situated within the highly reflective central echoes of the renal collecting system. The renal stones must reach a large enough size to produce acoustic shadowing before the diagnosis can be made. Another factor causing technical difficulty is that the kidney is situated deeper in the body than the gallbladder. This requires lower frequency and more deeply focused transducers. Therefore, an intravenous pyelogram or plain film of the abdomen is preferable to a sonogram when the diagnosis of renal stones is entertained.

Figure 7–61 is a coronal scan of the right kidney through an intercostal space. A renal stone (arrow) is noted to have increased echogenicity compared to the central collecting system echoes. The presence of acoustic shadowing confirms the diagnosis.

Figure 7–62 is a supine longitudinal scan of the right kidney showing an area of increased echogenicity in the central collecting system (arrow). The increased echogenicity may be secondary to through-transmission from a renal cyst (C). In this case the increased echogenicity is not a sufficient finding on which to base a diagnosis of renal stone because of the presence of through-transmission behind the renal cyst. The important ultrasound finding is acoustic shadowing, which makes the diagnosis of a renal calculus possible.

Figure 7–63 is a longitudinal scan of a right kidney. There is a highly reflective echo in the upper pole. Acoustic shadowing is noted deep to this echo, indicating the presence of a calcified renal calculus.

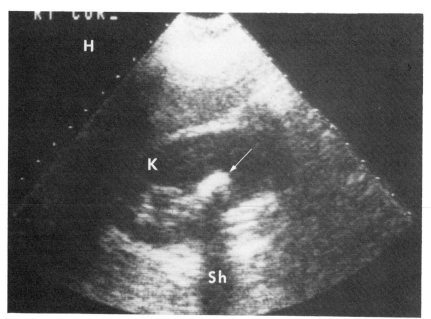

FIG 7–61.

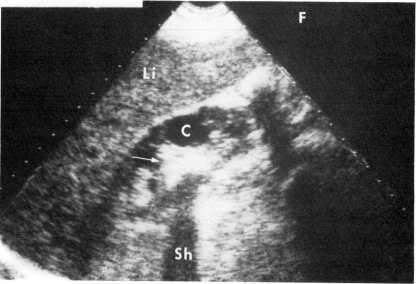

FIG 7–62.

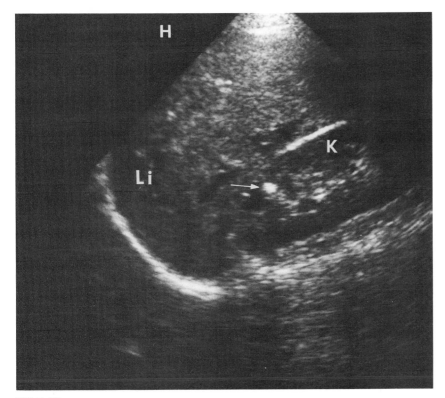

**FIG 7-63.**

Figure 7-64 is a longitudinal supine scan of the right kidney in which multiple strong echoes (arrows) are present within the renal pelvis. Some of these echoes are large enough to cause acoustic shadowing. With this ultrasound finding, the diagnosis of renal calculi can be made.

| | | |
|---|---|---|
| **Arrow** | = | Renal calculi |
| **C** | = | Simple cyst |
| **D** | = | Diaphragm |
| **F** | = | Foot |
| **GB** | = | Gallbladder |
| **H** | = | Head |
| **K** | = | Kidney |
| **Li** | = | Liver |
| **PV** | = | Portal vein |
| **Sh** | = | Acoustic shadowing |

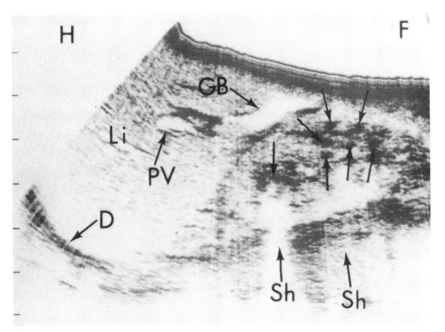

**FIG 7-64.**

## Renal Calcification

Ultrasound is not the procedure of choice in detecting renal stones. Figures 7–65 and 7–66 are longitudinal and transverse scans of a patient with renal calculi. This is an excellent example of a case in which the renal stones are lost in the highly reflective echoes of the central collecting system. The highly reflective stone is not visualized within the central echoes. The only clue that a stone is present is acoustic shadowing deep to the stone. Without this information, the diagnosis of renal calculi could easily be missed.

Figure 7–67 is a longitudinal scan through the left flank that shows a large, highly reflective region in the midportion of the left kidney. Acoustic shadowing is present deep to this region. The shadowing could represent an enlarged stone. However, it is secondary to calcification in an intrarenal hematoma. This was caused by a renal biopsy 4 years earlier. Ultrasound can not differentiate calcific entities such as this from renal calculi.

Figure 7–68 is a longitudinal scan through the right kidney of a patient who has nephrocalcinosis. When calcification is large enough, acoustic shadowing will be present. In this case, the calcification is too small to cause acoustic shadowing. The only ultrasound finding is increased central echoes, which could be misinterpreted as normal or sinus lipomatosis. Without acoustic shadowing, nephrocalcinosis will be missed on ultrasound. This case illustrates the shortcomings of ultrasound in diagnosing entities in which calcification may be present.

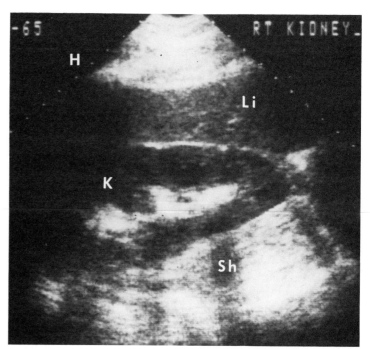

FIG 7–65.

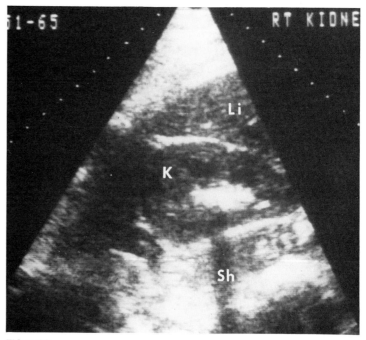

FIG 7–66.

Arrows = Nephrocalcinosis
F = Foot
H = Head
K = Kidney
Li = Liver
Sh = Shadowing

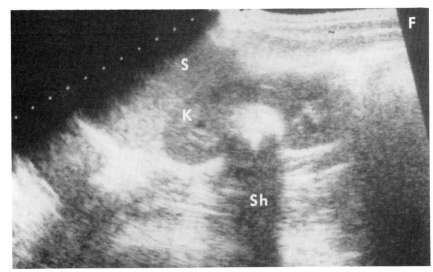

FIG 7–67.

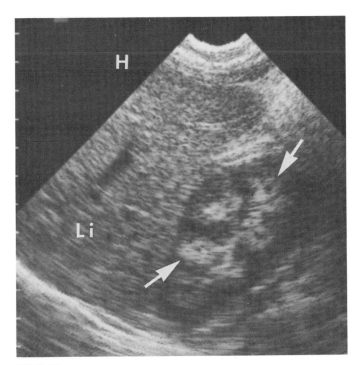

FIG 7–68.

## Renal Infections

Localized renal infection often causes disturbance in the renal parenchymal texture. This is usually manifested as an area of decreased echogenicity. In the examination of a patient thought to have intrarenal or perinephric infection, it is important to evaluate the kidney's mobility. This is performed using real-time equipment and patient respiratory movements. By having the patient inhale and exhale, the sonographer can evaluate renal mobility with real-time techniques. Excellent renal excursion usually rules out an inflammatory process. If severe inflammation is present, the patient will splint the involved kidney and do his breathing with the other diaphragm and thorax. This is a most helpful sign.

Figure 7–69 is a longitudinal scan with a renal carbuncle (arrow) in the upper pole of the right kidney in a patient suspected of having a perinephric abscess. The area was extremely difficult to visualize with the patient prone because of overlying ribs. Therefore, the patient was turned supine and the liver was used as an ultrasound window to visualize the upper pole of the right kidney. The area of the renal carbuncle is less echogenic than the surrounding renal parenchyma. A gallium scan demonstrated increased uptake in this region and confirmed the diagnosis of a renal carbuncle.

Figures 7–70 and 7–71 are scans from another patient who underwent ultrasonography to rule out a perinephric abscess. We can see marked asymmetry in the size of the kidneys, with the left kidney much larger than the right (Fig 7–70). The lateral portion of the left kidney is much less echogenic than the medial portion. Also, the large left kidney (arrows) has an inhomogeneous echo pattern to it. Figure 7–71 is a coronal scan with an uneven echo pattern throughout the left kidney. The large sonolucent area (arrows) in the periphery of the kidney establishes the ultrasound diagnosis of renal infection and abscesses. At operation numerous renal abscesses were found.

Figure 7–72 is a longitudinal scan

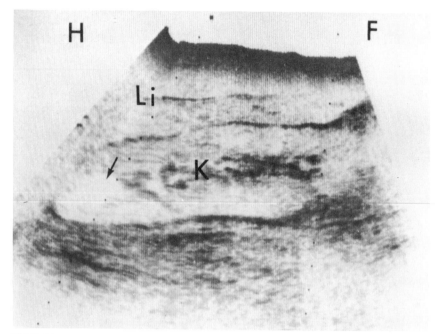

**FIG 7–69.**

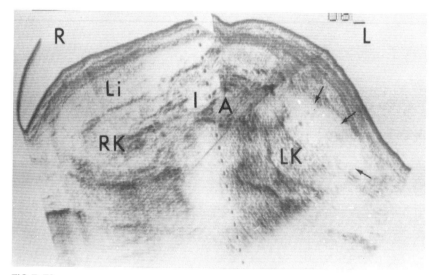

**FIG 7–70.**

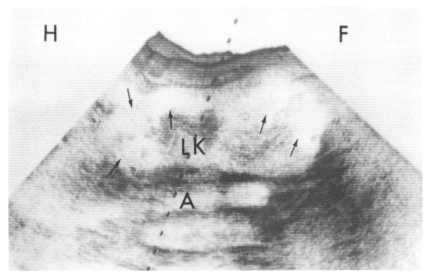

**FIG 7–71.**

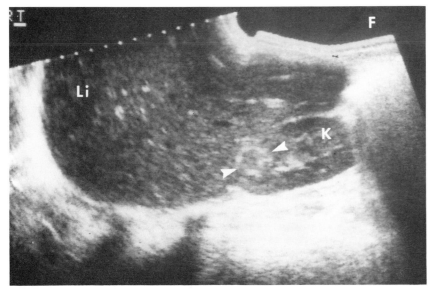

**FIG 7–72.**

of the right kidney in a 28-year-old woman admitted with acute right upper quadrant pain. Ultrasonography was performed to rule out gallbladder disease. The gallbladder was found to be normal, but there was an unusual appearance to the upper pole of the right kidney. The area of increased echogenicity was secondary to acute focal bacterial nephritis, which resolved with antibiotic therapy. A follow-up scan obtained several months later was normal. The renal inflammatory disease in this case has an unusual appearance: the involved area has increased rather than decreased echogenicity.

| **A** | = Aorta |
|---|---|
| **Arrow** | = Renal carbuncle (Fig 7–69) |
| **Arrows** | = Renal abscesses (Fig 7–71) |
| **Arrowheads** | = Focal bacterial nephritis |
| **F** | = Foot |
| **H** | = Head |
| **I** | = Inferior vena cava |
| **K** | = Kidney |
| **L** | = Left |
| **Li** | = Liver |
| **LK** | = Left kidney |
| **R** | = Right |
| **RK** | = Right kidney |

## Acute Pyelonephritis; Renal Vein Thrombosis

The inability to visualize one kidney on intravenous pyelography can be related to numerous factors. Ultrasound examination of the kidneys often will assist in narrowing the differential diagnosis. If no kidney is seen in the renal bed, the possibility of agenesis or ectopy should be considered. If a small shrunken kidney can be resolved, chronic infection or possible arterial disease should be considered. There will be instances in which the unseen kidney will be larger than the one on the normal side. Figures 7–73 and 7–74 are scans of a left kidney that is markedly enlarged compared to the normal right kidney. This turned out to be a case of acute pyelonephritis with the left kidney markedly swollen and nonfunctioning. Figure 7–74 is a longitudinal decubitus scan of the kidney; it appears more edematous and lucent than the normal right side.

Another cause of a nonvisualized large kidney is renal vein thrombosis. Figures 7–75 and 7–76 are scans obtained from a 23-year-old man who had recently been in an automobile accident. An intravenous pyelogram demonstrated nonfunctioning of the left kidney several days after the accident. In a prone transverse scan (Fig 7–75) the left kidney is approximately 2–3 times the size of the normal right kidney. In a longitudinal scan through the large left kidney (Fig 7–76) the pancreas is situated deep to the kidney. A venogram demonstrated left renal vein thrombosis. These entities should be considered when an ultrasound examination reveals a large unilateral nonfunctioning kidney.

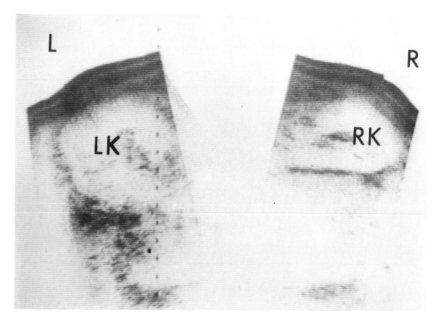

**FIG 7–73.**

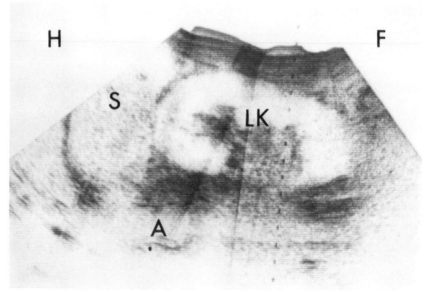

**FIG 7–74.**

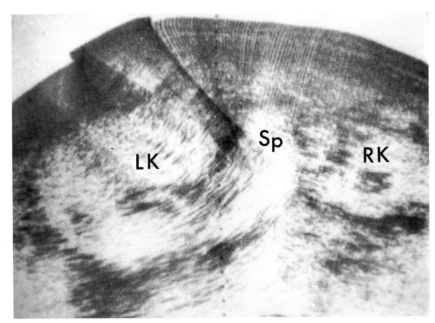

A  = Aorta
F  = Foot
H  = Head
L  = Left
LK = Left kidney
P  = Pancreas
R  = Right
RK = Right kidney
S  = Spleen
Sp = Spine

FIG 7–75.

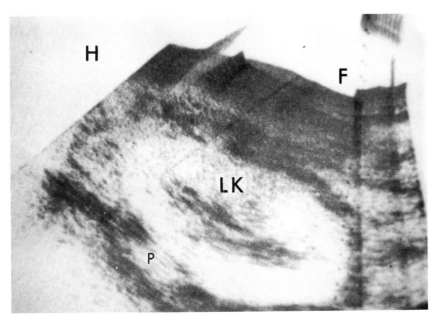

FIG 7–76.

## Chronic Renal Disease

Some patients with chronic renal disease have markedly elevated creatinine levels and intravenous pyelography would not be helpful. Therefore, ultrasound becomes an excellent means of initially examining these patients. For example, bilateral hydronephrosis can be easily ruled out.

When the renal parenchymal texture has increased echo amplitude, the diagnosis of chronic renal disease secondary to a variety of causes may be made if the kidneys appear smaller in size. It is important at this point to reemphasize the echo amplitude relationship of the upper abdominal organs. If there is no underlying disease in any of these organs, the pancreas and liver should have a higher amplitude echo than the kidney. Therefore, the renal parenchymal echo amplitude is the lowest of the three upper abdominal organs. This relationship is most easily evaluated between the liver and the right kidney, since they are in close proximity. It is difficult to evaluate chronic renal disease when scanning the left kidney. Usually chronic renal disease is bilateral, and information obtained about the right kidney can be assumed to apply to the left kidney as well. Also, the left kidney can be compared to the texture of the spleen. It is usually slightly lower in echo amplitude than the spleen.

Figure 7–77 is a longitudinal supine scan of the right kidney. It is a classic example of the ultrasound findings in chronic renal disease. The renal parenchyma is normally less echogenic than the liver. In Figure 7–77 the usual relationship between the liver and the kidney is reversed. The kidney is much more echogenic than the liver. Gallstones are present and block the view of the lower pole of the right kidney. However, the midportion and upper pole of the kidney are well seen and are of extremely high echo amplitude.

Another example of chronic renal disease is illustrated in Figure 7–78. The right kidney is of higher echo amplitude than the left. It is extremely important to evaluate the right kidney

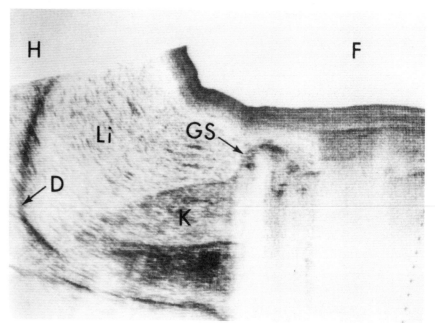

FIG 7–77.

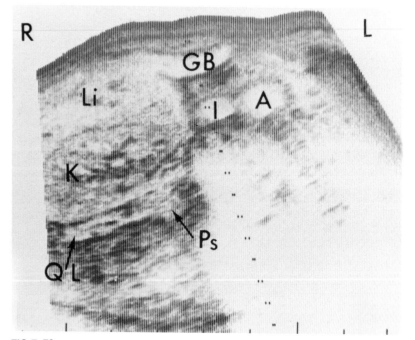

FIG 7–78.

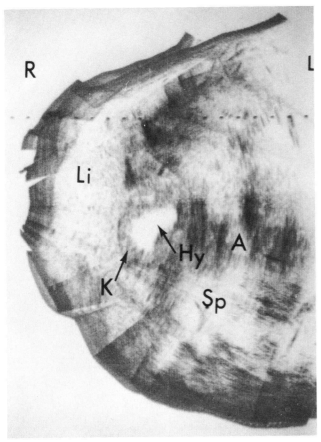

**FIG 7–79.**

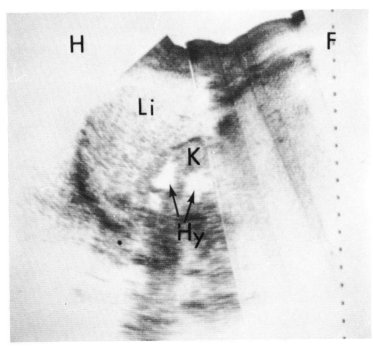

**FIG 7–80.**

through the liver when making this determination. If the right kidney is scanned through the gallbladder, the kidney will appear to be of increased echogenicity secondary to through-transmission enhancement of the gallbladder. Since chronic renal disease is usually bilateral, the right kidney can be evaluated in relation to the liver. Evaluation of the left kidney is less helpful.

In the examination of the patient with chronic renal disease, it is important to remember that associated pathology may be identified. Figures 7–79 and 7–80 are transverse and longitudinal scans of a patient with severe chronic renal disease. The disease is easily recognized from the highly echogenic right kidney compared to the normally echogenic liver. A sonolucent central region in the right kidney is secondary to hydronephrosis. Figure 7–79 is a transverse scan showing the dilated renal pelvis. Figure 7–80, a longitudinal scan obtained more peripherally in the kidney, shows areas of dilated calyces.

| | | |
|---|---|---|
| **A** | = | Aorta |
| **D** | = | Diaphragm |
| **F** | = | Foot |
| **GB** | = | Gallbladder |
| **GS** | = | Gallstone |
| **H** | = | Head |
| **Hy** | = | Hydronephrosis |
| **I** | = | Inferior vena cava |
| **K** | = | Kidney |
| **L** | = | Left |
| **Li** | = | Liver |
| **Ps** | = | Psoas muscle |
| **QL** | = | Quadratus lumborum muscle |

## Chronic Renal Disease

Ultrasound examination of a patient with chronic renal disease is a frustrating experience, especially for the novice. The kidneys are often small and contracted. Their irregular surfaces are difficult to image, compared to the excellent specular reflector of a normal renal capsule. The increased echogenicity in chronic renal disease causes further imaging difficulties. The right kidney is easier to image, since the liver is used as an ultrasound window. The left kidney is much more difficult to visualize than the right. If end-stage disease is present, often the left kidney cannot be found.

Figure 7–81 is a longitudinal scan of the right kidney in a 72-year-old man with chronic renal disease and a past history of multiple operations for removal of renal stones. The right kidney is of increased echogenicity and has a markedly irregular surface contour. An area of sonolucency (arrowheads) surrounds the right kidney. Figure 7–82 is a CT scan through both kidneys. A large amount of retroperitoneal fat is present bilaterally surrounding these small kidneys. The CT scan correlates well with the ultrasound findings. The lucent tissues surrounding the right kidney in Figure 7–81 is secondary to retroperitoneal fat.

Figure 7–83 is a longitudinal scan through the right kidney in a patient with long-standing renal disease. In this scan, the right kidney is very difficult to visualize because of its increased echogenicity. The surrounding retroperitoneal fat (arrowheads) is of increased echo amplitude, similar to the amplitude of the right kidney. A small cyst is present in the upper pole. This kidney was extremely difficult to visualize because of approximately equal echogenicity of the kidney and the surrounding retroperitoneal fat. The specular reflector of the renal capsule was the major factor permitting localization of the right kidney. The cyst in the upper pole also was quite helpful. Without the cyst or the specular reflector of the capsule, the right kidney could not be identified.

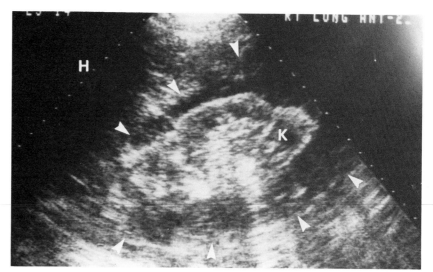

**FIG 7–81.**

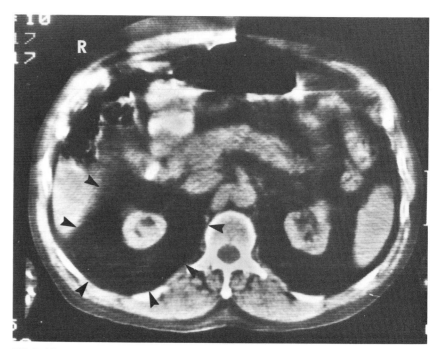

**FIG 7–82.**

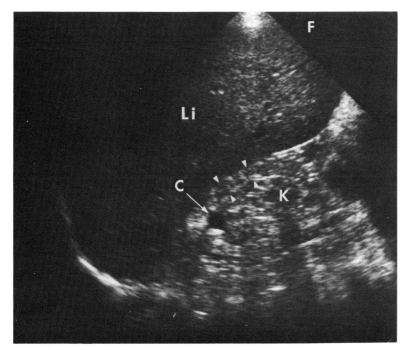

**FIG 7–83.**

Figure 7–84 is a longitudinal prone scan of the left kidney. It is difficult to distinguish the renal borders. The echogenicity of the left kidney is consistent with chronic renal disease, even without comparison to the liver. When there is difficulty in seeing the renal border, chronic pyelonephritis should be suspected. The irregular outer surface of the kidneys scatters the echoes, which do not return to the transducer. Therefore, there is extremely poor visualization of the renal borders. The left kidney is much more difficult to identify than the right kidney under these conditions. Often the splenic flexure or other bowel loops in the region of the left upper quadrant may be misinterpreted as the renal outline in such cases.

| **Arrowheads** | = Retroperitoneal fat |
|---|---|
| **C** | = Renal cyst |
| **F** | = Foot |
| **H** | = Head |
| **K** | = Kidney |
| **Li** | = Liver |

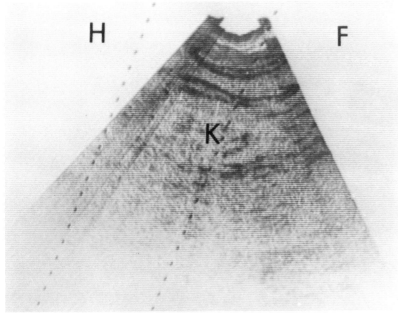

**FIG 7–84.**

## Increased Renal Echogenicity

On very rare occasions, normal-sized kidneys with markedly increased echogenicity may be encountered. These often have confusing and difficult to prove etiologies. Figure 7–85 is a longitudinal scan of the right kidney that is markedly increased in echogenicity. The right kidney is of extremely high echo amplitude compared to the liver. The confusing finding in this case is that the kidneys are not decreased in size but are normal or increased in size. At autopsy, performed about 2 weeks after the ultrasound examination, severe amyloidosis of both kidneys was found.

Figure 7–86 is a longitudinal scan through the right upper quadrant. The right kidney is of markedly increased echogenicity compared to the liver. The size of the kidney is normal. The patient had underlying renal disease secondary to long-standing heroin abuse.

Figure 7–87 is a longitudinal scan through the right kidney of another patient. There is dramatically increased echogenicity, but no evidence of a decrease in renal size. This kidney is normal in size and has a sharp contour. The echo amplitude relationship between the liver and kidney is dramatically reversed, as was noted in previous cases. The left kidney was similar in appearance and size. The patient had amyloidosis secondary to familial Mediterranean fever.

Figure 7–88 is a scan through the long axis of a renal transplant in a 15-year-old boy with systemic lupus erythematosus and end-stage renal disease. The transplant was performed approximately 6 months before this scan was obtained. Hydronephrosis developed and the ureter was reimplanted a few days before the scan. The renal pyramids are quite lucent compared to the highly echogenic cortex. There is a lucent rim of tissue surrounding the entire kidney. At surgery, the transplant was seen to be surrounded by a large amount of edematous reactive tissue. This explains the lucency noted on the pe-

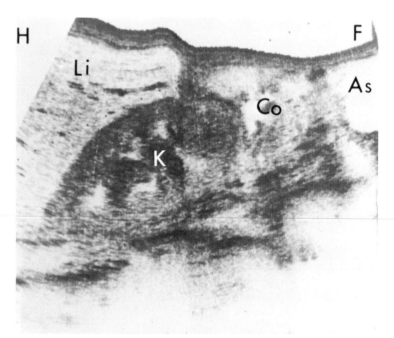

**FIG 7–85.**

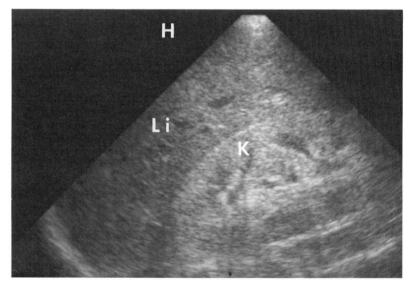

**FIG 7–86.**

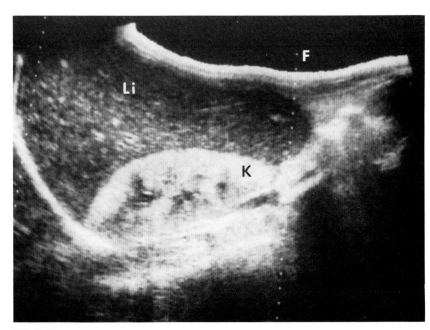

FIG 7–87.

riphery of the scan. The reason for the increased echogenicity of the cortex is unknown.

**As** = Ascites
**Co** = Colon
**F** = Foot
**H** = Head
**K** = Kidney
**Li** = Liver
**Py** = Renal pyramid

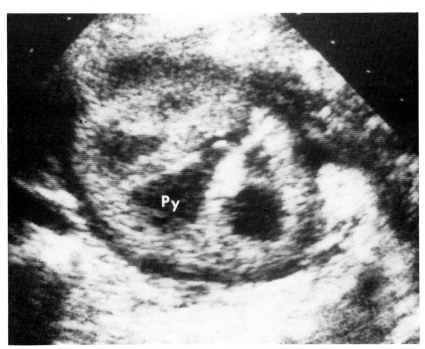

FIG 7–88.

## Sinus Lipomatosis

Fat is an extremely perplexing tissue to evaluate. It can present as either lucent or echogenic material on ultrasound examination, depending upon its location, and sometimes, its composition. There is great confusion as to how adipose tissue presents ultrasonographically. Figure 7–89 is an x-ray film of the kidneys following the injection of contrast material. The characteristic appearance of sinus lipomatosis on the left kidney is seen. The left kidney demonstrates a spider-like appearance to the collecting systems when compared with the right side. This is characteristic of sinus lipomatosis. A transverse prone scan of the same patient (Fig 7–90) shows a sonolucent central collection of tissue in the left kidney. The normal-appearing central echoes of the right kidney can be seen. The possibility of hydronephrosis arises. Figure 7–91, a longitudinal scan of the left kidney, also shows the central sonolucency. This case is a good demonstration of the sonolucent appearance to sinus lipomatosis which occurs in some patients.

Sinus lipomatosis can also be echogenic. Figure 7–92 is a longitudinal supine scan of the right kidney in another patient who had a similar radiographic appearance of sinus lipomatosis. Central echoes that are extremely echogenic are seen. It may be that a different amount of fibrotic tissue in certain cases will give an increased echogenicity. To date, however, there is no satisfactory answer as to why adipose tissue provides such a large spectrum of echogenic appearances. Therefore, sinus lipomatosis can occur anywhere on the spectrum, from extremely lucent to extremely echogenic.

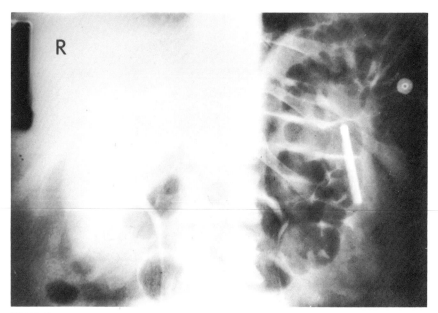

FIG 7–89.

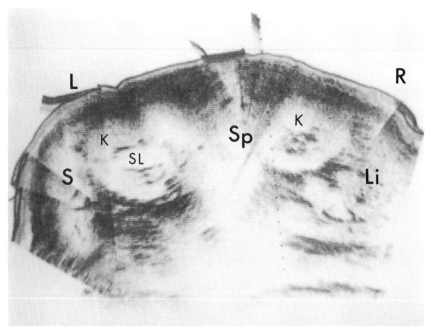

FIG 7–90.

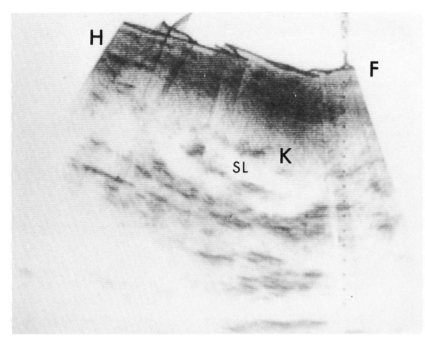

**FIG 7–91.**

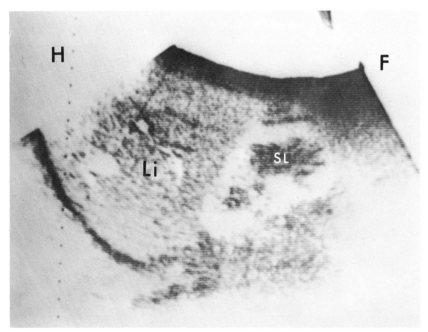

**FIG 7–92.**

F  = Foot
H  = Head
K  = Kidney
L  = Left
Li = Liver
R  = Right
S  = Spleen
SL = Sinus lipomatosis
Sp = Spine

## Renal Sinuses

The area of the renal sinuses can present a diagnostic problem on ultrasound. As noted in the section on imaging of normal kidneys, the central echoes are usually increased in echogenicity. In hydronephrosis and peripelvic cysts there is a central sonolucency separating the highly echogenic central echoes. Sinus lipomatosis may present as lucent or echogenic regions in the central echoes. In the case described here, magnetic resonance (MR) image played a helpful role in resolving problems associated with changes in the central echoes.

Figures 7–93 through 7–96 are renal images, obtained by various imaging modalities, in the same patient. The intravenous pyelogram in Figure 7–93 demonstrates splaying of the central collecting systems (M), suggestive of sinus lipomatosis or peripelvic cysts. The CT scan in Figure 7–94 shows low-density regions in the central portion of the kidneys, mainly consistent with sinus lipomatosis.

Figure 7–95 is a longitudinal scan of the right kidney. The central echoes are separated by a relatively sonolucent region with some soft internal echoes. The findings were thought to be secondary to sinus lipomatosis. The MR scan in Figure 7–96 indicates that low-density regions are present in the central areas of the kidneys. High-density fat is recognized throughout the remainder of the retroperitoneum, peritoneum, and subcutaneous regions. However, fat density is not present within the central regions of the kidney. The MR imaging study indicates that these areas are secondary to peripelvic cysts. Sonolucent regions on ultrasound in the central renal areas may be secondary to peripelvic cyst rather than sinus lipomatosis. MR imaging will be helpful in distinguishing these entities.

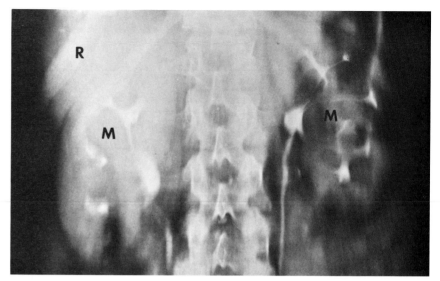

FIG 7–93.

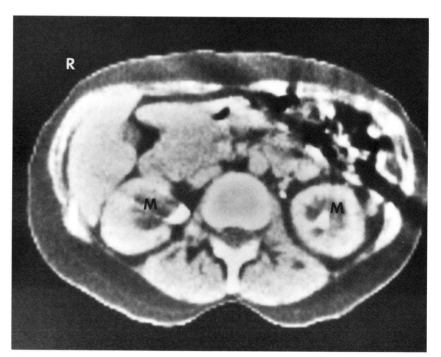

FIG 7–94.

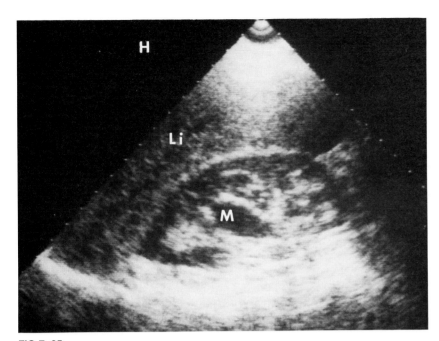

**FIG 7–95.**

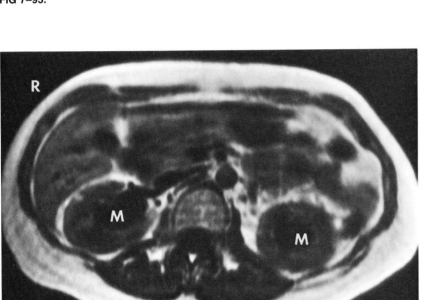

**FIG 7–96.**

**H**  =  Head
**Li**  =  Liver
**M**  =  Sinus lipomatosis
**R**  =  Right

## Angiomyolipoma

Angiomyolipoma presents an extremely confusing picture on ultrasound, if the examiner has never seen this entity previously. The highly reflective fat makes the renal fossae appear filled with bowel or retroperitoneal fat. These masses will cause the examiner to think of chronic renal disease or renal ectopy, since the kidneys are not readily identifiable.

Figure 7–97 is a longitudinal coronal scan of the left kidney which demonstrates a highly echogenic central portion with attenuation (arrows). The ultrasound appearance of this mass could be consistent with calcification in the kidney. It is, however, an angiomyolipoma with highly attenuating fat. Angiomyolipomas often yield highly echogenic masses that distort the renal architecture and parenchyma. When such a mass is visualized, CT should be performed. It will yield valuable information that will rule out entities other than angiomyolipoma. Because of the fat density, a CT scan will lead to the correct diagnosis.

Another example of an angiomyolipoma presenting as a highly echogenic mass is seen in Figure 7–98. This is a longitudinal scan of the left kidney. Only a small portion of normal renal parenchymal tissue can be identified. Marked attenuation deep to the highly reflective angiomyolipoma (arrows) is noted. Fatty tissue often attenuates the ultrasound beam quite dramatically, as in this case.

Figures 7–99 and 7–100 are two longitudinal scans through the right kidney of a patient with tuberous sclerosis. The kidneys contain numerous sonolucent areas that are secondary to renal cysts. Also present are several circular regions of increased echogenicity, which indicate fat in angiomyolipoma. The left kidney had a similar appearance. These findings are consistent with tuberous sclerosis in which bilateral renal cysts and angiomyolipomas are found in the kidneys. The patient also had adenoma sebaceum, mental retardation, and epilepsy, other aspects of this disease entity.

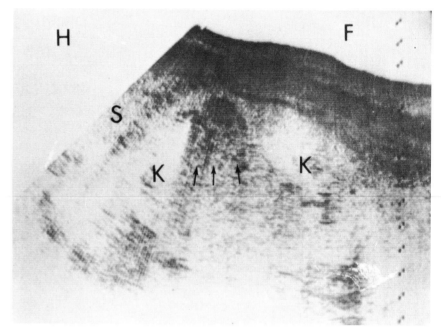

**FIG 7–97.**

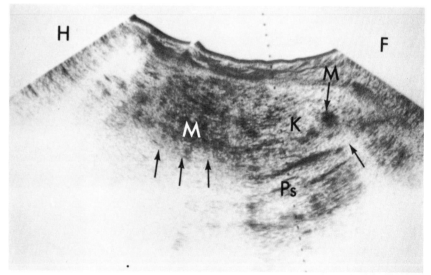

**FIG 7–98.**

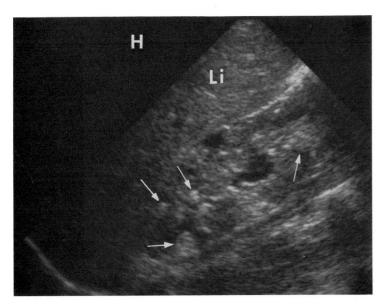

**FIG 7–99.**

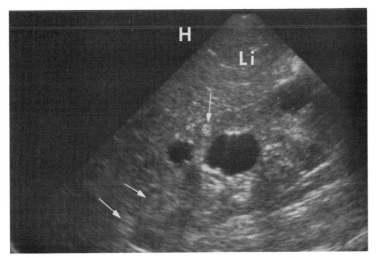

**FIG 7–100.**

| **Arrows** | = | Highly echogenic fatty areas of angiomyolipoma |
|---|---|---|
| **F** | = | Foot |
| **H** | = | Head |
| **K** | = | Kidney |
| **Li** | = | Liver |
| **M** | = | Angiomyolipoma |
| **Ps** | = | Psoas muscle |
| **S** | = | Spleen |

## Infiltrative Disease

Figure 7–101 is a tomogram from an intravenous pyelography study which demonstrates large kidneys with stretching and splaying of the renal collecting systems. Ultrasonography was performed to rule out polycystic kidney disease because of the suggestive findings on IVP. Polycystic renal disease is easily diagnosed by ultrasound. Numerous fluid-filled cystic masses spread throughout the renal parenchyma are present in polycystic renal disease. Figure 7–102 is a longitudinal scan of the left kidney in the same patient as in Figure 7–101. There is no evidence of any fluid-filled masses, as would be present in polycystic renal disease. Instead, the kidneys are diffusely filled with soft tissue masses. The collecting systems are difficult to see and consistent with the splayed appearance on IVP. Areas of the kidneys are completely filled with soft tissue regions. The patient was found to have diffuse lymphoma of the kidneys bilaterally.

Figure 7–103 is a transverse scan of the upper abdomen in a patient with two large masses. The masses are present in what appears to be the renal beds on this scan. They are well-defined, inhomogenous solid masses initially thought to be secondary to renal lymphoma. However, a longitudinal scan through the right abdomen (Fig 7–104) indicates that the masses are above the kidneys. The right kidney is displaced inferiorly and is mildly hydronephrotic. A similar finding is present on the left side. The patient was found to have lymphoma involving mainly the adrenal glands. A solid lymphomatous mass is also present in the right lobe of the liver, as can be seen in Figure 7–104. The initial transverse scan in Figure 7–103 could be thought to show renal lymphoma. However, the longitudinal scan confirms that the kidneys are displaced markedly inferiorly by the adrenal masses. What are structures 1, 2, and 3 in Figure 7–103?

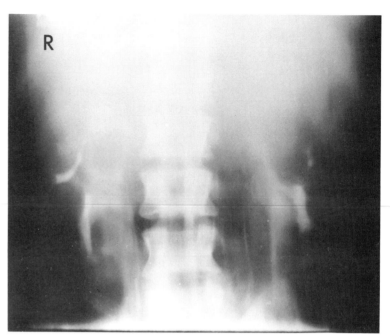

**FIG 7–101.**

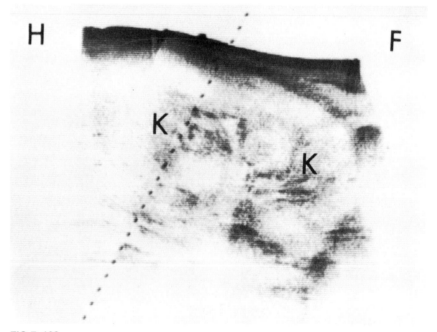

**FIG 7–102.**

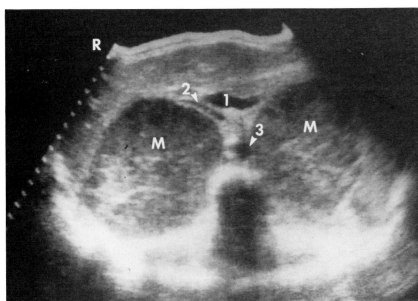

| F | = | Foot |
|---|---|---|
| H | = | Head |
| Hy | = | Hydronephrosis |
| K | = | Kidney |
| Li | = | Liver |
| M | = | Lymphomatous mass |
| R | = | Right |
| 1 | = | Splenic vein |
| 2 | = | Displaced inferior vena cava |
| 3 | = | Aorta |

FIG 7–103.

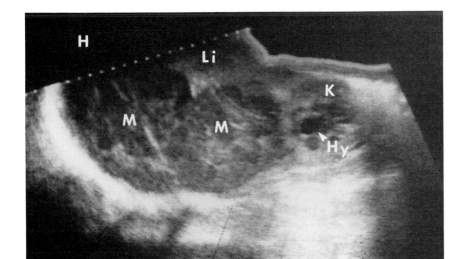

FIG 7–104.

## Leukemic Infiltrates

Infiltrative disease is often diffuse and involves the entire kidney. When this occurs, an infiltrative process can usually be suggested by ultrasound. When infiltrative disease is localized, the ultrasound findings are consistent with a focal mass lesion. Figures 7–105 and 7–106 are longitudinal and transverse scans of the right kidney with a focal sonolucent mass (arrowheads) in the anterior upper pole. This could represent a hypovascular renal carcinoma, transitional cell carcinoma, or focal bacterial nephritis. The mass in this case was secondary to focal leukemic infiltration of the right kidney. What are structures 1 and 2 in Figure 7–106?

Although most lymphoma and leukemic renal infiltrates will present as sonolucent masses on ultrasound, this is not always the case. Figures 7–107 and 7–108 are longitudinal and transverse scans of the right kidney in a patient who has renal infiltrative disease secondary to leukemia. Rather than numerous sonolucent regions, there are areas of mildly increased echogenicity spread throughout the kidney. This is an unusual ultrasound presentation for leukemic infiltrates.

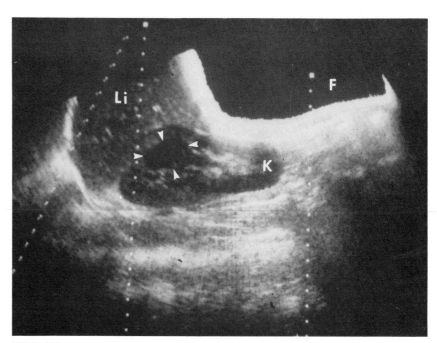

**FIG 7–105.**

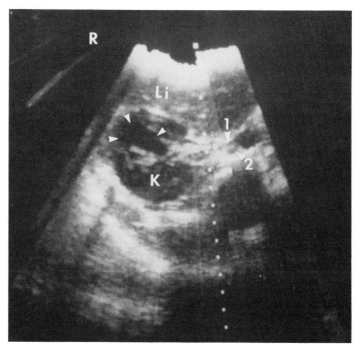

**FIG 7–106.**

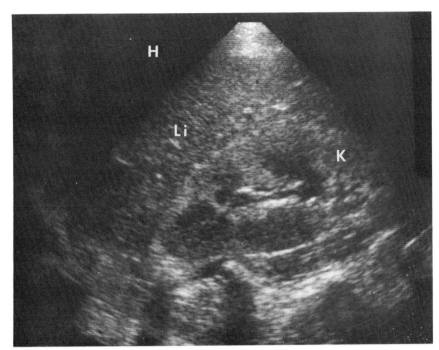

| Arrowheads | = | Focal leukemic infiltrate |
|---|---|---|
| F | = | Foot |
| H | = | Head |
| K | = | Kidney |
| Li | = | Liver |
| R | = | Right |
| 1 | = | Right renal artery |
| 2 | = | Crus of diaphragm |

FIG 7–107.

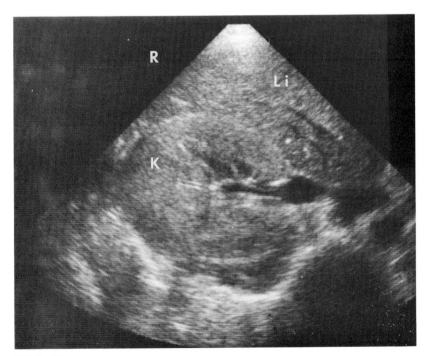

FIG 7–108.

## Echogenic Renal Carcinoma

Ultrasound evaluation of renal masses found on IVP can be extremely helpful in determining whether or not further studies should be performed. If a simple cyst is present on ultrasound examination and all of the ultrasound criteria have been met, the workup can stop at this point. If a thick-walled or septated cystic mass is present, cyst aspiration should be performed. Lesions that are solid on ultrasound necessitate further studies such as CT, MR imaging, and angiography, depending on available equipment and level of expertise.

Renal cell carcinomas can present with a variety of ultrasound appearances. They may be extremely echogenic, relatively sonolucent, or fluid-filled, in the case of necrotic tumors. Figure 7–109 is a longitudinal scan of the right kidney in a patient with recent hematuria. The upper pole was hydronephrotic secondary to obstruction by a large lower pole tumor. The renal mass is echogenic and consistent with a solid lesion of the lower pole of the kidney. A portion of the kidney is not visible because of overlying bowel air in the hepatic flexure. The liver was normal on examination at the time of initial diagnosis. At operation a large tumor of the right kidney was removed; the liver was thought to be normal.

A transverse scan of the liver (Fig 7–110) was performed approximately 1 year after the initial ultrasound examination and operation. The liver now contains several highly echogenic masses consistent with vascular metastatic lesions.

Figure 7–111 is an example of a small tumor of the lower pole of the right kidney. An increased echogenic region in the lower pole, approximately 2 cm in diameter, is seen. The remainder of the renal parenchyma is relatively sonolucent. The output and sensitivity of the unit were intentionally set to make the normal renal parenchyma extremely sonolucent. This technique brought out the marked discrepancy between the lower pole ech-

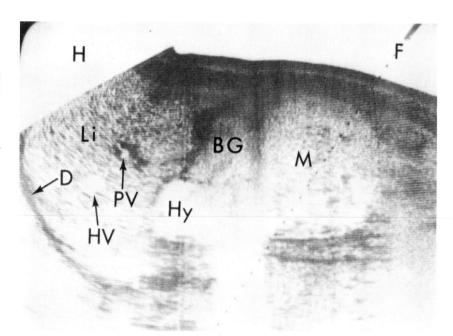

**FIG 7–109.**

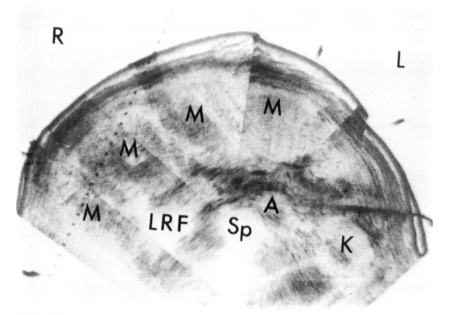

**FIG 7–110.**

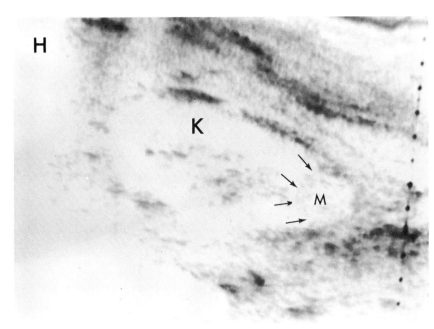

**FIG 7–111.**

ogenicity and the remainder of the normal renal parenchyma.

Figure 7–112 is an example of a hyperechoic neoplasm of the right upper pole. This is an extremely large mass that involves most of the right upper pole and extends posterior to the liver. Extremely vascular renal lesions will appear as highly echogenic lesions on ultrasound.

| | | |
|---|---|---|
| **A** | = | Aorta |
| **BG** | = | Bowel gas |
| **D** | = | Diaphragm |
| **F** | = | Foot |
| **H** | = | Head |
| **HV** | = | Hepatic vein |
| **HY** | = | Hydronephrosis |
| **K** | = | Kidney |
| **L** | = | Left |
| **Li** | = | Liver |
| **LRF** | = | Renal fossa |
| **M** | = | Echogenic tumor |
| **PV** | = | Portal vein |
| **R** | = | Right |
| **Sp** | = | Spine |

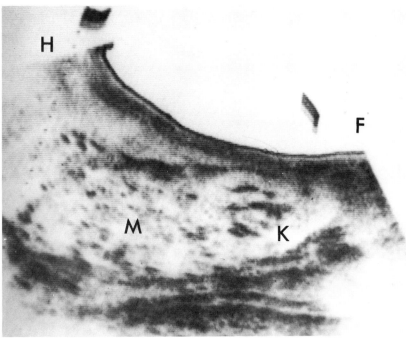

**FIG 7–112.**

## Hypoechoic Renal Neoplasms

Renal masses may also be decreased in echogenicity. This is usually true of hypovascular tumors. Close scrutiny of the central echoes on ultrasound is important in the evaluation of the kidney. A longitudinal scan of a left kidney (Fig 7–113) demonstrates marked distortion of the lower pole central echoes. The normal high echogenic central region is disrupted by a relatively lucent mass. The borders of this mass are irregular and are distorting the central echoes. This is a transitional cell carcinoma of the lower pole. Figure 7–114, another transverse scan of a left kidney, indicates distortion of the central echoes by an anterior mass. The mass is relatively hypoechogenic, as compared with the renal parenchyma. It was found to be a renal cell carcinoma and was somewhat hypovascular.

Figure 7–115, a longitudinal coronal scan of the left kidney, demonstrates a mass (arrows) situated on the lateral aspect of the kidney. Again, the important finding is distortion of the central echoes. Not only the architecture of the renal capsule and outline but also the central echoes must be closely examined during an ultrasound study. The only clue to renal pathology may be distortion of the central echoes, as these cases demonstrate.

Figure 7–116 is a longitudinal scan of the right kidney with a hypovascular mass adjacent to its upper pole. This mass could not be completely separated from the right upper pole. This is an extremely difficult area to evaluate because it is impossible to place the transmitted beam perpendicular to interfaces in this region. Several diagnostic possibilities, such as renal carcinoma or an adrenal lesion, exist. At surgery, it was found to be a benign renal adenoma arising from the upper pole of the right kidney.

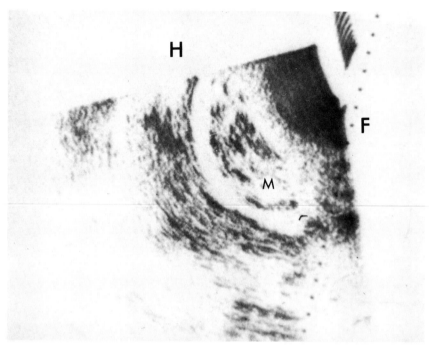

FIG 7–113.

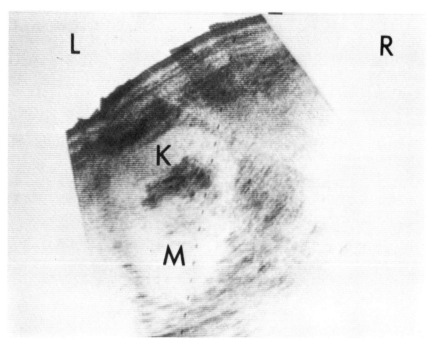

FIG 7–114.

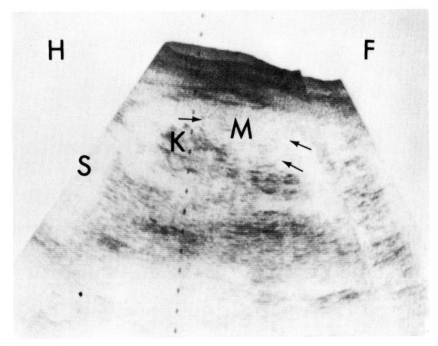

FIG 7–115.

| | | |
|---|---|---|
| **F** | = | Foot |
| **H** | = | Head |
| **K** | = | Kidney |
| **L** | = | Left |
| **Li** | = | Liver |
| **M** | = | Transitional cell carcinoma (Fig 7–113) |
| **M** | = | Hypovascular renal carcinoma (Fig 7–114) |
| **M** | = | Renal adenoma (Fig 7–116) |
| **M and arrows** | = | Hypernephroma (Fig 7–115) |
| **R** | = | Right |
| **RK** | = | Right kidney |
| **S** | = | Spleen |

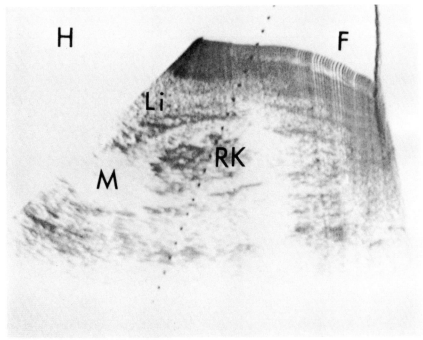

FIG 7–116.

## Renal Neoplasm

Renal neoplasm may present a variety of appearances on ultrasound. Masses may be hypoechoic, increased in echogenicity, or partially fluid filled in cases with necrosis. A systematic examination of the kidneys will usually avoid missing any of these masses. The renal contour in both longitudinal and transverse planes is examined to rule out any contour deformities. Exophitic renal masses are often missed on IVP. Ultrasound examination will usually be able to pick up such masses. Transverse scans of the renal contour are usually more helpful than longitudinal scans. The kidneys should be examined in transverse planes over the lower third, middle third, and upper third. These areas should be examined separately, and each area labeled and photographed for permanent records.

A second part of the examination entails close evaluation of the central renal echoes. Deformity of the central echoes should increase awareness of possible renal neoplasms. Sinus lipomatosis or the column of Bertin are normal anatomic findings that also distort the central renal echoes. These entities must be differentiated from neoplasm. Fluid-filled renal masses also present diagnostic difficulties. The diagnosis of a simple renal cyst versus other fluid-filled masses is important. If the criteria of a simple cyst are met, the diagnostic workup may stop with the ultrasound examination. However, any deviation from those criteria for a simple cyst will necessitate further examination.

Figure 7–117 is a longitudinal scan of the left kidney of a 82-year-old woman who developed hematuria after an accidental fall at home. Subsequently she experienced left flank pain. Ultrasound of the left upper quadrant was requested because of the hematuria and flank pain. The left renal contour is smooth, as can be seen in Figure 7–117. However, the central echoes are distorted (arrowheads) in the left lower pole. At operation the patient's left kidney was removed because of a transitional cell carcinoma.

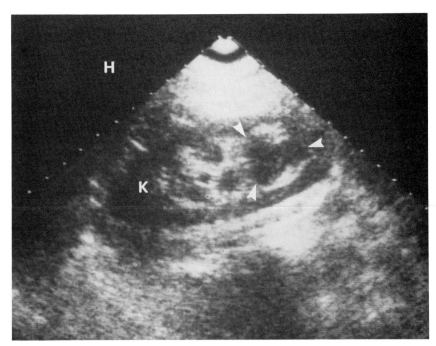

**FIG 7–117.**

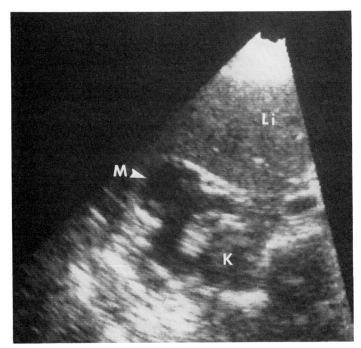

**FIG 7–118.**

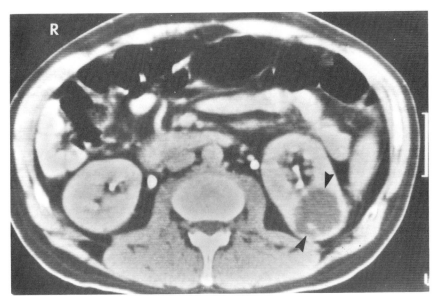

**FIG 7–119.**

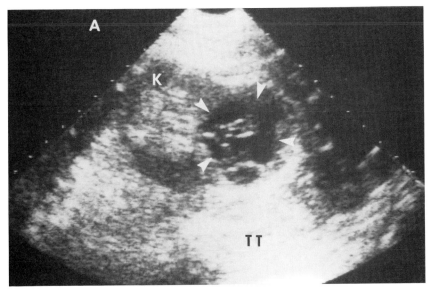

**FIG 7–120.**

Figure 7–118 is a transverse scan of the right kidney through an intercostal space. A solid mass causing a contour deformity is present over the middle to lower portion of the right kidney. An arteriogram indicated a hypovascular mass. At operation the right kidney was removed because of renal cell carcinoma. Although this mass was smooth in contour and hypovascular on arteriography, the ultrasound findings indicated a solid lesion.

Figure 7–119 is an abdominal CT scan that shows a cystic mass in the posterior aspect of the left kidney. There appears to be a single septum within the mass. A real-time ultrasound examination (Fig 7–120) demonstrates septations and internal echoes along with enhanced through-transmission. Although the mass is fluid, as indicated by the through-transmission, the criteria of a simple cyst have obviously not been met: there are numerous internal echoes. At operation the patient's left kidney was removed because of a hemorrhagic renal cell carcinoma.

| A | = Anterior |
| **Arrowheads** | = Renal neoplasm |
| H | = Head |
| K | = Kidney |
| Li | = Liver |
| M | = Mass |
| R | = Right |
| TT | = Through-transmission |

## Hypernephroma

Figures 7–121 and 7–122 are scans of a patient with renal cell carcinoma of the left kidney. The longitudinal scan of the left kidney (Fig 7–121) demonstrates marked distortion of the normal renal architecture. Visualization of the central echoes, as we see in the normal kidney, is not apparent. There are areas of increased echogenicity along with areas of decreased echogenicity (small arrows) noted throughout the kidney. This entire left kidney was filled with tumor. A longitudinal scan of the inferior vena cava of the same patient (Fig 7–122) delineates a large tumor within the lumen of the inferior vena cava. The inferior vena cava is markedly dilated due to partial obstruction by the tumor. There is also evidence of a tumor posterior to the inferior vena cava. The tumor mass extending from the left kidney is also seen in the caudal portion of the scan.

Figure 7–123 is a longitudinal scan in the midline of another patient with an unusual vascular finding. It demonstrates the aorta with the celiac axis and superior mesenteric artery arising from it. A markedly abnormal angulation to the superior mesenteric artery is noted. This is secondary to a massively dilated left renal vein. The patient has a large hypernephroma of the left kidney with marked arteriovenous shunting. The dramatically dilated left renal vein is secondary to increased blood flow. It is stretching and elevating the superior mesenteric artery.

Figure 7–124 is a transverse supine scan of the right kidney of another patient with a large tumor in the right renal bed. The tumor extends through the right renal vein to the inferior vena cava. The right renal vein is completely echo-filled; this is consistent with tumor deposits within it.

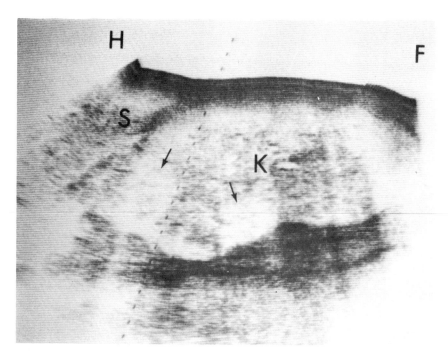

**FIG 7–121.**

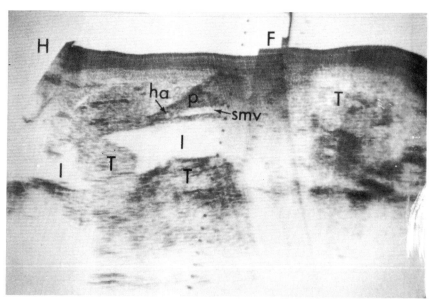

**FIG 7–122.**

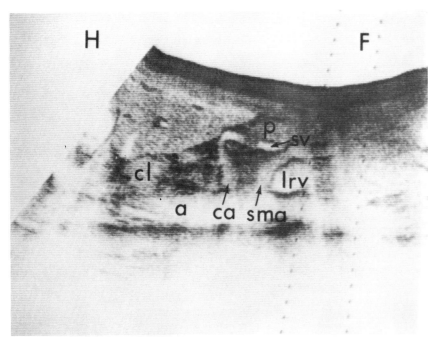

**FIG 7–123.**

| | | |
|---|---|---|
| **A** | = | Aorta |
| **a** | = | Aorta |
| **Arrows** | = | Hypoechogenic region of the tumor, (Fig 7–121) |
| **CA** | = | Celiac axis |
| **CL** | = | Caudate lobe |
| **Cr** | = | Crus |
| **F** | = | Foot |
| **H** | = | Head |
| **HA** | = | Hepatic artery |
| **I** | = | Inferior vena cava |
| **K** | = | Kidney |
| **L** | = | Left |
| **Li** | = | Liver |
| **LRV** | = | Left renal vein |
| **P** | = | Pancreas |
| **PV** | = | Portal vein |
| **R** | = | Right |
| **RRV** | = | Tumor in the right renal vein |
| **S** | = | Spleen |
| **SMA** | = | Superior mesenteric artery |
| **SMV** | = | Superior mesenteric vein |
| **SV** | = | Splenic vein |
| **T** | = | Tumor in the inferior vena cava and abdomen (Fig 7–122) |
| **T** | = | Hypernephroma of the right kidney (Fig 7–124) |

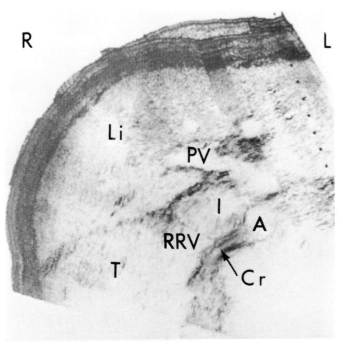

**FIG 7–124.**

## Septated Cystic Mass

Figures 7–125 through 7–128 are images made with various modalities of a renal mass in the right upper pole. Earlier case examples of a simple renal cyst considered the numerous criteria necessary to make the correct diagnosis of a simple renal cyst. First, the walls must be sharply identified when they are perpendicular to the beam path. Second, there must be no internal echoes except for noise or artifacts. Third, there must be prominent through-transmission. When these three criteria are met, the diagnosis of a simple renal cyst can be made on ultrasound examination. Often the workup will end at that point. However, if these criteria are not met, further imaging is necessary.

Figure 7–125 is a tomogram from an IVP study in which a well-marginated, low-density mass is present in the right upper pole (arrowheads). The mass is sharply demarcated and has the appearance of a renal cyst. Figure 7–126 is a CT scan of the right kidney in which we again see a low-density area in the lateral aspect of the right kidney. The borders of this fluid mass are slightly irregular but sharp. Figure 7–127 is a coronal scan obtained by MR imaging. The borders are not quite as sharp, and a low-density mass is present in the upper pole of the right kidney (arrowhead). Figure 7–128 is a transverse real-time ultrasound scan through an intercostal space. The fluid-filled mass has numerous septations within it. The septations are much more pronounced than in any of the images obtained by the other modalities. Because of the numerous septations, the diagnosis of a simple cyst could not be made. Even though the MR imaging and CT did not confirm the septations, the ultrasound appearance is highly suspicious. This could represent a septated cyst or a hemorrhagic neoplasm. Because of this finding, surgery was performed and a septated renal cyst was diagnosed. The workup must not stop with ultrasound unless the diagnosis of a simple cyst is made. If there is any question of septation or internal echoes, further examination must be

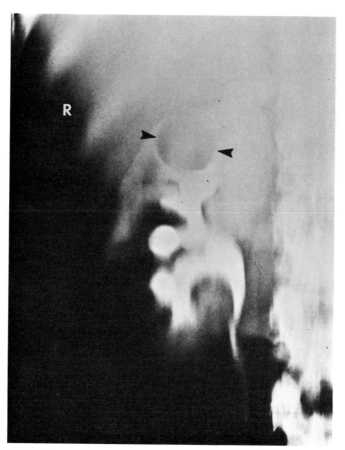

**FIG 7–125.**

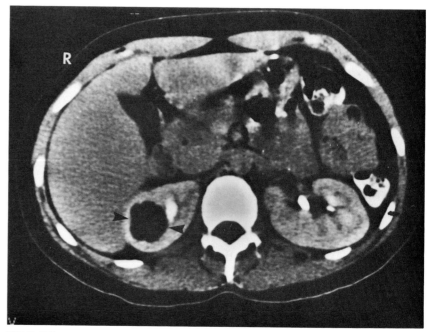

**FIG 7–126.**

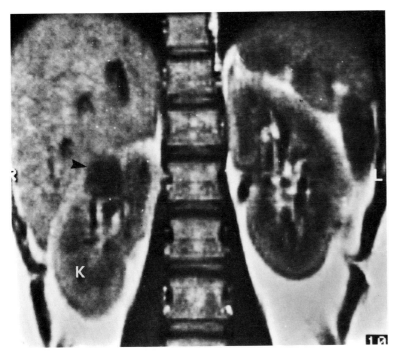

**FIG 7–127.**

undertaken. If other imaging modalities do not satisfactorily answer the question, needle biopsy or surgery is suggested. This is an excellent example of a septated renal mass which was highly suspicious for neoplasm. In this case, it turned out to be a septated renal cyst.

| | | |
|---|---|---|
| **Arrowheads** | = | Septated renal cyst |
| **K** | = | Kidney |
| **R** | = | Right |

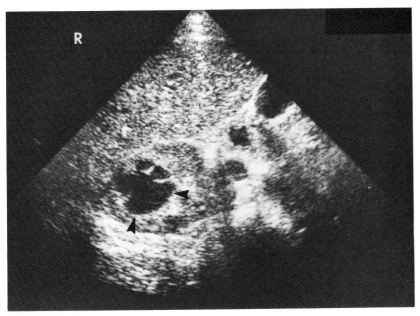

**FIG 7–128.**

## Renal Transplants

A longitudinal scan of a renal transplant in the right lower quadrant is seen in Figure 7–129. The strong central echoes are surrounded by the less echogenic renal parenchyma. A relatively lucent area is present within the renal parenchyma, secondary to a renal pyramid. The patient's right kidney is much more echogenic than the liver. This finding is consistent with chronic renal disease and warranted the renal transplant.

Figure 7–130 is an oblique longitudinal scan of a transplanted kidney undergoing rejection. Here we have difficulty visualizing the central echoes. The kidney is larger and thicker than usual. It is also somewhat less echogenic than normal. Renal transplants will enlarge in size when undergoing rejection.

Figure 7–131 is an example of a renal transplant in which hydronephrosis has developed. Hydronephrosis of a renal transplant is similar to that of a normally positioned kidney. We see a central sonolucency separating the central echoes. In this instance, the hydronephrosis extends into the calyceal region.

Figure 7–132 is another scan of a transplanted kidney in which we see mild hydronephrosis. The cause of the hydronephrosis, a renal stone, is visualized. Deep to the stone is acoustic shadowing.

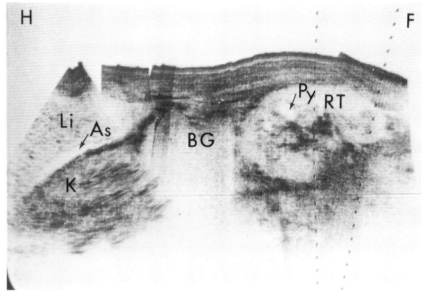

**FIG 7–129.**

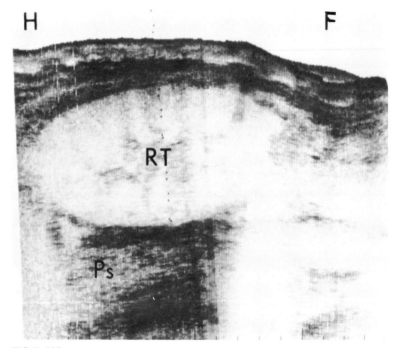

**FIG 7–130.**

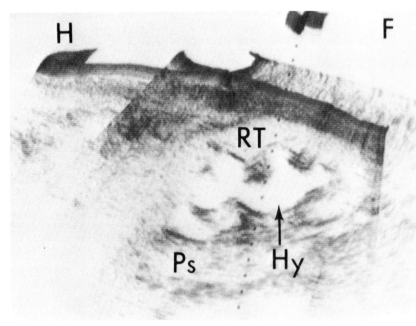

| | | |
|---|---|---|
| **As** | = | Ascites |
| **BG** | = | Bowel gas |
| **F** | = | Foot |
| **H** | = | Head |
| **Hy** | = | Hydronephrosis |
| **K** | = | Right kidney with chronic renal disease |
| **Li** | = | Liver |
| **Ps** | = | Psoas muscle |
| **Py** | = | Pyramid |
| **RT** | = | Renal transplant |
| **RT** | = | Renal transplant rejection (Fig 7–130) |
| **Sh** | = | Shadowing |
| **St** | = | Renal stone |

FIG 7–131.

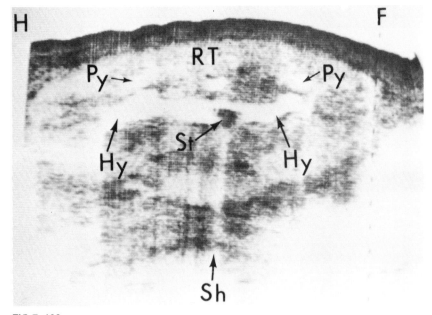

FIG 7–132.

## Renal Transplant Associated With Abscess and Urinoma

The perinephric region of a renal transplant is easily evaluated with ultrasound. An attempt should be made to visualize fluid collections around the transplanted kidney to rule out the possibility of abscesses, lymphoceles, hematomas, or urinomas. In a transverse section of a transplanted kidney (Fig 7–133), we see a relatively lucent mass on the lateral aspect of the kidney. This eventually was found to be a perinephric abscess (arrows). It was quite localized, and its expansion can be seen indenting the renal border.

Figure 7–134 is a scan of the transplanted kidney of another patient. A large fluid collection is seen surrounding both the upper and lower poles of the transplanted kidney. The fluid collection is not specific for any etiology, and at surgery it was found to be a large perinephric abscess that completely surrounded the transplanted kidney.

Figures 7–135 and 7–136 are scans from two different patients who also had fluid collections surrounding transplanted kidneys. In Figure 7–135, the fluid collection has some internal echoes within it. These could represent abscess, hematoma, urinoma with debris, or lymphocele with debris. At surgery, a urinoma was found. In Figure 7–136, a longitudinal scan of the abdomen demonstrates a transplanted kidney cephalad to a fluid-filled mass. Within the mass is a septum. This was also urinoma.

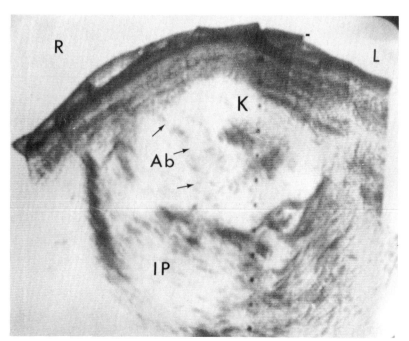

**FIG 7–133.**

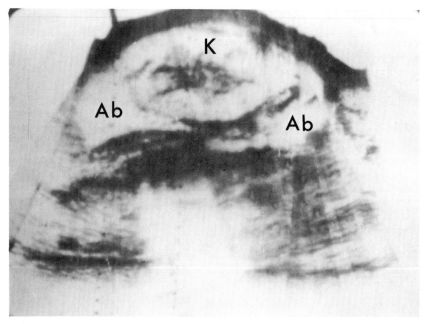

**FIG 7–134.**

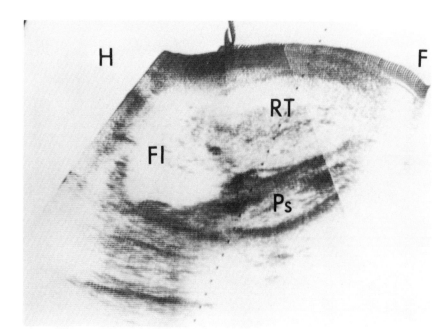

**FIG 7–135.**

SOURCE: Figures 7–133 and 7–136 are reproduced with permission from Cahill PJ, Cochran S, Sample WF: Conventional radiographic and ultrasonic imaging in renal transplantation. *Urology* 1977; 10(suppl): 33-42.

| | | |
|---|---|---|
| **Ab** | = | Perinephric abscess |
| **Arrows** | = | Abscess |
| **B** | = | Urinary bladder |
| **F** | = | Foot |
| **FI** | = | Urinoma |
| **H** | = | Head |
| **IP** | = | Iliopsoas muscle |
| **K** | = | Kidney |
| **L** | = | Left |
| **Ps** | = | Psoas muscle |
| **R** | = | Right |
| **RT** | = | Renal transplant |
| **S** | = | Septum in a urinoma |

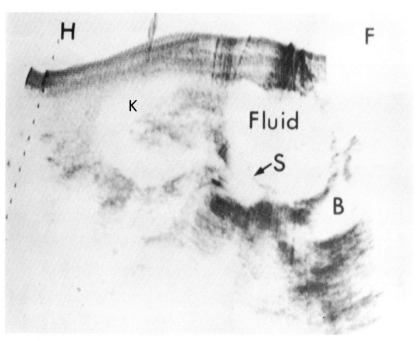

**FIG 7–136.**

## Renal Transplant
## With Lymphocele

The area around a renal transplant is examined to rule out any fluid collections or masses. Depending on their size and location, fluid collections may cause obstruction to the collecting system of the transplanted kidney. Lymphoceles will present as fluid-filled masses, with or without areas of septations.

The images in Figures 7–137 through 7–140 are all scans of the same patient, a middle-aged woman with a recent renal transplant. Figure 7–137 is a pelvic scan in which a fluid-filled mass is present cephalad to the urinary bladder. If the bladder were empty, this mass could be misdiagnosed for the urinary bladder since the mass is a single cystic structure. No septations are present within the mass.

Figure 7–138 is a longitudinal scan through the renal transplant obtained at the same time as the scan in Figure 7–137. Hydronephrosis is present in the transplant secondary to obstruction from the fluid-filled mass. The mass was tapped under ultrasound guidance and was found to be a lymphocele. However, the mass recurred quickly, and 1 month later the patient was operated on. The lymphocele was drained and a peritoneal window created to avoid further accumulation of the lymphocele.

Figure 7–139 and 7–140 are scans obtained after surgery. The pelvic scan in Figure 7–139 demonstrates disappearance of the lymphocele. The area cephalad to the urinary bladder does not demonstrate a fluid-filled collection. Figure 7–140 indicates that the hydronephrosis of the transplant has resolved after drainage of the lymphocele.

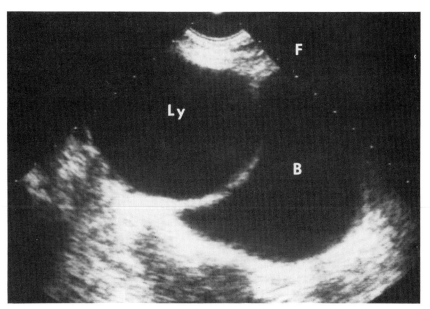

**FIG 7–137.**

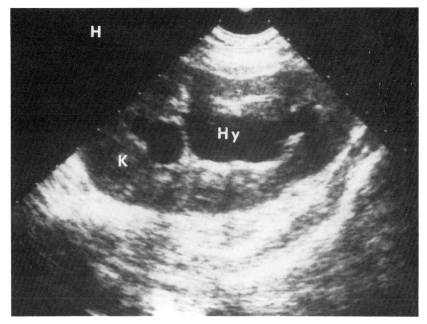

**FIG 7–138.**

B   =  Bladder
F   =  Foot
H   =  Head
Hy  =  Hydronephrosis
K   =  Kidney
Ly  =  Lymphocele
Ut  =  Uterus

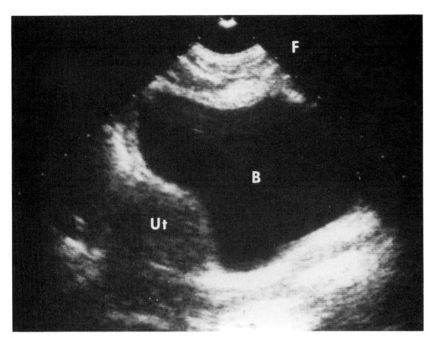

**FIG 7–139.**

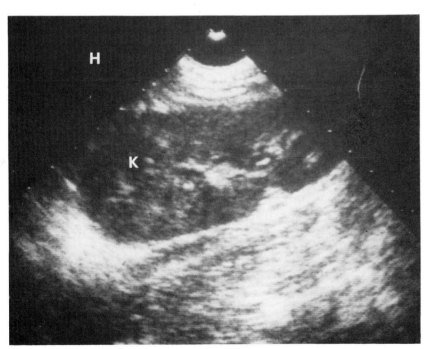

**FIG 7–140.**

## Renal Transplant With Lymphocele and Hematoma

Figure 7–141 is a longitudinal scan of the lower abdomen and pelvis in a patient with a recent renal transplant. Mild hydronephrosis of the transplanted kidney is present. A septated fluid-filled mass is noted in the pelvis, secondary to a lymphocele. The multiloculated cystic appearance is typical of a lymphocele. If the septations were not present, this lymphocele could easily be confused with the urinary bladder.

Figure 7–142 is a scan of the lower abdomen and pelvis in another patient with a renal transplant and hydronephrosis. Adjacent to the hydronephrosis is a large lymphocele. This was the cause of the hydronephrosis. Solid, echogenic components (arrowheads) are identified within the lymphocele. The mass was huge and measured 15 × 20 × 30 cm. The hydronephrosis was mild and surgery was not performed. The patient was examined 3 months later (Fig 7–143). Both the lymphocele and hydronephrosis had spontaneously resolved. Figure 7–143 is a scan through the long axis of the transplant showing a normal-appearing kidney.

Figure 7–144 is a scan through the iliac fossa over a renal transplant. A circumferential rind of increased echogenicity is seen surrounding the renal transplant. The patient had recently undergone renal biopsy, with the subsequent development of a perinephric hematoma. The kidney is compressed by the adjacent hematoma.

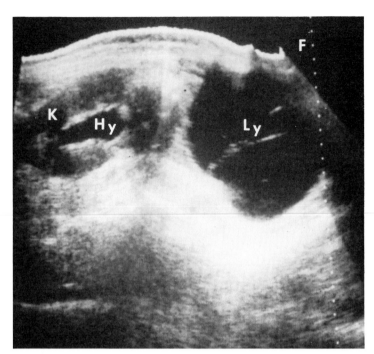

FIG 7–141.

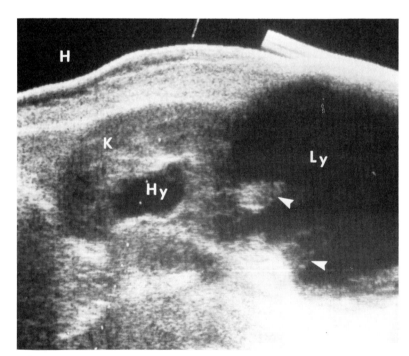

FIG 7–142.

arrows = Perinephric hematoma
F = Foot
H = Head
Hy = Hydronephrosis
K = Kidney
Ly = Lymphocele

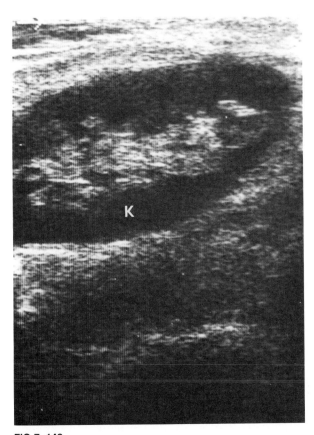

FIG 7–143.

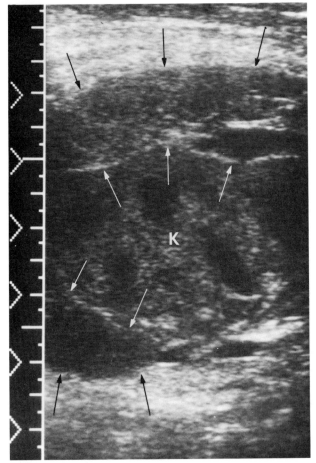

FIG 7–144.

# 8.
# Adrenal Ultrasonography

Nancy J. Worthen, M.D.

## Introduction

When the first edition of this book was published, adrenal sonography offered a noninvasive look at the adrenal region with better resolution than other available imaging modalities. At that time, Sample and Sarti reported similar diagnostic capabilities for second-generation computed tomography (CT) instruments and sonography in the evaluation of adrenal abnormalities. They reported a sensitivity of 82% for CT and 90% for sonography in imaging adrenal abnormalities, and a 95% specificity for each. As CT technology improved, however, a later prospective study comparing the imaging accuracy of sonography and CT found a dramatic diagnostic superiority for CT.[2] CT was reported to have a sensitivity of 84%, a specificity of 98%, and an accuracy of 90%; sonography was reported to have a sensitivity of 79%, a specificity of 61%, and an overall accuracy of 70%.

Ultrasound examination of the adrenal gland is technically difficult. It requires operator experience, special positioning of the patient, and a thorough knowledge of abdominal anatomy. CT is the imaging procedure of choice for the evaluation of adrenal glands to exclude pathology. In some instances, however, sonography is preferred for imaging a suspected adrenal lesion. These instances include children, pregnant women, thin adults, patients with known metastatic disease, and when CT is unavailable.

Many adrenal abnormalities, identified on sonograms will be incidental masses found on studies that have been performed for other clinical indications. The role of the sonographer in such instances is to define the sonographic characteristics and attempt to determine the origin of the lesion.

## Adrenal Anatomy

The adrenal glands are paired retroperitoneal structures. Each gland is contained within the perirenal space and is firmly attached to the renal fascia. This anatomic fusion prohibits motion of the adrenal glands during respiration or change in posture.

The right gland is suprarenal in location. It is situated between the right crus of diaphragm and the liver and is posterior to the inferior vena cava. The left gland is situated closer to and anterior to the upper pole of the left kidney. It is lateral to the left crus of the diaphragm and posterior to the tail of the pancreas. The esophagogastric junction is cephalad to the left gland. Caudad to it is the fourth portion of the duodenum.

The left adrenal gland is pyramidal or triangular in shape. The right gland tends to be more semilunar in shape. The average adrenal gland is normally 3–6 mm thick, 4–6 cm long, and 2–3 cm wide.

## Ultrasound Adrenal Imaging Technique

Large adrenal masses are easily imaged on routine longitudinal and transverse sonograms of the upper abdomen. The demonstration of smaller adrenal masses and normal adrenal glands requires specific scanning techniques and approaches. Sample was the first to describe specialized scanning of the adrenals using static B-mode scanning.[3, 4]

Transducer selection is based on patient size and depth of the adrenals. A 3.5-MHz transducer with a 13-mm face is used most frequently. A 5.0-MHz transducer may be used for imaging thinner adults and children.

The right adrenal gland is easier to scan than the left. The patient is placed in a decubitus position with the left side down. Transverse scans are performed via an intercostal approach using the liver as an acoustic window. The scanning plane is maintained with the transducer perpendicular to the planes of the medial border of the liver, the adrenal gland, and the crus of the diaphragm. Longitudinal scans can be performed from several approaches, depending on the liver size and its attenuation characteristics. A liver in which the left lobe crosses the midline may be scanned in an oblique longitudinal plane through the inferior vena cava (IVC). The right adrenal gland also may be imaged by scanning in a straight longitudinal plane through the right lobe of the liver and the IVC. When the liver is small or diseased, a more posterior longitudinal scan through the kidney may be used. Suspended respiration is best for longitudinal scanning, and occasionally a deep inspiration with suspended respiration will allow better separation of the adrenal and kidney.[3, 5] Sample reported an 85% visualization rate of the right adrenal gland and a 12% visualization rate of the right adrenal area using these techniques.[3, 4] The normal echogenicity of the adrenal is between that of the highly echogenic retroperitoneal fat and that of the mildly echogenic renal parenchyma.[3] Yeh also used static scanning for imaging the adrenals. He advocates the use of anterior transverse compound scanning with the patient in supine and semidecubitus positions to identify the right adrenal gland. He successfully identified the right adrenal gland in 78.5% of cases.[5]

The left adrenal gland is more difficult to scan. Sample described a coronal approach to the left adrenal through the spleen and kidney.[3, 4] Static scans are obtained with the patient in a left lateral decubitus position. The correct longitudinal scan plane is determined from initial transverse scans that define the axis of the left kidney and the position of the aorta. The resulting longitudinal scan is a posterior coronal scan with an oblique orientation. Using this approach, Sample reported visualization of the left adrenal in 85% of cases.[4] Yeh advocated using static compound scanning with the patient in a supine or semidecubitus position. Using anterior transverse and anterior longitudinal scans, he reported identifying the normal left adrenal in 44% of cases.[5]

Real-time scanning of the adrenals has historically received little attention. A single report confirmed Sample's original scanning techniques as the best approach for real-time evaluation of the adrenal regions.[6] The optimal real-time approach is to obtain intercostal transverse and longitudinal scans using a 3.5-MHz sector transducer. The transducer may be rocked back and forth in a rib space for complete visualization of the adrenal area. Gunther reported visualization of the adrenal area with real-time techniques but was unable to image the normal adrenal gland as a distinct structure. Failure to visualize the normal adrenal gland is probably related to the poor lateral resolution achievable with the real-time transducer, compared to resolution achievable with the focused static transducer. An advantage of real-time scanning may be its ability to resolve smaller adrenal lesions ($<$ 8 mm), compared to lesion resolution with static scanning ($>$ 12 mm).[5, 6] Both methods require the use of special views and an experienced operator for optimal results.

## Ultrasonographic Signs of Adrenal Disease

Adrenal masses are suspected when ultrasonography demonstrates a mass anterior and medial to the upper pole of either kidney. When the mass is found in the right adrenal area, it must be differentiated from a hepatic, renal, or retrocaval lymph node mass. The position of the right perirenal retroperitoneal fat has been used to identify the origin of the mass.[7] Hepatic and subhepatic masses will push the fat posteriorly, while adrenal and renal masses will displace the fat anteriorly. If the fat is wedged anteriorly near the upper pole of the right kidney, it is suggestive of an adrenal mass. A right adrenal mass may also cause anterior displacement or indentation of the posterior aspect of the IVC.[8-10] Kurtz specified that an adrenal mass should elevate only the upper hepatic portion of the IVC, i.e., that portion between the diaphragm and the portal vein. Right adrenal lesions larger than 5 cm may cause downward displacement of the right kidney.[11] Due to the orientation of the right renal capsule and the adrenal gland (both having curved ends), it is difficult to achieve separation of the glandular and capsular interface. Invasion of the kidney by an adrenal mass cannot be excluded unless a cleavage plane of the kidney and the adrenal area is seen on all scan planes.[9] Enlarged lymph nodes and other retroperitoneal masses in the same area of the adrenal gland are difficult to differentiate from adrenal masses.

Normal structures in the right upper quadrant that may simulate an adrenal mass on ultrasound scans are the crus of the diaphragm and the second portion of the duodenum.

A lesion in the region of the left adrenal must be differentiated from splenic, pancreatic, and renal lesions. Adrenal masses can be differentiated from pancreatic masses by the displacement of the splenic vessels. An adrenal mass will displace the splenic vessels anteriorly, while a pancreatic mass will displace them posteriorly.[11] Separation of an adrenal mass from a renal mass requires demonstration of an adrenal-renal interface.

Normal structures that may mimic a left adrenal mass on ultrasound scans include the esophagogastric junction, the stomach, the body of the pancreas, and the medial lobulation of the spleen.[12] Splenic vessels and the left renovascular bundle may also cause confusion. Real-time scanning with water ingestion and real-time scanning with Doppler techniques may help distinguish the normal bowel and vascular structures.

In general, tumors or masses of the adrenal should

sonographically appear as hypoechoic round masses.[6, 11] Adrenal cysts and/or adrenal calcifications have typical sonographic patterns.

## Ultrasound Imaging of Adrenal Pathology

### Cushing's Disease

Cushing's syndrome or hyperadrenocortism is the overproduction of steroid substances. Clinical signs are truncal obesity, buffalo hump, hypertension, abdominal striae, demineralization with hypercalcemuria, and psychoses in the advanced state.

The adrenal cortical hyperfunction of Cushing's disease is caused by either a primary pituitary malfunction (70%) or a functioning adrenal cortical neoplasm (30%), either a carcinoma or an adenoma.

Adrenal carcinoma can be identified as the etiology on the basis of chemical laboratory data. However, it is sometimes difficult to distinguish adrenal hyperplasia secondary to pituitary malfunction from an adrenal adenoma. Imaging of the adrenals in a patient with Cushing's disease may be performed preoperatively to determine the location of a possible adrenal neoplasm and to evaluate local extension and metastatic potential.

Because of the obesity associated with this syndrome, sonography is an ineffective imaging technique in identifying adrenal pathology. Sample evaluated four patients with Cushing's syndrome and successfully detected adrenal adenomas in each. Others have not reported such good results with the Cushing's disease patient.[2]

### Hyperaldosteronism

Hyperaldosteronism results from the increased production of the steroid aldosterone. Clinically, affected patients have hypertension associated with hypokalemia, hyperkaluria, and low plasma renin levels. Hyperaldosteronism is most frequently caused by adrenal cortical adenomas (90%) or diffuse focal adrenocortical hyperplasia (10%). Patients are thin to normal in size.

Imaging the adrenal area is useful in identifying an aldosteronoma within an adrenal gland. These tumors are usually small, ranging in size from 3 to 35 mm.

Most are between 8 and 20 mm in size.[13] Because of the slender body habitus of of affected patients, sonography has had some success in identifying the lesions.[2, 5, 6, 11] The smallest lesion diagnosed on static scanning was 1.3 cm,[11] and an 8-mm lesion was diagnosed on real-time scanning.[6] Sonographically, aldosteronomas are round and relatively anechoic.

## Adrenal Cysts

Cysts rarely develop in the adrenal glands. When they do occur, they are usually asymptomatic. Adrenal cysts may be secondary to hemorrhage or may be true cysts, such as retention cysts, cystic adenomas, or angiomatous cysts. No malignancies associated with adrenal cysts have been reported.[14] Sonographically the cysts appear as anechoic structures in the adrenal regions. They may mimic, and therefore must be distinguished from, renal cysts, hydronephrosis, splenic cysts or pancreatic pseudocysts.

## Pheochromocytoma

A pheochromocytoma is a functional tumor of the adrenal medulla that produces catecholamines which in turn cause hypertension. About 90% of pheochromocytomas are benign and 10% are malignant. These tumors are commonly located within the adrenal glands. In 10% of cases they are extra-adrenal, occurring in the thoracic or abdominal paraganglionic sympathetic chain. In 10% of cases they are found in both adrenals. Because of the bilateral and extra-adrenal locations of pheochromocytomas, accurate preoperative imaging is imperative.

Sonography has been successful in identifying adrenal pheochromocytomas. The lesions usually appear as a homogeneous mass with low level internal echoes. Yeh diagnosed 17 pheochromocytomas in the adrenal glands, four of which were bilateral. The tumors ranged in size from 2 to 7.2 cm. Yeh found no specific sonographic features that would differentiate a pheochromocytoma from other adrenal lesions.[5] Bowerman et al. described the sonographic features of eight pheochromocytomas. The larger tumors tended to have more hemorrhage and necrosis, resulting in sonographic heterogeneity and hypoechoic components. Acute hemorrhage tended to be echo-

genic.[15] Two cases of extra-adrenal pheochromocytoma diagnosed by ultrasound have been reported.[16] They were located in the renal hilum and resembled para-aortic nodal masses.

Ultrasound cannot locate extra-adrenal masses and therefore is of limited value in examining the patient with pheochromocytoma. In the abdomen, the para-aortic lymph node chain and the organ of Zuckerhandl are frequently obscured by bowel gas. Sonography is also of no value in evaluating the chest for extra-abdominal pheochromocytoma.

## Neuroblastoma

Neuroblastoma most frequently is a tumor of childhood. It usually arises in the adrenal medulla. Occasionally, like a pheochromocytoma, it may arise in an extra-adrenal location. Neuroblastomas tend to be highly echogenic tumors, probably because of hemorrhage, calcification, or necrosis.[17] The same limitations that apply to the sonographic detection of pheochromocytomas also apply to the detection of neuroblastomas.

## Myelolipomas

Myelolipomas of the adrenal gland are benign, rare, nonfunctioning tumors composed in varying proportion of fat and hematopoietic elements. Most patients are asymptomatic; however, some may complain of pain due to hemorrhage, necrosis, or pressure on adjacent structures.

Sonographically myelolipomas appear as highly echogenic lesions in the adrenal region.[18–20] The echo pattern is characteristic of a lipomatous lesion.[19, 21] When small these lesions may blend into the adjacent perirenal fat. Also, they may appear similar to angiomyolipomas of the kidney. There is some variability in their echogenicity, depending on their composition.[22] CT and fine needle biopsy are helpful in further characterizing a myelolipoma.

## Metastatic Disease

Many neoplasms can metastasize to the adrenal gland. The most frequent are tumors of the lung, breast, and melanomas.[23] Metastases to the adrenal gland seldom cause clinical symptoms. Sonography is useful in evaluating patients with known primary tumors for the progression of metastatic adrenal disease.[24]

The pattern of an adrenal metastasis is nonspecific and may be identical to that produced by primary adrenal tumors. The tumors appear solid, with varying degrees of echogenicity. The appearance of bilateral suprarenal masses on transverse scans has been reported to resemble the headlight of a car and may be characteristic of adrenal metastases.[25]

## References

1. Sample WF, Sarti DA: Computed tomography and gray scale ultrasonography of the adrenal gland: A comparative study. *Radiology* 1978; 128:377–383.
2. Abrams HL, Siegelman SS, Adams DF, et al: Computed tomography versus ultrasound of the adrenal gland: A prospective study. *Radiology* 1982; 143:121–127.
3. Sample WF: A new technique for the evaluation of the adrenal gland with gray scale ultrasonography. *Radiology* 1977; 124:463–469.
4. Sample WF: Adrenal ultrasonography. *Radiology* 1978; 127:461–466.
5. Yeh H: Sonography of the adrenal glands: Normal glands and small masses. *AJR* 1980; 135:1167–1177.
6. Gunther RW, Kelbel C, Lenner V: Real-time ultrasound of normal adrenal glands and small tumors. *JCU* 1984; 12:211–217.
7. Gore RM, Callen PW, Filly RA: Displaced retroperitoneal fat: Sonographic guide to right upper quadrant mass localization. *Radiology* 1982; 142:701–705.
8. Bernardino ME, Libshitz HI, Green B, et al: Ultrasonic demonstration of inferior vena caval involvement with right adrenal gland masses. *JCU* 1978; 6:167–169.
9. Bernardino ME, Goldstein HM, Green B: Gray scale ultrasonography of adrenal neoplasms. *AJR* 1978; 130:741–744.
10. Kurtz AB, Rubin C, Goldberg BB: Ultrasound diagnosis of masses elevating the inferior vena cava. *AJR* 1979; 132:401–406.
11. Yeh H, Mitty HA, Rose J, et al: Ultrasonography of adrenal masses: Usual features. *Radiology* 1978; 127:467–474.
12. Gooding GAW: The ultrasonic and computed tomographic appearance of splenic lobulations: A consideration in the ultrasonic differential of masses adjacent to the left kidney. *Radiology* 1978; 126:719.
13. Conn JW, Knopf RF, Nesbit KM: Clinical characteristics of primary aldosteronism from an analysis of 145 cases. *Am J Surg* 1964; 107:159.
14. Leder LD, Richter HJ, Stambohs C: Pathology of renal and adrenal neoplasms, in Lohr E (ed): *Renal and Adrenal Tumors.* New York, Springer-Verlag, 1979, pp 1–68.
15. Bowerman RA, Silver TM, Jaffee MH, et al: Sonography of adrenal pheochromocytomas. *AJR* 1981; 137:1227.
16. Yeh H, Mitty HA, Rose J, et al: Ultrasonography of adrenal masses: Unusual manifestations. *Radiology* 1978; 127:475–483.
17. Yeh H: Ultrasound and CT of the adrenals. *Semin Ultrasound* 1982; 3(2):97–113.
18. Behan M, Martin EC, Muecke EC, et al: Myelolipoma of the adrenal: Two cases with ultrasound and CT findings. *AJR* 1977; 129:993–996.
19. Scheible W, Ellenbogen PH, Leopold GR, et al: Lipomatous tumors of the kidney and adrenal: Apparent echographic specificity. *Radiology* 1978; 129:153–156.
20. Miller EI, Dickenson RW: Sonographic appearance of myelolipoma: Demonstration of adrenal and pelvic lesions. *JCU* 1983; 11:179–181.
21. Behan M, Kazam E: The echogenic characteristics of fatty tissues and tumors. *Radiology* 1978; 129:143–151.
22. Vick CW, Zeman RK, Mannes E, et al: Adrenal myelolipoma: CT and ultrasound findings. *Urol Radiol* 1984; 6:7–13.
23. Abrams HL, Spiro R, Goldstein N: Metastases in carcinoma: Analysis of 100 autopsied cases. *Cancer* 1950; 3:74.
24. Forsythe JR, Gosink BB, Leopold GR: Ultrasound in the evaluation of adrenal masses. *JCU* 1976; 5:31–34.
25. Zornoza J, Bernardino ME: Bilateral adrenal metastases: "Headlight" sign. *Urology* 1980; 15:91–92.

# CASES

Dennis A. Sarti, M.D.

## Normal Right Adrenal Gland

Ultrasound examination of the adrenal gland is best performed in thin patients. Excellent visualization of the adrenal gland is usually achievable in such patients. Obese patients are quite difficult to examine and CT is the method of choice. The right adrenal gland is usually easy to visualize, especially in thin patients. The reason is that the ultrasonic window of the liver allows good visualization of the adrenal gland.

The adrenal gland is situated between the liver and the crus of the diaphragm, posterior to the inferior vena cava and just cephalad to the right kidney. Retroperitoneal fat surrounds the right adrenal gland. The best scan plane for visualizing the right adrenal gland is through an intercostal space on the lateral aspect of the abdomen. The patient may be turned in a lateral decubitus position with the left side down for better visualization. In a lateral approach, axial resolution is utilized to visualize the right adrenal gland. Axial resolution is superior to lateral resolution.

The right adrenal gland usually appears as a linear or curvilinear structure situated within the highly reflective retroperitoneal fat. The acoustic texture of the adrenal gland is similar to that of the crus of the diaphragm. Transverse scans through the most appropriate intercostal space are initially performed in an attempt to visualize the right kidney. As scanning is continued cephalad, the upper pole of the right kidney will be visualized. During scanning of the right kidney, the inferior vena cava is identified. Once scanning continues just cephalad to the upper pole of the right kidney, the right adrenal gland will come into view. It is situated posterior to the inferior vena cava and medial to the crus of the diaphragm (Fig 8–1). The highly reflective fat provides a background against which the right

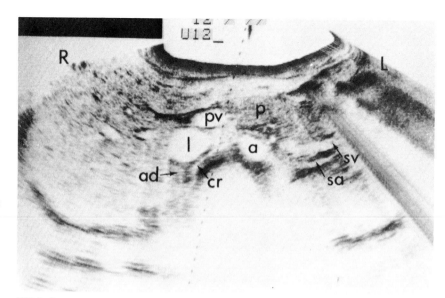

FIG 8–1.

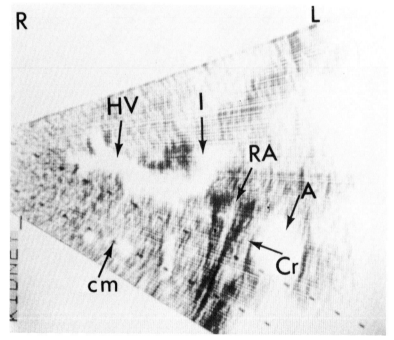

FIG 8–2.

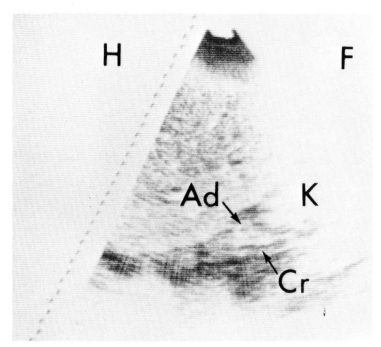

**FIG 8–3.**

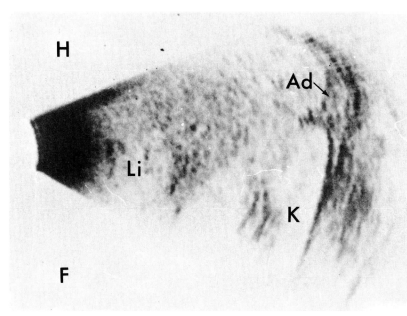

**FIG 8–4.**

adrenal gland stands out as a low-amplitude acoustic texture (Fig 8–2).

It is best to use real-time transducers with small acoustic heads in order to work within an intercostal space. Once the adrenal gland has been located on transverse scans, the transducer head is turned 90° to image the adrenal gland in a longitudinal coronal plane (Fig 8–3). This plane permits visualization of the upper pole of the kidney and the relationship of the adrenal gland to the upper pole (Fig 8–4). Because of attenuation and refraction of the sound beam by fat, obese patients are much more difficult to examine than thin patients. Obese patients are better examined by CT. The adrenal gland may also be difficult to visualize when liver pathology is present. Entities such as cirrhosis or fatty infiltration cause increased attenuation of the sound beam. Because of its typical appearance and consistent location, visualization of the right adrenal gland through the liver is usually not difficult.

SOURCE: Figures 8–2 and 8–4 are reproduced with permission from Sample WF: Adrenal ultrasonography. *Radiology* 1978; 127:461-466; Figure 8–3 is reproduced with permission from Callen PW, Filly RA, Sarti DA, et al: Ultrasonography of the diaphragmatic crura. *Radiology* 1979; 130:721–724.

| | | |
|---|---|---|
| **A** | = | Aorta |
| **a** | = | Aorta |
| **ad** | = | Right adrenal gland |
| **Ad** | = | Right adrenal gland |
| **cm** | = | Centimeter markers |
| **cr** | = | Crus of the diaphragm |
| **Cr** | = | Crus of the diaphragm |
| **F** | = | Foot |
| **H** | = | Head |
| **HV** | = | Hepatic veins |
| **I** | = | Inferior vena cava |
| **K** | = | Right kidney |
| **L** | = | Left |
| **Li** | = | Liver |
| **p** | = | Pancreas |
| **pv** | = | Portal vein |
| **R** | = | Right |
| **RA** | = | Right adrenal gland |
| **sa** | = | Splenic artery |
| **sv** | = | Splenic vein |

## Normal Left Adrenal Gland

Since a consistent acoustic window is not present on the left side, the left adrenal gland is much more difficult to visualize than the right. Attempts to visualize the left adrenal gland from an anterior approach are usually unsuccessful because of air in the stomach and colon. Therefore, the left adrenal gland is best visualized from a lateral or more often a posterior lateral approach. The patient is examined in the decubitus position with the right side down. A small-head real-time transducer is preferred since most scanning occurs in intercostal spaces. A large-head transducer is difficult to use because of the intercostal work space. Numerous scans are obtained at different levels in the intercostal region. The final scan plane is determined by the intercostal space that yields the best visualization of the region.

A lateral posterior approach is most often successful in visualization of the left adrenal gland. The proper scan plane lines up the left kidney and the aorta so that both can be visualized on the scan. The left adrenal gland is a triangular structure usually situated anterior to the upper pole of the left kidney (Fig 8–5). When this posterior lateral approach lines up the kidney and the aorta, the transducer is turned 90% so that a longitudinal plane of the left adrenal gland may be obtained. The left adrenal gland is situated between the upper pole of the left kidney and the aorta with the crus adjacent to the aorta (Fig 8–6).

If the spleen is quite prominent, a scan plane utilizing a coronal approach is suggested. The adrenal gland will be seen cephalad to the left kidney between the spleen and the crus of the diaphragm (Fig 8–7).

In those rare instances when the liver is markedly enlarged, the left adrenal gland may be visualized from an anterior approach. In this approach the liver functions as an acoustic window, just as it does in an examination of the right adrenal gland. Therefore, a large left lobe of the liver will permit visualization of the adrenal gland from an anterior approach (Fig 8–8). This

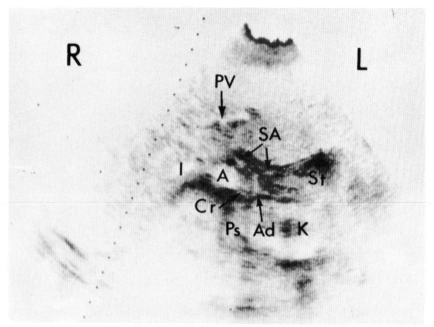

**FIG 8–5.**

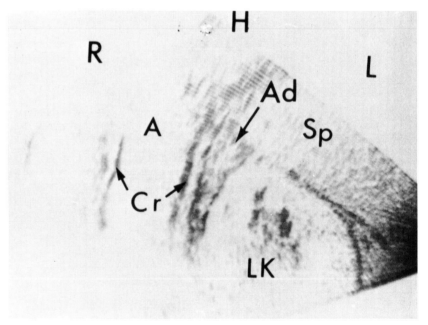

**FIG 8–6.**

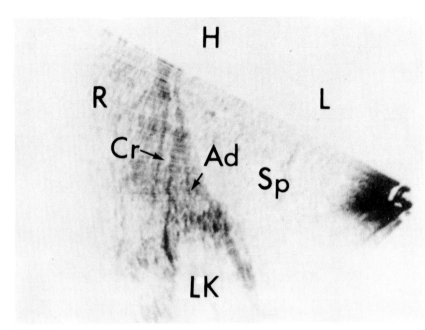

**FIG 8–7.**

situation is highly unusual. Because of the numerous anatomic structures in the vicinity of the left adrenal gland, it is more difficult to visualize than the right. Also, the left upper quadrant is always a more difficult ultrasonic examination because of the lack of good acoustic windows. Most successful scanning of this region is performed in the intercostal spaces utilizing the lateral or posterior lateral approach.

| | | |
|---|---|---|
| **A** | = | Aorta |
| **Ad** | = | Left adrenal gland |
| **Cr** | = | Crus of the diaphragm |
| **Du** | = | Duodenum |
| **F** | = | Foot |
| **H** | = | Head |
| **I** | = | Inferior vena cava |
| **K** | = | Left kidney |
| **L** | = | Left |
| **Li** | = | Liver |
| **LA** | = | Left kidney |
| **P** | = | Pancreas |
| **Ps** | = | Psoas |
| **PV** | = | Portal vein |
| **R** | = | Right |
| **SA** | = | Splenic artery |
| **Sp** | = | Spleen |
| **St** | = | Stomach |

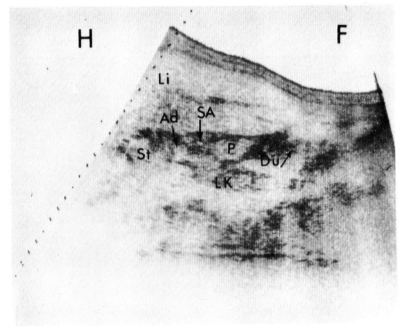

**FIG 8–8.**

## Pitfalls in Localization of the Left Adrenal Gland

Potential problems arise in visualization of the left adrenal gland because of the numerous anatomic structures found in the left upper quadrant. These anatomic structures are often confused with the left adrenal gland. The various structures located in the left upper quadrant include the esophagogastric junction, cardia of the stomach, duodenum, spleen, tail of the pancreas, splenic vessels, and left renal vessels. They can usually be differentiated from the left adrenal gland by their differing echo texture and contour. However, masses arising from any of the above-mentioned structures can be mistaken for left adrenal masses, or vice versa.

When the stomach is air filled, it is not mistaken for any adrenal masses since it obscures visualization of structures deep to it by its high reflectivity. However, in the collapsed state, the stomach can be confused with adrenal pathology (Fig 8–9). The usual clue that the stomach is the structure being imaged is the highly echogenic central mucosal lining. If there is any question, the patient can be given water to drink, and real-time examination will image the stomach.

The fourth portion of the duodenum sits adjacent to the aorta in the retroperitoneal region and quite close to the left adrenal gland. The duodenum can also be confused with a mass in the left adrenal gland (Fig 8–10). Again, the highly echogenic central mucosal echoes are the initial clue that the structure imaged is part of the GI tract. Real-time examination will often demonstrate peristalsis. If there is any question, the patient can be given water to drink.

The spleen is extremely variable in size and location. It may be situated quite cephalad underneath the right hemidiaphragm, or it may be laterally oriented against the costal margin. Any position between these two extremes is possible. The spleen may have lobulations and may be accompanied by accessory spleens. Medial lobulation of the spleen, as shown in

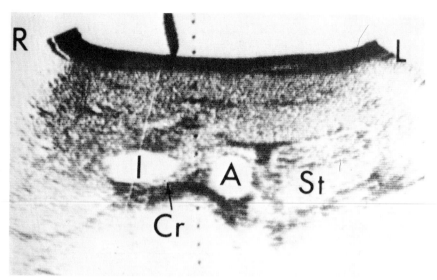

**FIG 8–9.**

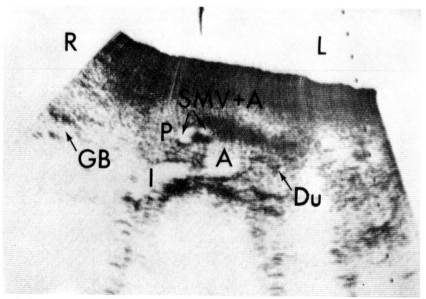

**FIG 8–10.**

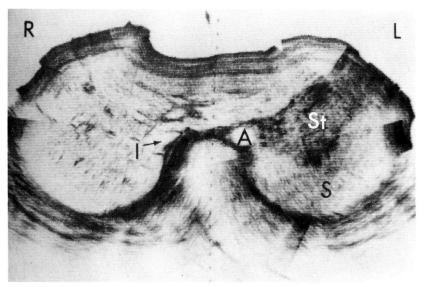

**FIG 8–11.**

Figure 8–11, indicates how the medial portion of the spleen can reside adjacent to the aorta. The sonographic picture may be quite confusing and may lead to an incorrect diagnosis of an enlarged left adrenal gland.

Numerous vessels are present in the upper left quadrant. These most often arise from the splenic artery and vein, which can be quite tortuous. Figure 8–12 shows prominent splenic veins cephalad to the left kidney; these veins may be mistaken for cysts in the adrenal gland. Recognizing the numerous anatomic structures in the left upper quadrant is most important in examining the left adrenal gland.

| | | |
|---|---|---|
| **A** | = | Aorta |
| **Ad** | = | Left adrenal gland |
| **As** | = | Ascites |
| **Cr** | = | Crus of the diaphragm |
| **Du** | = | Fourth portion of the duodenum |
| **GB** | = | Stones in the gallbladder |
| **H** | = | Head |
| **I** | = | Inferior vena cava |
| **K** | = | Left kidney |
| **L** | = | Left |
| **P** | = | Pancreas |
| **R** | = | Right |
| **S** | = | Spleen |
| **SMV** | = | Superior mesenteric vein |
| **SMA** | = | Superior mesenteric artery |
| **St** | = | Stomach |
| **SV** | = | Dilated splenic vein |

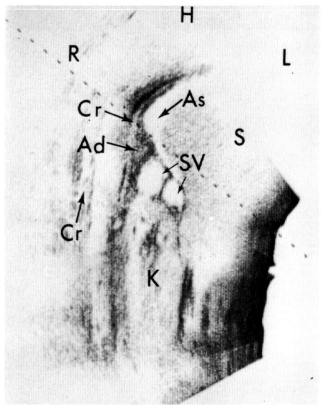

**FIG 8–12.**

## Adrenal Masses

As in any other part of the body, masses of the adrenal gland can be characterized by their ultrasound appearance. Pseudocysts of the adrenal gland are the most common type of adrenal cystic disease. They are usually the result of hemorrhage into or around the adrenal gland. They may be either secondary to trauma or, as in many cases, idiopathic. Ultimately, pseudocysts may form secondary to hemorrhage or necrosis into a tumor. A common form of adrenal pseudocyst occurs during the neonatal period and is related to adrenal hemorrhage in the gland. Pseudocysts appear as rounded, fluid-containing areas and usually have all the features of a fluid mass (Fig 8–13). In some cases, regions of calcification or dense clot retraction may persist and give some substance to the cyst wall or account for a solid projection within the fluid (Fig 8–14). In this instance, the solid component appears as a thickened portion to the wall in the deep aspect of the adrenal cyst.

Calcification of the adrenal gland has the same ultrasound appearance as calcification elsewhere in the body. Figure 8–15 shows a mass cephalad to the right kidney with a highly reflective border and acoustic shadowing. This scan was obtained in a 62-year-old woman with a history of tuberculosis. Calcification was noted in the right upper quadrant on a KUB study, and an ultrasound examination was ordered to localize the area of calcification. Figure 8–15 indicates the right adrenal gland as the site of origin. Figure 8–16 shows another example of calcification in the right adrenal gland. On this longitudinal scan a large right adrenal mass is present cephalad to the right kidney. A portion of the mass is calcified. The highly reflective borders and marked attenuation indicate calcification within a portion of the mass.

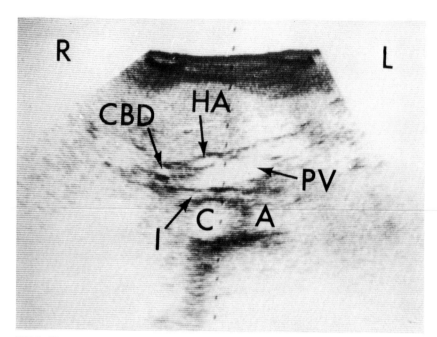

**FIG 8–13.**

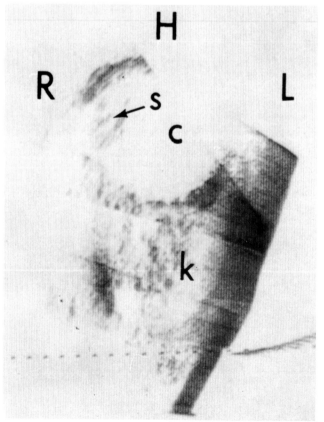

**FIG 8–14.**

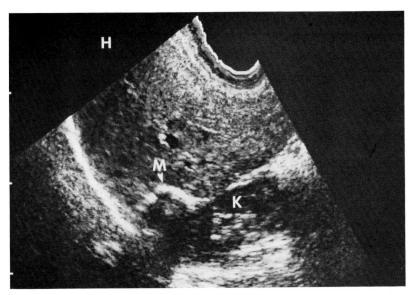

**FIG 8–15.**

| | | |
|---|---|---|
| **A** | = | Aorta |
| **Arrows** | = | Large adrenal mass |
| **C** | = | Cyst of the adrenal |
| **Ca++** | = | Calcification |
| **CBD** | = | Common bile duct |
| **D** | = | Diaphragm |
| **F** | = | Foot |
| **H** | = | Head |
| **HA** | = | Hepatic artery |
| **I** | = | Inferior vena cava |
| **K** | = | Kidney |
| **L** | = | Left |
| **M** | = | Calcified adrenal mass |
| **PV** | = | Portal vein |
| **R** | = | Right |
| **RK** | = | Right kidney |
| **S** | = | Solid component of adrenal cyst |

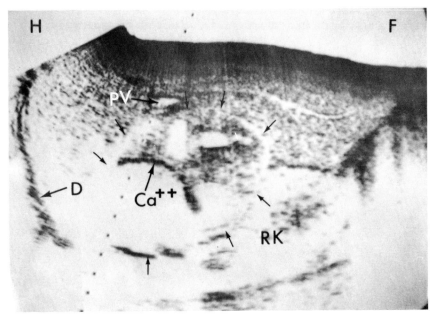

**FIG 8–16.**

## Adrenal Mass

In the discussion of the normal anatomy of the right adrenal gland, the relationship of the gland to the inferior vena cava was emphasized. The right adrenal gland is situated directly posterior to the inferior vena cava and just cephalad to the upper pole of the right kidney. Any distortion of the inferior vena cava will yield important clues to the site of origin of a right upper quadrant mass. If there is localized elevation and anterior displacement of the inferior vena cava in the region slightly cephalad to the right kidney, a right adrenal mass is the most likely site of origin. Figures 8–17 and 8–18 are transverse and longitudinal scans of a patient with pheochromocytoma of the right adrenal gland. The characteristic elevation of the inferior vena cava, the posteroinferior depression of the kidney with a clear margin between the mass and the right kidney, and draping of the right renal vein anteriorly over the mass properly localize the process to the right posterior retroperitoneum. Because of its location relative to the inferior vena cava and the right kidney, the site of origin is the right adrenal gland.

Figure 8–19 is the scan of another patient with pheochromocytoma. Again a retroperitoneal mass is seen to cause inferior displacement of the vena cava anteriorly. This displacement is very localized and compatible with a right adrenal mass. Note that the inferior vena cava has a normal appearance cephalad and caudad to the mass. When displacement of the inferior vena cava is very localized, as it is here, the diagnosis of a right adrenal mass can be made. If the inferior vena cava is displaced in a generalized manner over a larger length of the inferior vena cava, as in Figure 8–20, an adrenal mass is not the correct diagnosis. Figure 8–20 demonstrates generalized displacement of the inferior vena cava, which is surrounded by a mass over its entire length. This is an example of diffuse adenopathy surrounding the inferior vena cava rather than a localized adrenal lesion.

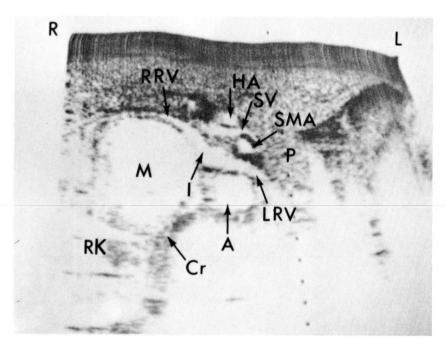

FIG 8–17.

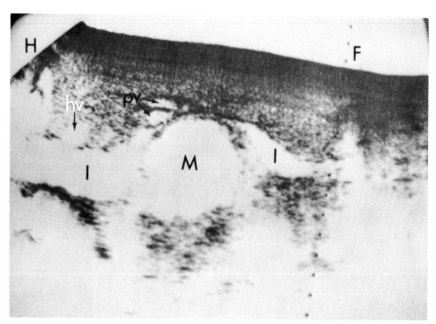

FIG 8–18.

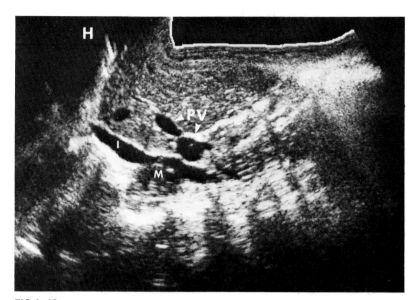

**FIG 8–19.**

| | | |
|---|---|---|
| **A** | = | Aorta |
| **Arrowheads** | = | Adenopathy around the inferior vena cava |
| **Cr** | = | Crus of the diaphragm |
| **F** | = | Foot |
| **H** | = | Head |
| **HA** | = | Hepatic artery |
| **hv** | = | Hepatic vein |
| **I** | = | Inferior vena cava |
| **L** | = | Left |
| **LRV** | = | Left renal vein |
| **M** | = | Adrenal mass (pheochromocytoma) |
| **P** | = | Pancreas |
| **PV** | = | Portal vein |
| **R** | = | Right |
| **RA** | = | Right renal artery |
| **RK** | = | Right kidney |
| **RRV** | = | Right renal veinn |
| **SMA** | = | Superior mesenteric artery |
| **SV** | = | Splenic vein |

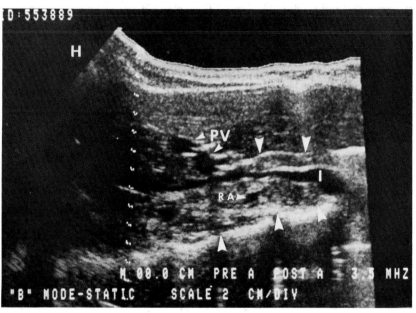

**FIG 8–20.**

## Adrenal Mass

Although ultrasound can identify an adrenal mass, it cannot discriminate the type of tumor imaged. The examiner must correlate the ultrasound appearance with clinical and laboratory data to determine the specific lesion that is imaged.

Aldosteronomas tend to be small and therefore challenge the imaging capabilities of both ultrasound and CT. Furthermore, the clinical syndrome may be secondary to nontumorous hyperplasia or a nodular form of hyperplasia. If the clinical syndrome is caused by a single adenoma, careful scanning in the adrenal areas with close attention to nearby anatomy will disclose a rounded mass, frequently only 1.5–2 cm in diameter. Figure 8–21 is a transverse scan through an intercostal space of a patient with a small aldosteronoma. Figure 8–22 is a CT scan of the same patient and made at approximately the same level as the ultrasound scan. Note the close correlation between the ultrasound and CT studies. CT will yield better visualization of the adrenal areas if the patient has adequate surrounding retroperitoneal fat. If very little fat is present, ultrasound is an excellent imaging modality.

Pheochromocytomas are generally medium-sized tumors, usually over 2 cm in diameter. Because of their size, they are usually readily visualized on ultrasound examinations when they occur in the adrenal or perirenal regions. The smaller tumors usually appear as rounded masses with low level echogenicity. Figures 8–23 and 8–24 are longitudinal and coronal scans of a teenage boy with hypertension. A well-circumscribed, poorly echogenic mass is present in the left adrenal region. This led to the diagnosis of pheochromocytoma. Since pheochromocytomas may occur bilaterally in 10% of patients, both adrenal areas must be scanned carefully.

Pheochromocytomas may occur in extra-adrenal locations such as the aortic region in either the chest or the abdomen or near the origin of the inferior mesenteric artery in the region of the organ of Zuckerkandl. These

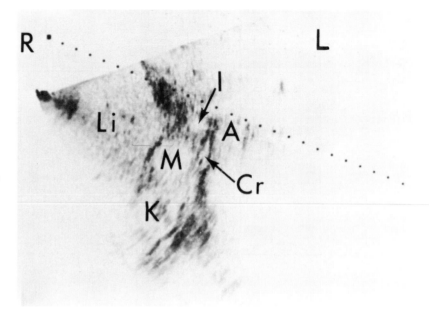

**FIG 8–21.**

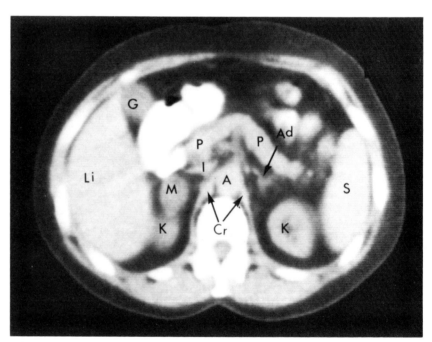

**FIG 8–22.**

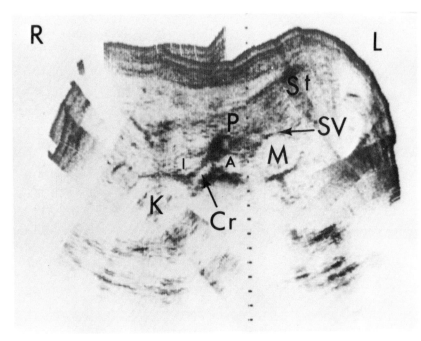

**FIG 8–23.**

latter locations are frequently not well visualized on sonograms because of overlying bowel gas. CT of this region usually yields adequate visualization of the retroperitoneum at the level of the aortic bifurcation.

| | | |
|---|---|---|
| **A** | = | Aorta |
| **Ad** | = | Adrenal |
| **Cr** | = | Crus of the diaphragm |
| **Du** | = | Duodenum |
| **F** | = | Foot |
| **G** | = | Gallbladder |
| **H** | = | Head |
| **I** | = | Inferior vena cava |
| **K** | = | Kidney |
| **L** | = | Left |
| **Li** | = | Liver |
| **M** | = | Adrenal mass |
| **P** | = | Pancreas |
| **R** | = | Right |
| **S** | = | Spleen |
| **Sp** | = | Spleen |
| **St** | = | Stomach |
| **SV** | = | Splenic vein |

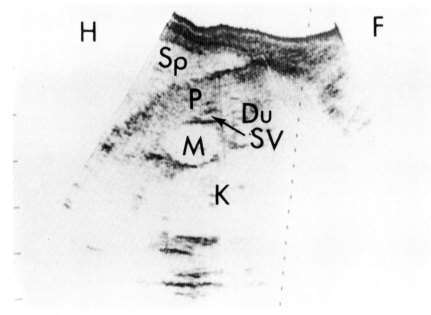

**FIG 8–24.**

## Adrenal Mass

Neuroblastoma is the adrenal malignancy of childhood, the second most common tumor of infancy. Approximately 50% of neuroblastomas originate in the adrenal medulla, but they may also be found in extra-adrenal locations related to the sympathetic ganglia. Although children are frequently asymptomatic, neuroblastoma often manifests as a palpable abdominal mass and must be differentiated from neonatal adrenal hemorrhage and hydronephrosis. The tendency toward microscopic calcification in neuroblastoma usually leads to a relatively solid-appearing echogenic mass on ultrasound (Fig 8–25). The tumors are frequently large and spread by extension to the lymph nodes. Metastases are frequently seen in the liver and bones.

An echogenic mass in the adrenal gland may be secondary to myelolipoma. This tumor is composed of varying amounts of fat and bone marrow elements. It is an uncommon tumor that previously had been reported as an incidental finding at autopsy. With modern-day imaging techniques, myelolipomas appear as echogenic masses on ultrasound and as fat densities on CT. Figure 8–26 is a longitudinal scan of the right upper quadrant in a 53-year-old woman. The echogenic mass in the right adrenal gland proved to be a myelolipoma composed of adipose tissue cells with small islands of hematopoietic tissue. (This case was contributed by Edward I. Miller, M.D.)

Localization of the right perirenal retroperitoneal fat can be helpful in identifying the site of origin of varying masses. If the kidney or adrenal gland is the site of origin, the highly echogenic fat plane will be displaced anteriorly. Figure 8–27 is a transverse scan of a patient with metastasis to the right adrenal gland. Note the highly reflective curvilinear line covering the adrenal mass. This line is displaced anteriorly, which helps the examiner localize the lesion in the right adrenal gland. If the mass is hepatic or subhepatic in origin, it will displace the fat plane posteriorly, as shown in

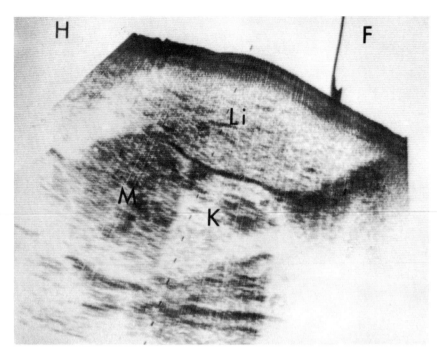

FIG 8–25.

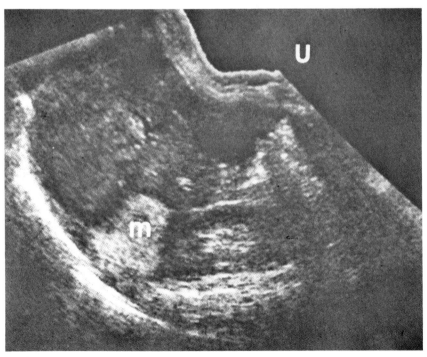

FIG 8–26.

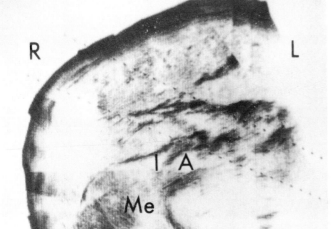

FIG 8–27.

Figure 8–28. Here a large liver abscess is displacing the fat plane (arrowheads) posteriorly.

Figure 8–26 is reproduced from Miller and Dickerson[20] by permission.

| | | |
|---|---|---|
| **A** | = | Aorta |
| **Ab** | = | Liver abscess |
| **Arrowhead** | = | Posterior displacement of the retroperitoneal fat line |
| **F** | = | Foot |
| **H** | = | Head |
| **I** | = | Inferior vena cava |
| **K** | = | Kidney |
| **L** | = | Left |
| **Li** | = | Liver |
| **m** | = | Myelolipoma |
| **M** | = | Neuroblastoma |
| **Me** | = | Adrenal metastasis |
| **R** | = | Kidney |
| **U** | = | Umbilicus |

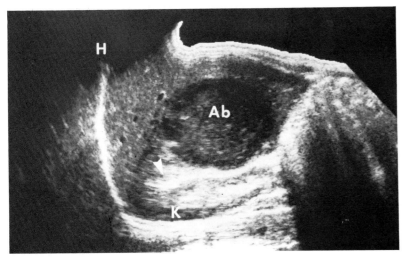

FIG 8–28.

# 9.
# The Retroperitoneum

Barbara Carroll, M.D.

## Anatomic Considerations of the Retroperitoneum

The retroperitoneum is that portion of the abdomen bounded by the parietal peritoneum and the transversalis fascia. The retroperitoneum is largest posteriorly but continues anteriorly as the properitoneal fat. Superficial to the transversalis fascia is the retrofascial space, which consistss predominantly of muscles. Although the retrofascial space is, strictly speaking, not part of the retroperitoneum, pathologic processes in this region can mimic retroperitoneal abnormalities and will be included in this discussion.

The retroperitoneum is bounded anteriorly by the posterior parietal peritoneum, laterally by the lateral fascia, and posteriorly by the transversalis fascia. The retroperitoneum is divided into a number of compartments by several fascial planes.[1, 2] The anterior pararenal space contains the ascending and descending colon, duodenal loop, pancreas, and mesenteric vessels. This space is delineated anteriorly by the posterior parietal peritoneum, laterally by the lateral conal fascia, and posteriorly by the anterior renal fascia. This space potentially communicates across the midline, although only pancreatic or lymph node abnormalities usually produce bilateral involvement. It also communicates with the bare area of the dome of the liver by way of the coronary ligament.

The anterior and posterior renal fasciae (Gerota's fasciae) surround the kidney and adrenal gland, creating the pararenal space. The anterior renal fascia fuses medially with dense fibrous tissue anterior to the prevertebral vessels (the aorta and inferior vena cava). Superiorly, the renal fascial layers fuse at the apex of the crus of the hemidiaphragm. Inferiorly the renal fascial layers are weakly fused or blend with the iliac fasciae. The posterior renal fascia fuses medially with the fascial coverings of the psoas muscle. Although prevertebral vessels are included in the pararenal space, communication across the midline does not occur.

The posterior pararenal space is invested by the transversalis fascia, the lateral conal fascia, and the posterior renal fascia. The posterior pararenal space contains only lymph nodes and vessels and extends from the diaphragm to the region of the iliac crest. This space is continuous with the properitoneal spaces anterolaterally and in the pelvis. Although the various fascial planes which subdivide the retroperitoneal spaces cannot usually be distinguished on ultrasonography, the echogenic retroperitoneal fat line separating peritoneal and retroperitoneal compartments can be visualized routinely.[3] Occasionally, one can distinguish the retrofascial spaces of the retroperitoneum on ultrasonography. A knowledge of the boundaries of the various compartments of the retroperitoneum will facilitate proper localization of pathologic processes and further understanding of the potential routes for disease spread.

## Retroperitoneal Scanning Techniques

Sonographic visualization of retroperitoneal structures is often impaired by bowel gas, bone, and extremely thick muscle or fatty layers. These natural impediments to sonographic imaging dictate an extremely flexible approach to the retroperitoneal space. Transverse and longitudinal scans performed with patients in the supine position usually outline major organs and aid the examiner in determining where the troublesome gas pockets are located. The high retroperitoneum is often well visualized, since the liver and spleen serve as acoustic windows. Adequate penetration of the ulltrasound beam should be confirmed by visualization of the diaphragmatic crura and prevertebral vessels. In the midabdomen, the pancreas, kidneys, duodenum, prevertebral vessels, and psoas muscles should be identified. In the lower abdomen, the prevertebral vessels, iliopsoas muscles, and quadratus lumborum muscles should be imaged on optimal scans. Transverse and longitudinal scans performed with the patient in a decubitis or prone position are useful to avoid bowel gas pockets or redistribute the bowel contents. Coronal scans performed with the patient in a decubitus or supine position also allow excellent visualization of the retroperitoneal space. Coronal scans of the supine patient may be of particular value, as gas within the ascending and descending colon will rise to a more anterior location, allowing visualization of the posterior retroperitoneum in many cases. Retroperitoneal structures such as the kidney or psoas muscle can be used in coronal projections as acoustic windows to visualize the retroperitoneal space. Such projections also allow visualization of segments of prevertebral vessels that are not seen on standard supine, sagittal, or transverse projections.

An additional benefit of coronal scanning of supine patients is that minimal patient manipulation and movement is required.[4, 5]

Patient preparation for retroperitoneal ultrasound examination is minimal. Although withholding food for 12 hours before the study may diminish gas, such preparation is not necessary. Attempts at pharmacologic reduction of bowel gas have not been sufficiently successful to warrant their routine use. However, patients may be given parenteral fluid or water enemas to displace gas and facilitate retroperitoneal imaging.[6] If possible, patients scheduled for barium studies should undergo the ultrasound examination before the barium examination, or the sonogram should be delayed until an abdominal radiograph demonstrates sufficient expulsion of barium.

## Signs of Retroperitoneal Disease

The most common sign of retroperitoneal disease is the presence of a mass.[7] Careful delineation of the boundaries of the mass, as well as the way in which it displaces normal organs and vasculature, can indicate not only the organ of origin, but occasionally the retroperitoneal compartment involved by disease. Masses can be further characterized with respect to their internal echogenicity. Sonography distinguishes cystic masses from solid or complex ones and defines patterns of internal echogenicity and wall characteristics. Echogenic areas with posterior shadowing suggest the presence of gas or calcification within a mass, which narrows the differential diagnosis. Evaluation of sound transmission by a retroperitoneal mass may be difficult when the mass abuts a bony structure or a loop of gas-filled bowel. Enhanced sound transmission is less-reliably detected at bone or air interfaces. Attention must be paid to the relative enhancement behind a mass vis-à-vis a known fluid-containing structure (i.e., the gallbladder) and to changes in sound transmission with increases or decreases of gain settings or changes in transducer frequency.

Abnormal displacement of normal structures is another manifestation of retroperitoneal disease. Anterior displacement of the aorta away from the spine or elevation of the inferior vena cava by retrocaval adenopathy may be the first indications of an infiltrative retroperitoneal process or mass. Retroperitoneal masses may obliterate the echogenic anterior wall of the abdominal aorta and create a "sonographic silhouette," another sign of retroperitoneal disease. Displacement or disruption of the echogenic retroperitoneal fat line is another indicator of retroperitoneal pathology. Direct invasion of retroperitoneal organs and structures by malignancies can be visualized as well. Occasionally, asymmetry of normal bilateral structures may be the only indication of the presence of retroperitoneal disease. This is especially true when tumors or inflammatory processes involve the muscles of the retrofascial space. In such instances, the patient should be questioned to determine whether this muscle asymmetry is related to neuromuscular or skeletal abnormalities or to differential use.

Loss of normal retroperitoneal detail may also indicate abnormality.[8] If poor penetration and suboptimal gain settings or scanning techniques can be excluded, a disease process should be suspected when normal retroperitoneal anatomy is obscured. Computed tomography (CT) should then be performed since the retroperitoneal fat, which degrades sonographic resolution, will enhance the CT evaluation of the retroperitoneum. In addition, gas usually does not degrade CT images.

## Indications for Retroperitoneal Sonography

Sonography is a noninvasive means of imaging the retroperitoneum. CT imaging of the retroperitoneum has a high overall diagnostic accuracy, because the retroperitoneal fat that impairs ultrasound imaging facilitates CT evaluation. In addition, bowel gas or shadowing behind bones impairs visualization of the retroperitoneum on ultrasound scans but not on CT scans. Nevertheless, ultrasound yields accurate images, is rapidly performed, and involves no ionizing radiation or exposure to contrast agents. For these reasons, it should be considered as the initial imaging procedure in very thin patients, in patients too ill to be moved to the CT suite, and in children and adolescents. In these patients, ultrasound can be used to detect the presence or absence of a malignancy, to define the extent of neoplastic involvement, and to detect retroperitoneal hematomas or abscesses.

Ultrasound combined with indium 111 white blood cell (WBC) scanning is useful in the workup of the patient with fever of unknown origin. Combined ultrasound and WBC scanning will detect most abdominal and retroperitoneal abscesses.[9] CT may also be necessary to define the extent of retroperitoneal abscesses. When other imaging techniques are suggested but do not clearly delineate a retroperitoneal mass, ultrasound may be useful in further patient evaluation. In addition, ultrasound can be used to confirm the presence of an abnormality and characterize its internal consistency, as it is superior to CT for distinguishing between cystic and solid masses. Finally, sonographic guidance for aspiration or biopsy of known masses is helpful, as is its use in radiation therapy treatment planning or follow-up.

## Retroperitoneal Pathology

### Lymphadenopathy

The sonographic appearance of lymphadenopathy is variable. Focal, discrete hypoechoic to anechoic masses are common. Alternatively, a hypoechoic mantle surrounding the prevertebral vessels may be seen. Although the retroperitoneal great vessels are usually discernible, para-aortic nodes frequently obscure the sharp anterior aortic vascular border and create the so-called sonographic silhouette sign. Such a finding may help distinguish para-aortic nodes from adjacent mesenteric nodes. The silhouetting produced by retroperitoneal pathology is usually more commonly seen in para-aortic nodes than with paracaval nodes.[5] Although adenopathy resulting from lymphoma is thought to be more sonolucent than the adenopathy resulting from metastatic disease, such diagnostic differentiation is unreliable.[5, 10] Technical factors, transducer frequency, DGC settings, and power output, as well as the location of nodal masses with respect to the focal zone of the beam, affect the internal echogenicity and sound transmission of lymphadenopathy. In addition, the amount of retroperitoneal fat or intervening bowel gas may alter the appearance of nodes. Totally anechoic nodal masses do occur in lymphoma and may resemble cystic structures. Careful attention to the sound transmission by the mass, its internal echogenicity at different gain settings, and the use of different transducer frequencies should allow one to distinguish cystic from solid masses.

Although adenopathy resulting from metastatic disease is usually more echogenic than the adenopathy associated with the majority of lymphomas, there is no reliable correlation between the sonographic characteristics of retroperitoneal masses and their histology. While patients with Burkitt's lymphoma rarely demonstrate the characteristic paravertebral mantle of nodes more commonly seen in Hodgkin's/non-Hodgkin's lymphoma,[11] and while patients with diffuse histiocytic lymphoma often have organ involvement in the absence of retroperitoneal adenopathy, the nodes and lymphomatous masses seen in these patients have sonographic features similar to those seen in other lymphomas.

Even though portions of the retroperitoneum may be obscured by bowel gas, and sonographic resolution is degraded by large quantities of retroperitoneal fat, ultrasound provides accurate, rapid, cost-effective imaging of retroperitoneal anatomy and pathology.[12, 13] The use of ultrasound as a primary imaging technique for detection of retroperitoneal disease can prevent unnecessary CT scans and lymphangiograms.[14] Lymph nodes as small as 0.5–1 cm can be visualized, making ultrasound a viable tool for imaging patients with suspected retroperitoneal adenopathy. It is important to remember that 10% of patients with nodal lymphomas will harbor disease in normal-sized nodes.[15] In such patients, lymphangiography will be necessary to determine the presence of disease. However, demonstration of abnormalities on ultrasound or CT scan may eliminate the need for lymphangiography in many instances. Sonography provides information about disease in areas not visualized on the lymphangiogram. These regions include the renal, hepatic, and splenic hili, the retrocrural area, and the mesentery. In addition to detection of nodal abnormalities, ultrasound can detect extranodal disease in such sites as the spleen, liver, and kidneys.

## Primary Neoplasms

Primary retroperitoneal tumors are uncommon and are usually mesenchymal sarcomas. These tumors often reach large sizes and outgrow their blood sup-

ply. In such cases the tumors have large cystic or echogenic components corresponding to regions of hemorrhage or necrosis. Liposarcomas are often highly echogenic retroperitoneal masses due to their high fat content. However, echogenic components may be seen in any of the sarcomas.[16] Calcifications can be identified in retroperitoneal sarcomas because of the posterior acoustic shadowing produced by these echogenic regions. Posterior shadowing may also occur behind retroperitoneal abscesses produced by gas-forming organisms. Shadowing produced by gas usually demonstrates characteristic reverberations within the shadow, or "dirty shadows," which helps distinguish it from shadows produced by calcific lesions. Primary retroperitoneal tumors may infiltrate throughout the retroperitoneum, distorting and displacing normal organs, so that it is difficult to determine the organ of origin of the mass. Because the appearance of these primary neoplasms is both variable and nonspecific, the examiner can only speculate as to the etiology of a retroperitoneal neoplasm by noting its location, the presence of a large necrotic component or calcification, and correlating ultrasound findings with the patient's history. In addition, sonography can be used to direct biopsies and monitor response to therapy.[16]

## Fluid Collections

A number of different fluid collections involve the retroperitoneum. These include hematomas, abscesses, urinomas, and lymphoceles. All of these fluid collections may have similar sonographic appearances. Most are round or oval masses. Abscesses and hematoma often have irregular, slightly thickened walls on ultrasonography, while urinomas and lymphoceles are more often smooth-walled and anechoic. Areas of acute bleeding may be uniformly echogenic, but they are readily distinguished from solid masses by their enhanced sound transmission. Furthermore, sequential examinations will reveal progressive liquefaction and clot retraction in hematomas. Abscesses are usually hypoechoic or anechoic processes. However, abscesses formed by gas-producing organisms contain microbubbles of gas, which may create an echogenic mass with decreased sound transmission. Abscesses, hematomas, complicated lymphoceles, or urinomas may contain septations. The orientation of dependent debris or fluid-solid interfaces may change with change in patient position. Such dynamic changes confirm the fluid nature of the mass. Ultrasound provides superior definition of the internal features and wall structure within predominantly cystic retroperitoneal masses and accurately distinguishes cystic from solid abnormalities. Aspiration of cystic masses or biopsy of sollid masses facilitates rapid diagnosis and the institution of appropriate therapy. Sonographic guidance for the placement of indwelling drainage tubes makes nonsurgical treatment of large abscesses possible, especially in patients too ill to be moved from their hospital bed.

### Retroperitoneal Fibrosis

Retroperitoneal fibrosis may be idiopathic, secondary to drugs, due to retroperitoneal bleeding or infection, or related to an infiltrative tumor. Sonographic findings in retroperitoneal fibrosis include the presence of a smooth-walled, hypoechoic to anechoic mantle that envelops the distal prevertebral vessels and may extend down to the level of sacral promontory.[8, 17] There is relatively little retroaortic extension of these masses, in comparison to that exhibited by malignant processes such as lymphoma. Occasionally retroperitoneal fibrosis may be a bulky, lobulated mass indistinguishable from lymphoma, sarcoma, or other malignancies.[5, 18] In addition, retroperitoneal fibrosis may resemble hemorrhage or infection. In these cases, ultrasound- or CT-guided biopsy will establish the definitive diagnosis. Retroperitoneal fibrosis may coexist with abdominal aortic aneurysms. In such cases, sonography is useful in separating the fibrotic process from the vascular abnormality. Real-time observation of vascular wall pulsations, as well as visible blood flow in saccular aneurysms, defines the vascular component of the mass. Use of Doppler ultrasound further substantiates flow within aneurysms. Associated unilateral or bilateral hydronephrosis may coexist. In the setting of profound uremia, minimal or absent hydronephrosis may be seen in retroperitoneal fibrosis.[19] Retrograde urograms may be necessary to confirm the presence of ureteral obstruction in such instances. When obstruction is documented, ultrasound can be used to place percutaneous nephrostomy tubes to relieve the obstruction. Sonography can also be used to follow regression of the fibrotic mass during steroid therapy.

### Pitfalls in the Diagnosis of Retroperitoneal Disease

One error in the evaluation of the retroperitoneum is to mistake an aberrantly located normal organ for a pathologic process. Ptotic kidneys, horseshoe or pelvic kidneys, or a low-lying pancreas (not uncommon in the elderly patient) account for frequent errors. Loops of aperistaltic bowel or adherent small bowel adjacent to the anterior retroperitoneal fascia may produce additional diagnostic dilemmas. Discerning the location of the superior mesenteric vessels relative to a mass should distinguish bowel from retroperitoneal processes. In addition, real-time observation of peristalsis with the passage of fluid or solid material along the bowel lumen confirms the nature of these structures. Fluid in the retroperitoneal portions of the colon and duodenum may also mimic pathologic collections. Parenteral administration of fluids or fluid enemas followed by appropriate repositioning of the patient will usually demonstrate the passage of microbubbles along the bowel lumen and associated peristalsis.

A prominent lobulated inferior crus of the right hemidiaphragm should not be mistaken for retroperitoneal adenopathy.[20] Although the crus may resemble adenopathy on transverse projection, real-time sagittal and coronal scans readily demonstrate the linear crus. A prominent quadratus lumborum muscle may mimic a retroperitoneal abscess or hematoma, but recognition of the solid, symmetric nature of these paired structures should allow the examiner to distinguish them from pathologic collections.[21] Because many pathologic processes involving the retroperitoneal space may have a similar appearance on ultrasonography, the correct diagnosis may only be possible after additional diagnostic or interventional procedures have been performed.

### References

1. Myers MA: The extraperitoneal spaces: Normal and pathologic anatomy, in Myers MA: *Dynamic*

*Radiology of the Abdomen.* New York, Springer-Verlag, 1976, pp 113–194.

2. Koenigsberg M, Hoffman JC, Schnur MJ: Sonographic evaluation of the retroperitoneum. *Semin Ultrasound* 1982; 3:79–95.

3. Gore RM, Callen PW, Filly RA: Displaced retroperitoneal fat: Sonographic guide to right upper quadrant mass localization. *Radiology* 1982; 142:701–705.

4. Magill HL, Tonkin ILD, Bada H, et al: Advantages of coronal ultrasonography in evaluating the neonatal retroperitoneum. *J Ultrasound Med* 1983; 2:289–295.

5. Carroll BA: Ultrasound of lymphoma. *Semin Ultrasound* 1982; 3:114–122.

6. Crade M, Taylor KJW, Rosenfield AT: Water distention of the gut in the evaluation of the pancreas by ultrasound. *AJR* 1978; 31:348–349.

7. Filly RA, Marglin S, Castellino RA: The ultrasonographic spectrum of abdominal and pelvic Hodgkin disease and non-Hodgkin lymphoma. *Cancer* 1976; 38:2143–2148.

8. Sanders RC, Duffy T, McLoughlin MG, et al: Sonography in the diagnosis of retroperitoneal fibrosis. *J Urol* 1977; 118:944–946.

9. Carroll BA, Silverman PM, Goodwin DA, et al: Ultrasonography and indium 111 white blood cell scanning for the detection of intra-abdominal abscesses. *Radiology* 1981; 140:155.

10. Hillman BJ, Haber K: Echographic characteristics of malignant lymph nodes. *JCU* 1980; 8:213–215.

11. Shawker TH, Dunnick NR, Head GL, et al: Ultrasound evaluation of American Burkitt's lymphoma. *JCU* 1979; 7:279–283.

12. Brascho DL, Durant JR, Green LE: The accuracy of retroperitoneal ultrasound in Hodgkin disease and non-Hodgkin lymphoma. *Radiology* 1977; 125:484–487.

13. Rochester D, Bowie JD, Kunzmann A, et al: Ultrasound in the staging of lymphoma. *Radiology* 1977; 124:483–487.

14. Beyer D, Peters PE: Real-time ultrasonography: An efficient screening method for abdominal and pelvic lymphadenopathy. *Lymphology* 1980; 13:142–149.

15. Goffinet DR, Warnke R, Dunnick WF, et al: Clinical and surgical laparotomy: Evaluation of patients with non-Hodgkin lymphoma. *Cancer Treat Rep* 1977; 61:981–992.

16. McLeod AJ, Lewis E: Sonographic evaluation of pediatric rhabdomyosarcomas. *J Ultrasound Med* 1984; 3:69–73.

17. Bowie JD, Bernstein JR: Retroperitoneal fibrosis: Ultrasound findings and case report. *JCU* 1977; 4:435–437.

18. Fagan CJ, Amparo EG, Davis M: Retroperitoneal fibrosis. *Semin Ultrasound* 1982; 3:123–138.

19. Curry N, Gobien R, Schabel S: Minimal-dilation obstructive nephropathy. *Radiology* 1982; 143:138.

20. Callen PW, Filly RA, Sarti DA, et al: Ultrasonography of the diaphragmatic crura. *Radiology* 1979; 130:721–724.

21. Callen PW, Filly RA, Marks WM: The quadratus lumborum muscle: A possible source of confusion in sonographic evaluation of the retroperitoneum. *JCU* 1979; 7:349–352.

## CASES

### Dennis A. Sarti, M.D.

### Normal Retroperitoneum

Ultrasonographic evaluation of the retroperitoneum is often very difficult because of overlying bowel air. Gentle pressure on the patient's abdomen may displace bowel gas and yield an adequate ultrasonic window. If a large mass is present, it will often displace bowel loops out of the way.

Figure 9–1 is an excellent illustration of the anatomy of the retroperitoneum. The anterior pararenal space is bounded anteriorly by posterior parietal peritoneum and posteriorly by the anterior renal fascia. This space contains the pancreas, retroperitoneal duodenum, and the ascending and descending colon. The middle space or perirenal space is bounded by the anterior and posterior layers of the renal fascia. These layers fuse superiorly with the diaphragm. The kidneys, ureters, and adrenal glands lie within the perirenal space. The aorta and inferior vena cava are located within this space. The connective tissue sheath of the aorta and inferior vena cava fuse with the renal fascia.

The posterior renal fascia and the transversalis fascia form the anterior and posterior borders of trhe posterior pararenal space, which is continuous from the diaphragm to the iliac crest. This space fuses medially over the psoas muscles.

Figure 9–2 is a transverse scan of the retroperitoneum that shows the characteristic sonolucencies of the aorta and inferior vena cava. Anterior to the right kidney is a fluid-filled duodenum. This should not be mistaken for a retroperitoneal mass. The head of the pancreas is situated anterior to the inferior vena cava. It yields a fairly characteristic echo pattern that will not be confused with any pathologic entity. Often, the fourth portion of the duodenum, situated to the left of the aorta, can be mistaken for a solid mass of the retroperitoneum. The patient may be given fluid, the patient's position changed, and real-time observations carried out before one can correctly diagnose fluid in the duodenum.

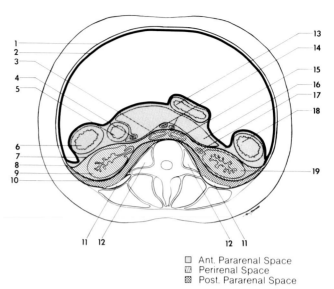

☐ Ant. Pararenal Space
▨ Perirenal Space
▩ Post. Pararenal Space

**FIG 9–1.**

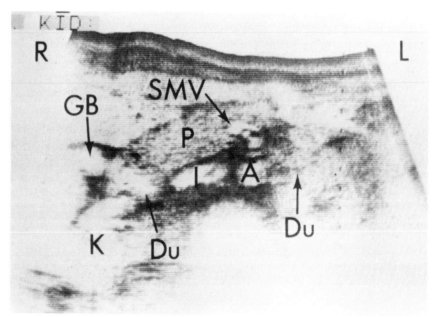

**FIG 9–2.**

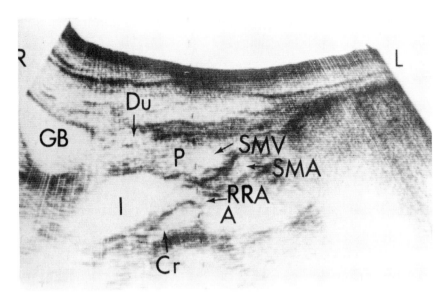

**FIG 9–3.**

Figure 9–3 is a transverse scan in which the inferior vena cava is seen as an extremely large sonolucent mass in the retroperitoneum. Deep to the inferior vena cava is the right renal artery, draping over an extremely thickened crus of the diaphragm on the right side. The crus of the diaphragm often is mistakenly interpreted as lymphadenopathy. Figure 9–4 is a transverse scan of the abdomen made at a lower level than the previous scans. In this scan two paraspinous masses are seen secondary to the iliopsoas muscles. The left iliopsoas muscle is larger than the right and could be mistaken for lymphadenopathy. The orientation of the spine is somewhat unusual. The patient has scoliosis, which explains the marked asymmetry of the iliopsoas muscles.

SOURCE: Figure 9–1 is reproduced with permission from Koenigsberg M, Hoffman JC, Schnur MJ: Sonographic evaluation of the retroperitoneum. *Semin Ultrasound* 1982; 3:79; Figure 9–2 is reproduced with permission from Sample WF, Sarti DA: Computed tomography and gray scale ultrasonography of the adrenal gland: A comparative study. *Radiology* 1978; 128: 377–383.

| | | |
|---|---|---|
| **A** | = | Aorta |
| **Cr** | = | Crus of the diaphragm |
| **Du** | = | Duodenum |
| **GB** | = | Gallbladder |
| **I** | = | Inferior vena cava |
| **IP** | = | Iliopsoas muscle |
| **K** | = | Kidney |
| **L** | = | Left |
| **P** | = | Pancreas |
| **QL** | = | Quadratus laborum muscle |
| **R** | = | Right |
| **RRA** | = | Right renal artery |
| **SMA** | = | Superior mesenteric artery |
| **SMV** | = | Superior mesenteric vein |
| **Sp** | = | Spine |

| | | |
|---|---|---|
| **1** | = | Transversalis fascia |
| **2** | = | Peritoneum |
| **3** | = | Inferior vena cava |
| **4** | = | Common bild duct |
| **5** | = | Duodenum |
| **6** | = | Ascending colon |
| **7** | = | Anterior renal fascia |
| **8** | = | Lateroconal fascia |
| **9** | = | Right kidney |
| **10** | = | Posterior renal fascia |
| **11** | = | Quadratus laborum muscle |
| **12** | = | Psoas muscle |
| **13** | = | Duodenum |
| **14** | = | Superior mesenteric artery and vein |
| **15** | = | Aorta |
| **16** | = | Pancreas |
| **17** | = | Ureter |
| **18** | = | Descending colon |
| **19** | = | Left kidney |

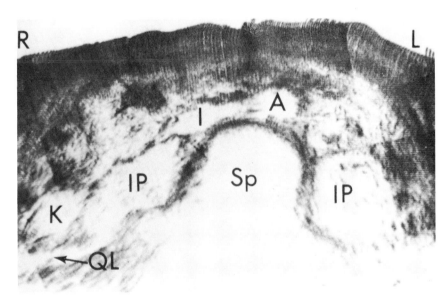

**FIG 9–4.**

## Normal Retroperitoneum

Ultrasonographic evaluation of the re-troperitoneum on longitudinal scans is more difficult than on transverse scans. Figure 9–5 is a parasagittal diagram through the right abdomen that illustrates the cephalocaudad boundaries of the spaces shown in Figure 9–1. The anterior pararenal space is bounded by the peritoneum and the anterior renal fascia. This space extends from the bare area of the liver to the pelvis. The perirenal space is bordered by the anterior and posterior layers of the renal fascia. This space extends from the dia-phragm to the iliac crest. The poste-rior pararenal space is bounded by the posterior renal fascia anteriorly and the transversalis fascia posteri-orly. This space also extends from the diaphragm to the iliac crest.

In Figure 9–6, a longitudinal scan of the retroperitoneal region, a fairly di-lated inferior vena cava can be seen. Anterior to the inferior vena cava are the main portal vein and the left portal vein. The sonolucent area draining into the inferior vena cava near the superior portion of the liver represents a hepatic vein. The lower portion of the inferior vena cava is extremely close to the skin surface. Near the umbilical level the inferior vena cava is only 2 cm from the skin surface.

Figure 9–7 is a longitudinal scan through an inferior vena cava which is less dilated than seen in Figure 9–6. Distensibility of the inferior vena cava is extremely variable from patient to patient. The right renal artery is seen as a circular lucency indenting the posterior aspect of the inferior vena cava in Figure 9–7. The high-ampli-tude echoes of the vertebral bodies are present posterior to the inferior vena cava. When retroperitoneal masses are present, they will displace the inferior vena cava away from the vertebral echoes.

Figure 9–8, a longitudinal scan of the retroperitoneum over the aortic re-gion, shows the common origin of the celiac artery and superior mesenteric artery. The tubular sonolucency ante-rior to the high abdominal aorta is secondary to the crus of the dia-

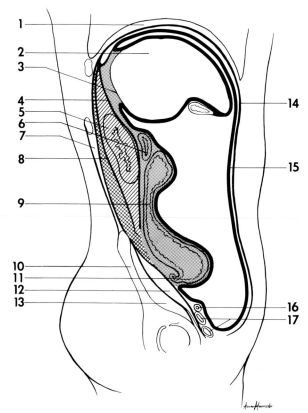

☐ Ant. Pararenal Space
▨ Perirenal Space
▩ Post. Pararenal Space

**FIG 9–5.**

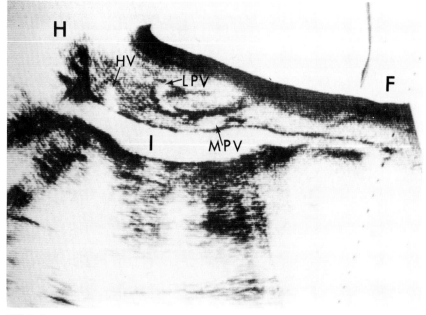

**FIG 9–6.**

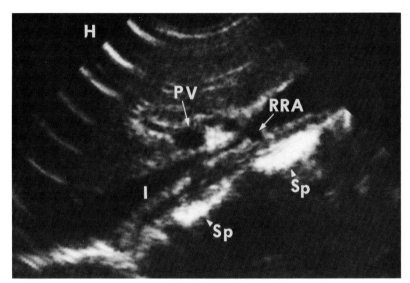

**FIG 9–7.**

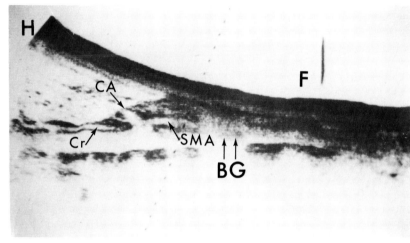

**FIG 9–8.**

phragm. This is a normal finding and should not be confused with lymphadenopathy. A portion of the aorta is obscured by bowel gas, which is common in an abdominal examination. The more caudal portion of the abdominal aorta is well visualized. Note that the aorta is not displaced away from the high-amplitude echoes of the vertebral bodies.

SOURCE: Figure 9–5 is reproduced with permission from Koenigsberg M, Hoffman JC, Schnur MJ: Sonographic evaluation of the retroperitoneum. *Semin Ultrasound* 1982; 3:79.

| | | |
|---|---|---|
| **BG** | = | Bowel gas |
| **CA** | = | Celiac artery |
| **Cr** | = | Crus of diaphragm |
| **F** | = | Foot |
| **H** | = | Head |
| **HV** | = | Hepatic vein |
| **I** | = | Inferior vena cava |
| **LPV** | = | Left portal vein |
| **MPV** | = | Main portal vein |
| **PV** | = | Portal vein |
| **RRA** | = | Right renal artery |
| **SMA** | = | Superior mesenteric artery |
| **Sp** | = | Spine |

| | | |
|---|---|---|
| **1** | = | Diaphragm |
| **2** | = | Liver |
| **3** | = | Bare area of the liver |
| **4** | = | Anterior renal fascia |
| **5** | = | Right kidney |
| **6** | = | Duodenum |
| **7** | = | Quadratus laborum muscle |
| **8** | = | Posterior renal fascia |
| **9** | = | Ascending colon |
| **10** | = | Iliac crest |
| **11** | = | Retrocecal appendix |
| **12** | = | Psoas |
| **13** | = | Iliacus |
| **14** | = | Transversalis fascia |
| **15** | = | Peritoneum |
| **16** | = | Ureter |
| **17** | = | Iliac vessels |

## Lymphadenopathy

Ultrasound examination of the retroperitoneum can detect lymphadenopathy. A great deal of the retroperitoneum is often obscured by bowel air. Computed tomography is the diagnostic procedure of choice in these situations. However, retroperitoneal masses can displace bowel enough to provide an ultrasonic window. Figure 9–9 is a transverse scan of the high retroperitoneum in which a large mass can be seen anterior to the aorta and inferior vena cava. The stomach is displaced anteriorly and is compressed. This lymphadenopathy, the result of a lymphoma, appears as a solid mass somewhat more lucent than the liver.

Figure 9–10 is an example of lymphadenopathy in the region of the porta hepatis. The aorta is in its normal location anterior to the spine. The inferior vena cava is displaced anteriorly relative to the aorta. Most of the lymphadenopathy is situated within the porta hepatis. Numerous relatively sonolucent masses can be seen surrounding the structures of the porta hepatis. The portal vein, hepatic artery, and common hepatic duct are displaced anteriorly by the enlarged nodes.

Figure 9–11, a longitudinal scan of the abdomen, illustrates tumor involving the caudate lobe of the liver and the high retroperitoneum. The important finding in this case is elevation of the superior mesenteric artery above the aorta by a mantle of nodes. The superior mesenteric artery is usually in close proximity to the anterior surface of the aorta. An increased distance between the superior mesenteric artery and the aorta indicate a retroperitoneal process.

Figure 9–12 is a longitudinal scan through the right upper quadrant of a 45-year-old man who had recently received a heart transplant. Ultrasound examination was performed because of fever and abdominal pain. The patient also had a poorly differentiated lymphocytic lymphoma. On the ultrasound scan a mass appears cephalad to the right kidney (arrowheads). This scan demonstrates invasion from the

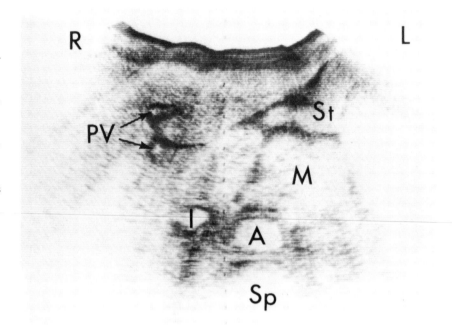

FIG 9–9.

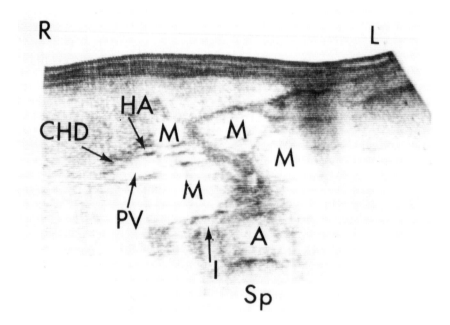

FIG 9–10.

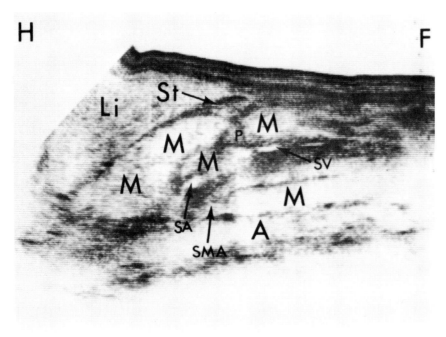

**FIG 9–11.**

retroperitoneum into the liver. The high-amplitude echoes in the center of the mass represent the echogenic retroperitoneal fat line. The mass has broken through this fat line and invaded the liver.

| | | |
|---|---|---|
| **A** | = | Aorta |
| **Arrowheads** | = | Lymphocytic lymphoma |
| **CHD** | = | Common hepatic duct |
| **F** | = | Foot |
| **H** | = | Head |
| **HA** | = | Hepatic artery |
| **I** | = | Inferior vena cava |
| **K** | = | Kidney |
| **L** | = | Left |
| **Li** | = | Liver |
| **M** | = | Lymphadenopathy |
| **P** | = | Pancreas |
| **PV** | = | Portal vein |
| **R** | = | Right |
| **SA** | = | Splenic artery |
| **SMA** | = | Superior mesenteric artery |
| **Sp** | = | Spine |
| **St** | = | Stomach |
| **SV** | = | Splenic vein |

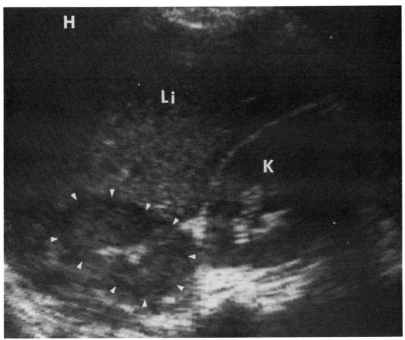

**FIG 9–12.**

## Retroperitoneal Lymphadenopathy

Normally, the inferior vena cava has a characteristic appearance on longitudinal ultrasound scans. It is quite distensible and in close proximity to the spine. The contour is usually smooth, without evidence of indentation from adjacent masses. Figures 9–13 through 9–16 illustrate examples of lymphadenopathy and the relationship of the masses to the inferior vena cava. Figure 9–13 is a longitudinal scan demonstrating a large lymph node on the posterior aspect of the inferior vena cava. The lymph node is actually situated posterior to the right renal artery. It is displacing this vessel and the inferior vena cava anteriorly. The lymph node appears highly localized and suggests an adrenal lesion. However, it is secondary to lymphadenopathy in the right renal hilum.

Figure 9–14 is a longitudinal scan demonstrating lymphadenopathy both anterior and posterior to the inferior vena cava. The inferior vena cava is narrowed and pinched between the enlarged lymph nodes. Again, the right renal artery is situated anterior to the lymphadenopathy.

An interesting case of testicular carcinoma is illustrated in Figure 9–15. Numerous enlarged lymph nodes surround the inferior vena cava. Near the caudal portion of the inferior vena cava, the lymph nodes markedly compress its lumen. Within the lumen of the inferior vena cava is an echogenic mass secondary to thrombus from tumor.

Figure 9–16 is another longitudinal scan in which the inferior vena cava is displaced anteriorly by retrocaval adenopathy. This is a case of lymphoma which was also surrounding the right renal artery.

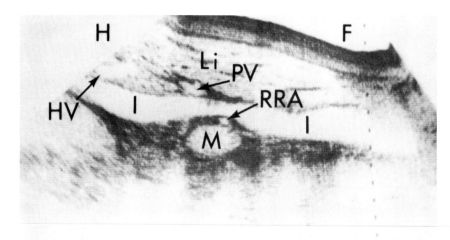

**FIG 9–13.**

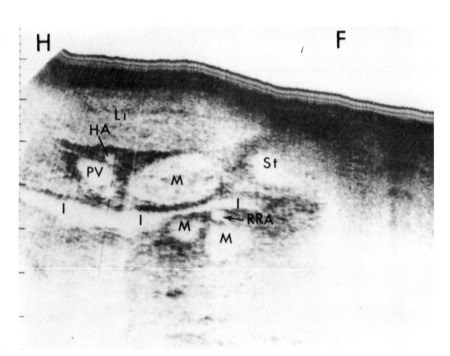

**FIG 9–14.**

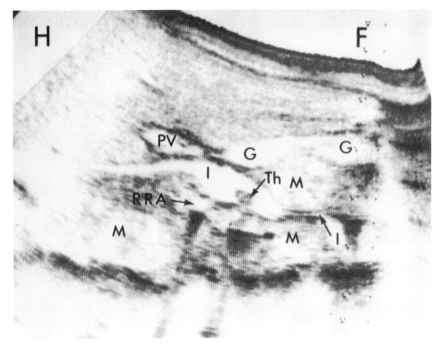

**FIG 9–15.**

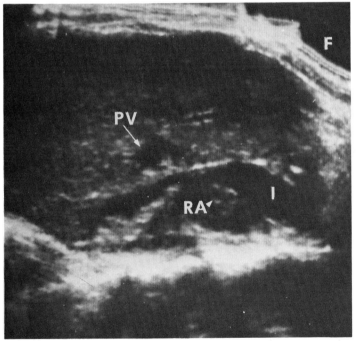

**FIG 9–16.**

| F   | = | Foot |
|-----|---|------|
| G   | = | Gallbladder |
| H   | = | Head |
| HA  | = | Hepatic artery |
| HV  | = | Hepatic vein |
| I   | = | Inferior vena cava |
| Li  | = | Liver |
| M   | = | Lymphadenopathy |
| PV  | = | Portal vein |
| RA  | = | Renal artery |
| RRA | = | Right renal artery |
| St  | = | Stomach |
| Th  | = | Tumor thrombus within the inferior vena cava |

## Retroperitoneal Adenopathy

The four figures in this section are transverse upper abdominal scans showing retroperitoneal lymphadenopathy. In Figure 9–17 a mass is situated posterior to the inferior vena cava. The larger component of the mass, however, is to the left of the aorta and posterior to the superior mesenteric artery. The mass is relatively sonolucent and consistent with retroperitoneal lymphadenopathy.

Figure 9–18 illustrates a similar case with a mass situated between the aorta and left kidney. The left renal vein is seen to be elevated as it drapes over the retroperitoneal lymphadenopathy. The left kidney is lateral to the mass. The mass can be seen between the kidney and the aorta.

Figure 9–19 is a transverse scan of the upper abdomen which shows distortion of the right renal echoes. The right kidney is involved with nodular mixed lymphoma. A mass (arrowheads) is also present in the right renal hilum and is displacing the inferior vena cava anteriorly and medially. The mass represents retroperitoneal lymphadenopathy. A tubular lucency (arrow) within the mass represents the right renal artery surrounded by adenopathy.

Figure 9–20 shows massive retroperitoneal adenopathy surrounding the aorta, above the left retroperitoneum, and in the region of the porta hepatis. The large sonolucent masses are consistent with lymph node enlargement. In this instance, it is difficult to visualize the lumen of the aorta because of the surrounding mass. The portal vein is surrounded anteriorly and posteriorly by lymphadenopathy. The left kidney is displaced posteriorly by a large left-sided retroperitoneal mass.

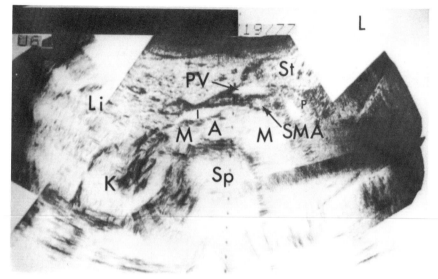

**FIG 9–17.**

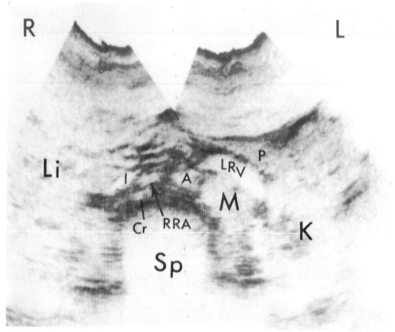

**FIG 9–18.**

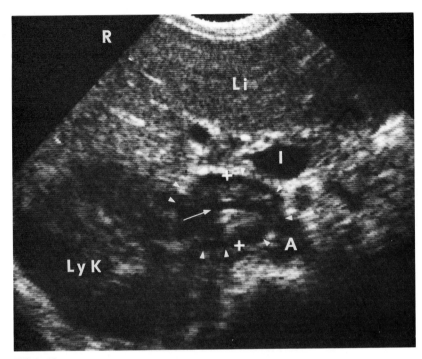

FIG 9–19.

| | |
|---|---|
| **A** | = Aorta |
| **Arrow** | = Right renal artery |
| **Arrowheads** | = Retroperitoneal lymphad-enopathy |
| **Bo** | = Bowel |
| **Cr** | = Crus of the diaphragm |
| **I** | = Inferior vena cava |
| **K** | = Kidney |
| **L** | = Left |
| **Li** | = Liver |
| **LRV** | = Left renal vein |
| **LyK** | = Lymphomatous involve-ment of the right kidney |
| **M** | = Adenopathy |
| **P** | = Pancreas |
| **PV** | = Portal vein |
| **R** | = Right |
| **RRA** | = Right renal artery |
| **S** | = Spleen |
| **SMA** | = Superior mesenteric artery |
| **Sp** | = Spleen |
| **St** | = Stomach |

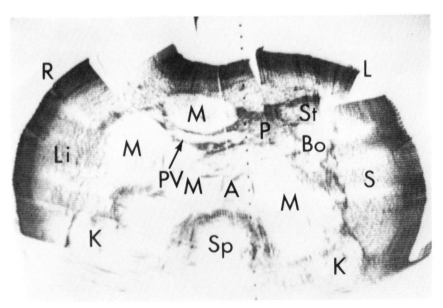

FIG 9–20.

## Retroperitoneal Lymphadenopathy

The transverse scan in Figure 9–21 demonstrates a large left-sided retroperitoneal mass displacing the aorta to the right. The left kidney is markedly displaced to the left side of the abdomen and in the usual position of the spleen. The spine is not in the middle of the patient's abdomen. This patient had marked asymmetry of the abdominal wall when scanned by ultrasound. The left side of the abdomen was massively enlarged secondary to lymphadenopathy.

Figure 9–22 is a slightly oblique transverse scan of the upper abdomen. A reniform mass is present anterior to the aorta and the inferior vena cava. Numerous entities could yield this ultrasound picture, including an ectopic kidney, a stomach or colon tumor, and pancreatic carcinoma. The patient had lymphoma with numerous enlarged mesenteric lymph nodes manifesting as a "pseudokidney" mass in the midabdomen.

Figures 9–23 and 9–24 are transverse and longitudinal scans of another patient with massive retroperitoneal adenopathy. The mass is mainly on the left side but is partially surrounding the aorta. Such masses can occasionally be confused with an abdominal aortic aneurysm. In this instance we see the aorta elevated off the spinal echoes in Figure 9–24. The transverse scan (Fig 9–23) demonstrates the left-sided soft tissue mass secondary to adenopathy.

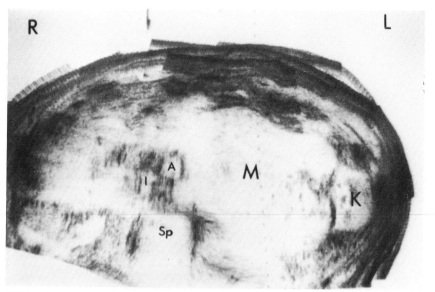

FIG 9–21.

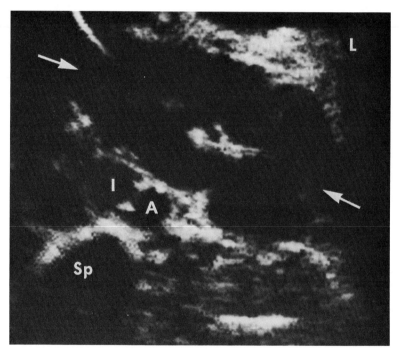

FIG 9–22.

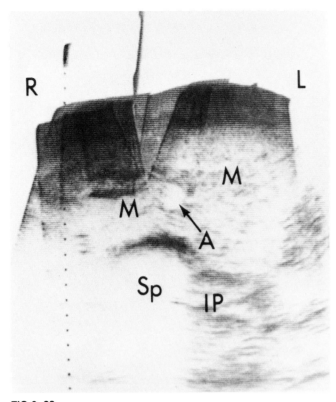

**FIG 9–23.**

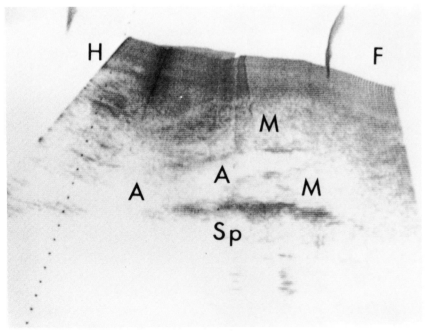

**FIG 9–24.**

| A | = Aorta |
| **Arrows** | = "Pseudokidney" secondary to mesenteric adenopathy |
| F | = Foot |
| H | = Head |
| I | = Inferior vena cava |
| IP | = Iliopsoas |
| K | = Kidney |
| M | = Adenopathy |
| R | = Right |
| Sp | = Spine |

## Lymphadenopathy

A transverse scan of the midabdomen (Fig 9–25) demonstrates multiple sonolucent masses on the left side. These are secondary to mesenteric adenopathy. The aorta is in its normal position, directly anterior to the spine. The lymphadenopathy was within the mesentery. Figure 9–26 is a transverse scan of the retroperitoneum near the bifurcation of the aorta. In this instance, the inferior vena cava is visualized. The massive lymphadenopathy, however, has obscured visualization of the aorta. This is consistent with the ultrasonographic silhouette sign.

One anatomic area that can be quite difficult to delineate on ultrasound examination is near the bifurcation of the aorta and the inferior vena cava. Since these two vessels bifurcate, numerous circular sonolucencies are visualized at this site. In a transverse scan (Fig 9–27) obtained near the bifurcation of the aorta, the inferior vena cava is visualized in its normal position and before it bifurcates. However, the two circular structures situated anterior and to the left of the inferior vena cava are secondary to the right common iliac artery and the left common iliac artery. An extra mass is present in this region. This represents lymphadenopathy. It is obvious how difficult this area can be to evaluate when these vessels begin to bifurcate.

Figure 9–28 is a transverse scan of the right lower quadrant showing lymphadenopathy anterior to the right iliopsoas muscle. We are often asked to examine this area to rule out an appendiceal abscess. In this instance, we did find a mass in this patient, secondary to lymphadenopathy.

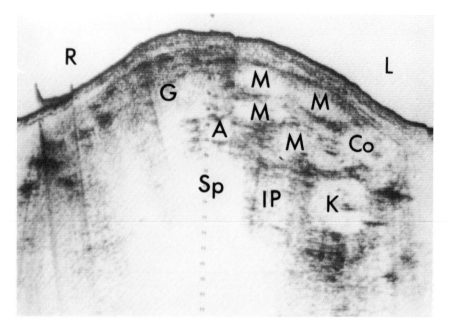

**FIG 9–25.**

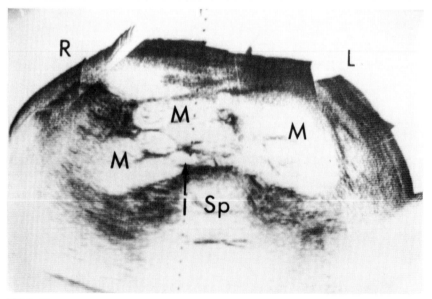

**FIG 9–26.**

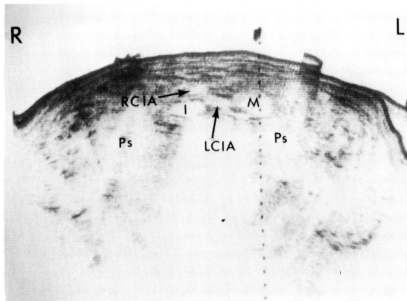

**A** = Aorta
**Co** = Colon
**G** = Bowel gas
**I** = Inferior vena cava
**IP** = Iliopsoas muscle
**K** = Kidney
**L** = Left
**LCIA** = Left common iliac artery
**M** = Lymphadenopathy
**Ps** = Psoas muscle
**R** = Right
**RCIA** = Right common iliac artery
**Sp** = Spine

FIG 9–27.

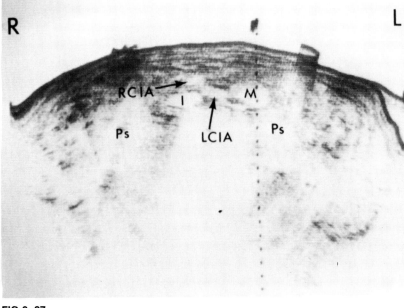

FIG 9–28.

## Retroperitoneal Tumors

Although masses arising from lymphadenopathy are the most common
cause of retroperitoneal solid masses
seen on ultrasound, solid tumors may
originate in other sites. Figure 9–29 is
a transverse scan of a 30-year-old
woman who was known to have extensive retroperitoneal neuroblastoma.
The scan shows a large echogenic
mass anterior to the aorta and the inferior vena cava. Two tubular structures within the mass represent the
hepatic and splenic arteries, which are
displaced anteriorly by the retroperitoneal mass. The mass is solid in nature, with numerous echoes noted
throughout and extensively involving
the upper abdomen. The portal vein is
displaced anteriorly by the mass,
along with the right lobe of the liver.

Figure 9–30 is a transverse scan of
a 60-year-old woman with a retroperitoneal liposarcoma. The mass is posterior to the portal vein. It is highly
echogenic, indicating its solid nature.
The portal vein is displaced anteriorly
as it drapes over the large retroperitoneal mass.

Figure 9–31 is a transverse scan of
a 55-year-old woman with a synovial
sarcoma of the lower extremity resected previously. Follow-up examinations revealed the development of a
large mass in the left upper quadrant,
which was eventually diagnosed as
metastatic synovial sarcoma. A transverse scan of the upper abdomen (Fig
9–31) shows a large mass in the left
upper quadrant. The extent of the
mass is indicated by the asymmetry of
the abdominal wall. It differs from the
previous two cases in that numerous
sonolucent areas are present within it.
These sonolucent areas are secondary to necrosis and liquefaction of the
solid tumor. It is common for extremely large masses to have sonolucent areas secondary to necrosis and
hemorrhage.

Figure 9–32 is a longitudinal scan
of a 55-year-old man who underwent
partial gastrectomy for a leiomyosarcoma. He was later found to have recurrent leiomyosarcoma. An ultrasound examination was done on the
left lateral abdomen. The longitudinal

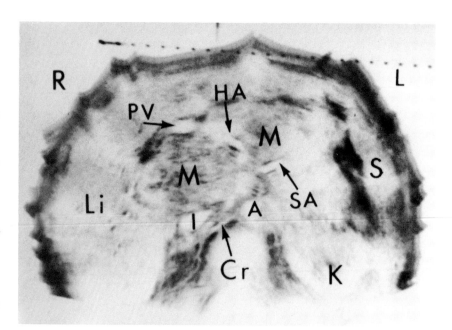

**FIG 9–29.**

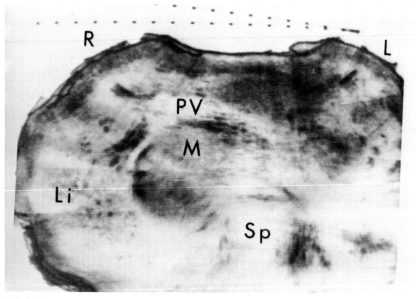

**FIG 9–30.**

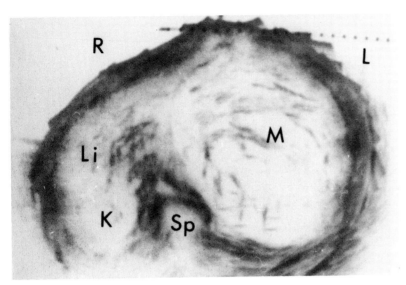

**FIG 9–31.**

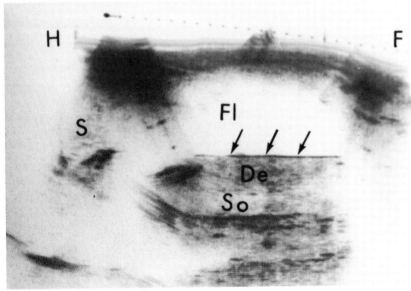

**FIG 9–32.**

scan shows a large mass caudal to the spleen. This mass has three components. The anterior portion is sonolucent secondary to fluid. Deep to the fluid area is a highly echogenic region, representing debris. A fluid level (arrows) is seen between the fluid and debris. Finally, the deep portion of the mass was solid. This large recurrent leiomyosarcoma shows the varied physical ultrasonographic appearance of large necrotic tumors.

SOURCE: Figures 9–29 through 9–32 are provided through the courtesy of B. Green, M.D.

| | | |
|---|---|---|
| **A** | = | Aorta |
| **Arrows** | = | Fluid level (Fig 9–32) |
| **Cr** | = | Crus of the diaphragm |
| **De** | = | Debris |
| **F** | = | Foot |
| **Fl** | = | Fluid |
| **H** | = | Head |
| **I** | = | Inferior vena cava |
| **K** | = | Kidney |
| **Li** | = | Liver |
| **M** | = | Solid retroperitoneal tumor |
| **PV** | = | Portal vein |
| **R** | = | Right |
| **S** | = | Spleen |
| **SA** | = | Splenic artery |
| **So** | = | Solid component to the tumor |
| **Sp** | = | Spine |

## Retroperitoneal Masses

The superficial borders of retroperitoneal masses usually have an irregular surface. The mass imaged in Figure 9–33 has a smooth surface on its anterior borders. Figure 9–33 is a longitudinal scan made over the middle to lower abdomen in a 39-year-old man with low-grade back pain and progressive renal failure. In the initial scan (Fig 9–33), a mantle of soft tissue echoes can be seen anterior to the aorta. These echoes are relatively symmetric in thickness. The superficial border is somewhat smooth and lacks the usual irregularity seen in retroperitoneal adenopathy. The hypoechoic mantle of tissue anterior to the aorta was found to be secondary to retroperitoneal fibrosis. High-dose steroid therapy was initiated, and 1 month after the initial study a longitudinal scan (Fig 9–34) was made of the abdominal aorta in its middle to lower portion. In this scan the aorta appears normal and without evidence of the mantle of soft tissue echoes, which disappeared completely with steroid therapy. Figures 9–33 and 9–34 illustrate the sonographic appearance of retroperitoneal fibrosis before and after steroid therapy.

Retroperitoneal tumors can displace retroperitoneal organs in a rather dramatic fashion. The mobility of retroperitoneal structures is never appreciated until a large retroperitoneal mass is identified and noted to displace these organs dramatically. Figure 9–35 is a transverse scan of a 50-year-old woman who had a history of left flank pain and increasing abdominal girth. The scan is difficult to interpret because no normal anatomic structures are readily identifiable. The only recognizable structure is the inferior vena cava anterior to the high-amplitude spinal echoes. The dominant feature of this scan is a large, highly reflective region involving most of the abdomen, especially on the left side. Bowel loops are displaced anteriorly, as is indicated by some shadowing just to the left of midline, along with a typical reverberation artifact.

Figure 9–36, a longitudinal scan of the same patient, shows a large,

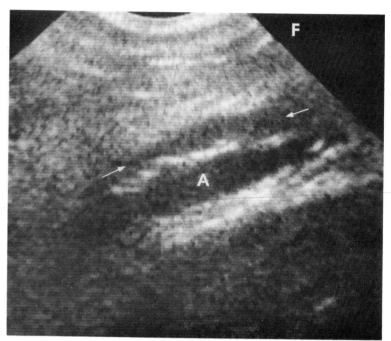

**FIG 9–33.**

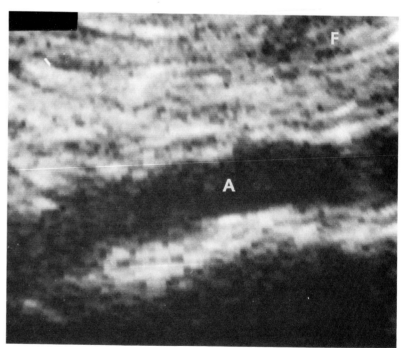

**FIG 9–34.**

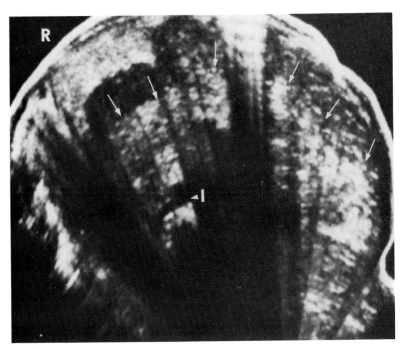

**FIG 9–35.**

highly reflective mass (arrows) anterior to the abdominal aorta and involving nearly the entire abdomen. An oval sonolucency is seen posteriorly over the lower abdomen, representing a markedly displaced left kidney. The large retroperitoneal mass was found to be liposarcoma, which was filling most of the abdomen. The mass was displacing the left kidney inferiorly and over the midline.

| | | |
|---|---|---|
| **A** | = | Aorta |
| **Arrows** | = | Retroperitoneal fibrosis (in Fig 9–33) |
| **Arrows** | = | Liposarcoma (in Figs 9–35 and 9–36) |
| **F** | = | Foot |
| **H** | = | Head |
| **I** | = | Inferior vena cava |
| **K** | = | Displaced left kidney |
| **R** | = | Right |

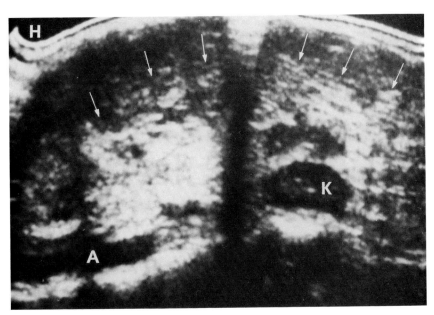

**FIG 9–36.**

## Retroperitoneal Abscesses

Large fluid-filled collections may be visualized on ultrasound studies of the retroperitoneum. The examiner must first rule out a fluid-containing loop of bowel. This can usually be excluded by real-time examination of the mass, with attention directed toward observing peristaltic activity. Once dilated bowel loops have been excluded, fluid-filled retroperitoneal masses are usually caused by abscesses, hematomas, urinomas, and lymphoceles. They are usually sonolucent masses with irregular borders and enhanced through-transmission. However, the ultrasonographic appearance may vary, depending on the internal consistency of the mass.

Figure 9–37 is a longitudinal scan showing a large psoas abscess inferior to the lower pole of the right kidney. This sonolucent mass could be consistent with other fluid-filled entities mentioned previously. The internal echoes on the back wall are highly suggestive of an abscess or a hematoma. Clinical findings and laboratory data usually allow the correct diagnosis to be made.

Figure 9–38, a transverse scan of a different patient, demonstrates an extremely unusual ultrasonographic finding. Two sonolucent masses are present in the left retroperitoneal region. These were found to be abscesses extending into both the psoas and the iliacus muscles on the left side.

Figures 9–39 and 9–40 are transverse and longitudinal scans of a patient with a long history of alcoholism. Seven days before admission he was kicked in the back. He presented with low-grade fever and left hip pain. X-ray studies of the hip were negative. Figure 9–39, a transverse scan of the abdomen, shows a large sonolucent mass with soft internal echoes markedly displacing the left kidney anteriorly. Figure 9–40 is a longitudinal scan that confirms the findings on the transverse scan. The kidney is also seen to be displaced in a cephalad direction on this scan. The mass was a large psoas abscess resulting from a hematoma following the initial trauma. Even though numerous internal

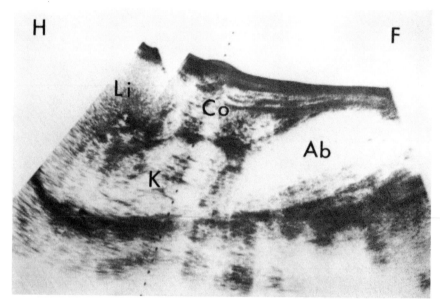

**FIG 9–37.**

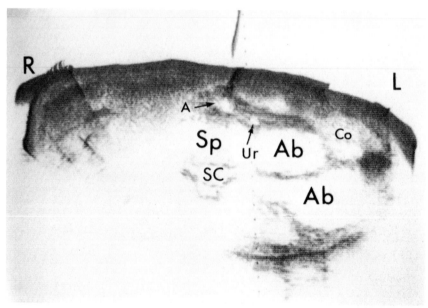

**FIG 9–38.**

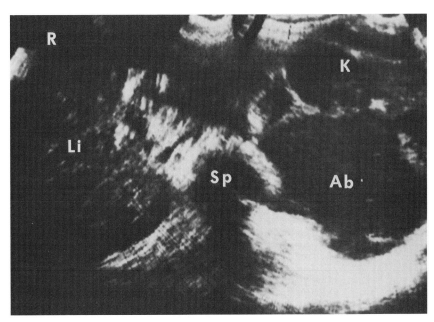

FIG 9–39.

echoes are present in the mass, this is a fluid-containing structure because of the enhanced through-transmission noted deep to the mass on both scans.

**A** = Aorta
**Ab** = Abscess
**Co** = Colon
**F** = Foot
**H** = Head
**K** = Kidney
**L** = Left
**Li** = Liver
**R** = Right
**SC** = Spinal canal
**Sp** = Spine
**Ur** = Ureter

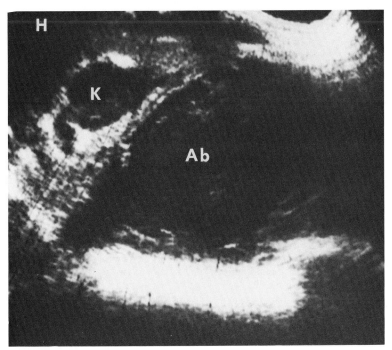

FIG 9–40.

## Retroperitoneal Abscess and Hematoma

Ultrasound is an excellent means of evaluating the perinephric region for any fluid collection. Figures 9–41 and 9–42 are scans obtained in an extremely unusual case with rather dramatic ultrasound findings. The patient was in an automobile accident approximately 2 weeks before admission. She noted a gradual increase in size of her abdomen on the right side over a 2-week period. Figure 9–41 is a transverse scan of the right abdomen obtained at the time of admission. A large, relatively sonolucent mass with marked through-transmission can be seen in the right abdomen. Asymmetry of the abdominal wall is indicated by the surface echoes. The spine is situated to the left of midline. Through-transmission is present along with internal echoes, indicating a fluid mass with some solid components. The findings are consistent with hematoma or abscess. At surgery, an infected hematoma was found. Figure 9–42 is a longitudinal scan over the midline with dramatic findings. The aorta is well seen, as are the splenic vein, pancreas, and superior mesenteric artery. Anterior to the pancreas is the right kidney, displaced over the midline by the large infected hematoma. Although the kidney and pancreas are retroperitoneal organs, it is amazing how far they can be displaced in the retroperitoneum.

Figure 9–43 is a transverse scan of a patient with a left perinephric abscess. The right kidney is in its normal position, adjacent to the spine. The left kidney is displaced anteriorly and laterally by a large perinephric collection.

Figure 9–44 is a longitudinal scan of the right upper quadrant in a patient with a bleeding diaphysis. The patient had a 1-week history of persistent right back pain and a dropping hematocrit. Figure 9–44 shows a sonolucent mass with enhanced through-transmission in the right subhepatic region. This was found to be a retroperitoneal hematoma.

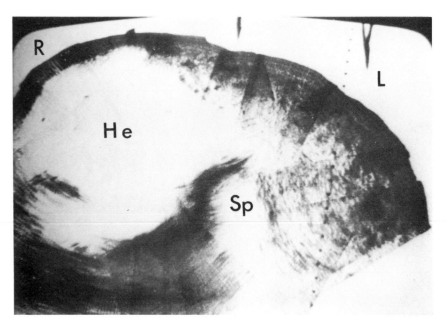

**FIG 9–41.**

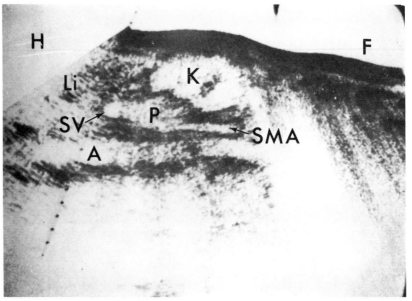

**FIG 9–42.**

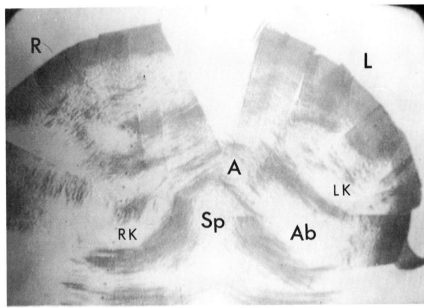

A   = Aorta
Ab  = Abscess
F   = Foot
H   = Head
He  = Hematoma
K   = Kidney
L   = Left
Li  = Liver
Lk  = Left kidney
P   = Pancreas
R   = Right
RK  = Right kidney
SMA = Superior mesenteric artery
Sp  = Spine
SV  = Splenic vein

FIG 9–43.

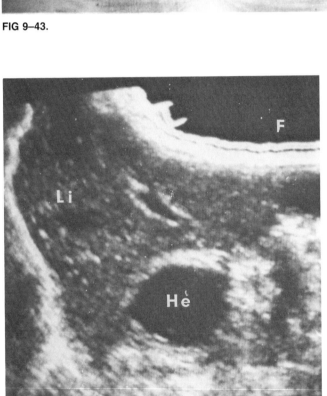

FIG 9–44.

## Retroperitoneal Lymphoceles

Lymphoceles usually present as fluid collections within the abdomen. Usually, they are basically echo free. They may, however, demonstrate echoes secondary to debris and fibrosis. Figures 9–45 and 9–46 are examples of large lymphoceles following retroperitoneal lymph node resection. In Figure 9–45, a large fluid collection is noted just beneath the umbilical level. A second fluid collection is present just above the urinary bladder. This lower fluid collection, however, has some echoes within it when compared to the more cephalad collection. Figure 9–46 is a transverse scan of the lymphocele in the umbilical region. The fluid is completely echo free, draping over the abdominal aorta.

Figure 9–47 is a lymphocele with multiple echoes within it. This would be difficult to distinguish from an abscess or hematoma. It did represent a lymphocele with debris. The lymphocele was causing hydronephrosis of the right kidney (Fig 9–48).

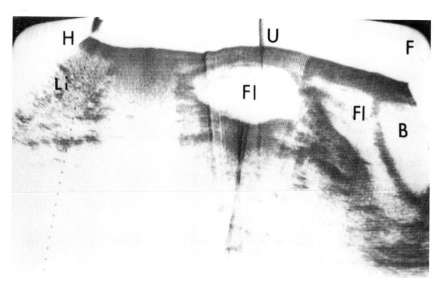

**FIG 9–45.**

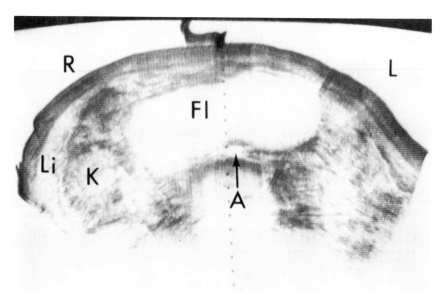

**FIG 9–46.**

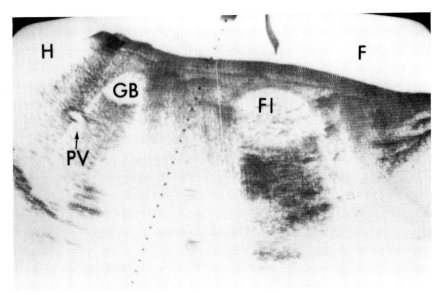

A   = Aorta
B   = Urinary bladder
F   = Foot
FI  = Fluid in the lymphocele
GB  = Gallbladder
H   = Head
Hy  = Hydronephrosis
K   = Kidney
L   = Left
Li  = Liver
PV  = Portal vein
R   = Right
U   = Umbilical level

FIG 9–47.

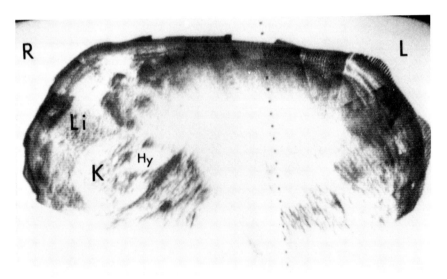

FIG 9–48.

# 10.
# Ultrasonography of the General Abdomen: Peritoneal Cavity, Bowel and Mesentery, and Abdominal Wall

Anthony A. Mancuso, M.D.

Despite a trend, since the late 1970s, toward performing computed tomography (CT) in the evaluation of abdominal masses and fluid collections, sonography retains an important place in the imaging approach to many of these cases. The widespread availability of real-time imaging equipment has added immeasurably to the speed and accuracy of the examination. We now must equivocate much less about "loops of fluid-filled bowel" masking or mimicking pathology. The real-time transducer virtually gives the experienced operator a "seeing hand" that can answer questions faster and more accurately than was possible only a few years ago with static scanning. The sonographer's major task is still to define the origin and extent of pathology, information that will direct the course of the remaining diagnostic evaluation.

An accurate differential diagnosis is possible with ultrasound, but often it depends more on clinical observations than on specific sonographic findings. A final diagnosis usually requires biopsy, aspiration, or other confirmatory studies. Often tissue or fluid sampling is guided or done by the sonographer. The intelligently aggressive use of ultrasound can often limit both morbidity and the cost of diagnosis. However, one must be careful not to make sonography cost additive in situations where other studies, such as CT or magnetic resonance (MR) imaging, may provide a more accurate or complete understanding of the problem at hand. We will consider the relative roles of all imaging options when appropriate in the following sections.

This chapter considers the role and technique of ultrasonography of the abdominal wall, the peritoneal cavity and spaces, the bowel and mesentery, and the diaphragm.

## Technique

### General Working Principles

A diagnostic imagery study is most useful when it is carried out to answer a specific, well-formulated question from the referring physician. Studies done as surveys or to "rule out pathology" tend to be much less informative. A flexible attitude toward the examination technique is also important. The examiner should never hesitate to change the patient's position to produce an adequate study. For example, decubitus views are extremely useful to determine whether a fluid collection is free, contained in bowel, or loculated.

While following the textual discussion and reflecting on the sonographic appearance of normal abdominal anatomy and pathologic changes, the reader may wish to keep in mind several basic questions as a useful framework for examination and interpretation:

1. What is the sonographic nature of the lesion? Does it indicate free fluid (simple or complex or localized abnormalities), simple cystic, mixed solid-cystic, or solid components?

2. Does the finding represent a significant abnormality, or is it a normal structure mimicking the appearance of pathology?

3. What is the origin and extent of the abnormality, using vector analysis?[1]

4. Are there any associated or specific findings that might help in the differential diagnosis?

5. How can I vary the technique of examination better to answer these questions?

6. Is CT, MR imaging, or diagnostic aspiration necessary?

The principles inherent in these questions are important to keep in mind while performing or interpreting any ultrasound examination. The following sections emphasize an overall approach while considering the limitations and pitfalls of the examination in individual areas.

## Patient Preparation

The preparation of the patient depends on the goals of the examination. If the patient is acutely ill and a specific question is raised, such as whether a subdiaphragmatic abscess is present, no preparation is needed, and the examination can be limited to the area designated. More often circumstances are not so acute, and some degree of preparation is possible and desirable. Routinely, the patients are kept without oral intake overnight, or at least are asked not to eat any fat-containing foods for approximately 12–18 hours before the study. This usually ensures visualization of the normal, distended gallbladder and may reduce gastrointestinal (GI) air content. If barium studies precede sonography within 2 days, bowel preparation is necessary. The barium-filled bowel may impair sound transmission or mimic an abnormal mass.[2]

Since gas poses a barrier to the transmission of sound, some attempt to reduce the volume of gas in the GI tract is a good idea. Investigators have met with some limited success in improving sound transmission with the use of oral methylcellulose preparations.[3,4] Water has been instilled in the stomach to reduce its gas content and produce a sonographic window for looking at the left upper quadrant. The water does not produce the desired sonographic window, because accompanying microbubbles of gas usually cause the sound to be dispersed.[5] Such a maneuver may, however, allow differentiation of the stomach from an abnormal left upper quadrant mass. A distended urinary bladder greatly facilitates examination of the pelvis because it displaces gas-filled bowel. A tap water enema may also prove useful in selected pelvic cases.

## Static Versus Real-Time Imaging

The articulated-arm contact scanner is not used when good real-time equipment is available. Real-time examination is preferred for several reasons in evaluating the abdominal cavity and GI tract:

1. Rapid examination of the abdomen is possible in 5–10 minutes by an experienced sonographer. Not only the viscera and spaces considered in this chapter but all of the organs in the abdominal cavity, retroperitoneum, and pelvis can be surveyed.

2. Ease of orientation allows rapid confirmation of pathologic conditions in two planes and is of great help in ultrasound-guided biopsy and aspiration.

3. Demonstration of physiologic motion aids in the evaluation of the diaphragm, blood vessels, and bowel. Much of the equivocation that was caused by bowel with the older static techniques can be avoided by careful observation with real-time instruments.

## Ultrasound Versus CT

In the abdominal cavity, mesentery, and GI tract, ultrasound suffers some serious limitations compared to CT. Some of these are clinical and others technical. However, ultrasound retains a primary diagnostic role in some instances and can be used in a highly efficacious manner if cases are selected appropriately. General indications for sonographic study of the abdominal cavity include (1) definition of the origin, extent, and character of a palpable mass lesion, 2) detection and characterization of intraperitoneal fluid collections, and (3) guided aspiration, biopsy, and drainage procedures.

The choice between ultrasound and CT (or MR imaging) as the initial examination often depends on subtle combinations of physician preference, the patient's age and condition, working diagnosis, and economics. Obviously we cannot provide an algorithm for all occasions. Some general guidelines we use include the following:

1. Ultrasound is the first choice in the following situations:
   a. To examine patients who are too sick to come to the department.
   b. To confirm or detect simple ascites.
   c. To rule out subphrenic abscess on the right and (if spleen is in) on the left.
   d. To evaluate abdominal wall masses.
   e. To guide procedures, when appropriate (to save cost of CT guidance).
2. CT is the first choice in the following situations:
   a. If the patient has numerous wounds, drains, etc. on the abdominal wall.
   b. If management decisions depend on a definitive anatomic study of other organs or sites (e.g., pancreas, mesentery).
   c. If a guided procedure cannot be done safely with ultrasound or fluoroscopic control alone.
3. MR imaging is reserved for special circumstances, at present. Its specific role with respect to other imaging modalities is still to be established. To date, we have exploited its multiplanar capabilities for determining the origin of large abdominal masses and its ability (sometimes) to differentiate tumor from posttreatment fibrotic residua.

## Guided Aspiration, Biopsy, and Drainage Procedures

Major advances in imaging have led to parallel developments in guided interventional procedures. In the abdomen these are done using a combination of ultrasound, CT, and fluoroscopy. Many excellent publications describing the details of these procedures are available.[6-11] In this discussion we will consider the

"basics." The presentation of the entire subject (i.e., clinical perspective, follow-up care, choice of catheter, etc.) is so good in the referenced publications that the reader is advised to conduct a thorough review of the subject before embarking on these often complex procedures.

### General Guidelines

The guiding principle for interventional procedures should be "physician, do no harm." Therefore, the physician must assume an active role in the preprocedure and postprocedure care of the patient. At least the following steps should be taken:

1. Review of all diagnostic imaging studies and carefully considered approach to the procedure.
2. A visit with the patient to obtain informed consent and allergy information.
3. Review of pertinent laboratory studies, especially bleeding parameters.
4. Postprocedure follow-up (this may be as simple as a single visit and progress notes or as complex as continuous monitoring of drainage catheters).
5. Must be available on a 24-hour basis for follow-up care or advice.
6. Must take primary responsibility for accurate handling of all diagnostic material (Table 10–1).

Several key clinical considerations in biopsy procedures include:

1. Likelihood of excessive bleeding: Check current prothrombin time, partial thromboplastin time, platelets, and bleeding time.
2. Antibiotic prophylaxis: Any work in a known or potentially infected field should be covered with broad-spectrum antibiotics.[6-11]
3. Premedication: Combinations of narcotics, barbiturates, diazepam, and phenothiazines may be employed. It is best if the person doing the procedure takes the responsibility for supervising the administration of these drugs.

### Choice of Guidance System

This section considers only some of the interventional procedures done today, namely, aspiration and biopsy of abdominal masses and fluid collections and drain-

**TABLE 10–1.**

**Clinical Characteristics of Aspirated Fluid***

| COLLECTION† | GROSS APPEARANCE | GRAM STAIN (ORGANISMS) | GRAM STAIN (WBCS) | CHEMISTRY | OTHER |
|---|---|---|---|---|---|
| Abscess | | | | | |
|   Pyogenic | Cloudy, purulent | + | + | | |
|   Sterile | Cloudy, yellow | − | + | | |
|   Amebic | "Anchovy paste" (wet mount) | + | + | | |
|   Fungal | Cloudy, purulent (hyphae, yeast) | + | + | | Special stains |
| Bowel | | | | | |
|   Large | Tan, brown | + | Few | | Odor |
|   Small | Yellowish | − | − | | |
| Hematoma | | | | | |
|   Bland | Red/dark red | − | Few | | |
|   Infected purulent | Red/dark red | + | + | | |
| Ascites | | | | | |
|   Bland | Clear, yellow | None | None | Protein + | |
|   Infected | Cloudy, yellow | + | + | Protein + | |
|   Sterile | Cloudy, yellow | − | + | Protein + | |
| Pseudocyst | | | | | |
|   Bland | Yellow | − | − | Amylase | |
|   Infected | Cloudy, yellow | + | + | Amylase | |
| Bile | | | | | |
|   In GB or biloma | Dark yellow/green | − | − | Bilirubin | |
|   Infected | Cloudy, green | + | + | Bilirubin | |
| Urinoma | Yellow, clear | − | − | Electrolytes like serum | Urinalysis |
| Lymphocele | Clear, yellow | − | − | | Fat globules |
| Necrotic tumor | Dark red/brown | − | − | | Cytology |

*Modified from Ferrucci et al.,[6] by permission.
†Bland means uncomplicated, noninfected, collection of a particular fluid.

age of abscesses or fluid collections in the peritoneal cavity. In the abdominal cavity the choice of a guidance system is usually between CT and ultrasound, either one then being used in combination with fluoroscopy whenever needed.[6–11] GI tract procedures are done under fluoroscopic control. The guiding principles here are safety, speed and flexibility, cost, and radiation exposure, of the physician as well as to the patient.

## BIOPSY

Ultrasound should be used if the lesion is clearly seen and the path is safe. In general, ultrasound in this setting is faster, less expensive, and less in demand than CT. The patient's safety must *never* be jeopardized for these reasons. One must be sure that the path will not cross the bowel (except for fine needle aspiration), the pleural space (lung), or a major blood vessel. In properly selected cases, real-time ultrasound is a very rapid and flexible guidance tool. Special biopsy transducers are available,[12, 13] but we find that scanning at right angles to the needle path with routine mechanical heads is sufficient. Jiggling the needle or injecting one to several tenths of a cubic centimeter of air can help in identifying the needle tip.[6–10, 14]

At times, gas may obscure a lesion previously seen on ultrasound. CT may be done to avoid repeated, unsuccessful sonographic localization. If detailed anatomic information is required for diagnosis or management, then CT should precede ultrasound guidance. This is especially true in solid masses of uncertain vascularity when a large bone cutting needle is used for sampling.[6–11]

Other advantages of CT include less operator dependence, lack of interference from gas, dressing, or bone, and the precise visualization of the needle tip, the last making CT preferred in deep-seated or small lesions.[6–11] If an angled approach or one near the pleural space is contemplated, fluoroscopy and CT should be used for needle placement.[15–17]

The choice of a specific thin (20–22 gauge) needle is a matter of personal preference. All have a wide margin of safety. The procedure may always be safely begun with a 22-gauge needle to identify the initial pathway. Multiple passes with a 20-gauge needle may then be done in a tandem fashion with little or no added risk.[6–11] Needle placement should be parallel to the transverse plane of the body whenever possible. Craniocaudal angulation complicates needle tip localization and almost always prolongs the study significantly. Chances of successful sampling also diminish. Medial or lateral angulation with the needle remaining in the chosen transverse plane may be done to avoid unfavorable paths.

### ASPIRATION OF FLUID COLLECTIONS

In large and superficial fluid collections, ultrasound is the preferred method of guiding the aspiration.[6–11] Return of fluid into the syringe confirms proper needle placement. If the tap is "dry" a change to CT may be indicated. Dedicated biopsy transducers or adaptors for standard mechanical sector heads are available.[6–10, 12, 13] We do not use these devices. If the lesion is suitable for ultrasound, it can usually be approached via a direct vertical path while the needle tip is followed with ultrasound from a location outside the sterile field. One must avoid bowel in aspiration of fluid collections to prevent infection of a previous sterile collection and to avoid contaminating the aspirate, which would yield a false positive diagnosis of abscess (see Table 10–1). If there is any question that the bowel may be entered, CT should be used for guidance.[6–11]

In the pelvis, left upper quadrant, and lesser sac, CT is almost always used because of variability of intervening bowel. Even more than in the case of biopsy one must not cross the pleural space.[6–10, 15–17] Contamination of a previously sterile space can be a serious complication, but it is almost always avoidable with careful planning and fluoroscopic or CT guidance. We are very conservative about using ultrasound in cases where the pleural space is nearby, especially in the left upper quadrant, where the presence of bowel and spleen increase the risks of the procedure.

Despite a fairly characteristic sonographic or CT appearance, a fluid collection may contain very tenacious material. This is true of relatively fresh hematomas and some abscesses (especially fungal). Aspiration should always start with a 22-gauge needle. If there is no return and if the needle is positioned in the center of the collection, progressively larger needles (20 and 18 gauge) or needle-sheath systems should be used. If aspiration through an 18-gauge sheath or needle is unsuccessful, the collection is either a very thick collection of pus, hematoma, or phlegmon. If a solid mass is a reasonable clinical consideration, biopsy may be done and the specimen sent for cytologic examination (see Table 10–1).

### Catheter Drainage of Fluid Collections and Abscesses

These procedures represent a major medical contribution of diagnostic imaging to patient care over the last 8–9 years. Percutaneous catheter drainage procedures have their foundation in both modern surgical and cross-sectional imaging techniques. Ultrasound plays a relatively minor role compared to CT and fluoroscopy in the therapeutic part of the algorithm. While ultrasound *can* be the imaging examination of choice in the initial search for and diagnostic aspiration of an abscess or fluid collection, there are significant limitations to its use in the planning, execution, and follow-up of the drainage procedure. The advantages of CT include (1) accurate planning of access routes (this is critical), (2) identification of additional collections perhaps remote from those most obvious on ultrasound or clinically, and (3) ease of follow-up in often critically ill patients with abdominal wounds and drains. Fluoroscopy is almost always used at some time in these patients. It has several key advantages, including the following (1) It allows visualization of the entire cavity as well as of fistulas to surrounding viscera with injection of contrast material. (2) It allows direct visual control of catheter and wire placement, side hole positioning, and selection of optimum course of dependent drainage. (3) It allows rapid assessment of the position of the diaphragm. (4) It facilitates follow-up studies (sinography, abscessography).

It should be clear even from this brief discussion that ultrasound guidance for drainage procedures is indicated only in a very small number of cases. A good example might be an abdominal wall collection. Small or deep-seated fluid collections require CT guidance and strict adherence to the surgical and clinical principles worked out over the last several years for safe and percutaneous successful drainage.[6-11, 15-17]

## Abdominal Anatomy

### Abdominal Wall

The abdominal wall and rectus sheath can be studied in detail with a 5- or 7-MHz short internal focus transducer. The time-gain compensation curve is set as if one were doing a thyroid study. This technique emphasizes the detail in the relatively superficial anatomy. The actual transducer chosen depends on the patient's habitus. The skin-transducer interface produces the initial "bang." Deep to this dark, linear echo is the relatively sonolucent subcutaneous plane, a fat and fibrous tissue zone producing variable amounts of low-level echoes. The exact appearance and thickness of this subcutaneous plane varies with fat content. The fascia surrounding the musculature of the abdominal wall produces strongly reflective surfaces, so that the musculofascial plane consists of a relatively thick, sonolucent muscular zone bracketed by two thin, very echogenic fascial interfaces.[17] The parietal peritoneum echoes blend with those of the deep fascia of the abdominal wall. Consequently, normal peritoneum is not seen as a distinct structure.[17, 18]

### Abdominal Cavity and Lesser Sac

The abdominal and pelvic cavities should always be considered a continuum; the pelvis represents the most dependent portion of this large space. For the purposes of discussion, however, we will consider the abdominal cavity to end inferiorly at the pelvic brim. Superiorly it is bounded by the diaphragm where the parietal peritoneum is firmly adherent to the diaphragmatic fascia.[18] Anteriorly and posteriorly, the parietal peritoneum is separated from the abdominal wall and retroperitoneum, respectively, by varying amounts of fat and connective tissue.[18]

Separation of the peritoneal cavity into several compartments produces a useful framework for understanding how the movement of fluid or spread of tumor and infection is channeled along the natural pathways the normal anatomy creates.[18-22] The transverse mesocolon divides the abdominal cavity into supramesocolic and inframesocolic spaces. The root of the small bowel mesentery runs obliquely from slightly to the left of midline at the ligament of Treitz to the cecum, thereby separating the inframesocolic compartment into two infracolic spaces. The right infracolic space is much smaller and does not communicate as readily as the left with the pelvis.[18-22]

The infracolic spaces are bound externally by paracolic gutters which may serve as communications between the pelvis and supramesocolic compartments. The degree of communication varies from side to side. On the right, the paracolic gutter is deeper and leads to the subhepatic space and its posterosuperior extension, the hepatorenal fossa (Morrison's pouch).[18-22] The hepatorenal fossa is a paravertebral space and the most fluid-dependent of the upper abdominal cavity spaces when the patient is supine.[18-22] These basically subhepatic spaces freely communicate with the right subphrenic space.[18-22]

The lesser peritoneal sac also communicates with the subhepatic spaces.[19-21] Anteriorly it is bounded by the lesser omentum. The right free edge of the lesser omentum forms the hepatoduodenal ligament and the anterior wall of the epiploic foramen (foramen of Winslow). The remainder of the lesser omentum spreads to join with the mesentery of the stomach, contributing to several ligaments between the stomach, liver, spleen, and diaphragm. This forms the anterior wall, the closed superior recesses, and the left lateral borders of the lesser sac.[18] The inferior border of the lesser sac is the transverse mesocolon. The very important relationship of the posteroinferior wall of the lesser sac to the pancreas must always be kept in mind.

The falciform ligament separates the right and left subphrenic spaces, though they may communicate anteriorly.[22] The left subphrenic and subhepatic spaces are in gross continuity and may be thought of as either entirely subphrenic or perihepatic. The phrenicocolic ligament attaches the colon to the left hemidiaphragm and forms an effective barrier between the relatively shallow left paracolic gutter and the perihepatic and perisplenic spaces.[19-22]

## Normal Bowel and Mesentery

The intestinal tract, from the stomach to the rectum, is usually distended with varying amounts of air. These highly reflective air–soft tissue interfaces are responsible for most of the artifacts encountered in abdominal scanning. Occasionally the intestinal tract is distended with fluid, in which case its appearance may mimic that of complex or simple fluid collections.

Various parts of the GI tract are often collapsed; the exact identification of the visualized, nondistended GI tract depends on the related anatomic landmarks. A good example is the collapsed gastric antrum lying anterior to the pancreas.[23–25] The pattern typical of collapsed portions of the GI tract consists of a central, highly reflective, usually linear echo representing mucus and admixed air.[23–25] If the bowel is fluid filled, it will have a central sonolucency surrounded by the high-level mucosal echoes. If it is not fluid filled, a peripheral sonolucency of varying thickness represents bowel wall which surrounds the collapsed lumen. This produces the normal "target" configuration. The sonolucent halo of the bowel wall is normally less than 2 cm thick.[25] This in turn is surrounded by a highly reflective interface representing the serosal surface of the bowel and closely related mesenteric attachments.[23, 24]

Perhaps the single most important contribution of real-time sonography in the general abdominal examination is that it allows the operator to more confidently distinguish normal bowel from abnormal masses or fluid collections in the peritoneal cavity. Real-time imaging will frequently show active peristalsis within the segment under study. At times water (or methylcellulose) is given to distend the stomach and help identify the proximal duodenum. This is sometimes augmented with scanning the patient in the upright position. Water enemas in pelvic sonography aid in excluding rectum or distal rectosigmoid as possible pelvic masses.

## Stomach

The gastroesophageal junction which lies just anterior to the aorta and is surrounded by the crura of the diaphragm produces a typical though somewhat elongated target configuration.[23, 24] The stomach's appearance is otherwise variable.[23–25] It usually contains enough air to obscure the left upper quadrant. At times, it contains fluid, food, and small amounts of air. It may mimic a complex mass lesion or lesser sac fluid collection. Often the gastric antrum is collapsed and can be seen lying immediately anterior to the pancreas. The central linear echo of the collapsed antrum and surrounding sonolucent stomach wall should not be mistaken for the pancreas and the pancreatic duct.[23, 24]

## Small Bowel

The duodenum, together with the gallbladder and proper vascular landmarks, forms a triad that helps to localize the pancreatic head.[23, 24] Although the duodenum is a useful landmark, it is also a source of serious artifacts. When it contains gas, reverberation artifacts can mimic pancreatic mass lesions. At times the highly reflective gas-filled duodenum mimics a gallbladder filled with calculi. Fluid-filled second and third portions of the duodenum create pseudomasses in the pancreatic or retroperitoneal areas. At the ligament of Treitz, fluid in the duodenum might mimic an adrenal mass or retroperitoneal lymphadenopathy.[23, 24]

The small bowel also has a variable appearance. When the bowel is distended with fluid, valvulae and bowel contents are sometimes visible within the obvious tubular structures. Even with its relatively small air content, the small bowel often obscures areas of interest within the abdomen. Collapsed small bowel without much air produces an amorphous echogenic pattern filling the middle to lower abdomen. Sometimes this collapsed bowel takes on a faint, serpiginous, or stacked appearance indicative of its origins.

## Large Intestine

The collapsed transverse colon will often be seen, especially on longitudinal scans, inferior to the plane of the pancreas and stomach. The gas-containing hepatic flexure may produce artifacts simulating gallbladder disease, much like the artifacts produced by the duodenum. Observing "dirty" versus "clean" shadowing patterns again may aid in differentiation. The splenic flexure can look like the left kidney.[26] The omentum and mesenteries are usually not distinctly visible unless they are diseased or a large amount of peritoneal fluid is present.

The important working principle is that the appearance of the bowel varies with bowel contents and degree of distention. Moreover, its appearance is often characteristic. As a source of artifacts the bowel may be responsible for abnormal findings such as localized fluid collections. As a useful anatomic landmark, it may result in a more accurate diagnosis.

## Pathologic Conditions in the Abdomen

### Pathology of the Abdominal Wall

Masses and fluid collections may arise in or involve the subcutaneous plane, musculofascial plane, peritoneal surface, or intra-abdominal compartment (Table 10–2). Following localization, the basic internal consistency of the abnormal area is considered, and it helps to rank differential possibilities (Tables 10–3 and 10–4). The clinical circumstances usually determine which is most likely. The differential diagnosis of predominantly cystic areas limited to the abdominal wall usually includes seroma, abscess, and hematoma.[27–30] Rarely, a cystic or necrotic tumor may be present. Ventral hernias, including spigelian type, with

**TABLE 10–3.**

**Characteristics of Abnormal Fluid Collections of the Abdomen**

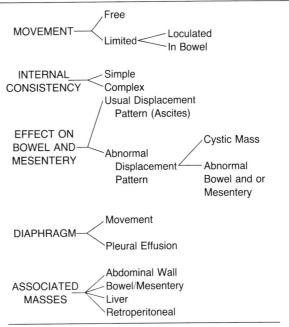

**TABLE 10–2.**

**Characteristics of Localized Abnormal Masses of the Abdomen**

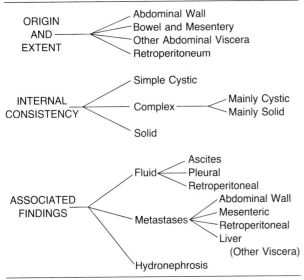

air- or fluid-filled bowel, are also included in the differential diagnosis when the clinical setting is appropriate.[31–33] Abdominal wall defects without herniated bowel may also be seen.[31] A solid mass with a homogeneous internal architecture may appear sonolucent and mimic the internal consistency of a fluid collection; through-transmission, however, will be absent. The differential diagnosis of predominantly solid processes includes tumor, clotted blood, and induration.[27–34] Desmoid tumor, malignant fibrous histiocytoma, and other sarcomas are possible.[34]

Of these masses, rectus sheath hematoma deserves special mention because its clinical presentation can mimic intra-abdominal pathology. This may occur in patients on anticoagulant therapy, but more often there is no such history. The hematoma is usually seen as a hypoechoic mass conforming at least in part to the shape of the rectus sheath but causing some bulging of its contour.[27–29] Aspiration can confirm the diagnosis.

Artifacts generated by the abdominal wall are mainly related to attenuation of the ultrasound beam by rib and loss of the acoustic coupling at the skin-transducer interface. Scars often cause a break in the skin-transducer couple. They attenuate sound because of their dense fibrous tissue content.

**TABLE 10–4.**

**Sonographic Characteristics as an Aid to Differential Diagnosis**

| | INTERNAL ECHOES | BORDERS | INCREASED THROUGH-TRANSMISSION | USUAL DIFFERENTIAL DIAGNOSIS | LESS COMMON DIAGNOSIS |
|---|---|---|---|---|---|
| **Free fluid collections*** | | | | | |
| Simple | No | Smooth, distinct | Yes | Ascites—transudate or exudate | Hematoma, abscess, fluid in bowel |
| Complex | Septated, debris | Irregular, thickened, indistinct (fuzzy) | Yes | Malignant ascites, inflammatory exudate with adhesions, simple ascites with preexisting adhesions | Bowel plus contents (ee complex), mainly cystic, localized abnormalities |
| **Localized abnormalities** | | | | | |
| Simple cystic | No | Smooth, regular distinct | Yes | Loculated ascites, cysts | Abscess, hematoma, fluid in bowel, pseudocyst, duplication or mesenteric cyst |
| Complex, mainly cystic | Septa, debris, fluid levels | Smooth, regular to irregular, thickened, indistinct | Yes, prominently | Abscess, hematoma, pseudocyst, bowel, loculated ascites, ovarian neoplasm | Lymphocele, duplication, mesenteric cyst, abnormal bowel, (infarcted, obstructed) |
| Complex, mainly solid | High-level calcium, air (microbubbles) septa, debris, solid elements, cystic foci | Regular and smooth to irregular, thickened, indistinct | Yes, often subtle | Pelvoabdominal neoplasm (lymphoma sarcomas, benign mesenchymal tumors) with necrosis | Abnormal bowel (infarcted), abscess, hematoma |
| Solid | High-level calcium, homogeneous and almost sonolucent, homogeneous and obvious internal architecture, variable gray tones | Regular, smooth to irregular and indistinct | No | Neoplasm, lymphoma, sarcoma, benign mesenchymal tumor | Barium in bowel, GI masses tumor, or intussusception, hematoma, abscess (none) |

*Loculated fluid; see localized abnormalities

*Fluid Collections in the Peritoneal Cavity*

The significance of a fluid collection is usually determined by the clinical setting and aspiration. The approach described below is useful because it makes the examiner think about what he is observing. It may provide clues about whether a collection needs to be aspirated, or perhaps that the diagnostic imaging evaluation may stop at sonography.

FREE FLUID—SIMPLE OR COMPLEX?

Fluid accumulations in the peritoneal cavity as seen on sonography may be free, loculated, or contained in bowel (see Table 10–3). Changing the patient's position and observing the movement of the fluid area will usually determine the nature of the accumulation. If not, it may be useful to wait several minutes or have the patient change position before rescanning the area. Real-time scanning is particularly valuable in this setting because it differentiates peristalsis from static extraluminal collections.

Free fluid may be either simple or complex in appearance (see Tables 10–3 and 10–4). Simple fluid collections have no internal echo pattern and form very smooth, well-defined interfaces with the surrounding tissues. Such fluid collections may be loculated. Complex fluid collections either have some sort of internal echo pattern, such as septae or floating debris, or form thickened and/or irregular interfaces with the surrounding anatomic structures.

Simple ascites is most often a transudate resulting from a metabolic disturbance; it may also originate from an inflammatory or neoplastic focus.[35] Complex ascites is more likely to be the result of an inflammatory or neoplastic process. These generalizations should not be carried too far. Any time free fluid is present, associated findings, such as localized masses or evidence of metastatic disease, should be sought to help clarify the etiology (see Table 10–4). In trauma cases the fluid may represent blood. Causes of hemorrhage such as subcapsular splenic or hepatic hematomas and/or fractures of the liver, spleen, or retroperitoneal viscera should be investigated. Occasionally, thickening of the peritoneal surfaces will indicate diffuse or localized tumor involvement.

FLUID MOVEMENT

The following factors influence the movement of fluid in the peritoneal cavity and its localization in various compartments:

1. The position of the patient
2. The amount of fluid[19–22, 35, 36]
3. The peritoneal organs, reflections, and ligaments (see Anatomy section)[19–22, 35, 36]
4. The presence of adhesions
5. Where the fluid originates[22, 35, 36]
6. What process is responsible for the presence of fluid[19–21]
7. Intraperitoneal pressure (movements secondary to changes in respiration and related changes in hydrostatic pressure)[19–23, 35]
8. Density of the fluid.[35]

Logical patterns of flow can be predicted by considering the patient's position in light of the previous anatomic discussion. These predicted flow patterns agree with those observed during cadaver studies on fluid movement within the peritoneal cavity and agree basically with the actual clinical experience.[19–22] Experimentally, fluid amounts as small as 100–200 ml can be detected sonographically.[22, 36] Clinically, small collections are typically seen in the right paracolic gutter, lateral and anterior to the liver, and in the subhepatic spaces.[22, 35] The sonolucency of preperitoneal fat anterior to the liver must not be interpreted as a fluid collection.

When right-sided fluid collections are large, they fill out the subhepatic space and hepatorenal fossa and extend to the right subphrenic space. Subhepatic space fluid may also enter the lesser sac. Flow across the midline may be restricted by the falciform ligament.[19–22, 35] Flow between the left supramesocolic space and paracolic gutter is limited on the left by the phrenicocolic ligament. Therefore, if fluid is present in the left subphrenic region, it most likely originated in the supramesocolic compartment.[19–21] There is free communication among the right upper and lower abdominal compartments via the deeper, unobstructed right paracolic gutter.[19–21]

*Ascites and Associated Effects on Bowel, Mesentery, and Liver*

Large ascitic collections present no problem in detection but do produce some interesting sonographic phenomena. Fluid in tense ascites will surround, compress, and displace the liver, causing it to have a more richly echogenic appearance than usual.[35] When the liver is surrounded by fluid, other peritoneal attachments such as the falciform ligament and the lesser omentum become visible.[35] Furthermore, the usual anatomic landmarks in the high retroperitoneum are obscured by the posteriorly and medially displaced bowel and mesentery.

As the ascites increases in volume, the normal mesentery tends to collect along the lines of its posterior peritoneal attachment, producing a highly reflective group of echoes in the middle and upper abdomen. With very fatty mesentery, the echo pattern tends to spread out more, because the mesentery is more buoyant and assumes a more vertical orientation. With a less fatty and less buoyant mesentery, the echoes tend to clump and collapse posteriorly.[35]

Normal bowel floats or sinks in ascitic fluid, depending on its relative air and fluid content. Bowel usually appears as echogenic clumps arranged in an arcuate fashion around the vertically oriented mesentery.[35] Occasionally bowel is seen in cross section as a rounded prominence at the end of a fingerlike mesenteric projection. Adhesions may be seen extending from bowel to the abdominal wall.[35]

### Localized Peritoneal Abnormalities

#### ULTRASOUND VERSUS CT

After the origin and extent of a peritoneal abnormality have been studied and it has been determined that the abnormality is most likely localized disease, the sonographic features of the localized mass or fluid collection can be scrutinized. Consideration of the internal consistency, borders, and associated findings aids greatly in weighing the differential diagnosis and directing further diagnostic evaluation.[37–41] Any classification of this type leads to overlapping of differential possibilities, so this categorization is intended only as a general aid to differential diagnosis (see Table 10–4). Again, ultrasound is carried out either to guide the clinician toward appropriate further studies or to outline the extent of disease for accurate planning of therapy. For instance, a perihepatic-subphrenic collection may be noninfected and due to an abscess elsewhere in the abdomen.

Ultrasound is best suited to the detection of fluid collections in the right subphrenic space, left subphrenic space (if the spleen is present), subhepatic spaces, paracolic gutters, and true pelvis. Abdominal wall and liver and splenic abscesses are also detected with 90%–95% accuracy on ultrasound.[42] The

middle and lower abdomen and other areas are best studied with CT. However, while detection rates are high, ultrasound often may not provide all the information necessary for management.[6, 7, 42]

Accurate, practical ultrasound examination requires real-time imaging as well as meticulous attention to detail. The gain settings must be scrupulously set when the examiner is searching for localized or small fluid collections. A fluid area with some internal debris may "fill in" and be missed if gain settings are too high.[37] Homogeneous solid abnormalities may be mistaken for fluid areas if gains are too low.[37, 41] Sometimes, examination at two different gain settings is required to avoid these pitfalls.[37] If high quality ultrasound is not available, it is probably wise to use CT as the screening examination.

#### LOCULATED ASCITES

Nonpyogenic inflammatory conditions (e.g., pancreatitis) produce fluid collections that spread as expected along existing anatomic pathways. Their inflammatory nature allows them to dissect along the large and small bowel mesenteries, which provide a direct path to any quadrant.[19–21] More often, the mesentery and the parietal and visceral peritoneum wall off these processes near their site of origin. Thus, whenever fluid becomes loculated, the differential diagnosis is shifted toward an inflammatory etiology, even when no internal echoes are present (see Table 10–4). Evaluation of the margins of the fluid area then becomes extremely important. At times, a fuzzy, irregular border may be the only differentiating characteristic between inflammatory or neoplastic exudate and simple ascites that has become loculated due to preexisting adhesions. In this setting, a fluid-filled loop of bowel must always be considered a possible source of the findings and excluded by changing the patient's position or by real-time examination.

#### ABSCESS

Abscesses present most often as complex, predominantly cystic masses.[6, 7, 37, 42, 43] Classically an abscess appears as an elliptical sonolucent mass with thick and irregular margins.[37] Abscesses tend to be under tension and displace surrounding structures.[37, 42–44] A septated appearance may result from previous or developing adhesions. Necrotic debris produces internal echoes and may be seen "floating" within the abscess. Occasionally, fluid levels are present secondary to layering, probably because of the setting of debris. Gas-containing abscesses present varying echo patterns. The general appearance is that of a densely echogenic mass with or without acoustic shadowing and otherwise increased through-transmission. Mixed, solid, and cystic calcium-containing mass lesions such as a teratoma may mimic the sonographic pattern of a gas-containing abscess, but the clinical history and plain film evaluation usuallly will exclude them from the diagnosis.[39] Occasionally a gas-containing or heavily debris-laden abscess will mimic a solid lesion. This is especially true if it lies in a position which makes it difficult to judge whether enhanced through-transmission is present.

Peritonitis and resultant abscess formation may be a generalized or localized process. Once such pathology has been discovered, its extent should be determined. Multiloculated abscesses or multiple collections should be documented and their size determined as accurately as possible to aid in planning drainage and for improved accuracy in follow-up studies.[6, 7, 42] Lesser-sac abscesses deserve some separate attention. The slitlike epiploic foramen usually seals off the lesser sac from inflammatory processes extrinsic to it.[19-21] If the inflammatory process begins within the lesser sac, such as with a pancreatic abscess, the sac may be involved in addition to other secondarily affected peritoneal and retroperitoneal spaces. Differential consideration of simple and complex lesser-sac collections should always include pseudocyst, pancreatic abscess, and gastric outlet obstruction. A normally fluid-filled stomach should always be excluded.

Subphrenic abscesses also present some unique diagnostic problems. The left upper quadrant is particularly difficult to examine.[6, 7, 42] Placing the patient in the right lateral decubitus position and scanning along the coronal plane of the body, as well as prone scanning using the spleen as a sonographic window, will ensure a more complete examination of the left upper quadrant. Pleural effusion should not be mistaken for subdiaphragmatic fluid collections. If clarification is necessary, the patient may be scanned upright, so that the pleural fluid, diaphragm, and subphrenic region relationships can be shown.[45, 46] The diaphragm must always be identified and its excursion quantitated when one is looking for subphrenic abnormalities.[45, 46] Subcapsular collections of fluid within the liver may mimic loculated subphrenic fluid. The intra-abdominal fluid may be differentiated by its smooth border and its tendency to conform to the contour of the liver while it displaces the liver medially, rather than to indent the border locally, as subcapsular fluid might. However, a tense subphrenic abscess can also displace the liver. Sometimes the differentiation of subphrenic abscess from localized simple ascites may be difficult. Often the margins of the fluid collection are the only clue to its inflammatory nature. Diagnostic aspiration is always done when abscess is a possible clinical consideration. Preperitoneal fat anterior to the liver may also mimic a localized fluid collection.

Diagnostic aspiration and percutaneous drainage were discussed earlier in this chapter. Gross appearance and Gram stain for organisms and white blood cells will exclude other diagnostic possibilities (see Table 10–1).

### HEMATOMA

Hematomas run the gamut of possible sonographic appearances (see Tables 10–3 and 10–4). The appearance of a hematoma at any given time depends on where the clot is in its natural course of organization from lysis to resorption stages.[47] The sonographic correlates of this process are roughly homogeneous solid to complex cystic to cystic. As a hematoma ages, it tends to appear as a complex fluid area containing echogenic clumps.[37, 47] Hematomas may become infected and at any stage may be sonographically indistinguishable from abscess. Hematomas in the hepatic or splenic subcapsular areas may mimic subphrenic fluid. During the first 24 hours CT will show increased attenuation in a fresh hemorrhage. After that period the density of the fluid collection decreases, diminishing the advantage of CT in this circumstance. Diagnostic aspiration will usually prove definitive (see Table 10–1).

### LYMPHOCELES

These fluid collections generally look like loculated, simple fluid collections, though they may have a more complex, usually septated morphology (see Table 10–4). Differentiation from loculated ascites is usually possible because the mass effect of a lymphocele that is under tension will displace the surrounding organs.[37, 38] Differentiation from other fluid collections is mainly made on clinical grounds and by aspiration. On microscopy, lymphoceles may contain distinctive fat globules.

OTHER MAINLY CYSTIC COMPLEX MASSES

Other possible etiologies for predominantly cystic complex masses must be considered in localized abdominal abnormalities (see Table 10–4). Multiple adherent loops of fluid-filled normal or "matted" abnormal bowel may look exactly like a complex predominantly cystic mass. Furthermore, ascites combined with adhesions and bowel has a similar appearance. Such abnormalities can be differentiated from masses arising from other pelvic and abdominal viscera or the retroperitoneum by determining the vector of the mass effect on the surrounding anatomy.[1, 35, 48] For example, large pelvoabdominal masses related to cystic ovarian tumors are notoriously difficult to differentiate from complex ascites with abnormal bowel unless the bowel is actually displaced posteriorly and superiorly by a mass. With massive complex pathology and possibly associated ascites, a definitive evaluation as to origin and extent may not be possible with ultrasound. In these circumstances, CT or MR imaging is done.

OTHER LOCALIZED PERITONEAL ABNORMALITIES

Predominantly solid and homogeneously solid masses may arise from the bowel and mesentery or from the peritoneal surfaces (see Tables 10–2 and 10–4). Abscess and hematoma are included in the morphologic group of complex, predominantly solid masses because of their occasional ultrasound appearance. However, this morphology is more often the result of primary neoplasms complicated by either necrosis or hemorrhage.

PERITONEUM

The peritoneal lining is not seen as a distinct structure during sonography unless it is thickened. Thickening is usually secondary to metastatic implants or to direct extension of tumor from the viscera or mesentery. Primary mesotheliomas occur rarely. In our experience, such processes are almost universally associated with malignant ascites when patients present for sonography. Such implants are only occasionally demonstrated by ultrasound or CT, even when many are discovered at surgery. By their nature they are usually small plaque-like "studs" that do not cause gross changes that are obvious except by direct inspection during surgery or peritoneoscopy. Thickening of the peritoneal lining may also be related to inflammation. In this case, the margin will become ill defined and thickened. The peritoneum also may form adhesions that help to limit the spread of inflammatory processes.

Bowel and Mesentery Pathology

Sonographically, bowel appears as amorphous, solid masses; mixed, solid, and cystic masses; complex fluid collections; and loculated fluid collections. It also produces many artifacts. For these reasons, abnormal and normal bowel enter the differential diagnosis of mass lesions and fluid collections in the abdomen and pelvis more often than expected.[25] Changing the patient's position often helps the examiner determine whether such findings are related to bowel. Examination with real-time capabilities is mandatory, for it allows direct observation of fluid movement in response to peristalsis. Consequently, although bowel enters the differential diagnosis more often than expected, it usually can be excluded. If any questions remain after a good real-time examination, CT is done. Also, if there is a chance of bowel lying in the pathway of a drainage procedure or diagnostic aspiration, CT is done.[6–11]

Perhaps the most exciting work in the sonographic diagnosis of GI tract abnormalities has been in congenital lesions. The antenatal diagnosis of many GI tract anomalies has become routine. The specifics of these are discussed elsewhere.

Mass Lesions

The ultrasound appearance of solid masses arising from various parts of the GI tract has been described by several authors.[25, 49–52] The pattern commonly described is a solid, basically sonolucent mass with a central, usually linear, echo. This pattern results from infiltration and resultant thickening of the bowel wall surrounding the lumen with its highly reflective mucus and gas content. This appearance is only an exaggeration of the pattern described for normal, collapsed bowel.[23–25] The expression "target-like" abdominal mass has been coined to describe these lesions. The "target-like" or "double ring" configuration is also seen in cases of intussusception.[52]

Fresh barium in the bowel will prevent through-transmission of sound.[2, 25] As the barium settles, its acoustic properties change and allow better transmission of the sound. The settled barium may then be mistaken for a pathologic echogenic, intraluminal mass lesion.[2] An abdominal x-ray study settles the issue.

It is rare that primarily cystic or mixed solid and cystic masses that arise from the bowel and mesentery can be seen on ultrasound.[47, 48, 53, 54] Duplications of the GI tract and biliary system should always be suspected in a primarily cystic lesion when it is adjacent to bowel or the biliary tree, respectively.[47, 54] Benign mesenchymal tumors and teratomas are also uncommon sources of primary mesenteric or bowel abnormalities seen on sonography. Ultrasound is nonspecific in the differential diagnosis of such an abnormality. In all of these possibly malignant abdominal masses, evidence of metastatic disease to the retroperitoneum or liver should always be sought (see Table 10–3).

If massive, complex ascites is present, it is often difficult to tell whether a mass plus the ascites is responsible for the image or whether the findings are due to fluid and related abnormal bowel and mesentery. If the bowel is displaced, a mass is more likely. If the bowel and mesentery are pathologically involved, their response to the pressure of intra-abdominal fluid will be altered. For example, when the mesentery is diffusely involved with metastatic disease, instead of floating or collapsing medially and posteriorly, it usually appears as a large echogenic mass surrounded by fluid.

*Obstruction*

Obstruction of the GI tract may produce sonographic patterns that appear quite bizzare until dilated.[25] The level of obstruction can, at times, be accurately predicted. The distended stomach is a prime example.[55, 56] When gastric outlet obstruction is suspected, other diagnostic possibilities, including lesser sac abscesses, pseudocyst, and a recent meal, should be excluded.

Numerous serpiginous fluid-filled loops of bowel may be clumped together or appear to be stacked one on another when a relatively distal obstruction is present. A closed-loop obstruction presents as a complex mass indistinguishable from an abscess.[37] Duodenal obstruction may produce a striking tubular sonolucency in the expected location.

Infarcted bowel produces an extremely amorphous, mixed, solid, and cystic sonographic pattern. At times

the infarcted bowel may take on the somewhat serpiginous character described for obstructed bowel. The appearance is nonspecific but should raise the index of suspicion for bowel infarction in the appropriate clinical setting.

The combination of a concentric ring sign and obstruction might lead to the suspicion of intussusception.[57] Ultrasound is not commonly used to evaluate some of these problems. Since it is used to evaluate patients with abdominal pain, it is helpful to recognize the morphology of abnormal bowel during the general abdominal survey so that appropriate studies can be done to confirm the diagnosis.

In general, abnormal and normal bowel enter the differential diagnosis of abdominal masses and fluid collections with great frequency. When abnormalities in the abdomen are encountered, bowel always should be considered as a possible origin. Usually it can be excluded as a source of the abnormal findings.

## References

1. Whalen JP, Evans JA, Shanser J: Vector principle in the differential diagnosis of abdominal masses: The left upper quadrant. *AJR* 1971; 113:104–118.
2. Sarti DA, Lazere A: Reexamination of the deleterious effects of gastrointestinal contrast material on abdominal echography. *Radiology* 1978; 126:231–232.
3. Sommer G, Filly RA: Patient preparations to decrease bowel gas: Evaluation by an ultrasonographic measurement. *JCU* 1977; 5:87–88.
4. Sommer G, Filly FA, Laing FC: Use of simethicone as a patient preparation for abdominal sonography. *Radiology* 1977; 125:219–222.
5. Yeh HC, Wolf BS: Ultrasonic contrast study to identify stomach tap water microbubbles. *JCU* 1977; 5:170–174.
6. Ferrucci JT, Wittenberg J, Mueller PR, et al: *Interventional Radiology of the Abdomen*, ed 2. Baltimore, Williams & Wilkins Co. 1985.
7. Clark RA, Towbin R: Abscess drainage with CT and ultrasound guidance. *Radiol Clin North Am* 1983; 21:445–459.
8. Gerzof SG, Robbins AH, Johnson WC, et al: Percutaneous catheter drainage of abdominal abscesses: A five-year experience. *N Engl J Med* 1981; 305:653–657.

9. Gerzof SG: Guided percutaneous catheter drainage of abdominal abscesses, in Pfister RC, Greene RE, et al (eds): *Interventional Radiology.* Philadelphia, WB Saunders Co, 1982, pp 557–567.

10. Gronvale S, Gammelgaard J, Haubek A, et al: Drainage of abdominal abscesses guided by sonography. *AJR* 1982; 138:527–529.

11. Haaga JR: CT-guided procedures, in Haaga JR, Alfidi RJ (eds): *Computed Tomography of the Whole Body.* St Louis, CV Mosby Co, 1983, pp 867–933.

12. Ohto M, Karasawa E, Tsuchiya Y, et al: Ultrasonically guided percutaneous medium injection and aspiration biopsy under a real-time puncture transducer. *Radiology* 1980; 136:171–176.

13. Lindgren PG: Ultrasonically guided punctures: A modified technique. *Radiology* 1980; 137:235–237.

14. Lee TG, Knochel JQ: Air as an ultrasound contrast marker for accurate determination of needle placement. *Radiology* 1982; 143:787–788.

15. van Sonnenberg E, Wittenberg J, Ferrucci JT Jr, et al: Triangulation method for percutaneous needle guidance: The angled approach to upper abdominal masses. *AJR* 1981; 137:757–761.

16. Neff CC, Mueller PR, Ferrucci JT, et al: Serious complications following trransgression of the pleural space in drainage procedures. *Radiology* 1984; 152:335–341.

17. van Sonnenberg E, Mueller PR, Ferrucci JT: Percutaneous drainage of 250 abdominal abscesses and fluid collections: Part I. Results, failures and complications. *Radiology* 1984; 151:337–341.

18. Hollinshead HW: *Textbook of Anatomy.* New York, Harper & Row Publishers, 1967.

19. Meyers MA: The spread and localization of acute intraperitoneal effusions. *Radiology* 1970; 95:547–554.

20. Meyers MA, Whalen JP, Peele K, et al: Radiologic features of extraperitoneal effusions. *Radiology* 1972; 104:249–257.

21. Meyers MA: *Dynamic Radiology of the Abdomen: Normal and Pathologic Anatomy.* New York, Springer-Verlag, 1982.

22. Proto AV, Lane EJ, Marangola JP: A new concept of ascitic fluid distribution. *AJR* 1976; 126:974–980.

23. Sample WF: Techniques for improved delinea-

tion of normal anatomy of the upper abdomen and high retroperitoneum with gray-scale ultrasound. *Radiology* 1977; 124:197–202.

24. Sample WF, Sarti DA: Computed body tomography and gray scale ultrasonography: Anatomic correlations and pitfalls in the upper abdomen. *Gastrointest Radiol* 1978; 3:243–249.

25. Fleischer AC, Muhletaler CA, James AE: Sonographic patterns arising from normal and abnormal bowel. *Radiol Clin North Am* 1980; 18:145–159.

26. Teele RL, Rosenfield AT, Freedman GS: The anatomic splenic flexure: An ultrasonic renal imposter. *AJR* 1977; 128:115–120.

27. Kaftori JK, Rosenberger A, Pollack S, et al: Rectus sheath hematoma: Ultrasonographic diagnosis. *AJR* 1977; 128:283–285.

28. Spitz HB, Wyatt GM: Rectus sheath hematoma. *JCU* 1977; 5:413–416.

29. Cervantes J, Sanchez-Cortazar J, Ponte RJ, Manzo M: Ultrasound diagnosis of rectus sheath hematoma. *Am Surg* 1983; 49:542–555.

30. Diakoumakis EE, Weinberg B, Selfe B: Unusual case studies of anterior abdominal wall mass as diagnosed by ultrasonography. *JCU* 1984; 12:351–354.

31. Spangen L: Ultrasound as a diagnostic aid in ventral abdominal hernia. *JCU* 1976; 3:211–213.

32. Thomas JL, Cunningham JJ: Ultrasonic evaluation of ventral hernias disguised as intra-abdominal neoplasms. *Arch Surg* 1978; 113:589–590.

33. Fried AM, Meeker WR: Incarcerated spigelian hernia: Ultrasonic differential diagnosis. *AJR* 1979; 133(1):107–110.

34. Yeh HC, Rabinowitz JG, Rosenblum M: Complimentary role of CT and ultrasonography in the diagnosis of desmoid tumor of abdominal wall. *Comput Radiol* 1982; 6:275–280.

35. Yeh HC, Wolf BS: Ultrasonography in ascites. *Radiology* 1977; 124:783–790.

36. Goldberg BB, Clearfield HR, Goodman GA, Morales JO: Ultrasonic determination of ascites. *Arch Intern Med* 1973; 131:217–220.

37. Doust BD, Thompson R: Ultrasonography of abdominal fluid collections. *Gastrointest Radiol* 1978; 3:273–279.

38. Fleischer AC, James AE, Millis JB, et al: Differential diagnosis of pelvic masses by gray scale sonography. *AJR* 1978; 131:469–476.

39. Kressel HY, Filly RA: Ultrasonographic appear-

ance of gas-containing abscesses in the abdomen. *AJR* 1978; 130:71–73.

40. Wicks JD, Silver TM, and Bree RL: Giant cystic abdominal masses in children and adolescents: Ultrasonic differential diagnosis. *AJR* 1978; 130:853–857.

41. Yeh HC, Wolf BS: Ultrasonography and computed tomography in the diagnosis of homogeneous masses. *Radiology* 1977; 123:425–428.

42. Mueller PR, Simeone JF: Intra-abdominal abscesses: Diagnosis by sonography and computed tomography. *Radiol Clin North Am* 1983; 21:425–443.

43. Taylor KJW, Sullivan DC, Wasson JFM, Rosenfield ART: Ultrasound and gallium for the diagnosis of abdominal and pelvic abscesses. *Gastrointest Radiol* 1978; 3:281–286.

44. Gerzof SG, Robbins AH, Birkett DH: Computed tomography in the diagnosis and management of abdominal abscesses. *Gastrointest Radiol* 1978; 3:287–294.

45. Haber K, Asher WM, Freimanis AK: Echographic evaluation of diaphragmatic motion in intra-abdominal diseases. *Radiology* 1975; 113:141–144.

46. Landay M, Harless W: Ultrasonic differentiation of right pleural effusion from subphrenic fluid on longitudinal scans of the right upper quadrant: Importance of recognizing the diaphragm. *Radiology* 1977; 123:155–158.

47. Wicks JD, Silver TM, Bree RL: Gray scale features of hematomas: An ultrasonic spectrum. *AJR* 1978; 131:977–980.

48. Haller JO, Schneider M, Kassner EG, et al: Sonographic evaluation of mesenteric and omental masses in children. *AJR* 1978; 130:269–274.

49. Kremer H, Lohmoeller G, Zollner N: Primary ultrasonic detection of a double carcinoma of the colon. *Radiology* 1977; 124:481–482.

50. Peterson LR, Cooperberg PL: Ultrasound demonstration of lesions of the gastrointestinal tract. *Gastrointest Radiol* 1978; 3:303–306.

51. Walls WJ: The evaluation of malignant gastric neoplasms by ultrasonic B-scanning. *Radiology* 1976; 118:159–163.

52. Weissberg DL, Scheible W, Leopold GR: Ultrasonographic appearance of adult intussusception. *Radiology* 1977; 124:791–792.

53. Goldberg BB, Capitanio MA, Kirkpatrick JA: Ultrasonic evaluation of masses in pediatric patients. *AJR* 1972; 116:677–684.

54. Teele RL, Henschke CI, Tapper D: The radiographic and ultrasonographic evaluation of enteric duplication cysts. *Pediatr Radiol* 1980; 10:9–14.

55. Boychuk RB, Lyons EA, Goodhan TK: Duodenal atresia diagnosed by ultrasound. *Radiology* 1978; 127:500

56. Teele RL, Smith EH: Ultrasound in the diagnosis of idiopathic hypertrophic pyloric stenosis. *N Engl J Med* 1977; 296:1149–1150.

57. Holt S, Samuel E: Multiple concentric ring sign in the ultrasonographic diagnosis of intussusception. *Gastrointest Radiol* 1978; 3:307–309.

## CASES

Dennis A. Sarti, M.D.

## Normal Anatomy

Ultrasound examination of the abdomen outside of the various organs has received relatively little attention. A thorough understanding of the anatomy is extremely helpful in doing a general search of the abdomen. Figure 10–1 is a schematic drawing which shows the relationship among the various peritoneal spaces. The mesenteric attachments of the large bowel form the major boundaries of the peritoneal cavity. Above the transverse mesocolon is the supramesocolic space. Inferior to the transverse mesocolon is the inferior mesocolic space. The root of the small bowel mesentery separates the inframesocolic spaces into right and left compartments. The right and left paracolic gutters are lateral to the ascending and descending colon, respectively. The phrenococolic ligament (arrows) limits communication among the left subphrenic, the perihepatic, and the perisplenic spaces and the paracolic gutter. Freer communication is present on the right side among the subhepatic space, the subphrenic space, and the lesser sac. Communication with the subhepatic space and the lesser sac occurs through the foramen of Winslow. The dotted lines in Figure 10–1 outline the pancreatic region situated posterior to the lesser sac.

Figure 10–2 is a sagittal view intended to depict the mesenteric relationships of bowel, retroperitoneum, and the peritoneal spaces. The lesser sac, a potential space, is bounded anteriorly by the stomach and its mesentery, inferiorly by the mesentery (arrow) of the transverse colon, and posteriorly by the retroperitoneal structures. The pancreas and the third portion of the duodenum are situated in the retroperitoneum deep to the lesser sac. The small bowel and its mesenteric attachment (arrow) are inferior to the lesser sac. The potential space of the lesser sac can enlarge and separate the distance between the stomach and the pancreas. When

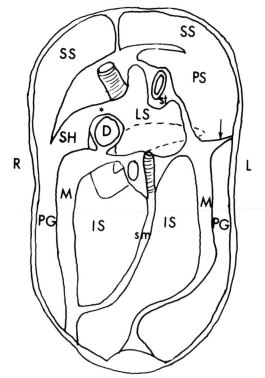

FIG 10–1.

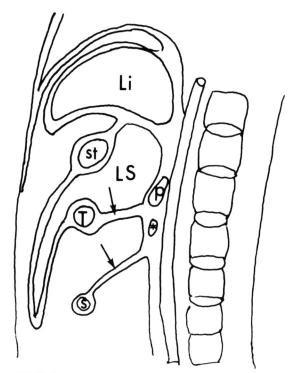

FIG 10–2.

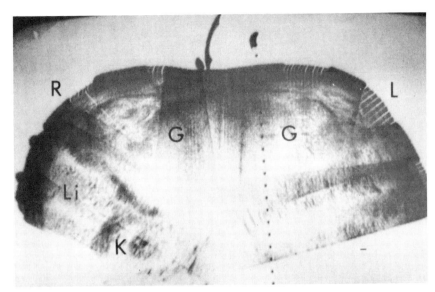

**FIG 10–3.**

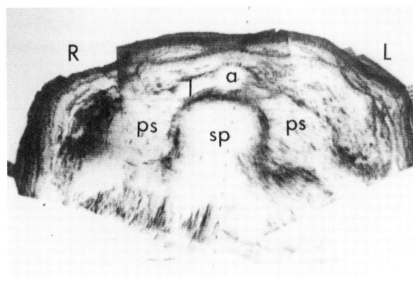

**FIG 10–4.**

an ultrasound examination is performed on a normal individual, the stomach rests directly on top of the pancreas in most instances.

Ultrasound examination of the abdomen is often obscured by bowel air. Figure 10–3 is a typical example of an air-filled study. Bowel gas yields a high-amplitude echo with no through-transmission. The abdominal cavity and retroperitoneal region cannot be evaluated when bowel gas is present. If large amounts of fluid were present in the potential spaces of the peritoneum, however, they would displace the bowel gas, and the ultrasound would yield important information. Figure 10–4 is a transverse scan of an airless abdomen. In this instance, we can see the aorta, inferior vena cava, psoas muscles, and spine. All of the structures anterior to the aorta represent collapsed and airless bowel.

| * | = | Foramen of Winslow |
|---|---|---|
| **A** | = | Aorta |
| **D** | = | Duodenum |
| **G** | = | Bowel gas |
| **I** | = | Inferior vena cava |
| **IS** | = | Inframesocolic space |
| **K** | = | Kidney |
| **L** | = | Left |
| **Li** | = | Liver |
| **LS** | = | Lesser sac |
| **M** | = | Mesenteric attachments of the large bowel |
| **p** | = | Pancreas |
| **PG** | = | Paracolic gutter |
| **PS** | = | Psoas muscle |
| **R** | = | Right |
| **S** | = | Small bowel |
| **SH** | = | Subhepatic space |
| **sm** | = | Small bowel mesentery |
| **Sp** | = | Spine |
| **SS** | = | Subphrenic space |
| **St** | = | Stomach |
| **T** | = | Transverse colon |

## Normal Anatomy of the Abdomen

Figure 10–5 is a schematic drawing of the abdominal wall with the skin as the superficial structure. Deep to the skin is the fibrofatty subcutaneous tissue which is extremely variable in thickness and causes great havoc to the passage of sound waves. Individuals with large amounts of subcutaneous fat scatter sound quite dramatically and yield extremely poor images. Deep to the subcutaneous fat is the musculofascial plane for which ultrasound can give a strong inner face. The peritoneum is then seen inferior to the muscle plane.

Figure 10–6 is an ultrasound scan demonstrating superficial structures. The skin surface coincides with the strong initial echo arising from the transducer-skin interface. Deep to the skin surface is the subcutaneous fat. This has a coarse echo appearance to it with areas of lucency separated by strong linear echoes. Deep to the subcutaneous fat is the rectus muscle and the peritoneal fat. The relationship of these structures can be seen quite well in Figure 10–6. The stomach gives a characteristic "bull's-eye" appearance of the bowel and structures deep to it can be visualized.

A longitudinal scan of the abdomen from the xiphoid to the symphysis pubis (Fig 10–7) shows the fairly characteristic appearance of the upper abdomen. Deep to the liver and the collapsed stomach, we can see the hepatic artery, superior mesenteric vein, and pancreas. Visualization of these structures is possible because of the collapsed stomach. The pelvic structures can also be visualized well because of the distended urinary bladder. The uterus is seen deep to the urinary bladder. The anatomy between the urinary bladder and the stomach, however, is completely obscured by the overlying bowel air.

The diaphragm and subhepatic space are also important areas for examination by ultrasound. The scan in Figure 10–8 was performed with the purpose of demonstrating diaphragmatic motion. This is relatively easy to do. Two scans are combined in the

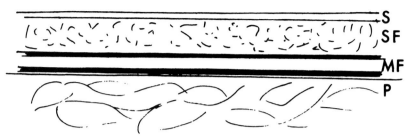

FIG 10–5.

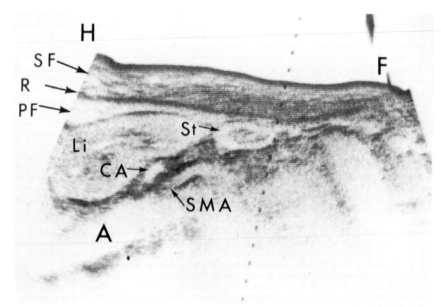

FIG 10–6.

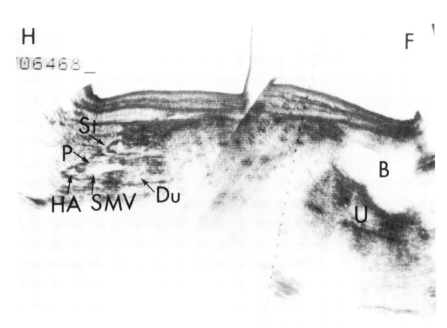

**FIG 10–7.**

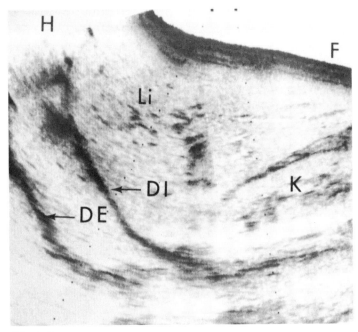

**FIG 10–8.**

same image. The first scan is performed in deep inspiration; the second, in deep expiration. The amount of diaphragmatic motion can then be documented. This procedure is extremely helpful in a patient with a pleural effusion on the right side. Fluoroscopy is not useful in this situation because of silhouetting of the diaphragm by pleural fluid.

We are, however, dealing with acoustic waves in ultrasound, and the diaphragm is readily visualized above the liver, whether or not a pleural effusion is present.

| | | |
|---|---|---|
| **A** | = | Aorta |
| **B** | = | Urinary bladder |
| **CA** | = | Celiac axis |
| **DE** | = | Diaphragm during expiration |
| **DI** | = | Diaphragm during inspiration |
| **Du** | = | Duodenum |
| **F** | = | Foot |
| **H** | = | Head |
| **HA** | = | Hepatic artery |
| **K** | = | Kidney |
| **Li** | = | Liver |
| **MF** | = | Musculofascial plane |
| **P (Fig 10–5)** | = | Peritoneal cavity |
| **P** | = | Pancreas |
| **PF** | = | Peritoneal fat |
| **R** | = | Rectus muscle |
| **S** | = | Skin |
| **SF** | = | Subcutaneous fat |
| **SMA** | = | Superior mesenteric artery |
| **SMV** | = | Superior mesenteric vein |
| **St** | = | Stomach |
| **U** | = | Uterus |

## Abdominal Wall Hematoma

Ultrasound is an excellent diagnostic tool for evaluation of masses within or adjacent to the abdominal wall. The subcutaneous fat appears most often as a relatively lucent area just beneath the skin surface. The rectus muscle in thin individuals will be a strong echogenic line. In more muscular individuals, both walls of the rectus muscle can be seen, with soft echoes of the muscle itself present within. Figures 10–9 and 10–10 are scans of a patient with a palpable mass in the left anterior abdomen after a traumatic episode. Ultrasound examination demonstrated a sonolucency within the rectus muscle. Figure 10–9 is a longitudinal scan through the midportion of the mass. A normal rectus muscle is seen above and below the mass. It is outlined by two strong linear echoes. The width of the rectus muscle is within normal limits both superior and inferior to the mass. In the midportion of the mass, a sonolucent region is noted that widens the area of the rectus muscle. This turned out to be a rectus hematoma. If widening of the rectus fascial planes can be demonstrated, a mass within the rectus sheath can be detected. This is the important finding on ultrasound. A transverse scan of the same patient (Fig 10–10) demonstrates the hematoma within the rectus muscle on the left side of the abdomen.

Figures 10–11 and 10–12 are transverse longitudinal scans of a 53-year-old man with a long history of alcoholism. He arrived at the emergency room with numerous areas of ecchymosis and a low hematocrit. Abdominal asymmetry was noted, and an ultrasound examination was ordered. Figure 10–11 is a transverse scan showing marked asymmetry of the abdominal wall with increased thickness on the right side. A large mass is noted over the right abdomen. Close examination reveals that this mass is anterior to the rectus muscle. The longitudinal scan in Figure 10–12 shows a large sonolucent mass anterior to the rectus muscle. The findings indicate a large subcutaneous hematoma rather than a rectus muscle he-

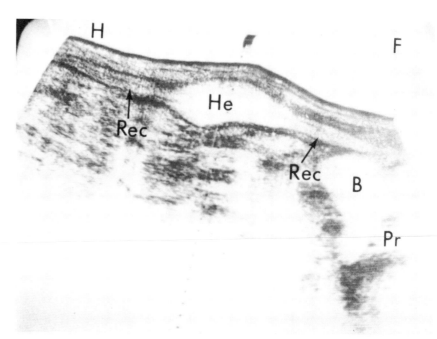

FIG 10–9.

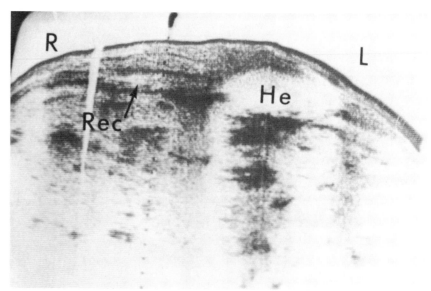

FIG 10–10.

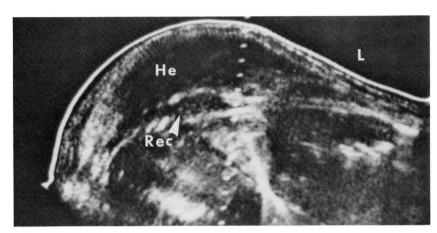

**FIG 10–11.**

matoma. By identifying the location of the rectus muscle and determining its relationship to various abdominal wall masses, the physician can accurately locate the mass on ultrasound. In this case a large subcutaneous hematoma was situated anterior to the rectus muscle.

| | | |
|---|---|---|
| **B** | = | Bladder |
| **F** | = | Foot |
| **H** | = | Head |
| **He** | = | Hematoma |
| **L** | = | Left |
| **Pr** | = | Prostate |
| **R** | = | Right |
| **Rec** | = | Rectus muscle |

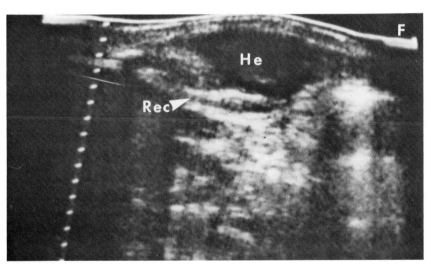

**FIG 10–12.**

## Abdominal Wall Mass

Figures 10–13 and 10–14 are transverse and longitudinal scans of the lower abdomen in a 23-year-old man with a recent history of abdominal trauma. Asymmetry of the abdominal wall is noted is Figure 10–13. The right side is markedly thickened compared to the left. An echogenic mass is present over the right abdomen, increasing the thickness to the abdominal wall. The mass appears to be mainly confined to the subcutaneous region. However, close examination to the rectus muscle reveals important information as to the site of origin. A comparison of the right and left rectus muscle reveals disparity between the two structures. The left rectus muscle (Fig 10–13) has sharp, well-demarcated boundaries both anteriorly and posteriorly. The borders of the right rectus muscle are less sharply defined. Notice that the anterior border of the right rectus muscle is weakly echogenic and poorly marginated (Figures 10–13 and 10–14). The right rectus muscle is also thicker than the left, and the posterior border of the right rectus muscle is disrupted. The findings indicate a right rectus hematoma with hemorrhage into the subcutaneous tissue. The hematoma's echogenicity is caused by an inhomogeneous internal architecture, most likely due to clot. What is structure 1 in Figure 10–14?

Figures 10–15 and 10–16 are transverse and longitudinal scans of a 28-year-old woman with acute myelogenous leukemia. She had recently undergone pelvic surgery for removal of a right chloroma. Lower abdominal pain with tenderness and fullness in the left lower quadrant developed. A persistent sonolucent area was identified in the subcutaneous region on ultrasound. This area was found to be a subcutaneous abscess. The rectus muscle is not identified in this patient. In some individuals, the rectus muscle is not seen because it is so thin.

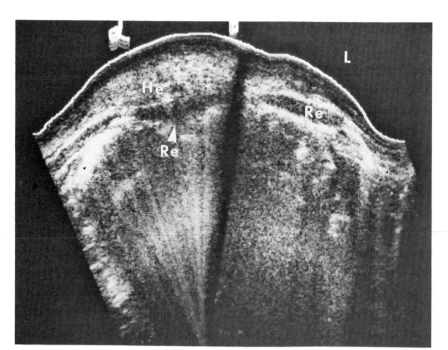

**FIG 10–13.**

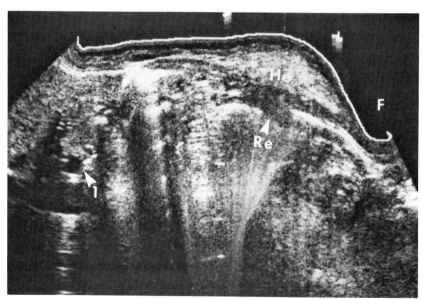

**FIG 10–14.**

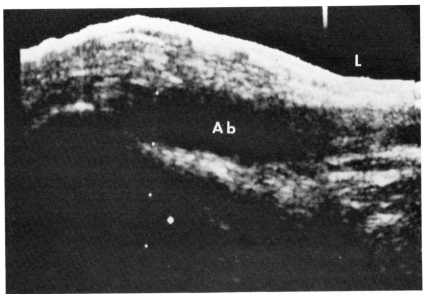

**FIG 10–15.**

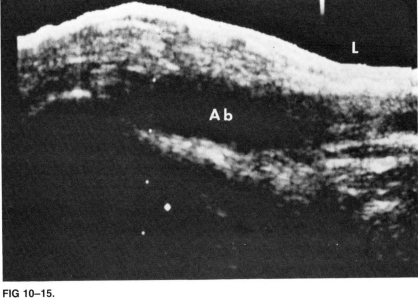

**FIG 10–16.**

| | | |
|---|---|---|
| **Ab** | = | Subcutaneous abscess |
| **F** | = | Foot |
| **He** | = | Hematoma |
| **L** | = | Left |
| **Re** | = | Rectus muscle |
| **1** | = | Portal vein |

## Superficial Abdominal Masses

When a mass is found in the abdominal wall, it may be difficult to make a specific diagnosis. By analyzing the ultrasound characteristics and clinical history, a fairly narrow differential diagnosis can be obtained. Figure 10–17 is a longitudinal scan of the right lower abdominal wall in a 49-year-old woman whose only finding was a superficial abdominal wall mass that had been present for years. There was no history of recent trauma, surgery, or infection. Ultrasound revealed an oval, 5 × 3-cm echogenic mass with a region of acoustic shadowing in its cephalad portion. The findings are fairly specific for a lipoma, which was documented at surgery. The clinical history and ultrasound characteristics led to the correct diagnosis.

Figure 10–18 is a transverse scan of the right midabdomen in a 50-year-old obese woman with a 5-year history of an umbilical hernia and a 1-day history of sharp lower abdominal pain. Ultrasound revealed a 3-cm cystic mass with a small echogenic region on its medial aspect. The mass was situated quite superficially. Through-transmission is present deep to the mass and confirms its fluid content. At surgery, an umbilical hernia with incarcerated omentum and a cystic sac enclosed by peritoneum was found.

Occasionally, sonolucent masses are seen adjacent to the muscle wall. Often it will be difficult to determine whether or not they are within the subcutaneous tissue, rectus muscle, or adjacent peritoneal cavity. However, close examination of the abdominal wall structures can usually localize the site of origin of many superficial masses. This is especially true if the rectus abdominis muscle can be identified.

Figures 10–19 and 10–20 are scans of a patient who had undergone previous surgery. Intraperitoneal abscess was suspected. Ultrasound examination revealed a sonolucent mass in the left upper abdomen. A transverse scan (Fig 10–19) shows the rectus muscle anterior to the mass.

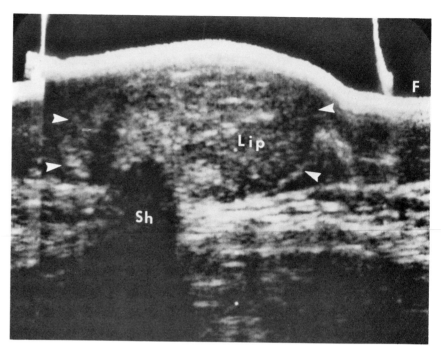

FIG 10–17.

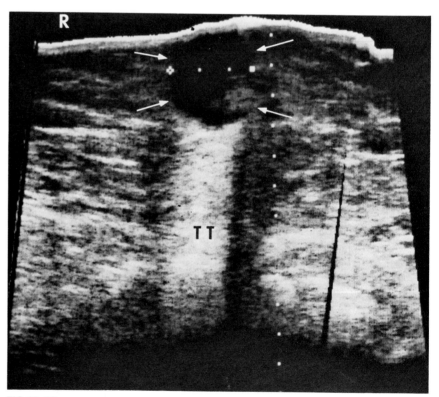

FIG 10–18.

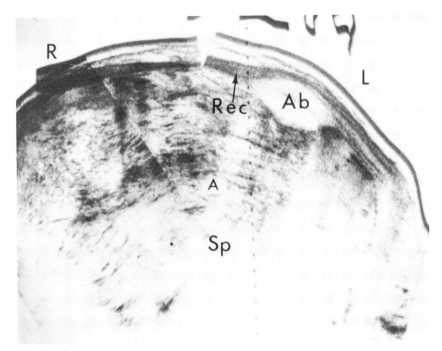

**FIG 10–19.**

The mass, therefore, is within the peritoneal cavity and is pushing the rectus muscle anteriorly. It is not situated within the rectus muscle since it does not spread apart both the muscles' borders. Figure 10–20 is a longitudinal scan through the abscess. The rectus muscle is again seen to be displaced anteriorly. At surgery, a loculated abscess with adherent edematous omentum was found.

| | | |
|---|---|---|
| **A** | = | Aorta |
| **Ab** | = | Abscess |
| **Arrows** | = | Incarcerated hernia |
| **Arrowheads** | = | Lipoma |
| **F** | = | Foot |
| **H** | = | Head |
| **L** | = | Left |
| **Lip** | = | Lipoma |
| **R** | = | Right |
| **Rec** | = | Rectus muscle |
| **Sh** | = | Shadow |
| **Sp** | = | Spine |
| **TT** | = | Through-transmission |

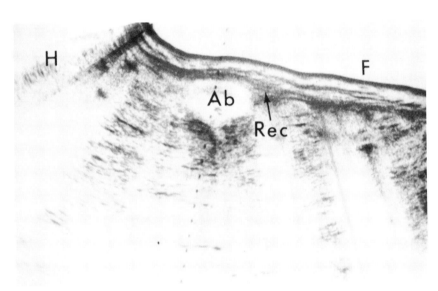

**FIG 10–20.**

## Abdominal Fluid Collections

Numerous clinical entities within the abdomen can yield a fluid-filled mass on ultrasound. Figures 10–21 and 10–22 are of a patient with vague abdominal pain. An ultrasound survey scan was performed. During the course of the examination, a small loculated fluid collection was noted in the right lower abdomen beneath the rectus muscle. Because of the vague abdominal pain, aspiration under ultrasound guidance was performed. The fluid that was collected was found to be serous. Cultures were negative. This sterile serous collection would have been almost impossible to detect and diagnose without the aid of ultrasound. The interesting point in this case is that we can see the serous collection just beneath the rectus muscle. We could not distinguish this from an abscess or loculated hematoma.

Often, we see numerous masses within the abdomen that represent fluid-filled or food-filled bowel. The stomach, duodenum, small bowel, and colon can be distended with something other than gas. These "massess" can be confused with pseudocysts, abscesses, or tumors. Therefore, it is important to recognize the potential mass-like appearance of normal bowel.

Figure 10–23 is an example of normal structures yielding a mass-like appearance. The gallbladder is easily seen on the right side of the abdomen and is not usually confused for a mass. The duodenum, however (Fig 10–23) may be mistaken for a mass near the head of the pancreas. It can appear as air-filled, fluid-filled, or food-filled. In this instance, it is fairly well collapsed and yields a circular or "bull's-eye" appearance very suggestive of normal bowel. Figure 10–23 also shows a mass over the anterior left abdomen which represents the stomach. Posterior to the stomach is the superior mesenteric artery and superior mesenteric vein. The stomach could be easily mistaken for an abscess or possible pseudocyst. There-

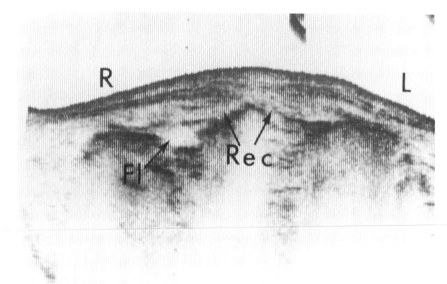

FIG 10–21.

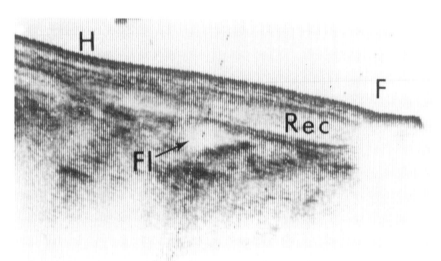

FIG 10–22.

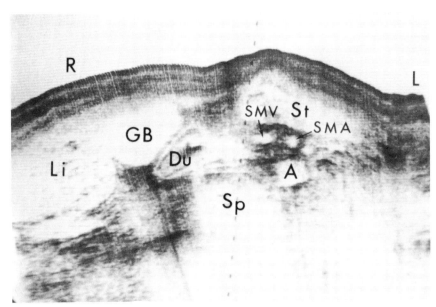

**FIG 10–23.**

fore, if there is any question it is important to perform the examination again 24 hours later after keeping the patient without oral intake overnight or use real-time ultrasound.

Infrequently, the large bowel will present difficulty on ultrasound examination. Figure 10–24 is an example of the presence of fluid and some feces in the descending colon. This could be easily misinterpreted as an abscess in the area. The patient had a history of diarrhea. Again, follow-up examination 24 hours later usually will remove any doubt as to whether or not a loop of bowel is masquerading as a pathologic entity.

| | | |
|---|---|---|
| **A** | = | Aorta |
| **Co** | = | Descending colon |
| **Du** | = | Duodenum |
| **F** | = | Foot |
| **Fl** | = | Sterile serous fluid collection |
| **G** | = | Bowel gas |
| **GB** | = | Gallbladder |
| **H** | = | Head |
| **K** | = | Kidney |
| **L** | = | Left |
| **Li** | = | Liver |
| **R** | = | Right |
| **Rec** | = | Rectus muscle |
| **SMA** | = | Superior mesenteric artery |
| **SMV** | = | Superior mesenteric vein |
| **Sp** | = | Spine |
| **St** | = | Stomach |

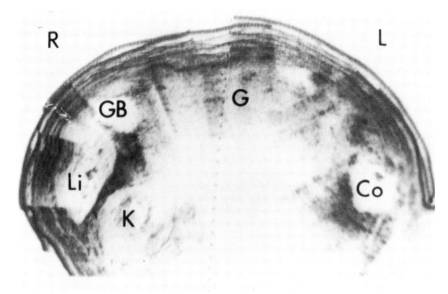

**FIG 10–24.**

## Ascites

Abdominal fluid can easily be detected on ultrasound. In fact, ultrasound is more sensitive to a minimal amount of fluid than is physical examination. Different kinds of fluid may be found in the abdominal cavity. These may include hematoma and abscess. However, the most common cause of diffuse fluid in the peritoneal cavity is ascites. Although ascites may loculate in unusual locations, there are certain anatomic areas in which it can be detected most easily, including the right subdiaphragmatic region, subhepatic region, hepatorenal angle, right paracolic gutter, lesser sac, perisplenic area, left upper quadrant, left paracolic gutter, pelvis, and the midabdomen. With systematic examination of these areas, small fluid collections will not be missed.

Figure 10–25 is a transverse scan of the right upper quadrant that shows a characteristic finding; the liver capsule (arrows) is displaced away from the right lateral abdominal wall by the ascitic fluid. The liver capsule is not normally visualized since it is in direct contact with the abdominal wall. With the sonolucent ascitic fluid adjacent to the abdominal wall, the strong echoes arising from the liver capsule are displaced medially and give a sharp, easily recognizable border.

Figure 10–26 is a transverse scan of the upper abdomen. Ascitic fluid is seen in the hepatorenal angle. This is a very common early site for ascitic fluid detection. Since this area is in the most dependent portion of the upper abdomen, ascitic fluid will often be noted here when it is not present in any other areas. Again we see the sharp, strong echo of the liver capsule (arrows), which is displaced away from the retroperitoneum adjacent to the right kidney.

Figures 10–27 and 10–28 are transverse and longitudinal scans showing fluid in the hepatorenal and subhepatic regions. Fluid is easily visualized in these areas because the liver acts as an ultrasound window. The right upper quadrant is the initial starting point for an abdominal scan to rule out fluid collections.

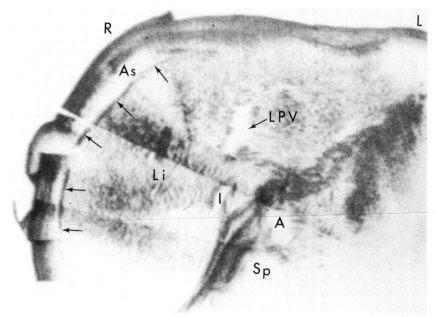

**FIG 10–25.**

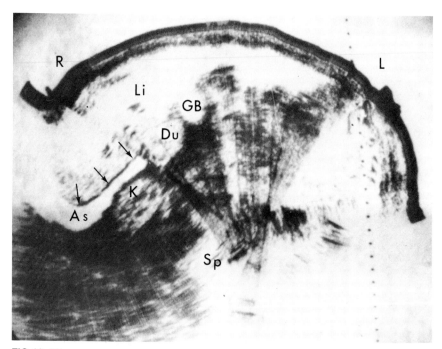

**FIG 10–26.**

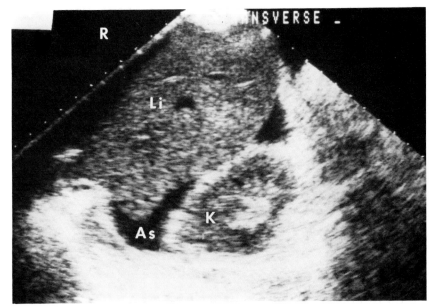

| A | = Aorta |
|---|---|
| **Arrows** | = Liver capsule |
| **As** | = Ascites |
| **Du** | = Duodenum |
| **GB** | = Gallbladder |
| **H** | = Head |
| **I** | = Inferior vena cava |
| **K** | = Kidney |
| **L** | = Left |
| **Li** | = Liver |
| **LPV** | = Left portal vein |
| **R** | = Right |
| **Sp** | = Spine |

**FIG 10–27.**

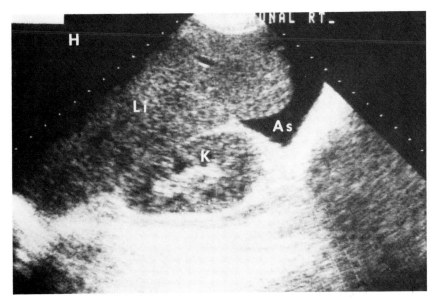

**FIG 10–28.**

## Ascites

The lesser sac is a potential space
that is visualized only when it contains
some material. Very small collections
of ascitic fluid can be seen in the
lesser sac. Figure 10–29 is an excellent example of ascitic fluid posterior
to the liver and anterior to the pancreas. This small linear lucency normally is not present. Whenever a
small sonolucency is seen adjacent to
the posterior aspect of the liver, loculated ascites, abscess, hematoma, or
pseudocysts should be considered. A
very smooth plane, separating the
liver from the pancreas and the stomach, is demonstrated. These findings
are highly consistent with a small loculated ascitic fluid collection in the
lesser sac.

Figure 10–30 is a transverse scan
of the upper abdomen. Again, ascitic
fluid is seen displacing the liver capsule (arrows) away from the right lateral abdominal wall. A similar finding
is also present in the left upper quadrant in the location of the spleen. The
splenic capsule also yields a highly
reflective interface when it is displaced
away from the left lateral abdominal
wall. Ascitic fluid is interposed between the left lateral abdominal wall
and the splenic capsule in a manner
similar to the liver.

After the upper abdomen has been
examined, the paracolic gutters and
pelvis should then be studied. Figure
10–31 is a longitudinal scan of the
right paracolic gutter showing ascitic
fluid displacing bowel loops. A triangular fluid area is seen in right lower
quadrant. Its borders are formed by
the abdominal wall, iliopsoas muscle,
and bowel loops. This characteristic
triangular fluid area indicates peritoneal fluid.

The next area to be examined is the
pelvis. Figure 10–32 is a characteristic picture of ascitic fluid situated in
the pelvis. The urinary bladder is
nearly completely collapsed with only
a small amount of urine present. Fluid
is seen in the pelvis with bowel loops
floating in the ascites. This should not
be confused with a distended urinary
bladder. The bowel loops give a characteristic circular indentation on the

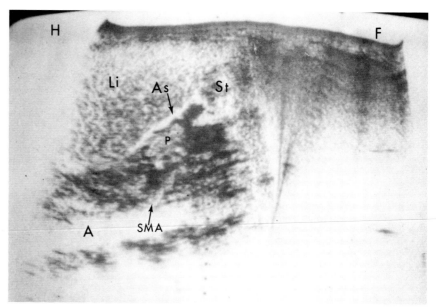

**FIG 10–29.**

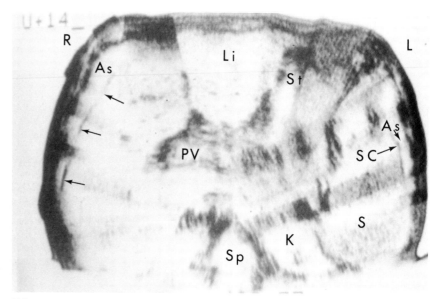

**FIG 10–30.**

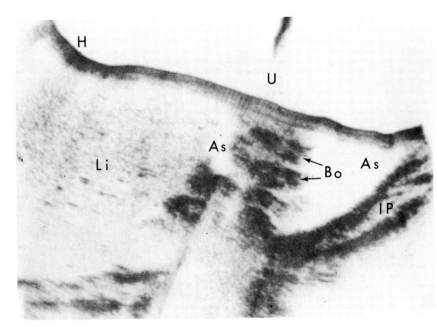

**FIG 10-31.**

ascitic fluid, which indicates the intra-peritoneal location of the fluid.

| | | |
|---|---|---|
| **A** | = | Aorta |
| **Arrows** | = | Liver capsule |
| **As** | = | Ascites |
| **B** | = | Bladder |
| **Bo** | = | Bowel loops |
| **F** | = | Foot |
| **H** | = | Head |
| **IP** | = | Iliopsoas muscle |
| **K** | = | Kidney |
| **L** | = | Left |
| **Li** | = | Liver |
| **P** | = | Pancreas |
| **PV** | = | Portal vein |
| **Pu** | = | Symphisis pubis |
| **R** | = | Right |
| **S** | = | Spleen |
| **SC** | = | Splenic capsule |
| **SMA** | = | Superior mesenteric artery |
| **Sp** | = | Spine |
| **St** | = | Stomach |
| **U** | = | Umbilicus |

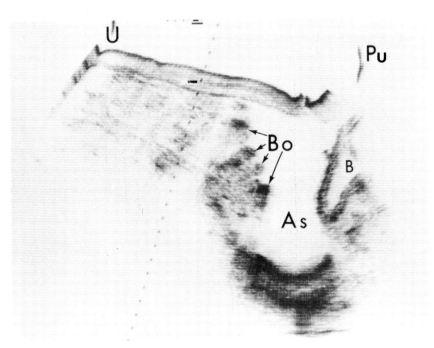

**FIG 10-32.**

## Massive Ascites

To identify small fluid collections, the anatomic regions noted in the previous cases must be systematically examined. Massive ascites, on the other hand, does not present any diagnostic difficulty and is readily evident on abdominal examination. If the ultrasonographer has never seen cases of massive ascites, it may be initially confused for large abdominal masses. However, there are certain anatomic findings that lead to the correct diagnosis of massive ascites.

Figures 10–33 through 10–36 are abdominal scans of different patients with massive ascites. Figure 10–33 is a transverse scan of the abdomen showing a characteristic echo pattern. Ascitic fluid is present laterally in the paracolic gutters, with bowel loops floating medially. A large amount of air is present centrally. This is similar to the x-ray finding in ascites, in which air is noted to collect in the central abdomen. The bowel loops give a characteristic rounded projection into the ascitic fluid, which is situated laterally in Figures 10–33 and 10–34. Figure 10–34 is a transverse abdominal scan in another patient with massive ascites. In this instance, more ascitic fluid is present and less air is noted centrally. Bowel loops are projecting into the ascitic fluid. The ascites in these two scans should not be confused with an abdominal or pelvic tumor. The findings indicating massive ascites are fluid collecting in the paracolic gutters, bowel loops projecting into the ascites, and central air.

Figure 10–35 is a transverse abdominal scan of a third patient with massive ascites. In this instance, ascites is so severe that bowel air is not seen centrally. The entire abdomen is filled with ascitic fluid. It is quite unusual to see ascites of this severity. Figure 10–36 is an abdominal scan in which bowel loops and their mesenteric attachments are noted to be floating within the ascitic fluid. Peristaltic activity can be identified on real-time examination. Such findings document the presence of retroperitoneal fluid.

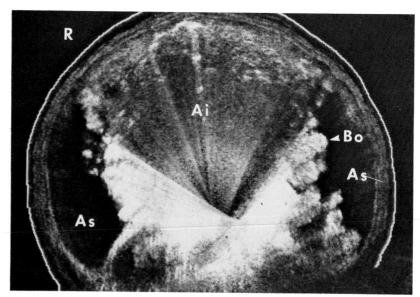

**FIG 10–33.**

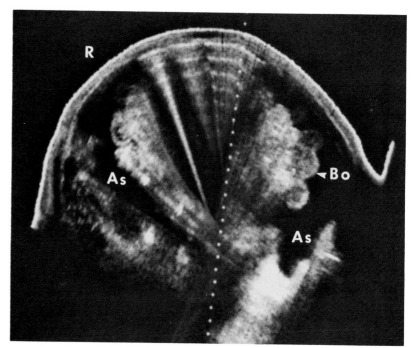

**FIG 10–34.**

Ai = Bowel air
As = Ascites
Bo = Bowel loops
Fl = Falciform ligament
GB = Gallbladder
L = Left
LC = Liver capsule
Li = Liver
R = Right

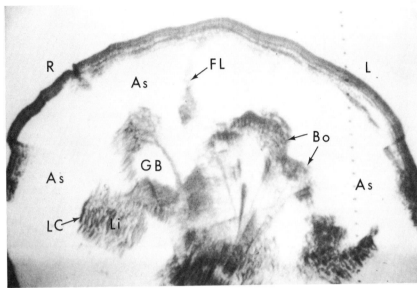

**FIG 10–35.**

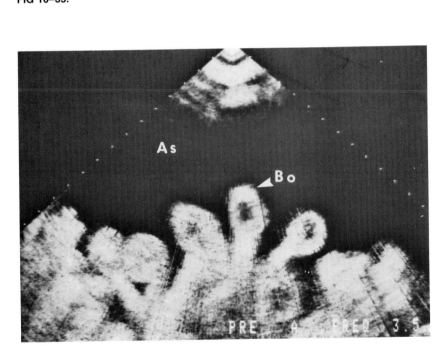

**FIG 10–36.**

## Malignant Ascites

Very often fluid is noted in the peritoneal cavity and is assumed secondary to ascites. However, clues indicate that this is not the typical ascites seen more commonly in chronic alcohol abuse. Figure 10–37 shows ascitic fluid in the lower abdomen and pelvis. It does not have the typical appearance of free-floating bowel loops. A soft tissue mass is present adjacent to the anterior abdominal wall and just superior to the urinary bladder. Findings of irregular soft tissue masses indicate malignancy. This, along with fluid in the pelvis, suggests malignant ascites. The patient had metastatic melanoma of the pelvis and anterior abdominal wall. The bowel loops are situated more centrally and are not floating as freely in the ascitic fluid as they usually would in uncomplicated ascites.

Figures 10–38 and 10–39 are transverse and longitudinal scans of a 62-year-old man who entered the hospital with an enlarging abdominal mass. Ultrasound examination demonstrated a strongly echogenic soft tissue mass adherent to the anterior abdominal wall. It was approximately 4–5 cm thick and had an irregular inner surface. Ascitic fluid is noted posterior to the mass. Bowel loops were seen floating within the ascitic fluid. A percutaneous biopsy of the mass revealed a diffuse adenocarcinoma. A barium examination revealed an "apple core" lesion of the transverse colon, indicating a primary colonic carcinoma. The patient had adenocarcinoma metastatic to the peritoneum and abdominal wall. This was an unusual case of soft tissue tumor adherent to the abdominal wall accompanied by malignant ascites.

Figure 10–40 is a longitudinal scan of the right abdomen in a 64-year-old man with gastric adenocarcinoma. Ascitic fluid is distending the abdomen and displacing the liver away from the abdominal wall. A large soft tissue mass is seen adhering to the anterior abdominal wall. The mass is secondary to metastatic implants. Bowel loops are present in the malignant ascites and are also adherent to meta-

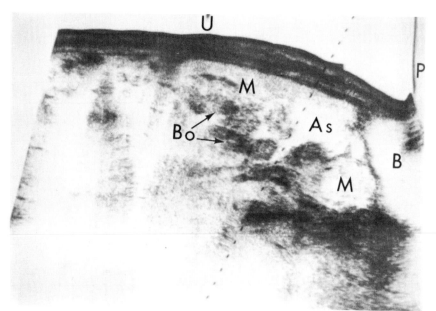

FIG 10–37.

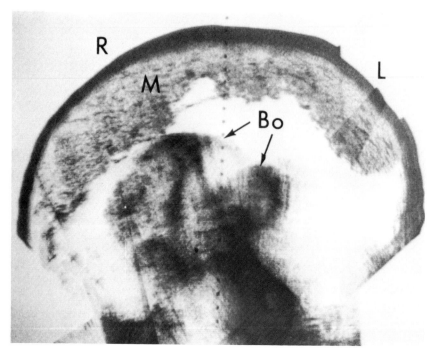

FIG 10–38.

static implants anteriorly. What is structure 1 in Figure 10–40?

| | | |
|---|---|---|
| **As** | = | Ascites |
| **B** | = | Bladder |
| **Bo** | = | Bowel loops |
| **F** | = | Foot |
| **L** | = | Left |
| **Li** | = | Liver |
| **M** | = | Metastatic implants |
| **P** | = | Symphisis pubis |
| **R** | = | Right |
| **U** | = | Umbilicus |
| **1** | = | Gallbladder |

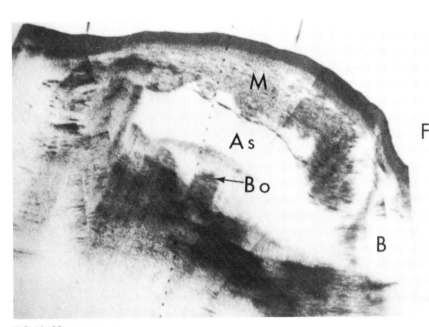

**FIG 10–39.**

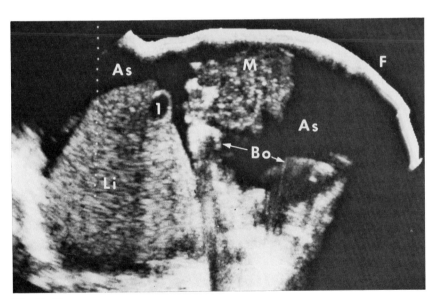

**FIG 10–40.**

## Dilated Bowel

Occasionally, numerous fluid-filled circular and tubular structures are seen within the abdomen. The possibility of obstructed bowel loops should always be considered. Figures 10–41 and 10–42 are scans of a patient with small bowel obstruction. Bowel loops can be visualized on both transverse and longitudinal scans. The transverse scans in Figure 10–41 show the bowel loops to be circular and oval in shape. There may be some confusion with an ovarian neoplasm. The longitudinal scan in Figure 10–42, however, shows a more tubular appearance suggesting bowel loops. These findings are highly consistent with obstructed fluid-filled loops, which can be confirmed by detecting peristaltic activity on real-time examination. By scanning the loops 90° to their circular appearance, one usually can see a tubular appearance in the case of bowel obstruction.

Figures 10–43 and 10–44 are transverse and longitudinal abdominal scans of a young man who had sustained a stab wound approximately 4 months earlier. He came to the emergency room complaining of acute abdominal pain. An abdominal ultrasound examination was ordered to evaluate the cause of pain. The ultrasound scan is characteristic, with numerous circular and tubular structures seen throughout the left abdomen, indicating bowel obstruction. Obstruction was confirmed by documenting numerous swirling, soft internal echoes, consistent with peristalsis, within the tubular structures on real-time examination. These echoes supported the diagnosis of dilated bowel loops rather than a multicystic abdominal mass.

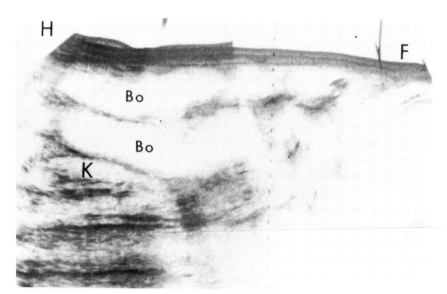

**FIG 10–41.**

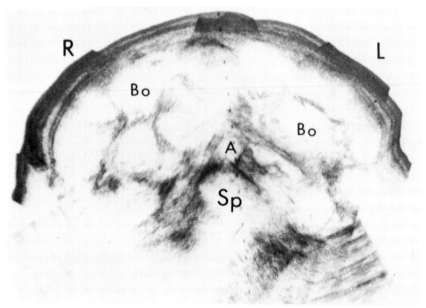

**FIG 10–42.**

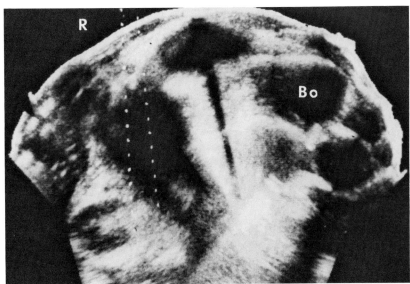

A   = Aorta
Bo  = Dilated bowel
F   = Foot
H   = Head
K   = Kidney
L   = Left
R   = Right
Sp  = Spine

FIG 10–43.

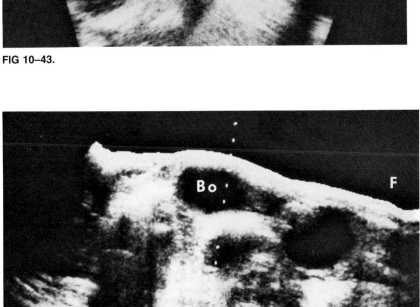

FIG 10–44.

## Dilated Bowel

Besides the characteristic circular and tubular appearance, dilated bowel loops may yield other ultrasound signs that lead to the correct diagnosis. A longitudinal scan (Fig 10–45) shows numerous tubular, fluid-filled bowel loops. These are due to a small bowel obstruction. The valvulae conniventes (arrows) can actually be seen within one of the loops of bowel. They appear as linear echoes crossing the bowel lumen. When these linear echoes are identified, one can be certain they are within bowel loops rather than other abdominal lesions.

Figure 10–46 is a transverse scan of the pelvis in which a multiloculated cystic mass is identified. Numerous polypoid protrusions into the lumen of the cystic regions are present that moved on real-time examination. These protrusions are characteristic of intestinal mucosa which is undergoing peristalsis and projecting into the fluid-filled intestinal lumen. When these findings are visualized, the correct diagnosis of bowel obstruction rather than ovarian tumor can be made.

Fluid-filled obstructed bowel loops usually have a fairly characteristic ultrasound appearance without a confusing etiologic picture. Figures 10–47 and 10–48 show the scans of a patient sent for a pelvic ultrasound examination because of lower abdominal and pelvic pain. The study revealed numerous sonolucent masses with very thick walls. These masses turned out to be infarcted bowel loops. At the time of examination, the possibility of ovarian mass was considered quite likely. Figures 10–47 and 10–48 show numerous circular sonolucencies with fluid centrally. The bowel walls were markedly thickened and edematous, which gives a picture different from the routine obstructed bowel noted in earlier cases. At operation, numerous bowel loops were present in the pelvis and not only were obstructed but also markedly thickened and edematous from infarction.

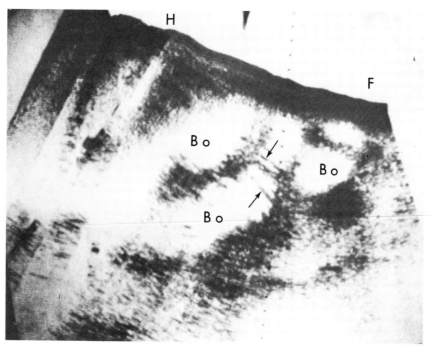

FIG 10–45.

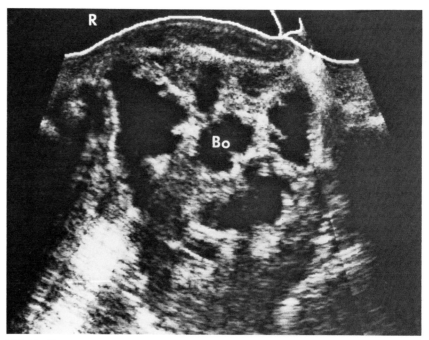

FIG 10–46.

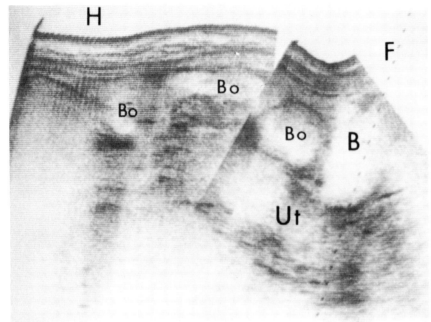

Arrows = Valvulae conniventes
B      = Bladder
Bo     = Bowel
F      = Foot
H      = Head
L      = Left
R      = Right
Ut     = Uterus

**FIG 10–47.**

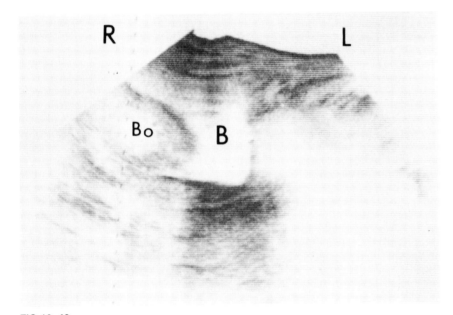

**FIG 10–48.**

## Bowel Masses

Figures 10–49 to 10–50 are scans of a patient who had previously undergone small bowel bypass for obesity. Because of intermittent abdominal pain, an ultrasound study was performed. A transverse scan of the midabdomen (Fig 10–49) shows a large mass draped over the spine. This mass has a lucent peripheral region surrounding a highly echogenic central portion. A longitudinal scan (Fig 10–50) gives a similar appearance. This is a common finding in bowel lesions. At operation intussusception of the blind loop segment was found. This large "target" or "bull's-eye" appearance has been reported in intussusception and GI tract tumors. When GI tract tumors are present, the echogenic central portion may often be eccentric in location. In intussusception or in the normal GI tract, the echogenicity is situated more centrally.

Figures 10–51 and 10–52 are ultrasound scans of a 17-year-old boy who was admitted with a 6-day history of abdominal pain. The scan shows a large mass with numerous internal echoes in the right upper quadrant. Through-transmission is noted posterior to the mass. These findings indicate a nonhomogeneous fluid-filled structure. The through-transmission is best seen on the longitudinal scan in Figure 10–52. At surgery, the mass was found to be a duplication cyst of the duodenum. The ultrasound appearance would be consistent with an abscess, hematoma, or peripancreatic pseudocyst with debris. There was nothing specific to suggest a diagnosis of duodenal duplication cyst. Other duplication cysts may be completely sonolucent without internal echoes.

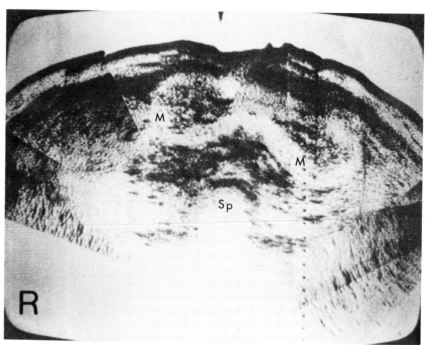

**FIG 10–49.**

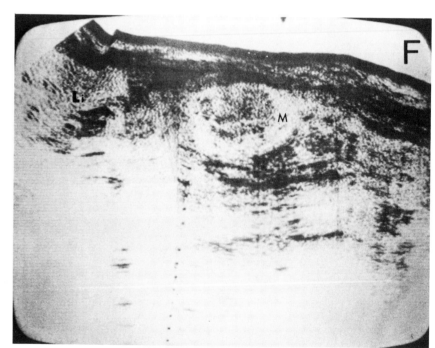

**FIG 10–50.**

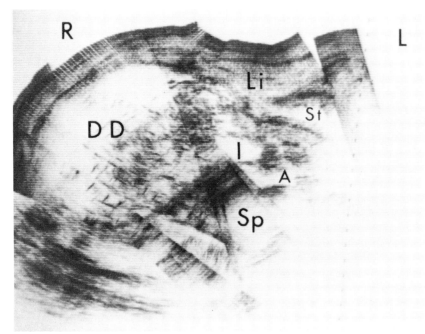

A  = Aorta
DD = Duodenal duplication cyst
F  = Foot
H  = Head
I  = Inferior vena cava
L  = Left
Li = Liver
M  = Intussusception
Sp = Spine
St = Stomach

**FIG 10–51.**

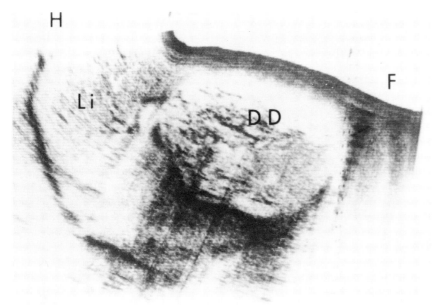

**FIG 10–52.**

## Peritonitis; Left Upper Quadrant Abscess

When ascites is present in the abdomen the fluid visualized on ultrasound is usually relatively echo free, unless there has been previous surgery. Other types of fluid may be present in the peritoneal cavity. When pus or blood is present, there often will be internal echoes noted within the fluid because of debris and fibrosis of clot formation. This is one general way of distinguishing ascites from other forms of fluid collection.

Figures 10–53 and 10–54 are scans of a patient with diffuse peritonitis secondary to bowel perforation. A longitudinal scan over the right abdomen (Fig 10–53) shows a fluid collection anterior to the right lobe of the liver. Within the fluid collection are numerous curvilinear echoes (arrows) which help to distinguish it from simple ascites. A longitudinal scan (Fig 10–54) of the right lower quadrant was obtained. Again we see numerous curvilinear echoes within the fluid. The patient has diffuse peritonitis. It is clear that the fluid collection is somewhat different than in the previous cases of ascites. There is much more evidence of debris within the fluid, and this is highly consistent with either pus or hematoma.

Figures 10–55 and 10–56 are scans of a patient with a large left upper quadrant abscess following surgery for colonic carcinoma. Figure 10–55 shows bowel loops floating within the fluid. The abscess shows evidence of linear echoes (arrows) within the fluid collection. A longitudinal scan of the left lateral abdomen (Fig 10–56) also shows numerous linear echoes within the abscess. Again, ascites tends to be relatively echo free as it displaces organs and bowel loops. Abscesses and hematomas within the abdomen tend to give more internal echoes.

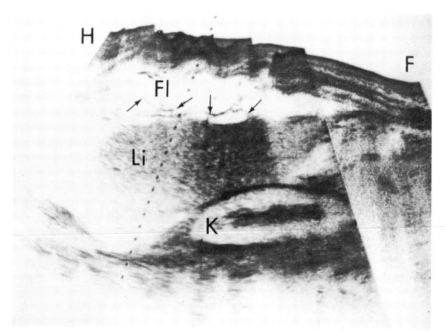

FIG 10–53.

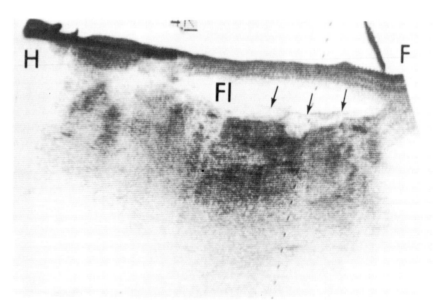

FIG 10–54.

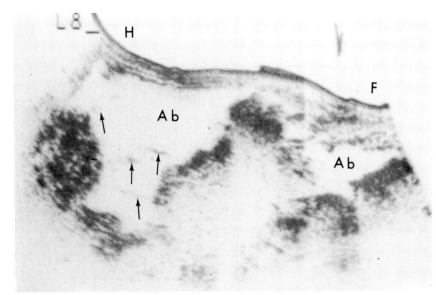

**FIG 10–55.**

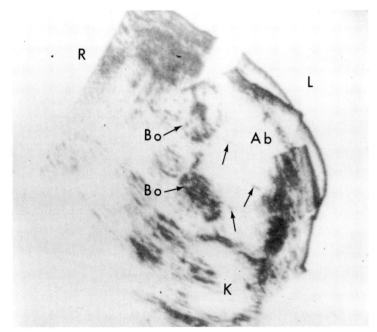

**FIG 10–56.**

| | | |
|---|---|---|
| **Ab** | = | Left upper quadrant abscess |
| **Arrows** | = | Internal echoes within the fluid, indicating debris |
| **Bo** | = | Bowel loops |
| **F** | = | Foot |
| **Fl** | = | Fluid secondary to peritonitis |
| **H** | = | Head |
| **K** | = | Kidney |
| **L** | = | Left |
| **Li** | = | Liver |
| **R** | = | Right |

## Intra-abdominal Abscesses

Ultrasound may be performed because of the provisional diagnosis of an intra-abdominal abscess. Ultrasound is an excellent means of visualizing intra-abdominal abscesses if no bowel air intervenes between the transducer and the mass. Abscesses can present with a variety of appearances. If the abscess is recent and suppurative, it will appear as a fluid-filled mass. If, however, the abscess is of a chronic nature, with a large amount of debris, it can present as a solid mass and be mistaken for a tumor. The scan shown in Figure 10–57 was made to rule out a right upper quadrant abscess. The longitudinal scan over the right upper abdomen demonstrates a subdiaphragmatic abscess anterior to the liver and just inferior to the right hemidiaphragm. It could also represent ascites, hematoma, or a bile leak. It is extremely difficult to distinguish among these entities by ultrasound. However, the clinical history often contributes to the ultrasound findings and leads to a correct diagnosis.

In an unusual case (Fig 10–58), a patient was examined for vague right upper quadrant pain. Initially the study was done to rule out cholelithiasis. During the course of the examination, a sonolucent mass in the lateral abdomen was noted. This decubitus transverse scan shows a sonolucent mass lateral to the liver. Because of this finding, associated with the vague right upper quadrant pain, the patient was operated on. Chronic appendicitis with a walled-off chronic abscess lateral to the liver at the location noted on ultrasound was found.

An abscess frequently will present with a large amount of debris and give the appearance of a solid mass on ultrasound. Figures 10–59 and 10–60 are scans of a patient found to have a subhepatic abscess at operation. The scans show a solid mass in the epigastric region beneath the left lobe of the liver. The numerous echoes within the abscess lead to the confusing picture of a solid lesion within the upper abdomen. This, however, was sec-

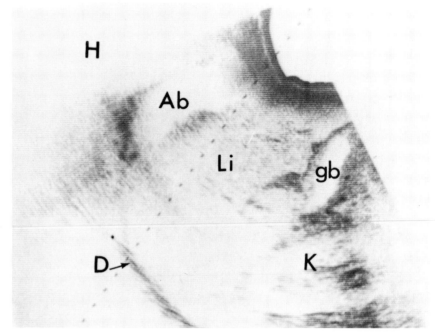

**FIG 10–57.**

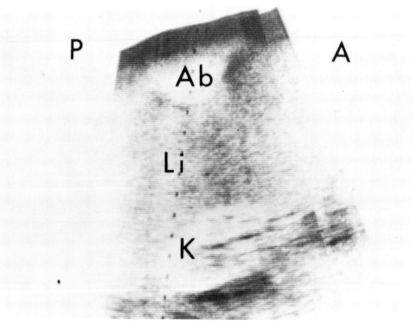

**FIG 10–58.**

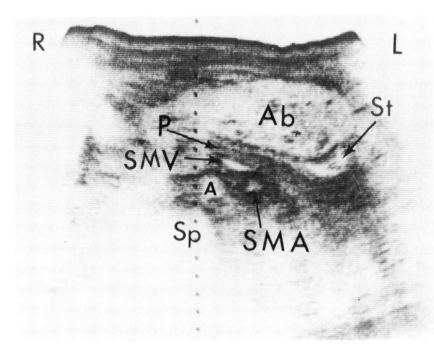

**FIG 10–59.**

ondary to a chronic abscess filled with a large amount of debris. It could also be misinterpreted as a stomach filled with food. The transverse scan in Figure 10–59, however, demonstrates a small amount of fluid within the stomach. The pancreas is seen posterior to the abscess and stomach. The longitudinal scan (Fig 10–60) shows the abscess to be in the subhepatic region.

| | | |
|---|---|---|
| **A** | = | Aorta |
| **A** | = | Anterior (Fig 10–58) |
| **Ab** | = | Abscess |
| **D** | = | Diaphragm |
| **F** | = | Foot |
| **GB** | = | Gallbladder |
| **H** | = | Head |
| **K** | = | Kidney |
| **L** | = | Left |
| **Li** | = | Liver |
| **P** | = | Pancreas |
| **P** | = | Posterior (Fig 10–58) |
| **R** | = | Right |
| **SA** | = | Splenic artery |
| **SMA** | = | Superior mesenteric artery |
| **SMV** | = | Superior mesenteric vein |
| **Sp** | = | Spine |
| **St** | = | Stomach |

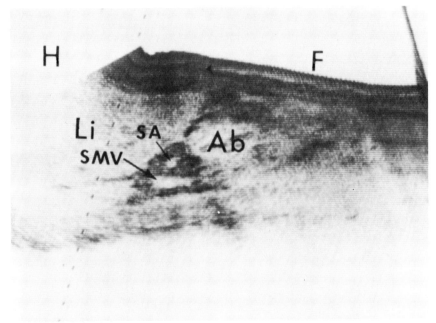

**FIG 10–60.**

## Abdominal Abscesses

Abdominal abscesses can be situated within an abdominal organ or within the peritoneal cavity. Intra-abdominal abscesses are found in those areas previously described in doing a fluid search in the abdomen. These areas include the right subdiaphragmatic area, subhepatic area, hepatorenal area, left upper quadrant, perisplenic area, lesser sac, right and left paracolic gutters, pelvis, and midabdomen at the root of the mesentery. With systematic examination, most intraperitoneal abscesses can be detected on ultrasound. Abscesses may present as sonolucent, echogenic, or mixed masses. Extremely high amplitude echoes will be seen in these masses if air is present.

Figures 10–61 and 10–62 are transverse and longitudinal scans of the right upper quadrant in a 63-year-old man who had recently undergone gallbladder surgery. Fever and an elevated right diaphragm developed. An ultrasound study was ordered to evaluate the elevated right diaphragm. In Figure 10–61 the right hemidiaphragm is seen to be thickened. Fluid collections representing a right pleural effusion and a subdiaphragmatic abscess are present posterior and anterior to the diaphragm. The important diagnostic finding is a region of extremely high echoes (arrowheads) medial to the diaphragm in Figure 10–61 and inferior to the diaphragm in Figure 10–62. This region represents air in a subdiaphragmatic abscess, which led to the correct diagnosis.

Ultrasound can be used to assist in the diagnosis of abdominal fluid by guiding percutaneous needle aspiration and drainage. Figures 10–63 and 10–64 are longitudinal and transverse scans of the right upper quadrant of an 18-month-old girl admitted for fever of unknown origin. Ultrasound revealed a mixed sonolucent mass in the posterior aspect of the liver near the hepatorenal angle. Under ultrasound guidance, a needle aspiration was performed and an abscess was documented. Figures 10–63 and 10–64 are scans obtained immediately after the needle aspiration. The high-

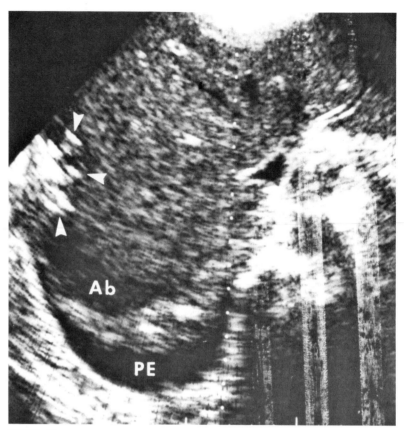

FIG 10–61.

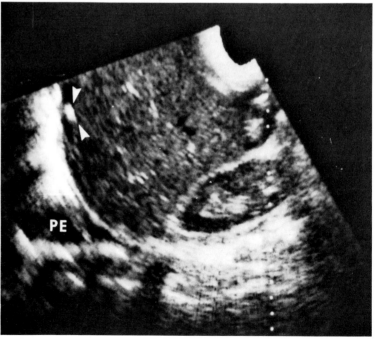

FIG 10–62.

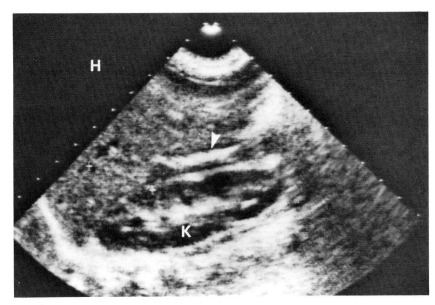

**FIG 10–63.**

amplitude region (arrowheads) represents air from the aspiration procedure. The patient was treated with appropriate antibiotics and showed marked improvement. Ultrasound assistance for percutaneous diagnoses and drainage is increasing. The ultrasonographer has a tremendous advantage since he can determine the best approach for the percutaneous procedure.

| | | |
|---|---|---|
| **Ab** | = | Abscess |
| **Arrowheads** | = | Air in abscess |
| **H** | = | Head |
| **PE** | = | Pleural effusion |
| **R** | = | Right |

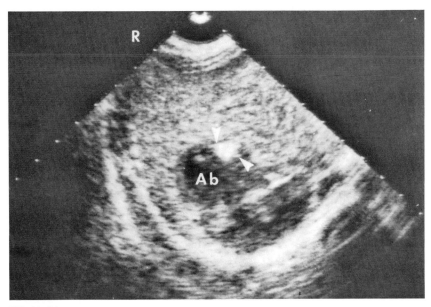

**FIG 10–64.**

## Pleural Effusions Presenting as Abdominal Masses

Figure 10–65 is a transverse scan of a patient with carcinoma of the left lung. Initially there appears to be a large fluid-filled mass in the left upper quadrant. The diagnostic possibilities include a pancreatic pseudocyst, ascites, abscess, or possibly a fluid-filled stomach with gastric outlet obstruction. The longitudinal scan, however (Fig 10–66) demonstrates a large pleural effusion. This scan was obtained in the right lateral decubitus position following the left axillary line. A completely filled left hydrothorax is seen. The diaphragm has been inverted by the large hydrothorax on the left side.

Pleural fluid frequently is confused for ascites. Figures 10–67 and 10–68 are scans of a 38-year-old man with a long history of alcohol abuse. He had a previous history of ascites and pleural effusion. The pleural effusion was negative on cytology and bacterial culture. A transverse scan of the right upper abdomen (Fig 10–67) shows ascitic fluid lateral to the liver. Posterior to the liver we see the pleural effusion in the posterior sulcus. The diaphragm can be visualized between the ascitic fluid and the pleural effusion. A longitudinal scan of the right upper quadrant (Fig 10–68) shows the pleural effusion superior to the diaphragm, while ascitic fluid is noted inferior to the diaphragm. Since pleural fluid is present in the right pleural space, we are able to see the posterior aspect of the thorax (arrows). Normally, this cannot be seen when air is present in the lungs. When visualizing the echoes of the thorax, fluid or a solid material has to be present superior to the diaphragm in order to demonstrate the posterior thorax this far cephalad.

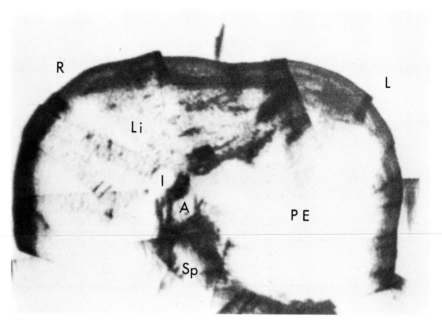

FIG 10–65.

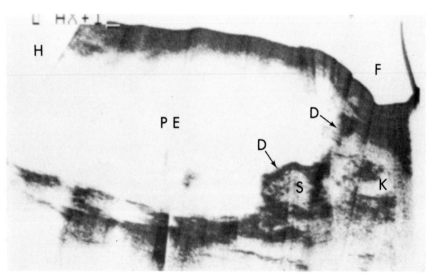

FIG 10–66.

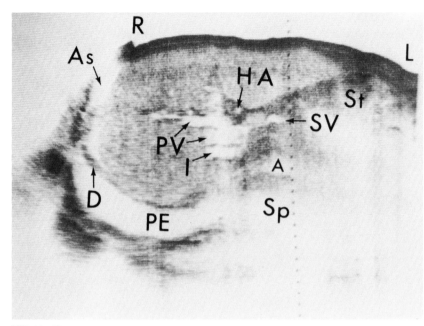

**FIG 10–67.**

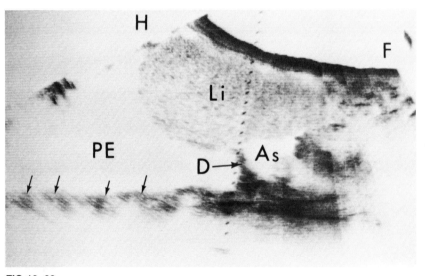

**FIG 10–68.**

| **A** | = | Aorta |
| **Arrows** | = | Posterior right thoracic wall |
| **As** | = | Ascites |
| **D** | = | Inverted diaphragm |
| **F** | = | Foot |
| **H** | = | Head |
| **HA** | = | Hepatic artery |
| **I** | = | Inferior vena cava |
| **K** | = | Kidney |
| **L** | = | Left |
| **Li** | = | Liver |
| **PE** | = | Pleural effusion |
| **PV** | = | Portal vein |
| **R** | = | Right |
| **S** | = | Spleen |
| **Sp** | = | Spine |
| **St** | = | Stomach |
| **SV** | = | Splenic vein |

## Abdominal Masses

Figures 10–69 and 10–70 are scans of a patient with an ultrasound picture highly consistent with a left upper quadrant abscess. However, at surgery, no abscess was found. The patient, a 62-year-old man, was admitted with the diagnosis of colonic cancer. He was operated on and a colostomy was performed. Three weeks after the operation there was a fever spike, and an ultrasound examination was performed. Figures 10–69 and 10–70 demonstrate a relatively sonolucent mass with some linear echoes present. It was situated superior, lateral, and anterior to the spleen. The finding was highly consistent with a left upper quadrant abscess. The patient underwent surgery and the left upper quadrant was explored. No abscess or hematoma was noted. The left upper quadrant had a large amount of edematous omentum which most likely had been viewed as this relatively lucent mass on ultrasound. We have seen other cases of edematous omentum presenting as sonolucent masses in the abdomen. If a mass is highly suggestive of an abscess or hematoma, the possibility of adherent edematous omentum should also be considered.

As noted in previous cases, GI structures have a "bull's-eye" appearance. The central, highly echogenic region is made up of mucosa with the surrounding lucent area secondary to the bowel wall. The normal airless GI tract usually has a very thin rim and a large, highly echogenic central region. We have previously shown a case of intussusception in which the wall was markedly thickened. When GI malignancy is present, not only is the lucent wall thickened, but the highly echogenic region is usually off center. Figure 10–71 is a transverse scan of the upper abdomen of a 67-year-old man with a bleeding gastric ulcer. The abdominal scan demonstrates a large soft tissue mass in the left upper quadrant. A highly echogenic, off-center region is noted. There is a large sonolucent rim of soft tissue. The patient had a 10-cm leiomyosarcoma of the stomach. The appearance of this

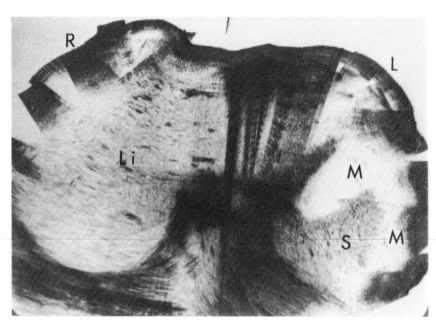

**FIG 10–69.**

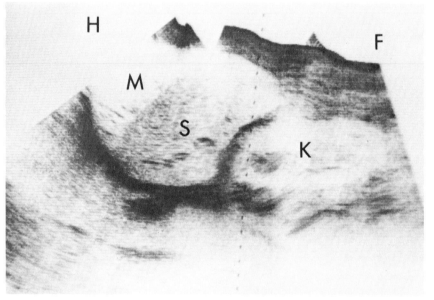

**FIG 10–70.**

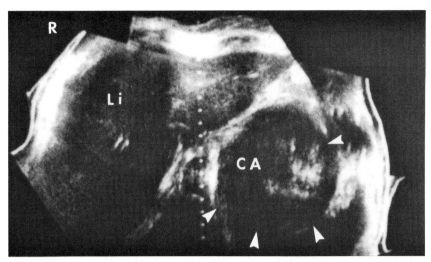

**FIG 10–71.**

mass is typical of GI malignancies.

Occasionally masses may be identified in the soft tissues of the abdomen, thigh, or buttocks. By scanning over the area of interest, some information may be obtained about the nature of such masses. Figure 10–72 is a scan of the right buttock in an elderly man who complained of tenderness over the region. A 6 × 8-cm soft tissue mass with a central fluid region is identified on ultrasound. The differential diagnosis would include abscess, hematoma, or necrotic soft tissue tumor. A biopsy with ultrasound guidance disclosed an abscess. The patient improved with appropriate therapy.

| | | |
|---|---|---|
| **Ab** | = | Abscess |
| **Arrowheads** | = | Leiomyosarcoma |
| **CA** | = | Leiomyosarcoma |
| **F** | = | Foot |
| **H** | = | Head |
| **L** | = | Left |
| **Li** | = | Liver |
| **M** | = | Edematous omentum |
| **R** | = | Right |
| **S** | = | Spleen |

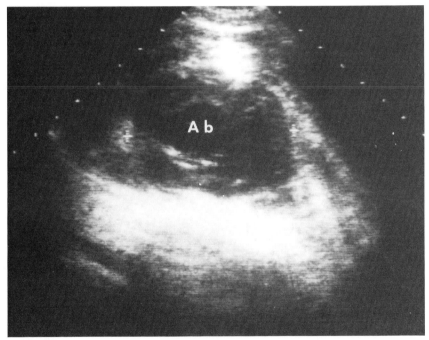

**FIG 10–72.**

## Abdominal Tumors

Previous cases demonstrated the ultrasound appearance in ascites. It is important to be able to distinguish ascites from fluid-filled multiloculated abdominal and pelvic masses. Figure 10–73 is a longitudinal scan of the midabdomen of a 52-year-old man with complaints of nausea, vomiting, and increasing abdominal girth. Three years earlier he had undergone resection of a leiomyosarcoma of the small intestine. Abdominal ultrasound now demonstrates a large multiloculated fluid-filled mass nearly filling the entire abdomen (arrowheads). This mass appears well circumscribed and not free in the intraperitoneal cavity. Such findings differ from ascites, in which bowel loops can be seen along with their mesenteric attachment. The patient was found to have metastatic leiomyosarcoma with hemorrhage causing the fluid-filled components of the mass.

Figures 10–74 and 10–75 are transverse and longitudinal scans of a 56-year-old man with a history of malignant mesothelioma. The ultrasound findings are dramatic and show a large retroperitoneal mass displacing the aorta and inferior vena cava anteriorly. This mantle of soft tissue is present anterior to the spine and is secondary to malignant mesothelioma. Figure 10–76 is a longitudinal scan of the right upper quadrant in a 64-year-old man with a history of metastatic melanoma to the lung and brain. The scan shows a mass near the dome of the liver. The important finding is disruption of the diaphragmatic echoes. The continuity of the diaphragm is interrupted (arrows) by a lung mass secondary to metastatic melanoma.

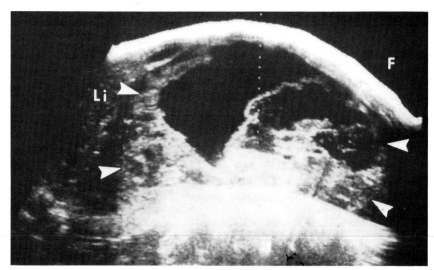

**FIG 10–73.**

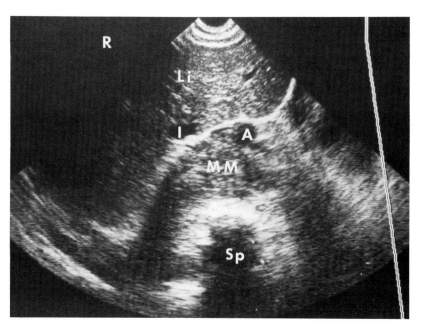

**FIG 10–74.**

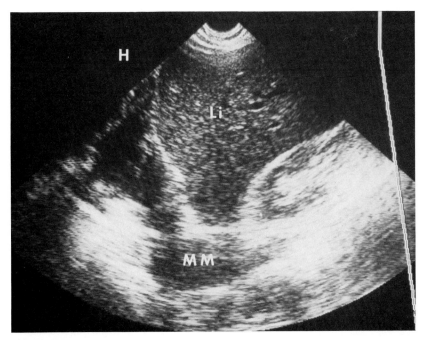

| A | = Aorta |
| Arrowheads | = Metastatic leiomyosar-coma |
| arrows | = Disruption of the dia-phragm |
| F | = Foot |
| GB | = Gallbladder |
| H | = Head |
| I | = Inferior vena cava |
| Li | = Liver |
| Me | = Metastatic melanoma |
| M | = Metastatic mesothelioma |
| R | = Right |
| Sp | = Spine |

FIG 10–75.

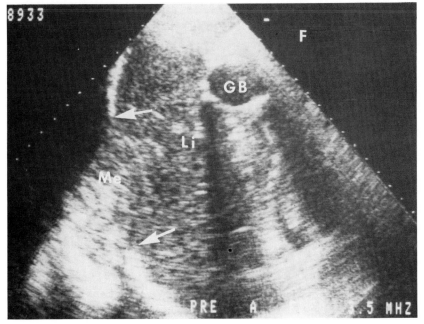

FIG 10–76.

## Abdominal Vessels

Abdominal vessels have been discussed in other chapters with the various organs with which they are closely associated. However, a few comments are in order about visualization of echoes within the vessel lumen. The output and sensitivity of an ultrasound unit can always be adjusted high to place artifactual echoes within the lumen of a vessel. Occasionally, intraluminal echoes arising from a catheter, thrombus, or tumor may be visualized within a vessel. These echoes often are difficult to separate from artifactual echoes. Figure 10–77 is a longitudinal scan of a 58-year-old woman with short bowel syndrome secondary to multiple bowel resections for ischemic disease. A tubular echo is noted within the lumen of the inferior vena cava. The echo represents a TPN catheter. Because of their high reflectivity, catheters are usually easy to visualize within a vessel lumen. They also yield a characteristic echo pattern, making their recognition easy.

Figure 10–78 is a longitudinal scan through the right upper quadrant of a 49-year-old woman with pancreatic carcinoma and leg edema of recent onset. On ultrasound, soft tissue echoes were noted within the inferior vena cava, consistent with thrombosis. The thrombotic area appears different from the catheter in Figure 10–77. The walls of the thrombus are not as sharply defined as those of the catheter. Also, there is the suggestion of soft tissue echogenicity rather than the marked, highly reflective echogenicity of the catheter.

Figures 10–79 and 10–80 are scans of a 64-year-old man with known hepatoma. In Figure 10–79, a transverse scan, soft tissue echoes are noted within the right portal vein. These echoes are more discrete than artifactual echoes. They represent tumor invading the right portal vein. Figure 10–80 is a longitudinal scan of the right upper abdomen in the same patient. Soft echoes secondary to tumor are again seen in the right portal vein. The caudad portion of the inferior vena cava is noted to be echo free.

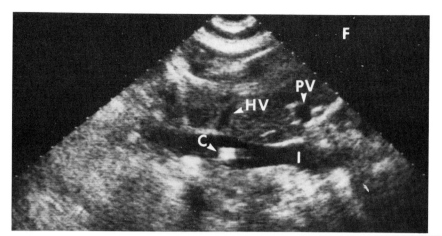

FIG 10–77.

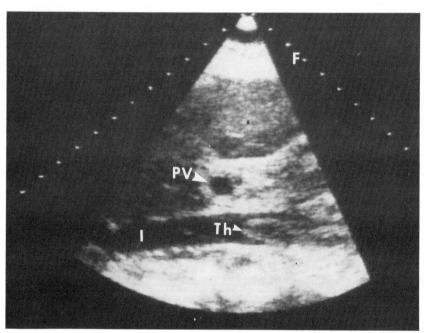

FIG 10–78.

However, soft echoes are present in the cephalad portion of the inferior vena cava, indicating tumor at this site.

C   = Catheter
F   = Foot
HV  = Hepatic vein
I   = Inferior vena cava
Li   = Liver
PV  = Portal vain
R   = Right
Sp  = Spine
Th  = Thrombus
T   = Tumor

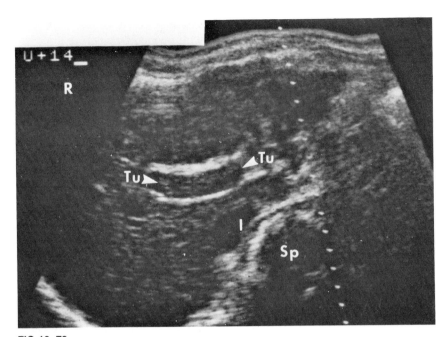

FIG 10–79.

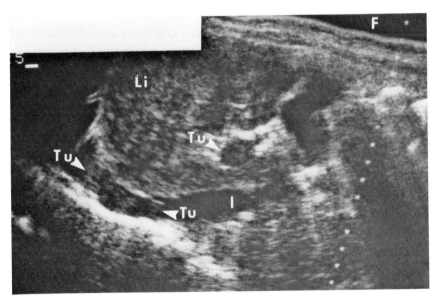

FIG 10–80.

# 11.
# Intraoperative Ultrasound

## William King III, M.D.

Technological advances in the basic sciences have historically been followed by incorporation of the technology into the practice of medicine. Imaging procedures are commonplace in the operating theater. Plain radiography, angiography, cholangiography, and cinefluoroscopy provide valuable information to the surgeon. Intraoperative ultrasound has become available to the surgical population over the last 6 years, with rewarding results. The positive response is primarily due to the development of portable real-time equipment with specialized transducers for near-field high-resolution studies. Intraoperative examinations of the brain and spinal cord, the gallbladder and biliary tree, the pancreas and liver, the kidneys and retroperitoneum, and vascular structures have been used to confirm pathology and guide biopsy and surgical procedures.

The first reported intraoperative ultrasound procedure was in 1961. A-mode one-dimensional technique was used for localizing renal calculi. This procedure was performed in conjunction with radiography and was primarily useful for detecting nonopaque calculi. Difficulties that arose in interpreting amplitude spikes and in differentiating stones from other tissue interfaces limited the application of this technique in the surgical community.[1] Image improvement resulting from bistable and subsequently gray-scale ultrasonography provided two-dimensional orientation and dynamic range, popularizing this procedure with the urologist in the mid-1970s.[2] The development of portable real-time equipment and smaller transducer heads in the late 1970s and early 1980s expanded the horizons of intraoperative imaging to the biliary system and pancreas,[3-5] vascular channels,[6-9] brain,[10-13] and spinal cord.[14-16]

The most obvious advantages are apparent in neurosurgical procedures, once the osseous elements protecting the brain and spinal cord were displaced surgically. Biopsy guide attachments and real-time visualization of biopsies and shunt placements increased the expertise and confidence in these procedures.[11, 13, 17] Dedicated intraoperative "neuro" sector scanners were manufactured for widespread application in several major medical centers. Special intraoperative transducers with high-resolution crystals (7.5–10.0 MHz) and smaller scan heads were designed by several manufacturers for use on existing ultrasound consoles.

The anatomic landmarks utilized in abdominal ultrasound have been well established. An understanding of neuroanatomy, as imaged on ultrasound, is crucial to the practicing neurosurgeon and attendant radiologist. Ultrasound investigations of brain anatomy and pathology in the developing fetus and in the neonate provided early impressions regarding gray-scale ultrasound images. Transfontanelle intracranial ultrasound by contact and real-time B-mode techniques,[18] popularized in pediatric intensive care units for the detection of congenital anomalies and intracranial bleeding episodes and their complications, provided a stimulus for intraoperative examinations of the brain.

Abdominal intraoperative ultrasound developed the advantage of direct surface contact scanning on tissues of interest. High-resolution images of the pancreas, kidney, liver, and biliary tree are now possible. A saline path can be used if a wider field of view is necessary for deep abdominal structures. Although ultrasound has not been widely used in abdominal surgery, it has been a useful adjunct to palpation by the sensitive fingertips of the surgeon and to standardized cholangiographic and radiographic techniques.

Incorporation of Doppler capabilities has further enhanced the usefulness of intraoperative ultrasound for the vascular surgeon.[19–20]

## Technique

Although dedicated intraoperative ultrasound units are available, most hospitals do not have a sufficient number of operative cases to justify the purchase of specialized equipment. Many manufacturers offer intraoperative transducer probes that can be attached to standard real-time equipment. These probes are expensive; however, certain features warrant their purchase. Thin probes can scan the brain through burr holes, eliminating the necessity of craniotomy for tissue biopsy of intracranial lesions. Thin probes can also reach into small areas intracranially and intra-abdominally. High-resolution probes (10.0 MHz) are necessary for fine detail, especially in vascular examinations. Elimination of near-field artifacts is important for the diagnosis of superficial lesions and direct contact scanning. If specially designed scanners and probes are not available, modifications of standard units and transducers can provide useful information. If near-field artifacts are a problem, a saline path can be interposed between the surface in the area of in-

terest and the transducer. If penetration is a problem, transducer selection should be questioned.

Whichever unit is used, clearance of the equipment for electrical safety by a bioengineer should be checked prior to its use in the operating theater. The unit should be scrubbed down with disinfectant each time it is used in the operating room.

The major modification for intraoperative ultrasound is sterile technique. This can be accomplished in many ways, depending on the needs of the surgeon and the ultrasonographer. In one method, the sonographer has scrubbed and is in sterile gown and gloves as a member of the surgical team. The circulating nurse passes a transducer and its cord into a sterile plastic or rubber sheath held by the scrub nurse with sterile gel inside the closed end of the sheath. Sterile rubber bands are placed around the sheath to secure the transducer.

Sterile plastic sheet can be placed over the control console for adjustments in scan technique. Touch-control buttons for time gain compensation (TGC), power, gain setting, and screen size can be used for adjustments in technique during the procedure by the person who has scrubbed. Alternatively, a technologist or assistant can adjust technique if touch-button controls are not present.

Different sterile techniques are possible. In one technique the transducer is placed in a large sterile plastic bag and the loose sides of the bag are twisted around the cord and then secured by sterile masking tape. In another technique the transducer and cord are passed through a sterile operating gown sleeve and into a sterile glove with sterile gel in the glove. The fingers of the glove are folded back and secured with sterile rubber bands. These methods allow the transducer to be in the sterile operative field.

A variation in technique uses a sterile plastic sheet placed over the operative field. The anatomic area of interest is then scanned through the sheet. Saline irrigant provides acoustic coupling on the sterile side of the sheet and gel is the coupling agent on the non-sterile side. This method allows the sonographer to scan without scrubbing and gowning. Once a lesion is localized, the sterile sheet is removed. A disadvantage with this technique is that a biopsy guide attachment cannot be attached for real-time biopsy guidance. This method does decrease the time required for the sonographer to scrub and gown. In many instances, a neurosurgeon asks for ultrasound guidance after the dura is open and a tumor mass is not visibly apparent. This sterile-drape technique has been useful and time-saving in these urgent situations.

## Biopsy Techniques

Ultrasound provides a planar method for tumor localization when tumors are neither palpable nor visible by the surgeon. A stereotactic apparatus can be fixed to the operative table which can hold the scanning transducer. Biopsy guides attached to the transducer can direct needle passage, verifying angle and depth.[21] Guides can be adjusted such that the angulation of the needle corresponds to a calculated depth of a tumor mass from the transducer. However, the stereotactic method is cumbersome, and hand-held transducers with biopsy guides are equally accurate.[22] Other guides have less variability in that a biopsy angle is prefixed and the transducer must be moved to coordinate the depth to this angle. This limitation causes difficulty when the operative defect is small.

Real-time visualization allows the physician to monitor the interaction of the biopsy needle with the tumor interface. Many tumors are encapsulated or have a tough, fibrous or rubbery outer border which can deflect a needle away from the tumor mass into normal tissue.

Free-hand techniques require greater skill and should be performed only when biopsy guide attachments are not available. The tumor is sited by real-time imaging and the depth is measured by ultrasound. The angle of the transducer and a three-dimensional visualization of the tumor location must be kept in mind once the transducer is removed from the tissue surface. The biopsy is then performed using visual coordinates. Verification of the biopsy can often be made by the observation of a needle track leading into the tumor or by positive pathology. Most biopsies will leave an echogenic needle track after removal of the needle. This is presumed to represent blood in the needle path.[23]

After a biopsy procedure, ultrasound can be used to evaluate for hemorrhage, cerebrospinal fluid leaks, and other complications. If tumor resection is the goal of the operation, residual tumor can be estimated. One problem during tumor resection is the introduction of air into the surrounding tissues, which creates unscannable defects. If this occurs, saline can be instilled into the resected area and the area rescanned for residual tumor. Artifacts can be produced by Gelfoam, laparotomy pads, clips, and other operative equipment.[24] If possible, such items should be removed before rescanning.

## Neurosurgical Procedures

A-mode ultrasound detection of cerebral neoplasms in postmortem brains was first reported in 1950.[25] A similar technique was attempted for the diagnosis of intracranial complications after head trauma in 1956, with limited results.[26] The development of bistable scanning was equally unsuccessful for evaluation of the intracranial contents, owing to the high acoustic impedance of overlying cranium.[27]

In 1951, brain tissue was scanned through a craniotomy defect; however, images were poor. Some improvement in image quality in 1970 allowed better anatomic correlation in patients scanned through postoperative defects.[28] The first study using B-mode gray-scale imaging through a craniotomy was not reported until 1975.[29] Application of gray-scale technique through the anterior fontanelle in infants proved that ultrasound was useful in providing detailed images of the intracranial contents and pathologic entities, such as hydrocephalus and intraventricular hemorrhages.[30–32] Further work through postsurgical craniotomy defects using 3.0- and 5.0-MHz transducers demonstrated residual tumors, cysts, and extracerebral fluid collections in 1981.[33]

The first reported intraoperative neurosonogram in 1965 using A-mode technique localized a brain tumor.[34] Limited application ensued until the early 1980s when numerous institutions simultaneously began using high-resolution real-time scanners.

Postoperatively, ventricular shunt catheters were easily visualized in hydrocephalic infants through transfontanelle techniques. It was quite natural to scan through the anterior fontanelle intraoperatively so that shunt placement could be accurately monitored and guided.[11, 13, 35, 36] The anterior fontanelle can be either outside or within the sterile field, depending on the surgeon's preference. The importance in placement of the tip of the shunt catheter in the anterior horn of the lateral ventricle is stressed. This decreases the possibility that the choroid plexus will occlude catheter sideholes. Furthermore, inadvertent placement of the catheter tip in the temporal horn precludes optimum ventricular drainage. Complicated shunts can also be monitored. Occasionally, intraventricular synechiae can develop following an intraventricular hemorrhage with resultant poor drainage from all horns of the lateral ventricle. In these situations, separate catheters must be placed in all undrained horns and intraoperative sonographic monitoring is very useful. Similarly, drainage of third ventricle cysts and brain abscesses can be guided by sonography through the anterior fontanelle.[37]

Brain tumors can be localized through craniotomy defects in children as well as adults for accurate guidance of biopsies or catheter placements.[38–42] Almost all brain pathology, with the exception of cysts and fluid collections, is echogenic compared to normal brain echogenicity. Most lesions are readily apparent and distinguishable from normal neural structures if proper technique is used and pitfalls are avoided.

Neurosurgical procedures are preempted by neuroradiologic and electroencephalographic examinations that confirm the presence of an intracranial or intraspinal abnormality in a specific location. Craniotomy and burr hole defects are directed over the area under suspicion. Attention to adjacent anatomic landmarks can help localize the lesion. In fact, the initial scans should provide a general orientation of brain anatomy, which can then be correlated with the preoperative studies. This is extremely important since it is often difficult to understand the position of the patient's skull beneath the surgical drapes. Once landmarks have been established, a search for pathology is simplified.

In general, brain tissue, with the exception of the cerebellum, is hypoechoic. Specular reflectors such as the junction of brain tissue with the cisterns and ventricles, the gyral folds, and the falx and tentorium create strong linear echoes. The folia of the cerebellar hemispheres and vermis have numerous interfaces in the adult, accounting for the echogenicity of the cerebellum. The choroid plexus also is echogenic, as are small pulsatile vascular structures in the gyral folds and the subarachnoid spaces. Cerebrospinal fluid, as expected, is sonolucent. Brain edema is often difficult to depict sonographically, although different authors describe edema as having either slightly increased[43] or decreased echogenicity.[10] Ultrasound has a distinct advantage over CT and MR imaging in its ability to depict lesions not detected by either modality, when each only reveals brain edema and no discrete lesion.[44] Rarely, sonography does not reveal pathology in an area of diffuse brain edema. In these instances, scans must be directed at the periphery of the surgical defect and high-resolution transducers must be used so that a lesion is not missed. Occasionally, a lesion might not be detectable and biopsy should be directed into the region of edema. A diffusely infiltrative glioma can present as just an edematous pattern on all imaging modalities; however, this situation is rare. Calcifications are echogenic and, if large enough, cause acoustic shadowing. Calcifications can be seen in oligodendrogliomas as well as in parasitic disorders.

The character of brain tumors can be assessed on ultrasound. Usually distinct margins are associated with low-grade primary brain neoplasms, metastasess, and abscesses. Indistinct and fading margins are seen in high-grade primary malignancies and in benign lesions that have hemorrhaged.

The extent of tumor can also be assessed transdurally. This is useful in evaluating meningiomas, which can invade the venous sinuses, especially the superior sagittal sinus.[10]

Solid intracranial lesions are echogenic and can be clearly differentiated from normal brain. Occasionally, sonolucent cystic lesions can be imaged as a component of a tumor mass or after radiation therapy. These lucencies may represent areas of necrosis. Abscesses can be either echolucent or echogenic. Hematomas, which are acute, are echogenic. Chronic hematomas can be liquefied, presenting as a sonolucent fluid collection. Needle tracks from a biopsy are echogenic and can be used to verify the site of biopsy. Continued monitoring can evaluate for subsequent bleeding. In cases of tumor resection, ultrasound can evaluate for residual tumor.

Intraoperative spinal sonography is performed in a slightly different fashion than brain sonography. The patient is placed in a prone position on the operating table and surgical dissection is carried out until the lamina overlying the dura is resected. Saline is then poured into the wound and the scans are performed through a water path. The scans will demonstrate the saline path as a sonolucent fluid collection overlying the linear echo of the dorsal aspect of the dural sac. The cerebrospinal fluid is also sonolucent. The anterior aspect of the dural sac appears as another linear echo on a sagittal scan. A transverse scan will reveal the circular dural sac as an echogenic ring. Epidural fluid can occasionally be seen on the ventral aspect of the dura. The spinal cord is echolucent, although a central linear echo can be seen emanating from the central canal. High-resolution scanners can demonstrate pulsations in the location of the anterior spinal artery.

Spinal tumors are imaged as echolucent or echogenic masses.[14, 16] Cystic components may be present.[45] The extent of tumor can be evaluated using intraoperative ultrasound and the precise location can be determined prior to opening the dura mater. Intraoperative studies in patients with spinal trauma can demonstrate the location of bone fragments, both extradurally and intradurally, as well as intramedullary hemorrhage.[46] Bone fragments and metallic fragments are echogenic and have acoustic shadowing. The adequacy of decompression can also be estimated prior to surgical closure. Myelomalacia shows a loss of surface detail, absence of a central canal, and increased echogenicity to the cord. Disk herniations can be seen transdurally, and loose fragments can be detected. Disk material is usually echogenic. The size of syrinxes, which are sonolucent fluid areas within the cord, is easily evaluated and the position of a syrinx shunt catheter can be monitored intraoperatively.[47, 48] Catheters can also be located in the postoperative shunt placement patient as the surgeon dissects toward the location of a failed shunt through fibrous scar tissue.

### Abdominal Procedures

Intraoperative abdominal sonography was initially used to detect renal calculi in 1961 using A-mode technique.[1] As in neurosonography, there was limited application of abdominal intraoperative sonography until the advent of B-mode gray-scale technique in 1977.[2] The advantages of a two-dimensional real-time imaging modality were apparent, and precise localization of an intrarenal calculus minimized surgical trauma to the kidney and inadvertent vascular damage and blood loss. Ultrasound is now a proved adjunct to the operative techniques of nephroscopy, operative radiography and fluoroscopy, and plasma coagulum studies.[49–53] High-resolution probes (6–10 MHz) can detect minute calculi, although penetration is limited.

Standard intraoperative cholangiographic techniques have been in use for many years in patients undergoing cholecystectomy and/or common bile duct exploration. Several authors have reported their experience with intraoperative sonography of the gallbladder and biliary tree, claiming impressive results, comparable to those of cholangiography.[34, 54] In vitro studies using different diameter tubes and varying concentrations of iodinated contrast showed that ultrasound was more sensitive for the detection of small filling defects and was independent of the concentration of the contrast material.[55] Small stones were distinguishable from tiny air bubbles. In a group of obese patients operated on for other problems, sonography detected cholelithiasis that was not diagnosed prior to surgery.[56]

Anatomic landmarks of the liver have been easily determined at surgery, including location of the hepatic venous structures.[57] This information is valuable in hepatic resections for malignancy.[58, 59] In addition, occult lesions and daughter lesions of primary malignancies are detectable intraoperatively with higher accuracy than preoperative studies.[60] Hepatic abscesses can be located, providing coordinates for real-time imaging-assisted drainage procedures.

The pancreas has been evaluated intraoperatively for both tumors and inflammatory processes. Islet cell tumors are difficult to diagnose preoperatively, often requiring multiple imaging studies and venous samplings. Lesions can be multiple. Intraoperative ultrasound is useful in detecting small tumors, using high-resolution transducers in contact with the surface of the pancreas. This technique is not possible transabdominally due to the deep location of the pancreas. The technique is advantageous in localizing these small tumors, which are sonolucent compared to the normal pancreatic parenchyma.[61–63] However, pancreatic carcinomas are difficult to distinguish from inflammatory processes of the pancreas. The primary usefulness in inflammatory conditions is in evaluating and localizing the pancreatic duct and peripancreatic fluid collections.[64, 65]

Many patients have had multiple abdominal operations, resulting in thick scar tissue and intraperitoneal adhesions. The possibility of cutting into adhered bowel is increased in these patients. Ultrasound guidance can be used to assist the laparotomy, evaluating the underlying tissues for air- or fluid-containing structures and peristaltic activity.

## Vascular Studies

Intraoperative real-time ultrasound of the carotid arteries and their intracranial branches has been used by both the vascular surgeon[8, 66] and the neurosurgeon.[67] The coronary arteries have been studied by the cardiac surgeon.[7, 68] High-resolution (10 MHz) transducers directly applied to the surface of exposed vessels demonstrate areas of stenosis, intimal flap formation, and thrombus. This has been especially useful following carotid endarterectomy. Preliminary investigations of Doppler imaging have been carried out in the intracranial branches of the carotid artery and bypass grafts from the superficial temporal artery.[69] Similar techniques are now available for flow studies after endarterectomy[70] and coronary bypass graft surgery and in portasystemic venous shunts.[9, 71]

## References

1. Schlegel JU, Diggdon P, Cuellar J: The use of ultrasound for localizing renal calculi. *J Urol* 1961; 86:367.
2. Cook JH III, Lytton B: Intraoperative localization of renal calculi during nephrolithotomy by ultrasound scanning. *J Urol* 1977; 117:543.
3. Lane RJ, Glazer G: Intra-operative B-mode ultrasound scanning of the extra-hepatic biliary system and pancreas. *Lancet* Aug 16, 1980.
4. Sigel B, Coelho JCU, Spigos DG, et al: Real-time ultrasonography during biliary surgery. *Radiology* 1980; 137:531–533.
5. Sigel B, Coelho JCU, Spigos DG, et al: Ultrasonic imaging during biliary and pancreatic surgery. *Am J Surg* 1981; 141:84–89.
6. Sigel B, Maschi J, Beitler JC, et al: Imaging ultrasound during vascular surgery. *Ann Radiol* 1982; 8:551–554.
7. Sahn D, Barrett-Boyes B, Graham K, et al: Ultrasonic imaging of the coronary arteries in open-chest humans: Evaluation of coronary atherosclerotic lesions during cardiac surgery. *Circulation* 1982; 66(5):1034–1044.
8. Lane RJ, Appleberg M: Real-time intraoperative angiosonography after carotid endarterectomy. *Surgery* 1982; 92:5–9.
9. Nichols WK, Lichti EL, Stephenson HE: Intra-operative determination of porto-systemic shunt patency. *Am Surg* 1982; 48:547–548.
10. Rubin JM, Dohrmann GJ, Greenberg M, et al: Intraoperative sonography of meningiomas. *AJNR* 1982; 3:305–308.
11. Rubin JM, Dohrmann GJ: Use of ultrasonically guided probes and catheters in neurosurgery. *Surg Neurol* 1982; 18(2):305–308.
12. Lange SC, Howe JF, Shuman WP, et al: Intraoperative ultrasound detection of metastatic tumors in the central cortex. *Neurosurgery* 1982; 11(2):219–222.
13. Shkolnik A, McLone DG: Intraoperative real-time ultrasonic guidance of ventricular shunt placement in infants. *Radiology* 1981; 141:515–517.
14. Dohrmann GJ, Rubin JM: Intraoperative ultrasound imaging of the spinal cord: Syringomyelia, cysts and tumors. A preliminary report. *Surg Neurol* 1982; 18(6):395–397.
15. Rubin JM, Dohrmann GJ: Work in progress: Intraoperative ultrasonography of the spine. *Radiology* 1983; 146:173–175.
16. Knake JE, Chandler WF, McGillicuddy JE, et al: Intraoperative sonography of intraspinal tumors: Initial experience. *AJNR* 1983; 4:1199–1201.
17. Collier BD, Seltzer SE, Kido DK, et al: Ultrasound directed placement of needles into the brains of rhesus monkeys. *Neuroradiology* 1980; 19:201.
18. Babcock DS, Han BK, LeQuesne GW: B-mode gray scale ultrasound of the head in the newborn and the young infant. *AJR* 1980; 134:457–468.
19. Gilsbach J, Hassler W: Intraoperative Doppler and realtime sonography in neurosurgery. *Neurosurg Rev* 1983; 7:199–208.
20. Tiberio G, Giulini SM, Floriani M, et al: Intra-operative control of carotid thromboendoarterectomy by Doppler spectrum analysis. *J Cardiovasc Surg* 1984; 25:361–364.
21. Tsutsumi Y, Andoh U, Inoue N: Ultrasound-guided biopsy for deep-seated brain tumors. *J Neurosurg* 1982; 57:164–167.
22. Knake JE, Chandler WF, Gabrielsen TO: Intraoperative sonography in the nonstereotaxic biopsy and aspiration of subcortical brain lesions. *AJNR* 1983; 4:672–674.
23. Rubin JM, Dohrmann GJ: Intraoperative neurosurgical ultrasound in the localization and char-

acterization of intracranial masses. *Radiology* 1983; 148:519–524.

24. Pasto ME, Rifkin MD: Intraoperative ultrasound examination of the brain: Possible pitfalls in diagnosis and biopsy guidance. *J Ultrasound Med* 1984; 3:245–249.

25. French LA, Wild JJ, Neal D: Detection of cerebral tumors by ultrasonic pulses: Pilot studies on post-mortem material. *Cancer* 1950; 3:705–708.

26. Leksell L: Echoencephalography: 1. Detection of intracranial complications following head injury. *Acta Chir Scand* 1956; 110:301–315.

27. de Vlieger M, Sterke A, de Molin CE, et al: Ultrasound for two-dimensional echoencephalography. *Ultrasonics* 1963; 1:148–151.

28. Fry FJ: Notes: Ultrasonic visualization of human brain structure. *Invest Radiol* 1970; 5(2):117–121.

29. Hoffman RB, Landau B: Ultrasound B-scan imaging of an intracranial lesion through a bone flap defect. *JCU* 1975; 4:125–127.

30. Haber K, Wachter RD, Christenson PC, et al: Ultrasonic evaluation of intracranial pathology in infants. *Radiology* 1980; 134:173–178.

31. London DA, Carroll BA, Enzmann DR: Sonography of ventricular size and germinal matrix hemorrhage in premature infants. *AJR* 1980; 135:559–564.

32. Silverboard G, Horder MH, Ahmann PA, et al: Reliability of ultrasound in diagnosis of intracerebral hemorrhage and posthemorrhagic hydrocephalus: Comparison with computed tomography. *Pediatrics* 1980; 66:507–514.

33. Gooding GAW, Bopggan JE, Bank WO, et al: Sonography of the adult brain through surgical defects. *AJNR* 1981; 2:449–452.

34. Tanaka K, Ito K, Wagai T: The localization of brain tumors by ultrasonic techniques. *J Neurosurg* 1965; 23:135–147.

35. Knake JE, Chandler WF, McGillicuddy JE: Intraoperative sonography for brain tumor localization and ventricular shunt placement. *AJR* 1982; 139:783.

36. Merritt CRB, Coulon R, Connolly E: Intraoperative neurosurgical ultrasound: Transdural and transfontanelle applications. *Radiology* 1983; 148:513–517.

37. Shkolnik A, McLone DG: Intra-operative real-time ultrasonic guidance of intracranial shunt tube placement in infants. *Radiology* 1982; 144:575–576.

38. Shkolnik A, Tomita T, Raimondi AJ, et al: Intraoperative neurosurgical ultrasound: Localization of brain tumors in infants and children. *Radiology* 1983; 148:525.

39. Chandler W, Knake J: Intraoperative use of ultrasound in neurosurgery. *Clin Neurosurg* 1983; 31:550–563.

40. Chandler WF, Knake JE, McGillicuddy JE, et al: Intraoperative use of real-time ultrasonography in neurosurgery. *J Neurosurg* 1982; 57:1547–1563.

41. Gooding GAW, Edwards MSB, Rabkin E, et al: Intraoperative real-time ultrasound in the localization of intracranial neoplasms. *Radiology* 1983; 146:459–462.

42. Grode ML, Komaiko MS: The role of intraoperative ultrasound in neurosurgery. *Neurosurgery* 1983; 12(6):624–628.

43. Rogers JV, Shuman WP, Hirsch JH, et al: Intraoperative neurosonography: Application and technique. *AJNR* 1984; 5:755–760.

44. Knake JE, Chandler WF, Gabrielsen TO, et al: Intraoperative sonographic delineation of low-grade brain neoplasms defined poorly by computed tomography. *Radiology* 1984; 151:735–739.

45. Hutchins WW, Vogelzang RL, Nelman HL: Differentiation of tumor from syringohydromyelia: Intraoperative neurosonography of the spinal cord. *Radiology* 1984; 151:171–174.

46. Montalvo BM, Quencer RM, Green BA, et al: Intraoperative sonography in spinal trauma. *Radiology* 1984; 153:124–134.

47. Knake JE, Gabrielsen TO, Chandler WF, et al: Real-time sonography during spinal surgery. *Radiology* 1984; 151:461–465.

48. Pasto ME, Rifkin MD, Rubenstein JB, et al: Real-time ultrasonography of the spinal cord: Intraoperative and postoperative imaging. *Neuroradiology* 1984; 26:183–187.

49. Thuroff JW, Alken P, Riedmiller H, et al: Doppler and real-time ultrasound in renal stone surgery. *Eur J Urol* 1982; 8:298–303.

50. Sigel B, Coelho JCU, Sharifi R, et al: Ultrasonic scanning during operation for renal calculi. *J Urol* 1982; 127:421–424.

51. Lytton B: Intraoperative ultrasound for nephrolithotomy. *J Urol* 1983; 130:213–217.

52. Rubin JM, Bagley DH, Lyon ES, et al: Intraoperative real time ultrasonic scanning for locating and recovering renal calculi. *J Urol* 1983; 130:434–437.

53. Marshall FF, Smith NA, Murphy JB: A comparison of ultrasonography and radiography in the localization of renal calculi: Experimental and operative experience. *J Urol* 1982; 126:576–580.

54. Lane R, Coupland G: Ultrasonic indications to explore the common bile duct. *Surgery* 1982; 91:268–274.

55. Machi J, Sigel B, Spigos DG, et al: Experimental assessment of imaging variables associated with operative ultrasonic and radiographic cholangiography. *J Ultrasound Med* 1983; 2:535–538.

56. Herbst CA, Mittelstaedt CA, Staab EV, et al: Intraoperative ultrasonography evaluation of the gallbladder in morbidly obese patients. *Ann Surg* 1984; 200(6):691–692.

57. Castaing D, Kunstlinger F, Habib N, et al: Intraoperative ultrasonographic study of the liver. *Am J Surg* 1985; 149:676–682.

58. Nagasue N, Suehiro S, Yakaya H: Intraoperative ultrasonography in the surgical treatment of hepatic tumors. *Acta Chir Scand* 1984; 150:311–316.

59. Igawa S, Kinoshita H, Sakai K: Clinical significance of intraoperative sonography on hepatectomy in primary carcinoma of the liver. *World J Surg* 1984; 8:772–777.

60. Sheu J, Lee C, Sung J, et al: Intraoperative hepatic ultrasonography: An indispensable procedure in resection of small hepatocellular carcinomas. *Surgery* 1985; 97(1):97–103.

61. Rueckert KF, Klotter HJ, Kummerle F: Intraoperative ultrasonic localization of endocrine tumors of the pancreas. *Surgery* 1984; 96(6):1045–1047.

62. Gunther RW, Klose KJ, Ruckert K, et al: Islet-cell tumors: Detection of small lesions with computed tomography and ultrasound. *Radiology* 1983; 148:485–488.

63. Charboneau JW, James EM, Van Heerden JA, et al: Intraoperative real-time ultrasonographic localization of pancreatic insulinoma: Initial experience. *J Ultrasound Med* 1983; 2:251–254.

64. Sigel G, Coelho JCU, Donahue PE, et al: Ultrasonic assistance during surgery for pancreatic inflammatory disease. *Arch Surg* 1982; 117:712–716.

65. Sigel B, Machi J, Ramos JR: The role of imaging ultrasound during pancreatic surgery. *Ann Surg* 1984; 200(4):486–493.

66. Sigel B, Flanigan DP, Schuler JJ, et al: Imaging ultrasound in the intraoperative diagnosis of vascular defects. *J Ultrasound Med* 1983; 2:337–343.

67. Hyodo A, Mizukami M, Tazawa T, et al: Intraoperative use of real time ultrasonography applied to aneurysm surgery. *Neurosurgery* 1983; 13:642–645.

68. Gunby P: Heart surgeons now using ultrasound intraoperatively. *JAMA* 249, No 10, March 1983.

69. Gilsbach JM, Hassier WE: Intraoperative Doppler and real time sonography in neurosurgery. *Neurosurg Rev* 1984; 7:199–208.

70. Tiberio G, Giulini SM, Floriani M, et al: Intraoperative control of carotid thromboendoarterectomy by Doppler spectrum analysis. *J Cardiovasc Surg* 1984; 25:361–364.

71. Nagasue N, Ogawa Y, Hirose S, et al: Intraoperative ultrasonography for detecting the renal vein during a distal splenorenal shunt procedure. *Am J Surg* 1983; 145:773–774.

## CASES

Dennis A. Sarti, M.D.

### Sterile Technique

There are different methods for utilizing sterile technique in the operating room. Figures 11–1 and 11–2 show a custom-made sterile sheath that can be used for intraoperative procedures. The ultrasound transducer is placed in the sterile sheath. Sterile acoustic gel is placed on the end of the ultrasound transducer so that when it is completely extended into the sheath there will be no air bubbles between the transducer and the sheath. Figure 11–2 shows the transducer completely within the sheath. Sterile rubber bands are used near the top of the transducer. The individual working the controls need not be sterile. A different individual can hold the end of the transducer and place the transducer in the operating field. Some units have touch-button controls. With such units, a sterile sheet can be placed over the controls and the individual handling the transducer can then also handle the controls.

If the specialized rubber sheath is not available, an operative sleeve can be used as shown in Figure 11–3. The transducer is placed in the operative sleeve, with the end of the transducer extending slightly out of the sleeve. The end of the transducer is coated with acoustic gel, then covered with a sterile surgical glove. Figure 11–4 shows the nonsterile individual holding the transducer wire as the sterile individual places the surgical glove over the end of the transducer. Figure 11–5 on page 552 shows the final step of placing sterile rubber bands over the transducer.

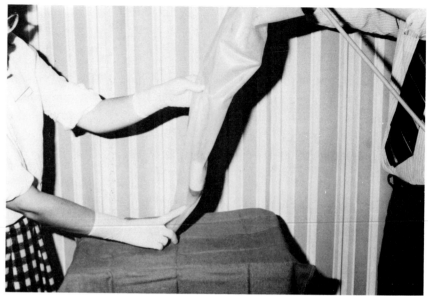

FIG 11–1.

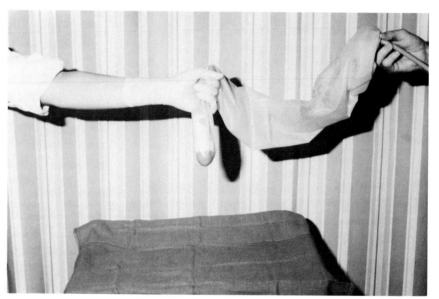

FIG 11–2.

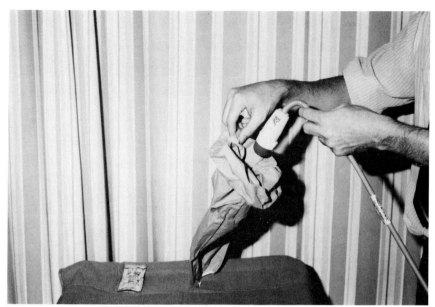

**FIG 11–3.**

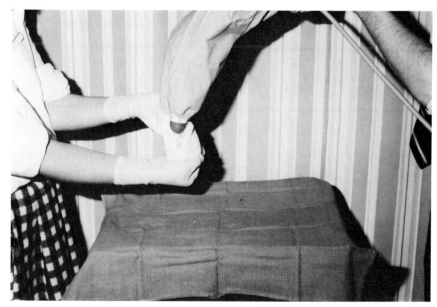

**FIG 11–4.**

## Sterile Technique and Normal Anatomy

Figure 11–5 is the final step in the procedure shown in Figures 11–3 and 11–4. Sterile rubber bands are applied over the sterile surgical glove and transducer head. Acoustic gel must be placed over the transducer face so that no air is present between the surgical glove and the transducer head.

Figure 11–6 illustrates another sterile technique. The transducer is placed on an exposed brain. Very often only a small window of exposed tissue is identified. It is usually quite difficult to get anatomically oriented. The various normal anatomic structures must be identified on preliminary scans before pathology can be definitely visualized.

Figures 11–7 and 11–8 are high transverse scans made through a parietal bone flap. Very often it is necessary to spend several minutes getting oriented. Attempts to visualize normal anatomic landmarks are quite helpful. Figure 11–7 demonstrates the frontal horns of the lateral ventricles (V). The septum pellucidum (S) is visualized between the two ventricles. Figure 11–8 is a transverse scan through the same bone flap made with a slightly more caudal orientation. The lateral ventricles appear smaller as we are over their inferior aspect. The highly echogenic posterior structure is the choroid plexus (C). Posterior to the choroid plexus are the fluid-filled occipital horns (O).

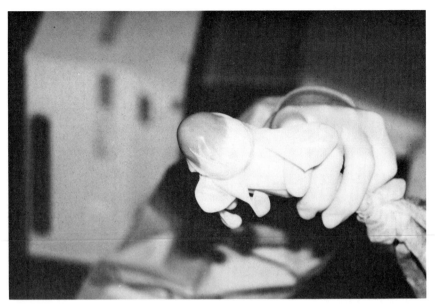

FIG 11–5.

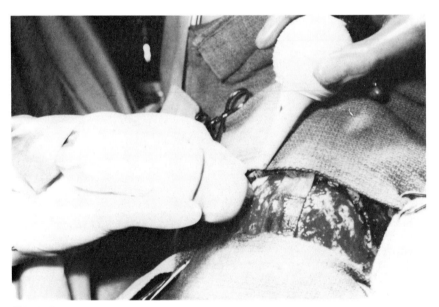

FIG 11–6.

C  =  Choroid plexus
O  =  Occipital horns
S  =  Septum pellucidum
V  =  Frontal horns of the lateral ventricles

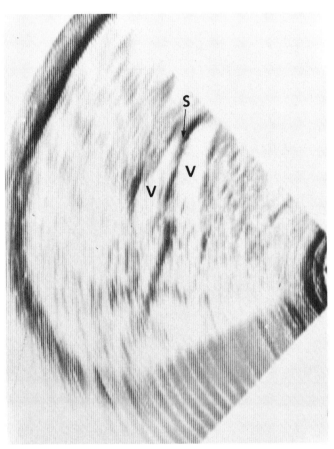

**FIG 11–7.**

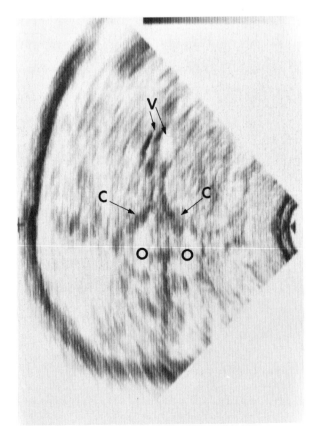

**FIG 11–8.**

## Normal Anatomy

Figures 11–9 through 11–12 are scans that continue illustrating the normal anatomy from Figures 11–7 and 11–8. The images are obtained through a parietal bone flap and are oriented cephalad to caudad from Figure 11–9 through Figure 11–12.

In Figure 11–9 the thalami are situated lateral to the third ventricle, which appears as a linear echo. The continuation of the posterior linear echo represents the posterior falx cerebri. Figure 11–10 is a scan made slightly more caudad, at the level of the midbrain. The circular echogenic region is the aqueduct. The choroid plexus is highly echogenic (C). This represents the region of the trigone. The linear posterior echo is the falx cerebri.

Figure 11–11 is slightly caudad scan made at the level of the belly of the pons. The aqueduct (A) is still visualized. An echogenic region is seen posterior to the aqueduct. The borders of this echogenic region are made up of the tentorium. The central portion of the echogenic region is secondary to the vermis of the cerebellum. A choroid plexus (C) is seen on this scan. The linear posterior echo is the posterior falx cerebri. The scan in Figure 11–12 represents a slightly more caudad view compared to Figure 11–11. The small lucent area represents the fourth ventricle (4). The vermis and tentorium are again seen, along with the posterior falx cerebri.

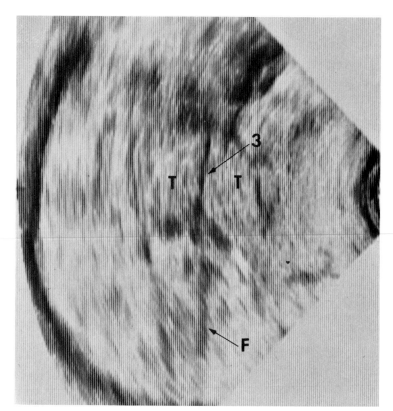

**FIG 11–9.**

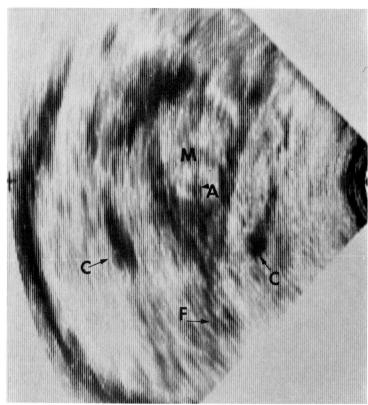

**FIG 11–10.**

A  =  Aqueduct
C  =  Choroid plexus
F  =  Posterior falx cerebri
M  =  Midbrain
P  =  Pons
T  =  Thalami (Fig 11–9)
T  =  Tentorium (Figs 11–11 and 11–12)
V  =  Vermis
3  =  Third ventricle
4  =  Fourth ventricle

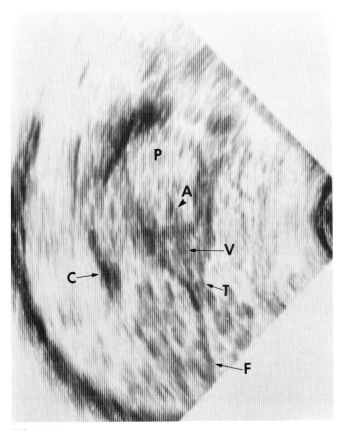

FIG 11–11.

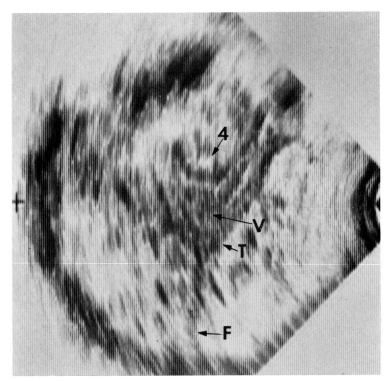

FIG 11–12.

## Biopsy Technique

Biopsy can be performed either free-hand or with transducer guides. Figure 11–13 shows transducer to which transducer guides are attached. The interrupted straight lines on the right side represent a fixed angle through which a needle can be passed. The needle will then be visualized on the image. This device can be used when the area of interest falls directly in the path of the lines noted on the television monitor. The dotted lines on the left side represent a variable angle through which the needle can be passed. As the area of interest is visualized, the angle can be adjusted appropriately. Different-sized holes are available to accommodate 18-, 20-, and 22-gauge needles. Even larger needles may be inserted in the left side through the variable angle.

Figures 11–14 and 11–15 are scans of an intraoperative biopsy performed using a transducer guide. Figure 11–14 is a scan made through a bur hole posteriorly. A cystic mass (M) is noted in the cerebellum (CB). The location and depth of the mass are indicated by the cursor in the midportion of the mass. In Figure 11–15 the needle passes through a biopsy angle guide. The needle (arrows) is visualized through the cerebellum and into the cystic mass. Reverberations are identified within the cystic mass, confirming the location of the needle tip.

Figure 11–16 illustrates the free-hand biopsy technique. This technique requires visualization of the area of interest and an approximation of the most appropriate angle. Once the best angle is determined, the needle is passed free-hand while the area of interest is visualized on ultrasound. Figure 11–16 illustrates biopsy of an area of edema in the frontal lobe. After the needle is removed, the echogenic needle tract (arrowheads) is visualized. This can determine the location of the biopsy.

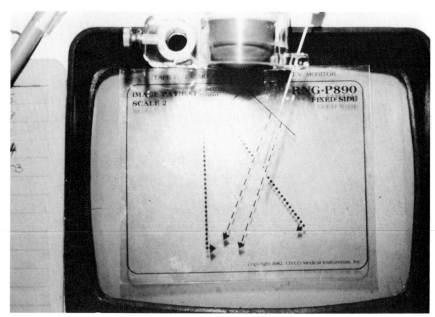

**FIG 11–13.**

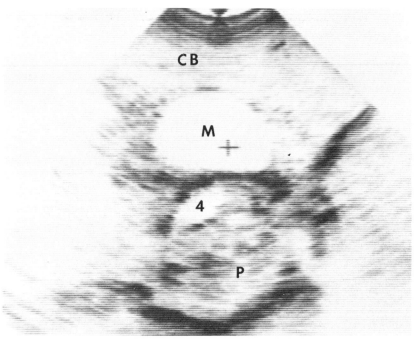

**FIG 11–14.**

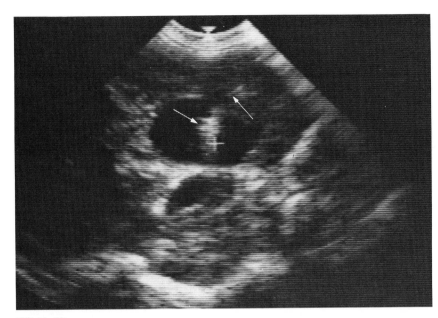

| **Arrows** | = | Biopsy needle |
| **Arrowheads** | = | Echogenic needle tract |
| **CB** | = | Cerebellum |
| **FC** | = | Falx cerebri |
| **M** | = | Cystic mass |
| **P** | = | Pons |
| **4** | = | Fourth ventricle |

**FIG 11–15.**

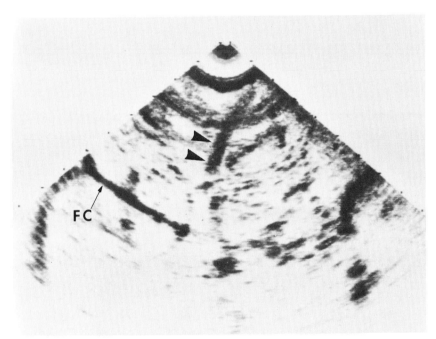

**FIG 11–16.**

## Reverberation Artifacts

Reverberation artifacts arise from the interface of the transducer with the brain substance. Often the reverberation artifacts may obstruct visualization of lesions that are close to the surface. If the lesions are situated deeper, they are usually more readily visible. It is also important to verify in two planes that a lesion is present.

Figure 11–17 is a coronal oblique scan obtained with a 5-MHz transducer through a parietal craniotomy. Reverberation artifacts (arrowheads) are noted close to the surface. There is an echogenic mass (M) present near the surface. This mass was very difficult to visualize initially. The reverberation artifacts (arrowheads) were a major problem in visualizing the area. Numerous scans were obtained before the image in Figure 11–17 was visualized.

Figure 11–18 shows an echogenic lesion situated slightly deeper in the brain substance. In this instance the reverberation artifacts (arrowheads) are not obstructing visualization of the echogenic mass (M). The mass is situated deep enough to be readily visible. Most brain tumors are echogenic.

Figure 11–19 is a CT scan showing a mass in the right frontal lobe. This mass has some associated edema, along with an echogenic region and a central low-density area. This was thought to be a necrotic tumor. Ultrasound revealed the lesion to be an echogenic mass with a lucent central area (Fig 11–20). Reverberation artifacts are noted superficially but are not interfering with visualization of the mass. The mass was localized on ultrasound and several biopsies were performed. No tumor tissue was identified. The mass was thought to be an old arteriovenous malformation in which there was a central hematoma.

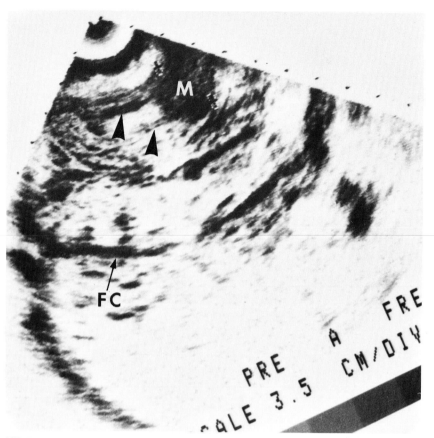

FIG 11–17.

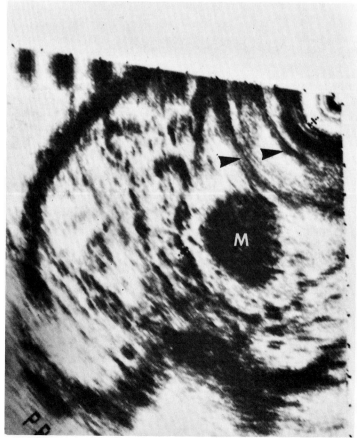

FIG 11–18.

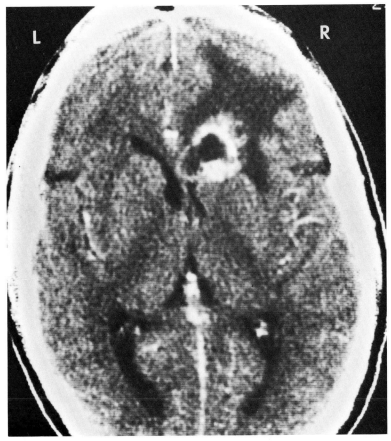

**FIG 11–19.**

| Arrowheads | = Reverberation artifact |
| --- | --- |
| **Fc** | = Falx cerebri |
| **L** | = Left |
| **M** | = Echogenic mass |
| **R** | = Right |

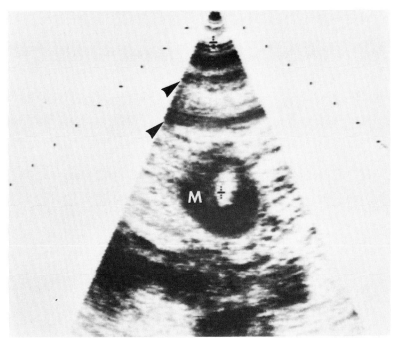

**FIG 11–20.**

## Astrocytoma

The case in Figures 11–21 through 11–24 is an example of a grade II astrocytoma. Figure 11–21 is an MR T1-weighted image (TE = 28 msec; TR = 500 msec). A low-intensity region is seen in the high parietal area on the left, indicating edema. Figure 11–22 is a transverse T2-weighted MR image (TE = 84 msec; TR = 1,984 msec). There is a large area of high intensity noted in the left parietal region. The CT scan in Figure 11–23 shows a vague area of low density (arrowheads) in the high parietal region. This area was seen only retrospectively.

Ultrasound was performed in the operating room. Nothing was seen with 3- and 5-MHz transducers. Only when a 7.5-MHz transducer was used did the echogenic mass (arrowheads) come into view. This echogenic mass was much smaller than the area noted on the MR images. The scans in Figure 11–21 and 11–22 show the area of edema. The echogenic mass itself was much smaller on the ultrasound scan. Adjacent to the mass was an echogenic sulcus (S). When this sulcus was scanned in a tangential plane, it initially appeared to be echogenic. However, by scanning at 90° it was confirmed to be a sulcus. The echogenic mass came into view adjacent to the sulcus and was visualized in two planes.

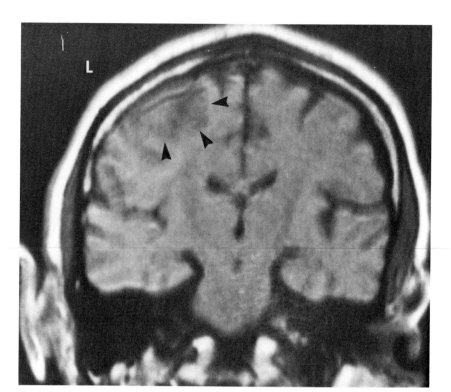

**FIG 11–21.**

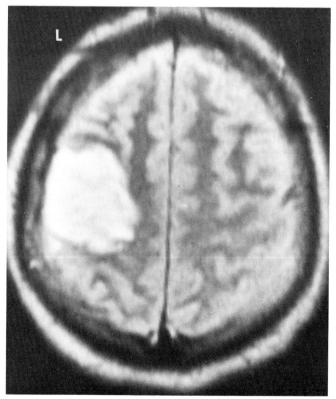

**FIG 11–22.**

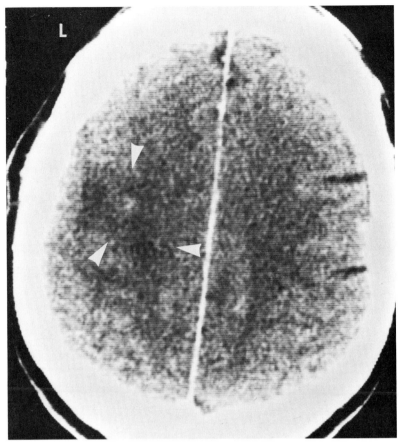

Arrowheads  = Grade II astrocystoma
L           = Left
S           = Sulcus

**FIG 11–23.**

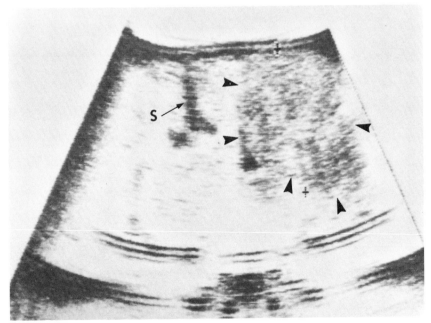

**FIG 11–24.**

## Astrocytoma

The patient had a grade II astrocytoma in the hypothalamic region. This was confirmed by needle biopsy. The patient received 5,000 rads to the area. The hypothalamic lesion became cystic after radiation therapy. Figure 11–25 is a scan through a frontal craniotomy. The anterior horns of both ventricles (V) are dilated. The echogenic posterior region is secondary to the choroid plexus. Figure 11–26 is a coronal scan through the right frontal craniotomy. A cystic mass (M) is noted in the midline slightly deep to the ventricles. The cystic mass was obstructing the foramen of Monro and causing dilatation of both lateral ventricles.

Using the free-hand technique, a catheter (arrowheads) was directed into the cystic mass (Fig 11–27). The catheter was passed through the frontal horn of the right lateral ventricle. The tip of the catheter was placed in the cystic tumor. Figure 11–28 is a scan made after the cystic mass had been decompressed and drained. The catheter was left in place for drainage.

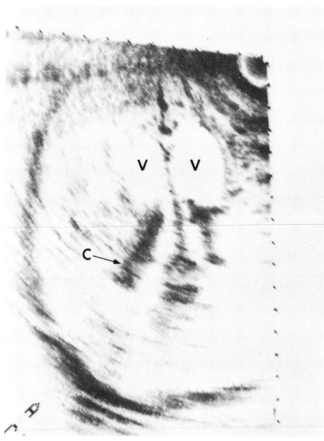

**FIG 11–25.**

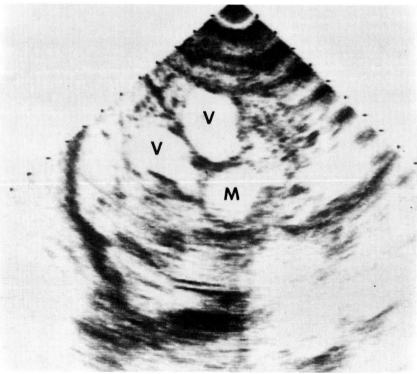

**FIG 11–26.**

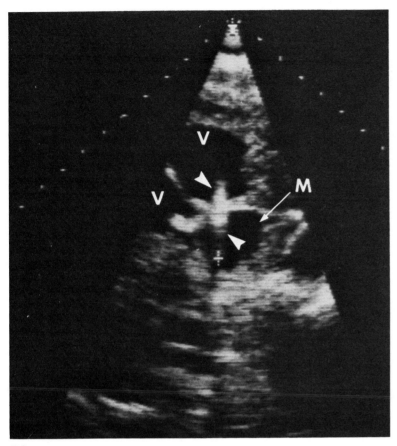

Arrowheads = Drainage catheter
C = Choroid plexus
M = Cystic astrocytoma
V = Dilated frontal horns

**FIG 11–27.**

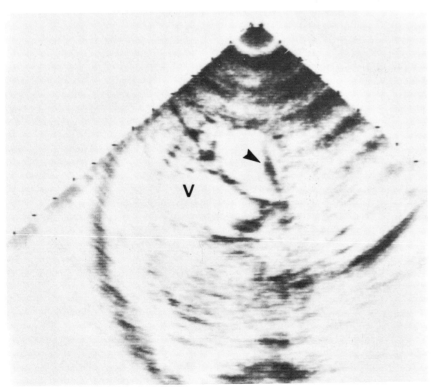

**FIG 11–28.**

## Shunt Placement

Figure 11–29 is a CT scan of an 8-month-old infant in whom hydrocephalus developed secondary to previous intraventricular hemorrhage. The right occipital horn was noted to be dilated. The left occipital horn (arrow) is decompressed, but there is dilatation of the left temporal horn.

Figure 11–30 is a coronal scan through the anterior fontanelle. The right lateral ventricle is dramatically enlarged compared to the left lateral ventricle (arrow). Both temporal horns (T) are dilated. The findings confirm the CT findings scan in Figure 11–29. A catheter was passed through a left temporal burr hole in Figure 11–31. The left temporal horn was visualized through the anterior fontanelle. The catheter was visualized in the left temporal horn (arrowheads). The catheter was slightly cephalad in position, and the left temporal horn did not drain. A second pass was attempted (Fig 11–32). The catheter (arrowheads) is now correctly positioned, and decompression of the left temporal horn occurred. A follow-up CT scan (Fig 11–33) shows decompression of the left temporal horn and a decrease in the size of the right lateral ventricle. This was because a separate shunt was placed in the right side. It is not visualized on the CT scan shown in Figure 11–33.

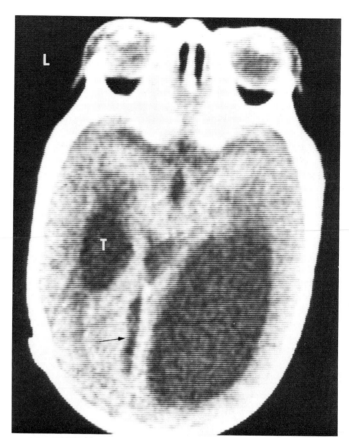

FIG 11–29.

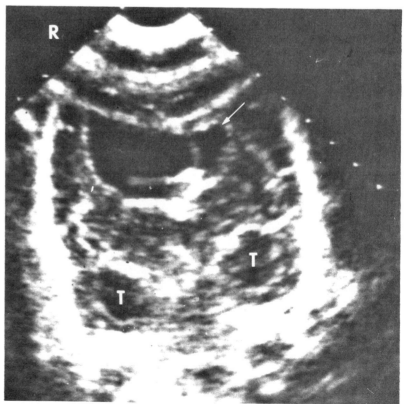

FIG 11–30.

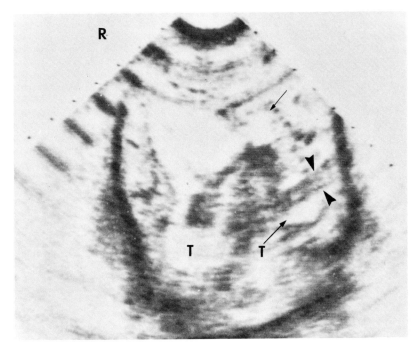

| **Arrow** | = Left anterior horn |
| **Arrowheads** | = Decompression shunt |
| **L** | = Left |
| **R** | = Right |
| **T** | = Temporal horn |

**FIG 11–31.**

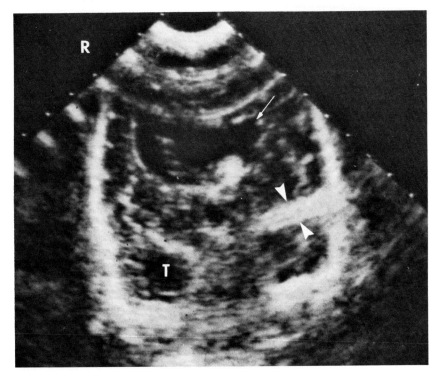

**FIG 11–32.**

## Ventricular Shunts

Figure 11–33 is a continuation of the case illustrated in Figures 11–29 through 11–32. This scan shows decompression of both ventricles bilaterally.

Figures 11–34 through 11–36 demonstrate intraoperative real time ultrasonic visualization of ventricular shunts. Figure 11–34 is a coronal scan of a 19-day-old infant with bilateral hydrocephalus. Shunts are seen in both ventricles (white arrows). The right ventricular shunt is noted to decompress the right ventricle. This shunt is well positioned, as is noted in Figure 11–36. Figure 11–36 shows the shunt situated in the frontal horn of the right ventricle. Figure 11–35 is a sagittal scan showing the left shunt situated in the anterior aspect of the temporal horn. The left ventricle remains dilated. The anterior extent of the choroid plexus (black arrow) is echogenic and does not represent the tip of the shunt.

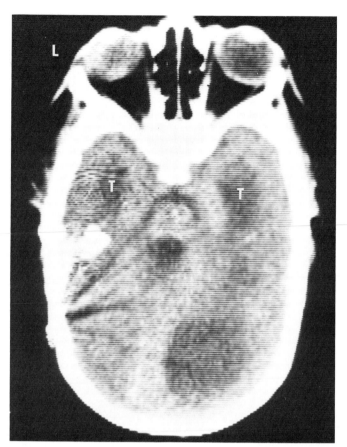

FIG 11–33.

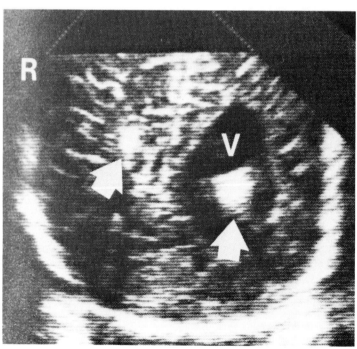

FIG 11–34.

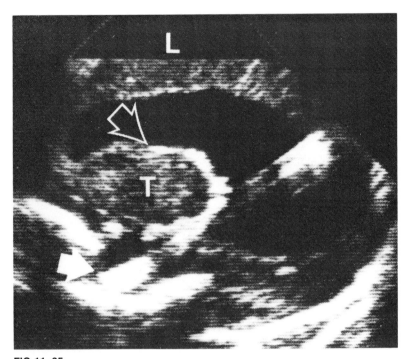

**FIG 11–35.**

SOURCE: Figures 11–34 through 11–36 are from Shkolnik A, McLone DJ: Intraoperative real time ultrasonic guidance of ventricular shunt placement in infants. *Radiology* 1981; 141:515. Reproduced by permission.

| White arrow | = | Ventricular shunt |
|---|---|---|
| **Black arrow** | = | Choroid plexus |
| L | = | Left |
| R | = | Right |
| T | = | Temporal horn (Fig 11–33) |
| T | = | Thalamus (Fig 11–35) |
| V | = | Dilated ventricle |

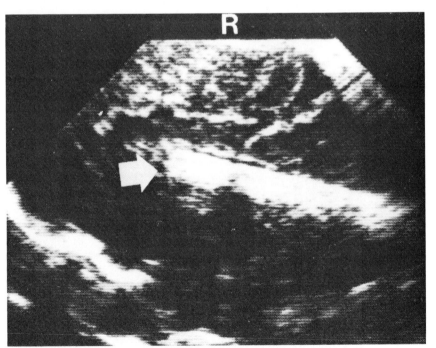

**FIG 11–36.**

## Intraoperative Spinal Sonography

Figure 11–37 is an anatomic drawing of intraoperative spinal sonography. After surgical removal of the posterior elements, a sterile liquid solution is placed in the surgical defect. With sterile technique, a 7.5- or 10-MHz transducer is placed in the solution and the spinal canal is examined.

Figure 11–38 is a scan of a patient who sustained a gunshot wound to T-4. At surgery, the thoracic spine was examined with ultrasound. The cord was noted to be atrophic with a large dorsal subarachnoid space (sas). The highly reflective cord surface (arrows) is difficult to distinguish from the substance of the cord. The findings are consistent with myelomalacia. A 1-cm intramedullary cyst (c) is noted within the cord.

Figure 11–39 is an intraoperative scan of a patient with old T-4 fracture. The scan shows two intramedullary cysts. The cephalad cyst (black arrow) appears unilocular. The caudal cyst (black and white arrows) appears to be multiloculated. Angulation of the bone (B) is noted between the two cystic regions.

Figure 11–40 is an intraoperative spinal scan of a patient who had a bullet fragment in the thoracic spine. The bullet fragment (B) is noted within the cord. Dural adhesions (between black arrows) are identified adjacent to the bullet fragment. There is increased echogenicity of the cord, compatible with myelomalacia. The spinal cord is atrophic (curved arrow) cephalad to the bullet fragment.

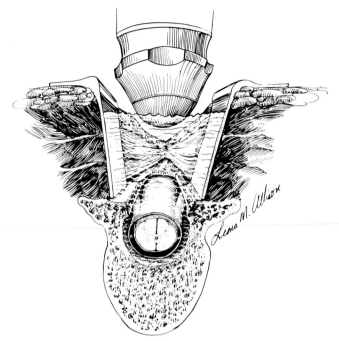

**FIG 11–37.**

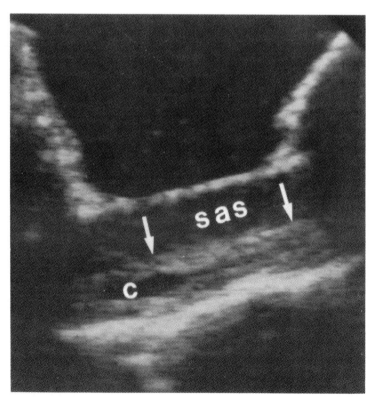

**FIG 11–38.**

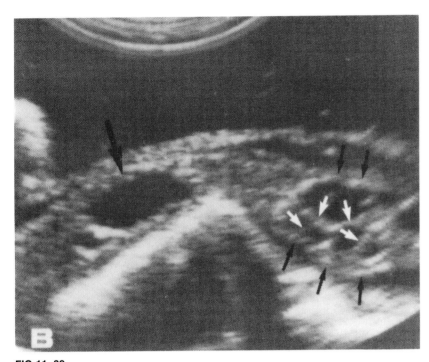

**FIG 11–39.**

Source: Figures 11–37 through 11–40 are from Montalvo BM, Quencer RM, Green BA, et al: Intraoperative sonography in spinal trauma. *Radiology* 1984; 153:125. Reproduced by permission.

| | | |
|---|---|---|
| **White arrow** | = | Spinal cord (Fig 11–38) |
| **Black arrow** | = | Unilocular cyst (Fig 11–39) |
| **White arrows** | = | Multiloculated cyst (Fig 11–39) |
| **Black arrows** | = | Dural adhesions (Fig 11–40) |
| **Curved arrow** | = | Atrophic cord (Fig 11–40) |
| **B** | = | Bony spinal elements (Fig 11–39) |
| **B** | = | Bullet fragment (Fig 11–40) |
| **c** | = | Intramedullary cyst |
| **sas** | = | Subarachnoid space |

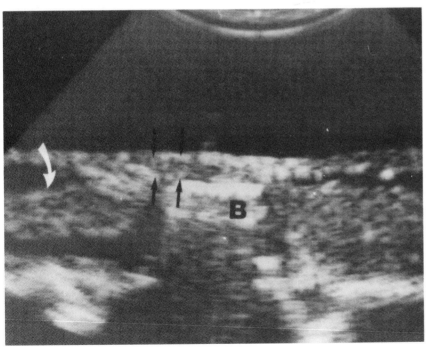

**FIG 11–40.**

# 12.
# Ultrasonography of the Scrotum

Barbara Carroll, M.D.

## Scanning Techniques

Ultrasound offers a rapid, noninvasive means for evaluating the scrotal contents. It readily distinguishes testicular from extratesticular pathology, a distinction which can be particularly difficult when a coexisting hydrocele obscures testicular palpation. This distinction is particularly important as most testicular masses are malignant, while most extratesticular masses are not. Early scrotal ultrasound examinations were contact scans performed using static, articulated-arm B-scanners and high-frequency transducers. The testes were cradled in a gloved hand or rested on a folded towel while contact scanning was performed. Testicular scans may also be performed with the testes immersed in a water or saline bath. Most scrotal ultrasound examinations are now performed using high-frequency real-time equipment and contact scanning. Such technique allows optimal anatomic positioning of the scrotal contents and real-time correlation of a palpable mass with an abnormality seen on the ultrasound image.[1] Indications for scrotal sonography include the evaluation of palpable scrotal masses, scrotal trauma, acute onset of scrotal pain, suspected occult testicular neoplasms, follow-up of patients with previous scrotal infections, evaluation of patients with a prior history of testicular neoplasms, leukemia, or lymphoma, evaluation of patients with undescended testes, evaluation of patients with chronic infertility syndromes, and evaluation of patients with metastatic germ cell tumors of unknown origin.[1-3]

## Scrotal Anatomy

The normal testis measures $3\frac{1}{2} \times 3$ cm and has uniform medium level echogenicity. Testicular asymmetry is normal. The normal testis contains 250 to 400 subdivisions, the lobulae testis, produced by fibrous septa extending from the mediastinum testis to the tunica albuginea. The mediastinum testis contains the testicular vessels. In this region the tunica albuginea invaginates into the testicular parenchyma, producing an echogenic linear structure that may be associated with refractory shadowing. Occasionally the echogenic septa of the testis will be visible as linear echogenicities within the testicular parenchyma. Other focal, nonlinear areas of increased echogenicity not associated with the mediastinum testis may be seen.

These focal echogenicities may produce posterior acoustic shadowing. Although their precise nature is not known, they are thought to represent either spermatic granulomas or phleboliths.

The normal epididymis is usually 7–8 mm thick and lies posterolateral to the testis. Its echogenicity is similar to that of the testes, although the parenchymal texture is somewhat coarser. The head, or globus major, lies adjacent to the superior pole of the testes and constitutes the joining of 10 to 15 efferent ducts from the rete testes into a single duct, the ductus epididymis. The body and tail of the epididymis course lateral and progressively inferior to the testes, where the tail of the epididymis or globus minor is invested with a muscular coat and ascends medially as the ductus deferens.

The testis is invested by several tissue layers referred to as the scrotum. The skin and tunica dartos form the outer scrotal layer. As the testes descend, they are invested with layers of tissue which correspond to the various layers of the abdominal wall musculature. The tunica vaginalis, derived from the peritoneum, accompanies the testis as the processus vaginalis in its descent into the scrotum and applies the testis to the posterior wall of the scrotum, forming an envelope around the organ. The tunica vaginalis represents two apposed layers of tissue, a visceral and a parietal layer, between which a potential space exists. This potential space may contain herniations and fluid accumulations in the form of hydroceles or hematoceles. The tunica albuginea is an echogenic fibrous covering that directly envelopes the surface of the testes. These individual layers are usually not visualized unless a hydrocele is present. Pathologic thickening and calcified plaques of the tunica can be seen in the presence of such fluid collections.

The spermatic cord contains testicular and deferential arteries and the pampiniform plexus of veins. It lies lateral to the testes and can be traced exiting the scrotum into the inguinal canal. Real-time scanning with Doppler techniques can demonstrate venous and arterial flow in the spermatic cord. The appendix testis and appendix epididymis can also be visualized lying between the epididymis and the superior pole of the testes when a hydrocele or adjacent fluid collection is present. It is not uncommon to see 1–2 mm of fluid within the potential space created by the tunica vaginalis. However, more than 2 mm of fluid is consistent with the diagnosis of a hydrocele.

## Testicular Masses

Separation of intratesticular and extratesticular pathology is the most valuable diagnostic clue provided by scrotal sonography. Improved resolution of real-time equipment, as well as enhanced diagnostic skills, allow this distinction to be made with an accuracy approaching 90%–95%. This distinction is particularly important since the overwhelming majority of intratesticular lesions will be malignant tumors. In fact, all intratesticular lesions should be considered potentially malignant until proved otherwise. On the other hand, most extratesticular lesions will be inflammatory, traumatic, or represent benign neoplasms. Ninety-five percent of primary testicular neoplasms are of germ cell origin. Seminomas, teratocarcinomas, and embryonal cell carcinomas comprise the majority of these. Although most tumors are unilateral, in 8% or more of patients a contralateral neoplasm may develop. These tumors account for less than 1% of all male malignancies and are most common in the 25–35-year-old age range. Testicular malignancies usually present as painless, testicular enlargement. From 4% to 14% of patients present with symptoms related to metastatic disease. Testicular neoplasms are usually focal, single, hypoechoic masses, but diffuse lesions can infiltrate the entire gland. Although most echogenic testicular masses will prove to be benign, secondary to infarctions or infectious processes, rarely echogenic or complex testicular neoplasms can occur.[1, 4–6] In appearance testicular neoplasms are indistinguishable from such processes as abscesses, infarctions, or hemorrhage. While homogeneous, echogenic testicular masses are usually benign and related to scar tissue or fibrosis, metastatic lesions and "burned-out" testicular tumors may present as focal echogenic scars. Thus, all intratesticular lesions must be considered potentially malignant until proved otherwise.

Seminomas account for 40%–50% of malignant testicular tumors and are more common in older patients (ages 30–40). These tumors are less aggressive than other germ cell tumors and are extremely radiosensitive. They are also the most common testicular tumor found in undescended testes. Sonographically, these tumors are usually homogeneously hypoechoic, as one would expect from their uniform histologic content with a paucity of necrosis or hemorrhage. Nonseminomatous elements can occur in seminomas. In these instances, the sonogram frequently shows a hypoechoic lesion that may contain scattered areas of increased echogenicity. Occasionally, seminomas may replace most of the testis, and the pseudocapsule which often appears to envelop these lesions may be difficult to visualize.

Embryonal cell carcinoma accounts for 20%–25% of germ cell tumors. It is a very aggressive tumor that frequently invades the tunica albuginea and distorts the testicular contour. Such tumors often contain areas of hemorrhagic necrosis or cystic change. The sonographic features reflect these changes, and the tumors frequently present as less well circumscribed, hypoechoic masses that are more inhomogeneous than seminomas. Teratocarcinomas are characteristically complex masses and may contain sonolucent and echogenic components reflecting their heterogeneous composition. Choriocarcinomas are rare germ cell tumors that frequently present with metastatic disease. These tumors usually contain areas of hemorrhage, necrosis, or calcification; not surprisingly, their sonographic appearance is that of a complex mass with cystic and calcific regions. While 60% of testicular neoplasms are made up of a single histologic type, 40% are of mixed histology. The mixed cell tumors are frequently aggressive and their sonographic appearance is that of an inhomogeneous mass.

Approximately 14% of patients with testicular neoplasms will present with signs or symptoms related to metastatic disease. In many the testes are normal on palpation. High-frequency ultrasound can detect these nonpalpable primary lesions, which may be as small as 3 or 4 mm in size.[8] Location of a primary tumor within the testes may facilitate appropriate surgical and medical management.

Testicular metastases are more common than germ cell tumors in patients over 50 years of age. These are often multiple bilateral lesions which are indistinguishable in appearance from primary testicular tumors. Such metastases commonly arise from the genitourinary tract, although metastases from other areas such as the lung, pancreas, or bowel have been observed. Lymphoma and leukemia can also involve the testes either as focal masses or as diffuse infiltrates. Lymphomatous involvement is more common with non-Hodgkin's lymphomas. Testicular leukemia may be the first manifestation of tumor relapse and often occurs in the presence of an otherwise normal hematologic profile. The testes appear to act as a "sanctuary organ" which may harbor leukemic or lympho-matous cells due to an apparent gonadal barrier which limits the concentration of chemotherapeutic agents. The sonographic manifestation of such leukemic or lymphomatous masses includes focal hypoechoic lesions or diffuse hypoechoic enlargement of the testes.[9]

Benign testicular lesions are much less common than malignant disease and in appearance are indistinguishable from malignant neoplasms. Testicular abscesses are usually a complication of epididymoorchitis, often occurring in a diabetic patient. Sonographically, abscesses are hypoechoic or complex masses that may rupture into the tunica vaginalis and lead to pyocele formation. Testicular infarcts can result from trauma, infections, torsion, or vascular lesions. These infarcts may present as focal hypoechoic masses or as diffusely hypoechoic, small testes. Occasionally echogenic areas representing focal fibrosis may occur following testicular infarction.[10] Other causes of benign testicular masses include Leydig cell tumors, testicular lipomas, Sertoli cell tumors, sarcoid, adrenal rests, and biopsy defects. Occasionally cysts of the tunica albuginea will indent the testes, mimicking an intratesticular lesion. These are classic cysts in direct continuity with the tunica albuginea. Their appearance suggests a benign lesion.

## The Acute Scrotum

The two major causes of an acutely painful and swollen scrotum are torsion of the testes and acute epididymitis. Differentiation between these two entities is important. There is a 60%–90% salvage rate for torsed testes if intervention occurs within 24 hours of the onset of pain, but less than a 20% salvage rate if intervention occurs later. The combined use of high-resolution sonography, Doppler ultrasound, and radionuclide scanning frequently allows the clinician to make this distinction in a reliable fashion.

Testicular torsion results from torsion of the spermatic cord as the result of abnormal testicular development. In such cases the testis is not applied to the posterior wall of the scrotum by the tunica vaginalis, but rather is suspended within the processes vaginalis as the clapper is suspended within the bell.[11] Sonographic changes occur early after testicular torsion. Hricak et al. performed serial sonography of testes in dogs after torsion.[12] Testicular and epididymal enlargement with decreased echogenicity, loss of spermatic cord Doppler findings, scrotal thickening, and the appearance of hydroceles were seen 1 hour after the onset of torsion. The sonographic findings in dogs are similar to those reported in humans by Bird et al.[11] Doppler ultrasound is able to detect flow in spermatic cord vessels. Flow may persist in a decreased fashion following testicular torsion, making the value of Doppler ultrasound greatest when combined with high-frequency imaging. Radionuclide examinations provide additional diagnostic information in this clinical setting. In cases of torsion, decreased radionuclide perfusion is seen on the affected side, and there is a "cold area" in the region of the nonperfused testis. These findings are quite different from those seen in epididymitis, in which increased perfusion is present on the affected side. Performing an initial ultrasound study allows one to accurately evaluate the scrotum for the presence or absence of extratesticular and intratesticular masses, which facilitates a more accurate radionuclide diagnosis.

Sonographic changes seen in epididymitis include an enlarged, hypoechoic epididymis associated with an otherwise normal testis. As many as 20% of patients with epididymitis may show focal hypoechoic areas of testicular orchitis or testicular enlargement. Such patients should be followed up with ultrasound to observe for the subsequent development of abscess. Chronic epididymitis may result in an enlarged, echogenic epididymis.

Testicular trauma with resultant rupture of the testes can be corrected in up to 90% of cases if surgery is performed within 72 hours after the trauma. Sonography provides valuable diagnostic information by detecting such abnormalities associated with testicular rupture as focal areas of increased and decreased echogenicity, inhomogeneity of the entire testes, failure to identify normal testicular anatomy, and, infrequently, visualization of the testicular fracture plane.[13, 14] Testicular rupture after trauma may occur without an accompanying hematocele. When hematoceles are present they frequently have a characteristic appearance which includes septations and dependent debris within the fluid collection.[15]

## The Undescended Testes

Approximately 3%–4% of mature infant males have undescended testes. Testicular descent may stop at any point along the path from the retroperitoneum to the scrotum. However, 80% of undescended testes lie in the region of the inguinal canal.[16] The undescended testis is often oval or elongated and is smaller than the normally positioned gland, but of similar echogenicity.

Cryptochordism may be bilateral in 10% of cases. Localization of the undescended testis is important for two reasons: first, if the testis is surgically moved into the scrotum by age 6, normal maturation and relatively normal fertility will result; second, because undescended testes are almost 50 times more likely than descended testes to harbor testicular malignancies, particularly seminomas, it is important to position the gland where it may be readily palpated. Sonography accurately locates undescended testes and should be the initial examination performed since patient exposure to ionizing radiation and sedation are unnecessary. If ultrasound fails to locate the undescended testis, a computed tomographic examination will be necessary.

## Extratesticular Lesions

The potential space created by the two layers of the tunica vaginalis may be filled with accumulations of serous fluid, blood, infectious debris, or urine. Such collections are confined to the anterolateral portions of the scrotum because the tunica applies the testes to the posterior scrotum, preventing fluid accumulations in this region. The most common fluid collections are hydroceles, which are most often idiopathic. These are usually anechoic fluid collections that provide an ideal acoustic window for evaluating the testis suspected of harboring a mass. Approximately 10% of testicular neoplasms have an associated hydrocele. Other causes of hydroceles include trauma, infection, infarction, and torsion. Hematoceles and pyoceles are less common. Hematoceles occur after trauma, surgery, atherosclerotic disease, or neoplasms. Pyoceles follow rupture of an abscess into a coexisting hydrocele or directly into the space between the two layers of the tunica vaginalis. Hematoceles often contain septations and loculations with dependent debris. While pyoceles and hematoceles may have a similar ultrasound appearance, the clinical situation should enable the examiner to distinguish between these conditions.

Varicoceles are dilated veins of the pampiniform plexus and usually lie posterolateral to the testis. They are present in up to 15% of adult men and have been implicated as a cause of infertility.[17, 18] Varicoceles are more common on the left side and normally decompress when the patient is recumbent and distend when the patient is upright or performs a Valsalva maneuver. Varices that do not behave in this manner often are the result of retroperitoneal tumors or venous thrombosis.[1] Normal veins in the pampiniform plexus are no greater than 2 mm in caliber, while varicoceles may distend to 5 or 6 mm in diameter. Visible particulate flow can be seen in these distended veins on high-frequency real-time ultrasound imaging; in addition, duplex ultrasound with Doppler capability can detect venous flow. Varices can be traced as they exit into the inguinal canal, whereas spermatoceles usually are located within the scrotal sac in the region of the head of the epididymis. Such findings readily distinguish varices from spermatoceles.

Spermatoceles are most common in the region of the globus major and arise in the rete testis. Spermatoceles are cysts filled with fluid containing spermatozoa, lymphocytes, fat globules, and cellular debris. They range in size from a few millimeters to centimeters and occasionally are septated. Epididymal cysts are much less common than spermatoceles and may occur anywhere along the course of the epididymis. Like spermatoceles, epididymal cysts are cystic masses that may contain septations. Occasionally, epididymal cysts or spermatoceles become large enough to indent the testes and mimic intratesticular lesions.

Extratesticular neoplasms are rare. The most common is the adenomatoid tumor, which usually arises in the region of the globus minor of the epididymis. Such tumors may be echogenic or hypoechoic solid masses. Their appearance is indistinguishable from that of leiomyomas, fibromas, adrenal rests, and lipomas of the spermatic cord. Spermatic granulomas may arise either within the testes or in the extratesticular space. When extratesticular, these granulomas may mimic intratesticular lesions. Spermatic granulomas are usually hypoechoic solid masses. Sarcoidosis may produce focal epididymal enlargement and hypoechoic masses that may be difficult to distinguish from primary testicular lesions.[19] Chronic epididymitis may also produce persistent epididymal enlargement with focal areas of nodularity. Thus a variety of inflammatory and granulomatous processes and benign tumors account for the majority of extratesticular masses. Malignant tumors in this area are rare and include such entities as metastatic disease and sarcomas.

Scrotal hernias are usually clinically obvious; however, the diagnosis may occasionally be in question. Ultrasound scanning of the scrotum and inguinal canal facilitates the diagnosis by allowing identification of bowel or omentum in these areas. The characteristic sonographic appearance of valvulae conniventes or haustra, or the detection of peristalsis in herniated bowel loops, readily facilitates the ultrasound diagnosis of inguinal hernias, which may often be associated with hydroceles.[20]

High-frequency real-time ultrasound allows rapid, noninvasive imaging of the scrotum. It accurately localizes scrotal masses, detects lesions that are not readily palpable, and is a quick, noninvasive method for evaluating inflammatory, neoplastic, and traumatic scrotal pathology.

## References

1. Carroll BA, Gross DM: High-frequency scrotal sonography. *AJR* 1983; 140:511–515.
2. Arger PH, Mulhern CB, Coleman BG, et al: Prospective analysis of the value of scrotal ultrasound. *Radiology* 1981; 141:763–766.
3. Leopold GR, Woo VL, Scheible FW, et al: High-resolution ultrasonography of scrotal pathology. *Radiology* 1979; 131:719–722.
4. Blei L, Sihelnik S, Bloom D, et al: Ultrasonographic analysis of chronic intratesticular pathology. *J Ultrasound Med* 1983; 2:17–23.
5. Vick CW, Bird KI, Rosenfield AT, et al: Scrotal masses with a uniformly hypoechoic pattern. *Radiology* 1983; 148:209–211.
6. Abul-Khair MH, Arafa NM, Sobeih AM, et al: Sonographic of bilharzail masses of the scrotum. *JCU* 1980; 8:239–240.
7. Shawker TH, Javadpour N, O'Leary T, et al: Ultrasonographic detection of "burned-out" primary testicular germ cell tumors in clinically normal testes. *J Ultrasound Med* 1983; 2:477–479.
8. Glazer HS, Lee JKT, Melson GL, et al: Sonographic detection of occult testicular neoplasms. *AJR* 1982; 138:673–675.
9. Lupetin AR, Kint III W, Rich P, et al: Ultrasound diagnosis of testicular leukemia. *Radiology* 1983; 146:171–172.
10. Bird K, Rosenfield AT: Testicular infarction sec-

ondary to acute inflammatory disease: Demonstration by B-scan ultrasound. *Radiology* 1984; 152:785–788.

11. Bird K, Rosenfield AT, Taylor KJW: Ultrasonography and testicular torsion. *Radiology* 1983; 147:527–534.

12. Hricak H, Lue T, Filly RA, et al: Experimental study of the sonographic diagnosis of testicular tortion. *J Ultrasound Med* 1983; 2:349–356.

13. Lupetin AR, King III W, Rich PJ, et al: The traumatized scrotum. *Radiology* 1983; 148:203–207.

14. Jeffrey RB, Laing FC, Hricak H, et al: Sonography of testicular trauma. *AJR* 1983; 141:993–995.

15. Cunningham JJ: Sonographic findings in clinically unsuspected acute and chronic scrotal hematoceles. *AJR* 1983; 140:749–752.

16. Wolverson MK, Houttuin E, Heiberg E, et al: Comparison of computed tomography with high resolution real-time ultrasound and the localization of the impalpable undescended testes. *Radiology* 1983; 146:133–136.

17. Wolverson MK, Houttuin E, Heiberg E, et al: High-resolution real-time sonography of scrotal varicocele. *AJR* 1983; 141:775–779.

18. Rifkin MD, Foy PM, Kurtz AB, et al: The role of diagnostic ultrasonography in varicocele evaluation. *J Ultrasound Med* 1983; 2:271–275.

19. Rifkin MD, Kurtz AB, Goldberg BD: Epididymis examined by ultrasound: Correlation with pathology. *Radiology* 1984; 151:187–190.

20. Subramanyam BR, Balthazar EJ, Raghavendra BN, et al: Sonographic diagnosis of scrotal hernia. *AJR* 1982; 139:535–538.

## CASES

Dennis A. Sarti, M.D.

### The Normal Scrotum

Examination of the normal scrotum can be easily performed with conventional contact scanners. The scrotum is supported on a rolled towel and is gently scanned in the transverse planes without stabilization (Figs 12–1 and 12–2). The median raphe is an area of high attenuation. On either side the finely granular echogenicity of the glandular elements of the testes can be seen. The ductus deferens is visualized along the posterior medial aspect of each testis as a relatively circular echo-free area. Five-MHz transducers with a short internal focus are usually used. The slightly increased level of echogenicity at the focal plane can frequently be appreciated on the scans (Fig 12–2).

Longitudinal scans of the testes are usually best performed with a contact scanner after the palpable epididymis has been aligned directly posterior to the glandular elements of the testes. The scrotum is stabilized in this position, and the longitudinal scan is performed (Fig 12–3). High-resolution real-time systems with a built-in water delay have become available. The field of view is considerably smaller (3 × 4 cm), but the degree of detail is rather remarkable (Fig 12–4). The superficial scrotal areas can be appreciated, and the potential space created by the tunica vaginalis can often be seen as an echogenic line. The fine homogeneous texture of the glandular elements of the testes is even more evident.

In an evaluation of the scrotum, symmetry is the key, as in any paired organ. Most of the time, the testes are symmetric unless there has been atrophy related to a previous insult such as a mumps orchitis or trauma.

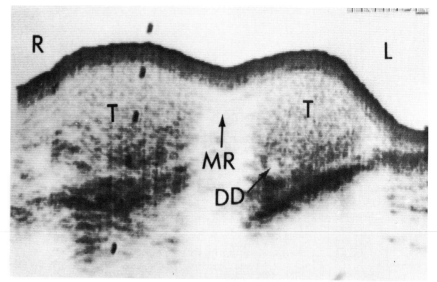

**FIG 12–1.**

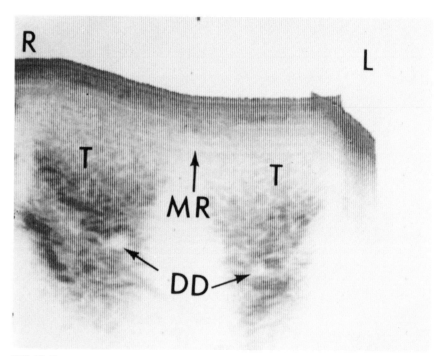

**FIG 12–2.**

DD  = Ductus deferens
F   = Foot
H   = Head
L   = Left
MR  = Median raphe
R   = Right
T   = Testis
TV  = Tunica vaginalis

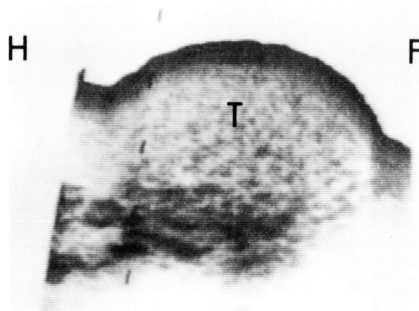

**FIG 12–3.**

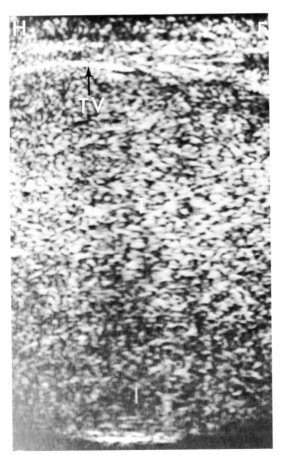

**FIG 12–4.**

## Normal Scrotum

High-resolution real-time equipment has made testicular examination much easier and more thorough. Examination with B-scanners may miss small lesions. Real-time studies permit easy visualization of the entire testis in a relatively short period of time. Five-, 7.5-, and 10-MHz real-time transducers are used in scrotal examinations. Some transducers have a built-in water path distance that permits placement of the testis within the focal zone. Other real-time transducers have dynamic focusing which permits focusing and improved resolution in the near field.

The testicular parenchymal echo pattern is even and similar in appearance to that of the thyroid. Discrete intratesticular masses stand out quite easily against the normal parenchymal pattern. The cases that pose present diagnostic difficulties are tumors diffusely involving the entire testis. Such tumors can occasionally yield an even parenchymal pattern that may be misinterpreted for a normal testis. I routinely begin a scrotal examination by starting with the uninvolved side. This permits the examiner to set up the equipment correctly for that specific patient. Once the normal side has been studied, the suspicious area can be examined with confidence and compared to the normal side.

Figure 12–5 is a longitudinal scan of a normal testis performed using a scanner with dynamic focusing. The testicular parenchymal pattern is even throughout the entire gland. The small posterior tubular lucency represents the normal epididymal region. Figure 12–6 is a longitudinal scan through the midportion of a normal testis. Cephalad to the gland is the head of the epididymis. A small amount of fluid is present anterior to the head of the epididymis. Small hydroceles are commonly seen on normal examinations.

Figure 12–7 shows an echogenic tubular structure in the midportion of the testicular parenchymal echoes. The increased tubular echoes arise from the tunica vaginalis and mediastinum testis, which contain testicular

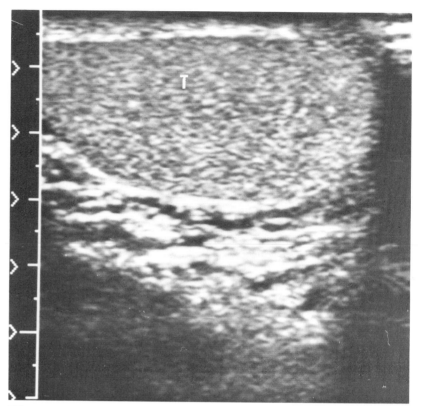

**FIG 12–5.**

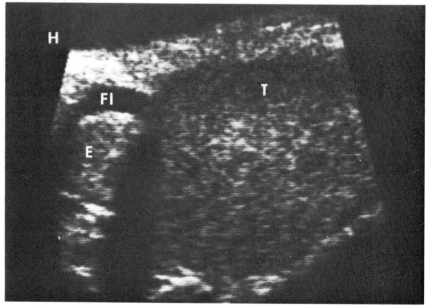

**FIG 12–6.**

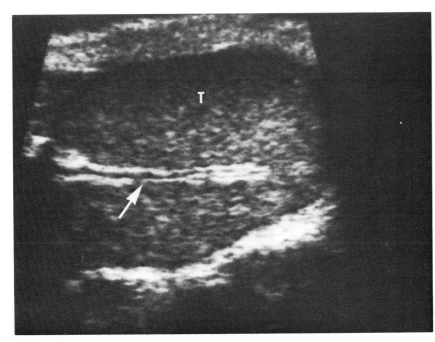

**FIG 12–7.**

vessels running through the midportion of the gland.

Figure 12–8 is a longitudinal scan of the right inguinal region performed using a real-time scanner with a built-in water path. A right testis was not identified during scrotal examination, so ultrasound of the right inguinal region was performed. Figure 12–8 demonstrates the typical testicular echo texture and confirms the diagnosis of an undescended testis.

| | | |
|---|---|---|
| **Arrow** | = | Mediastinum tesits |
| **E** | = | Head of the epididymis |
| **FI** | = | Hydrocele |
| **H** | = | Head |
| **T** | = | Testis |

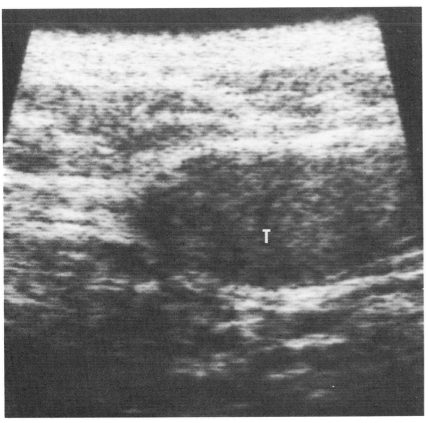

**FIG 12–8.**

## Testicular Tumors

When performing a scrotal examination, the major concern of the ultrasonographer is whether or not there is a testicular mass. All efforts should be directed toward answering this basic question. As noted in the previous discussion, it is important to adjust the ultrasound unit during imaging of the normal side so that the area of concern can be examined with maximum efficiency. The great majority of testicular tumors are hypoechoic masses. Some of these masses may be small and nonpalpable and ultrasound is the only means of detection. Testicular tumors are neoplasms of germ cell origin. Seminomas, embryonal cell carcinomas, and teratocarcinomas account for the majority of testicular tumors.

Figures 12–9 and 12–10 are longitudinal scans of two different patients with small hypoechoic masses less than 1 cm in size. The masses are slightly decreased in echogenicity compared to the remainder of the normal testicular parenchymal texture. The mass in Figure 12–10 has a small amount of attenuation posterior to it.

Figure 12–11 is a longitudinal scan of the left testicle in a 40-year-old man who was admitted for a seizure disorder. Physical examination by several physicians established the possible presence of a testicular mass. Ultrasonography was performed to determine whether or not a mass was present. An oval hypoechoic mass (arrowheads) is seen in the upper pole of the left testis. With incorrect gain setting, sensitivity, and TGC setting, the mass could easily be missed. A 1.5-cm seminoma was found at surgery. Ultrasound played a major role in the correct diagnosis in this patient.

Figure 12–12 is a longitudinal scan of the right testis of a patient who had noted recent scrotal enlargement. The left side was examined first and found to be normal. There is a large hypoechoic tumor with a fairly even parenchymal pattern. Note the normal testicular parenchymal pattern compressed peripherally. The tumor involves nearly the entire gland. Enough normal testicular echoes are

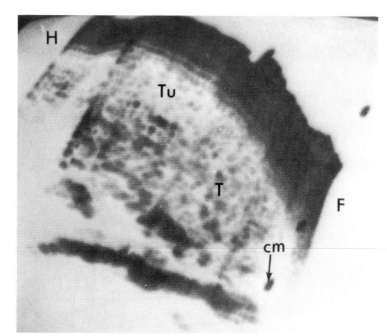

FIG 12–9.

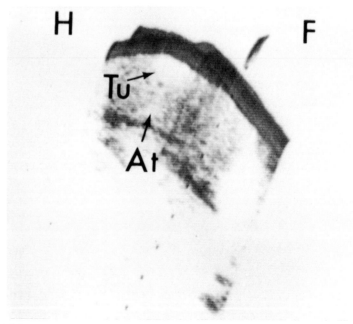

FIG 12–10.

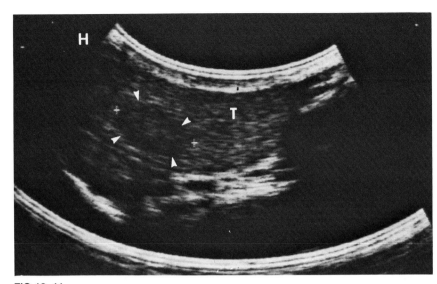

**FIG 12–11.**

present that the tumor stands out separate from normal tissues. Whenever a lesion involves the entire gland and has a fairly even parenchymal pattern, it can easily be missed. This case is helpful because it shows the hypoechoic tumor adjacent to a small amount of the normal testis.

SOURCE: Figure 12–9 is reproduced with permission from Sample WF, Gottesman JE, Skinner DG, et al: Gray scale ultrasound of the scrotum. *Radiology* 1978; 127:225–228.

| | | |
|---|---|---|
| **Arrowheads** | = | Testicular tumor |
| **At** | = | Attenuation |
| **cm** | = | Centimeter markers |
| **F** | = | Foot |
| **H** | = | Head |
| **T** | = | Normal testis |
| **Tu** | = | Tumor |

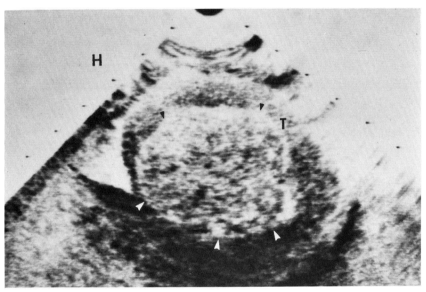

**FIG 12–12.**

## Testicular Tumors

Intratesticular masses may be secondary to entities or conditions other than neoplasms, such as infection and trauma. However, the main concern of the ultrasonographer is to determine whether or not an intratesticular mass is present. If such a mass is identified, the possibility of a testicular neoplasm must always be considered. The clinical history may assist in establishing the correct diagnosis.

Figure 12–13 is a longitudinal scan of the left testicle of a 36-year-old man. The patient first noted enlargement of the left testicle approximately 5 weeks earlier. There was no associated trauma or pain. A longitudinal scan of the left testicle shows a large hypoechoic mass replacing nearly the entire gland. A small amount of normal testicular parenchymal texture is evident in the upper pole. A left testicular seminoma was found at surgery.

Figure 12–14 is a longitudinal scan of the right testicle in a young man with a similar history of painless, nontraumatic enlargement of the testicle. The scan demonstrates increasing size of the testicle with a diffusely uneven texture. This mass is hypoechoic compared to the expected normal texture. It is important to keep in mind the appearance of the normal testicle during imaging for possible abnormalities.

Figures 12–15 and 12–16 are longitudinal scans of two different patients in which there is generalized enlargement to the testicles. The key ultrasound feature in these scans is inhomogeneity of the acoustic texture with areas of increased and decreased echogenicity throughout.

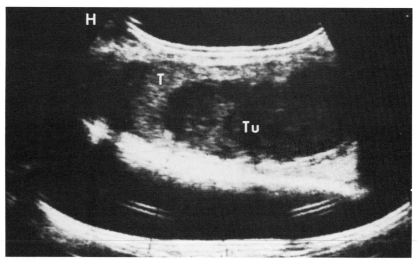

**FIG 12–13.**

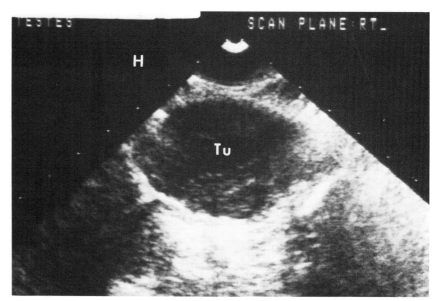

**FIG 12–14.**

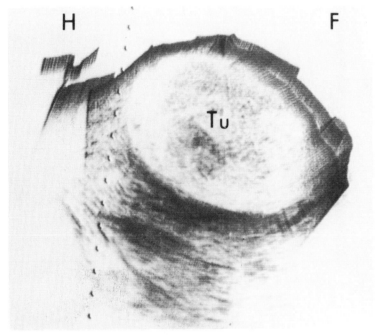

**FIG 12–15.**

F  = Foot
H  = Head
T  = Normal testicle
Tu = Tumor

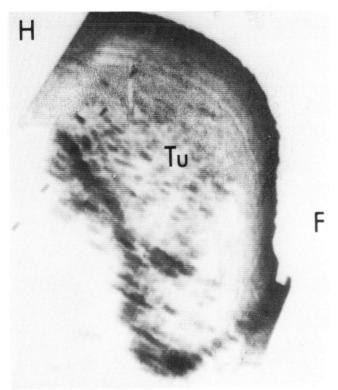

**FIG 12–16.**

## Testicular Tumors

Diffuse testicular tumors may have an even parenchymal pattern that may be incorrectly interpreted as normal unless the normal side is scanned for comparison. The cases discussed in this section illustrate abnormal scrotal texture compared to the normal texture.

Figure 12–17 is a transverse scan of the scrotum in which the right testis is slightly larger than the left. Without the normal left testis for comparison, the abnormal right side could be considered uninvolved. If the study was initially begun on the right side and the instrument setting was established for a normal testis, the right gland would appear to have even parenchymal texture because of the fairly homogeneous appearance of the tumor. Such cases emphasize the importance of starting the examination on the uninvolved side. A transverse scan showing both testes is also helpful. Since testicular tumors are usually hypoechoic lesions, the right side was involved with tumor.

Figure 12–18 is a transverse scan of another patient. Asymmetry in echo amplitude is noted when the two sides are compared. The right testis is normal in size and echogenicity. A small lucent rim is present around the right testis, consistent with a small hydrocele. The left testis is increased in size and decreased in echo amplitude. The parenchymal texture pattern of the left side is fairly even in echo distribution. The left testis is diffusely involved with lymphoma.

Figure 12–19 is a transverse scan through both testes and Figure 12–20 is a longitudinal scan through the right testis in a young man in his early 20s. He noted slight enlargement of the right side which he thought was secondary to a recent sports incident. The transverse scan in Figure 12–19 demonstrates a marked difference in echo amplitude between the two sides. The left testis has a normal, even appearance. On the right side a hypoechoic mass is seen involving the entire gland. A longitudinal scan (Fig 12–20) shows nearly complete replacement with tumor. Only a small

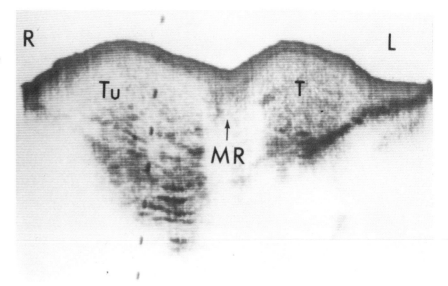

FIG 12–17.

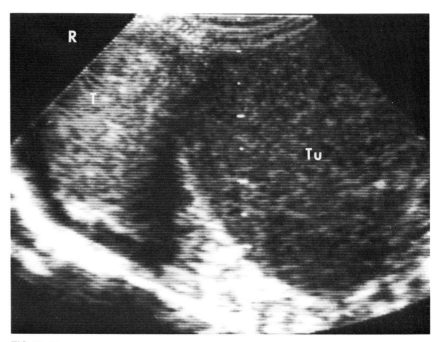

FIG 12–18.

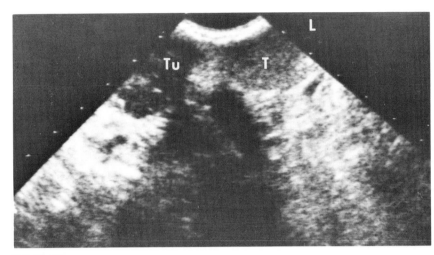

**FIG 12–19.**

area of normal-appearing testicular texture is noted over the lower pole. At operation the right gland was found to be involved with seminoma.

| | | |
|---|---|---|
| **L** | = | Left |
| **MR** | = | Median raphe |
| **R** | = | Right |
| **T** | = | Normal testis |
| **Tu** | = | Tumor |

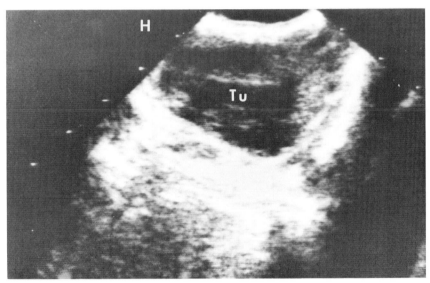

**FIG 12–20.**

## Testicular Tumors

In previous examples, testicular neoplasms have been described as mainly hypoechoic soft tissue tumors on ultrasound. This is generally the case. However, variations are found. When these masses are demonstrated, the differential diagnosis includes infection and trauma. Figure 12–21 is a longitudinal scan through the testis in a patient with metastatic embryonal cell carcinoma to the retroperitoneum and mediastinum from an unknown primary. The patient received radiation therapy and chemotherapy. After this treatment was concluded, an ultrasound examination of the testicles was performed. Figure 12–21 shows a small "burned-out" embryonal cell carcinoma cnsisting of a small hypoechoic component (Tu) and a dense echogenic component with posterior acoustic shadowing. It is unusual to see cases of calcification and shadowing in tumors. The appearance is most likely secondary to the therapy.

Figure 12–22 is a longitudinal scan of the left testis in a 21-year-old man. The lower pole of the gland is involved with tumor. This portion has decreased echo amplitude compared to the normal upper pole. Numerous small sonolucent circular regions are noted surrounding the solid component of the tumor. These areas are secondary to necrosis.

Usually testicular tumors appear solid on ultrasound. The above case illustrates early necrotic changes. Figure 12–23 is a longitudinal scan of another patient in which the testis is mainly fluid filled secondary to necrotic changes. Only a small portion of normal testicular echo texture is noted over the lower pole. The remainder of the gland is cystic, secondary to a necrotic tumor. However, the ultrasound findings could be secondary to trauma or infection in a different clinical setting.

Figure 12–24 is a longitudinal scan of the right scrotum in 33-year-old man with painless scrotal swelling of 1 month's duration. The scan shows a loculated fluid collection surrounding the testis. There is slightly uneven

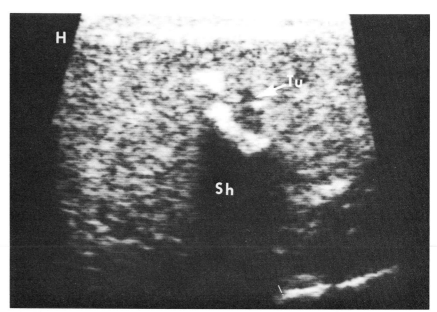

FIG 12–21.

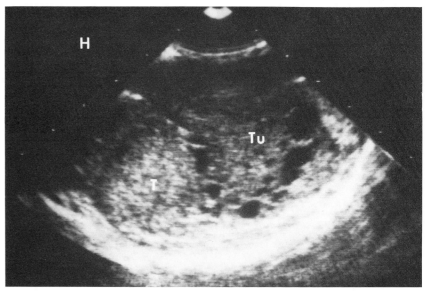

FIG 12–22.

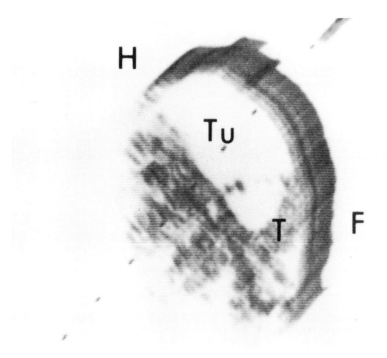

**FIG 12–23.**

echo texture in the lower pole of the gland which is also minimally hypoechoic compared to the upper pole. If a history of trauma or infection were present, the ultrasound findings could be consistent with either entity. However, painless scrotal swelling in the absence of a history of trauma or infection most likely represents tumor. At operation an embryonal cell carcinoma with hematocele was found.

SOURCE: Figure 12–23 is reproduced with permission from Sample WF, Gottesman JE, Skinner DG, et al: Gray scale ultrasound of the scrotum. *Radiology* 1978; 127:225–228.

| | | |
|---|---|---|
| **F** | = | Foot |
| **H** | = | Head |
| **He** | = | Hematocele |
| **Sh** | = | Acoustic shadowing |
| **T** | = | Normal testicle |
| **Tu** | = | Tumor |

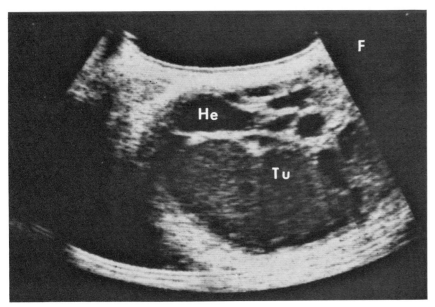

**FIG 12–24.**

## Epididymitis

In cases of acute epididymitis, the clinical setting is often helpful in leading to the correct diagnosis. However, the ultrasonographer must keep in mind that the major function of an ultrasound study is to rule out an intra-testicular mass. Most often, a normal testis will be identified in cases of epididymitis. If an abnormal testicular texture is present, the possibility of orchitis versus tumor must be considered. The patient should be studied after antibiotic therapy to see that the testicular texture returns to normal. If it does not return to normal, neoplasm cannot be entirely excluded. Figure 12–25 is a longitudinal scan of the testis in a patient with uncomplicated acute epididymitis. The ductus deferens and epididymis are enlarged as a result of the inflammatory process. In addition, the epididymal area loses echogenicity. The epididymis appears as a relatively sonolucent cord running along the underside of the normal testicular glandular elements. Careful scanning is required to ensure that a tissue plane is present between the epididymis and testis.

Figure 12–26 is a longitudinal scan of the testis in another patient with acute epididymitis. The epidymis is increased in size and sonolucency. It is situated posterior and inferior to the testis. The inferior and superior poles of the testis are often very difficult to visualize. A texture change between the testis and epididymis can be noted in cases of epidymitis. Meticulous scanning is necessary to identify the upper and lower poles.

Figure 12–27 is a longitudinal scan through the upper pole of the left testis in a 28-year-old man with a 1-week history of a tender, erythematous left scrotum. The ultrasound scan shows a hypoechoic, enlarged head and body of the epididymis, associated with a small reactive hydrocele. The upper pole of the testis is normal in echogenicity and is the critical finding on ultrasound. This scan demonstrates the ability of ultrasound to differentiate the thickened epididymis from the upper pole of the testis.

Chronic epididymitis frequently pre-

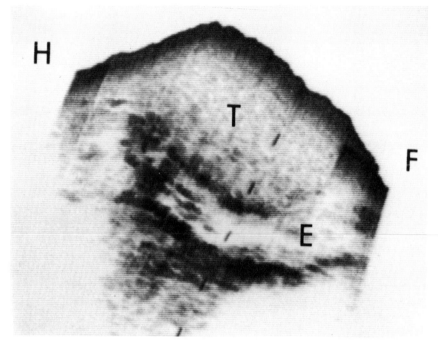

FIG 12–25.

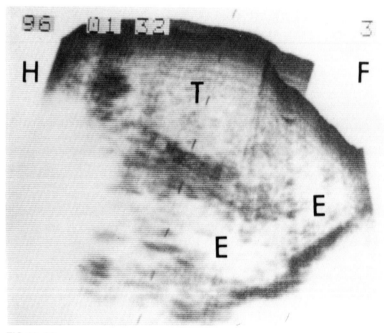

FIG 12–26.

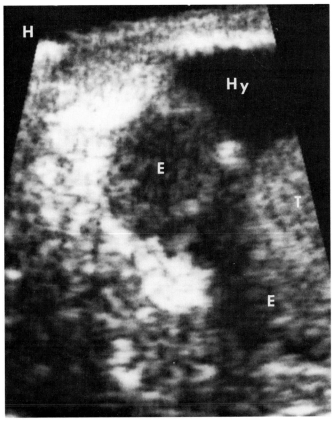

FIG 12–27.

sents as enlargement of the scrotum. The extratesticular nature of the process can be determined from ultrasound examination. In chronic epididymitis, focal or generalized thickening of the epididymis is usually present. Figure 12–28 is a longitudinal scan of a patient who was found to have a rock-hard mass in the lower pole of the testis on physical examination. Ultrasonography was performed to confirm the diagnosis of a testicular tumor. A cleavage plane between the epididymis and glandular elements of the testis is preserved in Figure 12–28. Because of this finding, a testicular tumor was excluded. If a cleavage plane is not seen on the sonogram, an underlying occult neoplasm cannot be ruled out. Uncomplicated chronic epididymitis usually presents as a solid region of epididymal thickening. The patient whose scan is shown in Figure 12–28 was found to have chronic epididymitis and was treated accordingly. This case illustrates the important role of ultrasound in leading to the correct diagnosis. As mentioned earlier, the major role of scrotal ultrasound imaging is to determine whether a mass is intratesticular or extratesticular.

| | | |
|---|---|---|
| **E** | = | Epididymitis |
| **F** | = | Foot |
| **H** | = | Head |
| **Hy** | = | Hydrocele |
| **T** | = | Testis |

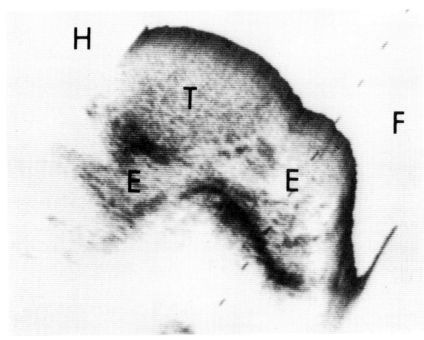

FIG 12–28.

# Epididymitis and Hydrocele

Small hydroceles may be seen normally without any underlying pathology as a cause. When a pathologic condition such as a neoplasm, infection, or trauma is present, reactive hydrocele can be visualized during scrotal examination. Figures 12–29 through 12–32 are transverse and longitudinal scans of four different patients who have epididymitis associated with reactive hydroceles.

In Figure 12–29, a transverse scan, a small hydrocele is visible. This is not an unusual finding in cases of epididymitis. A few llinear echoes are noted within the hydrocele, and infection cannot be excluded. Figure 12–30 illustrates another case of hydrocele accompanying epididymitis. However, the scrotum was quite tense in this patient. Massive hydroceles can occasionally be confused with large solid masses. Ultrasound demonstrates fluid as the major cause of the scrotal enlargement. No echoes are noted within this hydrocele, and infection within the fluid is unlikely.

Figure 12–31 is a longitudinal scan in which a small fluid collection is visible inferior and superior to the testis. No internal echoes are identified within the fluid. In Figure 12–32 there is the suggestion of a few linear echoes within the hydrocele. In these instances the possibility of infection in the fluid must be considered.

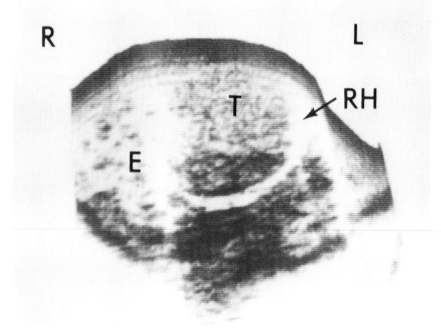

FIG 12–29.

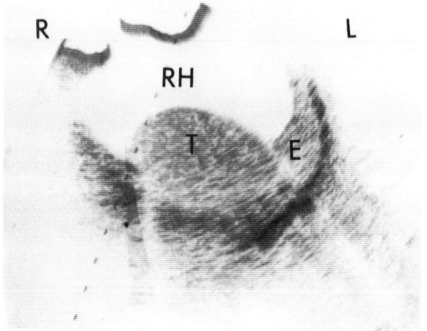

FIG 12–30.

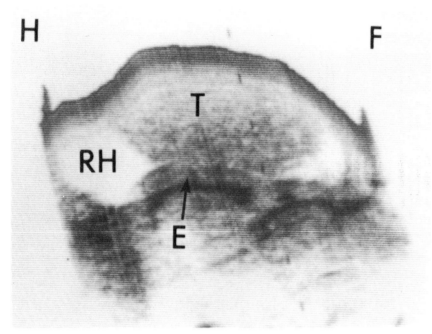

FIG 12–31.

SOURCE: Figure 12–32 is reproduced with permission from Sample WF, Gottesman JE, Skinner DG, et al: Gray scale ultrasound of the scrotum. *Radiology* 1978; 127:225–228.

| | | |
|---|---|---|
| **E** | = | Epididymitis |
| **F** | = | Foot |
| **H** | = | Head |
| **L** | = | Left |
| **R** | = | Right |
| **RH** | = | Reactive hydrocele |
| **T** | = | Testis |

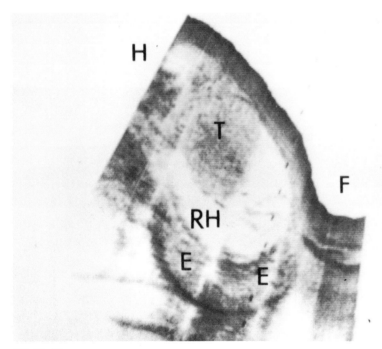

FIG 12–32.

## Infection

Figure 12–33 is an oblique transverse through the right scrotum of a 77-year-old man with a history of chronic alcoholism and a recent prostatectomy secondary to prostatic carcinoma. On physical examination the right scrotum was enlarged, warm, erythematous, and tender. The scan shows an increased epididymis lateral and cephalad to the testis. A septated fluid collection is present within the scrotal sac, compatible with an infected hydrocele. Figure 12–34 is a longitudinal scan through the fluid area only. Multiple septations along with soft internal echoes indicate that the entity is not a simple reactive hydrocele. The patient was treated with intravenous antibiotics, and symptoms resolved.

Figure 12–35 is a transverse scan of a man in his mid-60s who underwent ultrasound examination because of an enlarging, tender scrotum. The patient was diabetic. Figure 12–36 is a longitudinal scan through the left scrotum. This case differs from the previous one in that the hydrocele is echo free and without evidence of internal echoes. The testes are normal in texture and there is no evidence of intratesticular masses. The dominant feature is the markedly thickened size of the soft tissue structures of the scrotum. The ultrasound findings indicate severe cellulitis of the scrotum. The patient was treated with antibiotics, with marked improvement in symptoms. Later, ultrasound examination demonstrated a decrease in size of the scrotal swelling.

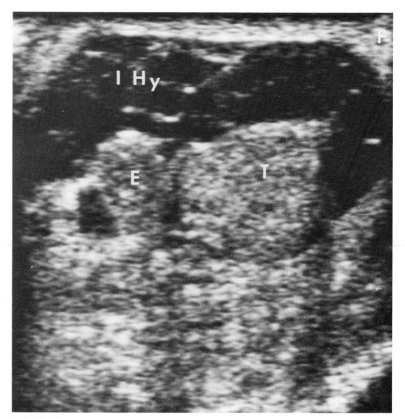

**FIG 12–33.**

**FIG 12–34.**

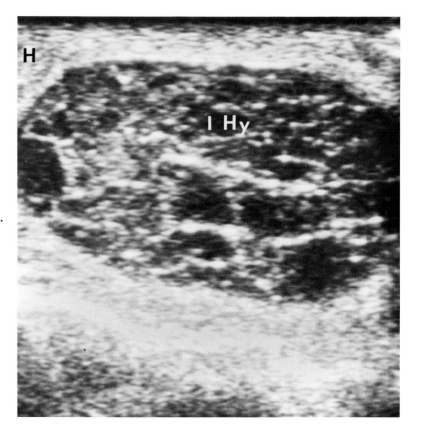

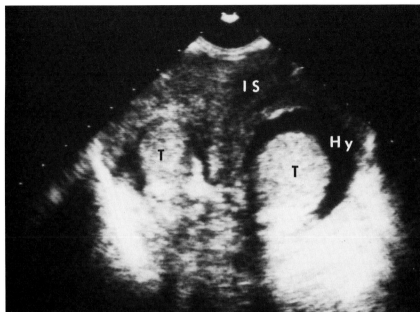

E   = Epididymitis
H   = Head
IHy = Infected hydrocele
IS  = Infected scrotum
T   = Testis

FIG 12–35.

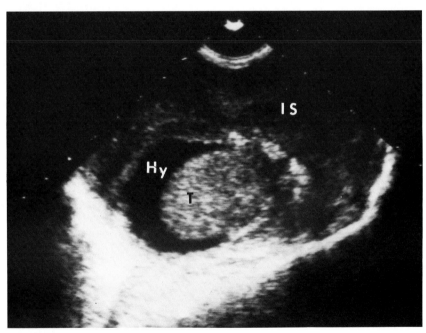

FIG 12–36.

## Infection

Infection of the testicle presents a confusing ultrasound picture since neoplasm must be considered. When there is a change in testicular architecture, neoplasm cannot be ruled out until this architectural change is resolved. Figure 12–37 is a transverse scan of the scrotum in a patient with acute epididymal orchitis. The right testis is normal in size and texture. The left testis is enlarged and hypoechoic. The possibility of a diffusely infiltrative neoplasm must be considered. A helpful finding in this case is enlargement of the epididymis, suggesting the diagnosis of inflammation, which is consistent with the clinical history.

In some patients, a focal area of orchitis may develop adjacent to the epididymis (Fig 12–38). This pattern is indistinguishable from an occult neoplasm, which may be the underlying cause of the epididymitis. These two entities can be distinguished only after serial examinations following antibiotic therapy. In the case of acute epididymitis associated with focal orchitis, the echogenicity of the epididymal region and the glandular elements will often return to normal.

Figure 12–39 is a longitudinal scan of a testis. A high-amplitude echo with acoustic shadowing is present in the epididymal region. The patient had chronic epididymitis with calcification.

In Figure 12–40, a longitudinal scan, epididymitis is noted posterior and inferior to the testis. The fluid collection cephalad to the testis is secondary to a spermatocele. Spermatoceles appear as cystic accumulations of sperm, usually in a ductule leading from the epididymis to the testis near the head of the epididymis. These accumulations may arise as a result of trauma or secondary to chronic epididymis (Fig 12–40). In the latter case, findings of chronic epididymitis will frequently be present. Spermatoceles are usually round and do not deform the glandular elements of the testis.

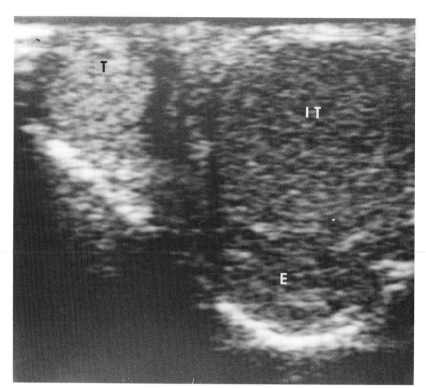

**FIG 12–37.**

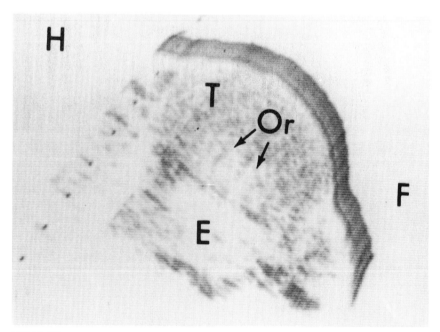

**FIG 12–38.**

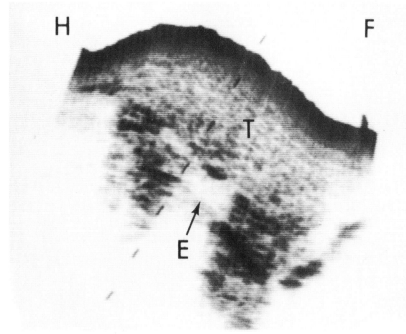

E = Epididymitis
F = Foot
H = Head
IT = Infected testis
Or = Orchitis
Sp = Spermatocele
T = Testis

**FIG 12–39.**

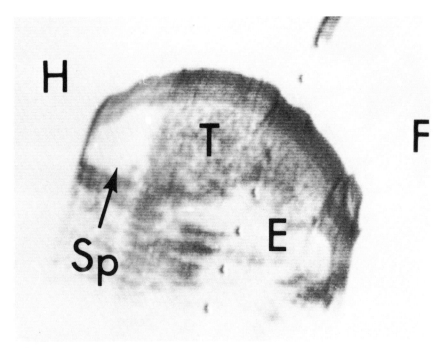

**FIG 12–40.**

## Acute Scrotal Torsion and Trauma

Two frequently encountered pathologic conditions in the differential diagnosis of the acutely enlarged scrotum are acute torsion and acute scrotal trauma. Acute torsion of the testes may have a number of patterns on ultrasound. In some cases the entire scrotal contents are abnormal in organization and texture (Fig 12–41). All layers of the scrotum seem involved, and a reactive hydrocele may be present. In addition, the acoustic texture of the glandular elements of the testes is usually abnormal. This picture may mimic that of a testicular abscess.

In other cases of acute torsion the actual twisted vascular pedicle can be resolved (Fig 12–42). The consistent abnormality in torsion of the testes is a lack of attachment of the epididymis to the scrotal tissues. This provides a pedicle upon which torsion can occur. The typical features of involvement of the entire scrotum, a reactive hydrocele, and an abnormal acoustic texture to the glandular elements of the testes again are seen.

In the evaluation of acute trauma to the scrotum, the viability of the testes must be established. Careful comparative scanning of the scrotum in the case of a viable testis with a hemorrhagic hydrocele demonstrates the complex mass surrounding the glandular elements of the testis. This mass represents the hemorrhagic hydrocele. In addition, the two testes appear equal in size and acoustic texture (Figs 12–43 and 12–44). If any abnormality in testicular texture is noted, the probability of damage to the glandular elements of the testes is increased.

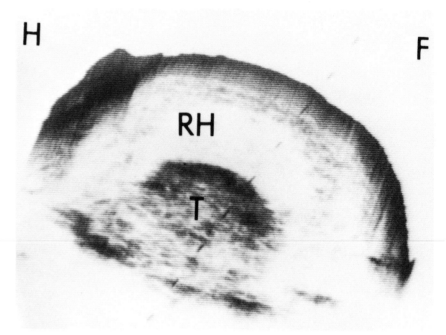

FIG 12–41.

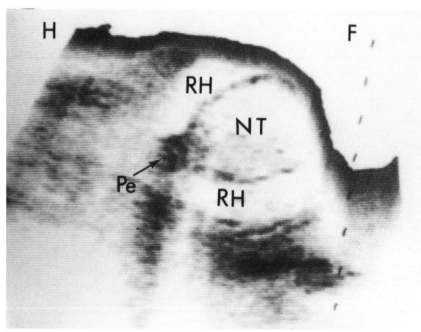

FIG 12–42.

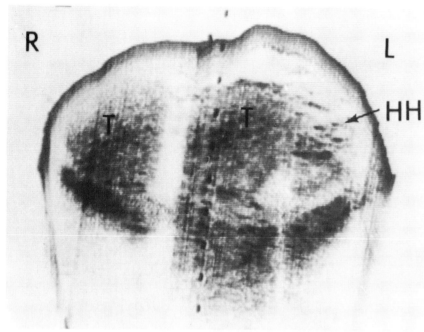

F = Foot
H = Head
HH = Hemorrhagic hydrocele
L = Left
NT = Necrotic testis
Pe = Vascular pedicle
R = Right
RH = Reactive hydrocele
T = Glandular elements of testis

**FIG 12–43.**

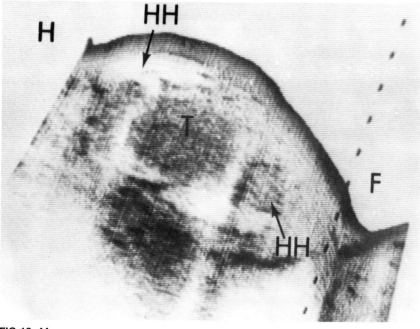

**FIG 12–44.**

## Scrotal Torsion and Trauma

In various stages, subacute and chronic torsion may appear as mixed fluid and solid masses that may involve the testis. The ultrasound picture may be bizarre and suggest infection or necrotic neoplasm. Correlation with Doppler and radionuclide studies will reveal decreased perfusion. Figure 12–45 is a transverse scan of an enlarged right scrotum in a patient with chronic torsion. On the ultrasound scan a fluid mass is seen with thickened solid components. These findings would be consistent with a scrotal abscess in the appropriate clinical setting. The patient suffered from chronic torsion with resulting necrosis of the testis.

Figure 12–46 is a longitudinal scan of the left testis in a patient from whom the right testis had previously been removed because of embryonal cell carcinoma. Three weeks before the scan in Figure 12–46 was made, the patient underwent open testicular biopsy of the left gland because of a suspected second primary tumor. No tumor was found. An ultrasound examination because of scrotal pain. Figure 12–46 shows a complex mass in the upper pole of the left testis that is secondary to a hemorrhage biopsy defect.

Figure 12–47 is a longitudinal scan of the scrotum of a patient who had sustained trauma to the scrotum approximately 2 weeks before the ultrasound examination. This scan of the upper pole of the testis demonstrates a septated fluid mass secondary to a hematocele. The testis and epididymis were slightly hypoechoic secondary to infarction. The ultrasound appearance of the hematocele is similar to that of an abscess. However, the clinical setting is consistent with hemorrhage. Another entity that may appear as a complex scrotal mass involving the extratesticular elements is a hernia (Fig 12–48). When the hernia contains fat, which may cause high reflectivity and attenuation, the resulting ultrasound picture can be quite distorted and confusing. Differentiation from in-

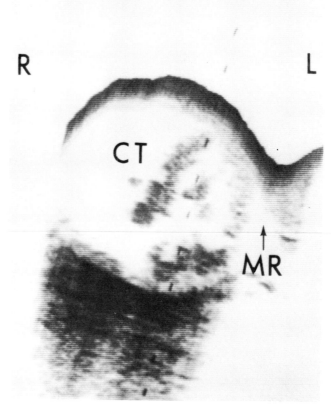

FIG 12–45.

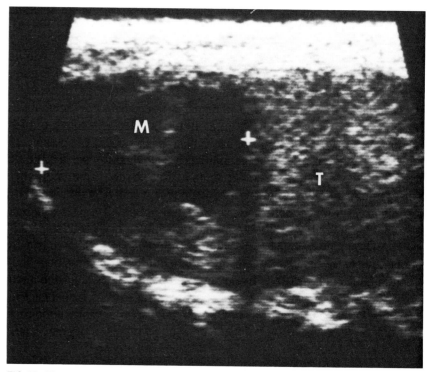

FIG 12–46.

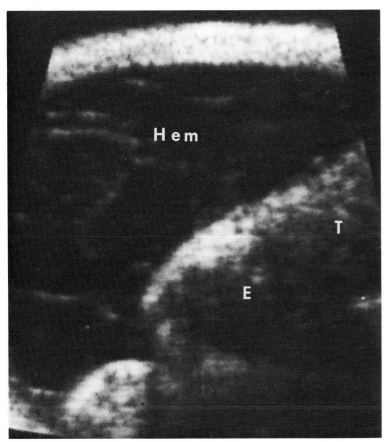

**FIG 12–47.**

fection and trauma can be difficult, especially if real-time equipment is not available. However, peristaltic activity can be identified on real-time imaging. Once this is noted, the diagnosis of herniation can easily be made.

Source: Figure 12–48 is reproduced with permission from Sample WF, Gottesman JE, Skinner DG, et al: Gray scale ultrasound of the scrotum. *Radiology* 1978; 127:225–228.

| **CT** | = Chronic torsion |
|--------|-------------------|
| **E** | = Epididymis |
| **F** | = Foot |
| **H** | = Head |
| **He** | = Herniation |
| **Hem** | = Hematocele |
| **L** | = Left |
| **M** | = Biopsy hematoma |
| **MR** | = Median raphe |
| **R** | = Right |
| **T** | = Testis |

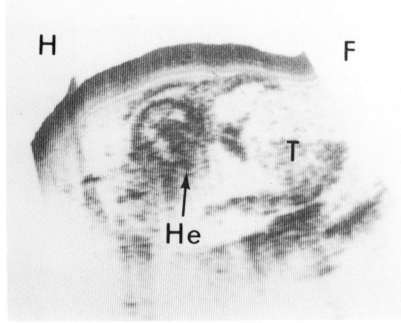

**FIG 12–48.**

## Hydrocele

Hydroceles are probably the most commonly encountered scrotal masses. Frequently the simple fluid nature of the mass can be ascertained by transillumination. However, a number of hydroceles does not transilluminate. This can make clinical distinction quite difficult and necessitate an ultrasound examination. Small accumulations of scrotal fluid may be present for no apparent reason. The hallmark of a simple hydrocele on ulltrasound is the presence of a simple fluid collection surrounding the testes. The only area that is not surrounded by fluid is the attachment of the region of the epididymis to the scrotum (Fig 12–49 and 12–50). Since hydroceles may be idiopathic or associated with prior trauma, infection, or neoplasm, careful examination of the acoustic texture of the testes is important.

Large hydroceles are often associated with trauma, infection, or neoplasm. On rare occasions, hydroceles may be so large that they present clinically as rock-hard masses and may be thought to be neoplasms. It is always surprising to find a large fluid collection when examining these rock-hard masses. Figure 12–51 is an example of a large hydrocele thought to be a tumor on clinical grounds. Note the compressed appearance of the testis posterior to the hydrocele.

Figure 12–52 is a longitudinal scan of the right scrotum in which a small fluid collection is present cephalad to the right testis. This may be a spermatocele. However, the fluid is secondary to a small hydrocele. The diagnosis of a hydrocele was confirmed by moving the testis, which allowed the fluid to change position within the scrotal sac.

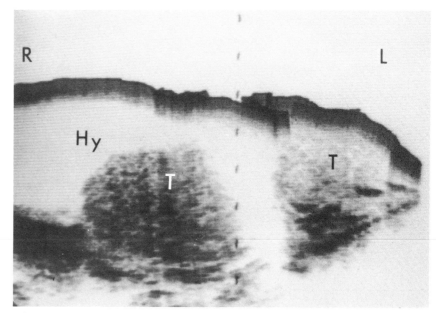

**FIG 12–49.**

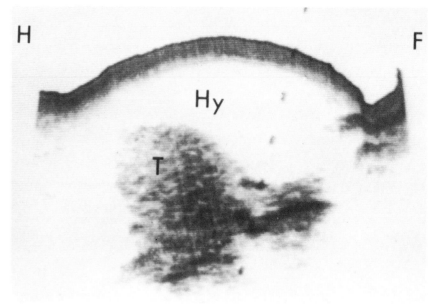

**FIG 12–50.**

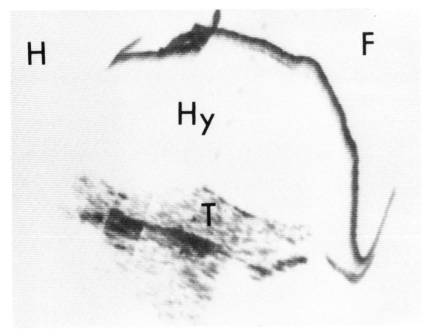

**FIG 12–51.**

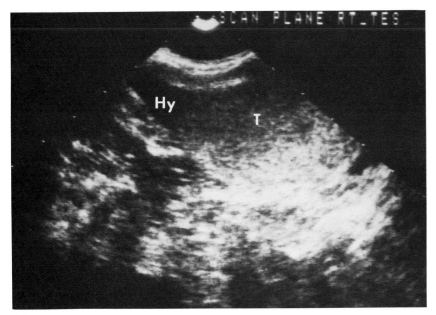

**FIG 12–52.**

F = Foot
H = Head
Hy = Hydrocele
L = Left
R = Right
T = Testis

## Scrotal Fluid

Fluid collections within the scrotum can usually be correctly identified on the basis of their appearance and location. Hydroceles are fluid collections within the potential space of the scrotal sac. Fluid collections cephalad to the upper pole of the testis may be loculated hydroceles but are more likely to be secondary to spermatoceles. If the position of the testis is changed, the fluid collection will change shape and location if it is secondary to a hydrocele. This is not true of a spermatocele. As mentioned previously, spermatoceles are cystic dilations secondary to accumulation of sperm, usually arising near the head of the epididymis. Figures 12–53 and 12–54 are typical scans of spermatoceles, which appear as round to oval cystic structures cephalad to the testis. They do not usually indent or impinge upon the testicular elements. Changing the position of the testis does not change the location of the spermatocele, as is the case in hydroceles.

Figure 12–55 is a transverse scan of the left scrotum in a patient who underwent ultrasound examination because of left testicular pain and mass. The patient was clinically thought to have a testicular tumor. The ultrasound scan reveals a well-circumscribed cystic mass within the confines of the testis and impinging on the parenchymal echoes of the testis. The fluid nature of this mass is evident from the prominent enhanced through-transmission deep to it. A small hydrocele is also present. At operation a cyst of a tunica albuginia was found. No testicular tumor was evident.

Figure 12–56 is a longitudinal scan of the testis in which there is a high-amplitude echo with acoustic shadowing on the anterior surface of the testis. This is secondary to a calcified plaque of the tunica vaginalis.

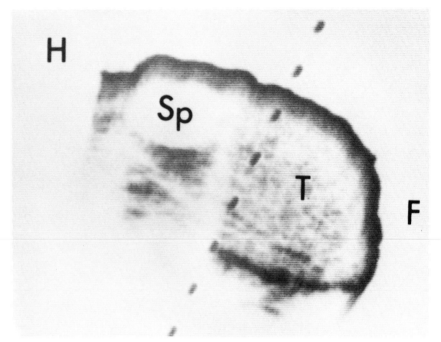

FIG 12–53.

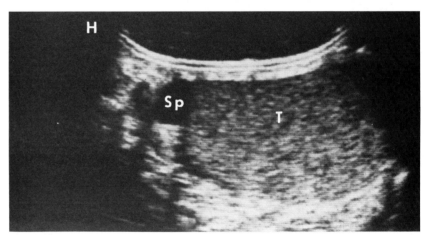

FIG 12–54.

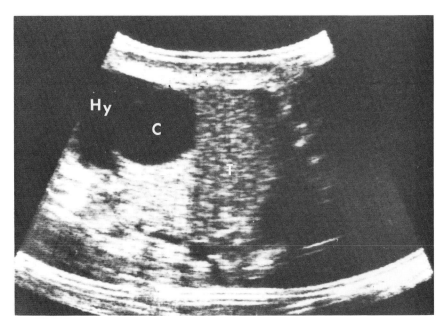

Arrow = Calcified plaque
C     = Cyst of the tunica albuginia
F     = Foot
H     = Head
Hy    = Hydrocele
Sp    = Spermatocele
T     = Testis

**FIG 12–55.**

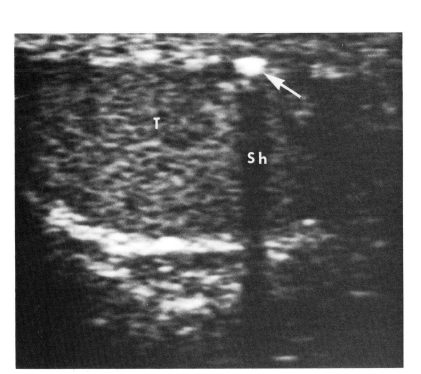

**FIG 12–56.**

## Varicocele

Varicoceles may present clinically as palpable masses with scrotal pain. They are secondary to dilated veins within the spermatic cord. The important task of the ultrasonographer is to rule out an intratesticular mass. Figures 12–57 and 12–58 are longitudinal scans of two different patients that show numerous dilated, serpiginous tubular structures posterior to the testes. The ultrasonographic appearance rules out intratesticular neoplasms. The lucent areas posterior to the testes could be interpreted as epididymitis. However, these dilated tubular lucencies have a more structured appearance than is present in epididymitis. In epididymitis usually the epididymal region is increased in size but ill defined in architecture owing to inflammation. In Figures 12–57 and 12–58, the beaded tubular structures have a more organized appearance and are suggestive of varicoceles.

Figures 12–59 and 12–60 are transverse and longitudinal scans of the left scrotum of a patient with a palpable testicular mass. Ultrasound was performed to rule out testicular neoplasm. No intratesticular lesions were seen in the testis. Numerous circular lucencies are seen posterior to the testis on the transverse scan (Fig 12–59). The longitudinal scan (Fig 12–60) indicates that these circular areas are really beaded, tubular structures consistent with varicoceles.

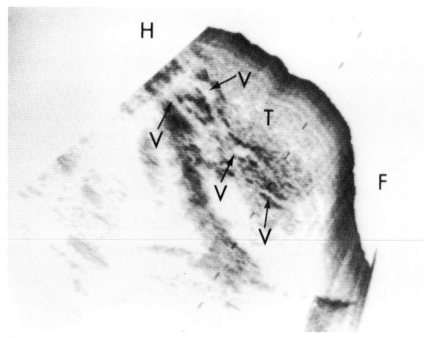

FIG 12–57.

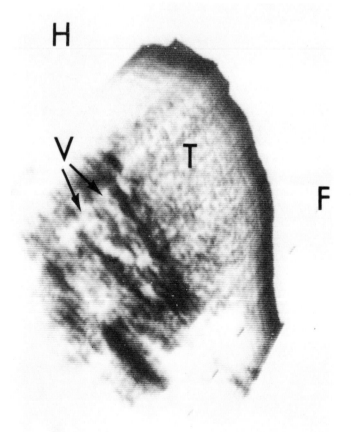

FIG 12–58.

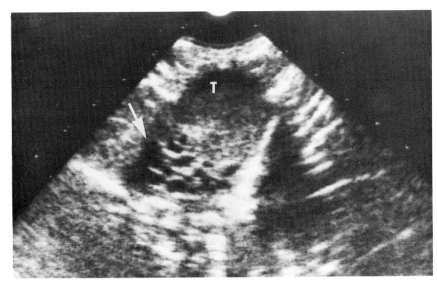

**Arrow** = Varicoceles
**F**     = Foot
**H**     = Head
**T**     = Testis
**V**     = Varicoceles

**FIG 12–59.**

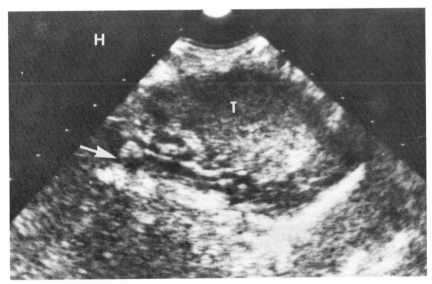

**FIG 12–60.**

## Varicoceles

Figure 12–61 is a transverse scan through the upper portion of the left scrotum cephalad to the left testis. Ultrasound was performed because the patient had a large scrotal mass, thought possibly to be a neoplasm. Other scans demonstrated a normal left testis. Cephalad to the testis was a large, 6 × 3-cm collection of tubular and circular lucencies.. These were secondary to numerous varicoceles. Figure 12–61 shows the numerous circular cystic regions.

Figure 12–62 is a transverse scan of the scrotum in another patient with a palpable scrotal mass. On other scans the testis was normal. Figure 12–62 shows a hydrocele anterior to numerous tubular structures that represent varicoceles. Note the organized structured appearance to the varicoceles.

Figures 12–63 and 12–64 are longitudinal scans of the left scrotum in a patient with a palpable mass. The upper pole of the left testis is normal in appearance, as was the remainder of the gland. Numerous circular lucent areas are seen cephalad to the testis. These may represent spermatoceles or varicoceles. The patient was asked to perform a Valsalva maneuver during the examination, and the cystic areas were observed with real-time scanning. Figure 12–64 was scanned during the Valsalva maneuver. The largest cystic region is increased in size and tense in appearance, compared to Figure 12–63. This change in size was consistently noted on real-time examination when the Valsalva maneuver was performed. These findings indicate the presence of varicoceles.

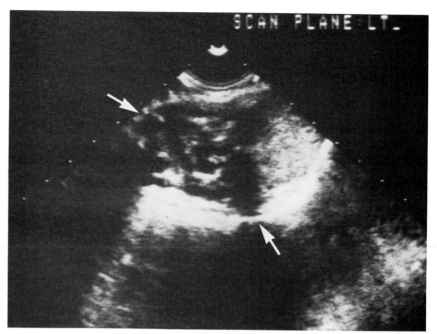

FIG 12–61.

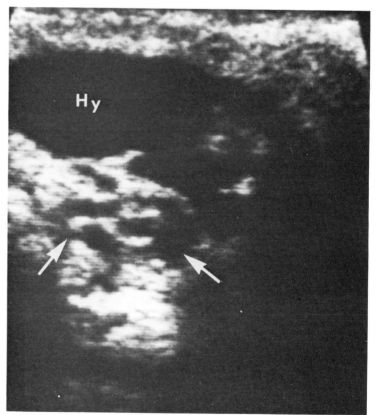

FIG 12–62.

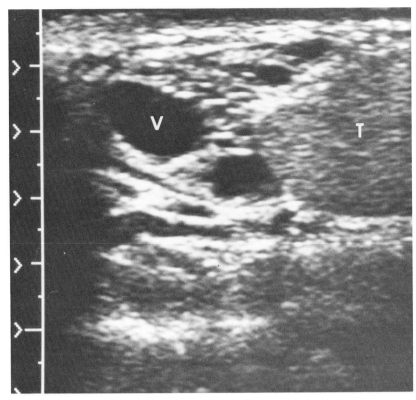

Arrows  = Varicoceles
Hy      = Hydrocele
T       = Testis
V       = Varicoceles

**FIG 12–63.**

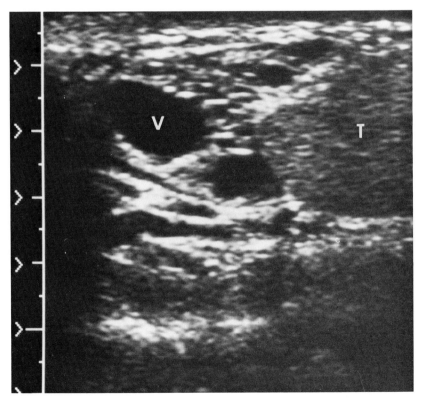

**FIG 12–64.**

# 13.

# Ultrasonography of Thyroid, Parathyroid, and Neck Masses

## Catherine Cole-Beuglet, M.D.

### Introduction

The development and widespread use of high-resolution equipment have resulted in a reappraisal of the indications for ultrasonography of thyroid, parathyroid, and neck masses (Table 13–1).[1,2] The majority of patients referred for ultrasound evaluation of the thyroid gland are initially seen with a palpable nodule in one lobe of the gland. A palpable thyroid nodule is estimated to occur in 3%–4% of the population of North America.[3] Clinically, focal thyroid enlargement warrants an investigation of the function of the gland with a radionuclide examination. Demonstration of iodine trapping and organification indicates that a nodule has a low risk of malignancy. However, a nonfunctioning or hypofunctioning "cold" nodule is estimated to have a 20% risk of malignancy in patients undergoing surgery for removal of a cold nodule.[4] Ultrasound examination of solitary cold nodules was initially used to differentiate cystic from solid or complex lesions. Approximately 20% of the cold nodules so examined proved to be cystic, and thus of low malignant potential.[4,5] The majority of cold nodules represent solid or complex lesions. No specific ultrasound characteristic differentiates benign from malignant lesions. Percutaneous aspiration and/or biopsy is required to establish the diagnosis. These studies can be performed with ultrasound monitoring to select a site for tissue sampling that is remote from areas of degeneration.[4,6]

The use of high-frequency (7.5– and 10–MHz) transducers has resulted in improved resolution and the detection of cystic and solid masses as small as 2–4 mm within the thyroid gland.[7] In the series reported by Scheible et al., an additional thyroid nodule or abnormality was detected in 40% of patients referred with the diagnosis of a solitary nodule as established by palpation or radionuclide scan.[1]

The probability that a cold nodule in a multinodular gland is malignant is approximately 1%–6%.[4] Thus, the primary indication for sonography of the thyroid is detection of a multinodular gland when only one nodule is apparent clinically or by scintigraphy.[2] One exception is the patient who received irradiation to the head, neck, and upper portion of the chest in childhood. A single cold nodule on the radionuclide scan of a patient with a history of head and neck irradiation has approximately a 30% probability of malignancy, which increases to 40% when there are multiple cold nodules.[8,9]

**TABLE 13–1.**

**Indications for Thyroid Sonography**

PRIMARY

    Detection of a multinodular gland

    Detection of occult carcinoma

    Detection of recurrent carcinoma after thyroidectomy

    Monitoring aspiration-biopsy procedures

SECONDARY

    Determination of size and volume of the gland

    Determination of size and volume of a nodule

    Monitoring the size of a nodule under treatment

    Screening patients with histories of head and neck irradiation

    Preoperative evaluation of contralateral lobe

    Determining the nature of a neck mass when its origin is uncertain (i.e., thyroglossal duct cyst)

    Evaluation of the hypothyroid infant

## Anatomy of the Thyroid Gland

The thyroid, an endocrine gland, develops as a median diverticulum from the floor of the primitive pharynx at the level of the first pharyngeal pouch. It has been identified in a 2-mm embryo (17 days old). It becomes a solid mass at the base of the tongue and with fetal growth migrates caudally and rests in front of the larynx in the 14- to 15-mm embryo (7th week). It retains its connection with the pharyngeal floor until the 7-mm stage (5½ weeks), with its point of origin manifest as the foramen caecum. The stalk between the tongue and thyroid is the thyroglossal duct, and if any portion of it persists in postnatal life, cysts, sinuses, fistulas, or accessory thyroids may occur. If the stalk migrates further caudally, thyroid tissue can be found in the superior mediastinum in a retrosternal position. If the inferior portion of the thyroglossal duct below the hyoid bone fails to atrophy, a pyramidal lobe may develop.

The thyroid gland is composed of two lateral lobes with a connecting isthmus between their bases, forming a U or a low-slung H in front of the larynx and trachea. The isthmus lies across the third and fourth tracheal cartilaginous rings. It varies in size from a thin band to a broad thick band, or it may be absent. Occasionally an extra lobe, the pyramidal lobe, extends upward from the isthmus in the midline. The apex of each lateral lobe extends between the sternothyroid and inferior constrictor muscles of the pharynx. The lateral surface is covered by the infrahyoid muscles, the sternothyroid, sternohyoid, and omohyoid muscles. The medial surface rests on the trachea, the inferior constrictor muscle of the pharynx, and the esophagus. The recurrent laryngeal nerve runs between these tubular passages. The posterior surface is in contact with the paired parathyroid glands, the prevertebral muscle, the longus colli, the sympathetic trunk, and the carotid sheath. This sheath contains the common carotid artery medially, the internal jugular vein laterally, and the vagus nerve between them posteriorly. The gland is covered by a thin fibrous capsule that is adherent to it and a sheath from the pretracheal layer of deep cervical fascia.[10]

The size and weight of the thyroid are variable. In general, the gland is larger in females than in males, larger with age, and larger in inland populations than in coastal populations. The average weight is 25–35 gm. The lateral lobes measure approximately 5–8 cm vertically and up to 2.5 cm in anteroposterior diameter (Table 13–2).[11]

The gland is highly vascular, with four constant paired superior and inferior thyroid arteries and a single thyroid ima artery. Venous drainage accompanies the arterial pattern in reverse direction.

The thyroid lobes move upward approximately 2 cm when a person swallows.[12] Partial or total aplasia may occur. The isthmus is the structure most frequently affected in aplasia (5%). Aplasia of a lobe occurs most frequently on the left side. Hypoplasia of the thyroid is rare.[13]

A recent application of high-resolution real-time scanning of the thyroid is in the evaluation of the hypothyroid infant. In the neonatal period hypothyroidism may be caused by agenesis of the gland, a nonfunctioning thyroid gland, a gland suppressed by maternal medication, and the "sick" euthyroid gland in prematurity. Infants found to have rare agenesis of the thyroid gland can be started on replacement therapy immediately without fear of suppressing a hypo-

**TABLE 13–2.**

**Dimensions of Thyroid and Parathyroid Glands**

| AGE | TRANSVERSE (CM) | VERTICAL (CM) | ANTEROPOSTERIOR (CM) |
|---|---|---|---|
| *Thyroid Gland* | | | |
| Newborn to 2 yr | 1–1.5 | 2–3 | 0.18–1.2 |
| Adult | | | |
|    Lobe | 2–4 | 5–8 | 1–2.5 |
|    Isthmus | 2 | 2 | 0.2–0.6 |
| *Parathyroid Gland* | | | |
| Newborn | 1.9–2.4 | 3 | 1.2–1.4 |
| Adult | 3–4 | 4–15 | 1.5–2 |

functioning gland. In the neonate or infant whose mother is known to be taking thyroid suppressant medication, visualization of a normal-appearing thyroid gland allows the clinician to observe the infant for the expected slow rise in thyroid function.[14]

## Equipment

With the advent of gray-scale imaging techniques, thyroid sonography became an established clinical examination. Gray-scale recording of low-level amplitude information from the internal structure of the gland facilitated the differentiation of normal from pathologic conditions.[15] Contact scanning of the angular neck contour became technically easier when transducer with smaller diameters were developed. The subsequent development and use of high-resolution (7.5- and 10-MHz) transducers has resulted in improved resolution: less than 1 mm in the axial plane and 1–2 mm laterally. Real-time imaging with enclosed water bath, high-frequency transducers allows the examiner to rapidly survey the internal tissue texture and pulsations of thyroid and neck masses at the time of examination. The field of view of these scanners is 3–6 cm, so the use of linear-array or contact scanners with linear motions results in maximal gland imaging. Sector scanners with their pie-shaped image may require a water delay system to image the superficial layers. When a large mass lesion is present in the neck, the examiner may use a lower frequency transducer (5- or 3.5-MHz) with short internal focal ranges to image the extent of the tumor and the adjacent neck anatomy.

## Examination Technique

Patients are examined in the supine position with the shoulders positioned on a folded pillow to hyperextend the neck. The head may be turned away from the side being scanned. It is important to palpate the gland and if necessary outline on the patient's skin surface with a felt-tipped pen the location of the nodules designated as nonfunctioning on a prior isotope study. Contact solution, either water-soluble gel or mineral oil, is applied to the skin.

Transverse scans of the entire gland from the supraclavicular fossa cephalad are performed in a continuous motion with real-time equipment and at 1-cm intervals with contact B-mode scanners. Bilateral longitudinal views are obtained by moving from the greater vascular bundle medially. Multiple oblique and angled projections may be necessary, especially when examining a multinodular gland.

Landmarks to be identified on every thyroid scan are the anterior wall of the trachea in the midline, the carotid sheath laterally, and the strap muscles of the neck. Air in the trachea reflects the sound beam and results in a midline shadow under the strong anterior trachea-wall interface. Reverberation echoes often occur within this acoustic shadow. The carotid sheath along the posterior lateral margin of the thyroid contains the common carotid artery. Its walls image as strongly echo-reflective surfaces. On a transverse single-sweep contact scan they may appear as two parallel echoes, whereas on a compound scan, a circle is imaged when the lateral walls reflect the sound beam. On longitudinal scans, the demonstration of two parallel strongly echo-reflective surfaces at the posterior lateral margin of the gland identifies the walls of the carotid artery, which mark the lateral boundary of the thyroid lobe. The fluid-filled artery lumen acts as an echo-free reference standard to be compared with echo-free spaces within the thyroid gland. The walls of the external jugular vein give weaker echo reflections than the artery. The echo-free vein varies in size with respiration, attaining maximum diameter with a Valsalva maneuver. The strap muscles of the neck appear anterior and lateral to the gland and are relatively echo free compared to the gland.

Visualization of the prevertebral muscles posteriorly indicates adequate penetration for visualization of the entire thyroid gland area. Real-time imaging allows identification of the pulsations of the common carotid artery and numerous small vessels running through the thyroid gland, especially at the periphery. Changes in caliber of the internal jugular veins with respiration are also visualized. These reference landmarks aid the examiner in distinguishing between intrinsic mass pulsations and the transmitted pulsations from adjacent vessels.[16]

The use of high-resolution real-time equipment with its limited penetration and small field of view (4–6 cm) may result in segments of the thyroid gland not being imaged in any one view. The typical anatomic landmarks may be absent. Thus, it is important that the person doing the final reporting be present during the examination.

The normal thyroid gland has a homogeneous medium gray-level echo texture. The parenchyma images through diffuse reflections, and is thus independent of the angle of inclination of the ultrasound beam.[15] In a series of 28 cadaver thyroids scanned in vitro with 7.5- and 10-MHz transducers, Katz et al. demonstrated thin echogenic lines within the normal thyroid gland, which represented fibrous septa. They also observed occasional 3- mm-diameter oval echo-free spaces with no acoustic enhancement, which represented dilated colloid follicles within normal glands.[17] The fibrous tissue capsule of the thyroid gland is not imaged unless it is thickened.

## Pathology

Enlargement of the thyroid gland may be diffuse or nodular. Graves' disease, acute and subacute thyroiditis, lymphadenoid goiter, and Riedel's struma cause diffuse enlargement of both lobes and the isthmus of the gland.[18] In acute conditions the thyroid appears enlarged on ultrasound scans and is hypoechoic compared to the normal thyroid. In subacute thyroiditis (de Quervain's thyroiditis) or chronic thyroiditis (Hashimoto's disease), discrete nodular areas of increased and decreased echogenicity can be imaged. In Hashimoto's thyroiditis the echo pattern is diffusely abnormal and the gland is enlarged. The diagnosis is based on clinical and laboratory studies, as ultrasound findings cannot be used to differentiate chronic thyroiditis from multinodular goiter.[2] As the acute changes resolve, the gland decreases in size and the echogenicity increases, presumably because of the development of fibrous tissue and calcification within the gland.

Repeated involvement of the thyroid gland by hyperplasia and involution causes alternating enlargement and regression of the thyroid tissue. This results in a multinodular configuration developing in the gland, with individual nodules measuring 1–4 cm in diameter. Hemorrhage or degenerative changes occur within the nodules and appear on sonograms as central, predominantly fluid-filled areas with dispersed, low-level, scattered echoes or irregular solid septations. These adenomatous nodules have an incomplete fibrous tissue capsule and contain areas of dystrophic calcification. The overall glandular configuration is distorted as the gland enlarges, and no recognizable normal thyroid parenchyma may be imaged.[2, 17] Large glands may extend into the upper thorax and mediastinum. Computed tomography (CT) is indicated to image intrathoracic goiters.[19] Ultrasound examination of a patient with a multinodular goiter cannot distinguish malignant nodules from benign. Rapid growth of a thyroid mass in a preexisting goiter is the most common manifestation of anaplastic carcinoma of the thyroid.[20] Fine-needle aspiration biopsy under ultrasound guidance is recommended to select a site of sampling for histologic evaluation and avoid areas of hemorrhage and necrosis.[4, 10]

### Mass Lesions

Follicular adenomas are the most frequently occurring solid nodules in the thyroid gland.[21] On a sonogram they exhibit variable echogenicity. Most are hypoechoic relative to the normal thyroid, although a few are of the same echogenicity as the normal thyroid and a few are hyperechoic. The majority are solitary and totally surrounded by a 0.5-mm fibrous capsule. On a sonogram a 1- to 2-mm uniform echo-poor rim at the periphery of a nodule, the "halo" sign, represents the fibrous capsule and adjacent inflammatory changes.[16, 22] The halo sign is seen in approximately 60% of follicular adenomas.[2] Small adenomas are initially contained within the thyroid lobes. As they grow they compress the adjacent thyroid tissue and bulge outward along the periphery of the gland. Many of the adenomas contain a small amount of fluid due to internal hemorrhage and necrosis. The majority do not contain as much fluid as the adenomatous nodules of multinodular goiters. The occasional pure follicular carcinoma of the thyroid may be ultrasonographically indistinguishable from a benign follicular adenoma.[2] The presence of a capsular "halo" has been reported in both benign and malignant nodules.[2, 22]

When a palpable cold nodule images as a solid mass, the physician may elect to follow up the patient clinically to evaluate the response of the mass to suppression therapy. This therapeutic approach is based on the effectiveness of administration of thyroid hormone in doses sufficient to suppress endogenous thyroid-stimulating hormone (TSH). If ultrasonographic evaluation shows a decrease in size or disappearance of the thyroid nodule, the nodule is designated TSH dependent and is likely a benign adenoma. Follow-up clinical and ultrasound studies at monthly intervals have shown a 50% decrease in size of an adenoma within 3 months.[6] This change in size has been observed with nodules designated as solid on ultrasound examination. If the nodule has a complex appearance, with evidence of hemorrhage or degeneration, then only slight or no decrease in size with suppression therapy is likely. Both the solid nodule, which is not suppressed, and the complex nodule require fine-needle aspiration or biopsy to determine if the nodule is malignant.[21]

Irradiation of the head and neck region, usually of low dosage, results in an increased frequency of thyroid, parathyroid, and salivary gland tumors. Papillary or mixed papillary-follicular carcinoma is the commonest type of thyroid carcinoma.[8, 23] One study reported that parathyroid adenomas were the most frequent tumor in patients with primary hyperparathyroidism and mucoepidermoid carcinoma was the commonest salivary gland tumor.[9] A latent period of 10–25 years following irradiation, both in children and in adults, is typical before the appearance of tumors. Occasionally a tumor may develop at more than one of the above sites. There is an association between hyperparathyroidism and malignant thyroid tumors (1.2%–11.4%) which may be related to previous irradiation.[9]

*Thyroid Cancer*

Carcinoma of the thyroid is relatively rare, compared to benign adenoma. It accounts for less than 0.5% of cancer deaths per year.[24] This neoplasm has a slow growth pattern and remains within the confines of the thyroid gland for many years. The major presenting symptoms include a lump in the neck, a history of an enlarging goiter, hoarseness, pressure symptoms, and pain. The major presenting signs are a solitary thyroid nodule, a multinodular gland, and a lateral neck mass.[25] Extension beyond the thyroid capsule frequently results in metastasis to the lateral lymph nodes in the neck, which may bring the patient to the attention of a clinician. At some centers the patient may be spared bilateral thyroidectomies if a preoperative ultrasound examination discloses a unilateral lesion. The primary lesion, particularly papillary carcinoma, may be too small to detect clinically or by scintigraphy within the gland. Malignant lesions in the 5-mm range have been imaged with high-resolution real-time techniques.[1, 2] The majority of thyroid carcinomas image as hypoechoic solid masses relative to the normal gland. The margins between the tumor

and the normal thyroid parenchyma are usually distinct; however, they may be irregular or exhibit a halo sign. Predominantly papillary carcinoma occurs in the fourth and fifth decades of life and is three times more frequent in women than in men. The majority of papillary carcinomas are solid hypoechoic masses, though cystic papillary carcinomas do occur.[2] Needle aspiration biopsy under ultrasound guidance is a sensitive method to distinguish cystic papillary carcinoma from cystic degeneration within a benign nodule.[26] Follicular thyroid carcinoma occurs in approximately 18% of thyroid malignancies. Unless there is extension outside the thyroid capsule, these lesions may be ultrasonographically indistinguishable from benign follicular adenomas. Hemorrhage and cystic degeneration are not as prominent within carcinomas as within adenomas. Most thyroid carcinomas are of the mixed papillary-follicular type. Other histologic types include medullary carcinomas (3%), anaplastic carcinomas (3%), lymphomas (2%), and sarcomas (1%).[24]

Microcalcifications (< 1 mm diameter) are most commonly associated with papillary carcinomas as psammoma calcifications. On a sonogram, microcalcifications may appear as punctate or linear echogenic foci. A roentgenogram of the area is usually more definitive. Microcalcifications may also be imaged in follicular and undifferentiated carcinomas; however, they are not found in normal thyroid tissue. Calcifications found in medullary carcinoma are granular and lie within the fibrous stroma or within amyloid masses, which are present in more than 50% of tumors. The majority of calcifications imaged within the thyroid gland occur in benign conditions (e.g., adenomas, multinodular goiter, postinflammatory thyroiditis, and posthemorrhagic necrosis). Benign calcifications have a coarse appearance and tend to be located within the center of the masses. Acoustic shadowing is frequently noted posterior to the coarse calcifications, which image as bright echogenic areas. Calcifications in benign adenomas are rare. They are curvilinear and are often present at the periphery of the nodule.[27] Peripheral eggshell calcifications also occur in the wall of thyroid cysts.

Ultrasound examinations have been used to detect recurrent thyroid carcinoma in patients who have been previously operated on for thyroid malignancy. Both palpation and reexploration are difficult in these patients because of scarring. Malignant masses, particularly hypoechoic papillary tumors, may be imaged in the thyroid bed.[2]

Primary malignant tumors from other sites may metastasize to the thyroid gland. The patient typically presents with an enlarging thyroid nodule that fails to trap radioiodine. An ultrasound examination of the mass confirms its location, either within the thyroid lobes or in an extraglandular location. There are no reliable criteria to differentiate primary or secondary thyroid malignancy from benign tumors; thus biopsy is generally required.[3, 6, 28] Since follicular thyroid carcinoma can image as an intraluminal mass when angioinvasion occurs, evaluation of the jugular vein and superior vena cava should be performed.[29] Metastatic hypernephroma to the thyroid may also spread via tumor extension along the thyroid veins to produce a tumor thrombus within the internal jugular vein.[30]

Ultrasound examination shows a fluid-filled area in 11%–20% of patients referred for ultrasonographic evaluation of a cold nodule detected on radionuclide studies.[6] True epithelial-lined cysts of the thyroid gland are rare. The majority of fluid-filled regions within the gland represent hemorrhagic or colloid degeneration within adenomas. Acute hemorrhagic cysts appear spontaneously as rapidly enlarging neck masses. On sonograms they appear as predominantly cystic areas with irregular borders and multiple internal septations.

An anteriorly located neck mass on a line from the base of the tongue to the sternal notch usually represents a thyroglossal duct remnant. Thyroglossal duct cysts occasionally develop along the duct remnant. They may enlarge suddenly secondary to infection or hemorrhage. On sonograms they appear as fluid-containing areas with multiple bright internal echoes.[10, 20]

## Salivary Glands

In a study of 20 volunteers, Bartlett and Pon found the submandibular gland could be imaged using 5- and 10-MHz linear-array and small parts scanners.[31] The gland is located in the submandibular fossa and lies between the mandible laterally and the mylohyoid muscle medially and superiorly. A deep portion of the gland curves around the posterior border of the mylohyoid muscle and extends anteriorly between the mylohyoid and hypoglossus muscles. The duct exits from the deep portion of the gland and extends anteriorly to its termination in the floor of the mouth along the plica sublingualis. The mylohyoid muscle is a constant landmark superficial to the duct anteriorly and deep to

the submandibular gland on sagittal scans along the ramus of the mandible.

On a sonogram the parenchyma of the gland is moderately echogenic and homogeneous, similar to the ultrasound appearance of the thyroid gland. In 57% of the examinations the extraglandular ductal elements were imaged at the hilum or anteriorly and measured less than 2 mm in diameter. In one patient the duct lumen increased to 3 mm after the patient sucked on a lemon. A calculus appeared as a bright echogenic focus with posterior acoustic shadowing within a dilated submandibular duct. Enlargement of the gland, whether from inflammation or tumor, can be imaged and differentiated from enlarged cervical lymph nodes.[31]

The parotid gland, located at the angle of the mandible, can be scanned with contact or real-time equipment in sagittal and coronal planes.[32] The gland images with homogeneous medium gray-level echoes similar to the thyroid gland. It enlarges with inflammatory disease, acute parotitis, and tumor. Acute parotitis images with decreased echogenicity. Abscesses can occur distal to obstructed ducts and appear as focal echo-poor regions with irregular margins. Calculi within the parotid gland appear on sonograms as bright echogenic foci with distal shadowing.[33] Parotid tumors are well-circumscribed hypoechoic solid masses. As they enlarge, hemorrhage or myxoid degeneration and calcifications occur. Sonography can be useful in determining whether palpable neck masses are within the salivary glands or extrinsic, within adjacent lymph nodes.[34]

## Extrathyroidal Neck Masses

Branchial cysts appear to develop from remnants of the cervical sinus, an internal sinus connecting the branchial pouches and clefts. High-lying cysts of second cleft origin are found anterior to the internal carotid artery (derived from the third branchial arch). Cysts of third cleft origin are found posterior to the internal carotid artery. The typical lower lying cyst is found anterior to the common carotid artery along the anterior border of the sternocleidomastoid muscle.

The infant or patient presents with a lateral neck mass. On a sonogram the mass is predominantly cystic and contains some low-level internal echoes, which may assume a dependent layer with change of position. The mass may show minimal wall irregularity and exhibit good through-transmission. It is separate from the thyroid gland, anterior and lateral to the carotid sheath, and anterior to the sternocleidomastoid muscle. Branchial cleft cysts are solitary, typically unilateral, and can be differentiated from cystic hygroma, which is multiloculated and normally found in children less than 2 years old.[35] A simple abscess in the lateral neck may be indistinguishable from a branchial cleft cyst, as both may appear anechoic with internal debris. Adenopathy, either inflammatory or neoplastic, appears as relatively anechoic lateral neck masses on a sonogram. Typically, several confluent masses are imaged with adenopathy, and their walls appear as bright echogenic septations within a larger lesion.[36] Calcifications can occur in cervical lymph nodes containing metastatic disease.

Nodal metastases of head and neck carcinomas and lymphomas are the most frequent cause of malignant lateral neck adenopathy. Metastatic disease and Hodgkin's disease image as enlarged nodes (> 1 cm in diameter) with a heterogeneous echo pattern. Non-Hodgkin's disease shows a homogeneous low-level echo pattern in the enlarged nodes.[28] The position and condition of the neck vessels can be evaluated with real-time imaging. Enlarged nodes may cause thrombosis of veins, whereas the arterial trunks are usually displaced.

## Parathyroid

Currently, the diagnosis of hyperparathyroidism is based on clinical and chemical criteria. Widespread clinical use of automated biochemical screening profiles has identified a population of patients with asymptomatic hypercalcemia.[37] Over 90% of patients with hypercalcemia who have hyperparathyroidism can be diagnosed from the results of serum parathyroid hormone (PTH) assay. In the remaining 5%–10% and in the few patients with overt malignancy, hypercalcemia and slightly elevated serum PTH levels along with sonographic or CT localization of parathyroid enlargement may confirm the diagnosis. Imaging can demonstrate enlarged parathyroid glands. The traditional demonstration of skeletal, soft tissue, renal, and gastrointestinal lesions is now less significant in the diagnosis of hyperparathyroidism. PTH assay is independent of thyroid pathology, previous surgery, or ectopic glands.

### Preoperative Parathyroid Localization

Clinicians request parathyroid localization to determine the site of enlarged glands before surgery in patients with the diagnosis of hyperparathyroidsm. Parathyroid glands, whether normal or abnormal, are found in the neck near the thyroid gland in 90% of patients.[38] The standard surgical technique is primary neck exploration to examine both sides of the neck and expose at least four parathyroid glands. In the hands of experienced surgeons this technique has a 95% success rate.[39] Wang has advocated unilateral neck exploration with removal of a single enlarged gland and identification of one normal gland for adenomas as the incidence of multiple adenomas is low, approximately 4.5%.[38, 48] In patients with hyperplasia he advocates removal of three and one-half glands, or excision of all glands and transplantation of parathyroid tissue into the muscles of the forearm with cryopreservation of remaining tissue. Correct preoperative localization and unilateral neck exploration can save 2–3 hours of operative time, and there is a lower rate of post-operative symptomatic hypocalcemia.

In approximately 5%–10% of patients with hyperparathyroidism the glands are located ectopically, either in the neck or in the mediastinum.[38] Searching for ectopic adenomas during an operation is time-consuming and difficult. Following initial surgery, a small percentage of patients remain hypercalcemic or redevelop hyperparathyroidism, and further surgery is necessary. Noninvasive preoperative localizing procedures are important in these patients. Methods include scintigraphy, superselective angiography and/or venous sampling, digital subtraction angiography, sonography, and CT of the neck and mediastinum.[41–44]

### Parathyroid Anatomy

Two pair of parathyroid glands are normally located in the neck along the posterior medial surface of the lateral thyroid lobes in close proximity to the minor neurovascular bundle containing the superior and inferior thyroid arteries and the recurrent laryngeal nerve. There are usually four glands. There may be two to ten glands. The normal glands are small, approximately 5 mm in longest diameter, although they have a range of sizes (see Table 13–2). The average weight of a single gland is 30–40 mg.[38] Each gland is flat and discoid, and the echo texture is similar to that of the overlying thyroid gland. For this reason normal-sized glands are rarely imaged on sonography, even with the use of high-frequency transducers. Enlarged glands (> 5 mm dimension) have a decreased echo texture and appear sonographically as elongated masses between the posterior longus colli muscle and the anterior thyroid lobe. The glands are surrounded by an echogenic line thought to represent the fibrous tissue capsule and fascia separating them from the thyroid gland. The parathyroids usually lie outside the thyroid capsule but may rest within it and be adjacent to the posterior thyroid tissue. If a parathyroid adenoma is within the thyroid gland, it typically has an echogenic margin which aids in the distinction from an adenomatous thyroid gland. However, the diagnosis of intrathyroid masses is difficult when thyroid gland abnormalities are also present.[45]

The location of the glands is variable. Approximately 5% will be found in other regions of the neck or in a substernal position.[13, 38] The superior parathyroid glands originate from the dorsal aspect of the fourth branchial pouch. Their location is usually close to the superoposterior thyroid lobes. Enlarged glands have been found behind the esophagus, between the trachea and thyroid, within the thyroid, and in the posterosuperior mediastinum.

The inferior parathyroid glands originate from the dorsal aspect of the third branchial pouch. They usually lie close to the posterior medial inferior surface of the lateral thyroid lobes. Enlarged glands have been located within the carotid sheath, behind the esophagus, in the anterior mediastinum, within or adjacent to the thymus, and adjacent to the aortic arch and pericardium.[13] If an enlarged gland is located in an ectopic position it assumes a spherical shape.[45]

A dual tracer imaging technique using two isotopes (thallium 201 and technetium 99m) and computer subtraction of the images has a high sensitivity and specificity for localization of parathyroid adenomas.[46] False positive studies can occur with overlying thyroid gland abnormalities. Thallium imaging alone may detect uptake in adenomas located in ectopic positions in the mediastinum or pericardium.

High-resolution CT of the neck and mediastinum with the bolus injection of contrast agent has a reported sensitivity of 76% and a specificity of 89% in the detection of enlarged glands.[47] Tumor size was related to the diagnostic sensitivity. Enlarged glands

must be differentiated from enlarged lymph nodes, which are usually located laterally. In patients with allergies to intravenous contrast agents or poor renal function, lymph nodes or tortuous vessels may be a problem. CT scans in patients with previous surgery may be difficult to interpret due to distorted anatomy, postsurgical fibrosis, and streak artifacts from metallic clips.

Sonography using high-frequency scanners has resulted in the detection of 85% of enlarged glands in the neck (Table 13–3). A literature review of 10-MHz parathyroid ultrasound shows a sensitivity of 65%–88% and a specificity of 94%–98%.[2, 43, 47–49] In a series of patients with persistent or recurrent hyperparathyroidism after surgery, use of 10-MHz sonography resulted in a sensitivity of 82% for the detection of abnormal glands in the neck.[50] The mediastinum cannot be evaluated by sonography due to the bony thoracic cage. If the sonographic examination of the neck is negative, other localizing studies such as scintigraphy and CT are indicated to search for a mediastinal gland.[47]

### Scan Technique

The patient is placed supine with the neck slightly hyperextended. High-resolution (7.5- and 10-MHz) transducers are used to record transverse and longitudinal scans through the thyroid gland. The lower pole of the thyroid may be elevated from the bony thorax by asking the patient to swallow during real-time observation to detect inferiorly located parathyroid glands. The normal parathyroid glands are seldom identified.[48]

### Pathology

Most large series report single parathyroid adenomas as being responsible for primary hyperparathyroidism

**TABLE 13–3.**
**Primary Indications for Parathyroid Sonography**

Patients newly diagnosed with hyperparathyroidism who are undergoing neck exploration
Patients undergoing repeat neck exploration
Patients with severe hypercalcemia, in search of a parathyroid adenoma
Monitoring aspiration-biopsy procedures

in approximately 80% of cases. Hyperplasia of the glands accounts for 13.5% of cases of primary hyperthyroidism, multiple adenomas for 4.5%, and carcinoma for less than 2%.[42]

Secondary hyperparathyroidism due to chronic renal disease can result in mild enlargement of the parathyroid glands that may be difficult to image on a sonogram. In most cases all the glands are involved in the hyperplasia. However, there are reports of patients with only a single gland involved in hyperplasia.[39]

On a sonogram parathyroid tumors image as discrete, sharply marginated solid nodules. Their echogenicity varies from homogeneous to an inhomogeneous pattern. There are no distinguishing characteristics to identify an adenoma versus hyperplasia or carcinoma.

The presence of a single enlarged gland favors the diagnosis of an adenoma. When multiple enlarged glands are imaged, hyperplasia is the commonest etiology, although multiple adenomas occur in 4.5% of cases of hyperparathyroidism.[40] Hyperplastic glands may be within the normal parathyroid size range, or minimally enlarged. In the series reported by Stark et al., high-resolution sonography was superior to CT for the detection of multiple hyperplastic glands because these tumors were relatively small and sonography is less dependent on tumor size than is CT.[47] Cystic degeneration occurs occasionally within large parathyroid adenomas; however, it is not as common as within thyroid adenomas.

Misinterpretation of normal structures in the neck is not uncommon as they may mimic parathyroid enlargement. The minor neurovascular bundle (inferior thyroid artery and the recurrent laryngeal nerve) has a maximum diameter of 5 mm and can be confused with a normal parathyroid gland.[48] Asymmetry of the longus colli muscles can be mistaken for a parathyroid mass on a single transverse image; however, imaging the area in two planes will outline the longitudinal extent of the muscle. The collapsed esophagus may image on either side at the tracheothyroid junction. Having the patient swallow water will distend the esophagus, and peristalsis can be observed with real-time scanning. Lymph node groups are typically present along the lateral surface of the thyroid and major neurovascular bundle. Slight enlargement of lymph nodes can be mistaken for an ectopically located parathyroid gland. Posteriorly located thyroid nodules which do not exhibit the halo sign may also be mistaken for an enlarged parathyroid gland.

Parathyroid cysts are rare and may be mistaken for an adjacent thyroid cyst on sonography. The aspirate of a parathyroid cyst is clear and reveals elevated PTH levels.[57] If the patient's serum calcium level is normal, indicating nonfunction, surgery is not required, as no carcinoma has been described in a nonfunctioning parathyroid cyst.[51]

Parathyroid carcinoma typically presents in patients with hyperparathyroidism with a palpable neck mass and spontaneous vocal cord paralysis. The diagnosis is often not made until surgery or pathologic review of excised tissue. Local recurrence is more frequent than distal metastasis. Ultrasound examination shows a hypoechoic mass posterior to the thyroid. If fibrosis is present, the mass may exhibit a greater degree of acoustic attenuation than benign adenomas. Ultrasound has been utilized to guide fine-needle aspiration biopsy of parathyroid tumors.[52]

## References

1. Scheible W, et al: High resolution real-time ultrasonography of thyroid nodules. *Radiology* 1979; 133:413–417.
2. Simeone JF, et al: High resolution real-time sonography of the thyroid. *Radiology* 1982; 145:431–435.
3. Brown CL: Pathology of the cold nodule. *Clin Endocrinol Metab* 1981; 10:235–245.
4. Walfish PG, Hazani E, Strawbridge HTG: Combined ultrasound and needle aspiration cytology in the assessment and management of hypofunctioning thyroid nodule. *Ann Intern Med* 1977; 87:270–274.
5. Rosen IB, Walfish PG, Miskin M: The ultrasound of thyroid masses. *Radiol Clin North Am* 1979; 59:19–33.
6. Ashcraft MW, Van Herle AJ: Management of thyroid nodules. *Head Neck Surg* 1981; 3:216–227.
7. Carroll BA: Asymptomatic thyroid nodules: Incidental sonographic detection. *AJR* 1982; 138:499–501.
8. Favus MJ, et al: Thyroid cancer occurring as a late consequence of head and neck irradiation. *N Engl J Med* 1976; 294:1019–1025.
9. Palmer JA, Mustard RA, Simpson WJ: Irradiation as an etiologic factor in tumors of the thyroid, parathyroid and salivary glands. *Can J Surg* 1980; 23:39–42.

10. Wang CA: Management of thyroid disease based on needle biopsy pathology. *Clin Endocrinol Metab* 1981; 10:293–298.

11. Mortensen JD, et al: Gross and microscopic findings in clinically normal thyroid glands. *J Clin Endocrinol Metab* 1955; 15:1270–1280.

12. Shawker TH, Paling MR, Weintraub B: Dysphagia due to thyroid immobilization: Value of real-time sonography. *AJR* 1981; 136:601–602.

13. Hunt PS, Poole M, Reeve TS: A reappraisal of the surgical anatomy of the thyroid and parathyroid glands. *Br J Surg* 1968; 55:63–66.

14. Pasto MEP, et al: High resolution scanning of the thyroid in infancy: The sonographic spectrum in hypothyroidism. *J Ultrasound Med* 1984; 3:116.

15. Jellins J, et al: Ultrasonic gray-scale visualization of the thyroid gland. *Ultrasound Med Biol* 1975; 1:405–410.

16. Hassani SN, Bard RL: Evaluation of solid thyroid neoplasms by gray scale and real-time ultrasonography: The "halo" sign. *Ultrasound Med* 1977; 4:323–328.

17. Katz JF, et al: Thyroid nodules: Sonographic-pathologic correlation. *Radiology* 1984; 151:741–745.

18. Blum M, et al: Thyroid echography of subacute thyroditis. *Radiology* 1977; 125:795–798.

19. Barhit B, Ellis K, Gold RP: Computed tomography of intrathoracic goiters. *AJR* 1983; 140:455–460.

20. Suen KC, Quenville NF: Fine needle aspiration biopsy of the thyroid gland: A study of 304 cases. *J Clin Pathol* 1983; 36:1036–1045.

21. Mazzaferri EL: Solitary thyroid nodule: Selective approach to management. *Postgrad Med* 1981; 70:107–109.

22. Propper RA, et al: The nonspecificity of the thyroid halo sign. *JCU* 1980; 8:129–132.

23. Schneider AB, et al: Characteristics of 108 thyroid cancers detected by screening in a population with a history of head and neck irradiation. *Cancer* 1980; 46:1218–1227.

24. Rosen IB: Diagnostic studies of thyroid cancer. *J Surg Oncol* 1981; 16:233–250.

25. Wanebo HJ, Andrews W, Kaiser DL: Thyroid cancer: Some basic considerations. *Cancer* 1983; 33:87–98.

26. Muller N, et al: Needle aspiration biopsy in cystic papillary carcinoma of the thyroid. *AJR* 1985; 144:251–253.

27. Ciatti S, et al: Microcalcifications and malignancy in cold thyroid nodules detected by ultrasound. *J Fr Echographie* 1983; 8:26–27.

28. Sirota DK, Segal RL: Primary lymphomas of the thyroid gland. *JAMA* 1979; 242:1743–1746.

29. Perez D, Brown L: Follicular carcinoma of the thyroid appearing as an intraluminal superior vena cava tumor. *Arch Surg* 1984; 119:323–326.

30. Chatzkel S, et al: Ultrasound diagnosis of a hypernephroma metastatic to the thyroid gland and external jugular vein. *Radiology* 1982; 142:165–166.

31. Bartlett LJ, Pon M: High-resolution real-time ultrasonography of the submandibular salivary gland. *J Ultrasound Med* 1984; 3:433–437.

32. Gooding GAW: Gray-scale ultrasound of the parotid gland. *AJR* 1980; 134:469–472.

33. Pickrell KL, Trough WS, Shearin JC: The use of ultrasound to localize calculi within the parotid gland. *Ann Plast Surg* 1978; 1:543–546.

34. Gooding GAW, et al: Ultrasonic assessment of neck masses. *JCU* 1977; 5:248–252.

35. Kittredge RD, Finby N: The many facets of lymphangioma. *AJR* 1965; 95:56–66.

36. Badami JP, Athey PA: Sonography in the diagnosis of branchial cysts. *AJR* 1981; 137:1245–1248.

37. Heath H, Hodgson SF, Kennedy MA: Primary hyperparathyroidism: Incidence, morbidity and potential impact in a community. *N Engl J Med* 1980; 302:189–193.

38. Wang CA: The anatomic basis of parathyroid surgery. *Ann Surg* 1976; 183:271–275.

39. Edis AJ, et al: Conservative versus liberal approach to parathyroid neck exploration. *Surgery* 1977; 82:466–473.

40. Carnevale N, Samson R, Bennett BP: Multiple parathyroid adenomas. *JAMA* 1981; 246:1332–1333.

41. Doppman JL, et al: Aspiration of enlarged parathyroid glands for parathyroid hormone assay. *Radiology* 1983; 148:31–35.

42. Duffy P, et al: Parathyroid sonography: A useful aid to preoperative localization. *JCU* 1980; 8:113–116.

43. Scheible W, Deutsch A, Leopold G: Parathyroid adenoma: Accuracy of preoperative localization

by high-resolution real-time sonography. *JCU* 1981; 9:325–330.

44. Simeone J, et al: High resolution real time sonography of the parathyroid. *Radiology* 1981; 141:743–751.

45. Moreau JP, et al: Localization of parathyroid tumors by ultrasonography. *N Engl J Med* 1980; 302:582–583.

46. Park CH, et al: Dual tracer imaging for localization of parathyroid adenomas. *Radiology* 1984; 153:35.

47. Stark DD, et al: Parathyroid imaging: Comparison of high resolution CT and high-resolution sonography. *AJR* 1983; 141:633–638.

48. Sample WF, Mitchell SP, Bledsoe RC: Parathyroid ultrasonography. *Radiology* 1978; 127:485–490.

49. Reading CC, et al: High resolution parathyroid sonography. *AJR* 1982; 139:539–546.

50. Reading CC, et al. Postoperative parathyroid high-frequency sonography: Evaluation of persistent or recurrent hyperparathyroidism. *AJR* 1985; 144:399–402.

51. Clark OH: Parathyroid cysts. *Am J Surg* 1978; 135:395–402.

52. Solbiati L, et al: Ultrasonically guided fine-needle aspiration biopsy of parathyroid tumors. *Ultrasound Med Biol* 1982; 8:181–189.

# CASES

## Dennis A. Sarti, M.D.

### Normal Thyroid

Figure 13–1 is an anatomic drawing of the neck in the region of the thyroid gland. The lobes of the thyroid are situated on each side of the trachea. A small isthmus of the thyroid is seen anterior to the trachea. On ultrasound examination, the trachea will appear as a strong echo posterior to the isthmus. Deep to the trachea will be a shadow secondary to air. The lobes of the thyroid are situated on each side of the trachea and are usually fairly symmetric. Posterior to the trachea is the esophagus. We usually do not see the esophagus on an ultrasound examination, since it is situated posterior to the air-filled trachea. Lateral to the lobes of the thyroid are the common carotid artery and the deep jugular vein. This major neurovascular bundle also includes the vagus nerve. The carotid artery and the jugular vein can be visualized and the jugular vein can be visualized on ultrasound. Posterior to the lobes of the thyroid are found the inferior thyroid artery and the recurrent laryngeal nerve, together known as the minor neurovascular bundle. The minor neurovascular bundle is extremely important in attempting to evaluate parathyroid adenomas. Posterior to the esophagus and trachea are the muscles situated anterior to the cervical vertebrae. The longus colli muscles are also important ana-

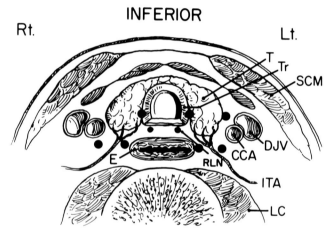

FIG 13–1.

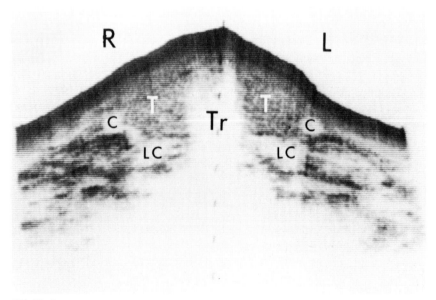

FIG 13–2.

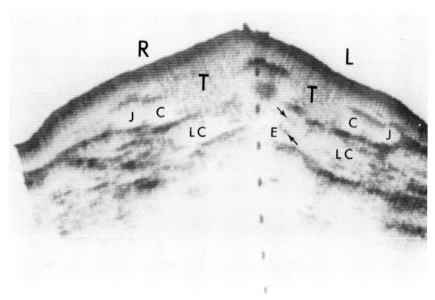

**FIG 13–3.**

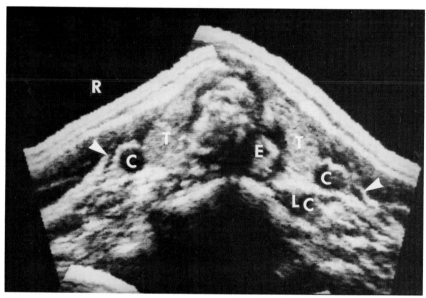

**FIG 13–4.**

mately 5 mm thick or less. We cannot distinguish the normal parathyroid from the minor neurovascular bundle. Therefore, anything 5 mm thick or smaller is considered within normal limits. If a mass situated between the lobe of the thyroid and the longus colli muscle and larger than 5 mm is consistent with a parathyroid adenoma.

Lateral to the lobes of the thyroid are circular sonolucencies, representing the carotid arteries and jugular veins. Figures 13–2 to 13–4 show variation in the appearance of the jugular veins. In Figure 13–3 both the carotid arteries and jugular veins are well seen. In Figures 13–2 and 13–4, the jugular veins are not identified. They appear as slit-like lucent areas in Figure 13–4 and are not even visible in Figure 13–2. This tremendous variability can cause diagnostic problems. If there is any question at all of the location of the jugular vein, a Valsalva maneuver can be performed. This maneuver will markedly distend the jugular vein, allowing identification of its location.

It is important to recognize the esophagus on scans of the thyroid. The esophagus is usually seen posterior to the left lobe of the thyroid. Unless it is recognized as a normal anatomic structure, a thyroid or parathyroid lesion may be wrongly diagnosed. Figures 13–3 and 13–4 demonstrate a normal-appearing esophagus. There is usually a central echogenic region representing mucosa, surrounded by a lucent rim representing the muscle wall. With high-resolution real-time examination, the patient can swallow or be given water. Air and water can be seen bubbling through the esophagus, confirming the correct diagnosis.

| | | |
|---|---|---|
| **Arrowheads** | = | Collapsed jugular vein |
| **C** | = | Carotid artery |
| **CCA** | = | Common carotid artery |
| **DJV** | = | Jugular vein |
| **E** | = | Esophagus |
| **ITA** | = | Inferior thyroid artery |
| **J** | = | Jugular vein |
| **L** | = | Left |
| **LC** | = | Longus colli |
| **Lt** | = | left |
| **R** | = | Right |
| **RLN** | = | Recurrent larygneal nerve |
| **SCM** | = | Sternocleidomastoid |
| **T** | = | Thyroid |
| **Tr** | = | Trachea |

tomical landmarks in the evaluation of the thyroid and parathyroid.

The parathyroid glands are situated posterior to the lobes of the thyroid. Four parathyroid glands are usually present. The upper-pole parathyroid glands are fairly consistent in location, situated just deep to the thyroid lobes. The parathyroid glands can be mistaken for the minor neurovascular bundle on an ultrasound examination.

Figures 13–2 to 13–4 are transverse scans in the region of the thyroid gland. In Figures 13–2 and 13–4 the lobes are symmetric, but in Figure 13–3 the right thyroid lobe is larger

than the left. This is not an unusual finding in an ultrasound examination.

The thyroid lobes usually have an even homogeneous echo pattern throughout. Situated between the thyroid lobes is the strong echo and shadow of the trachea. There is no sound passing through the trachea because it is air filled. Deep to the lobes of the thyroid are the longus colli muscles. These are extremely important landmarks in an evaluation of the parathyroid region. The parathyroid area is situated between the thyroid and longus colli muscles. The normal parathyroid gland is approxi-

## Normal Thyroid

Figures 13–5 to 13–8 are longitudinal scans through the lobes of the thyroid. The scans in Figures 13–5, 13–6, and 13–8 are all angled medially. The scan in Figure 13–7 is angled laterally. Medial angulation of the transducer usually provides the best skin contact because of the contour of the neck. It also lines up the thyroid and the longus colli muscles. In Figure 13–5 a small tubular lucency can be seen between the thyroid and the longus colli muscle. This lucency is secondary to the minor neurovascular bundle.

The scan in Figure 13–7 was made with lateral angulation of the transducer. The thyroid gland can be seen anterior to the carotid artery. This relationship is usually not visualized with medial transducer angulation, as was done with the other three scans shown here.

All four scans show an even parenchymal pattern to the lobes of the thyroid. In Figure 13–5 there is some difficulty visualizing the upper and lower poles of the thyroid. Both poles are well seen in Figure 13–6, and the lower pole is well seen in Figure 13–8. If the examiner has difficulty visualizing the lower pole on a routine scan, the patient can be asked to swallow. On real-time examination, the lower pole will come into view as the patient swallows. This is very helpful in evaluating lower lobe lesions and parathyroid pathology.

The high-amplitude echoes (arrowheads) in Figure 13–6 are secondary to the cervical vertebrae posterior to the longus colli muscle. In Figure 13–8, there is a different lucent appearance anterior to the vertebral bodies. This is secondary to the esophagus. The high-amplitude echoes of the esophageal lumen distinguish the esophagus from the longus colli muscle. If there is any confusion, the patient can be asked to swallow. Swallowing will introduce air into the esophagus, which is visualized on real-time examination.

Most thyroid ultrasound examinations are performed with high-frequency transducers ranging from 5 to

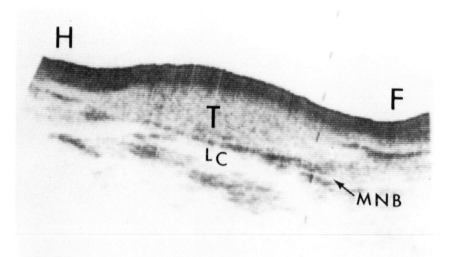

**FIG 13–5.**

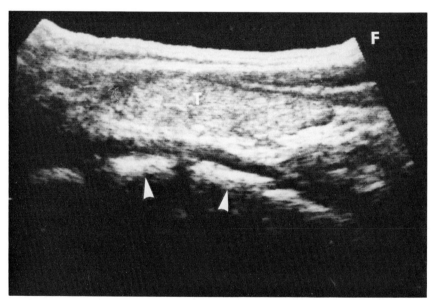

**FIG 13–6.**

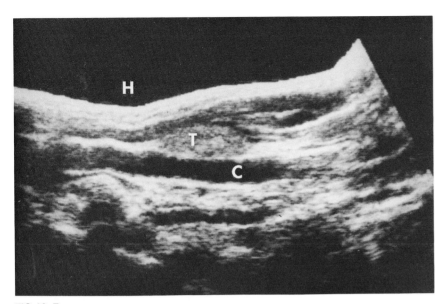

**FIG 13–7.**

10 MHz. Both B-mode and real-time studies may be performed. The increased resolution enables detection of small lesions.

| **Arrowheads** | = | Anterior cervical vertebrae |
| **C** | = | Carotid artery |
| **E** | = | Esophagus |
| **F** | = | Foot |
| **H** | = | Head |
| **LC** | = | Longus colli muscle |
| **MNB** | = | Minor neurovascular bundle |
| **T** | = | Thyroid |

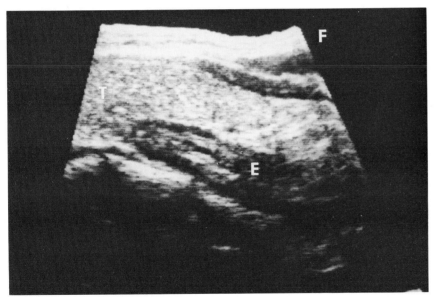

**FIG 13–8.**

## Thyroid Cyst

Ultrasound examination of the thyroid is most commonly performed to examine a cold nodule found on isotope study. The role of the ultrasonographer is to determine whether or not a thyroid cyst is present. If a cyst is detected as the cause of the cold nodule, a follow-up study or a cyst puncture is the next step. If a solid lesion is detected, however, surgery must be considered.

Figure 13–9 is a transverse scan of a patient with a large cyst in the left lobe of the thyroid. The cyst is sonolucent with fairly sharp walls; it is situated medial to the carotid artery and jugular vein. The right lobe of the thyroid has a normal echogenic appearance. Figure 13–10 is a longitudinal scan of another patient with a cyst off the lower pole of the thyroid. The cyst is situated anterior to the longus colli muscle. As in other parts of the body, it has the characteristic of a fluid-filled structure; through-transmission (arrows) is present. The mass is also completely sonolucent and has fairly sharp borders.

Figure 13–11 is a transverse scan of another cyst with through-transmission manifested by increased echogenicity of the left lobe of the thyroid compared with the right. If thyroid tissue is deep to a cyst, through-transmission can be assessed. If the cyst is situated anterior to the vertebral bodies, however, through-transmission cannot be assessed as in other parts of the body. Whenever a fluid-filled mass is situated anterior to a bone or air interface, the amount of through-transmission is difficult to assess because of the high-amplitude echo arising from the bone or air interface.

Figure 13–12 is a longitudinal scan of another thyroid cyst situated in the lower pole of the thyroid. The cyst is anterior to the longus colli muscle. There is excellent visualization of through-transmission (arrows) as the thyroid deep to the cyst has higher amplitude echoes, as does the longus colli muscle.

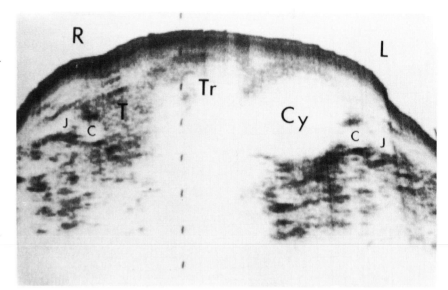

**FIG 13–9.**

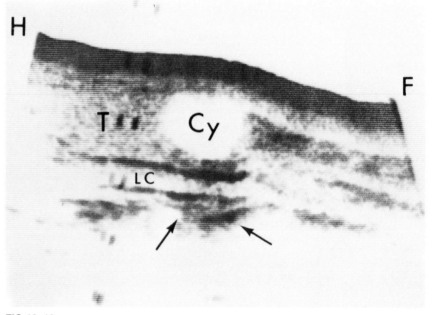

**FIG 13–10.**

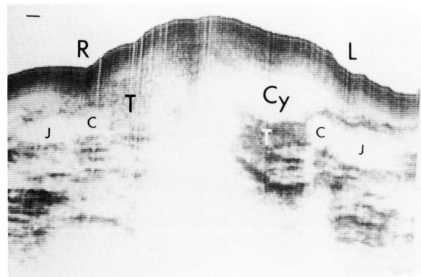

**FIG 13–11.**

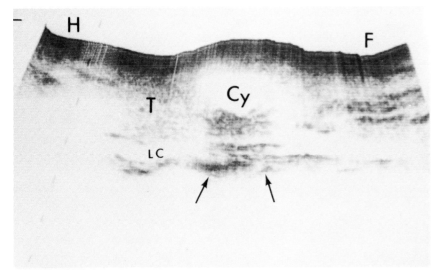

**FIG 13–12.**

| | | |
|---|---|---|
| **Arrows** | = | Through-transmission |
| **C** | = | Carotid artery |
| **Cy** | = | Thyroid cyst |
| **F** | = | Foot |
| **H** | = | Head |
| **J** | = | Jugular vein |
| **L** | = | Left |
| **LC** | = | Longus colli muscle |
| **R** | = | Right |
| **T** | = | Thyroid |
| **Tr** | = | Trachea |

## Thyroid Cyst; Hemorrhagic Cyst

Figure 13–13 is a transverse scan through both lobes of the thyroid. The left lobe of the thyroid has an even-textured echo pattern throughout. In the center of the right lobe of the thyroid is a small 4-mm sonolucent area with prominent through-transmission deep to it. These findings satisfy the ultrasound criteria of a cyst. Even though the lesion is quite small, we are able to identify through-transmission because of the high-frequency transducers that are used in thyroid ultrasound. Usually 5, 7.5-, or 10-MHz transducers are used to evaluate the thyroid. The through-transmission is easily identified on this scan. What are structures 1 and 2?

Figure 13–14 is a longitudinal scan through the right lobe of the thyroid. Thyroid texture is well visualized and is even throughout except for two sonolucent areas. There is a small cyst in the midportion of the lobe of the thyroid. A small amount of through-transmission is identified deep to this structure, indicating that it is a cystic mass. The walls are well circumscribed, and no internal echoes are identified. A second smaller lucent area is seen in the lower posterior aspect of the lobe of the thyroid. In this instance, through-transmission is not identified, for several reasons. The cyst is only 1–2 mm in anteroposterior diameter. Even at high frequencies, through-transmission cannot be identified in such small lesions. A certain volume of fluid is necessary to bring out the ultrasound characteristics of through-transmission. If a lesion is too small for the specified transducer frequency, through-transmission will not be noted. Therefore, an evaluation by the ultrasonographer of the size of the lesion is necessary. A second reason for lack of through-transmission is that the cyst is situated directly against a high-amplitude reflector, the cervical vertebrae. It is always difficult to evaluate enhanced through-transmission when the lesion is abutting a bone or air reflector.

Occasionally a cystic mass will be encountered that gives an extremely

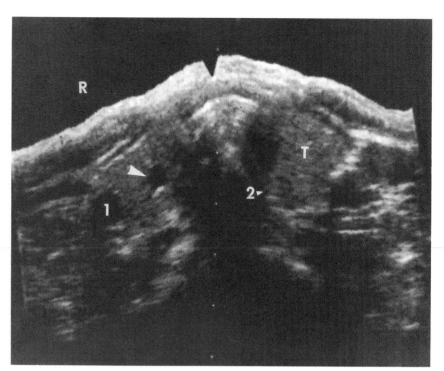

FIG 13–13.

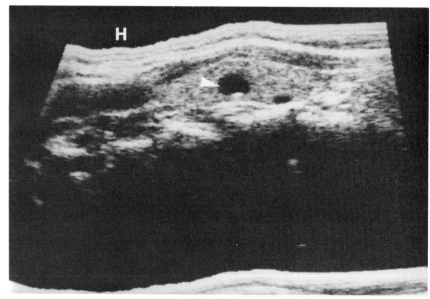

FIG 13–14.

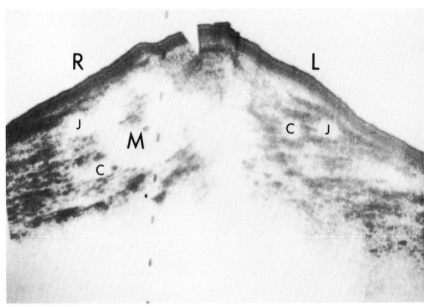

**FIG 13–15.**

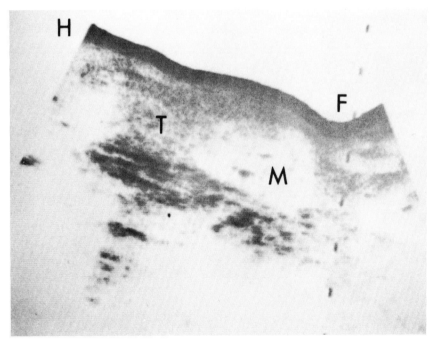

**FIG 13–16.**

confusing ultrasonographic picture. Figures 13–15 and 13–16 are examples of a thyroid cyst which was thought to be a solid mass on ultrasound examination. At surgery, it was found to be a cyst filled with clotted blood. The hemorrhagic cyst is seen in the right lobe of the thyroid (Fig 13–15). The right carotid artery is displaced posteriorly and the right jugular vein is displaced laterally by the mass. A longitudinal scan (Fig 13–16) shows the hemorrhagic cyst in the lower pole of the thyroid. Numerous echoes are noted within the mass. No enhanced through-transmission is identified deep to the mass. These are the reasons why the diagnosis of a solid lesion was made on ultrasound examination.

| Arrowheads | = Cysts |
|---|---|
| C | = Carotid artery |
| F | = Foot |
| H | = Head |
| J | = Jugular vein |
| L | = Left |
| M | = Hemorrhagic cyst |
| R | = Right |
| T | = Thyroid |
| 1 | = Carotid artery |
| 2 | = Esophagus |

## Thyroid Adenoma

Thyroid adenomas present as solid lesions within the thyroid. They may have a lucent periphery on ultrasound. Figures 13–17 and 13–18 are scans obtained from a patient with a large thyroid adenoma found at surgery. The mass is seen on the left side of the thyroid. It is mainly echogenic in its central portion. A longitudinal scan (Fig 13–18) demonstrates a lucent periphery which is casting a shadow deep to it. The shadowing may be due to the velocity change and critical angle phenomenon discussed in the first chapter. The major portion of the mass, however, is echogenic. The effect of the mass on the skin can be seen (Fig 13–18) as the mass is protruding beneath the skin surface.

Figure 13–19 is a transverse scan of the thyroid. A large thyroid adenoma is seen in the right lobe. It has the distinguishing feature of a surrounding lucent halo. When such a well-circumscribed halo is seen, the diagnosis is most often (though not always) a thyroid adenoma. Note the thyroid texture anterior and lateral to the adenoma. It has a slightly different parenchymal pattern than the adenoma itself. What is structure 1 in Figure 13–19?

Figure 13–20 is a transverse scan of the thyroid in a different patient. A subtle texture change in the posterolateral aspect of the left lobe of the thyroid (arrowheads) can be detected. The texture change represents a small solid lesion of the thyroid. At surgery a thyroid adenoma was found that measured 6 × 8 mm. With high-resolution ultrasound, very small lesions within the thyroid parenchyma can be identified. This is an excellent example of such a case: the parenchymal texture change makes the lesion stand out relative to the parenchymal pattern of the thyroid. What is structure 2?

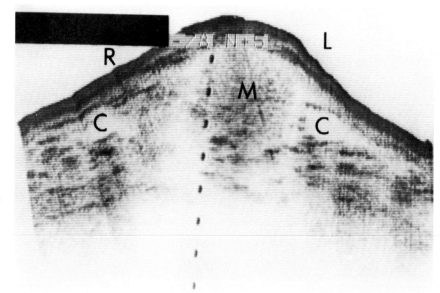

**FIG 13–17.**

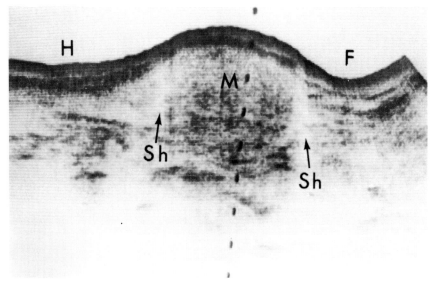

**FIG 13–18.**

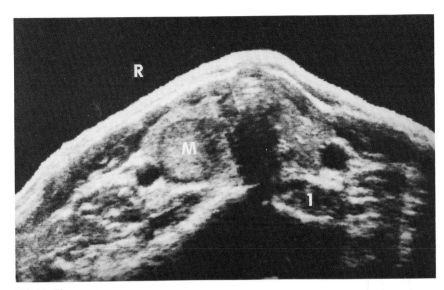

**FIG 13–19.**

| | | |
|---|---|---|
| **Arrowheads** | = | Small thyroid adenoma |
| **C** | = | Carotid artery |
| **F** | = | Foot |
| **H** | = | Head |
| **L** | = | Left |
| **M** | = | Thyroid adenoma |
| **R** | = | Right |
| **Sh** | = | Shadowing behind the lucent periphery of a thyroid adenoma |
| **1** | = | Left longus colli muscle |
| **2** | = | Left jugular vein (note collapsed right jugular vein) |

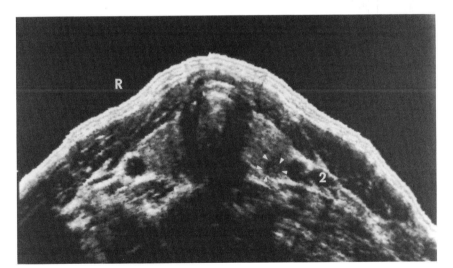

**FIG 13–20.**

## Thyroid Adenoma

The images shown here are from four different patients and illustrate various presentations of thyroid adenomas. Figure 13–21 is a longitudinal scan of patient with two thyroid adenomas of the left lobe found at surgery. A normal portion of the thyroid is seen in the superior region of the left lobe. Two thyroid adenomas (arrows) are seen in the middle and lower poles. A surrounding sonolucent rim is evident in both adenomas. Centrally, there is a highly echogenic region, which is characteristic of a thyroid adenoma.

The central echogenicity does not have any necrotic portion in Figure 13–21. However, Figure 13–22 is a longitudinal scan obtained from another patient which shows a large adenoma with a surrounding sonolucent rim (arrows). Within the sonolucent rim is a highly echogenic area. In the central portion of that echogenic region is a smaller sonolucency that may represent an area of early necrosis.

Figure 13–23 is a transverse scan of another patient with a thyroid adenoma of the right lobe. Again we visualize a surrounding sonolucent rim (arrows) with a more echogenic central portion. In this case, fluid is present within the central highly echogenic region, indicating necrosis and hemorrhage. In Figure 13–24 a large amount of necrosis associated with a thyroid adenoma is visualized. The normal thyroid is situated in the upper left lobe. In the lower left lobe is an echogenic area surrounded by fluid, and a second fluid component inferior to it. This is an example of severe degeneration in a thyroid adenoma.

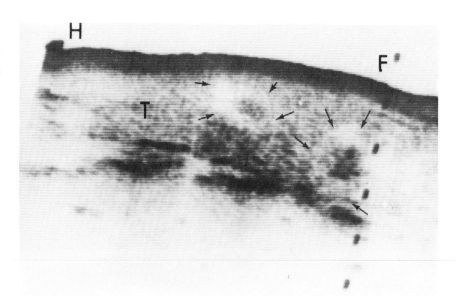

**FIG 13–21.**

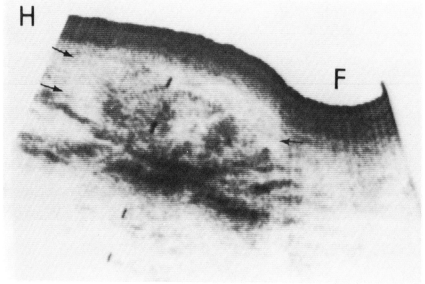

**FIG 13–22.**

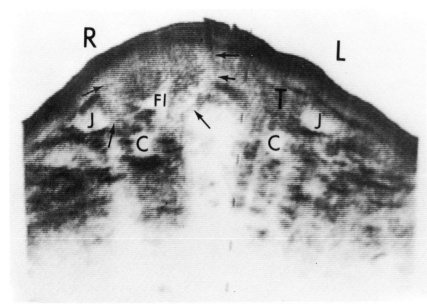

| Arrows | = | Thyroid adenoma |
| C | = | Carotid artery |
| F | = | Foot |
| FI | = | Fluid indicating degeneration and necrosis |
| H | = | Head |
| J | = | Jugular vein |
| L | = | Left |
| M | = | Solid portion within a degenerating thyroid adenoma |
| R | = | Right |
| T | = | Thyroid |

**FIG 13–23.**

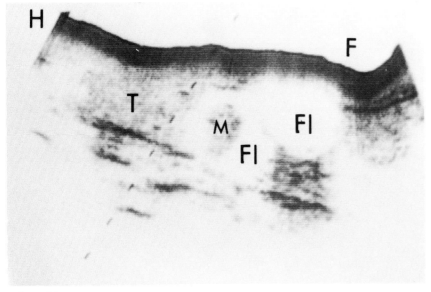

**FIG 13–24.**

## Thyroid Adenoma

When an isotope study is performed and a cold nodule is demonstrated, ultrasound examination is the next procedure to be considered. The main function of the ultrasonographer is to determine whether or not the nodule represents a cystic or solid mass. Occasionally the thyroid mass may have a mixed appearance with both cystic and solid components. This most often is secondary to degeneration.

Figure 13–25 is an isotope scan of the thyroid showing a cold lesion in the lateral aspect of the right lobe. The patient was a 68-year-old woman who had had a palpable nodule in the right lobe for 3 years. The nodule had not changed size in the interim. Because of the cold nodule, ultrasound examination was performed. Figure 13–26 demonstrates a multiloculated cystic lesion in the right lobe of the thyroid. Figure 13–27 is a longitudinal scan through the area. The ultrasound findings were secondary to a degenerating thyroid adenoma with multiple areas of hemorrhage and necrosis. What is structure 1 in Figure 13–26?

Figure 13–28 is the scan of another patient with a thyroid adenoma in the lower pole of the left lobe. The adenoma has a large cystic area with two satellite cystic components present posteriorly. These represent areas of hemorrhage and necrosis. What is structure 2 in this scan?

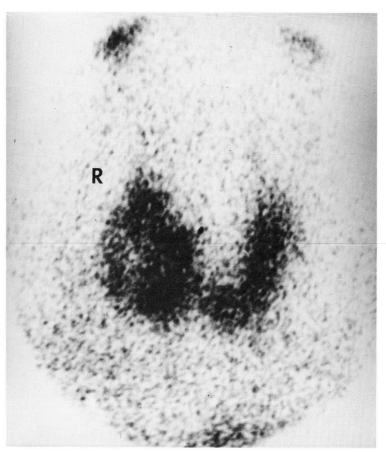

FIG 13–25.

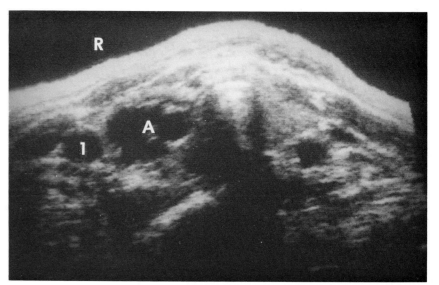

FIG 13–26.

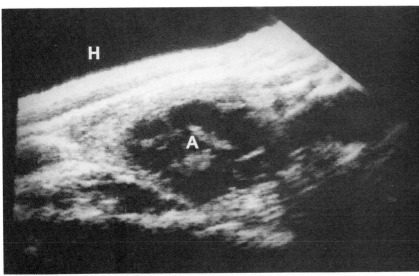

**FIG 13–27.**

A = Degenerating thyroid adenomas
H = Head
R = Right
1 = Right carotid artery
2 = Distended right jugular vein

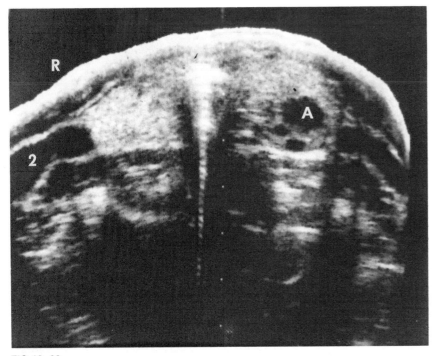

**FIG 13–28.**

## Thyroid Adenomas

Detection of small lesions in the thyroid is made possible by the use of high-frequency transducers. Figures 13–29 and 13–30 are scans obtained with 10-MHz transducers in two different patients. Figure 13–29 is a B-mode scan obtained with a 10-MHz transducer. The patient had a palpable thyroid isthmus, which is more prominent than usual in this scan. In the midportion of the isthmus is an uneven parenchymal pattern with some areas having a more subtle lucency than the left lobe of the thyroid. At operation a thyroid adenoma was found. The isthmus of the thyroid is usually not so prominent. The change in parenchymal texture indicates pathology in the area.

Figure 13–30, a scan obtained with a 10-MHz real-time unit, demonstrates capsular "halo" sign. This capsular sign is thought to be secondary to the fibrous capsule of a thyroid adenoma. It is most often associated with a benign lesion of the thyroid. However, there have been reports of malignant thyroid lesions that are well encapsulated. Therefore, a halo sign is not necessarily indicative of a benign lesion. The oval lucent area in the central portion of this lesion represents the region of central necrosis, which is commonly seen in thyroid adenomas.

Figures 13–31 and 13–32 are scans of the same patient. Figure 13–31 is a longitudinal scan through the right lobe of the thyroid. In the middle and lower portions of the right lobe are two separate lesions. The more cephalad lesion has the "halo" appearance of a typical thyroid adenoma. Inferior to this lesion is a multicystic lesion with the typical appearance of a degenerating thyroid adenoma. Figure 13–32 is a transverse scan through the more inferior lesion. This case is an excellent illustration of two thyroid adenomas with markedly different ultrasound appearances. The inferior adenoma has the typical appearance of a degenerating process with multiple sonolucent areas secondary to hemorrhage and necrosis. The superior lesion has the

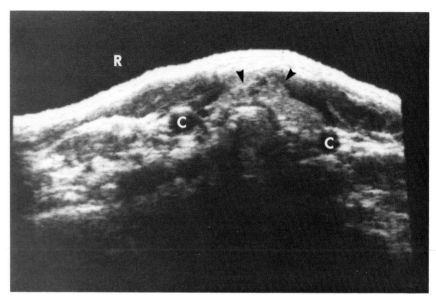

FIG 13–29.

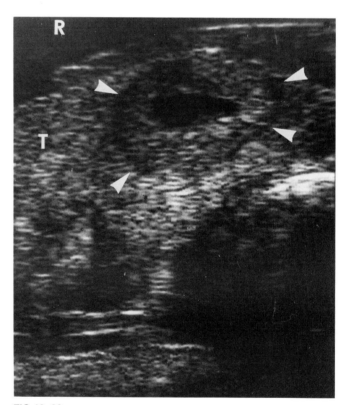

FIG 13–30.

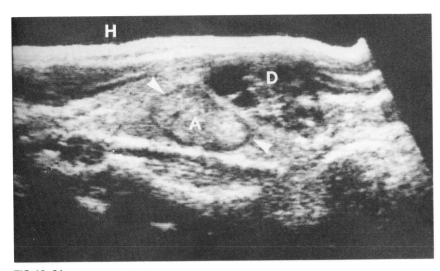

**FIG 13–31.**

typical appearance of a well-encapsulated thyroid adenoma with the "halo" sign.

| | | |
|---|---|---|
| **A** | = | Adenoma |
| **Arrowheads (black)** | = | Adenoma of thyroid isthmus |
| **Arrowheads (white)** | = | "Halo" sign of the capsule about a thyroid adenoma |
| **C** | = | Carotid arteries |
| **D** | = | Degenerating thyroid adenoma |
| **H** | = | Head |
| **R** | = | Right |
| **T** | = | Thyroid |

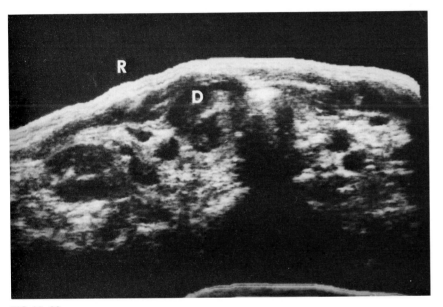

**FIG 13–32.**

## Calcified Thyroid Adenomas

Figures 13–33 and 13–34 are transverse and longitudinal scans of a 37-year-old woman with a small papable cold nodule in the left lobe. Scans were performed using a 7.5-MHz transducer. The most important finding on these scans is the high-amplitude region causing an acoustic shadow posteriorly. Surrounding the high-amplitude area is a relatively lucent rim. The sonographic findings are consistent with calcification. Acoustic shadowing arising from the center of a high-amplitude echo is most consistent with calcification. Such a finding in the thyroid lesion suggests calcification of a thyroid adenoma. What is structure 1 in Figure 13–33? Note the appearance of the esophagus on longitudinal scan. The central echoes of the esophagus arise from the mucosa. What is structure 2 in Figure 13–34?

Figures 13–35 and 13–36 are longitudinal scans of two different patients. On both scans a high-amplitude echo is the source of acoustic shadowing. The sonographic findings are consistent with calcification of a thyroid adenoma, and are highly specific. It is important to make sure that the high-amplitude echo arises from the central portion of the lobe of the thyroid. Occasionally, one can scan the thyroid obliquely and run into the high-amplitude echo and shadowing of the trachea. However, both longitudinal and transverse scans will document the location of the high-amplitude echo. As long as it arises within thyroid tissue, the diagnosis of a calcified thyroid adenoma can be suggested.

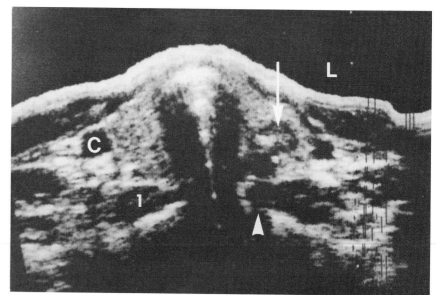

FIG 13–33.

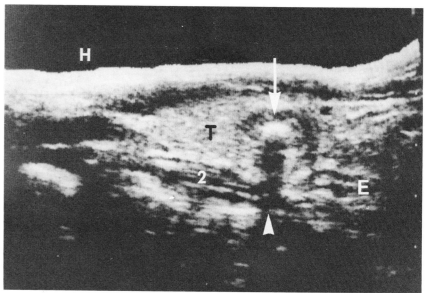

FIG 13–34.

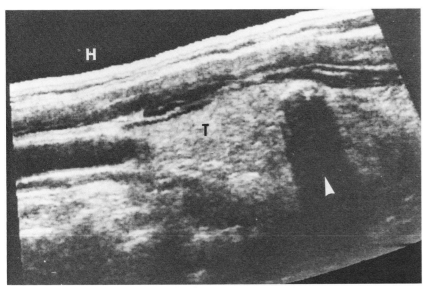

| Arrow | = Calcified adenoma |
| **Arrowhead** | = Shadowing posterior to the calcified adenoma |
| C | = Carotid artery |
| E | = Esophagus |
| H | = Head |
| L | = Left |
| T | = Thyroid |
| 1 | = Longus colli muscle on transverse scan |
| 2 | = Longus colli muscle on longitudinal scan |

FIG 13–35.

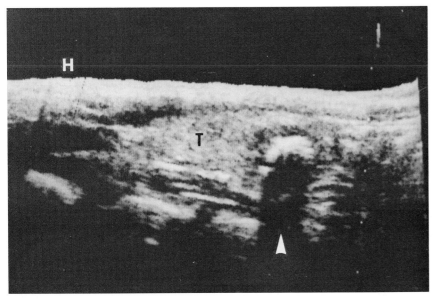

FIG 13–36.

## Goiter

Diffuse enlargement of the thyroid consistent with a goiter gives an ultrasonic appearance of a solid echogenic mass throughout the thyroid. The echo pattern from a goiter is usually uneven and more coarse than seen in a normal thyroid examination. Figure 13–37 is a transverse scan obtained from a patient who had diffuse enlargement of the thyroid due to a goiter. Both lobes of the thyroid are enlarged. The goiter has an uneven coarse echo pattern. A small fluid collection is noted in the midportion of the massively enlarged isthmus.

Figure 13–38 is a scan of a patient with a goiter which involves predominantly the right lobe of the thyroid. This marked asymmetry would be difficult to distinguish from a large adenoma or carcinoma. A goiter presents as an echogenic mass which cannot be diagnosed as malignant or benign. Figures 13–39 and 13–40 are scans of a patient with a goiter undergoing necrosis and degeneration. The enlarged goiter presents as an uneven echogenic mass. Within the mass is a sonolucent fluid collection which indicates an area of necrosis.

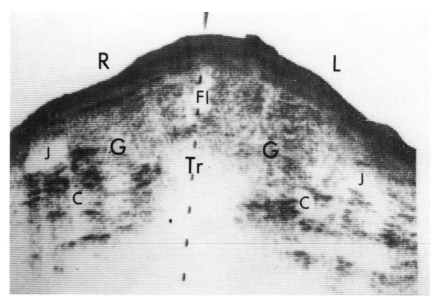

FIG 13–37.

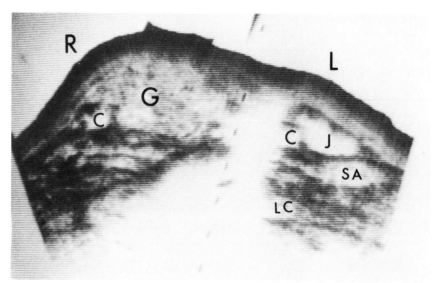

FIG 13–38.

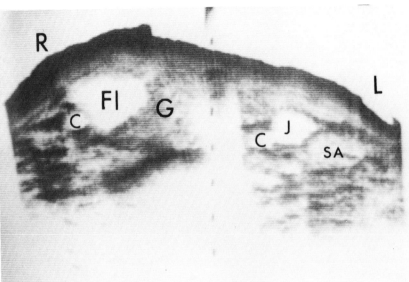

C   = Carotid artery
F   = Foot
Fl  = Fluid consistent with necrosis and
        degeneration
G   = Goiter
H   = Head
J   = Jugular vein
L   = Left
LC  = Longus colli muscle
R   = Right
SA  = Scalenus anterior muscle
Tr  = Trachea

**FIG 13–39.**

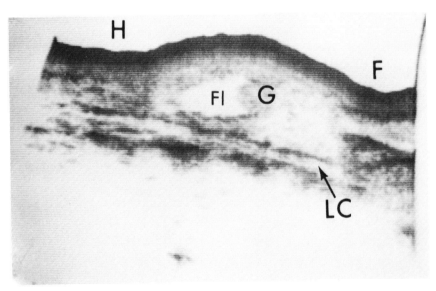

**FIG 13–40.**

## Thyroid Carcinoma

Thyroid carcinomas usually present as solid masses on ultrasound examination. Their echo pattern is often uneven and irregular. Usually a thyroid carcinoma is less echogenic than surrounding thyroid. Figure 13–41 is a transverse scan of the neck of a 24-year-old man who noted right neck swelling approximately 5 months prior to admission. This was disregarded until the patient noted some tenderness. He finally saw a physician and was admitted to the hospital. A large mass in the region of the right thyroid is seen in Figure 13–41. It has an uneven echo pattern. Although it is relatively sonolucent, echoes are noted within it. No enhanced through-transmission is present. The findings are indicative of a large solid lesion of the right lobe of the thyroid. A relatively sonolucent, though solid, mass lateral to the carotid artery is also demonstrated. At surgery it was diagnosed as a metastatic lymph node. The larger mass was found to be a papillary carcinoma of the thyroid. Numerous metastatic lymph nodes were also present.

Thyroid carcinomas are usually irregular in their echo pattern and less echogenic than the normal thyroid gland. In Figure 13–42, however, we see a mass in the right lobe of the thyroid that is extremely echogenic. This mass was found at surgery to be a papillary adenocarcinoma. It is somewhat unusual in its high echogenicity.

Figure 13–43 is a transverse scan of a 62-year-old man who had a history of previous goiter. A mass in the right lobe has an irregular echo pattern. Although the mass is relatively sonolucent compared to normal thyroid tissue, it does have numerous internal echoes, indicating its solid nature. There is no evidence of any well-circumscribed capsule. At surgery, this mass was found to be a mixed papillary follicular adenocarcinoma.

Figure 13–44 is a transverse scan of the thyroid region obtained using a 7.5-MHz transducer. What is the cystic structure labeled 1 in the lateral aspect of the right side of the neck?

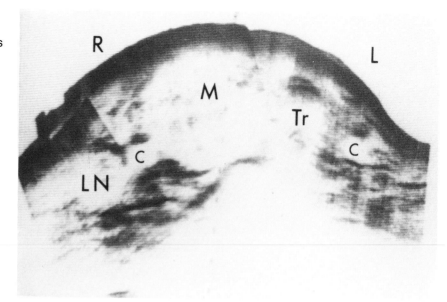

FIG 13–41.

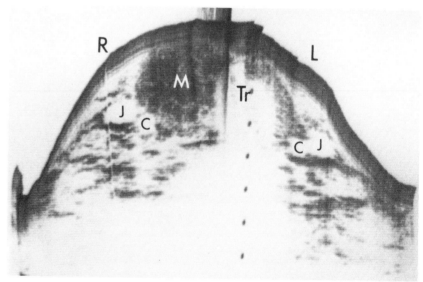

FIG 13–42.

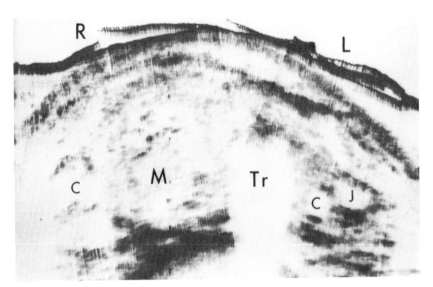

**FIG 13–43.**

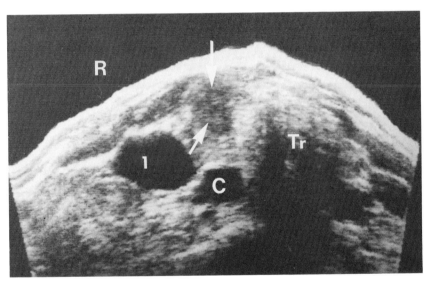

**FIG 13–44.**

Note that the trachea is displaced to the left side by a moderately sized mass in the right thyroid region (arrows). There is a subtle echo texture change within the mass, indicating its solid nature. This hypoechoic mass in the anterior right lobe bulges the thyroid anteriorly and displaces the trachea to the left. At surgery, the mass was found to be mixed papillary-follicular carcinoma of the right lobe of the thyroid.

The large cystic structure labeled 1 in Figure 13–44 is a markedly distended jugular vein. As mentioned earlier, the jugular vein may vary tremendously in its size and appearance in different patients and at different times in the same patient. Note the large difference in size of the right and left jugular veins. In this instance, the jugular vein could be mistaken for a cystic mass of the neck.

| **Arrows** | = | Papillary-follicular adenocarcinoma of the thyroid |
|---|---|---|
| **C** | = | Carotid artery |
| **J** | = | Jugular vein |
| **L** | = | Left |
| **LN** | = | Metastatic lymph node |
| **M** | = | Thyroid carcinoma |
| **R** | = | Right |
| **Tr** | = | Trachea |
| **1** | = | Dilated jugular vein |

## Thyroid Carcinoma; Thyroid Metastases

Figure 13–45 is a longitudinal scan through the right lobe of the thyroid obtained using a 7.5-MHz real-time transducer. A cold nodule was noted involving the lower pole of the right lobe of the thyroid on isotope study. The thyroid ultrasound texture of the middle and upper pole of the right lobe is even and normal in appearance. A sonolucent mass is noted in the lower pole. This mass contains very few echoes. The attenuation of sound deep to the mass indicates its solid structure. Often relatively hypoechoic masses are mistaken for cystic structures. However, marked attenuation such as is present in this case indicates the solid nature of the mass. The mass turned out to be a mixed papillary-follicular adenocarcinoma of the right lobe of the thyroid.

Rarely, solid lesions of the thyroid may be secondary to metastatic disease from other primary sites. Figure 13–46 is a transverse scan of the thyroid showing a moderately large solid mass in the right lobe and isthmus (arrows). The trachea is displaced to the left by the mass. The patient was a 67-year-old man with a palpable nodule in the right lower neck. Fifteen years earlier he had undergone thyroid lobectomy for a benign adenoma; 4 years earlier he had had a right pneumonectomy for bronchogenic carcinoma. A radionuclide scan showed no uptake over the right side of the neck. Therefore, this solid lesion does not represent thyroid tissue but rather metastatic disease from the primary lung tumor.

Figures 13–47 and 13–48 are transverse and longitudinal scans of a 60-year-old man who had undergone nephrectomy 13 years earlier for renal carcinoma. He had been relatively symptom free until the recent development of a mass in the left neck. An isotope study demonstrated decreased activity in the inferior left lobe of the thyroid. Figure 13–47 is a transverse scan obtained using a 7.5-MHz transducer. The left lobe of the thyroid is markedly enlarged (arrowheads). Note that the trachea is dis-

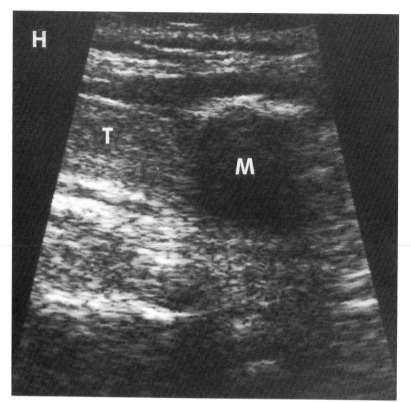

**FIG 13–45.**

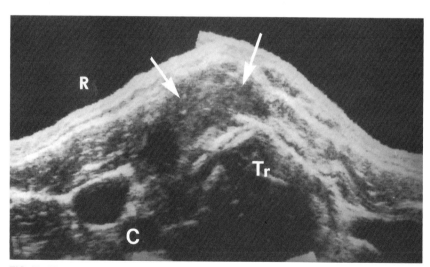

**FIG 13–46.**

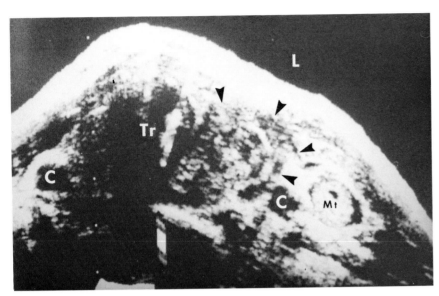

**FIG 13–47.**

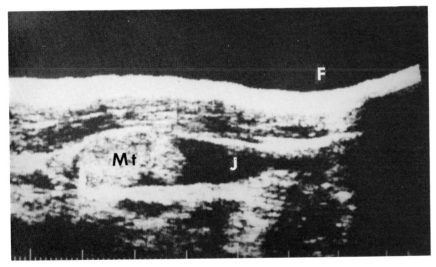

**FIG 13–48.**

placed to the right by this large mass. Lateral to the left carotid artery is an unusual echogenic region with a lucent periphery. A longitudinal scan through this region is shown in Figure 13–48. This case is an unusual one because of the metastatic lesions to the left neck from the tumor removed 13 years earlier. The mass in the left neck is a metastatic hypernephroma with a tumor thrombus in the jugular vein. The longitudinal scan in Figure 13–48 demonstrates the patent portion of the jugular vein inferior to the metastatic thrombus.

| | |
|---|---|
| **Arrows** | = Metastasis from bronchogenic carcinoma |
| **Arrowheads** | = Metastasis from hypernephroma |
| **C** | = Carotid artery |
| **F** | = Foot |
| **H** | = Head |
| **J** | = Jugular vein |
| **L** | = Left |
| **M** | = Papillary-follicular carcinoma |
| **Mt** | = Metastatic thrombus in the jugular vein |
| **R** | = Right |
| **T** | = Thyroid |
| **Tr** | = Trachea |

## Thyroiditis

In thyroiditis the ultrasonographic findings are similar to findings in other organs involved with diffuse inflammatory changes. Figures 13–49 and 13–50 are transverse and longitudinal scans of a patient with chronic thyroiditis. Diffusely enlarged thyroid lobes are visualized in Figure 13–49. The lobes themselves have a decreased echogenic appearance. The diffuse sonolucent involvement of the thyroid is highly suggestive of inflammatory disease. Figure 13–50 is a longitudinal scan of the right lobe of the thyroid anterior to the longus colli muscle. Compared with the normal echogenic appearance of the thyroid seen in previous cases, the thyroid lobes in this case are much less echogenic than expected. The curvature of the skin (Fig 13–50) indicates thyroid enlargement.

Figure 13–51 is a transverse scan of a patient who also was diagnosed to have thyroiditis. In this instance, the thyroiditis is much more localized. Figure 13–51 shows a large sonolucency on the right side that is displacing the trachea to the left. Within this sonolucent area is a fluid level (arrows). Aspiration of the cystic region yielded cholesterol crystals, which are consistent with the diagnosis of thyroiditis. Thyroiditis in this case cannot be differentiated from a hemorrhagic cyst based on ultrasound findings alone. Clinical history and aspiration were necessary for the correct result.

Figure 13–52 is a transverse scan of the thyroid region in a middle-aged woman. Both lobes of the thyroid are markedly enlarged. An uneven parenchymal pattern is present bilaterally. The thyroid lobes are seen medial to the carotid arteries. The patient was diagnosed as having Hashimoto's thyroiditis. The ultrasound characteristics of Hashimoto's thyroiditis cannot be distinguished from those of multinodular goiter. Hashimoto's thyroiditis is a clinical diagnosis in which the ultrasound findings may be of assistance. Basically, the thyroid is enlarged bilaterally with an uneven parenchymal pattern. In this case, hypoechoic

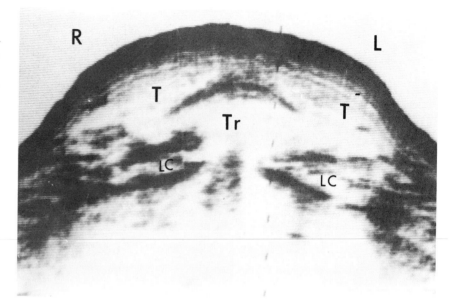

**FIG 13–49.**

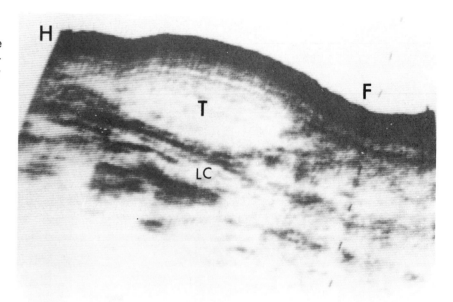

**FIG 13–50.**

areas are noted anteriorly and more echogenic thyroid tissue is present posteriorly.

| Arrows | = | Fluid level |
|--------|---|-------------|
| C | = | Carotid artery |
| F | = | Foot |
| H | = | Head |
| J | = | Jugular vein |
| L | = | Left |
| LC | = | Longus colli muscle |
| R | = | Right |
| T | = | Thyroid |
| Tr | = | Trachea |

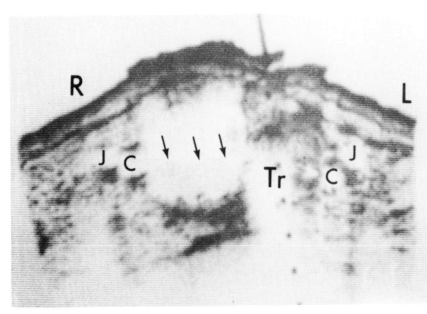

**FIG 13–51.**

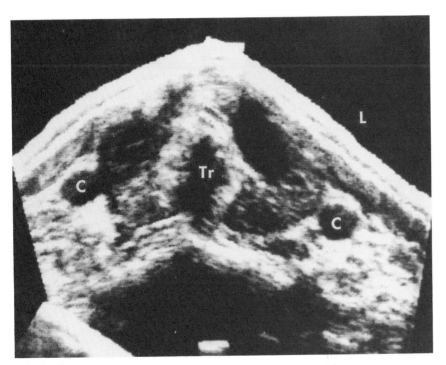

**FIG 13–52.**

## Parathyroid Adenomas

Earlier in this chapter, in the section on normal anatomy, the relationship between the lobe of the thyroid, carotid artery, and the longus colli muscle was outlined (see Figs 13–1 through 13–8). This triangular relationship is extremely important in a parathyroid examination. There should be no mass greater than 5 mm in diameter between the lobe of the thyroid and the longus colli muscle. The minor neurovascular bundle, which is comprised of the recurrent laryngeal nerve and the inferior thyroid artery, is present in this location. If the size of such a mass is 5 mm or less, however, it is considered to be within normal limits. When a lesion is greater than 5 mm, we have ultrasonic criteria for the diagnosis of a parathyroid adenoma. Figures 13–53 and 13–54 are examples of a parathyroid adenoma deep to the superior pole of the thyroid. In Figure 13–53, the relationship of the thyroid to the carotid artery and the longus colli muscle is seen. On the right side, there is a lucent area between the lobe of the thyroid and the longus colli muscle. At surgery, this lucent area proved to be a parathyroid adenoma of the superior right side. The adenoma measures approximately 7–8 mm, which is above our criterion for normal. Figure 13–54 is a longitudinal scan of the same patient with the parathyroid adenoma deep and superior to the thyroid. In this plane, it is approximately 8–9 mm, which is well above the 5-mm criterion.

Figures 13–55 and 13–56 are transverse and longitudinal scans of a patient who has a parathyroid adenoma posterior to the inferior portion of the left thyroid lobe. The adenoma is anterior to the longus colli muscle, medial to the carotid artery, and posterior to the left lobe of the thyroid. It would be difficult to make the diagnosis from the transverse scan (Figure 13–55) because of a collapsed jugular vein (arrowhead). Real-time study confirmed the location of the carotid artery on the basis of arterial pulsation. Once the carotid artery was identified, the jugular vein could be made

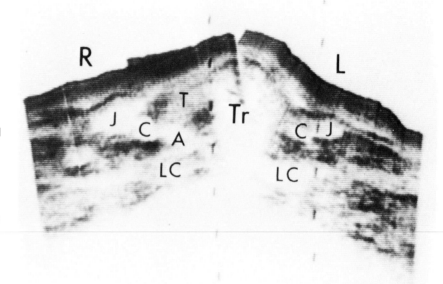

FIG 13–53.

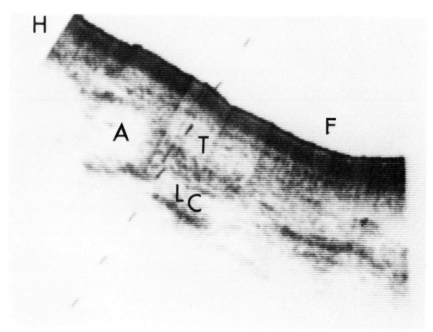

FIG 13–54.

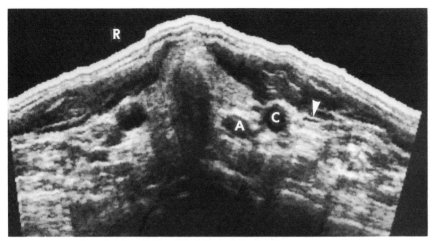

**FIG 13–55.**

to stand out more clearly with a Valsalva maneuver. When these two vessels were located, the third sonolucency is identified medial to the carotid artery. This may be the esophagus. By having the patient swallow, one can ascertain whether or not this structure is the esophagus. Therefore, this sonolucency on the transverse scan was highly suspicious of a parathyroid adenoma. The longitudinal scan in Figure 13–56 confirms the oval appearance of the sonolucent mass. The two studies together indicate the location of a parathyroid adenoma.

| **A** | = Parathyroid adenoma |
|---|---|
| **Arrowhead** | = Collapsed left jugular vein |
| **C** | = Carotid artery |
| **F** | = Foot |
| **H** | = Head |
| **J** | = Jugular vein |
| **L** | = Left |
| **LC** | = Longus colli muscle |
| **R** | = Right |
| **T** | = Thyroid |
| **Tr** | = Trachea |

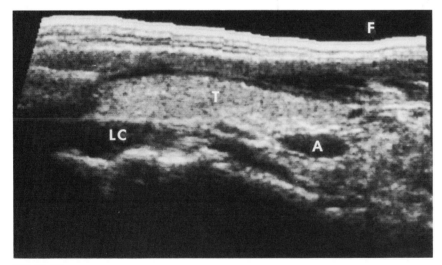

**FIG 13–56.**

## Parathyroid Adenomas

In the examination of a patient with suspected parathyroid adenoma, it is important to visualize any lesion in both transverse and longitudinal planes. A correct identification of anatomic structures is more likely if two planes are used in the diagnosis. Figure 13–57 is a longitudinal scan of a patient with a rather large parathyroid adenoma that did not pose any difficulties. In this instance, a relatively sonolucent parathyroid adenoma, measuring 12 × 20 mm, is seen deep to the inferior pole of the thyroid and anterior to the longus colli muscle. A transverse scan of the same patient (Fig 13–58) confirms this finding. Figure 13–58 demonstrates the lucent parathyroid adenoma on the left side of the neck, compared with the normal echogenicity of the right lobe of the thyroid. The parathyroid adenoma is situated anterior to the longus colli muscle. In this scan, the normal minor neurovascular bundles can be visualized bilaterally. The minor neurovascular bundles, composed of the recurrent laryngeal nerve and inferior thyroid artery, measure approximately 3 mm in thickness on these scans. It becomes clear, especially on the right side, how the minor neurovascular bundle may pose a diagnostic problem when a patient is scanned for a parathyroid adenoma. Presently, only the size criterion of greater than 5 mm gives the ultrasound diagnosis of a parathyroid adenoma.

A sonolucent parathyroid adenoma slightly greater than 5 mm is seen in Figure 13–59. In this instance, the parathyroid adenoma is approximately 6–7 mm thick. It is situated between the longus colli muscle and the lobe of the thyroid. The minor neurovascular bundle is superior to the parathyroid adenoma and measures only 2 mm in thickness.

Figure 13–60 shows an adenoma small enough to lead to a false negative diagnosis on ultrasound examination. A small parathyroid adenoma is situated between the thyroid and longus colli muscle. It is slightly medial to the carotid artery. The thickness of the adenoma, however, is only 2–3 mm.

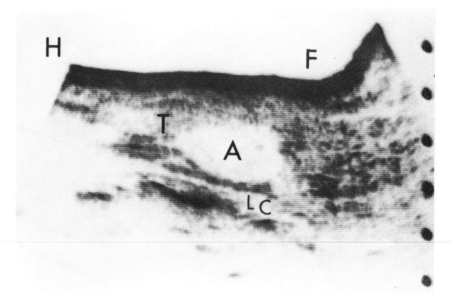

**FIG 13–57.**

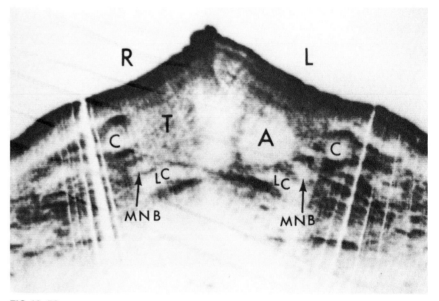

**FIG 13–58.**

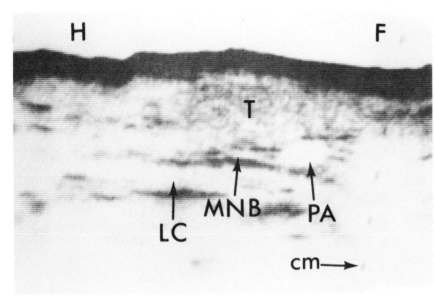

**FIG 13–59.**

This was below our criterion and therefore was called normal on ultrasound examination. At surgery, however, a parathyroid adenoma was found in this location, approximately 3 mm thick but 1 cm long. This misdiagnosis by ultrasound was caused by the size of the adenoma in its anteroposterior dimension.

| A | = | Parathyroid adenoma |
|---|---|---|
| C | = | Carotid |
| cm | = | Centimeter markers |
| F | = | Foot |
| H | = | Head |
| L | = | Left |
| LC | = | Longus colli muscle |
| MNB | = | Minor neurovascular bundle |
| PA | = | Parathyroid adenoma |
| R | = | Right |
| SCM | = | Sternocleidomastoid muscle |
| T | = | Thyroid |
| Tr | = | Trachea |

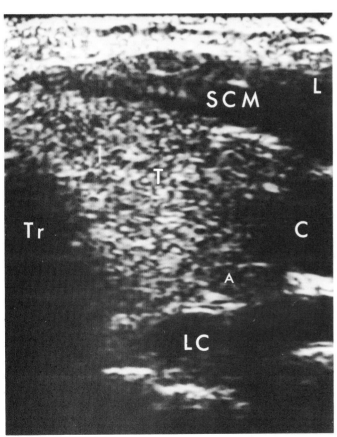

**FIG 13–60.**

## Parathyroid Adenoma

Figures 13–61 and 13–62 are transverse and longitudinal scans of the left side of the neck. The findings indicate a parathyroid adenoma posterior to the lower pole of the left lobe of the thyroid. Figure 13–61 is an excellent example of the anatomic relationship of the jugular vein, carotid artery, and the esophagus. If this normal anatomic relationship is understood, parathyroid adenomas will not be missed. The jugular veins are bilaterally collapsed (arrowheads). As mentioned earlier, the jugular veins can be variable in size. With a Valsalva maneuver, the jugular veins will distend on real-time examination.

On the left side of the neck in Figure 13–61, four structures come into view posterior to the left lobe of the thyroid. The most medial structure with an echogenic center is the esophagus. The echogenic center is the mucosal echoes. Having the patient swallow will increase the amplitude of the echoes within the esophagus, and movement will also be identified. Just lateral to the esophagus is the left parathyroid adenoma. This can be mistaken for the carotid artery if care is not taken during the course of the examination. Lateral to the adenoma is the carotid artery. Real-time examination can disclose arterial pulsations. Lateral to the left carotid artery is the collapsed jugular vein (arrowhead). There is excellent anatomic correlation of these four structures. The parathyroid adenoma is confirmed by the longitudinal scan in Figure 13–62. The adenoma appears as a pear-shaped, relatively hypoechoic mass posterior to the lobe of the thyroid and anterior to the longus colli muscle. It is not tubular in shape as the carotid artery or esophagus would be. It did not pulsate on real-time examination. There was no evidence of any change in appearance when the patient swallowed. All of these findings are necessary to confirm the diagnosis of parathyroid adenoma.

Figures 13–63 and 13–64 are transverse and longitudinal scans of another patient with a large lower pole

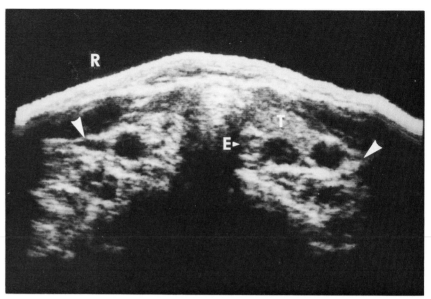

**FIG 13–61.**

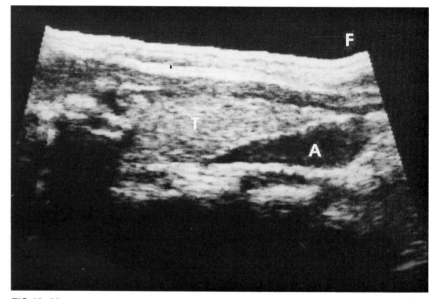

**FIG 13–62.**

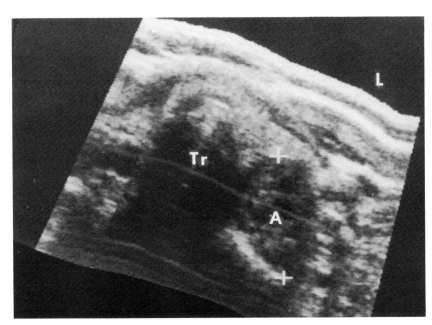

**FIG 13–63.**

parathyroid adenoma. The parathyroid adenoma stands out quite easily as a hypoechoic mass with some internal echoes. Such a large mass could be confused with an adenoma of the thyroid. The right clinical setting and laboratory findings are necessary for the diagnosis. It is especially difficult to separate the parathyroid adenoma from thyroid tissue in the longitudinal scan (Fig 13–64).

| | | |
|---|---|---|
| **A** | = | Parathyroid adenoma |
| **Arrowheads** | = | Collapsed jugular vein |
| **E** | = | Esophagus |
| **F** | = | Foot |
| **H** | = | Head |
| **L** | = | Left |
| **LC** | = | Longus colli |
| **R** | = | Right |
| **T** | = | Thyroid |
| **Tr** | = | Trachea |

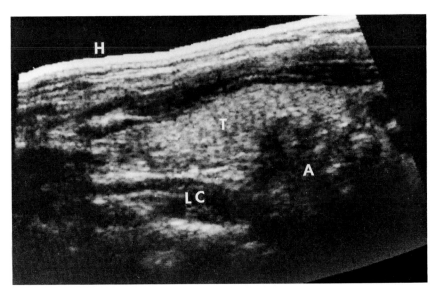

**FIG 13–64.**

## Other Neck Masses

Ultrasound of the neck is usually performed for thyroid and parathyroid pathologic conditions. However, palpable masses arising from other regions may also be examined by ultrasound. Figure 13–65 is a longitudinal scan obtained in the midline. A mass is seen slightly superior to the thyroid. The mass is sonolucent, and there is the suggestion of through-transmission. However, through-transmission is difficult to evaluate since the mass is directly anterior to the trachea. Evaluation of through-transmission is always difficult when a mass is situated anterior to bone or air. This lesion was a thyroglossal cyst in the midline anterior to the trachea.

Figure 13–66 is a transverse scan of the neck in a middle-aged woman. The patient experienced sudden enlargement of an anterior neck mass with accompanying pain and discomfort. The scan was obtained using a 5-MHz transducer. The mass is relatively sonolucent with soft echoes scattered in the dependent region. Prominent through-transmission is noted deep to the mass, indicating its fluid-filled nature. The ultrasound findings are suggestive of either hemorrhage or infection because of the dependent debris. This patient turned out to have a thyroglossal duct cyst in which hemorrhage had occurred.

Figure 13–67 is a longitudinal oblique scan of the neck in a 6-day-old infant. The infant was noted to have a mass in left lateral neck region. This area was scanned with a 5-MHz real-time transducer. A 4-cm mass was identified that is sonolucent anteriorly and has soft echoes in its deep portion. There is a sharp demarcation (arrowhead) between the sonolucent and echogenic area. When the patient was scanned in an upright position, the echogenic area moved slowly into a dependent position. This real-time ultrasound finding is often seen in masses with debris or hemorrhage. The infant was diagnosed to have a branchial cleft cyst that was filled with debris. Aspiration revealed cholesterol within the fluid. If a fluid or debris level is suspected, the patient

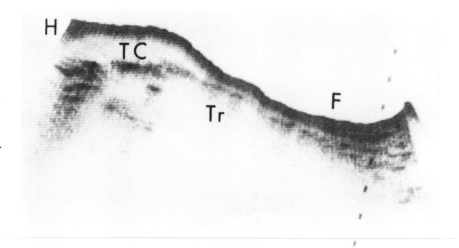

FIG 13–65.

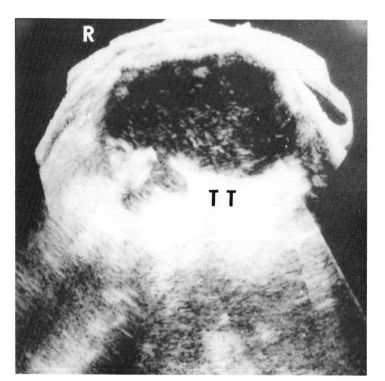

FIG 13–66.

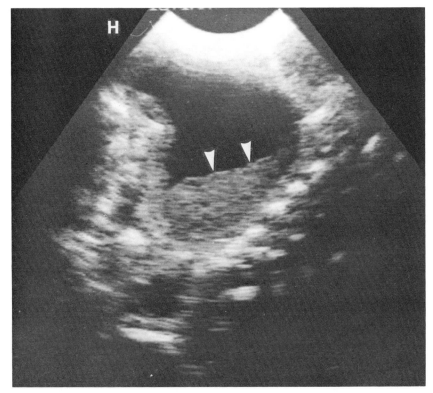

FIG 13–67.

should be examined with real-time equipment. By placing the transducer over the mass and changing the patient's position, the examiner can visualize movement of the dependent debris on real-time sonography.

Figure 13–68 is a longitudinal scan over a right neck mass in a 55-year-old man with a history of chronic alcholism. The mass was tender and red and was situated near the angle of the mandible on the right side. The contour of the skin is markedly deformed. There are three components to the mass. Superficially, the mass is basically echo free. In the midportion some soft echoes are noted, suggestive of debris. In the deeper portion the mass has a solid component. Finally, deep to all of these structures is prominent through-transmission, indicating the fluid-filled nature of the mass. These ultrasound findings are fairly typical of either hemorrhage or inflammation. Hemorrhage into a lesion or an abscess cannot be distinguished on ultrasound. In this instance, the ultrasound findings were secondary to an abscess within the parotid gland. The abscess was drained surgically.

| **Arrowheads** | = Fluid-debris level |
| **F** | = Foot |
| **H** | = Head |
| **R** | = Right |
| **TC** | = Thyroglossal duct cyst |
| **Tr** | = Trachea |
| **TT** | = Through-transmission |

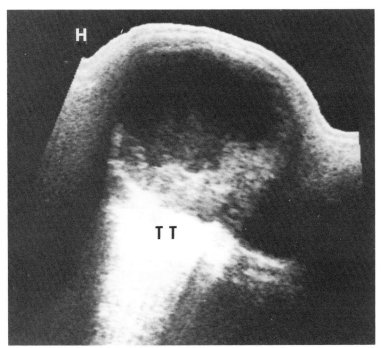

FIG 13–68.

## Other Neck Masses

Ultrasound may be requested to evaluate palpable neck masses unrelated to the thyroid. Figures 13–69 and 13–70 are scans of a patient who had recently had catheterization of the left jugular vein. The transverse scan (Fig 13–69) shows a mass surrounding the jugular vein on the left side. The carotid and jugular vein on the right side are in the normal location and are normal in size. The jugular vein on the left is markedly enlarged. There is a circumferential mass (arrows) surrounding the lumen of the jugular vein. Figure 13–70 is a longitudinal scan of the left jugular vein. Again, the lumen of the jugular vein is seen to be surrounded by a large soft tissue mass (arrows). The mass was due to a jugular vein hematoma.

Figure 13–71 is a transverse scan of a patient with a large palpable mass on the right side of the neck. The mass proved to be metastatic squamous cell carcinoma. Figure 13–72 is a transverse scan of another patient who had a palpable mass on the left side of the neck. The mass represented tumor recurrence from a thyroid carcinoma. Ultrasonography can be used to evaluate mass lesions within the neck to determine whether they are fluid-filled or solid, and thereby narrow the differential diagnosis.

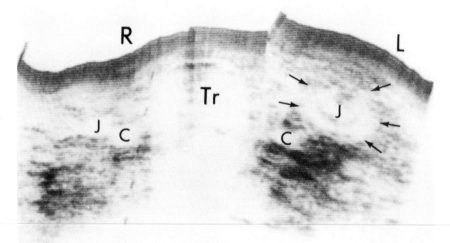

**FIG 13–69.**

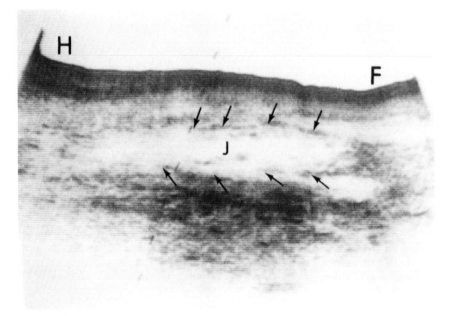

**FIG 13–70.**

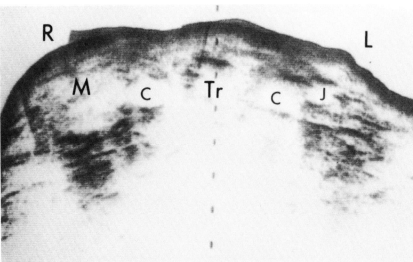

FIG 13–71.

Arrows = Jugular vein hematoma
C      = Carotid artery
F      = Foot
H      = Head
J      = Jugular vein
L      = Left
M      = Solid mass in the neck
R      = Right
Tr     = Trachea

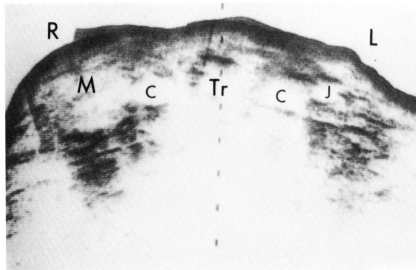

FIG 13–72.

## Other Neck Masses

Figure 13–73 is a transverse scan of a patient who underwent ultrasonography for evaluation of a left neck mass. The right lobe of the thyroid has a normal echo texture. In the region of the left lobe of the thyroid is a large sonolucent mass. There are no echoes identified within the mass. However, the mass is unquestionably a solid lesion because of the poor through-transmission. Even though no echoes are present, it is the lack of through-transmission that indicates its solid nature. A cystic structure of this size would have great deal of sound transmitted deep to it. The mass was a homogeneous solid lesion found at surgery to be a granular cell myoblastoma.

Figure 13–74 is a transverse scan in the midline of the neck that shows a suprasternal notch mass. The anterior portion of the mass is echo free, with through-transmission noted deep to it. This is the fluid-filled portion of the mass. However, within the mass is an echogenic area, indicating a solid component. At surgery the mass was found to be a benign cystic teratoma. This is an unusual site for a cystic teratoma. However, the ultrasound characteristics are somewhat typical. Benign cystic teratomas have a mixed ultrasound appearance, with both fluid and solid components.

Figure 13–75 is a transverse scan of the neck of a 40-year-old man with bilateral palpable masses. A 4-cm mass is present on a right side and a 2-cm mass on the left side. Some soft echoes are present within both masses. The patient has a history of lymphoma. The masses represent lymph nodes enlargement secondary to Hodgkin's lymphoma.

Figure 13–76 is a transverse scan of another patient with lymphoma. This middle-aged woman presented with a large mass in the left neck inferior to the mandible. The lymph node is markedly sonolucent without evidence of any internal echoes. If this represented a cystic mass, prominent through-transmission would be seen deep to the mass. However, there is no evidence of through-transmission.

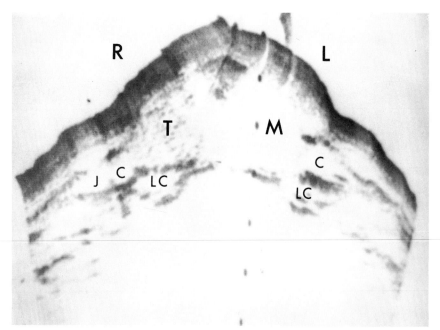

FIG 13–73.

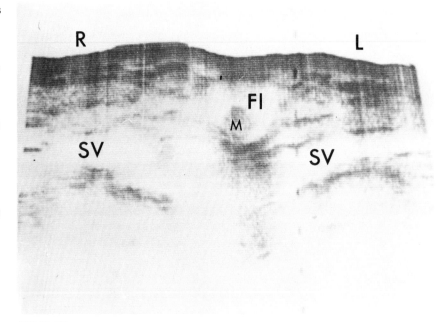

FIG 13–74.

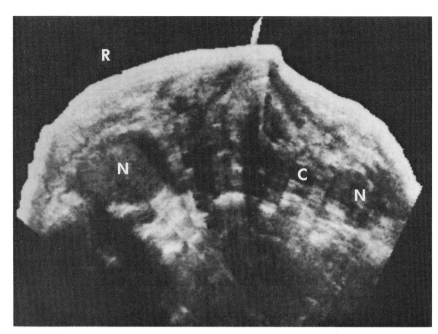

**FIG 13–75.**

Lymph nodes can be quite sonolucent. They are often mistaken for cysts because of their lack of internal echoes. However, in this instance, the relatively poor through-transmission for the size of the mass indicates its solid nature.

| | | |
|---|---|---|
| **C** | = | Carotid artery |
| **Fl** | = | Fluid |
| **J** | = | Jugular vein |
| **L** | = | Left |
| **LC** | = | Longus colli muscle |
| **M** | = | Solid mass of the left neck (Figure 13–73) |
| **M** | = | Solid component (Fig 13–74) |
| **N** | = | Enlarged lymph nodes |
| **R** | = | Right |
| **SV** | = | Subclavian vessels |
| **T** | = | Thyroid |

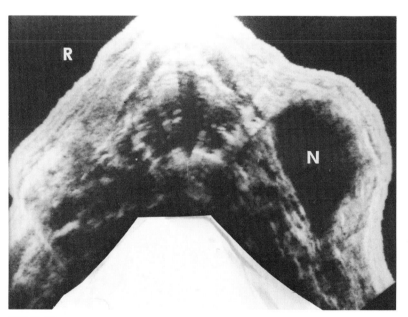

**FIG 13–76.**

# 14.
# Breast Ultrasound

Lawrence W. Bassett, M.D.
Richard H. Gold, M.D.
Carolyn Kimme-Smith, Ph.D.

## Introduction

The breast was one of the first organs examined by ultrasound when, over 30 years ago, Wild and Reid[1] and Howry et al.[2] demonstrated the potential usefulness of A-mode technique for differentiating cystic from solid palpable masses. Later, Kratchowil and Kaiser[3] reported that B-mode equipment was useful in the evaluation of palpable masses. Subsequently, dedicated whole-breast automated ultrasound units were developed by DeLand,[4] Jellins, Kossoff, et al.,[5] Kobayashi,[6] and Kelly-Fry.[7]

## Clinical Applications

The most important clinical use of breast ultrasound continues to be the differentiation of cysts from solid masses. In this endeavor, accuracy rates of 96%–100% have been reported for ultrasound, far exceeding the accuracy of mammography or physical examination.[8–10] However, needle aspiration of palpable masses is easy to perform and usually therapeutic as well as diagnostic. Sonography, therefore, is more useful for evaluation of a nonpalpable, mammographically detected, indeterminate mass, for which aspiration is unlikely to be successful. Ultrasound is also recommended for the evaluation of a patient with breast cysts so numerous as to make aspiration impractical. Breast ultrasound is a useful adjunct to mammography in three clinical situations: when palpable masses have indeterminate mammographic features; when nonpalpable, mammographically detected masses have indeterminate features; and when dense parenchymal tissue limits the mammographic evaluation of an entire breast or a localized site of suspected abnormality.[11]

Automated whole-breast ultrasound has at various times been proposed as a method for breast cancer screening. However, its sensitivity and specificity in the detection of breast cancer are far lower than the figures reported for mammography.[12] The limitations of ultrasound in breast cancer detection are (1) poor results in fatty breasts, (2) inability to depict microcalcifications, often the earliest sign of breast cancer, (3) inconsistent identification of solid lesions less than 1 cm in diameter, and (4) unreliability in distinguishing benign from malignant solid masses. Ultrasonography is most accurate in breasts that have little or no fat and that are radiographically dense, limiting film-screen and xeromammographic evaluation. The combined use of mammography and ultrasound has been shown to improve the detection rate for breast cancer.[13] Ultrasound-guided aspiration biopsy of nonpalpable lesions has been shown to be effective, and the method has also been advocated for prebiopsy needle localization of nonpalpable masses.[14]

## Technical Considerations

Breast sonography differs from other types of ultrasound imaging in several ways. First, breast tissue is unusually heterogeneous, so that while the ultrasound beam may need to traverse a tissue thickness of only 3–5 cm, the amplitude of the beam rapidly diminishes due to the impedance mismatches of the many tissue interfaces. The resulting extensive refraction, combined with the high-frequency attenuation of dense glandular tissue, leads to beam defocusing.[15] Therefore, tightly focused large-aperture, high-frequency transducers should be used whenever possible in order to depict small structures that may represent significant pathology.

Because breast abnormalities may be present only a short distance beneath the skin, transducers with a water path or fluid offset are required to depict structures that otherwise might be lost in the near field. The size, shape, and margin of a breast mass may be distorted when it is imaged in the near or far field of the focal zone.[16]

Cystic/solid differentiation is the most important task of breast ultrasound, and an accurate determination depends on the use of appropriate technical factors and instruments. For example, enhancement of distal echoes, a characteristic feature of cysts, depends on selecting the correct time gain compensation (TGC) and appropriate gray scale map (matched to the preamplifier), and the location of the mass (echoes are harder to appreciate when a cyst is adjacent to the chest wall). Absence of interior echoes is another characteristic feature of cysts, but artifactual echoes can result from gain settings that are too high. In addition, artifactual echoes may be seen when the cyst is out of the section thickness direction focal zone.

When a phased-array transducer is used, artificial echoes may be due to grating lobes. A fluid offset distance may reverberate within the breast and create the false appearance of a septum in a cyst.

## Instrumentation

Breast ultrasound can be performed with either high-frequency real-time hand-held units or automated dedicated breast units.

### Hand-Held Real-Time Units

Hand-held units are most commonly used. Hand-held instruments fall into three types: mechanical sector scanner, phased-array scanners, and hybrid units with an annular phased-array that mechanically rocks to provide a sector or linear format type of image.

If a water offset is not included with the ultrasound unit that is to be used for breast imaging, it should be improvised in the form of a water bag that can be placed on the breast, with acoustic gel covering the breast and transducer surfaces. A water offset is particularly important when a phased-array unit is used to image superficial breast lesions. When a water-filled plastic bag is used for the offset, the sonographer adjusts the thickness of the water bag with one hand while scanning with the other hand.

Dynamic focusing annular array units are required to avoid section thickness artifacts that may result in false echoes within cysts. Individual transducers should be tested in a nonattenuating medium containing thread targets to evaluate noise generated by side and grating lobe artifacts, which can also create false echoes within a cyst.[17] Unfortunately, refocusing reduces the total area that is in sharp focus, leading to a rapid divergence of the beam and subsequent elongation and loss of detail of the deeper breast structures in the far field.

### Automated Breast Imaging Units

An advantage of automated water path instruments is the long water offset that is built into these systems. This allows the use of a less curved lens transducer that produces less distortion of details in the far field. Thus, a section of the entire breast and adjacent chest wall can be clearly depicted in a single image. Three manufacturers have marketed dedicated breast ultrasound equipment—Labsonics, Ausonics, and Technicare.

**Labsonics.**—This unit is similar to an automated B-mode instrument. The supine patient is scanned using a rectilinear pattern with either a 4-MHz or 7.5-MHz transducer. A built-in TGC is matched to the intensity profile of a wide-aperture, tightly focused transducer. The technologist places the transducer and water bag over the area of interest. The transducer moves back and forth over this area, and can be raised or lowered to adjust the focal zone.

**Ausonics.**—With this unit the patient lies prone with the breast dependent in a heated, chlorinated water bath, while up to four matched transducers produce sector scans of the breast. The water offset varies from 3 to 12 cm, depending on breast size and focal zone placement in the breast. Because of the large water offset, the transducer frequency is limited to 4.5 MHz. This unit is the only one that can produce acceptable images without breast compression, an advantage for depicting superficially located architectural distortions or skin thickening.

**Technicare.**—Although this water path instrument is no longer manufactured, many are still in clinical use. Two 4.2-MHz transducers are focused at different depths in the dependent, compressed breast of the prone patient. The TGC can be selected by the technologist, and a video camera in the water tank can be used for patient positioning and biopsy localization.

*Hand-Held versus Automated Breast Ultrasound*

High-resolution hand-held units are superior to automated breast scanners when attention can be directed to a specific area of interest. Hand-held units are also useful for ultrasound-guided aspiration or prebiopsy needle localization. The disadvantages of hand-held units are uneven penetration of breast tissue, lack of consistent anatomic labeling, and decreased resolution near the transducer. Although water-path instruments permit systematic examination of the entire breast, a theoretical advantage in searching for nonpalpable and mammographically occult le-

sions, the yield of nonpalpable cancers is almost nil. The disadvantages of current automated units are lower resolution than is available with hand-held instruments, higher cost, greater space requirements, the need for specially trained technologists, and the relatively long time required for the examination. Since the major use of ultrasound is to evaluate localizable, palpable or mammographically visible masses, hand-held units remain preferable in most settings.

**Ultrasonography of the Normal Breast**

The breast is composed of fat, lactiferous ducts and lobules (collectively called the parenchyma), and connective tissue. The amount of each of these tissues varies with age and parity and among women of the same age and parity. Therefore, there is considerable variation in the appearance of the normal breast. For purposes of evaluating the ultrasound examination, the breast can be conveniently divided into four distinct anatomic regions: (1) the region composed of the skin, nipple, and subareolar structures, (2) the subcutaneous region, (3) the parenchymal region, and (4) the retromammary region.[18] The subcutaneous region is composed of fat lobules and distal extensions of the suspensory ligaments of Cooper. The cone-shaped parenchymal region includes the functional elements (mammary lobules and ducts), connective tissue, suspensory ligaments, and varying amounts of fat. The retromammary region, a thin layer of fat, separates the parenchyma from the fascia overlying the pectoralis muscles.

The breast is composed of fatty, parenchymal, and connective tissues. Of these, the acoustic impedance of fat is lowest, that of parenchymal tissue is intermediate, and that of connective tissue is highest. Dense connective tissue attenuates the ultrasound beam more than does loose connective tissue. These differences in attenuation are an important factor in the production of the breast ultrasound image.

The skin appears as a thick, uniform, highly reflective line 0.5–2 mm thick on ultrasound. The nipple contains a large amount of connective tissue which, in combination with the dense connective tissue surrounding the subareolar ducts, can lead to acoustic shadowing sufficient to prevent the depiction of an underlying mass. Nipple shadowing may be reduced by applying sufficient compression so that the nipple does not protrude beyond the contour of the breast surface. The ducts cast narrow cylindrical shadows because of the acoustic attenuation of the surrounding dense connective tissue. Subareolar ducts are normally dilated and can be identified as sonolucent tubular structures 2–8 mm in diameter.

Because of differences in acoustic impedance, the interface between the subcutaneous fat and the dense parenchymal connective tissue is readily visualized. The amplitude of the echoes at the interface is affected by the incident angle of the ultrasound beam, being brightest where the beam is 90° to the interface. The subcutaneous region usually shows fine, weakly echogenic reflections from fat lobules, interspersed with strong echoes from the suspensory ligaments of Cooper. These ligaments can produce suspicious shadowing when the angle of incidence of the beam is such that considerable sound wave refraction occurs. The shadowing is reduced when the ligaments are flattened and made more perpendicular to the incident beam by breast compression.[17]

The retromammary parenchymal tissue assumes a triangular configuration. The sonographic appearance of the parenchyma depends on the relative amounts of fat and connective tissue within it. Ultrasound breast parenchymal patterns have been correlated with mammographic patterns.[18–20]

In the fatty breast, sonolucent fat lobules replace nearly all of the parenchymal tissue, producing a relatively anechoic, loose, lace-like ultrasound pattern. While ideally suited to x-ray mammography, the fatty breast is poorly suited to ultrasound, since fat does not transmit sound well and fat lobules may simulate breast masses.

Dense, fibrous breasts are filled with connective tissue that produces strong coalescent echoes similar to those in the skin. The subcutaneous layer is often very thin, and no fat lobules are visible in the parenchyma. Beam attenuation may be severe, and compression is required for the sound beam to penetrate to the chest wall. However, sonolucent masses are easily identified. Because mammography is extremely limited in these cases, breast ultrasound is an important adjunct in the evaluation of palpable abnormalities. Some advocates of breast ultrasound believe it is more effective than mammography for breast cancer screening in this type of breast.

With increasing age and with child-bearing, the parenchyma involutes and is replaced by fat. When fat lobules are admixed with dense parenchymal tissue, it is difficult to differentiate a focus of fatty replacement from a sonolucent breast mass. In this situation the importance of correlating the x-ray and sonographic examinations cannot be overemphasized.

Sonographic depiction of the retromammary region is evidence of adequate penetration of the breast tissue. The layer of fat in the retromammary region is thinner than that in the subcutaneous region. The underlying pectoral muscle is easily recognized because of the strongly echoic interface between the retromammary fat and the connective tissue of the fascia overlying the muscle.

The pregnant breast has a uniform "snowy" ultrasound appearance of weak, poorly defined echoes, attributable to relatively small differences in acoustic impedance at multitudinous tissue interfaces resulting from the proliferation of ducts and lobules throughout the breast.

### Benign Disorders

*Cysts*

Cysts, the most frequent mass lesions of the breast in women aged 35–50 years, are believed to develop from dilatation of the terminal ducts. The fluid-filled masses may be solitary or multiple, unilateral or bilateral. Ultrasound is the most reliable noninvasive method for the detection of cysts, including some as small as 2 mm in diameter. Sonograms have been reported to be approximately 98% accurate in this endeavor.[21] The characteristic ultrasound features of cysts are well-circumscribed margins, including a definite posterior wall; round or oval contour; absence of internal echoes; and enhanced distal echoes.[22] The anterior and posterior margins of a cyst should be clearly depicted. However, the curvature of the cyst may make it impossible to visualize the lateral edges, which are specular reflectors. Therefore, the lateral walls frequently product posterior refractive shadows beyond the true lateral boundaries of the cyst. Cysts are round or oval and may change shape when compression is applied. They may be multiloculated. At times, a septum may be observed within the cyst.

The homogeneity of the cyst fluid provides an anechoic interior, the single most important sonographic feature of a cyst. However, debris in the fluid of a chronic cyst may cause confusing echoes. The debris is usually found in the most dependent portion of the cyst and may shift with patient repositioning. Excessively high power settings may result in false echoes in the periphery of the cyst interior.

Enhancement of the echoes beyond the cyst results from the lower acoustic absorption coefficient of the cyst relative to that of the surrounding tissues. This "tadpole tail" sign[22] is usually present, even in association with cysts as small as 2 mm. As the cyst enlarges, it may compress the surrounding parenchymal tissue, which then takes on a stronger than usual echo pattern.

A multinodular breast may contain many cysts of varying size. Ultrasound is an excellent method for the follow-up of such patients since it can depict changes in the size of cysts in response to medical therapy and can be repeated as often as necessary without concern over ionizing radiation. Although mammography is often of limited value in these patients because of the increased density of their breasts, regular mammographic screening is still useful for the detection of occult carcinomas, which may be detectable solely by virtue of microcalcifications.

### Fibroadenoma

Fibroadenoma is the most frequent breast mass in women less than 25 years of age. The mass is usually solitary, but may be multiple in 15% of cases. Histologically, fibroadenoma is well encapsulated and composed of a proliferating fibrous connective tissue stroma, ducts, and acini. Clinically, it presents as a discrete, nontender, firm to rubbery, movable mass. During pregnancy, fibroadenomas may rapidly grow to a large size. In postmenopausal women fibroadenomas involute, often resulting in the pathognomonic mammographic sign of popcorn-like calcifications.

Fibroadenomas tend to have the following sonographic features: smooth, well-circumscribed margins; round, oval, or lobulated shape; and uniform internal echoes of equal or weaker intensity than the echoes of the surrounding parenchymal tissue.[23] Echoes distal to the fibroadenoma may be decreased or enhanced.[24]

The margins are smooth, well demarcated, and sometimes lobulated. Approximately 20% of fibroadenomas show distal refractive shadowing.[23] This refractive shadow sign results from nonspecular refraction at the lateral aspects of the capsule of the fibroadenoma. The internal echoes are attributed to the regularly spaced cleft-like ducts in the tumor. Jackson et al. reported that only 12 of 76 biopsy-proved fibroadenomas had the classic sonographic appearance.[24] Atypical findings that are reported to occur in many fibroadenomas include border irregularity, lobulation, and inhomogeneity of internal echo texture.

### Cystosarcoma

Cystosarcoma phylloides is a fibroepithelial tumor similar to, and perhaps derived from, fibroadenoma. Cystosarcomas are usually benign, but rarely have been reported to metastasize. Histologically, cystosarcoma manifests an excessively cellular, often sarcoma-like stroma, in comparison to the hypocellular stroma of fibroadenoma. Although the sonographic features are usually similar to those of fibroadenoma, cystosarcoma may show anechoic cystic spaces within the tumor and secondarily enhanced acoustic transmission.[25]

### Abscess

The clinical history may include breast tenderness, an enlarging mass, and fever. Abscesses are usually located in the subareolar area. Since abscesses contain fluid, their sonographic features may be similar to those of cysts. Typically they have a thick, irregular wall. Their interior is hypoechoic or anechoic, and may contain septations.

### Galactocele

Arising within a lactating breast, the galactocele represents a localized accumulation of milk secondary to an obstructed duct. It may be detected long after nursing has been terminated. Sonographic features are similar to those of cysts: well-defined margins and an oval shape that may be altered by compression.

However, the milk content gives multiple low-level echoes. Posterior enhancement, if at all present, is moderate.

### Hematoma

A hematoma is usually characterized by a poorly defined focus of architectural disruption containing weak internal echoes. Often there is a history of preceding surgery or trauma. The hematoma may liquify within 2 or 3 hours after the trauma,[26] resulting in the sonographic appearance of a fluid-filled area. Blood cells and serum may separate, resulting in a fluid-sediment level.

### Postsurgical Changes

In addition to the formation of a hematoma, a biopsy may also result in changes in skin and parenchymal texture. The skin may be thickened and retracted at the biopsy site. Skin retraction and parenchymal scars may result in attenuation of the ultrasound beam that may mimic a shadowing lesion or obscure an underlying abnormality. It is important, therefore, to be aware of the sites of previous biopsies when interpreting an ultrasound examination.

### Augmentation Mammoplasty

Although saline or silicone gel-filled implants tend to limit the usefulness of both mammography and breast ultrasound, sonography sometimes depicts more of the displaced parenchyma. The prosthesis appears as a relatively echo-free area in the center of the breast. However, it is not unusual to see echoes representing debris within the implant bag.[27]

## Malignant Lesions

The ultrasound appearances of the various types of breast carcinoma are not sufficiently consistent to use as a basis for predicting histologic type. Rather, breast carcinoma has a broad range of sonographic features. Infiltrating ductal carcinoma tends to have the most distinctive features, while medullary carcinoma tends to have features similar to those of benign solid masses.

### Poorly Circumscribed Cancers

Infiltrating ductal carcinoma, the most common breast malignancy, usually forms a mass that has poorly defined margins. Grossly, the tumor has irregular margins. On mammograms, it may be associated with microcalcifications and adjacent parenchymal and skin changes. Histologically infiltrating ductal carcinoma contains a preponderance of fibrous connective tissue and a far lesser amount of epithelial tumor cells.[28]

The sonographic features are irregular margins, a moderately sharp anterior boundary, a poor or absent posterior boundary, weak inhomogeneous internal echoes, and attenuation of posterior echoes.[28-30] Secondary signs include alteration of surrounding echoes, thickening or straightening of Cooper's ligaments, skin thickening and retraction, and alteration of the echoes in the subcutaneous fat.[31] Microcalcifications, often the key mammographic feature of this tumor, are only rarely imaged on sonograms. Thus mammography is far more effective for early diagnosis.

The boundary of the tumor is jagged and uneven. The boundary is usually intermediate in brightness anteriorly but weak to absent posteriorly. The sonographic depiction of the margins of the tumor depends both on the nature of the mass and the incidence of the ultrasound beam. The lateral borders are usually better visualized than the anterior and posterior ones.

Internal echoes may vary in number and intensity from one lesion to the next, but generally are of a low level, similar to those of fatty tissue, and lower than those of breast parenchymal tissue. The internal echoes tend to be nonuniform in size and intensity.

Attenuation of echoes distal to the tumor is a helpful sign, but only occurs in approximately two thirds of cases. The sign has been termed posterior shadowing, distal shadowing, distal attenuation, retrotumorous shadowing, and acoustic middle shadowing. The degree of attenuation of distal echoes will depend also on the nature of the mass, the scanning technique, and instrumentation. Posterior shadowing is believed to be due to the high absorption of ultrasonic energy by the tumor, and depends directly on its fibrous connective tissue content.[28, 29]

Skin changes resulting from carcinoma are best depicted in examinations performed with water-path automated scanners. Bilateral asymmetry in ultrasonic penetration of the breasts is another important secondary sign that may be appreciated in water-path examinations.[32] Lack of adequate penetration of an area of one breast should be viewed with suspicion, and a further attempt should be made to depict the region by increasing sonic power and/or by using breast compression. Focal abnormalities in the fat overlying a carcinoma include increased echogenicity and loss of the normally well demarcated fat-parenchymal interface.

### Well-circumscribed Carcinomas

Approximately 10% of carcinomas have a well-circumscribed margin on ultrasound images and are difficult or impossible to differentiate sonographically from benign solid masses. The sonographic features of these carcinomas are smooth margins with moderately strong anterior and posterior boundaries, homogeneous internal echoes, and variable distal echoes. Carcinomas that typically show well-circumscribed margins on mammography and ultrasound include the medullary, papillary, and colloid histologic types. Infiltrating ductal carcinomas are sometimes well marginated. Intracystic papillary carcinoma is rare and tends to occur in older women. Sonographically it may have a mixed cystic and solid echo pattern.[33]

### Cancer Metastatic to the Breast

Tumors metastatic to the breast from extramammary malignancies are uncommon, but may originate from almost any primary tumor. The metastases may be single or multiple. They tend to be well circumscribed on mammograms, albeit with a slightly irregular or fuzzy border.[34] On ultrasound they show smooth margins and varying distal echo effects.

### Sarcomas

Sarcomas of the breast are relatively rare. Grant et al. reported an angiosarcoma of the breast that was characterized by a multilobulated mass manifesting both low- and high-level internal echoes and no significant attenuation of distal echoes.[35]

## Potential Errors

Errors may result from faulty interpretation, suboptimal performance of the examination, or limitations of the ultrasound instrument.

Knowledge of the patient's history and physical examination and mammographic findings is essential when interpreting the sonogram. For example, in women under 30 years of age almost all well-circumscribed solid masses are fibroadenomas. Awareness of the location of previous trauma or surgery is essential when interpreting the examination, since these episodes may result in skin thickening or retraction, asymmetric acoustic attenuation, architectural changes, shadowing, or mass (hematoma, or lipid-filled cyst secondary to fat necrosis). Lumpectomy and radiation therapy may lead to localized architectural abnormalities and skin thickening.[36]

Sonography should not be used as a substitute for mammography. Ultrasound is particularly inaccurate in the detection of cancers less than 1 cm in diameter, cancers within a fatty breast, and cancers manifested mammographically only by malignant calcifications. In one prospective study of 1,000 women, ultrasound detected only 8% of cancers less than 1 cm in diameter, compared to 92% detected by mammography.[9] Ultrasound frequently fails to depict a cancer in a fatty breast even when it is obvious on clinical and mammographic examinations; ultrasound images of fatty breasts are generally unsatisfactory because of poor penetration of the sound beam due to reflection and distortion by multiple interfaces of fat with Cooper's ligaments, ducts, vessels, and parenchymal tissue. Although mammography reliably depicts microcalcifications, ultrasound usually does not detect this important sign of early breast cancer.

An isolated island of fat may mimic a solid mass, particularly in a predominantly glandular or fibrous breast. Correct identification of the fat lobule depends on careful serial evaluation to determine that it merges with and has a texture identical to that of the adjacent fatty tissue. Correlation with mammograms is important since mammography is very accurate in fatty breasts.

Benign conditions may on occasion present with the typical sonographic features of malignancy: irregular margins, diminished sound transmission distally, thickened or retracted skin, and architectural changes. Decreased sound transmission can be seen behind such normal structures as the nipple and Cooper's ligaments, and behind any focus of increased fibrous tissue such as a scar or a nodule of sclerosing adenosis.

Inadequate sound penetration of breast tissue may result in a false negative examination. The center of the breast may be poorly imaged due to nipple shadowing, dense parenchyma, increased amounts of connective tissue around the more central lactiferous ducts, or increased prominence of Cooper's ligaments. Methods for improving penetration include the use of greater power, changing transducers, and compression of the breast.

The use of excessive power may result in artifactual echoes in a cyst. Debris within a fluid-filled mass will also produce echoes, but these can be shown to be gravity dependent by repositioning the patient. It may be difficult to show enhancement of echoes distal to a cyst that is adjacent to the chest wall. This problem can be overcome by repositioning the patient so that she is oblique or by redirecting the ultrasound beam from the side. This will often cause some of the parenchyma, and hence distal echo enhancement, to appear behind the cyst.

Different types of real-time or automated ultrasound equipment may produce vastly different images of the same breast. Furthermore, the same machine operated by different technologists may yield varying images. It is important to learn the advantages and disadvantages of specific instruments.[17]

## References

1. Wild JJ, Reid JM: Further pilot echographic studies on the histologic structure of the living intact human breast. *Am J Pathol* 1952; 28:839.
2. Howry DM, Stott DA, Bliss WR: The ultrasonic visualization of carcinoma of the breast and other soft tissue structures. *Cancer* 1954; 7:354.
3. Kratchowil A, Kaiser P: Die Darstellung der Erkrankungen der weiblichen Brust im Ultraschallschnitt-bildverfahren, in Bock J, Ossoining K (eds): *UltrasonoGraphia Medica.* Vienna, Verlag der Weiner Medizinischen Akademie, 1969, vol 3, pp 119–126.
4. Deland FH: A modified technique of ultrasonography for the detection and differential diagnosis of breast lesions. *AJR* 1969; 105:446.
5. Jellins J, Kossoff G, Buddee FW, et al: Ultrasonic visualization of the breast. *Med J Aust* 1971; 1:305.
6. Kobayashi T: Ultrasonic diagnosis of breast cancer. *Ultrasound Med Biol* 1975; 1:383.
7. Kelly-Fry E: Breast imaging, in Sabbagha RE (ed): *Ultrasound Applied to Obstetrics and Gynecology.* New York, Harper & Row, 1980, pp 327–350.
8. Rosner D, Weiss L, Normal M: Ultrasonography in the diagnosis of breast disease. *J Surg Oncol* 1980; 14:83.
9. Sickles EA, Filly RA, Callen PW: Benign breast lesions: Ultrasound detection and diagnosis. *Radiology* 1984; 151:467.
10. Fleischner AC, Muhletaler CA, Reynolds VH, et al: Palpable breast masses: Evaluation by high frequency, hand-held real-time sonography and xeromammography. *Radiology* 1983; 148:813.
11. Rubin E, Miller VE, Berland LL, et al: Hand-held real-time breast sonography. *AJR* 1985; 144:623.
12. Sickles EA, Filly FA, Callen PW: Breast cancer detection with ultrasonography and mammography: Comparison using state-of-the-art equipment. *AJR* 1983; 140:843.
13. Texidor HS, Kazam E: Combined mammographic-sonographic evaluation of breast masses. *AJR* 1977; 128:409.
14. Kopans DB, Meyer JE, Lindfors KL, et al: Breast sonography to guide cyst aspiration and wire localization of occult solid lesions. *AJR* 1984; 143:489.
15. Kossoff G, Jellins J: The physics of breast echography. *Semin Ultrasound* 1982; 3:5.
16. Kimme-Smith C, Hansen M, Bassett LW et al: Ultrasound mammography: Effects of focal zone placement. *RadioGraphics* 1985; 5:955.
17. Bassett LW, Gold RH, Kimme-Smith C (eds): *Hand-Held and Automated Breast Ultrasound.* New Jersey, Slack, 1985.
18. Schneck CD, Lehman DA: Sonographic anatomy of the breast. *Semin Ultrasound* 1982; 3:13.
19. Rubin CS, Kurtz AB, Goldberg BB, et al: Ultra-

sonic mammographic parenchymal patterns: A preliminary report.

20. Cole-Beuglet C: Ultrasound, in Bassett LW, Gold RH (eds): *Mammography, Thermography, and Ultrasound in Breast Cancer Detection.* New York, Grune & Stratton, 1982, p 151.

21. Jellins J, Kossoff G, Reeve TS: Detection and classification of liquid-filled masses in the breast by gray scale echography. *Radiology* 1977; 125:205.

22. Kobayashi T, Takatani O, Hattori N, et al: Differential diagnosis of breast tumors. *Cancer* 1974; 33:940.

23. Cole-Beuglet C, Beique RA: Continuous ultrasound B-scanning of palpable breast masses. *Radiology* 1975; 117:123.

24. Jackson VP, Rothchild PA, Kriepke OT, et al: The spectrum of sonographic findings of fibroadenoma of the breast. *Invest Radiol* 1986; 21:34.

25. Cole-Beuglet C, Soriano R, Kurtz AB, et al: Ultrasound, x-ray mammography and histopathology of cystosarcoma phylloides. *Radiology* 1983; 146:481.

26. Cutler M: *Tumors of the Breast.* Philadelphia, JB Lippincott Co, 1962, p 83.

27. Cole-Beuglet C, Schwartz G, Kurtz AB, et al: Ultrasound mammography for the augmented breast. *Radiology* 1983; 146:737.

28. Cole-Beuglet C, Soriano RZ, Kurtz AB, et al: Ultrasound analysis of 104 primary breast carcinomas classified according to histopathologic type. *Radiology* 1983; 147:191.

29. Kobayashi T, Takatani O, Hattori K: Differential diagnosis of breast tumors. *Cancer* 1974; 33:940.

30. Jellins J, Reeve TS, Kossoff G, et al: The ultrasonic characterization of breast malignancies, in Levi S (ed): *Ultrasound and Cancer.* Amsterdam, Excerpta Medica, 1983, p 283.

31. McSweeney MB, Murphy CH: Whole-breast sonography. *Radiol Clin North Am* 1985; 23:157.

32. Kopans DB, Meyer JE, Steinbock RT: Breast cancer: The appearance as delineated by whole breast water-path ultrasound scanning. *JCU* 1982; 10:313.

33. Reuter K, D'Orsi CJ, Reale F: Intracystic carcinoma of the breast: The role of ultrasonography. *Radiology* 1984; 153:233.

34. Derchi LE, Rizzatto G, Giuseppetti GM, et al: Metastatic tumors in the breast: Sonographic findings. *J Ultrasound Med* 1985; 4:69.

35. Grant EG, Holt RW, Chun B, et al: Angiosarcoma of the breast: Sonographic, xeromammographic, and pathologic appearance. *AJR* 1983; 141:691.

36. Grant EG, Richardson JD, Citgay OS, et al: Sonography of the breast: Findings following conservative surgery and irradiation for early carcinoma. *Radiology* 1983; 147:535.

## CASES

Lawrence W. Bassett, M.D.

### Instrumentation

Figure 14–1 illustrates a breast examination with a hand-held transducer.
This requires a methodical scanning
pattern. The patient is placed supine
and then slightly rotated by means of
a towel behind her back on the side of
the breast being examined. The nipple
should be centered and the ipsilateral
arm ideally should be abducted to
help spread out the breast tissue and
allow greater access to the axillary
tail. A water bag placed between the
breast and the transducer may be
used to place objects that are close to
the surface of the breast within the focal zone of the transducer. Acoustic
gel is placed in the interfaces between
the water bag, breast, and transducer.
Note that one hand holds the water
bag and adjusts its thickness.

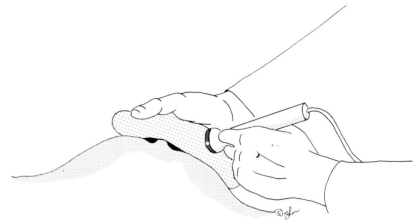

**FIG 14–1.**

Figures 14–2 through 14–4 show
three automated breast scanning units
currently in use. The word "automated" is not precise because considerable skill and experience on the part
of the technologist are required for operation, positioning, and selecting the
imaging parameters.

Figure 14–2 shows the Labsonics
unit. The patient is examined supine.
The scanning arm is moved by a re-
mote-controlled motor in a linear pattern over the compressed breast. Manipulation of the body position in
conjunction with angulation and
compression of a water-filled polyeth-
ylene bag attached to the scanning
arm is used to achieve the optimal angle of entrance of the sound beam. A
4-MHz or 7.5-MHz transducer submerged in the water bag forms transverse, diagonal, or longitudinal sections at intervals of 1 mm or greater.

Figure 14–3 depicts the relationship
of the breast and the four transducers
of the Ausonics unit. The patient lies
prone with one breast at a time submerged in the water bath; the breast
is scanned by one to four of the transducers, currently 3.9 MHz or 4.5 MHz.
The breast can be examined free-
hanging or compressed, but most

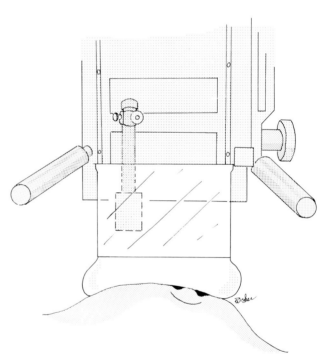

**FIG 14–2.**

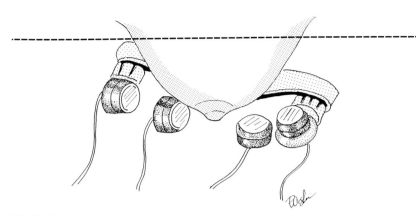

**FIG 14–3.**

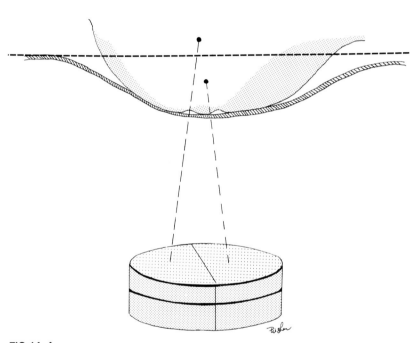

**FIG 14–4.**

breasts require compression for complete penetration. The mount for the transducers can move up or down in the tank, thus moving the focal zone to the most appropriate level.

Figure 14–4 illustrates the relationship of the breast and transducers in the Technicare instrument. The patient imaged is prone with one breast at a time submerged in a water tank. The breast is always imaged while compressed. The two transducers, each occupying one half of a round cylinder, are focused at different depths. This unit is the easiest to operate and requires the least time for a complete examination. However, because of its inflexibility, it lacks some of the diagnostic capabilities of the other machines.

## Normal Anatomy

Figures 14–5 through 14–8 illustrate normal breast anatomy. In Figure 14–5 a midline transverse section of the noncompressed breast is shown in a line drawing, and in Figure 14–6, made with an Ausonics instrument, a whole-breast ultrasound image is shown in transverse section. The breast can be divided into four distinct regions: (1) the region of the skin, nipple, and subareolar tissues, (2) the subcutaneous region, which is composed of subcutaneous fat and Cooper's ligaments, (3) the parenchymal region, and (4) the retromammary region, which is composed of a layer of fat between the parenchyma and the chest wall. With adequate penetration, the pectoral muscles can be identified deep to the breast. In Figure 14–6 the deeper tissue is not penetrated because of insufficient power combined with acoustic attenuation by the nipple, ducts, and parenchymal tissue.

Figure 14–7 is a transverse ultrasound image of the same breast with compression. The deeper tissue is now well penetrated. However, the lateral aspects of the breast are not penetrated because of critical angle refraction at the skin and fat-parenchymal interfaces.

Figure 14–8 is a sagittal ultrasound image of the whole breast of the same patient. The same anatomic structures are depicted. In addition, the ribs are seen as sonolucent structures posterior to the breast.

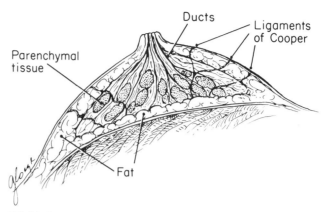

**FIG 14–5.**

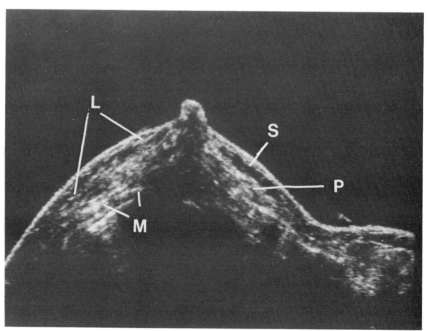

**FIG 14–6.**

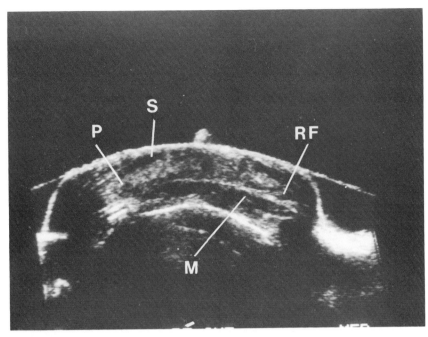

**FIG 14–7.**

SOURCE: Figure 14–5 is reproduced with permission from Bassett LW, et al: *Hand-Held and Automated Breast Ultrasound.* NJ, Slack, 1985, p 64.

L = Ligaments of Cooper
S = Subcutaneous fat
P = Parenchymal tissue
M = Muscle
RF = Retromammary fat
R = Rib

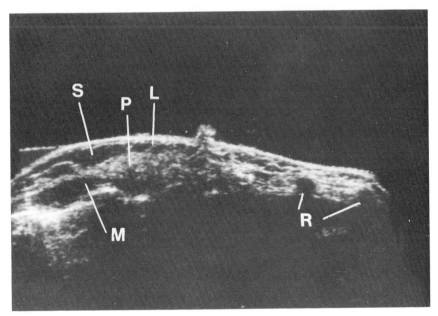

**FIG 14–8.**

## Cysts

Figure 14–9 presents the typical ultrasound features of a breast cyst (arrowhead): well-circumscribed margins, including a definite posterior wall; round or oval contour; absence of internal echoes; and enhancement of echoes distal to the center of the mass ("tadpole tail" sign). Echoes distal to the lateral aspects of the mass are attenuated due to lateral edge refraction.

Figure 14–10 shows flattening of a cyst (arrowhead) against the adjacent chest wall, a result of compression during scanning. In this case the chest wall attenuated the ultrasound beam so that distal echo enhancement is difficult to appreciate. Scanning from the side of the breast with the patient prone may allow the demonstration of enhanced echoes in the distal parenchymal tissue.

Figures 14–11 and 14–12 demonstrate an important use of ultrasound: evaluation of a nonpalpable, mammographically detected mass. The cephalocaudal mammogram in Figure 14–11 shows a small, well-defined mass (arrowhead) deep in the breast. In Figure 14–12, hand-held real-time ultrasound directed over the area in the mammogram shows a cyst (arrowhead) with well-circumscribed anterior and posterior margins, anechoic interior, and enhanced distal echoes.

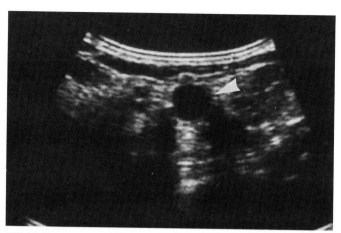

**FIG 14–9.**

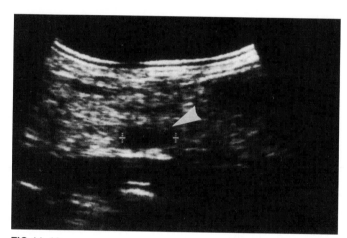

**FIG 14–10.**

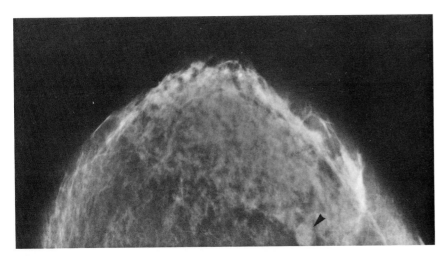

FIG 14–11.

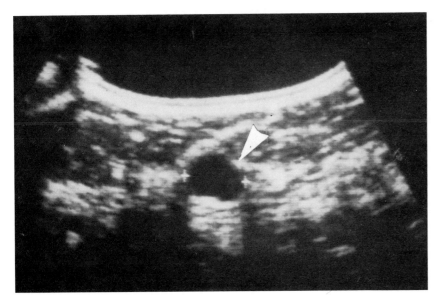

FIG 14–12.

## Cysts

Figures 14–13 and 14–14 are images of the same patient made with different transducers. Figure 14–13 is a sagittal whole-breast section obtained with a water bag and a 7.5-MHz polyvinyldene flouride transducer (Labsonics). Two nonpalpable cysts (arrowheads) are seen in the superior aspect of the breast. The larger cyst measures 4 mm. Figure 14–14 shows the same cysts (arrowheads) examined with a hand-held water-offset 10-MHz PZT transducer (Diasonics). In both studies the cysts are well depicted, but through-transmission is difficult to appreciate, because (1) the beam of these high-frequency transducers is already significantly attenuated at this depth within the breast, (2) the cysts are small, and (3) the underlying chest wall absorbs much of the remaining transmitted sound.

Figures 14–15 and 14–16 are ultrasound images of another patient with multiple lumps in both breasts. The mammograms showed very dense parenchyma, and were therefore of limited usefulness. Figure 14–15 is a transverse section from an automated whole-breast examination (Ausonics). The most lateral cyst in this section is septated (arrowhead). In Figure 14–15, compression of the lateral septated cyst (arrowhead) is demonstrated during a hand-held real-time examination.

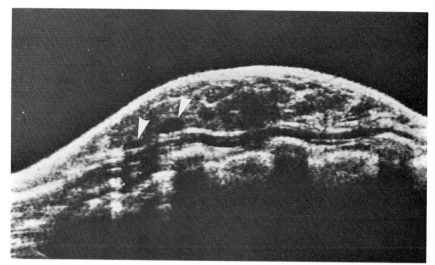

**FIG 14–13.**

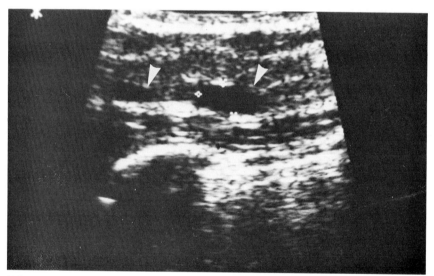

**FIG 14–14.**

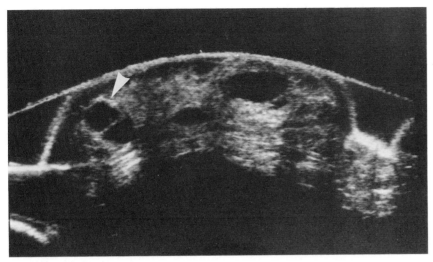

FIG 14–15.

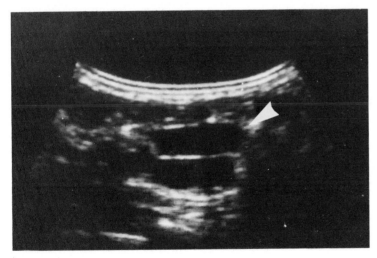

FIG 14–16.

## Fibroadenomas

Figure 14–17 shows a typical fibroad-enoma examined by hand-held ultra-sound equipment. The mass is well circumscribed, contains low-level echoes (less than surrounding paren-chyma), and results in enhancement of distal echoes.

In Figure 14–18 a fibroadenoma (arrowhead) is depicted in a whole-breast sagittal section obtained with automated equipment (Labsonics). The mass is well circumscribed and contains very low-level echoes. Unlike a cyst, it does not change shape even though it is compressed against the chest wall.

Figure 14–19 shows a fibroaden-oma of pregnancy. The patient felt a firm mass in her breast during the second trimester. The whole-breast transverse image shows that the large mass (arrowheads) is well circum-scribed and contains homogeneous medium-level echoes throughout. The surrounding breast echoes have a uniform "snowy" texture, characteristic of the pregnant breast.

Figure 14–20 is an example of a cystosarcoma of the breast, a fibroepi-thelial tumor similar to and possibly derived from fibroadenoma. The mass is well circumscribed and contains medium-level echoes. The fluid-filled spaces (arrowheads) identified in this scan (hand-held equipment) are typi-cal of cystosarcoma and may contrib-ute to the enhanced through-transmis-sion of sound characteristic of this tumor.

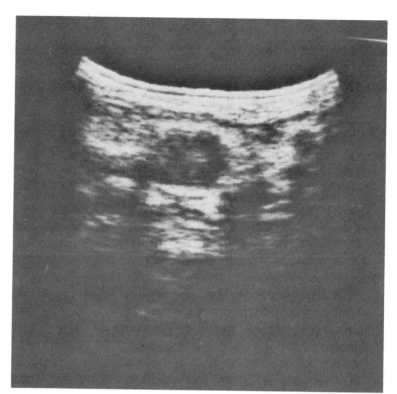

FIG 14–17.

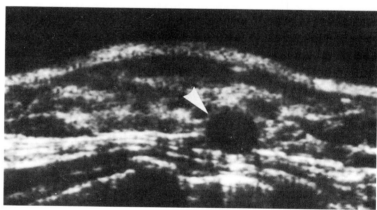

FIG 14–18.

Source: Figure 14–18 is reproduced courtesy of Joel Sokoloff, M.D.

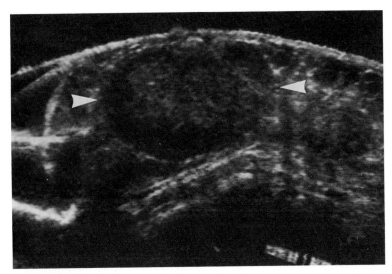

FIG 14–19.

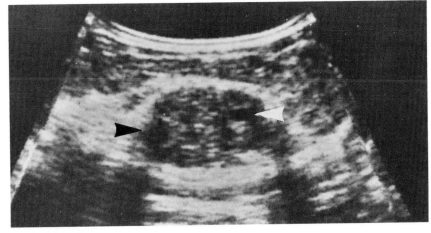

FIG 14–20.

## Other Benign Conditions

Figure 14–21 shows a breast abscess. The patient complained of pain and tenderness. The ultrasound scan reveals thick walls (arrowheads) and an anechoic interior except for two septae (arrows).

Figure 14–22 is an image from a hand-held examination of a woman 6 months post partum. A soft mass (arrowhead) is seen in the subareolar region. Aspiration revealed milky material, diagnostic of a galactocele. The ultrasound features are even echoes, relatively well-defined margins, and compressibility.

Figure 14–23 shows an image of a palpable hematoma identified 3 weeks after a breast biopsy. The margins of the mass (M) are irregular. The hand-held examination, performed with the patient supine, reveals a line of demarcation (arrowhead) between the clear fluid above and the debris-filled fluid below that has settled to the dependent portion of the hematoma.

Figure 14–24 is a sagittal section from a whole-breast examination of a patient with a silicone gel implant (Ausonics). The implant is mostly anechoic with a few scattered echoes. The surrounding parenchymal tissue is well depicted.

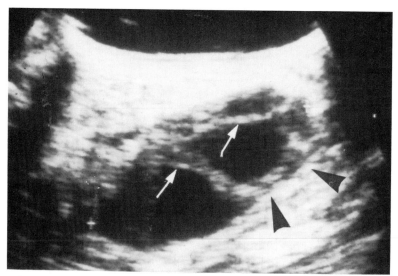

FIG 14–21.

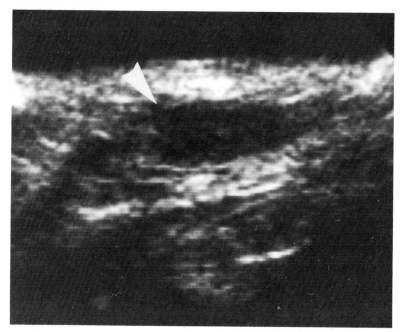

FIG 14–22.

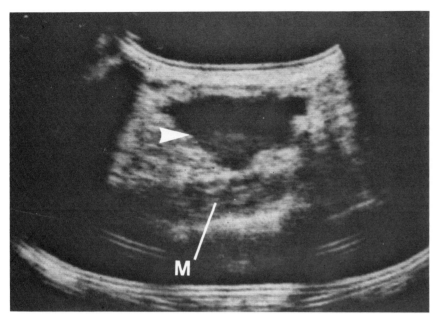

FIG 14–23.

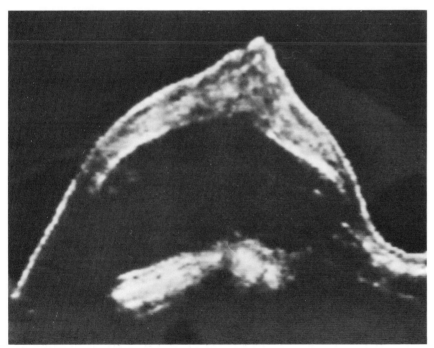

FIG 14–24.

## Breast Malignancy

Figures 14–25 and 14–26 show classic features of poorly circumscribed ductal carcinomas, taken from examinations of two patients, performed with hand-held equipment. The carcinoma in Figure 14–25 is a poorly circumscribed hypoechoic mass (arrowhead) with a poorly defined anterior wall and no sonographic indication of the posterior wall. The echoes distal to the tumor are strikingly attenuated. In Figure 14–26 the sonolucent hypoechoic mass (arrowhead) is slightly better defined anteriorly but the posterior wall is not clearly seen. There is considerable shadowing distal to the mass. The oval carcinomatous mass and the enlarging shadow distal to it combine to form a "keyhole" appearance.

Figures 14–27 and 14–28 illustrate the detection of breast carcinoma in a routine ultrasound examination. The patient, a 47-year-old woman, had no palpable or mammographic abnormalities. Ultrasound was performed because the breasts were lumpy and difficult to examine by palpation. In Figure 14–27, a film-screen cephalocaudal mammogram reveals scattered calcifications, but the excessively dense parenchyma is responsible for a suboptimal examination. A transverse section from an automated whole-breast ultrasound examination (Ausonics) (Fig 14–28) discloses a sonolucent mass (arrowhead) containing a few low-level echoes and relatively well-circumscribed margins anteriorly and posteriorly. In addition, there is lateral edge refraction. Biopsy revealed a relatively well-circumscribed ductal carcinoma.

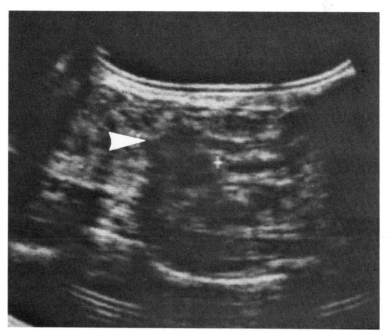

**FIG 14–25.**

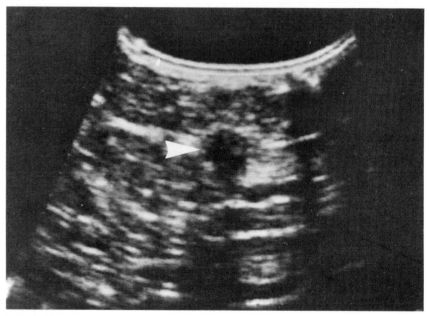

**FIG 14–26.**

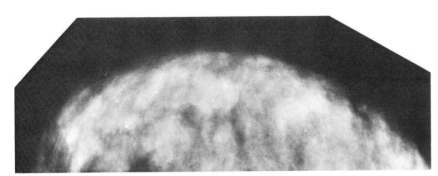

FIG 14–27.

SOURCE: Figures 14–27 and 14–28 are reproduced with permission from Bassett LW, et al (eds): *Automated and Hand-Held Breast Ultrasound.* NJ, Slack, 1985, p 179.

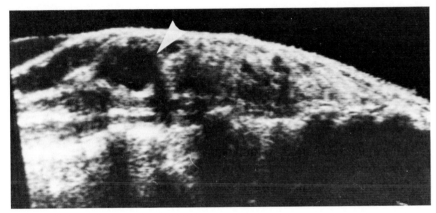

FIG 14–28.

## Breast Malignancy

Figures 14–29 through 14–32 show examples of well-circumscribed malignancies that serve as reminders that the "typical" signs of malignancy are not always reliable in differentiating benign from malignant solid masses. For example, attenuation of echoes distal to a mass is typical of malignancy; however, the carcinomas shown in Figures 14–29 through 14–31 all show *enhancement* of posterior echoes.

Figures 14–29 reveals a medullary carcinoma. The hypoechoic tumor (arrowhead) is lobulated, the anterior and posterior margins are both visible, and there is enhanced transmission of distal echoes.

Figures 14–30 is the ultrasound scan, obtained with hand-held equipment, of a 79-year-woman with a palpable mass that was well demarcated on mammograms. The tumor (arrowhead) has well-circumscribed margins, a smooth contour, hypoechoic echoes, and enhanced transmission of echoes beyond the tumor.

Figure 14–31 shows a well-circumscribed colloid carcinoma (arrowheads) that is difficult to differentiate from the surrounding fatty tissue. However, the posterior wall is clearly seen and there is marked enhancement of posterior echoes, signs usually associated with a benign mass.

Figure 14–32 shows a lesion metastatic to the breast (arrowhead) from a primary lung carcinoma. Note the high- and medium-level internal echoes, lobulated well-circumscribed margins, and slight posterior echo enhancement.

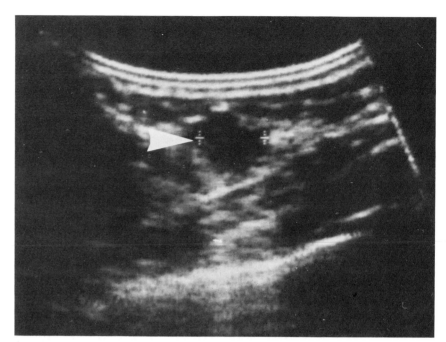

**FIG 14–29.**

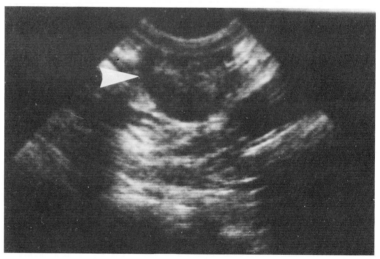

**FIG 14–30.**

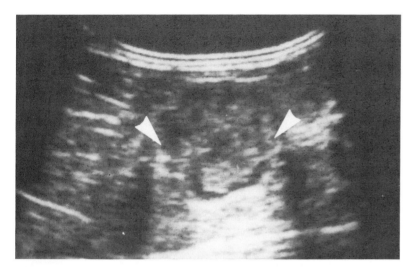

FIG 14–31.

SOURCE: Figure 14–32 is provided courtesy of Valerie Jackson, M.D.

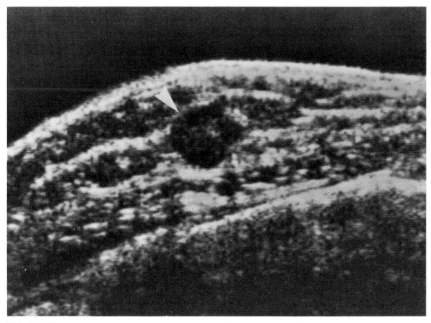

FIG 14–32.

## Potential Errors

The scans shown here illustrate potential errors in the interpretation of ultrasound images of the breast.

A localized shadow may represent malignancy. However, a shadow may also result from attenuation of the ultrasound beam by breast interfaces and Cooper's ligaments when the beam strikes them at the critical angle. Figure 14–33 illustrates shadowing (arrowhead) arising from retracted skin at the site of a previous biopsy. In the image shown in Figure 14–34, the shadowing (arrowheads) was secondary to an air bubble on the surface of a breast suspended within the water tank of an automated unit (Ausonics).

Figures 14–35 and 14–36 illustrate a frequent problem, the difficulty of distinguishing a mass from the surrounding fat. The mammogram in Figure 14–35 depicts a mass (arrowhead). The parenchymal pattern consists of fat interspersed with dense tissue. In the automated ultrasound examination (Technicare) shown in Figure 14–36, the sonolucent mass (arrowhead) is difficult to differentiate from the surrounding fat lobules.

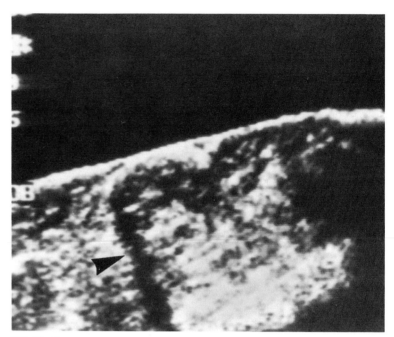

FIG 14–33.

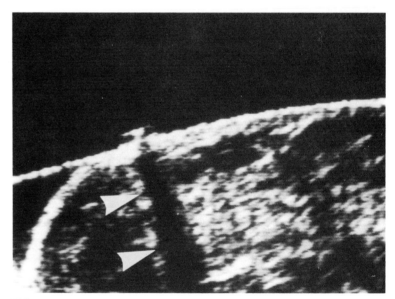

FIG 14–34.

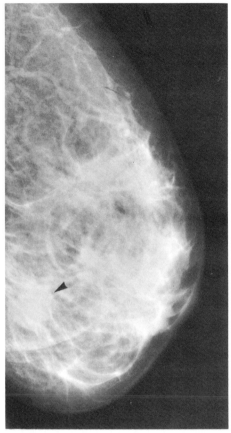

**FIG 14–35.**

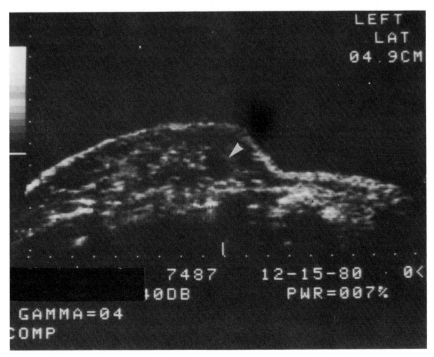

**FIG 14–36.**

# 15.
# Pelvic Ultrasonography

George R. Leopold, M.D.

## Introduction

It is not surprising that the study of gynecologic masses was one of the earliest applications of B-scan ultrasonography. In addition to the fact that Dr. Ian Donald, an obstetrician and gynecologist, was among the first users, the anatomic considerations suggest that the pelvis is an ideal area for investigation. The position of the urinary bladder, which, when distended, displaces bowel and provides a reference fluid, is particularly fortuitous. It is this feature that renders ultrasound so successful in studies of the developing fetus. In addition, gynecologic masses are frequently large and fluid filled, making them ideal targets for sonography.

In recent years, the scope of sonography has been greatly widened in the study of pelvic pathology.[1] Improved resolution real-time instrumentation now permits evaluation of much smaller structures (e.g., ovaries, seminal vesicles). A wide range of studies in the male patient has also evolved and is providing greater diagnostic capability. It should also be remembered that in addition to the male and female genitourinary tract, the pelvis is also home to the anterior abdominal wall, the tissues of the pelvic sidewall, the large and small bowel, and the bony pelvis.[2] Pathologic conditions involving these structures may also present on pelvic sonography and increase the diagnostic challenge (and reward).

## Examination Techniques

Although air-filled bowel may degrade ultrasound images of the upper abdomen, this is almost never the case in pelvic sonography. Significant advantages accrue from distention of the urinary bladder. Ingestion of several glasses of water 30–40 minutes before the examination will usually be satisfactory. If more rapid filling is desired, intravenous diuretics are occasionally used. In some patients, retrograde filling of the bladder through a catheter is a suitable alternative.

In some situations significant bladder filling is impossible. In those patients who have undergone cystectomy, the usual advantages are lost (but ultrasound can still provide useful information). When pelvic masses are large, the patient will have difficulty filling the bladder. This accounts for the very prominent symptom of urinary frequency. Fortunately, this is not a severe problem, as the mass itself achieves the goal of upward displacement of the bowel.

In performing such studies, the sonographer should recall that the examination is accompanied by some discomfort, particularly if undue pressure is exerted on the transducer. It is therefore imperative that the diagnostic information be obtained as quickly as possible. In many cases the patient may be allowed to void either partially or completely after scanning has visualized the lowest recesses of the pelvis. Such scanning also has diagnostic utility as it will occasionally disclose that the fluid-filled pelvic mass in question is the urinary bladder itself. If the kidneys are to be examined to detect hydronephrosis or other pathology, this should be done after the patient has voided, as many normal patients show distention of the renal pelvis when the bladder is full.

The choice of equipment for pelvic studies is quite varied. Both static scanning and real-time methods have strong advocates. Static scans with their more global views are preferred by many, particularly if those interpreting the study are not present when it is performed. Proponents of real-time scanning point out the advantage of being able to recognize peristalsis within fluid-filled small bowel loops, which distinguishes them from pathologic masses. In addition, real-time scanning is essential if a water enema is being used to confirm the relationship of the rectum and sigmoid colon to an observed abnormality. More recently, some have recommended combining the real-time scanning with digital examination to increase diagnostic accuracy.[3]

In general, instruments that produce images in sector format are more satisfactory for these applications. The ability to angle these transducers caudad from behind the symphysis pubis is a significant advantage. Also, in scanning the pelvic sidewalls, the smaller apertures are better suited to the angled approach from the opposite side of the pelvis necessary for optimum demonstration.

A complete survey of the area in question is required. In the transverse (axial) plane the scans must extend from the umbilicus to the symphysis or as far caudad as possible. In the sagittal plane, the scans must be carried from one side of the true pelvis to the other. The distal portion of the iliopsoas muscle forms a convenient landmark indicating the boundary between true and false pelvis. At times, oblique planes

are necessary to establish relationships between structures seen in different scan planes. For example, oblique planes are quite useful in determining whether a mass arises from the uterus (connects with the cervix) or from the adnexal structures.

## Normal Pelvic Anatomy

### General Considerations

#### URINARY BLADDER

The most consistent anatomy in the pelvis easily identified on sonography is the fluid-filled urinary bladder. Its shape on transverse scans is somewhat variable, but when completely distended it has an amazingly rectangular shape. Urine volume may be accurately estimated by using a variety of elaborate planimetric methods, but this is unnecessary for most clinical purposes. In the dependent portion of the bladder, a collection of low-level echoes is frequently seen and is believed to represent sediment. This is to be differentiated from the band of echoes seen in the bladder when a scan is made close to its border with surrounding soft tissue. This band of echoes is usually referred to as "slice thickness artifact" and arises from the width of the transducer beam, similar to the partial volume effect observed on computed tomography (CT) scans. These artifacts may be differentiated from true echoes by their disappearance when the same area is examined in a scan made at a 90° angle to the first scan. Similarly, commonly seen echoes just deep to the interface between the skin and the anterior aspect of the bladder represent reverberation echoes from the marked mismatch in acoustic impedance that occurs at that site.

In the sagittal plane, the bladder shape looks considerably different. Its apex (cephalad) is often pointed, a feature believed to be related to its embryologic connection with the urachus.

#### PELVIC MUSCULATURE

On high transverse scans, the iliopsoas muscles are noted in their characteristic position along the pelvic sidewall. These muscles are flame-shaped in outline and possess a dense central echo which represents the division between the iliacus and psoas portion of the muscle. In this groove run the neurovascular structures that supply the muscle. Farther caudad, the thinner obturator internus muscles are seen covering the pelvic sidewalls—usually oriented in a direct anteroposterior plane. Posteriorly and coursing transversely, the piriform muscles may also be identified. Between the anteriorly located bladder and the piriform muscles, the rectum is a prominent feature. On sonograms it is easily recognized by the shadowing effect that comes from air admixed with stool in the rectum. Anterior to the urinary bladder, the symmetric halves of the rectus abdominis muscle are easily visualized if proper care in scanning is observed.

### Male Pelvis

The prostate and seminal vesicles are easily recognized by utilizing the distended bladder technique. In both transverse and sagittal planes, the prostate is best seen by angling the transducer caudally from a position just above the symphysis pubis. The normal prostate appears as rectangular structure with rounded corners at the base of the bladder. The portion best seen on suprapubic sonography is the median lobe. With high-resolution instruments, the prostatic urethra may be seen as an echogenic dot in the center of the gland. Ordinarily low-level echogenicity is noted, but in older patients, strong punctate echoes with shadowing are often noted from the calcifications that commonly occur.

The seminal vesicles lie just cephalad and slightly posterior to the prostate. On transverse scans they can be seen by angling the transducer slightly cephalad from the prostate. In this plane, the "bowtie" configuration of these glands is quite distinctive. On sagittal scans a slightly oblique orientation is necessary to demonstrate both the prostate gland and one of the seminal vesicles on a single scan. The normal glands have a texture very similar to that of the prostate.

Other ultrasonographic approaches to these structures have been advocated by many. The prostate and seminal vesicles may be studied in greater detail by introducing a probe into the rectum and advancing it to the appropriate level.[4] Contact with the rectal mucosa is achieved by covering the transducer with a water-filled balloon. Such images may be generated by the use of transducers that rotate 360° (circular image) or by linear array transducers (square or rectangular images).[5] A third endoscopic approach is a small rotational transducer mounted on a cystoscope used in conventional manner. The advantage of both the urethral and rectal methods is the decreased distance the sound must travel from the transducer to the target. This allows the use of probes of higher frequency and correspondingly improved resolution. While such devices have been slow to be accepted, they continue to increase in favor with urologists for solving specific problems.

### Female Pelvis

Since the normal uterus is closely applied to the surface of the bladder, it is an easy target for sonography. Because its long axis is chiefly in the sagittal plane, images made in this projection more completely demonstrate the organ. Before the onset of puberty, the uterus is seen as a uniform block of tissue in the expected location. It is only with the onset of menses that it assumes the characteristic pear-shaped configuration.[6] The uterine cervix is directly posterior to the bladder and often forms a distinct angle with the fundus of the uterus. In most patients the fundus folds anteriorly, a condition referred to as anteflexion. If it folds posteriorly (retroflexed), a normal variant, many patients will be referred with the suspicion of an adnexal mass in the cul-de-sac detected on bimanual examination. On sonography, retroflexion is easy to detect. Such uteri often appear to be slightly larger than normal, leading to many presumptive diagnoses of uterine myomas. If the entire uterus is deviated (as opposed to just the fundus), the terms anteversion and retroversion are sometimes used. Criteria for the size of the normal uterus at all ages have been published.[7] Estimation of uterine size (and shape) is quite important in many gynecologic conditions.

The muscular portions of the normal uterus possess uniform intermediate echogenicity. The endometrial cavity, also better visualized in the sagittal plane, is a highly echogenic structure. Recent studies indicate cyclic changes of the endometrial echoes.[8-10] Near the time of menses, this echo complex broadens considerably. In the postmenopausal patient, the cavity is atrophic and prominent endometrial echoes are distinctly abnormal.

On sagittal scans continued inferiorly, the vagina may be recognized beneath the base of the bladder as a highly reflective structure, probably because of the echogenic nature of its mucosa.[11] Posterior to the uterus, in the region of the pouch of Douglas, a small amount of free fluid may normally be seen at midcycle. Aspiration of this fluid has confirmed that this represents an ovarian transudate and not blood, as was previously suspected.[12]

Demonstration of the ovaries requires that the bladder be maximally distended. In this situation, the ovaries are pressed against the posterolateral pelvic sidewalls and are more easily seen. Although visible in both transverse and sagittal planes, the long axis is usually better seen in sagittal projection. Some use the ovarian arteries to localize the ovaries. The ovaries are approximately 3 × 2 × 1 cm in the adult patient, but there is considerable variation in size and shape, depending on the age of the patient. If pelvic ascites is present, visualization of the ovaries, is usually enhanced. The ovaries closely resemble the myometrium in echo texture. Since they are quite mobile, a great variety of positions is possible, particularly with incomplete distention of the bladder. On transverse scans it is common to see one ovary tightly tucked against the side of the uterus while the other is separated from it by 5–6 cm, often with the rectum interposed. Such variability makes it difficult to specify precisely which ovary is being imaged when only one can be identified.

Recently, attention has been directed to the use of intravaginal transducers at the tip of the examining finger.[13] Such an approach allows the use of higher ultrasound frequencies and results in images of improved resolution. This has been particularly helpful in performing follicle studies. Evaluation of follicle size has become critical in the workup and therapy of infertility patients.[14] With the improved resolution of modern instruments, developing follicles can be seen when they reach a diameter of 1–2 mm. Ovulation generally occurs when the follicles are at a diameter of about 25 mm, and the changes observed ultrasonographically correlate well with the hormonal levels that are usually monitored simultaneously. In measuring follicles, either averaged diameters or actual volumetric calculations may be used to account for shape distortions produced by the distended urinary bladder.

In addition to diagnostic evaluation, sonography is now being used to assist in the harvesting of oocytes for in vitro fertilization procedures.[15] This may be done through transducers with biopsy guides or simply by looking from a site remote from the actual needle insertion site.[16] Such needles have been introduced through the anterior abdominal wall, the urinary bladder (via catheter), and the vagina. In many centers these procedures have replaced laparoscopic methods for oocyte retrieval.[17]

## Pathologic Conditions of the Pelvis

### Urinary Bladder

A considerable spectrum of pathology involving the bladder is demonstrable. Intravesical processes are easily seen because of the natural contrast provided by urine. Included among these are tumors, calculi, blood clots, ureteroceles, and bladder diverticula.

#### TUMOR

Ordinary bladder cancers arise from the transitional epithelium and present as polypoid masses projecting into the lumen of the bladder.[18] They are often irregular in shape and appear pedunculated. Since sonography is capable of examining the entire periphery of the bladder, one sometimes encounters lesions that cannot easily be seen on cystoscopy.[19] Such polypoid lesions are often noted as incidental findings on sonography done for other reasons, which emphasizes the need for careful inspection of the bladder on all studies. When these masses arise from the base of the bladder, there may be some confusion as to whether the source is the prostate or the bladder. Early workers hoped that thickening or rigidity of the wall of the bladder at the base of the tumor might permit better staging of these neoplasms. To date this has remained a difficult task. Greater promise is provided by intravesical sonography with improved resolution. When bladder masses are discovered, the pelvic sidewalls and adjacent supporting soft tissues must be carefully studied to detect extension of disease outside the bladder. This determination is complicated by the fact that not all enlarged lymph nodes (one of the principal means of spread) will contain tumor. Even more distressing, microscopic involvement of the nodes is routinely overlooked, causing underestimation of the extent of disease. Most workers now favor CT for complete evaluation of malignancies of the bladder, prostate, and cervix, but the problem of small diseased nodes is a serious drawback to both methods.

## CALCULI AND CLOTS

Bladder calculi and blood clots present no special problem in diagnosis. Both appear as dependent echogenic structures that shift position rapidly as the patient's position is altered. They may be differentiated from each other by the acoustic shadowing accompanying stones. Since stones often occur in situations in which bladder outlet obstruction or neuromuscular problems are present, it is not surprising that mucosal thickening is also present in a high percentage of cases (analogous to that seen on the urograms of such patients). Calcifications involving the bladder wall show acoustic shadowing, but are not displaced with positional maneuvers. They result from several conditions. Schistosomiasis is a common cause in areas where the disease is endemic. These patients eventually develop bladder cancer in the great majority of cases. More recent literature calls attention to the calcified bladder plaques and pseudopolyps that occur in patients being treated with Cytoxan therapy.

## URETEROCELES

Intrusions of the ureter into the bladder are commonly encountered. In the simple ureterocele, the urine-filled mass is found in the vicinity of the trigone, while in the ectopic ureterocele (childhood) the mass may be found in a wide variety of locations.[20] In the latter condition, careful search of the kidneys is mandatory, since many ectopic ureteroceles will be associated with an obstructed upper pole collecting system. On occasion, ectopic ureteroceles are large enough to produce obstruction of the bladder neck or of the opposite (normal) ureter, resulting in bilateral hydronephrosis.

## DIVERTICULA

Urine-filled outpouchings of the bladder are easy to recognize. Such lesions usually arise from the posterolateral aspect of the bladder. In some patients, diverticula will not empty with voiding and are therefore seen on postvoiding scans. Since stasis of urine within diverticula is common, stones are frequently identified and may be a source of persistent infection. Diagnostic confusion occasionally arises when the divertculum is very large. In this situation, it is often mistaken for the bladder itself, or an incorrect diagnosis of duplication of the bladder is suggested. In male patients, diverticula may be mistaken for cysts of the seminal vesicles if strategically placed.

## Bowel

Those performing pelvic sonography must constantly be aware of the possibility of bowel pathology presenting in this location. Both tumor and inflammatory processes may complicate the analysis of such scans.

## TUMOR

Carcinoma of the rectum presents as a solid mass with variable local spread and involvement of the regional lymph nodes. As with bladder cancer, most workers now use CT for staging purposes, but recent reports with endoscopic probes suggest that the degree of involvement of the bowel wall can be accurately predicted. Carcinoma of the cecum or sigmoid may also present as a pelvic mass. As is usual with lesions involving the bowel in circumferential fashion, a target lesion (pseudokidney sign) consisting of a hypoechoic rim and an echogenic center is produced. Although numerous loops of small bowel are found in the pelvis, tumors are relatively rare, and this diagnosis is almost never correctly suggested.

## INFLAMMATORY PROCESSES

These conditions produce collections of pus causing pelvic peritonitis. Their appearance varies from a complicated, irregular, fluid-filled mass (common) to a nearly solid tumor-like phlegmon (less common). When the right half of the pelvis is involved, appendicitis with rupture is often the inciting cause. Left-sided presentation should prompt a search for diverticulitis with abscess formation. Occasionally, other disorders such as Crohn's disease or Meckel's diverticulitis may produce identical findings.

## Upper Abdominal Organs in the Pelvis

The presence of upper abdominal organs in the pelvis may cause confusion for the unwary sonographer. On occasion, the liver and spleen may be massively enlarged and provoke this confusion. The spleen also enters the pelvis in two additional ways. In the first, sometimes termed "wandering spleen," the organ is permitted to prolapse into this area because of a very long and lax mesenteric attachment. In this situation, the spleen derives its blood supply in normal fashion from the celiac axis. Alternatively, the spleen may be truly ectopic, in which case it will be supplied by branches of the iliac artery.

The most confusing situation is the presence of renal tissue in the pelvis. Embryologically this is easy to understand, since this is their primitive location. While some of these masses have a shape and internal appearance like that of normal kidney, others have a much more bizarre appearance and defy diagnosis. As a result, any strange solid pelvic mass should prompt investigation of the normal renal locations. Absence of one or both kidneys then suggests that the pelvic mass represents ectopic renal tissue. Recognition of these kidneys is important in preventing surgical misadventures.

*Other Pelvic Structures*

Masses arising from the remaining soft tissues of the pelvis are common, and because of their extensive variety, the differential diagnosis list is very long. As mentioned above, lymph node enlargement is a common finding. In addition, tumors of the supporting muscles and skeleton occasionally are detected on pelvic sonograms. Aneurysms of the pelvic arteries can present as cystic collections—more easily recognized on real-time imaging by their pulsations. More recently, duplex Doppler instruments have aided in their evaluation. Varicosities of the adnexa are common in multiparous patients but may also be seen in patients with portal hypertension, where they serve as collaterals between the protal and systemic veins.

Posteriorly, masses such as anterior meningocele and sacrococcygeal teratoma may present as complex masses and cause considerable diagnostic confusion. Anteriorly, hemorrhage into the rectus abdominis muscle can result from a myriad of causes. These fluid-filled lesions do not cross the midline and have a rather characteristic appearance. On physical examination they are frequently confused with masses involving the more deeply located structures.

## Pathology of the Male Pelvis

*Prostate*

Considerable attention has been devoted to the ultrasonographic study of the prostate. Several approaches are possible. There is general agreement that sonography can provide an excellent estimate of the size of the gland, whether by suprapubic or by transrectal examination. Such determinations may be crucial in deciding between transurethral and suprapubic resection in cases of benign prostatic hypertrophy (BPH). One of the most valuable aspects of this study is that sonography demonstrates best the median lobe of the prostate, which is the most difficult part to palpate on rectal examination.

Attempts at differentiating prostatic cancer and BPH have been less successful.[21] Similarly, invasion beyond the capsule of the prostate is of interest but is still difficult to ascertain with current instrumentation. It is clear that sonography can increase the yield of prostatic biopsies, just as it has with biopsy of the liver and other organs.[22] One innovative approach is the use of a linear array intrarectal probe to guide perineal biopsies of the gland. If the needle is directed to a suspicious focus (usually a hypoechogenic area), the percentage of positive biopsies is significantly increased.

Following transurethral prostatectomy, the characteristic defect of the posterior urethra often observed on radiographic studies is also readily apparent on sonography.

*Seminal Vesicles*

These structures are important in a number of clinical settings. With reference to prostatic cancer, they are often involved by direct extension of the tumor. While this is occasionally noted on sonography,[23] most now believe that CT is superior in detecting tumorous seminal vesicles. More recent studies suggest that obliteration of the fat plane between the prostate and seminal vesicles on CT is considerably less reliable than was first believed.

Inflammatory processes involving the seminal vesicles are relatively common. In such cases, sonography may show a spectrum of findings ranging from diffuse enlargement to focal abscess formation. Congenital cysts are also relatively common. When such a lesion is discovered, careful examination of the kidneys is warranted, since there is a very high incidence of anomalies, particularly unilateral renal agenesis.

## Pathology of the Female Pelvis

### *Uterus*

#### INTRAUTERINE CONTRACEPTIVE DEVICES

Localization of these devices is a common reason for referral to an ultrasound laboratory. Although retraction of the attached string into the uterus is by far the commonest cause, perforation does occur and can cause serious sequelae. Sonography is a rapid and accurate method of confirming the intrauterine location of the device. Currently the copper devices are the most frequently used. Sonographically they appear as strong linear echoes in the expected position of the endometrial cavity. Differentiation from prominent endometrial cavity echoes may be made by recognition of the separate entrance and exit echoes.[24] If perforation has occurred, recognition of its extrauterine location may be quite difficult (due to bowel gas or a distant location). Therefore, if the sonographic study does not confirm an intrauterine location, plain film radiography is recommended to prove that the patient has not unknowingly extruded the device with menstruation.

Sonographers should be aware of the fact that patients with IUDs are far more susceptible to ectopic pregnancy and pelvic infections of all types.[25] In fact, the production of low-grade endometritis may well be the mechanism by which pregnancy is prevented. Such infection may be confined to the endometrium or may spread via the tubes to the peritoneal cavity. Tubo-ovarian abscesses produced in this fashion are frequently unilateral, in contrast to the usual situation. Most believe that this is due to obstruction of one tube by the tip of the device. The organisms responsible for pelvic infection with IUDs include the usual pathogens as well as more indolent organisms such as *Actinomyces* and *Chlamydia*.

#### CONGENITAL ABNORMALITIES

One of the common anomalies frequently encountered by sonographers is due to the presence of imperforate hymen.[26] In this situation, the abnormality is often not discovered until the time of menarche. Accumulated menstrual blood behind the membrane may cause massive dilatation of the vagina (hematocolpos) or of both the vagina and uterus (hematometrocolpos). Such cases produce characteristic findings and are easily diagnosed by recognizing the position of the large fluid-filled masses. Interestingly, some cases present in the newborn period, or even in late fetal life. Here the impacted secretions probably result from maternal hormonal stimulation. It must also be remembered that not all cases of hydrocolpos are due to vaginal obstruction. In some cases fistulous connections between the bladder and vagina will present identical sonographic findings.[27]

Abnormal division of the uterus is a common anomaly. The degree of division ranges from a ridge at the top of the endometrial cavity (bicornuate uterus) to a complete duplication of the uterus, cervix, and vagina (uterus didelphys).[28] Intermediate forms are also present and can cause confusion in diagnosis. In general it is helpful for the sonographer to know that if two cervices are present, a complete duplication must be present. Thus, careful scans to demonstrate the cervix in relationship to the uterine mass(es) are necessary.

In the nonpregnant state, congenital malformations may be difficult to demonstrate. If recognized at all, they are detected from mild enlargement of the uterus, usually best seen in the transverse plane. Differentiation from minimal involvement by leiomyomas may be extremely difficult. If sagittal scans show that both solid masses in the expected location of the uterus connect with the cervix (or cervices), the diagnosis of one of these disorders may be suggested. Better evidence is provided by noting two distinct endometrial cavities in transverse section. Scans performed late in the menstrual cycle when endometrial echoes are more abundant may be diagnostic.

More often, duplication anomalies will be discovered during pregnancy.[28] In this situation, depending on the degree of division, both horns may share the pregnancy (bicornuate uterus with partial septum), or the uninvolved horn may present as an enlarging solid mass alongside the pregnant horn. The key to differentiating this from a fibroid is the presence of a prominent endometrial echo. This prominence and the growth of the uninvolved horn are caused by the hormonal stimulation of the co-existing pregnancy. In cases where the pregnancy is shared between the two horns, it is particularly important to note the site of placental attachment, since implantation on the avascular septum has a strong association with abruption and subsequent pregnancy loss. As a result of the abnormal uterine musculature, dystocic labor is common and often leads to the performance of cesarian section.

## ABNORMALITIES OF SIZE AND SHAPE

Standards for uterine size at varying ages have been established. At about the time of menarche, the uterus assumes its characteristic pear-shaped configuration. If this appearance is noted in a very young child, the sonographer should suspect abnormal production of female hormones, and the ovaries should be carefully inspected. After menopause, the uterus becomes atrophic and may even be difficult to recognize. Indeed, an enlarged uterus in this period of life should be carefully evaluated to exclude the possibility of endometrial carcinoma.

## INFLAMMATORY CONDITIONS

Endometritis, almost always occurring in a setting of generalized pelvic inflammatory disease, has a variable sonographic appearance. It is common to see small collections of fluid within the uterine cavity, usually creating diagnostic confusion with both intrauterine and ectopic pregnancy. More commonly, the endometrial canal will simply appear more prominent without a definite fluid collection. In the immediate postpartum period, the presence of retained tissue is difficult to distinguish from inflammatory debris.[30] Such tissue may in fact be the nidus upon which endometritis develops.

Some authors report findings of cystic masses within the myometrium just deep to the endometrial cavity as evidence of adenomyosis. Generally considered to be "endometriosis of the uterus," this should probably be considered a different disease. Unlike endometriosis, it is usually associated with prior pregnancy and is believed to be an infolding of bits of endometrium. In any event, the finding is seen so inconsistently that it is generally of little diagnostic help.

Careful scanning in the region of the uterine cervix often discloses one or two tiny (1–2-mm) cysts within its. These represent nabothian cysts and are thought to be secondary to retention of mucus formed in the healing phases of chronic cervicitis.[31] They are of no clinical significance unless superinfection is present.

## TUMORS OF THE UTERUS

**Leiomyoma.**—The incidence of all other tumors of the uterus is dwarfed by leiomyoma (fibroid). These lesions are extremely common, particularly among black females, in whom they are also seen at a much earlier age than in the general population. Although benign, they are important because of their mass effect if large (i.e., displacement of surrounding structures, often causing bowel and bladder symptoms). In addition, they may be important during pregnancy for a variety of reasons, and their presence should be carefully noted by the sonographer. These lesions may be mucosal (deforming the endometrial cavity), mural (deforming the body of the uterus), or serosal (hanging off the exterior of the uterus). To make matters more confusing, they may be totally separate from the uterus and exist in locations such as the leaves of the broad ligament or even in the retroperitoneum. As might be expected, appearance varies widely with location. With mucosal lesions, the only observed change might be generalized enlargement of the uterus. Mural lesions, often eccentric, cause localized deformity of the uterine contour. Serosal fibroids may have a pedunculated appearance, and careful scanning is necessary to establish the connection with the uterus.

Most fibroids have an internal echo texture that is quite similar to that of the uterus itself.[32] Larger lesions may be difficult to penetrate, requiring a lower frequency transducer for demonstration. Even if such masses are markedly hypoechoic, lack of through-transmission should serve to distinguish them from cystic adnexal pathology. Focal areas of increased echogenicity usually correspond to calcification, which is commonly present. If the degree of calcification is marked, acoustic shadowing may be present and also provides a clue to the diagnosis. The literature frequently mentions enlargement of fibroids during pregnancy, but more careful studies suggest that these changes may be more apparent than real. What does occur is increased sonolucency of the mass, probably secondary to vascularity changes that accompany pregnancy. Necrosis of fibroids during pregnancy is a common cause for first-trimester pain, which on occasion may be quite severe.

Rarely, leiomyomas may undergo malignant transformation. Although the internal texture of the lesion may change, there is unfortunately no typical picture by which the sonographer may reliably predict malignancy. The best indicator of malignant transformation is very rapid growth of the lesion, so that serial studies are of considerable benefit.

**Endometrial carcinoma.**—As was previously noted, the presence of an enlarged uterus in the postmenopausal patient should arouse suspicion of endometrial carcinoma (most leiomyomas atrophy during this period of life). Many cases present with abnormal echogenic foci representing blood clots and/or tumor mass in the area of the endometrial cavity.[33, 34] Another common observation in this disorder is hematometrium or pyometrium caused by tumor stenosis of the lower uterine segment. Any of these findings should strongly suggest the diagnosis of cancer and promote further diagnostic workup. Sonography can also be of benefit in the staging of such lesions. It has been clearly demonstrated that uterine size at the time of diagnosis has a clear relationship to eventual outcome. In the past, such estimates have been made by passing of progressively larger sounds into the uterine cavity to determine its length. Not only is this procedure grossly inaccurate, it carries a significant risk of perforation. Noninvasive sonography is therefore clearly advantageous.[35]

**Carcinoma of the cervix.**—Unfortunately, this disease is still occasionally discovered by the sonographer. It is detected by the presence of a variable-sized mass involving the cervix and is often accompanied by extension into the vagina and adnexae. Since obstruction of the ureters is common, evaluation of the kidneys should be routine in these situations. The dilated ureter may often be visualized on sagittal scans of the pelvis. On transverse scans, it is easily confused with other cystic adnexal pathology. Although most cases are not discovered at a much earlier stage, careful inspection of this portion of the uterus should be done on every examination. This is particularly important in pregnancy, for the disease progresses quite rapidly and the consequences for both the mother and the fetus are profound.

*Ovary*

Both benign and malignant masses involving the ovaries are very common. They arise in many diverse clinical situations and range from cystic to solid in consistency. Precise diagnosis on the basis of the ultrasound scan alone is usually impossible. Consideration of the ultrasound scan with the results of history, physical, and laboratory diagnosis will often, however, permit an accurate assessment of pathology.[36] For purposes of discussion, these lesions will be divided into primarily cystic, a complex mixture of cystic and solid elements, and those that are predominantly solid.

CYSTIC (CYST-LIKE) MASSES

Normal follicular cysts are frequently seen and should not be mistaken for pathology. Incidental cysts less than 2 cm in diameter in a premenopausal patient may safely be watched. A subsequent scan after the next menstrual period usually shows disappearance of the lesion. At times, after ovulation, the corpus luteum of the ovary undergoes hemorrhagic change which causes it to enlarge (3–4 cm). These bodies are properly termed corpus luteum cysts. They are particularly common during the first trimester of pregnancy and require no special therapy. Rarely, as with other ovarian masses in pregnancy, they may undergo torsion and cause an acute surgical emergency.[37] Case reports also exist of such masses becoming trapped in the pelvis by the rapidly enlarging uterus and thereby preventing vaginal delivery.

Sonography may also be of benefit in the evaluation of the polycystic ovary (Stein-Leventhal) syndrome. In this condition, infertility and virilization are the most outstanding clinical features.[38] Both ovaries tend to be symmetrically enlarged and filled with multiple tiny cysts. Caution is recommended in diagnosing the syndrome on the basis of the ultrasound study alone, as many normal women tend to have very similar findings.[39] Multiple follicles are also present in the newborn and are believed to be a response to circulating maternal hormones. In premenarchal children, their presence is abnormal and should raise a suspicion of hypothyroidism.[40]

Normal ovaries may also respond to increased levels of circulating hCG by exploding into large, cystic, multiseptated masses. Since they are hormonally mediated, these cysts are bilateral. Termed theca lutein cysts, they are most frequently seen in association with forms of molar pregnancy (20%–30%). Similar changes occur in some patients being treated with infertility drugs, particularly menotropins (Pergonal). In such cases, the drug must be stopped to prevent further complications such as rupture with hemoperitoneum. If the patient does become pregnant at this time, the result is a multiple gestation with its attendant poor obstetric outcome. Occasionally, theca lutein cysts are seen in normal pregnancy, usually regressing as the patient approaches term. Because normal hCG levels are usually found in this situation, it is presumed that the ovaries are for some reason unusually sensitive to the hormone.

Other primarily cystic lesions may include dermoid cysts (although their appearance is usually more complex), endometriosis, and pelvic inflammatory disease (ovarian or tubo-ovarian abscess). Based on ultrasonographic appearance, there is little to differentiate these lesions.

In the postmenopausal patient, benign cystic lesions of the ovary are quite rare and must be considered malignant until proved otherwise. The common form of ovarian cancer occurs predominantly in older women and consists of cystic masses with varying degrees of septation and solid mural nodules. These tumors are often asymptomatic until very late in the course of the disease when they have metastasized widely to the peritoneum. In later stages, ascites is almost always present and may be loculated in nature. Because of this, precise definition of the pelvic mass is difficult. In such cases, CT may offer additional advantages, but it often suffers from the same difficulties as sonography. The cure rate for such lesions is quite poor. There is little doubt that survival in this dismal disease could be improved by earlier diagnosis of the mass, either by sonography or by physical examination.[41]

Occasionally cystic adnexal masses that arise from paramesonephric tissue or wolffian duct remnants are encountered on sonograms. It is impossible to differentiate these masses from those of primary ovarian origin. Usually referred to as parovarian cysts, they can become quite large and are subject to the same complications as their ovarian counterparts. Some pathologic series claim that parovarian cysts may account for 10%–20% of all adnexal tumor-like conditions.[42]

COMPLEX MASSES

Included here are a wide variety of lesions. Although they are generally indistinguishable from each other, there are often clues which in conjunction with the history provide an accurate diagnosis.

In premenopausal women, dermoids (benign cystic teratomas) are quite common and may be bilateral in as many as 20% of cases. As their name suggests, these tumors contain elements of ectoderm, mesoderm, and endoderm. It is therefore not unusual to find fat, hair, bone, keratin, and an assortment of other tissues within. Their sonographic appearance depends greatly on which elements predominate.[43] If significant bone or teeth formations are present, acoustic shadowing will be present. Some authors have claimed that the "classic" appearance of such lesions is a peripheral plug of solid material in an otherwise cystic mass.[44] While dermoids can clearly assume this appearance, it is not frequent in studying the entire spectrum of the disorder. In addition, other ovarian pathologic conditions such as serous cystadenoma or cystadenocarcinoma can present with identical findings. Fluid/fluid or fluid/solid levels are frequently encountered. These may be confirmed by the use of decubitus scanning. Unfortunately, this finding is also nonspecific, as it may be seen in pelvic abscesses and endometriomas as well. Finally, some have stated that a location just cephalad to the fundus of the uterus is typical for dermoid. In fact, this is a common location for all types of ovarian pathology and is in no way diagnostic. Although dermoids have no known malignant potential, they are usually removed surgically to confirm the diagnosis. Cases of rupture of dermoid and development of ascites and/or peritonitis have been reported but are rare.[45]

Of all the complex lesions, endometriosis is by far the most underdiagnosed. Gynecologists are consistently surprised to find implants from this disorder widely disseminated throughout the pelvis at the time of laparoscopy or laparotomy performed for other reasons. While careful questioning of such women may disclose symptoms that could be attributed to the disorder, they are apparently so mild that patients do not seek medical attention. Abnormal tissue may attach to virtually any structure (including bowel and ureters) and cause significant clinical problems. One of the most common complaints is infertility secondary to involvement of the ovaries and tubes. At times, the implants form cysts which can be quite sizable. It is in these patients that sonography may play a role in recognition of the disease. Although sometimes they are totally cystic, it is far more common to find a diffuse low-level echogenicity representing old blood. On gross examination endometriotic implants frequently resemble, and are called "chocolate cysts" because of the discolored blood. Alternatively, they may contain fluid/fluid levels due to different degrees of organization of the hemorrhage. More commonly with endometriosis, there are no cysts but rather a diffuse disorganization of the pelvic anatomy, often making it difficult to recognize either the uterus or the ovaries.[46] This appearance is quite similar to that seen in diffuse pelvic inflammatory disease and chronic ectopic pregnancy. A recent study comparing sonography and laparoscopy concluded that sonography is relatively insensitive and nonspecific in diagnosing this important disorder, particularly in its early phases.[47]

In pelvic inflammatory disease, a variety of appearances is also possible.[48] A common presentation is diffuse obliteration of the tissue planes within the pelvis. At laparoscopy such patients will be found to have widespread adhesions throughout the pelvis. Localized abscesses may involve the pelvis generally, the ovary alone, or in the form of a tubo-ovarian collection.[49] Tubo-ovarian collections are usually bilateral and are believed to arise from tubal infection, primarily of gonococcal origin. Unilateral tubo-ovarian abscesses are more frequently seen in association with intrauterine contraceptive devices. It should also be noted by sonographers that not all pelvic infection comes from the reproductive organs, and the possibility of appendiceal and diverticular abscesses should be considered.

Because abscesses contain much echogenic material, they may be easily overlooked or may even appear solid in consistency. Examination of the area behind such lesions, however, will reveal the characteristic enhancement of a cystic lesion. Correlation with plain films, barium studies, nuclear medicine examinations, and CT is often necessary. While some decry the use of multiple modalities to make this diagnosis, it should be kept in mind that this is an entirely treatable disorder which, if left untreated, is associated with extensive morbidity and high mortality. It therefore seems justified to use as many tests as necessary to confirm or exclude this diagnosis.

Ovarian carcinomas may also have a complex appearance. In general, these tumors are mostly cystic but contain varying amounts of solid tissue. Two types are widely recognized. In mucinous cystadenocarcinoma (benign form, mucinous cystadenoma), thin internal septations are commonly observed. This form previously was called "pseudomucinous" because of failure to recognize the material within as true mucin. In the other form, serous cystadenocarcinoma (benign form, serous cystadenoma) clumps of solid tissue frequently line the cyst. Pure serous cystadenocarcinoma has a somewhat poorer prognosis, and sonographers have therefore made an effort to distinguish between the two.[50] For the most part this effort has been unsuccessful, since the two forms commonly coexist in the same tumor and are probably just different ends of the spectrum a single disorder.

While peritoneal implants (metastases) and ascites are quite common with these disorders, the former are only rarely visualized on sonography or CT because of their small size. In contrast to the usual serous ascites seen with liver disease, the fluid collections are frequently asymmetric or loculated. Detection of these loculations is important if peritoneal chemotherapy is being considered. Sonography is also of use in the placement of catheters to instill chemotherapeutic agents. When the bowel becomes matted together by tumor on its serosa or within the mesentery, all diagnostic imaging methods are generally useless. Late in the course of the disease, liver metastases may be noted on sonograms. More frequently, and at an earlier stage, lesions are seen on the surface of the liver where it is covered by peritoneum; lesions here are difficult to distinguish from intrahepatic involvement. Metastases from ovarian carcinoma can have a strikingly cystic appearance much like that of the primary lesion.

SOLID MASSES

Entirely solid ovarian masses are far less common than the cystic variety. In younger patients, the presence of such a lesion often indicates dysgerminoma. These tumors are essentially all malignant in nature, but are usually indolent. Also included in the differential diagnosis are a plethora of rarer tumors including fibroma, thecoma, and combinations of the two.[51] Interestingly, the coma may appear in a variety of ways. The literature reports cases in which the coma presented as a lesion that was very difficult to penetrate, almost as if it were surrounded by a rim of calcium.[52] In other reports the tumor has been easily seen and entirely echo free. Such cases are difficult to distinguish from cysts unless careful attention is paid to the lack of increased sound transmission posterior to the mass. Metastatic disease to the ovary occurs from a variety of tumors and usually is solid in nature. "Drop" metastases from tumors of the stomach and colon are common and frequently bilateral. Such lesions are referred to as Krukenberg tumors and are often associated with ascites.[53] Central necrosis of these masses may occur and thereby produce a more complex appearance.

## References

1. Fleischer AC, Walsh JW, Jones HW III, et al: Sonographic evaluation of pelvic masses: Method of examination and role of sonography relative to other imaging modalities. *Radiol Clin North Am* 1982; 20:397–412.
2. Kurtz AB, Rubin CS, Kramer FL, et al: Ultrasound evaluation of the posterior pelvic compartment. *Radiology* 1979; 132:677–682.
3. Bluth EI, Ferrari BT, Sullivan MA: Real-time pelvic ultrasonography as an adjunct to digital examination. *Radiology* 1984; 153:789–790.
4. Harada K, Tanahashi Y, Igari D, et al: Clinical evaluation of inside echo patterns in gray scale prostatic echography. *J Urol* 1980; 124:216–220.
5. Rifkin MD, Kurtz AB, Choi HY, et al: Endoscopic ultrasonic evaluation of the prostate using a transrectal probe: Prospective evaluation and acoustic characterization. *Radiology* 1983; 149:265–271.
6. Orsini LF, Salardi S, Pilu G, et al: Pelvic organs in premenarcheal girls: Real-time ultrasonography. *Radiology* 1984; 153:113–116.
7. Sample WF, Lippe BM, Gyepes MT: Gray-scale ultrasonography of the normal female pelvis. *Radiology* 1977; 125:477–483.
8. Brandt TD, Levy EB, Grant TH, et al: Endometrial echo and its significance in female infertility. *Radiology* 1985; 157:225–229.
9. Fleischer AC, Pittaway DE, Beard LA, et al: Sonographic depiction of endometrial changes occurring with ovulation induction. *J Ultrasound Med* 1984; 3:341–346.
10. Hall DA, Hann LE, Ferrucci JT, et al: Sonographic morphology of the normal menstrual cycle. *Radiology* 1979; 133:185–188.
11. McCarthy S, Taylor KJW: Sonography of vaginal masses. *AJR* 1983; 140:1005–1008.
12. Koninckx PR, Renaer M, Brosens IA: Origin of peritoneal fluid in women: An ovarian exudation product. *Br J Obstet Gynaecol* 1980; 87:177–183.
13. Schwimer SR, Lebovic J: Transvaginal pelvic ultrasonography. *J Ultrasound Med* 1984; 3:381.
14. Mendelson EB, Friedman H, Neiman HL, et al: The role of imaging in infertility management. *AJR* 1985; 144:415–420.
15. Lenz S: Ultrasonically guided aspiration of human oocytes. *Ultrasound Med Biol* 1984; 10:625–628.
16. Wikland M, Nilsson L, Hansson R, et al: Collection of human oocytes by the use of sonography. *Fertil Steril* 1983; 39:603–608.
17. Lewin A, Margalioth EJ, Rabinowitz R, et al: Comparative study of ultrasonically guided percutaneous aspiration with local anesthesia and laparoscopic aspiration of follicles in an in vitro fertilization program. *Am J Obstet Gynecol* 1985; 151:621–625.
18. Abu-Yousef MM, Narayana AS, Franken EA Jr, et al: Urinary bladder tumors studied by cystosonography. *Radiology* 1984; 153:223–226.
19. Cronan JJ, Simeone JF, Pfister RC, et al: Cystosonography in the detection of bladder tumors: A prospective and retrospective study. *J Ultrasound Med* 1982; 1:237–241.
20. Friedman AP, Haller JO, Schulze G, et al: Sonography of vesical and perivesical abnormalities in children. *J Ultrasound Med* 1983; 2:385–390.
21. Abu-Yousef MM: Benign prostatic hyperplasia: Tissue characterization using suprapubic ultrasound. *Radiology* 1985; 156:169–173.
22. Rifkin MD, Kurtz AB, Goldberg BB: Sonographically guided transperineal prostatic biopsy: Preliminary experiences with a longitudinal linear-array transducer. *AJR* 1983; 140:745–757.
23. Abu-Yousef MM, Narayana AS: Prostatic carcinoma: Detection and staging using suprapubic US. *Radiology* 1985; 156:175–180.
24. Callen PW, Filly RA, Munyer TP: Intrauterine contraceptive devices: Evaluation by sonography. *AJR* 1980; 135:797–800.
25. Burkman RT: Association between intrauterine device and pelvic inflammatory disease. *Obstet Gynecol* 1981; 57:269–276.
26. Comstock CH, Boal DK: Pelvic sonography of the pediatric patient. *Semin Ultrasound CT NMR* 1984; 5:54–67.
27. Schaffer RM, Taylor C, Haller JO, et al: Nonobstructive hydrocolpos: Sonographic appearance

and differential diagnosis. *Radiology* 1983; 149:273–278.

28. Worthen NJ, Gonzalez F: Septate uterus: Sonographic diagnosis and obstetric complications. *Obstet Gynecol* 1984; 64:34S–38S.

29. Pennes DR, Bowerman RA, Silver TM: Congenital uterine anomalies and associated pregnancies: Findings and pitfalls of sonographic diagnosis. *J Ultrasound Med* 1985; 4:531–538.

30. Lee CY, Madrazo B, Drukker BH: Ultrasonic evaluation of the postpartum uterus in the management of postpartum bleeding. *Obstet Gynecol* 1981; 58:227–232.

31. Fogel SR, Slasky BS: Sonography of nabothian cysts. *AJR* 1982; 138:927–930.

32. Gross BH, Silver TM, Jaffe MH: Sonographic features of uterine leiomyomas: Analysis of 41 proven cases. *J Ultrasound Med* 1983; 2:401–406.

33. Breckenridge JW, Kurtz AB, Ritchie WGM, Macht EL Jr: Postmenopausal uterine fluid collection: Indicator of carcinoma. *AJR* 1982; 139:529–534.

34. Johnson MA, Graham MF, Cooperberg PL: Abnormal endometrial echoes: Sonographic spectrum of endometrial pathology. *J Ultrasound Med* 1982; 1:161–166.

35. Requard CK, Wicks JD, Mettler FA Jr: Ultrasonography in the staging of endometrial adenocarcinoma. *Radiology* 1981; 140:781–785.

36. Walsh JW, Taylor KJW, Wasson JF McI, et al: Gray-scale ultrasound in 204 proved gynecologic masses: Accuracy and specific diagnostic criteria. *Radiology* 1979; 130:391–397.

37. Graif M, Shalev J, Strauss S, et al: Torsion of the ovary: Sonographic features. *AJR* 1984; 143:1331–1334.

38. Hann LE, Hall DA, McArdle CR et al: Polycystic ovarian disease: Sonographic spectrum. *Radiology* 1984; 150:531–534.

39. Parisi L, Tramonti M, Derchi LE, et al: Polycystic ovarian disease: Ultrasonic evaluation and correlations with clinical and hormonal data. *JCU* 1984; 12:21–26.

40. Lindsay AN, Voorhess ML, MacGillivray MH: Multicystic ovaries in primary hypothyroidism. *Obstet Gynecol* 1983; 61:433–437.

41. Heintz APM, Hacker NF, Lagasse LD: Epidemiology and etiology of ovarian cancer: A review. *Obstet Gynecol* 1985; 66:127–135.

42. Alpern MB, Sandler MA, Madrazo BL: Sonographic features of parovarian cysts and their complications. *AJR* 1984; 143:157–160.

43. Laing FC, Van Dalsem VF, Marks WM, et al: Dermoid cysts of the ovary: Their ultrasonographic appearances. *Obstet Gynecol* 1981; 57:99–104.

44. Quinn SF, Erickson S, Black WC: Cystic ovarian teratomas: The sonographic appearance of the dermoid plug. *Radiology* 1985; 155:477–478.

45. Stern JL, Buscema J, Rosenshein NB, et al: Spontaneous rupture of benign cystic teratomas *Obstet Gynecol* 1981; 57:363–366.

46. Walsh JW, Taylor KJW, Rosenfield AT: Gray scale ultrasonography in the diagnosis of endometriosis and adenomyosis. *AJR* 1979; 132:87–90.

47. Friedman H, Vogelzang RL, Mendelson EB, et al: Endometriosis detection by US with laparoscopic correlation. *Radiology* 1985; 157:217–220.

48. Sample W: Pelvic inflammatory disease in Sanders R, James A Jr (eds): *Ultrasonography in Obstetrics and Gynecology.* New York, Appleton Century-Crofts, 1977, pp 357–385.

49. Swayne LC, Love MB, Karasick SR: Pelvic inflammatory disease: Sonographic-pathologic correlation. *Radiology* 1984; 151:751–755.

50. Moyle JW, Rochester D, Sider L, et al: Sonography of ovarian tumors: Predictability of tumor type. *AJR* 1983; 141:985–991.

51. Stephenson WM, Laing FC: Sonography of ovarian fibromas. *AJR* 1985; 144:1239–1240.

52. Diakoumakis E, Vieux U, Seife B: Sonographic demonstration of thecoma: Report of two cases. *Am J Obstet Gynecol* 1984; 150:787–788.

53. Athey PA, Butters HE: Sonographic and CT appearance of Krukenberg tumors. *JCU* 1984; 12:205–210.

## CASES

Dennis A. Sarti, M.D.

### Normal Longitudinal Scans

When the urinary bladder is well distended, the uterus is easily visualized posterior to it. With some caudal angulation, the vagina is well seen (Fig 15–1). When more cephalad, the cervix and the uterus come into view. Figure 15–1 is a scan showing the normal pear-shaped appearance of the uterus with fairly even echoes throughout the myometrium. No internal echoes are seen within the uterus on this scan. The rectum and bowel loops are noted posterior to the uterus and vagina.

Figures 15–2 through 15–4 are longitudinal scans of the uterus with a linear echo seen within the myometrial echoes of the uterus. This linear echo is secondary to visualization of the endometrial cavity. This is normally seen during menstruation. The linear echo is not markedly thick and has a characteristically high-amplitude echo to it. In Figure 15–4 sonolucency is seen secondary to fluid within the vagina. This is due to urine in the vagina, which is not unusual to see with marked bladder filling.

Usually, indentation of the posterior bladder wall by the fundus of the uterus can be seen. In all of these scans we see the uterine indentation on the bladder wall in the longitudinal scans.

Figure 15–1 also suggests a large mass posterior to the uterus. However, this is merely a pseudomass, which is very commonly seen in pelvic studies. It is due to a duplication artifact off the urinary bladder (see chapter 1).

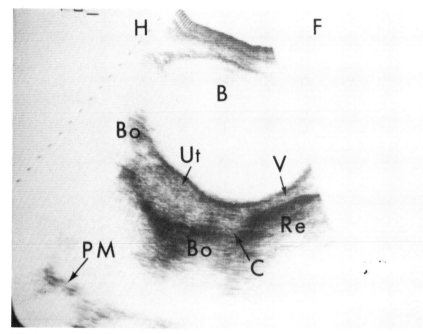

FIG 15–1.

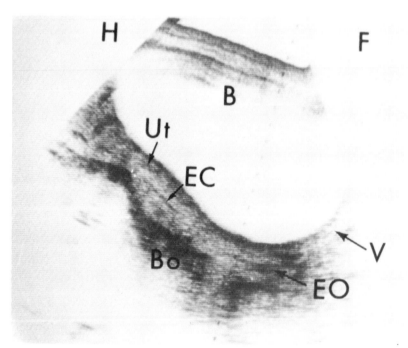

FIG 15–2.

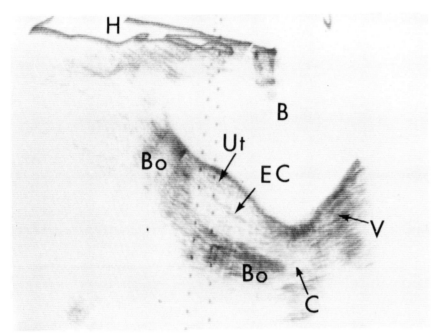

**FIG 15–3.**

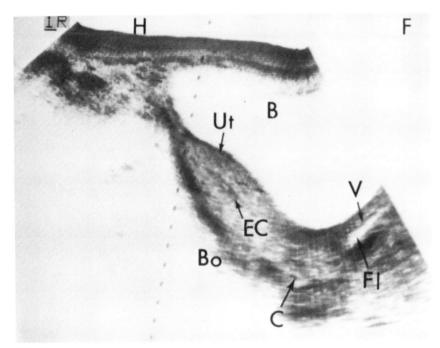

**FIG 15–4.**

| | | |
|---|---|---|
| **B** | = | Urinary bladder |
| **Bo** | = | Bowel |
| **C** | = | Cervix |
| **EC** | = | Endometrial cavity |
| **EO** | = | External os |
| **F** | = | Foot |
| **FI** | = | Fluid in the vagina |
| **H** | = | Head |
| **PM** | = | Pseudomass |
| **Re** | = | Rectum |
| **Ut** | = | Uterus |
| **V** | = | Vagina |

## Normal Longitudinal Scans

Figure 15–5, a longitudinal scan, demonstrates a linear echo within the uterus, secondary to visualization of the endometrial cavity. Around the endometrial cavity is a relatively sonolucent region (arrows). This region usually can be visualized just prior to menstruation and may represent some edema of the uterine mucosa. A strong linear echo is also noted in the cervical region, representing the external cervical os.

Occasionally, while scanning the uterus in the midline, the sonographer may see an ovary in the cul-de-sac, posterior to the cervical region of the uterus. Figure 15–6 shows an ovary in this location.

In Figure 15–7 an ovary is seen in the midline. This time, however, it is situated superior to the fundus of the uterus. It has caused indentation (arrows) on the superior aspect of the urinary bladder. Indentation of the bladder by the uterus and ovaries is a normal occurrence. It is very important to become familiar with this indentation on the bladder wall, because it may be the only clue that a pelvic mass is present.

Figure 15–8 is an example of a questionable mass in the cul-de-sac region. However, it has a strongly echogenic center and a relatively lucent periphery that is consistent with bowel.

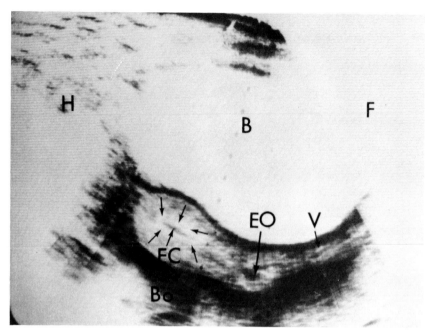

FIG 15–5.

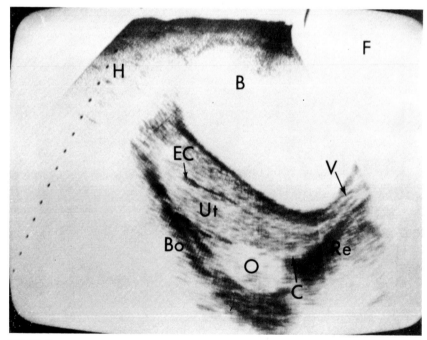

FIG 15–6.

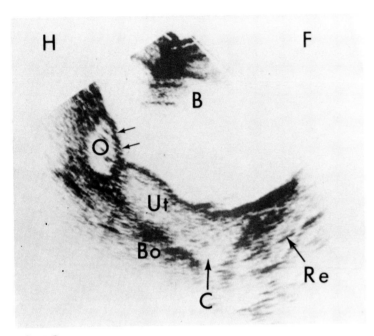

| **Arrows** | = | Lucencies surrounding the en- |
| | | dometrial cavity |
| **B** | = | Urinary bladder |
| **Bo** | = | Bowel |
| **C** | = | Cervix |
| **EC** | = | Endometrial cavity |
| **EO** | = | External os |
| **F** | = | Foot |
| **H** | = | Head |
| **O** | = | Ovary |
| **Re** | = | Rectum |
| **Ut** | = | Uterus |
| **V** | = | Vagina |

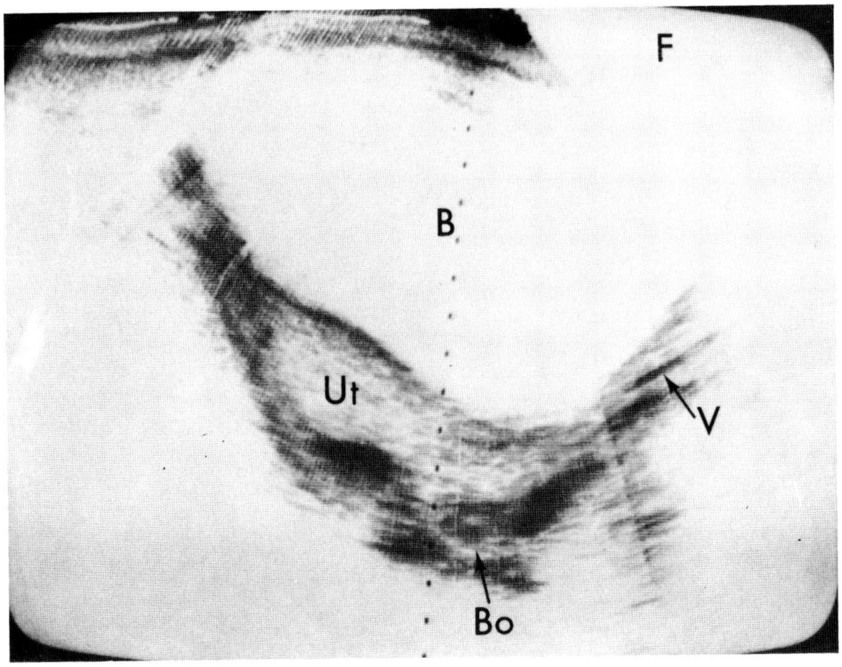

**FIG 15–7.**

**FIG 15–8.**

## Longitudinal Scans of the Normal Ovary

When examining the normal ovary, it is important to scan through the urinary bladder from the opposite side of the pelvis. For example, when the right ovary is scanned, the transducer should be over the left lower abdomen and pelvis, angled toward the posterior right side of the bladder. This will yield the best visualization of the ovary on a longitudinal scan.

Figure 15–9 is a longitudinal scan of the right ovary. Here we see the soft echoes of the ovary situated posterior to the urinary bladder. It is important to note the indentation (arrows) of the ovary on the posterior bladder wall. This is a normal finding. As mentioned previously, indentation on the urinary bladder is important in detecting a pathologic condition. Just deep to the ovary, we will see an echogenic region secondary to the piriform muscle.

In Figures 15–10 through 15–12, several tubular structures are seen deep to the ovary. These tubular structures represent the internal iliac vessels. They are important landmarks and can be visualized fairly routinely. The ovary is situated anterior to them. In Figure 15–12 another tubular structure is seen deep to the ovary. This structure is the ureter. The ovary has an oval appearance and gives a fairly homogeneous echo pattern that is often slightly less echogenic than that of the uterus.

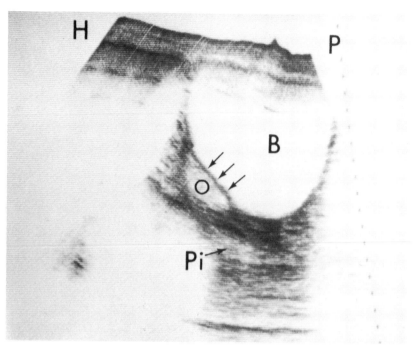

FIG 15–9.

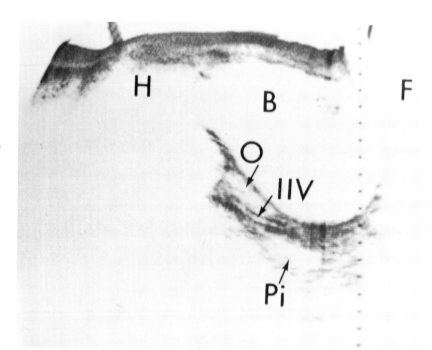

FIG 15–10.

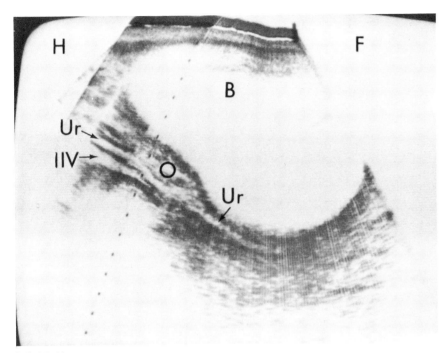

**FIG 15–11.**

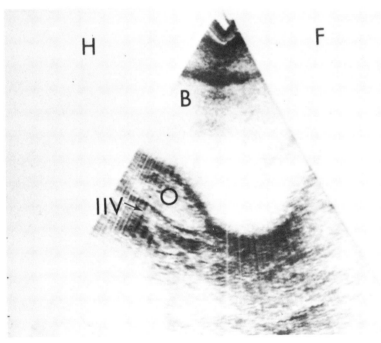

**FIG 15–12.**

SOURCE: Figures 15–10, 15–11, and 15–12 are reproduced with permission from Sample WF: Normal anatomy of the female pelvis: Computed tomography and ultrasonography, in Rosenfield AT: *Genitourinary Ultrasonography* (Clinics in Diagnostic Ultrasound Series, vol 2). New York, Churchill Livingstone, Inc, 1979.

| | | |
|---|---|---|
| **Arrows** | = | Indentation of the ovary on the urinary bladder wall |
| **B** | = | Urinary bladder |
| **F** | = | Foot |
| **H** | = | Head |
| **IIV** | = | Internal iliac vessels |
| **O** | = | Ovary |
| **P** | = | Level of the symphysis pubis |
| **Pi** | = | Piriform muscle |
| **Ur** | = | Ureter |

## Normal Transverse Scans

When attempting to visualize the vagina in a transverse plane, a caudal angulation of the transducer is necessary. Figures 15–13 and 15–14 are scans in which the vagina is visualized posterior and deep to the urinary bladder. The vagina appears as a strong linear central echo surrounded by a sonolucent rim. The strong echogenic area in the vagina is due to opposition of the vaginal mucosa. Deep to the vagina are echoes often seen arising from the rectum. Scanning more cephalad, the uterus is visualized (Figs 15–15 and 15–16). Transverse scans through the uterus are made with the transducer angled more cephalad. This places the transducer beam perpendicular to the body of the uterus.

Figure 15–15 demonstrates linear echoes on the lateral pelvic wall, lateral to the urinary bladder. These echoes arise from the obturator internus muscle. They should not be confused with echoes arising from the ovary.

The ovary will come into view as a soft echogenic mass situated in the adnexa lateral to the uterus (Fig 15–16). On the left side of the uterus (Fig 15–16) is a highly echogenic region secondary to bowel loops, most likely the sigmoid colon. It is important to recognize the muscle planes in the pelvis so as not to confuse them with the ovary. The obturator internus muscles seen in Figures 15–15 and 15–16 usually do not cause problems, because they are fairly thin and parallel the lateral urinary bladder wall.

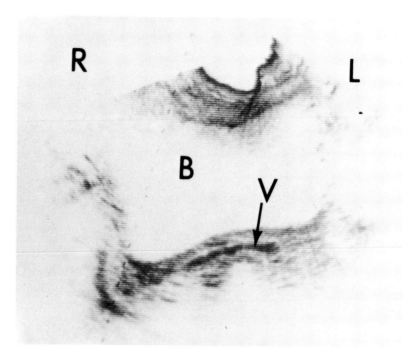

FIG 15–13.

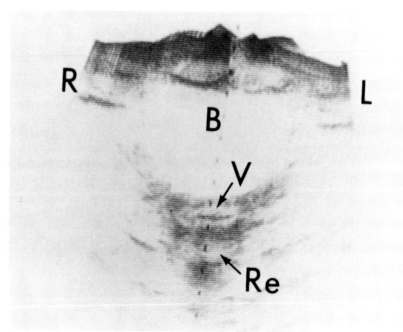

FIG 15–14.

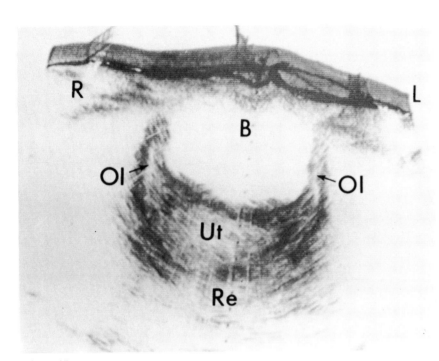

**FIG 15–15.**

SOURCE: Figures 15–14, 15–15, and 15–16 are reproduced with permission from Sample WF: Normal anatomy of the female pelvis: Computed tomography and ultrasonography, in Rosenfield AT: *Genitourinary Ultrasonography* (Clinics in Diagnostic Ultrasound Series, vol 2). New York, Churchill Livingstone, Inc, 1979.

| | | |
|---|---|---|
| **B** | = | Urinary bladder |
| **Bo** | = | Bowel |
| **L** | = | Left |
| **O** | = | Ovary |
| **OI** | = | Obturator internus muscle |
| **R** | = | Right |
| **Re** | = | Rectum |
| **Ut** | = | Uterus |
| **V** | = | Vagina |

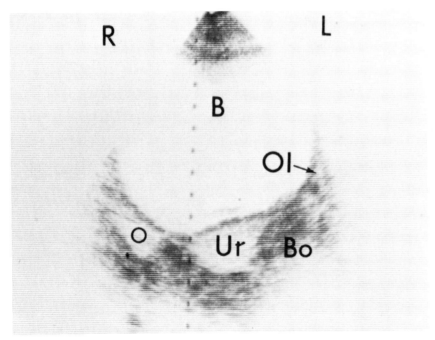

**FIG 15–16.**

## Normal Transverse Scans

As mentioned previously, it is important to recognize the various muscle bundles within the pelvis. Figure 15–17 demonstrates the right obturator internus muscle lateral to the urinary bladder. Just medial to this muscle, the right ovary can be seen to the right of the uterus. The ovary is situated just medial to the obturator internus muscle in this case.

Figure 15–18 shows two muscle groups which occasionally may be confused with the ovary or ovarian masses. The iliopsoas muscle is seen more anterior to the left ovary in Figure 15–18. A characteristically strong central echo is present within the iliopsoas muscle, and this makes it fairly easy to recognize. A lucent region is also noted anterior to the iliopsoas muscle; this represents the external iliac vessels. In Figure 15–18 the piriform muscle can be visualized posterior to the left ovary. It is this muscle that is usually mistaken for the ovary.

Figure 15–19 demonstrates the right piriform muscle posterior to the fallopian tube and the uterus. The piriform muscle often will be confused with the ovary. Usually symmetry between the piriform muscles can be seen, but the rectum and sigmoid will occasionally obscure the left piriform muscle, allowing visualization only of the right side. This may be confused with the ovary. If there is any question, a longitudinal scan over the region will determine whether the ovary or the muscle is visualized.

Figure 15–20 demonstrates a mass posterior to the uterus and secondary to an ovary which has slipped into the region of the cul-de-sac. This is a common site for the ovary. We also see the fallopian tube draping along the lateral right aspect of the uterus. Again, the characteristic appearance of the iliopsoas muscle, with the strong central echogenic center, is seen.

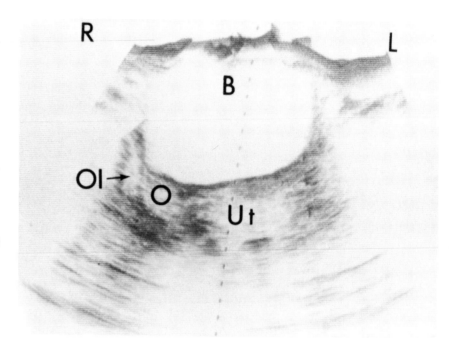

**FIG 15–17.**

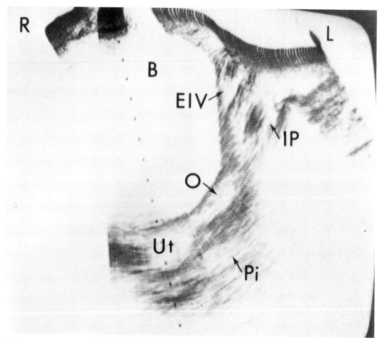

**FIG 15–18.**

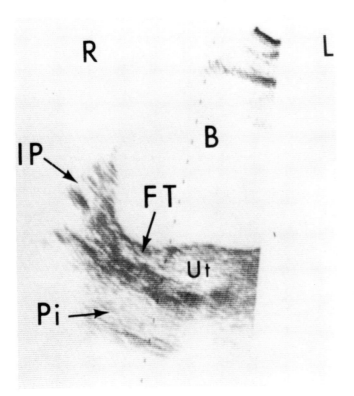

FIG 15–19.

SOURCE: Figures 15–17, 15–18, and 15–20 are reproduced with permission from Sample WF: Normal anatomy of the female pelvis: Computed tomography and ultrasonography, in Rosenfield AT: *Genitourinary Ultrasonography* (Clinics in Diagnostic Ultrasound Series, vol 2). New York, Churchill Livingstone, Inc, 1979.

**B** = Urinary bladder
**EIV** = External iliac vessels
**FT** = Fallopian tube
**IP** = Iliopsoas muscle
**L** = Left
**O** = Ovary
**OI** = Obturator intermus muscle
**Pi** = Piriform muscles
**R** = Right
**Re** = Rectum
**Ut** = Uterus

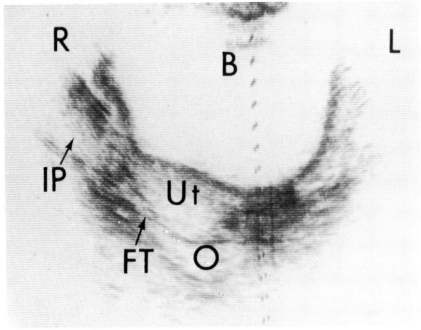

FIG 15–20.

## Retroverted and Retroflexed Uterus

When the uterus is in a neutral or anteverted position, there is excellent parenchymal texture to the uterine fundus, body, and lower segment on ultrasound imaging. The even parenchymal pattern facilitates the diagnosis of fibroids. When the uterus is retroverted or retroflexed, a technical problem arises because the deep portion of the uterus is often more lucent than anticipated. This usually leads to an overdiagnosis of uterine fibroids. A uterus is retroverted when the entire uterus is angled posteriorly relative to the vagina. A uterus is retroflexed when the fundal portion of the uterus is bent posteriorly relative to the lower uterine segment.

Figure 15–21 is the scan of a markedly retroflexed uterus. The curvilinear line (arrow) represents the interface between the body of the uterus and the lower uterine segment. This interface often assists in determining the severity of retroflexion. The fundal region of the uterus is slightly more lucent than anticipated and a fibroid could be interpreted. In Figure 15–22, a transverse scan of the same patient, the fundus of the uterus appears larger than anticipated. Fibroid is often included in the differential diagnosis. These scans show only a normal anatomic variant in which severe retroflexion is present.

Figure 15–23 shows an example of mild retroversion in which the entire uterus is tipped posteriorly. In this instance, the fundal portion of the uterus is more lucent than anticipated. The diagnosis of a fundal fibroid could readily be made in this case. However, this is a common finding and should be looked for in such cases.

Figure 15–24 shows an example of retroflexion. The uterine cavity is filled with increased echoes (arrowheads), and curves posteriorly in the fundal region. This is an excellent example of what happens to the uterus in retroflexion. On physical examination such a uterus will often present a diagnostic problem as a posterior mass will be palpated. The ultrasound findings are extremely helpful in eliciting the cause

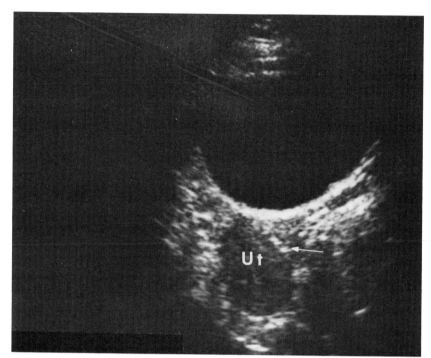

FIG 15–21.

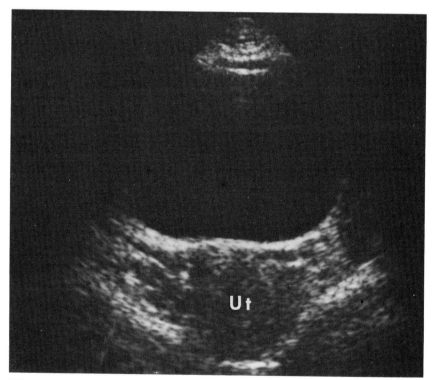

FIG 15–22.

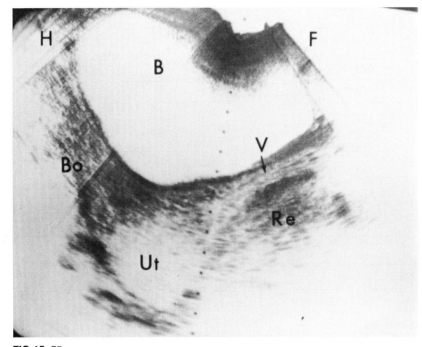

FIG 15–23.

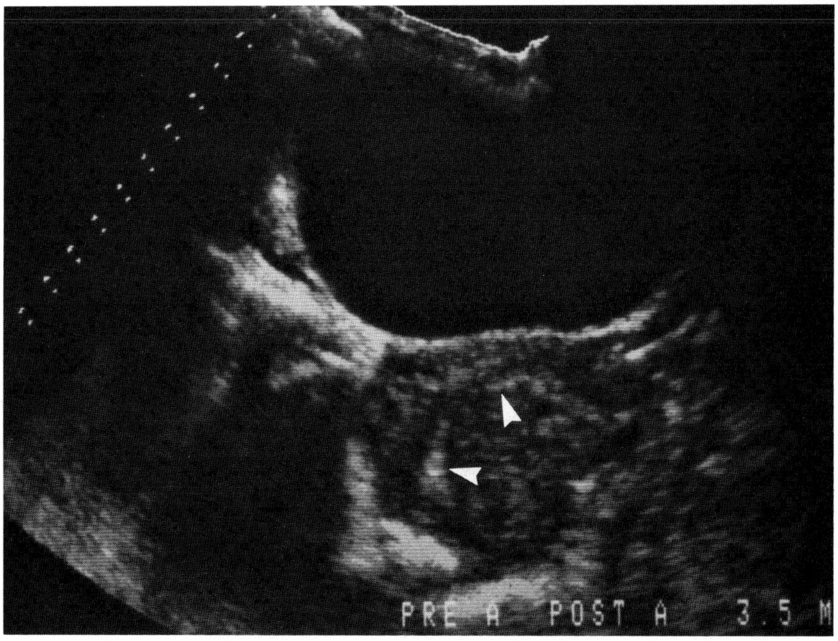

of such masses. It is easier to diagnose a retroflexed uterus when the uterine cavity is filled with echoes, such as during menstruation.

| **Arrow** | = Retroflexed uterus |
| **Arrowheads** | = Uterine cavity in a retroflexed uterus |
| **B** | = Bladder |
| **Bo** | = Bowel |
| **F** | = Foot |
| **H** | = Head |
| **Re** | = Rectum |
| **Ut** | = Uterus |
| **V** | = Vagina |

FIG 15–24.

## Absent Uterus

The pelvis is always examined with the urinary bladder filled to displace bowel loops out of the pelvis. When the bladder is well filled, the uterus is easily visualized deep to the urinary bladder. Occasionally no uterus may be identified. This may be secondary to congenital absence or may occur in an elderly woman. Most commonly, however, if the uterus is not visualized the woman has had a previous hysterectomy. In such instances, the urinary bladder will be well distended but no soft tissue mass consistent with the uterus will be visualized deep to the urinary bladder. Instead, high-amplitude echoes will be noted adjacent to the bladder surface. Acoustic shadowing will be present deep to these high-amplitude echoes secondary to air in bowel loops.

The longitudinal scan in Figure 15–25 of a patient with a previous hysterectomy is fairly characteristic. It shows a vagina continuing posteriorly and ending abruptly without evidence of a uterus. Superior to the vagina, only bowel air is visualized. Occasionally a small cervical cuff may be present and may be mistaken for a small uterus, especially in the elderly patient.

Figures 15–26 and 15–27 are also scans of women who have undergone hysterectomy. No uterus is identified cephalad to the vagina. Only bowel air is seen superior to the urinary bladder. In these two scans, fluid is present in the vagina secondary to reflux of urine into the vaginal lumen. Note that the vagina ends abruptly, with no evidence of the uterus cephalad to its end.

Figure 15–28 is a longitudinal scan of a male pelvis. The male pelvis can be differentiated from the female pelvis by the presence of the prostate gland (P) in the caudal inferior aspect. This is a typical longitudinal scan of the male pelvis. No soft tissue mass is identified cephalad to the urinary bladder, as it would be in the pelvis of a woman who has had a hysterectomy.

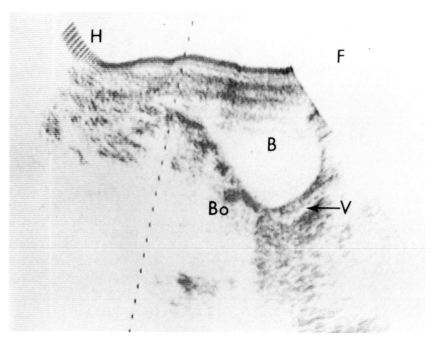

FIG 15–25.

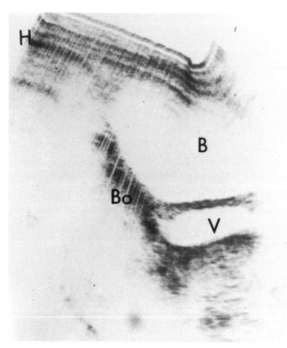

FIG 15–26.

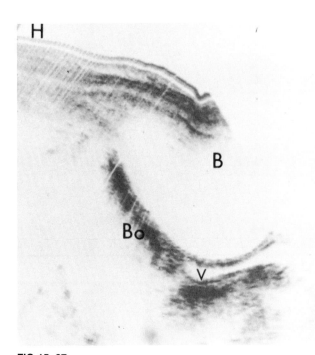

B  = Urinary bladder
Bo = Bowel
F  = Foot
H  = Head
P  = Prostate
V  = Vagina

**FIG 15–27.**

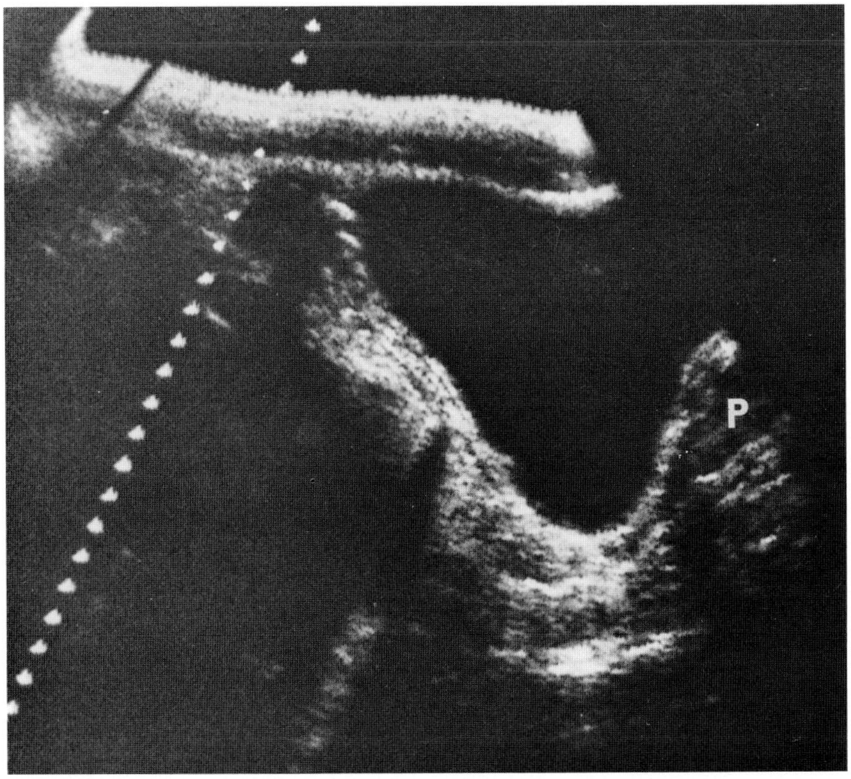

**FIG 15–28.**

## Bicornuate Uterus

The scans in Figures 15–29 through 15–32 are of a 27-year-old woman who had had three pregnancies ending in a first or second trimester abortion. Because of this history, an ultrasound examination was performed, followed by hysterosalpingography. The diagnosis of a bicornuate uterus was made. The transverse scans (Figs 15–29 and 15–30) demonstrate myometrial echoes in the right and left pelvis consistent with a bicornuate uterus. Figure 15–30 is a slightly more cephalad transverse scan that shows further separation of the bicornuate uterus. The indentation on the bladder wall (arrows) by the uterus is noted. This is a normal finding in the pelvis. Posterior to the uterus are the piriform muscles, which should not be mistaken for ovaries.

   Figure 15–31 is a longitudinal scan through the long axis of the right uterus. Here we see some reverberations off the anterior wall of the urinary bladder, which is a normal finding in the pelvis. A longitudinal scan lining up the long axis of the left-sided uterus (Fig 15–32) demonstrates echoes within the endocervical cavity on this side. A hysterosalpingogram confirmed the diagnosis of bicornuate uterus. This is a fairly characteristic appearance of this entity; it is best diagnosed on transverse scans made through the cephalad portion of the uterus.

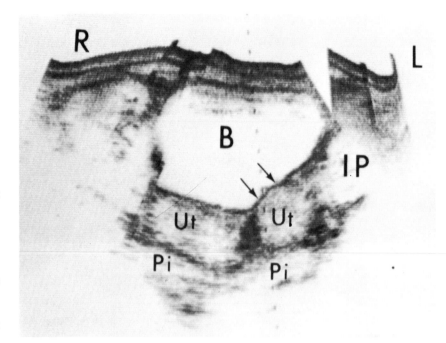

**FIG 15–29.**

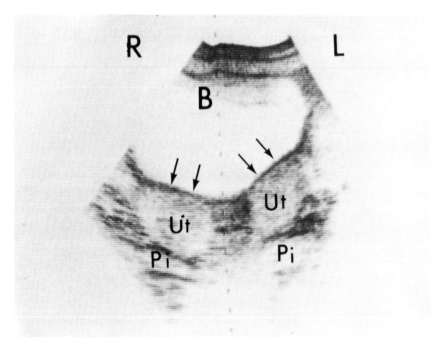

**FIG 15–30.**

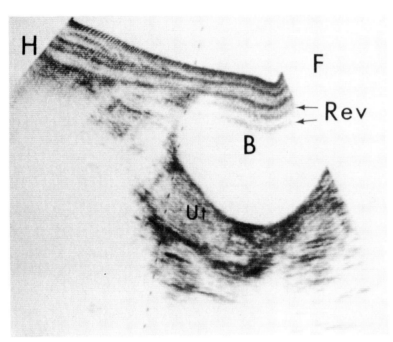

**FIG 15–31.**

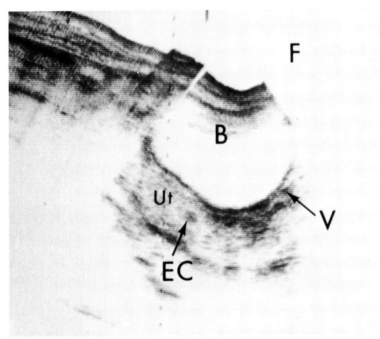

**FIG 15–32.**

| **Arrows** | = | Indentation of the uterus on the urinary bladder wall |
|---|---|---|
| **B** | = | Urinary bladder |
| **EC** | = | Endometrial cavity |
| **F** | = | Foot |
| **H** | = | Head |
| **IP** | = | Iliopsoas muscle |
| **L** | = | Left |
| **Pi** | = | Piriform muscle |
| **R** | = | Right |
| **Rev** | = | Reverberation artifacts in the urinary bladder |
| **Ut** | = | Uterus |
| **V** | = | Vagina |

## Uterine Anomalies

Various degrees of uterine duplication can be visualized on ultrasound. These are most easily diagnosed in very early pregnancy when a gestational sac is present. In the nonpregnant uterus the diagnosis can be difficult. It is most helpful to study such patients during menstruation. The menstrual echoes will be highly echogenic and will establish the location of the uterine cavity. If an anomalous uterus is studied when the patient is not menstruating, the diagnosis is much more difficult. Figures 15–33 and 15–34 are transverse scans of a patient with a bicornuate uterus. A small right ovarian cyst (C) is noted in the right adnexal region. The high-amplitude echoes of the uterine cavity (arrows) are identified on the scan. Figure 15–33 is the more cephalad of the two scans, and the central echoes of the uterine cavity are farther apart than in Figure 15–34. Figure 15–34 is a more caudad transverse scan. The high-amplitude echoes of the uterine cavity are closer together. These two scans confirm the diagnosis of the bicornuate uterus. As the echoes of the uterine cavity approach each other near the uterine body, the diagnosis can be made.

Figures 15–35 and 15–36 are transverse scans of a patient with complete duplication of the uterus. This is a difficult diagnosis to make since the lower uterine segment is often difficult to visualize. Figure 15–35 is a transverse scan through the fundal region of the duplicated uterus. A right and left uterus (Ut) are identified in this scan. Figure 15–36 is a caudad scan over the cervical region. The high-amplitude echoes (arrowheads) of the two cervices are clearly seen, confirming the diagnosis of uterus didelphys.

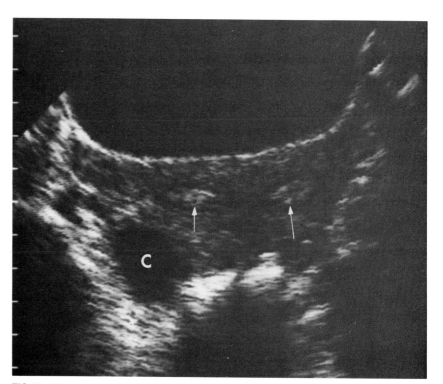

**FIG 15–33.**

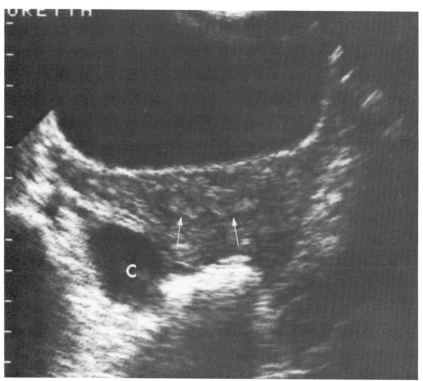

**FIG 15–34.**

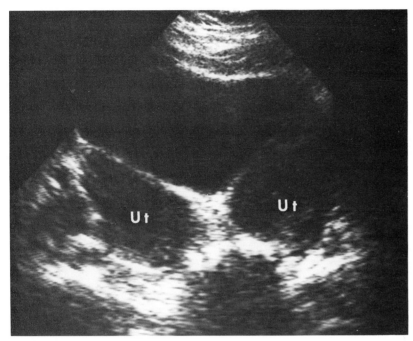

| Arrows | = Uterine cavity |
| Arrowheads | = Cervix |
| C | = Right ovarian cyst |
| Ut | = Uterus |

**FIG 15–35.**

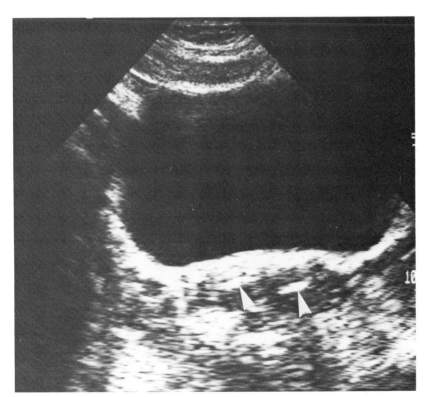

**FIG 15–36.**

## Intrauterine Devices

The various intrauterine devices give fairly characteristic echo patterns within the endometrial cavity.

Figure 15–37 is a longitudinal scan through the uterus. The echoes arising within the endometrial cavity have a step-like appearance that is characteristic of a Lippe's loop. Posterior to the central echoes is evidence of shadowing.

A longitudinal scan of the uterus (Fig 15–38) demonstrates a strong central echo arising from a Dalkon shield. This device presents an uninterrupted echogenic appearance without evidence of the step-like echoes noted in a Lippe's loop.

Figures 15–39 and 15–40 are longitudinal and transverse scans of a uterus containing a Copper 7 intrauterine device. Copper 7's and Copper T's have a fairly characteristic appearance of a circular echo on transverse scans through the uterus. Longitudinal scans through the uterus show a fairly strong linear echo suggesting a small tubular structure approximately 2-3 mm in diameter.

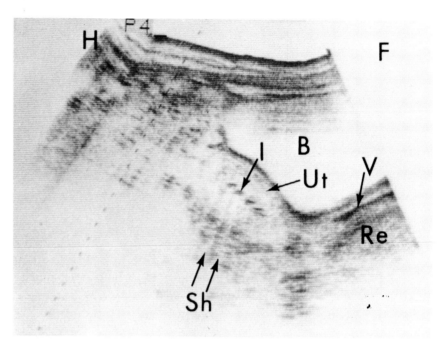

**FIG 15–37.**

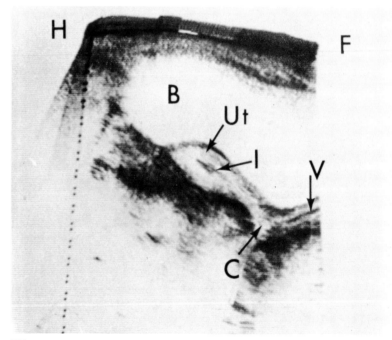

**FIG 15–38.**

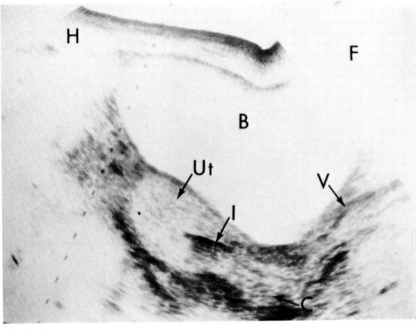

**FIG 15–39.**

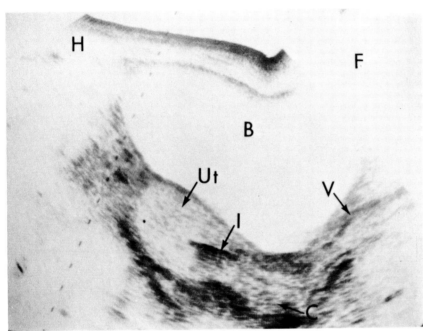

**FIG 15–40.**

B  = Urinary bladder
C  = Cervix
F  = Foot
H  = Head
I  = Intrauterine device
IP = Iliopsoas muscles
L  = Left
O  = Ovary
R  = Right
Sh = Shadowing
Ut = Uterus
V  = Vagina

## Intrauterine Device

Intrauterine devices image as high-amplitude echoes within the uterine cavity. Occasionally, a confusing ultrasound picture may merge on pelvic examinations. Figure 15–41 is a transverse scan of the pelvis in a patient with a Copper 7 intrauterine device in place. It appears on this scan that two intrauterine devices (arrows) are present within the uterine cavity. This can initially be confusing to the novice scanner. However, the abdominal wall musculature and fat can create duplication artifacts secondary to refraction (see chapter 1). Figure 15–42 is a scan of the same patient as in Figure 15–41, but made with the patient in a slightly different position. This scan shows a single intrauterine device in the uterine cavity. A duplication artifact arising from the abdominal wall can create some diagnostic difficulties. This case is an example of a duplication artifact in the presence of a uterine device. Very early gestational sacs can also be accompanied by a duplication artifact and a mistaken diagnosis of a twin gestation may be made. If the position and angulation of the transducer are changed slightly and the patient is rescanned, the diagnosis of a duplication artifact can be made.

Very often localization of an intrauterine device may be requested in a pregnant woman. One can usually detect an intrauterine device very early in pregnancy, from 5 to 10 menstrual weeks. Later in pregnancy, the location of an intrauterine device is quite difficult to ascertain, because of the high-amplitude echoes that arise from the fetal interfaces. Figure 15–43 is a longitudinal scan of the uterus at approximately 10 weeks' gestation. A high-amplitude echo is noted adjacent to the uterine cavity (arrow). This echo arises from a Copper 7 intrauterine device. Note the acoustic shadowing distal to the Copper 7 device, which confirms the diagnosis of an intrauterine device. Later in the pregnancy it would be almost impossible to detect the intrauterine device. It is important to let the referring physicians know

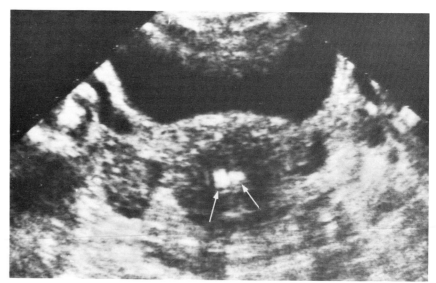

**FIG 15–41.**

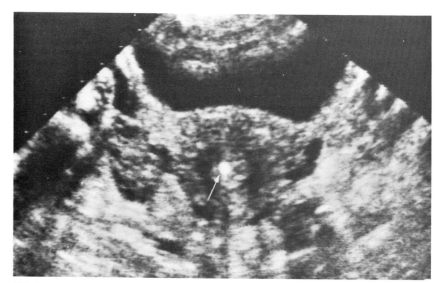

**FIG 15–42.**

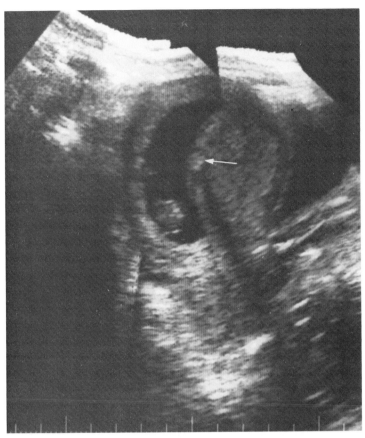

FIG 15–43.

that detection of an intrauterine device is easiest in very early pregnancy.

Figure 15–44 is a longitudinal scan in a 37-year-old woman who presented with recent pelvic pain. A Copper 7 intrauterine device had been recently inserted. Physical examination did not reveal the location of the intrauterine device, and the patient was sent for ultrasound and x-ray examination of the pelvis. An x-ray film revealed the location of the Copper 7 device in the pelvis. The ultrasound examination indicates that the intrauterine device is not in the expected location. In this instance, the intrauterine device is seen near the fundus of the uterus (arrow). Only a small portion of the intrauterine device was identified. The findings were consistent with penetration of the intrauterine device through the uterine wall. At surgery, the Copper 7 device was found to have perforated through the uterus and was embedded in omentum just cephalad to the uterus. The ultrasound findings led to the correct diagnosis.

**Arrows** = Intrauterine device

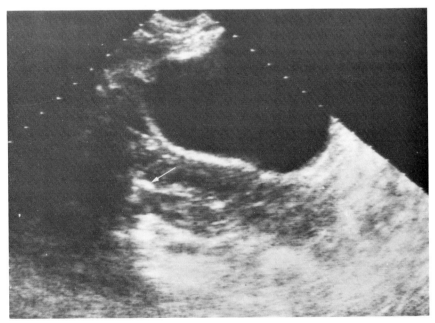

FIG 15–44.

## Fibroid Uterus

Leiomyomas of the uterus are fairly common. Their appearance varies, depending mainly on their size and internal consistency. Figures 15–45 and 15–46 are scans of a patient with a myoma in the posterior fundal region of the uterus. The difference in echogenicity between the myoma and the normal myometrium arising from the uterus and cervix is notable. The myoma is less echogenic than the normal myometrial echoes. A word of caution is in order when evaluating the fundal region of the uterus. Often the fundus of the uterus appears less echogenic than the middle and lower uterine segments. However, this is extremely dependent on the degree of bladder filling. When the urinary bladder is not well filled, the fundal region of the uterus often will appear less echogenic, because a distended urinary bladder is not present anterior to it. We must remember that the through-transmission from the urinary bladder increases the level of echoes arising from the uterus. Therefore, a misdiagnosis of a fundal myoma is very common when the urinary bladder is only partially filled.

Figures 15–47 and 15–48 are scans of a myoma that contains calcification. Calcifications are often present within a myoma. They give very strong echoes that are often accompanied by shadowing. The myoma in these scans has a less echogenic appearance than the normal myometrial echoes arising within the uterus. The transverse scan in Figure 15–48 shows that the myoma is somewhat pedunculated and situated off the posterior left aspect of the uterus.

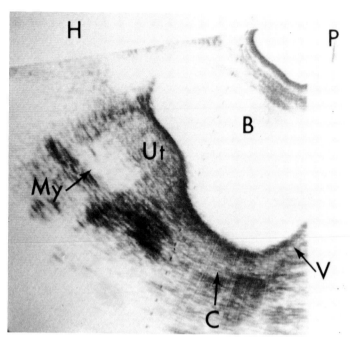

FIG 15–45.

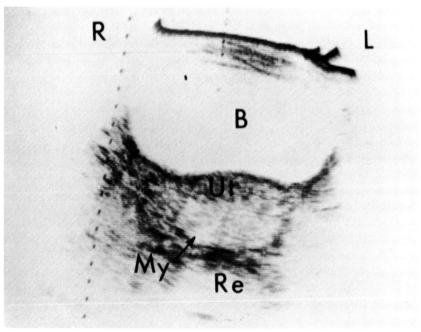

FIG 15–46.

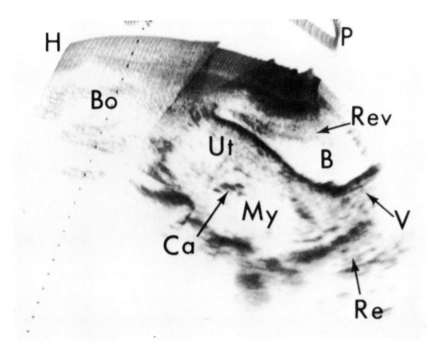

B   = Urinary bladder
Bo  = Bowel
C   = Cervix
Ca  = Calcification
H   = Head
L   = Left
My  = Myoma
P   = Level of the symphysis pubis
R   = Right
Re  = Rectum
Rev = Reverberation artifacts
Ut  = Uterus
V   = Vagina

**FIG 15–47.**

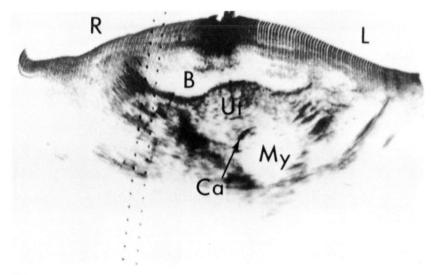

**FIG 15–48.**

## Uterine Fibroids

Uterine fibroids may cause a contour deformity of the uterus along with an abnormal textural change compared to the normal myometrium. Often both findings are present. Figure 15–49 is a longitudinal midline scan of a uterus with fundal fibroid (M). There is a subtle texture change between the fibroid and the remaining portion of the uterus. Note that the echoes within the fibroid are slightly more irregular in echogenicity and distribution than the echoes of the normal myometrium in the uterine body and cervix. There is also evidence of a slight contour deformity in the fundal region of the uterus. The fundal region appears larger than anticipated, and the usual contour of the fundus of the uterus is not present. These two findings indicate the presence of a fundal myoma.

Fibroids are often present in pregnancy. Figure 15–50 is a longitudinal midline scan in which we see a gravid uterus with the embryo (arrows) of approximately 10–11 weeks' gestational size. The echogenic placenta is noted in the fundal portion of the uterus. Cephalad to the uterus and urinary bladder is a large echo-free mass (M). Evaluation of the transmission of this mass indicates that very little sound is penetrating through this lucent mass. The findings indicate that even though there are no echoes within this mass, it does represent a solid lesion. Novice ultrasonographers may misdiagnose such a lucent mass as a cystic structure. However, the mass is so large that prominent through-transmission should be present if it represented a cystic lesion. Instead, very little sound is transmitted through the mass, confirming its solid nature. These findings are typical of a homogeneous fibroid, which the mass turned out to be. The patient underwent surgery early in pregnancy to remove the fibroid. This is an example of a sonolucent mass that is attenuating sound. Remember this mass when we describe the appearance of ovarians cysts in later cases in this chapter. Ovarian cysts are as sonolucent, but they also have enhanced through-transmission.

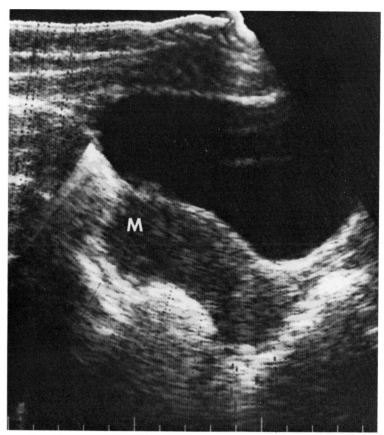

**FIG 15–49.**

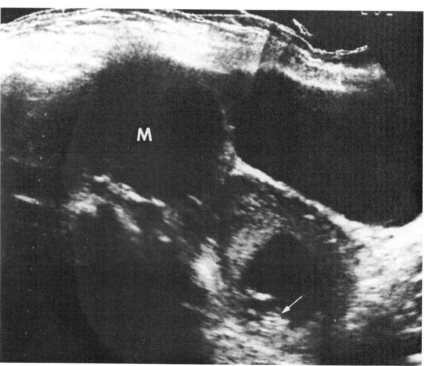

**FIG 15–50.**

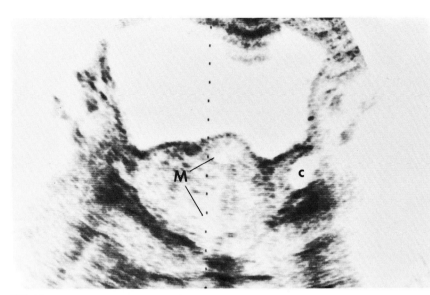

**FIG 15–51.**

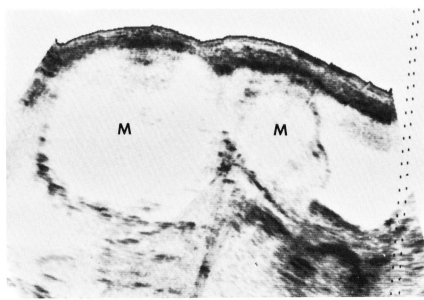

**FIG 15–52.**

Figure 15–51 is a transverse scan of a patient with multiple fibroids within the body and fundus of the uterus. The texture of the uterine echoes is markedly abnormal. There are relatively lucent areas present within the uterus, compatible with myomas (M). A sonolucent mass in the left adnexal region represents an ovarian cyst. Note the increased echoes deep to the ovarian cyst, confirming its fluid-filled nature.

Figure 15–52 is a longitudinal scan of a patient in whom a large abdominal mass was palpable. In reality, two large masses are present. A 15-cm pedunculated fibroid is present cephalad to the uterus. This myoma (M) is relatively sonolucent with a few internal echoes. Very little sound is being transmitted through this large sonolucent mass, confirming its solid nature. A second myoma (M) is present in the fundal region of the uterus and is indenting the urinary bladder. This is a typical appearance of uterine fibroids.

| | | |
|---|---|---|
| **Arrow** | = | Embryo |
| **C** | = | Left ovarian cyst |
| **M** | = | Myomas |

## Uterine Fibroids

Earlier examples of uterine fibroids demonstrated that they were mainly relatively sonolucent masses. When the uterine myoma is homogeneous, very few interfaces are present, and this type presents as a sonolucent mass on ultrasound. However, when necrosis or degeneration occurs, the ultrasound appearance will demonstrate increased echogenicity to the uterine fibroids. Figure 15–53 is a longitudinal midline scan of a patient in early pregnancy. The conceptus is seen in the fundal region of the uterus. Inferior to the conceptus is a large mass with numerous internal echoes. The possibility of a molar pregnancy could be considered in this instance. However, the texture of the mass is coarser than that seen in molar pregnancy. The findings are compatible with a degenerating myoma of the lower uterine segment. Note that the internal architecture in this mass is less homogeneous than was noted in the previous cases of sonolucent fibroids.

Figure 15–54 is a longitudinal scan of another patient in which a myoma (M) is noted to have numerous internal echoes. This myoma is situated posterior to the uterus and is compressing the uterus against the urinary bladder. A strong linear echo is noted in the uterine cavity. The increased echoes within the uterine myoma indicate degeneration and necrosis.

Figures 15–55 and 15–56 are longitudinal and transverse scans of a 41-year-old woman who came to the emergency room complaining of vaginal bleeding for several weeks. On admission, her hematocrit was 38%. Two days after admission, the hematocrit had dropped to 32%. Ultrasound examination revealed a mixed pattern, with areas of increased and decreased echogenicity (arrowheads) within the midportion of the uterus. The differential diagnosis of such a mass would include a molar pregnancy, uterine cancer, and a degenerating fibroid. Vaginal bleeding continued and increased. A hysterectomy was performed, and a large submucous myoma was removed. There

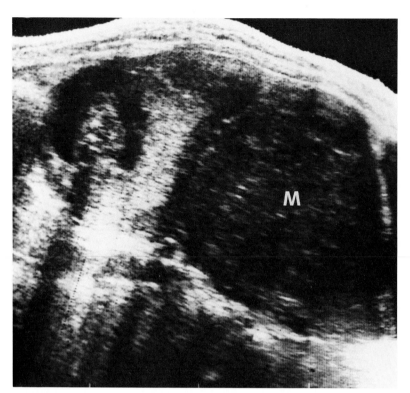

FIG 15–53.

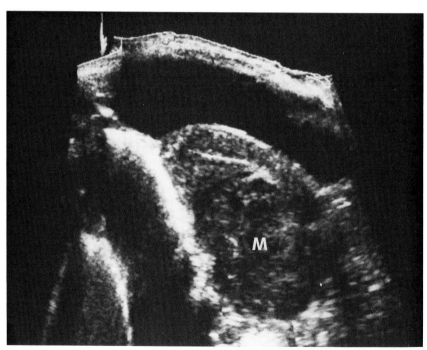

FIG 15–54.

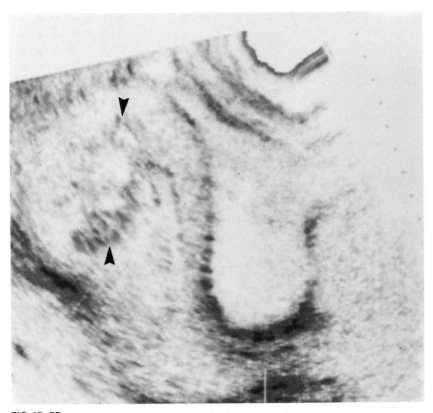

**FIG 15–55.**

was evidence of severe necrosis and hemorrhage within the myoma. The findings on ultrasound indicate a diffusely mixed echo pattern. Degenerating fibroids are often worrisome because uterine malignancies can have a similar appearance.

**Arrowheads** = Degenerating uterine fibroid
**M** = Uterine fibroid

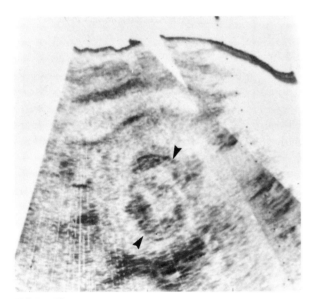

**FIG 15–56.**

## Fibroid Uterus

Figure 15–57, a longitudinal scan, shows nearly the entire fundal region of the uterus containing a large myoma. The only normal appearing uterine echoes arise from the cervical region and the lower uterine segment. The myoma has a fairly homogeneous, relatively sonolucent appearance which is characteristic of a fibroid uterus.

Another longitudinal scan (Fig 15–58) demonstrates a uterus containing a large myoma. In this case, however, numerous echoes are present within the myoma. This is an instance of a fibroid uterus undergoing some degeneration. This can occur to such a severe degree that the uterus may occasionally be mistaken for a hydatidiform mole. The echoes are more irregular in a degenerating fibroid uterus than in a mole.

Figures 15–59 and 15–60 are scans of a patient with a large fibroid uterus, part of which was undergoing degeneration. The longitudinal scan (Fig 15–59) shows the myomatous uterus involving much of the entire abdomen. Again, the only normal-appearing myometrial echoes are in the cervical region. There is relatively poor through-transmission on the posterior aspect of the myoma, and this is another characteristic of fibroid lesions within the uterus. Figure 15–60 is a transverse scan of a myomatous mass with attenuation on the right side. The portion of the mass on the left side, however, does have some through-transmission with a relatively sonolucent central area. This is due to fluid within a degenerating fibroid uterus. When severe degeneration occurs, a myoma may appear relatively echo-free with through-transmission secondary to fluid within its central portion.

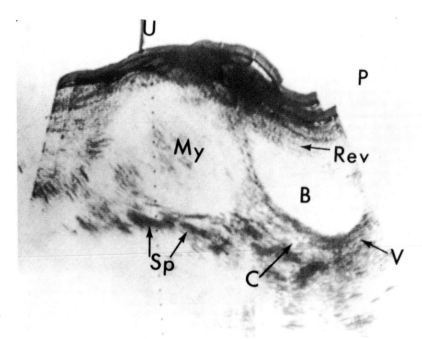

FIG 15–57.

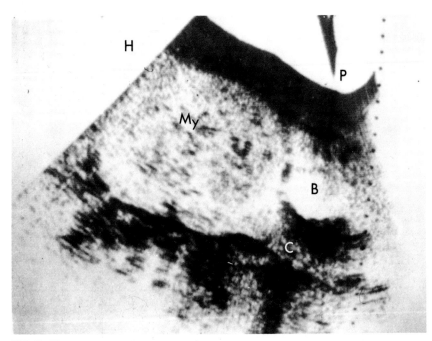

FIG 15–58.

B    = Urinary bladder
C    = Cervix
F    = Foot
f    = Fluid in a degenerating fibroid
H    = Head
L    = Left
M    = Myoma
My   = Myoma
P    = Level of the symphysis pubis
Rev  = Reverberations
S    = Spleen
Sp   = Spine
U    = Umbilical level
V    = Vagina

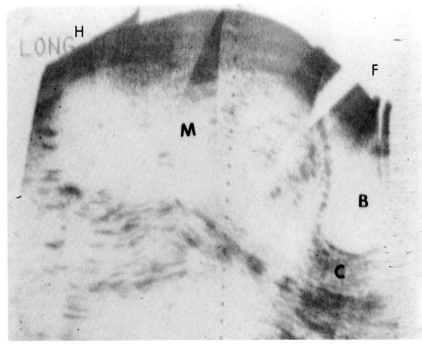

FIG 15–59.

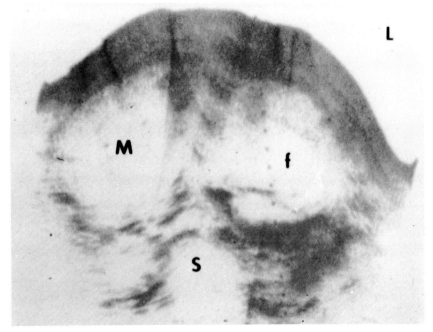

FIG 15–60.

## Uterine Masses

Most masses within the uterus are solid in nature. However, certain uterine masses have a cystic appearance. Often small, well-circumscribed cystic areas are identified on ultrasound in the cervical region of the uterus. Figure 15–61 is a longitudinal scan in which a 1-cm cyst is present in the cervix (arrow). This is secondary to a Nabothian cyst. Nabothian cysts are benign lesions of the cervix and are thought to result from chronic cervicitis. They are commonly seen on ultrasound and usually do not pose any diagnostic difficulties.

Figures 15–62 and 15–63 are longitudinal and transverse scans of the pelvis of a 42-year-old woman who had experienced increasing pelvic pain in the last several months. The ultrasound picture is very confusing. The uterine body and fundus were noted to be enlarged. There are regions of sonolucency, but also areas of high echogenicity. Through-transmission is identified, indicating the fluid-filled nature of this process. The uterine wall appears to be well circumscribed, and the mass was thought to be within the uterine cavity. The ultrasound findings were compatible with hemorrhage within the uterine cavity. At operation a 13-cm uterus was removed. The uterus was filled with hemorrhage and fresh clotted blood. The findings indicated a degenerating fibroid along with adenomyosis with bleeding in an area consistent with a chocolate cyst. The hemorrhage within the uterus was secondary to degeneration of a fibroid and adenomyosis.

Figure 15–64 is a longitudinal scan of a young girl who experienced delayed menarche. An ultrasound examination was requested to evaluate various possibilities. Figure 15–64 is a longitudinal midline scan in which large relatively lucent mass is noted in place of the uterus. Some internal echoes are present, along with enhanced through-transmission. The findings are consistent with hematocolposis. This condition results from an imperforate hymen and is usually discovered at menarche when men-

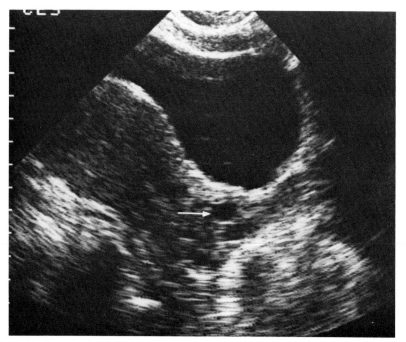

FIG 15–61.

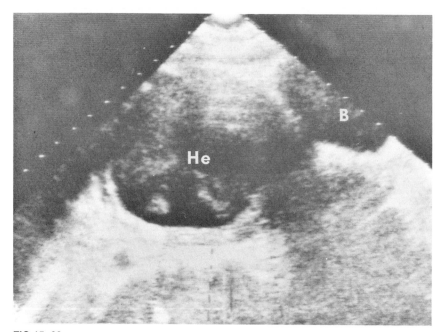

FIG 15–62.

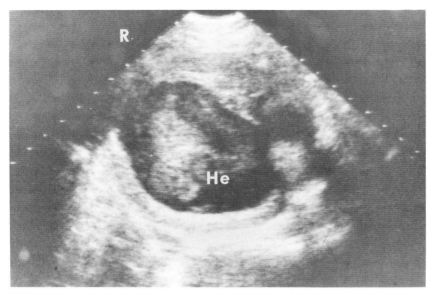

**FIG 15–63.**

strual flow is absent. Ultrasound is an excellent means for diagnosing this entity since the enlarged blood-filled uterus stands out quite easily. The uterine cavity is filled with hemorrhage (He). The uterine cavity is dilated down in the endocervical canal and even into the vagina to the imperforate hymen.

**Arrow** = Nabothian cyst
**B** = Urinary bladder
**He** = Hemorrhage in the uterine cavity
**R** = Right

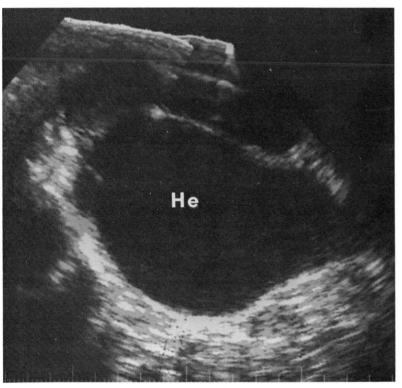

**FIG 15–64.**

## Cervical Carcinoma

The ultrasound findings of cervical carcinoma usually indicate a relatively lucent mass in the region of the cervix. Although ultrasound can identify cervical carcinoma, it does not estimate the extent of disease as well as does pelvic CT. Figures 15–65 and 15–66 are transverse and longitudinal scans in a patient with cervical carcinoma. The difference in echogenicity between the uterus and the cervix can be noted. The cervix is markedly enlarged with somewhat irregular borders and decreased echo amplitude. Figure 15–66 is a transverse scan through the region of cervical carcinoma in which a portion of the decreased echo amplitude is identified.

Figure 15–67 is a longitudinal scan in the pelvis of another patient with cervical carcinoma. Note the similar appearance to the echogenicity of the lesion. The region of carcinoma (C) is much more sonolucent than the normal myometrial echoes in the body and fundus. There is also evidence of a mass effect in the region of the cervix, as is demonstrated by indentation on the urinary bladder.

Figure 15–68 is a longitudinal scan of a 39-year-old woman with cervical carcinoma. She was admitted to the emergency room because of extensive vaginal bleeding. An emergency ultrasound examination demonstrated the region of cervical carcinoma (C). Also noted were high-amplitude echoes in the cervical canal and vagina. These high-amplitude echoes (arrowhead) were secondary to massive hemorrhage. The region of cervical carcinoma again has a characteristic appearance. The area is less echogenic than the body and fundus of the uterus. There is also evidence of indentation on the posterior aspect of the urinary bladder. This case differs from the other two in that high-amplitude echoes secondary to hemorrhage are evident in the endocervical canal.

Cervical carcinoma cannot be distinguished from cervical fibroids on ultrasound examination. A cervical myoma can have a similar appearance in that it is decreased in echo-

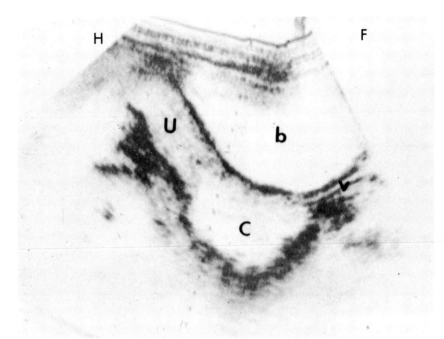

FIG 15–65.

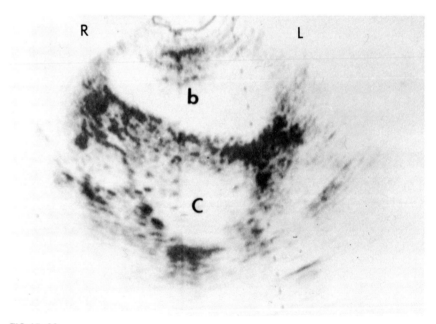

FIG 15–66.

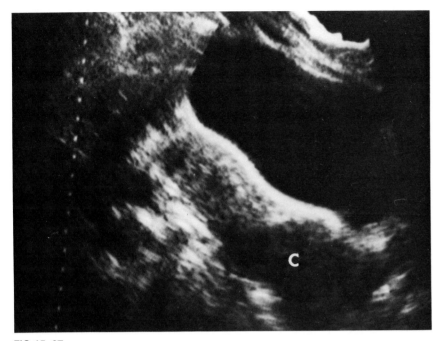

FIG 15–67.

genicity and deforms the posterior aspect of the urinary bladder.

**Arrowhead** = Hemorrhage
**b** = Urinary bladder
**C** = Cervical carcinoma
**F** = Foot
**H** = Head
**R** = Right
**U** = Uterus
**V** = Vagina

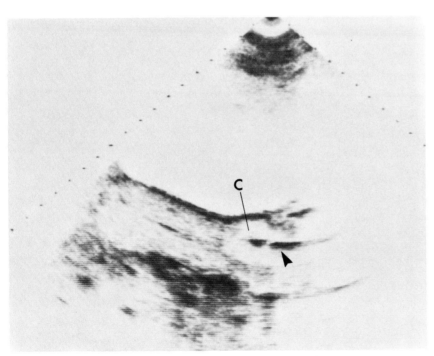

FIG 15–68.

## Uterine Neoplasms

Uterine neoplasms usually give a mixed echo appearance with areas of fluid and solid tissue present. They cannot be distinghished from degenerating fibroids. In fact, when the diagnosis of degenerating fibroids is made, the possibility of uterine neoplasms should also be considered. A nondegenerating fibroid that is mainly sonolucent and attenuating is usually not worrisome for neoplasm. However, when necrosis and hemorrhage are present within a fibroid, the possibility of uterine neoplasm must always be raised.

Figures 15–69 and 15–70 are scans of a 66-year-old woman with lower abdominal pain and a palpable pelvic mass. Ultrasound examination revealed a large mass within the pelvis and lower abdomen. The echogenic portion of this mass was posterior to a sonolucent segment that was thought to be fluid. At operation, adenocarcinoma of the endometrium was found. The ultrasound examination revealed evidence of tumor necrosis, with fluid anteriorly and through-transmission present. The solid component is the posterior echogenic area. Uterine carcinoma is difficult to distinguish from necrotic fibroids. When a fluid component is evident in a solid lesion, the possibility of uterine neoplasm must always be considered.

Figure 15–71 is a transverse scan of the pelvis in which another necrotic mass is identified in the uterine bed. There is a sonolucent area centrally, along with solid components posteriorly and in the left lateral aspect. These findings indicate a necrotic or hemorrhagic solid lesion. This can represent a degenerating fibroid. However, the most likely possibility is uterine neoplasm because of the large amount of hemorrhage and necrosis that is present. This mass was secondary to tumor involvement of the lower uterine segment. This was found to be endometrial carcinoma.

Figure 15–72 is a longitudinal scan of the pelvis in which a large pelvic and lower abdominal mass is present. This mass also has a mixed appear-

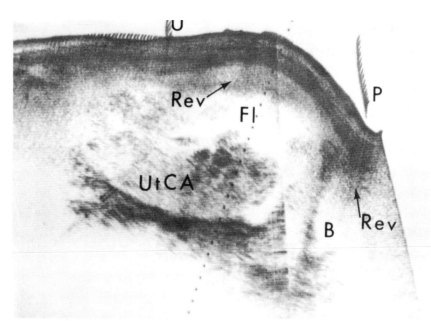

**FIG 15–69.**

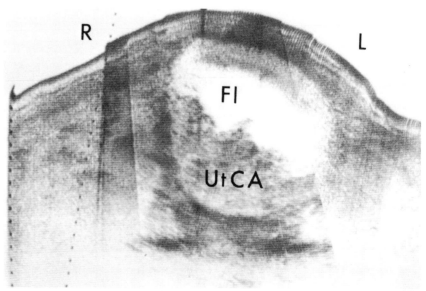

**FIG 15–70.**

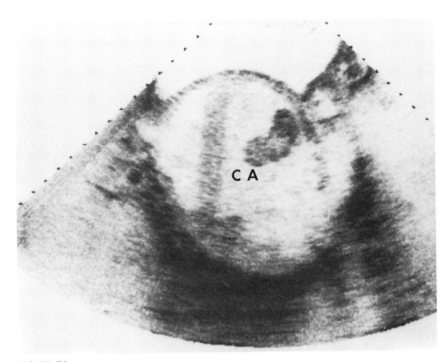

**FIG 15–71.**

ance in which sonolucent and solid components are identified. This mass turned out to be a leiomyosarcoma. Ultrasound cannot distinguish between the various forms of neoplasms. There is no way to distinguish a leiomyosarcoma from a uterine carcinoma. The ultrasound appearances are similar in that solid tumors with areas of necrosis and hemorrhage are identified.

SOURCE: Figure 15–71 is provided courtesy of Stanley Nakamoto, M.D., Orange, Calif.

| | | |
|---|---|---|
| **B** | = | Urinary bladder |
| **CA** | = | Endometrial carcinoma |
| **FI** | = | Necrotic fluid |
| **L** | = | Left |
| **LS** | = | Leiomyosarcoma |
| **P** | = | Symphysis pubis |
| **R** | = | Right |
| **Rev** | = | Reverberation |
| **U** | = | Umbilical level |
| **Ut CA** | = | Adenocarcinoma of the uterus |

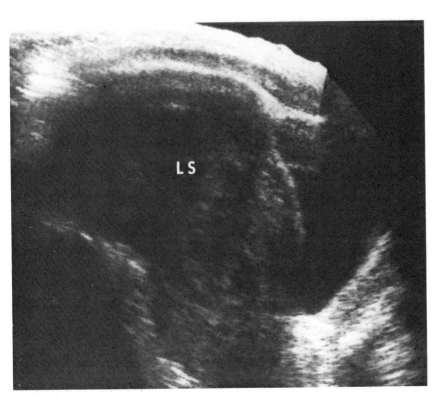

**FIG 15–72.**

## Follicular Cyst

Ultrasound has been used to evaluate foilicle size in the workup and therapy of fertility patients. The diameter of a follicular cyst can be determined with ultrasound. Ovulation usually occurs when the average diameter of the follicular cyst is in the range of 2–2.5 cm.

Figures 15–73 and 15–74 are transverse and longitudinal scans of a patient with a follicular cyst in the right ovary. The follicular cyst is smooth-walled, and echo-free, with enhanced through-transmission. The cyst may be circular to oval in appearance. If the bladder is markedly filled, there may be some distortion in the contour of the follicular cyst. Because of this, the average of the three diameters is obtained.

Figure 15–75 is a longitudinal scan of an ovary which has a follicular cyst (C) in its inferoposterior portion. Notice the normal echogenicity of the ovary. The cyst grows at a rate of approximately 2 mm/day and can be followed quite accurately with ultrasound. At the time of ovulation, fluid can be noted in the cul-de-sac. Figure 15–76 is a scan showing fluid in the cul-de-sac (Fl) after recent ovulation. The through-transmission deep to the fluid confirms its nature.

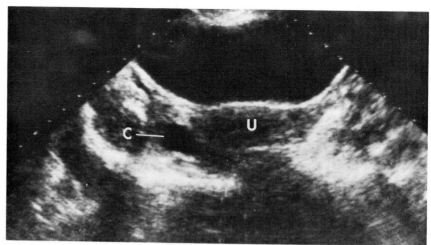

FIG 15–73.

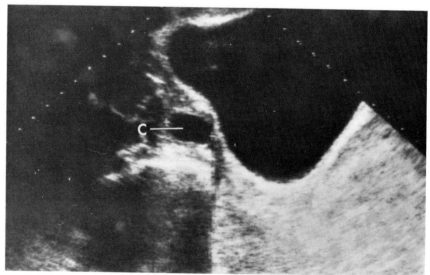

FIG 15–74.

C  = Follicular cyst
FI = Pelvic fluid
U  = Uterus

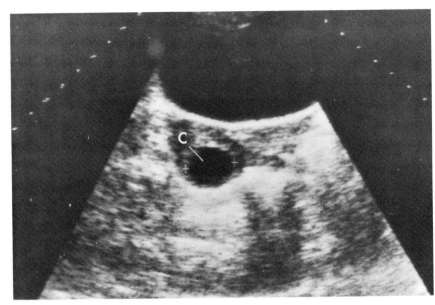

FIG 15–75.

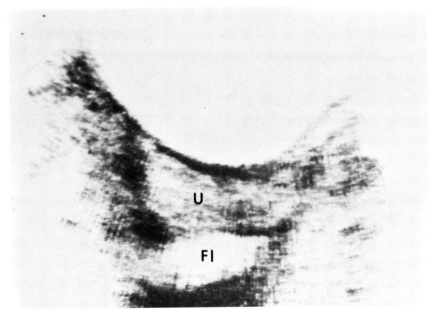

FIG 15–76.

## Follicular Cyst

By following the development of follicular cysts, ovulation can be documented. Ovulation often occurs when the cyst reaches 2–2.5 cm in diameter. After ovulation, the follicular cyst will decrease in size and fill in with soft echoes. Figures 15–77 and 15–78 are transverse scans of the same patient obtained at the same examination. Figure 15–77 is an earlier transverse scan in which a 2.4-cm cyst is present in the left ovary. The cyst is well distended and has sharp walls. No fluid is present posterior to the uterus in Figure 15–77. During the course of the examination, a change in the appearance of the pelvis was noted: fluid (arrowheads) accumulated in the cul-de-sac, as is noted in Figure 15–78. The left cyst was also noted to decrease slightly in size and to have a less tense appearance. This case is an example in which we visualized ovulation with fluid accumulation in the cul-de-sac during the course of an examination.

In the workup of an infertility patient, multiple cysts may be visualized in the ovary when exogenous hormones are given. Figure 15–79 is a longitudinal scan of the right ovary in a patient who was administered Clomid. Four measurable cysts are identified in the lower pole of the right ovary. There are also three smaller cysts noted just anterior to cyst 1. These cysts are too small to measure. This is a typical finding in an ovary which is being stimulated for follicular development.

Figure 15–80 is a longitudinal scan in a patient with an unusual ultrasound finding. Initial scan obtained a month earlier did not demonstrate any cystic development in the ovaries. There may have been a few small 2–3-mm cysts identified. At examination 1 month later the ovaries were noted to have enlarged, with multiple cysts (1–5). After further questioning, it was found that the patient had been taking exogenous hormone on her own. This led to the development of multiple follicular cysts within the ovaries.

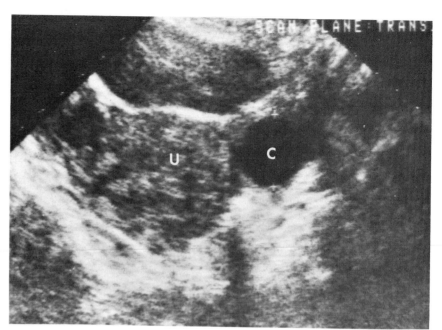

**FIG 15–77.**

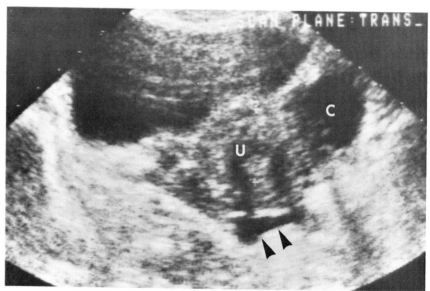

**FIG 15–78.**

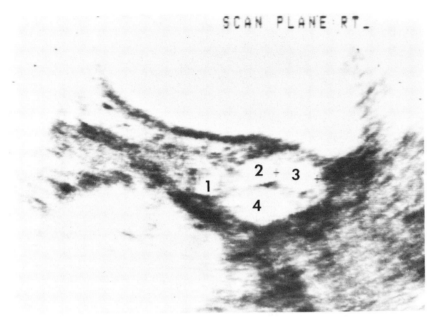

Arrowheads = Fluid in the cul-de-sac
C = Follicular cyst
U = Uterus
1–5 = Follicular cysts

**FIG 15–79.**

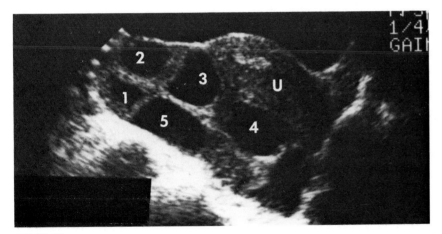

**FIG 15–80.**

## Ovarian Cyst

A nonfunctioning cyst of the ovary cannot be distinguished from functional cysts except by following them serially. Nonfunctioning cysts can get quite large. Simple ovarian cysts have sharp borders, no internal echoes, and prominent through-transmission. They can range in size from a few millimeters to large masses. They are usually characteristic in appearance and do not cause any diagnostic problems. Ovarian cysts are unlikely to be confused with such entities as abscesses, hematomas, or necrotic tumors. The walls are very sharp and no internal echoes are identified. By following an ovarian cyst serially, and noting that it does not change in size or rupture, the diagnosis of a nonfunctioning ovarian cyst can be made. Figure 15–81 is a longitudinal scan of the right ovary in which a small ovarian cyst (OC) is noted to arise from the superior pole of the right ovary (O). Figure 15–82 is a transverse scan in which a left ovarian cyst (OC) is identified. Through-transmission is noted deep to the cyst. There is also evidence of sharp borders and no internal echoes. Figure 15–83 is a longitudinal scan of the same patient in Figure 15–82. The ovarian cyst is seen to involve the superior pole of the left ovary. High-amplitude echoes deep to the ovarian cyst indicate through-transmission. It is often difficult to evaluate through-transmission in the pelvis because of the strong echoes that arise from air-filled bowel.

Figure 15–84 is a longitudinal scan of the right pelvis in a patient with a 5-cm ovarian cyst. A small portion of the uterus (U) is noted anterior to the ovarian cyst (C). High-amplitude echoes are present deep to the ovarian cyst, indicating through-transmission (TT). Enhanced through-transmission confirms the fluid-filled nature of the cystic masses.

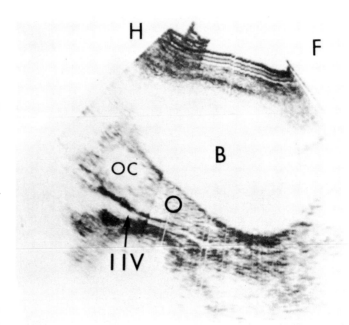

**FIG 15–81.**

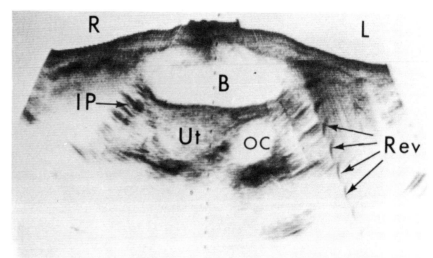

**FIG 15–82.**

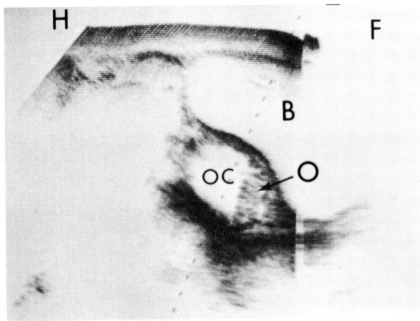

B = Bladder
C = Ovarian cyst
F = Foot
H = Head
IIV = Internal iliac vessels
IP = Iliopsoas muscle
L = Left
O = Ovary
OC = Ovarian cyst
R = Right
Rev = Reverberation
TT = Through-transmission
U = Uterus
Ut = Uterus

FIG 15–83.

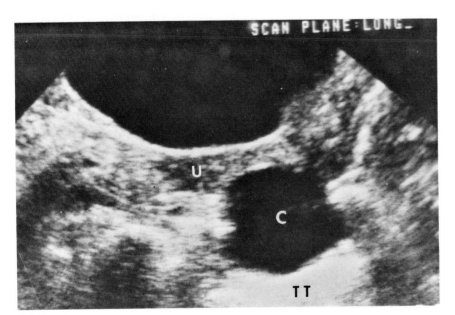

FIG 15–84.

## Hemorrhagic Cyst and Torsion

Patients are commonly sent for ultrasound examination because of the sudden onset of pelvic pain. Very often a characteristic ultrasound picture will be present. Figure 15–85 is a longitudinal scan of the left pelvis in a patient who had previously undergone hysterectomy. She experienced the onset of lower abdominal and pelvic pain 3 days before the ultrasound examination. The ultrasound study revealed an enlarged left adnexa that measured approximately 6 cm in diameter. There was an oval, sonolucent, 4-cm mass in the superior aspect of the left ovary. This mass had enhanced through-transmission, indicating its fluid-filled nature. However, numerous soft internal echoes were present within the mass, indicating that it was simply a fluid-filled cyst. Note the indentation on the urinary bladder. At operation a hemorrhagic cyst was removed. This is a typical appearance of a hemorrhagic cyst. Soft echoes are present within the mass along with enhanced through-transmission. Other entities that may have a similar ultrasound appearance are abscess, endometriosis, and necrotic tumors.

Figure 15–86 is a transverse scan of another patient who had torsion of an ovarian cyst. A similar finding is present in the right adnexa, where a mass (M) is identified. The mass had internal echoes, suggesting it may be a solid lesion. However, there is the through-transmission deep to the mass. Enhanced through-transmission suggests that the mass is fluid in nature. The internal echoes within the mass suggest entities such as hemorrhage and clot, abscess, and necrosis. The important finding is the enhanced through-transmission deep to the mass, which confirms its fluid-filled nature. Such cases are generally surgical emergencies. This turned out to be torsion of the right ovary with hemorrhage into the region.

Figures 15–87 and 15–88 are longitudinal and transverse scans of a patient who had a large mass in asso-

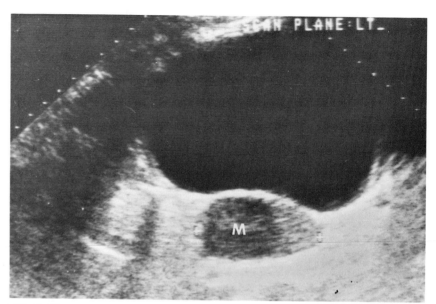

FIG 15–85.

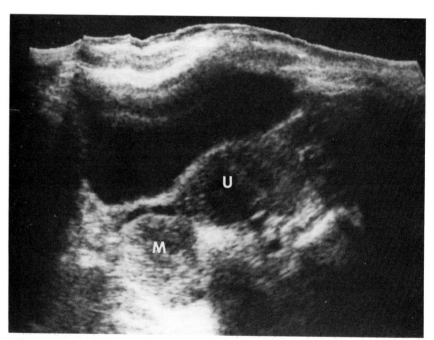

FIG 15–86.

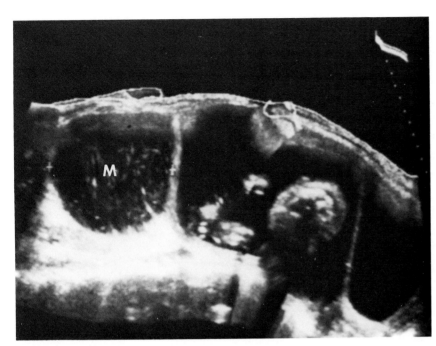

**FIG 15–87.**

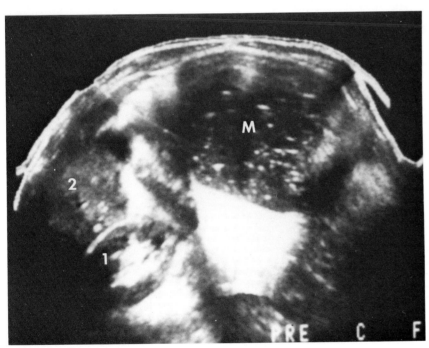

**FIG 15–88.**

ciation with pregnancy. The conceptus is identified cephalad to the urinary bladder in Figure 15–87. Cephalad to the conceptus is a large mass (M). Figure 15–88 is a transverse scan through the mass. This lesion has enhanced through-transmission, indicating its fluid-filled nature. However, the mass is not echo free. There are numerous echoes within it. The mass represented torsion of a large ovarian cyst in association with pregnancy. Torsion usually presents as a relatively lucent mass with numerous internal echoes, enhanced through-transmission, and pelvic pain. The ultrasound findings along with the clinical picture usually lead to the correct diagnosis.

What are structures 1 and 2 in Figure 15–88?

M = Torsion of the ovary with hemorrhage
U = Uterus
1 = Right kidney
2 = Right lobe of the liver

## Theca Lutein Cysts

Theca lutein cysts present as large, multiloculated and multiseptated cystic masses situated bilaterally. Theca lutein cysts result from increasing levels in hCG, causing the ovaries to enlarge into multicystic masses. Theca lutein cysts are most often associated with molar pregnancy. Figure 15–89 is a transverse scan of the lower abdomen in which hydatidiform mole (M) is present within the uterus. Bilateral multicystic masses are present (C), representing theca lutein cysts. These cysts can reach extremely large size, filling nearly the entire abdomen. When a molar pregnancy is present, the adnexal region should be examined for the presence of theca lutein cysts.

Occasionally, theca lutein cysts can be present in association with a normal singleton pregnancy. Figure 15–90 is a transverse scan of the abdomen in which a single intrauterine pregnancy is present. The placenta is posterior on the right side (P). Multiloculated cystic masses are seen bilaterally (C). Figure 15–91 is a tangential scan through one of the cysts showing the multiloculated and multiseptated appearance. Usually, theca lutein cysts are not present in a normal singleton pregnancy. However, occasionally normal ovaries may respond to slightly increased levels of hGC in this manner. Theca lutein cysts are more often seen in twin or triplet gestations than in singleton gestations. They may also be seen when the patient is given medication for infertility.

Figure 15–92 is a transverse scan of the abdomen in a 24-year-old woman whose uterus had been recently evacuated for a hydatidiform mole. One week after evacuation an ultrasound examination was performed. Figure 15–92 shows two large multiloculated masses filling nearly the entire abdomen. Theca lutein cysts may persist for several months after evacuation of a hydatidiform mole. When they reach this size, they are often painful.

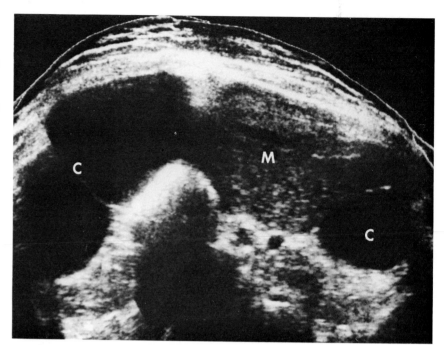

FIG 15–89.

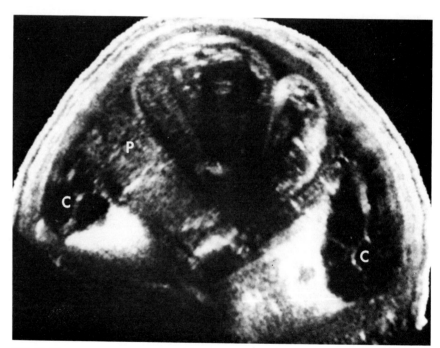

FIG 15–90.

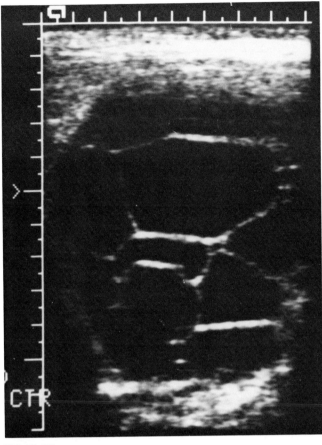

**FIG 15–91.**

SOURCE: Figure 15–92 is provided courtesy of Barry Green, M.D.

**C** = Theca lutein cysts
**L** = Left
**M** = Hydatidiform mole
**P** = Placenta
**R** = Right
**Sp** = Spine

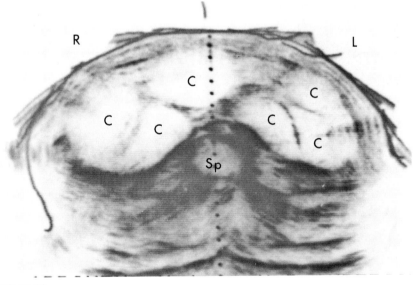

**FIG 15–92.**

## Polycystic Ovaries

Figures 15–93 through 15–96 are pelvic ultrasound scans of a 16-year-old girl referred for secondary amenorrhea. Examination was concentrated on the ovaries to determine their size and echogenicity. A longitudinal scan in the midline (Fig 15–93) shows the uterus to be of normal size and stimulated. A stimulated uterus has a fundal region that is usually thicker and larger than the cervical region. The unstimulated uterus will have a small, thin fundus with a smaller diameter than the cervical region.

A large sonolucent mass is also present posterior to the urinary bladder. This is a false mass (arrows) and secondary to an artifact. The duplication artifact of the urinary bladder can present as a false mass. This is a fairly common occurrence, and care must be taken not to misdiagnose an extremely large sonolucent mass in the pelvis. The patient must return with varying bladder filling if any question of a false mass has been created by bladder duplication. In trying to find the ovaries, we can often follow the uterus until the fallopian tubes are visualized. A transverse scan (Fig 15–94) shows the fallopian tubes quite well bilaterally. The piriform muscles could be confused for the ovaries in this patient. They are, however, situated somewhat posterior to the uterus and are fairly symmetric in appearance. We see only the anterior and posterior borders of the piriform muscles, not the lateral borders.

Following the fallopian tubes, the ovaries can finally be identified bilaterally. A transverse scan (Fig 15–95) that is actually cephalad to the fundus of the uterus shows the uterus to be no longer in the central portion of the scan. Bowel gas is seen. If the fallopian tubes had not been followed, the piriform muscles in Figure 15–94 might have been misinterpreted as the ovaries. In Figure 15–95 we see the ovaries bilaterally. The right ovary is anterior to the internal iliac vessels. On this transverse scan the ovaries have a much coarser appearance than was noted in previous examples.

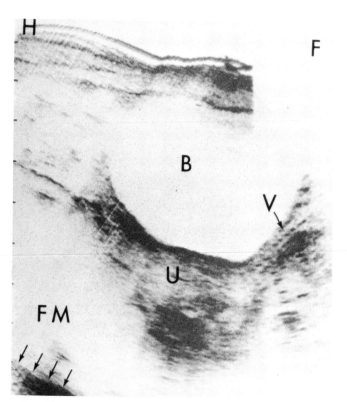

FIG 15–93.

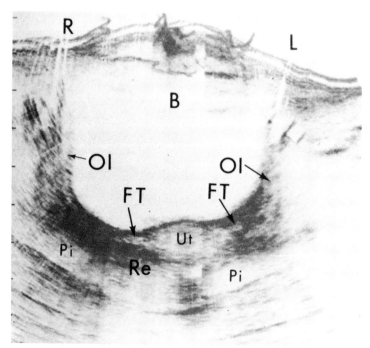

FIG 15–94.

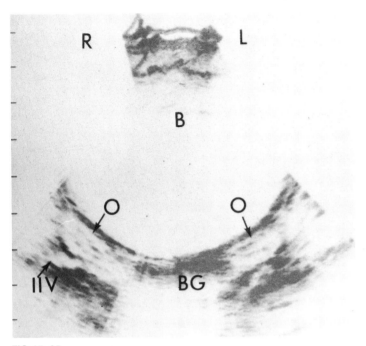

**FIG 15–95.**

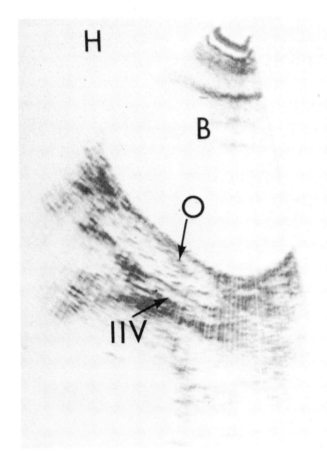

**FIG 15–96.**

Numerous strong linear echoes are present within them.

Figure 15–96 is a longitudinal scan of the right ovary, which is seen anterior to the internal iliac vessels. Again, numerous curvilinear strong echoes within the ovary are noted. These are consistent with the walls of the numerous small cysts in these polycystic ovaries. The cysts are quite small in size. The lumen cannot actually be visualized but the sharp echogenic walls are demonstrated. This is fairly characteristic of polycystic ovaries. The patient also had hormonal levels which confirmed the diagnosis of polycystic disease.

| | | |
|---|---|---|
| **B** | = | Urinary bladder |
| **BG** | = | Bowel gas |
| **F** | = | Foot |
| **FM and arrows** | = | False mass due to bladder duplication artifact |
| **FT** | = | Fallopian tubes |
| **H** | = | Head |
| **IIV** | = | Internal iliac vessels |
| **L** | = | Left |
| **O** | = | Ovaries |
| **OI** | = | Obturator internus muscles |
| **Pi** | = | Piriform muscles |
| **R** | = | Right |
| **Re** | = | Rectum |
| **U** | = | Uterus |
| **Ut** | = | Uterus |
| **V** | = | Vagina |

## Polycystic Ovaries (Stein-Leventhal Syndrome)

Polycytic ovaries (Stein-Leventhal syndrome) have a clinical presentation of infertility and virilization. The ultrasound findings usually indicate bilateral ovarian enlargement. The ovaries are not only enlarged but have a tense appearance. Multiple small cysts are noted in both ovaries. Normal women may have multiple small 5-mm cysts within their ovaries. However, in polycystic ovaries, the ovarian contour is increased in size and very tense in appearance. The ultrasound findings can confirm the clinical suspicion. Figures 15–97 and 15–98 are two transverse scans in a patient with polycystic ovaries. Both ovaries are enlarged. Note the size of the ovaries relative to the uterus. They are approximately equal or greater in size compared to the transverse diameter of the uterus. This is an unusual finding and suggestive of polycystic ovaries. Numerous sharp linear echoes are identified in each ovary outlining the numerous tiny small cysts. The left ovary is indenting the urinary bladder, confirming its increased size. This constellation of findings is consistent with bilateral ovarian enlargement and polycystic ovaries.

Figures 15–99 and 15–100 are transverse and longitudinal scans in another patient with polycystic ovaries. In Figure 15–99, we see the left ovary adjacent to the uterus. The left ovary is increased in size and more lucent than usual. The reason for the increased lucency is the presence of multiple small cysts, which are outlined by high-amplitude linear echoes. The right ovary was positioned in the cul-de-sac region, as is noted in Figure 15–100. This longitudinal scan shows a large right ovary, more lucent than anticipated, situated posterior to the uterus. Numerous high-amplitude linear echoes are present within the ovary, confirming the presence of multiple small cysts.

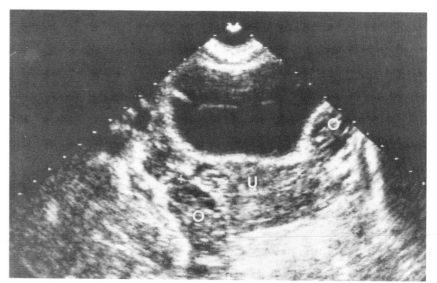

**FIG 15–97.**

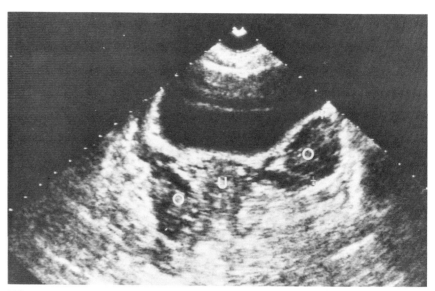

**FIG 15–98.**

O  =  Polycystic ovaries
U  =  Uterus

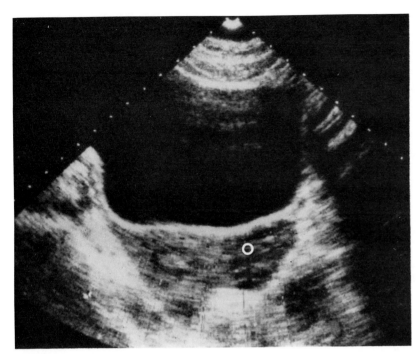

**FIG 15–99.**

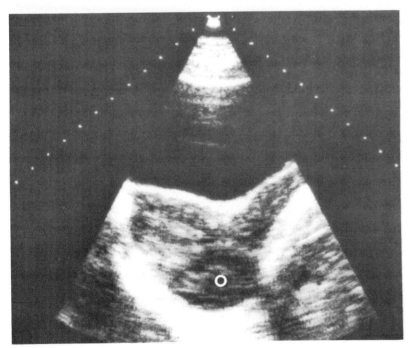

**FIG 15–100.**

## Cystadenoma

Ovarian lesions may have a varied ultrasound appearance. When a multiloculated, multiseptated cystic structure is identified in the adnexal region, the possibility of cystadenoma or cystadenocarcinoma should be considered. Generally, there are two types of lesions in this category. A mucinous cystadenoma tends to have thin internal septations. A serous cystadenoma tends to have more solid-appearing components. However, there is broad overlap between the two entities. Ultrasound cannot distinguish between a benign cystadenoma and cystadenocarcinoma. It is generally thought that the more solid-appearing lesions are more likely to be cystadenocarcinomas. However, this distinction cannot be made with certainty. The diagnosis of a mass should always raise the possibility of a cystadenocarcinoma, even though a great majority will be benign cystadenomas. Figure 15–101 is a longitudinal scan of the left ovary in a patient with a palpable pelvic mass. The mass is mainly fluid-filled with enhanced through-transmission. Several small linear septations are present in the midportion of the mass. At operation a mucinous cystadenoma was found. Figure 15–102 is another example of a mucinous cystadenoma. This has the appearance of a multiloculated cystic mass in the right ovary. The septations are quite sharply identified.

Figure 15–103 is a longitudinal scan of the right abdomen and pelvis. A multiloculated cystic is filling nearly the entire abdomen. A few small thin septations are identified. The mass is so large that it is resting in the right lower quadrant anterior to the iliac wing (I). These masses can reach dramatic size.

Figure 15–104 is a transverse scan of the pelvis in which we see a large cystic mass with prominent through-transmission. On the left lateral border of the cystic mass is a solid component (arrow). This turned out to be a serous cystadenoma. The distinction between a cystadenoma and a cystadenocarcinoma is not possible in any of the above-mentioned cases. Ultra-

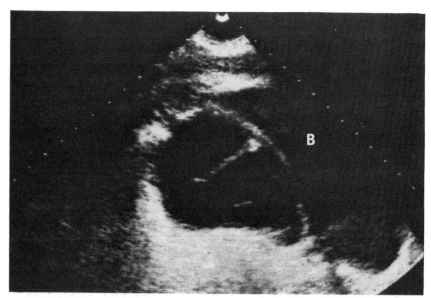

**FIG 15–101.**

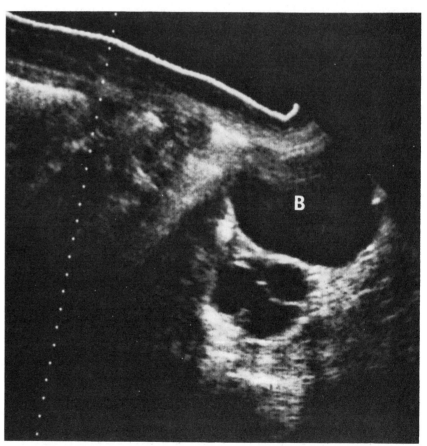

**FIG 15–102.**

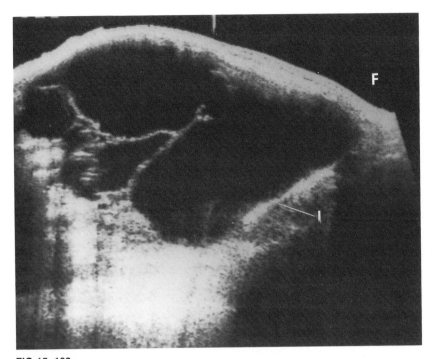

**FIG 15–103.**

sound cannot differentiate between benign and malignant forms.

**Arrow** = Solid component of serous cystadenoma
**B**      = Urinary bladder
**F**      = Foot
**I**      = Iliac wing

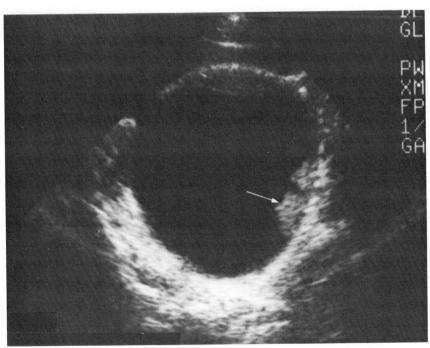

**FIG 15–104.**

## Cystadenoma and Cystadenocarcinoma

The four images shown here illustrate three cases of cystadenoma and cystadenocarcinoma. All of the masses have a similar appearance. There is no way to ascertain whether these masses are malignant from ultrasound criteria alone. Therefore, a mass can be diagnosed from ultrasound findings, but no attempt should be made to describe it as benign or malignant.

Figure 15–105 is a transverse scan over the abdomen of a 59-year-old woman who had previously undergone abdominal hysterectomy. She now had a 4-month history of slowly increasing abdominal girth. Anorexia and weight loss, along with a 4-day history of constipation, led to an emergency room visit. At that time a large abdominal mass was palpable and a pelvic ultrasound examination was ordered. A huge multiloculated mass was noted in the abdomen and pelvis. The findings were consistent with a cystadenoma or cystadenocarcinoma. At operation an ovarian mucinous cystadenoma of borderline malignancy was removed.

Figure 15–106 is a transverse scan of the abdomen in an 83-year-old woman who reported increasing abdominal girth over the last 8 months. She also complained of progressive constipation. Physical examination revealed a 20 weeks' size uterus. An ultrasound examination revealed a 30 × 20 × 20 cm multiloculated cystic mass consistent with a cystadenoma or cystadenocarcinoma. At operation a benign, mucinous cystadenoma of the ovary was removed.

Figures 15–107 and 15–108 are transverse and longitudinal scans of a 62-year-old woman with increasing abdominal girth. The scans disclose a large multiloculated mass filling the entire pelvis and lower abdomen. The findings are similar to those in the previous two cases. All of these lesions are remarkably similar in their ultrasound appearance. At operation a large 20-cm mass was removed. The diagnosis was mucinous cystadenocarcinoma. In this instance, multiple

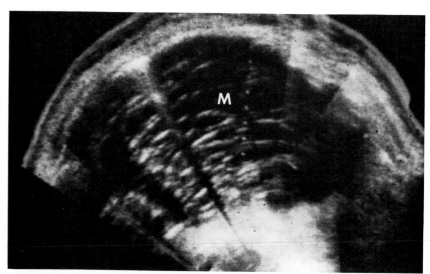

FIG 15–105.

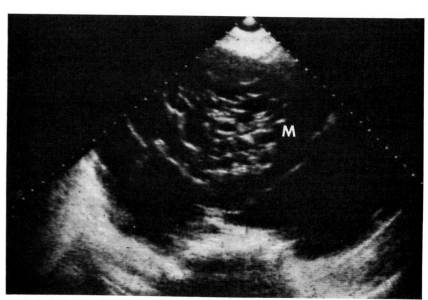

FIG 15–106.

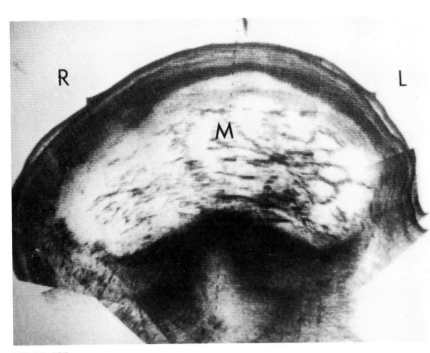

**FIG 15–107.**

metastatic implants were noted throughout the abdomen with nodules present over the diaphragm, liver, gallbladder, right kidney, stomach, and omentum. As can be seen from the three cases, the ultrasound appearance will not yield suggestive evidence whether or not a lesion is benign or malignant.

**L** = Left
**M** = Multiloculated mass
**P** = Symphysis pubis
**R** = Right
**U** = Umbilicus

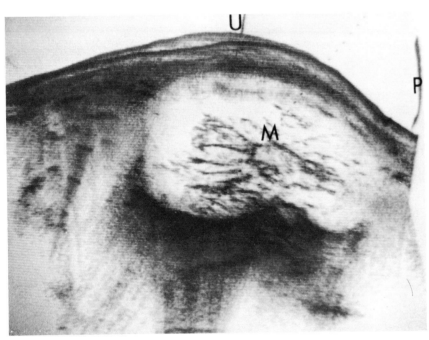

**FIG 15–108.**

## Cystadenoma and Cystadenocarcinoma

Figure 15–109 is a transverse scan of the abdomen in which a large mass is identified. Initially, it has the appearance of a hydronephrotic kidney. There is central sonolucency with a large soft tissue rim indicating a large solid component. The mass was found in a 68-year-old woman in whom lower abdominal mass was palpated on routine examination. The ultrasound examination indicated a solid-appearing lesion with central lucencies. The solid component was so large that a cystadenocarcinoma was suspected. At operation a mucinous cystadenocarcinoma was removed.

Figure 15–110 is a longitudinal scan showing a cystic mass (M) associated with an intrauterine pregnancy. The placenta is identified anteriorly, along with some fetal extremities. The cystic mass was quite low in the pelvis. It appeared to be a unilocular cyst with sharp walls. This lesion appeared quite innocent but proved to be a serous cystadenocarcinoma. It is extremely unusual that such a smooth-walled cyst will turn out to be malignant. But it proves the point that ultrasound cannot determine the difference between malignancy and benignity.

Occasionally, cystadenomas can reach enormous size, filling the entire abdomen. Figures 15–111 and 15–112 are transverse and longitudinal scans of a 57-year-old woman with a 2-year history of increasing abdominal girth. By the time she sought medical attention, her abdomen was nearly filled by a large cystic mass. This can easily be differentiated from ascites since no bowel loops are seen floating within the fluid-filled structure. The mass turned out to be a benign mucinous cystadenoma of the right ovary. These masses may enlarge dramatically in a patient who refuses to see a physician.

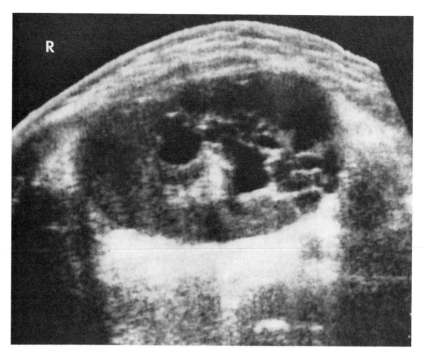

FIG 15–109.

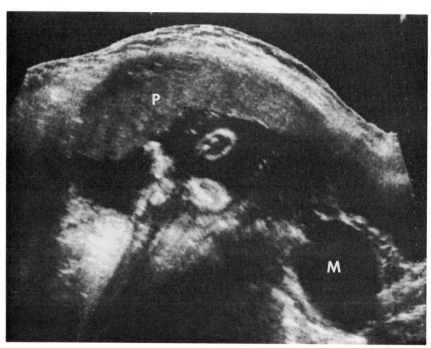

FIG 15–110.

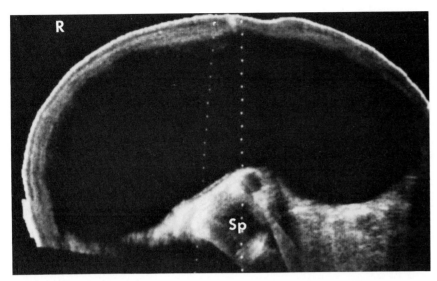

F  = Foot
IM = Iliacus muscle
M  = Serous cystadenocarcinoma
P  = Placenta
R  = Right
Sp = Spine

**FIG 15–111.**

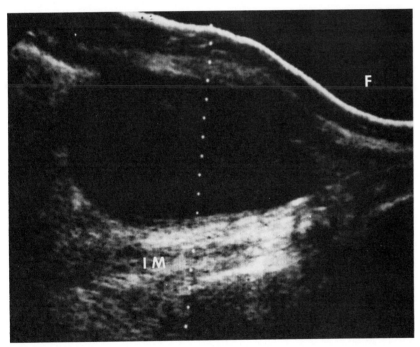

**FIG 15–112.**

## Papillary Cystadenocarcinoma

Figures 15–113 through 15–116 are scans of a 14-year-old girl with increasing abdominal girth. An intravenous pyelogram was initially obtained and suggested small bowel obstruction with areas of decreased density noted over the abdomen. Because of this, an ultrasound examination was done. This case is quite interesting in that it shows the various presentations of a cystadenocarcinoma. Figure 15–113 is a longitudinal scan of the abdomen and pelvis from the xyphoid to the symphysis pubis. Ascitic fluid is seen beneath the liver and in the pelvis. In Figure 15–116, ascitic fluid is seen in the pelvis surrounding the uterus. Also noted in Figures 15–113 and 15–116 is a large echogenic mass just above the ascitic fluid in the pelvis. It has a fairly homogeneous echogenic component to it, indicating the solid nature of this tumor.

A second component in this mass, however, has a more characteristic appearance of a cystadenocarcinoma. This is in the middle and upper abdomen. In Figures 15–113, 15–114, and 15–115, numerous curvilinear echoes surrounding fluid-filled regions are noted. A transverse scan (Fig 15–115) of the midabdomen demonstrates the solid component of the mass along with the fluid and curvilinear echoes. In fact, the fluid-filled areas are highly suggestive of bowel loops, with which this entity could be confused. In papillary cystadenocarcinoma, however, the fluid-filled masses appear somewhat more irregular and disorganized than bowel loops. Examples of bowel obstruction are presented in the general abdomen chapter. Also noted in Figures 15–114 and 15–115 is ascitic fluid in the right lateral gutter of the abdomen. At surgery, this mass was found to be a papillary cystadenocarcinoma. It had a large solid component in its inferior portion and a more characteristic fluid-filled component in the cephalad region.

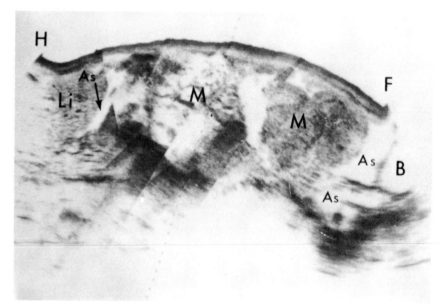

FIG 15–113.

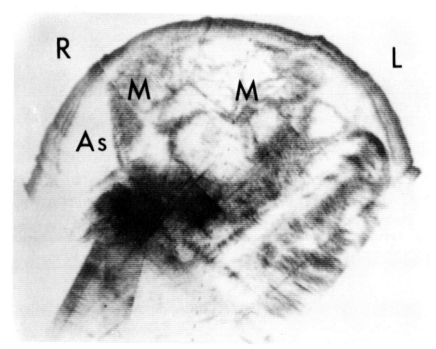

FIG 15–114.

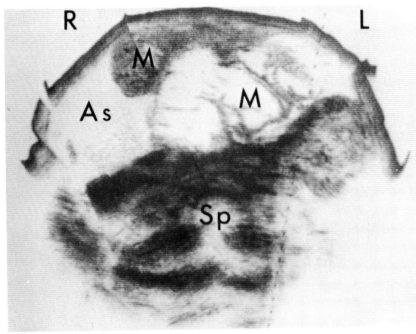

**As** = Ascites
**B** = Urinary bladder
**F** = Foot
**H** = Head
**L** = Left
**Li** = Liver
**M** = Papillary cystadenocarcinoma
**R** = Right
**Sp** = Spine
**Ut** = Uterus

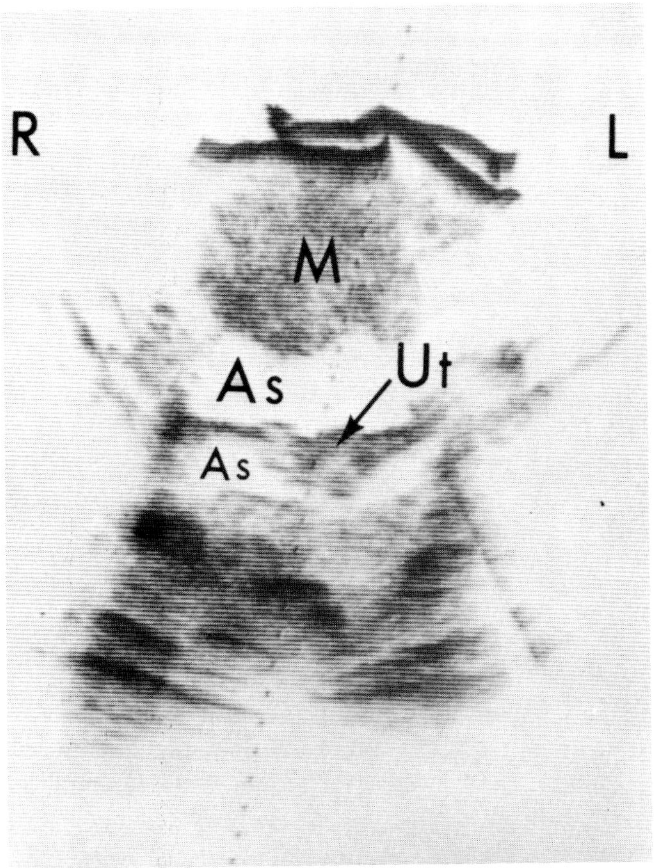

**FIG 15–115.**

**FIG 15–116.**

## Solid Ovarian Tumors

Solid ovarian tumors give an ultra-sound appearance of large echogenic masses within the pelvis. The ultra-sound appearance, however, is not very helpful in distinguishing one type of tumor from another. The major difficulty with a pelvic ultrasound examination of a solid ovarian tumor is the inability to distinguish it from the uterus. If a complete separation of the uterus from the solid mass can be shown, an adnexal lesion can be diagnosed. If the lesion cannot be separated entirely from the uterus, however, the possibility of a uterine growth must be considered.

Figure 15–117 is a longitudinal scan showing a large mass superior to the uterus. The mass is markedly attenuating (arrows). The posterior wall of the mass is difficult to see because of this marked attenuation. The possibility of a pedunculated fibroid off the fundus of the uterus cannot definitely be ruled out. A fairly good interface is seen between the mass and the uterus. This case turned out to be a fibrosarcoma of the ovary. Fibrous tumors of the ovary may have an ultrasound appearance similar to that of fibroids of the uterus. The architecture of the tumor is usually fairly sonolucent with marked attenuation and poor through-transmission, as is seen in a fibroid of the uterus.

Figure 15–118 is a longitudinal scan of a 10-year-old girl with a pelvic mass. A large sonolucent mass is seen separate from the uterus. Although the mass is extremely sonolucent, there is very poor through-transmission deep to it. This may be confused with a cystic lesion. The lack of an extremely sharp posterior border and through-transmission, however, indicates its solid nature by ultrasound. At exploration, a 10 × 5 × 3 cm, solid lobulated mass of the left ovary was found. It was diagnosed as a fibrosarcoma of the left ovary. Again, fibrous lesions of the ovary can be fairly sonolucent masses with poor through-transmission, similar to fibroid lesions of the uterus.

Figure 15–119 is a longitudinal scan of the pelvis of an 8-year-old girl

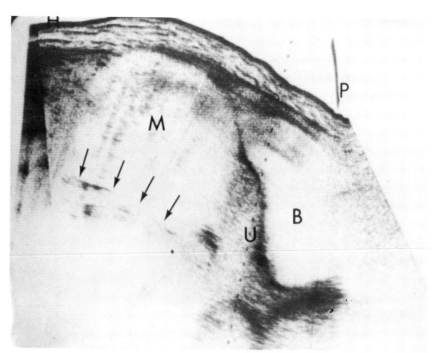

**FIG 15–117.**

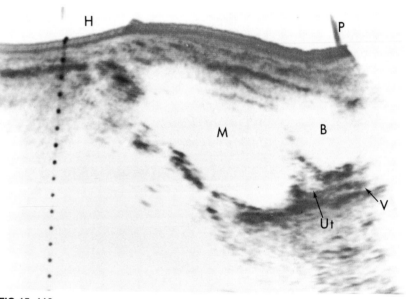

**FIG 15–118.**

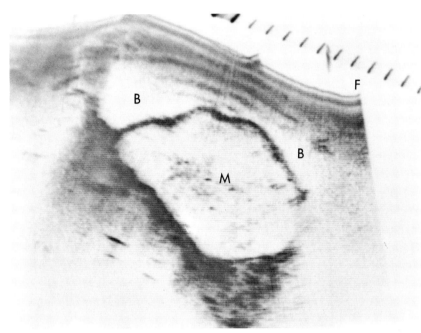

**FIG 15–119.**

with acute lymphocytic leukemia. A large, relatively lucent mass is seen posterior to the urinary bladder. A marked irregular indentation on the posterior wall of the urinary bladder is also noted. Diffuse echoes are present within the mass, indicating the solid nature of this lesion. It turned out to be leukemic ovarian infiltrates.

Figure 15–120 is a longitudinal scan of the pelvis of a 27-year-old woman with increasing abdominal girth. Ultrasound demonstrated a large echogenic mass in the pelvis and abdomen. The distention of the abdominal wall by this mass can be seen. The solid nature was confirmed by numerous internal echoes and a poorly defined posterior wall with a lack of through-transmission. This was found to be a dysgerminoma of the ovary. These rapidly growing tumors of the ovary cannot be distinguished by their ultrasonic appearance.

SOURCE: Figures 15–118 and 15–119 are provided through the courtesy of Barry Green, M.D.

| | | |
|---|---|---|
| **A** | = | Aorta |
| **Arrows** | = | Lack of through-transmission |
| **B** | = | Urinary bladder |
| **F** | = | Foot |
| **H** | = | Head |
| **M** | = | Solid ovarian mass |
| **P** | = | Level of the symphysis pubis |
| **U** | = | Uterus |
| **Ut** | = | Uterus |
| **V** | = | Vagina |

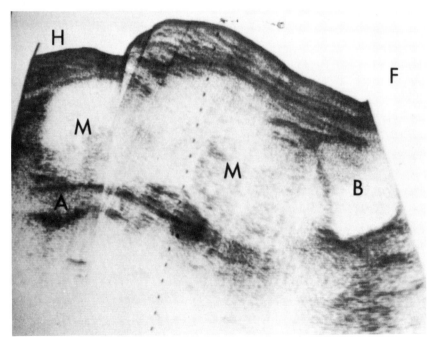

**FIG 15–120.**

## Ovarian Neoplasms

Solid ovarian neoplasms are less common than the cystic types previously described. When solid ovarian enlargement is present, the possibility of ovarian neoplasm is most likely. Figure 15–121, a transverse scan, shows an unusual-appearing solid lesion of the right ovary. The right ovary is extremely sonolucent. There are no internal echoes identified within the mass. The important finding is the lack of through-transmission deep to the mass, indicating that the ovarian lesion is solid rather than cystic. The mass was an extremely homogeneous thecoma of the right ovary. Despite its sonolucent appearance, the lesion was entirely solid. The lack of enhanced through-transmission confirmed the solid nature of this lesion and indicated that surgery was necessary. If the mass had been misinterpreted as an ovarian cyst, surgery may have been deferred.

Figure 15–122 is a longitudinal midline scan in which a large, relatively sonolucent mass is noted cephalad to the uterus. The mass may represent a pedunculated fibroid. There is no way to distinguish a pedunculated fibroid from a solid ovarian lesion. The mass turned to be a large ovarian fibroma. The lack of through-transmission deep to the mass indicates its solid nature.

Krukenberg tumors of the ovary arise from gastrointestinal malignancies with metastasis to ovaries. Figure 15–123 is a longitudinal midline scan in a young patient who had gastric carcinoma with metastasis to both ovaries. Only one ovary is identified on this scan and is cephalad to the uterus (U). This metastatic lesion (M) has a sonolucent central portion and a solid periphery. Ascites is also present, both anterior and posterior to the uterus. Ascites is common in such cases.

Figure 15–124 is a scan of the right upper quadrant in a patient who had ovarian carcinoma. Ascites is noted in the hepatorenal angle. Also present are two round soft-tissue nodules (arrows) that are secondary to peritoneal metastasis from the ovarian carcinoma. Usually peritoneal metastases

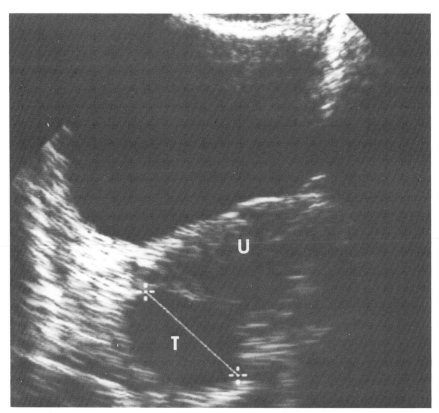

FIG 15–121.

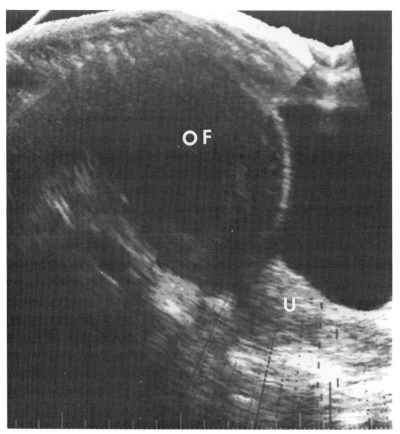

FIG 15–122.

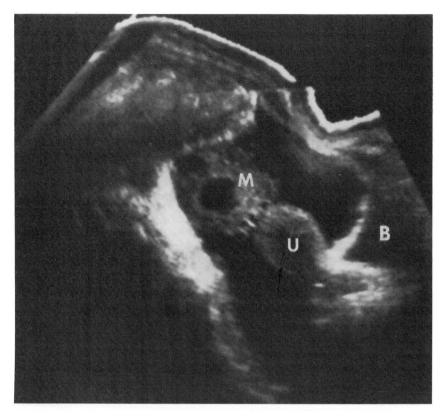

**FIG 15–123.**

are too small to be visualized on ultrasound. Even though they are small, ascites is usually present.

| Arrows | = Peritoneal metastasis |
| --- | --- |
| **B** | = Bladder |
| **F** | = Foot |
| **M** | = Ovarian metastasis from gastric carcinoma |
| **OF** | = Ovarian fibroma |
| **T** | = Thecoma |
| **U** | = Uterus |

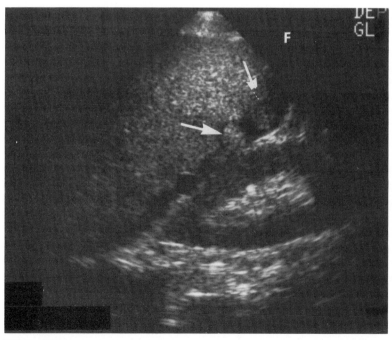

**FIG 15–124.**

## Dysgerminoma

Figures 15–125 and 15–126 are ultrasound scans of a 15-year-old girl with increased abdominal girth. A large solid mass is seen in the pelvis and abdomen. The anterior abdominal wall is distended secondary to the size of the mass. Within the mass are numerous strong echoes (arrows) of very high amplitude. An abdominal film revealed scattered calcifications throughout the abdomen, corresponding to these highly echogenic regions within the mass. At operation a dysgerminoma was found. These tumors can grow extremely rapidly. They have the ultrasound appearance of a solid lesion within the pelvis and abdomen.

Figures 15–127 and 15–128 are scans of a patient with dysgerminoma. This 13-year-old girl had had a large 20-cm dysgerminoma removed from the right ovary 1 year previously. Figure 15–127 is a transverse scan of the patient several months after surgery. The uterus is seen deviated slightly to the right. A mass in the left adnexal region represents the left ovary. The posterior left wall of the urinary bladder has a normal contour. The echogenicity of the ovary was somewhat worrisome at that time. It was decided to follow the patient serially with ultrasound examinations.

Figure 15–128 is a transverse scan of the same patient obtained later approximately 4 months. We now see an enlargement of the left adnexal mass. Indentation on the left posterior urinary bladder wall (arrows) is also noted. Evaluation of the bladder wall is an excellent means for detecting pelvic masses or changes in any pelvic masses. Although this depends on the degree of bladder filling, it can provide important diagnostic information. The left ovary is now enlarged (Fig 15–128). An irregular echo pattern throughout it indicates a solid lesion. The patient was also found to have a dysgerminoma of the left ovary.

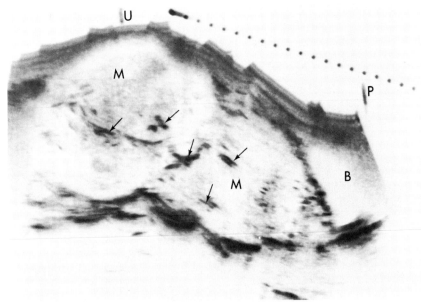

**FIG 15–125.**

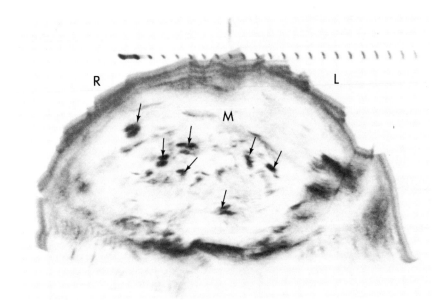

**FIG 15–126.**

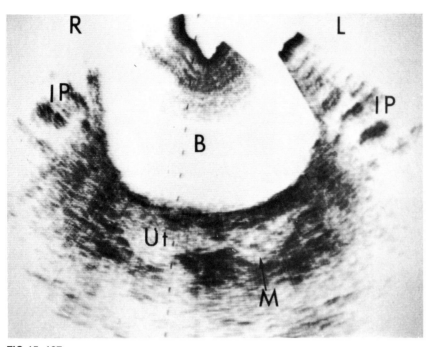

**FIG 15–127.**

SOURCE: Figures 15–125 and 15–126 are provided through the courtesy of Barry Green, M.D.

| | | |
|---|---|---|
| **Arrows** | = | Areas of calcification in the dysgerminoma (Figs 15–125, 15–126) |
| **Arrows** | = | Indentation on the bladder wall (Fig 15–128) |
| **B** | = | Urinary bladder |
| **IP** | = | Iliopsoas muscle |
| **L** | = | Left |
| **M** | = | Dysgerminoma |
| **P** | = | Level of the symphysis pubis |
| **R** | = | Right |
| **U** | = | Umbilical level |
| **Ut** | = | Uterus |

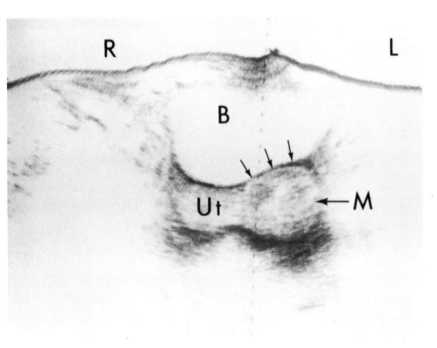

**FIG 15–128.**

## Dermoids

Dermoids contain elements of ectoderm, mesoderm, and endoderm. Because of this variety of elements, dermoids will present a spectrum of appearances on ultrasound. Depending on which of these elements are present within the dermoid, the ultrasound appearance will vary greatly. For this reason, dermoids are often difficult to identify unless the ultrasonographer is familiar with their appearances. The numerous following cases will demonstrate the large variety of dermoids.

Mural nodules have been considered to be the classic appearance of dermoids. Mural nodules are sometimes seen in a dermoid but certainly not in a high percentage of cases. The cases shown here demonstrate solid mural components to mainly cystic dermoids. Figures 15–129 and 15–130 are transverse and longitudinal scans in a patient with a large pelvic and abdominal mass. The mass is mainly fluid filled in its posterior portion. Round, solid, echogenic regions are present on the right anterior wall of this dermoid.

Figure 15–131 is a longitudinal midline scan in another patient who has a large cystic mass up to the umbilical level. In the inferior portion of the cystic mass is an echogenic solid region (arrow) representing a solid mural nodule. Figure 15–132 is a transverse scan of the pelvis of a separate patient in which we see a left cystic mass. On the posterior aspect of this mass is an echogenic solid region (arrow). In each of these cases the dermoid is mainly fluid filled. However, a portion of the wall has a nodular solid component suggesting the diagnosis of a dermoid. Although the findings are most consistent with dermoids, the possibility of an ovarian neoplasm cannot be entirely excluded.

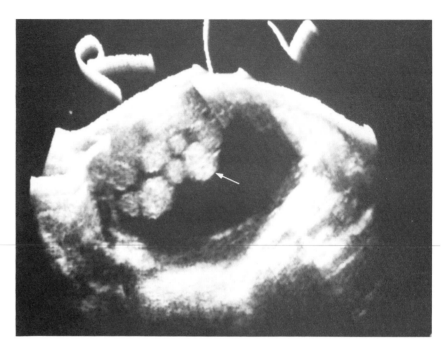

**FIG 15–129.**

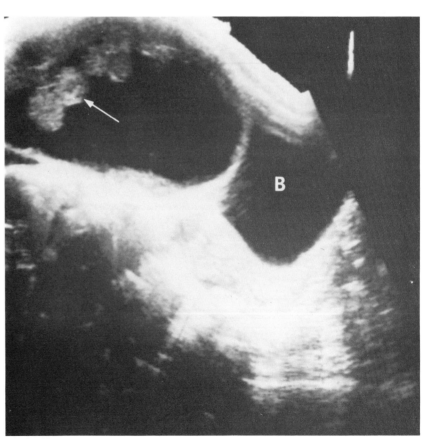

**FIG 15–130.**

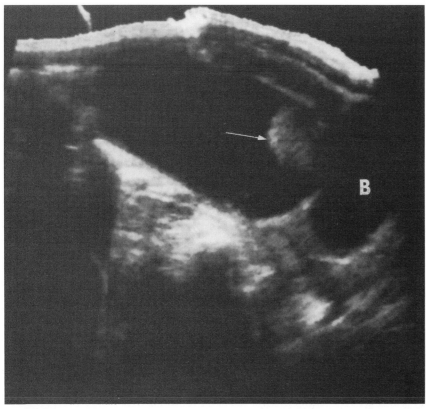

**Arrow** = Solid mural component to the dermoid
**B** = Urinary bladder

**FIG 15–131.**

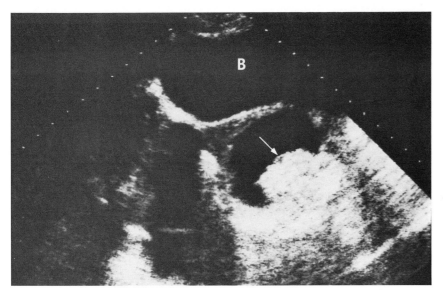

**FIG 15–132.**

## Dermoids With Calcification

Another characteristic finding in the presence of dermoids are high-amplitude echoes with acoustic shadowing. The findings are secondary to teeth within the lesion. When these areas of high-amplitude echoes and acoustic shadowing are noted on ultrasound, a pelvic x-ray film should be obtained for confirmation. Figure 15–133 is a longitudinal scan of the right pelvis in a 27-year-old woman who had recently experienced the onset of lower abdominal pain. Physical examination revealed a 5 × 8 cm mass in the right pelvis. An ultrasound study confirmed the presence of a large mass. In the inferior border of the mass in Figure 15–133 is a high-amplitude echo (arrowhead). Acoustic shadowing (S) is noted deep to the region of increased echogenicity. This finding is highly consistent with a dermoid. Because of the ultrasound finding, a pelvic x-ray film was obtained (Fig 15–134). Teeth are noted in the right pelvis (arrowhead). The pelvic x-ray and ultrasound findings confirm the diagnosis of a dermoid.

Figure 15–135 is a longitudinal scan in the right lower abdomen and pelvis of a 23-year-old woman. Ultrasound examination, performed because of a suspected ovarian cyst, revealed an 8 × 6 cm mass (arrows) which had a mixed appearance. There was a large area of increased echogenicity near the cephalad portion of this mass. Acoustic shadowing (S) was noted deep to this area of increased echogenicity. Because of the ultrasound findings, a dermoid was suspected. A pelvic x-ray film was obtained for confirmation. The x-ray film confirmed the presence of teeth and fat, consistent with a dermoid.

Figure 15–136 is a transverse scan of a 22-year-old woman also thought to have a cyst of the left ovary. The ultrasound scan shows a mixed solid-appearing mass (arrows) in the left pelvis. An area of high echogenicity is identified in the midportion of the mass. Acoustic shadowing (S) is noted deep to this area of increased echogenicity. Note the curved lucent

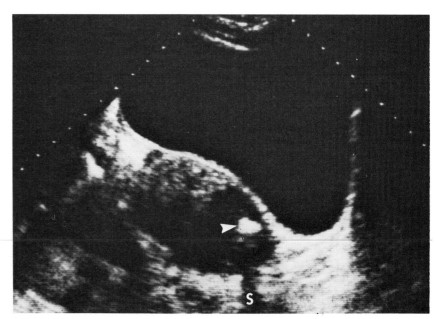

FIG 15–133.

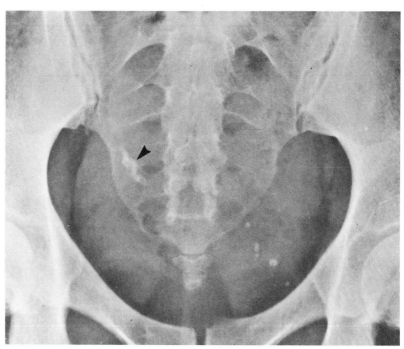

FIG 15–134.

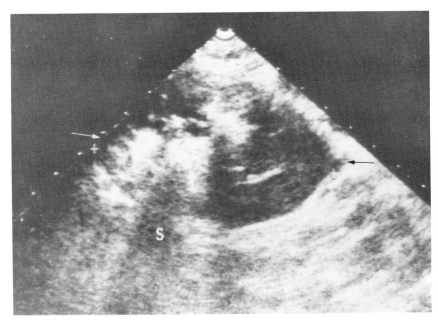

**FIG 15–135.**

rim around the area of increased echogenicity. This is often visualized in the presence of dermoids. Again, because of the ultrasound findings, a pelvic x-ray film was obtained. The x-ray film revealed several small areas of calcification consistent with a dermoid.

**Arrows** = Dermoid
**Arrowhead** = Teeth
**S** = Acoustic shadowing

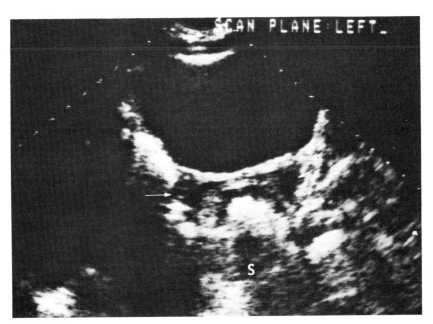

**FIG 15–136.**

## Dermoids

Figure 15–137 is a longitudinal scan of the pelvis and abdomen in a young woman with a large abdominal mass. The uterus is displaced posteriorly by the mass, which also impinges on the urinary bladder. Both solid and fluid components are present within the mass. At operation a large dermoid was found. Dermoids may contain numerous elements, which can yield a mixed ultrasound pattern. Cystadenoma or cystadenocarcinoma would be included in the differential diagnosis in this case.

Figure 15–138 is a transverse scan of the pelvis in a patient with a palpable pelvic mass. The mass (M) was difficult to visualize on ultrasound. In Figure 15–138, we see the uterus displaced anteriorly by an echogenic region in the cul-de-sac. The mass has ill-defined borders and is difficult to see. Note the indentation on the entire posterior aspect of the urinary bladder, an important diagnostic clue. Because of the ultrasound findings, a pelvic x-ray film was obtained and is shown in Figure 15–139. A large fatty density is present in the pelvis, confirming the diagnosis of a dermoid. At operation a 13-cm right dermoid was removed.

Figure 15–140 is a transverse scan in another patient who had a dermoid that was extremely difficult to visualize on ultrasound. However, one should keep in mind the varying appearances of such lesions. An ill-defined, relatively lucent mass is present in the right adnexa (arrows). Very little sound is being transmitted through the mass. This is an important diagnostic clue to the attenuation of such a lesion. At operation an 8-cm dermoid was removed from the right adnexa.

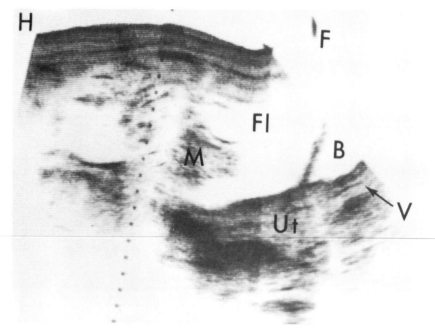

FIG 15–137.

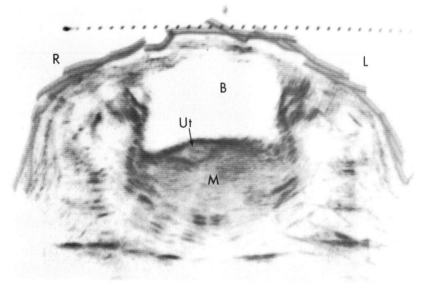

FIG 15–138.

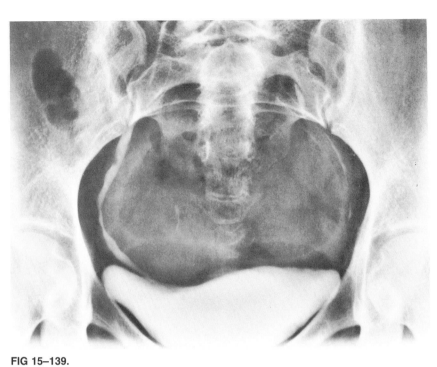

**FIG 15–139.**

| **Arrows** | = | Dermoid |
|---|---|---|
| **B** | = | Urinary bladder |
| **F** | = | Foot |
| **Fl** | = | Fluid component to the dermoid |
| **H** | = | Head |
| **L** | = | Left |
| **M** | = | Dermoid |
| **R** | = | Right |
| **U** | = | Uterus |
| **Ut** | = | Uterus |
| **V** | = | Vagina |

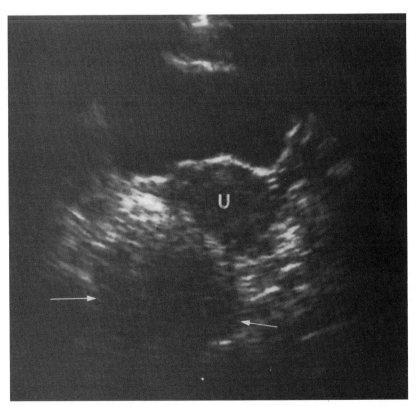

**FIG 15–140.**

## Echogenic Dermoids

One of the most difficult lesions to detect on ultrasound is an extremely echogenic dermoid. Frequently, dermoids with high-amplitude echoes will be missed because these echoes blend in with the surrounding high-amplitude echoes of bowel. Certain clues, however, help in detecting these echogenic lesions. If the referring physician palpates a large mass in the adnexa and no lesion can be identified, it is extremely important to look for an echogenic dermoid. Also, evaluation of the urinary bladder contour will provide important clues.

Figure 15–141 is a transverse scan of a patient in whom a left adnexal mass was palpated by the referring physician. This scan demonstrates the extremely important sign of bladder wall indentation (arrows). It is the most important clue to correct identification of a left adnexal mass. The size of the mass can be measured from the bladder wall (arrows) to the piriform muscle on the left side. The mass could easily have been missed except for the bladder wall contour deformity. At surgery, a 7-cm dermoid was found. It contained a large amount of subaceous material along with hair and fat.

Figure 15–142 is another example of a echogenic dermoid that could easily be missed. The referring physician palpated a mass on the right side. Again, the important sign of bladder wall indentation (arrows) is the initial clue to the correct diagnosis. An echogenic mass is situated posterior to the region of bladder wall contour deformity. It is obvious how easily this mass might be lost in the high-amplitude echoes of a normal pelvis. Once this region was identified, a longitudinal scan through the right adnexal was obtained (Fig 15–143). Better delineation of the dermoid (M) is now noted. The bladder contour deformity is again identified on longitudinal scan (arrows). Cephalad to the echogenic portion of the dermoid is a slightly lucent rim of tissue. At operation a right dermoid was removed.

Figure 15–144 is a transverse scan in a 25-year-old woman thought on

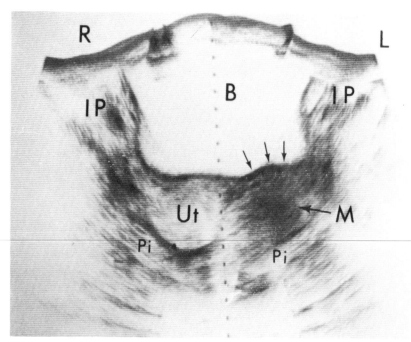

**FIG 15–141.**

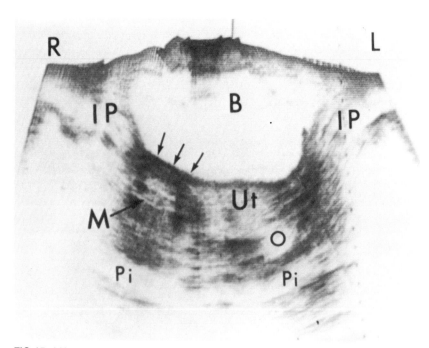

**FIG 15–142.**

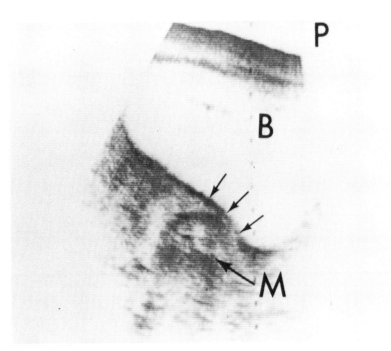

**FIG 15–143.**

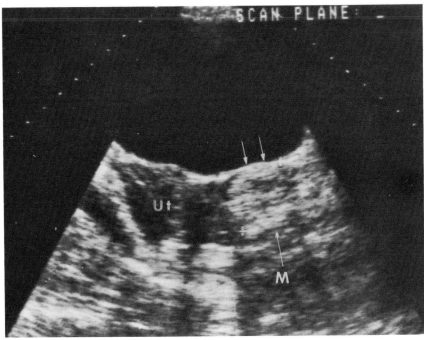

**FIG 15–144.**

clinical grounds to have a cyst in the left ovary. Ultrasound examination demonstrated a 4-cm echogenic mass in the left adnexal region (M). The initial clue was again the slight bladder contour deformity (arrows). Deep to the bladder contour deformity is a round echogenic region with acoustic shadowing noted posterior to it. These findings indicate the presence of a echogenic dermoid. A 4-cm dermoid was removed surgically.

If the referring physician believes there is a large mass in the pelvis and no mass is identified on ultrasound, an echogenic dermoid must always be considered. It is extremely important to evaluate the contour of the urinary bladder wall. This may provide the only clue that a mass is present. It is also necessary to evaluate high-amplitude echoes in the region surrounding the uterus, ovaries, and pelvic musculature. If a region of increased echogenicity is present deep to an area of bladder contour deformity, the possibility of an echogenic dermoid should be considered.

| **Arrows** | = | Indentation of the urinary bladder wall |
| **B** | = | Urinary bladder |
| **IP** | = | Iliopsoas muscle |
| **L** | = | Left |
| **M** | = | Echogenic dermoid |
| **O** | = | Ovary |
| **Pi** | = | Piriform muscle |
| **R** | = | Right |
| **Ut** | = | Uterus |

## Echogenic Dermoid

Echogenic dermoids may have an associated lucent rim of tissue surrounding the echogenic area. This can often be very helpful in leading to the correct diagnosis. Figure 15–145 is a longitudinal scan of the right pelvis in a young woman. The ultrasound examination demonstrates a 4-cm mass in the right adnexa. The inferior portion of the mass is echogenic. Deep to the echogenic region is an area of acoustic attenuation. The cephalad portion of the mass is slightly more sonolucent. Because of the ultrasound findings, a pelvic x-ray film was obtained (Fig 15–146). A round, fat density (arrowheads) was identified on the pelvic x-ray film, confirming the presence of a right dermoid. This small lesion could have easily been missed on ultrasound examination.

Figure 15–147 is a transverse scan of the pelvis in a 26-year-old woman who was admitted to the hospital for swallowing difficulties. During a routine physical examination, a pelvic mass was noted in the right adnexal area. The patient was sent to ultrasound to determine the etiology of the pelvic mass. A large right adnexal mass (arrowheads) is present impinging on the posterior urinary bladder. The echogenic region is surrounded by a lucent rim. This lucent rim is often characteristically seen in the presence of a echogenic dermoid. At operation a 6-cm echogenic dermoid of the right ovary was removed.

Figure 15–148 is a transverse scan in a 18-year-old woman thought to have a left ovarian cyst. An echogenic mass was noted in the left adnexa (arrowheads). In this instance, a lucent rim completely surrounds the echogenic region. This finding is highly consistent with a dermoid. At operation a 4.5-cm left dermoid was removed.

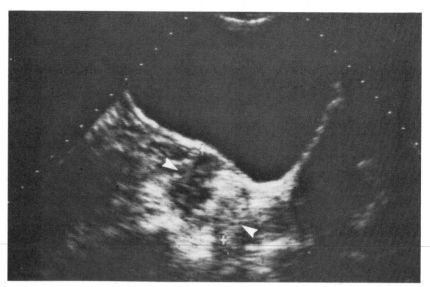

**FIG 15–145.**

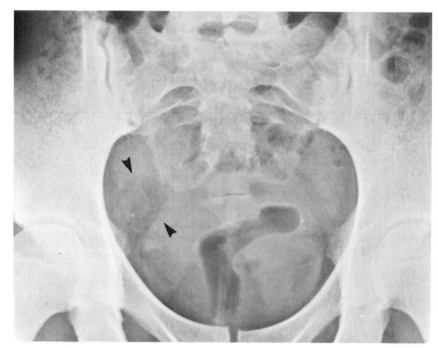

**FIG 15–146.**

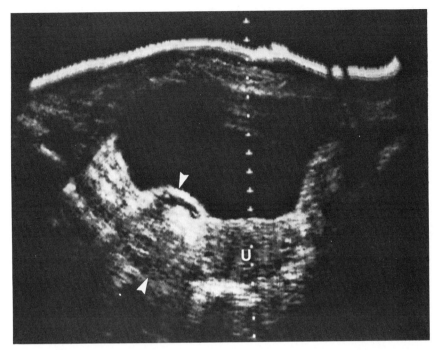

Arrowheads = Dermoid
U = Uterus

FIG 15–147.

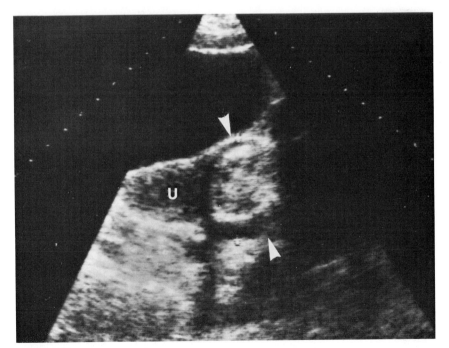

FIG 15–148.

## Changing Dermoid, Simulating Pelvic Kidney

Figures 15–149 and 15–150 are scans of the same patient; the scans demonstrate the occasionally documented changing nature of dermoids. Figure 15–149 is a longitudinal scan of the patient before pregnancy. A dermoid (arrowheads) is present posterior to the uterus in the region of the cul-de-sac. There is a soft echogenic center with a lucent periphery. This could be confused for a pelvic kidney. Early in the pregnancy a longitudinal scan was obtained (Fig 15–150). A gestational sac is identified in the fundal region of the uterus. Posterior to the uterus in the cul-de-sac is the previously noted dermoid (arrowheads). On this scan, the echogenic center is more eccentric in nature. It is now more readily visible and higher in echogenicity than on the previous study. There is also a fluid component present posteriorly and inferiorly.

Previous examples of dermoids demonstrated that they may have a lucent periphery surrounding an echogenic rim. In the previous cases the lucent periphery was quite small and thin. However, dermoids may occasionally have a larger periphery surrounding an echogenic center. Figure 15–151 is a longitudinal scan of the pelvis in which a dermoid (arrowheads) simulates a pelvic kidney. The highly echogenic central region has the appearance of the collecting system of the kidney. The thick lucent periphery appears to be the renal cortex. The smooth, sharp border to the dermoid could be confused for a pelvic kidney. When such a finding is identified, the renal fossae should then be examined to document the normal appearance and location of both kidneys. If both kidneys are normal in appearance, then the likelihood of a pelvic dermoid could be considered. Occasionally bowel lesions may have a similar appearance.

Figure 15–152 is a longitudinal scan of the pelvis in a 43-year-old woman who had lower abdominal pain for 1 year before hospitalization. There was a suggestion of a mass in

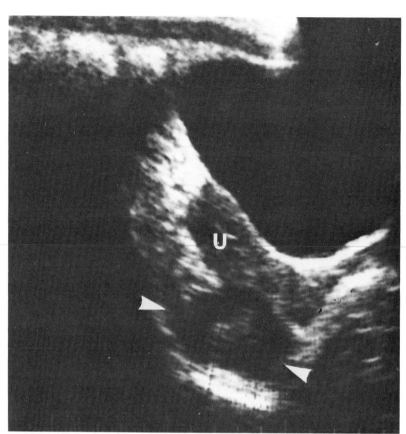

**FIG 15–149.**

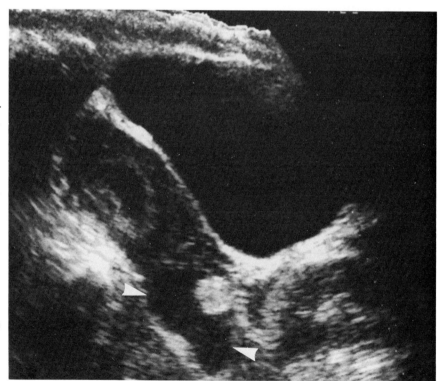

**FIG 15–150.**

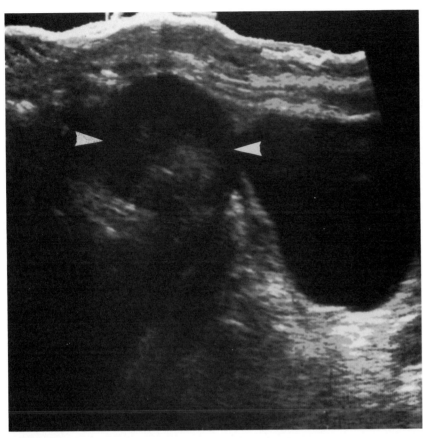

**FIG 15–151.**

the right pelvis. An ultrasound examination revealed a mass cephalad to the uterus. This mass has a bull's-eye appearance suggestive of a pelvic kidney. Both renal areas were examined and found to be normal. Because of this finding, a dermoid was quite likely. At operation a 7 × 7 cm right dermoid was removed.

**Arrowheads** = Dermoid
**U** = Uterus

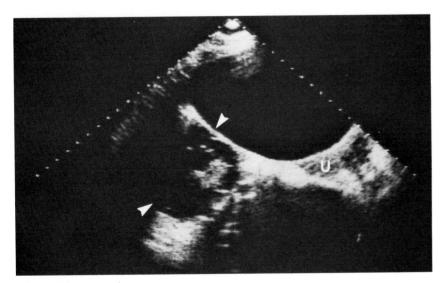

**FIG 15–152.**

## Dermoids With Fluid Levels

Since dermoids can contain numerous types of tissues, fluid levels can be identified on ultrasound examination. Figures 15–153 and 15–154 are transverse and longitudinal scans of a 36-year-old woman with a palpable mass in the right adnexal region. On ultrasound the mass appeared to be mainly cystic. However, a persistent linear echo was noted in the midportion of the mass (arrowhead). When the patient was turned into the decubitus position, the echo leveled out. The findings indicated a fluid-fluid level within the mass. At operation a right dermoid was removed. Fluid-fluid levels are sometimes suggestive of dermoids. However, other entities such as hemorrhagic cysts and hydrosalpinx may have fluid-fluid levels.

Figure 15–155 is a longitudinal scan in a patient with a large abdominal mass. This mass was noted to extend from the level of the symphysis pubis to nearly the xiphoid. A mixed echo pattern is present throughout the mass. In the midportion of the mass is a highly echogenic region anteriorly with some acoustic shadowing deep to it. Near the cephalad region of the mass is a fluid level (arrowhead). A transverse scan was obtained through the region of this fluid level (Fig 15–156). The superior portion of the mass had an area of anterior echogenicity layering out on a sonolucent fluid component posteriorly. The mass turned out to be a large 25-cm dermoid with numerous tissue components throughout.

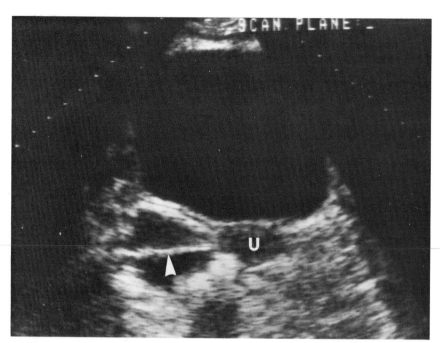

FIG 15–153.

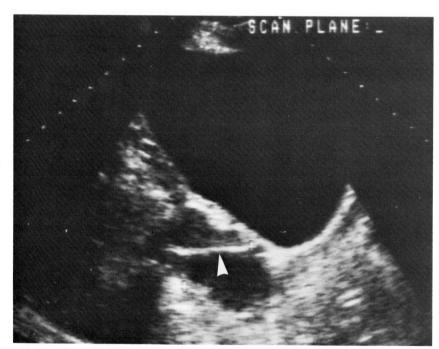

FIG 15–154.

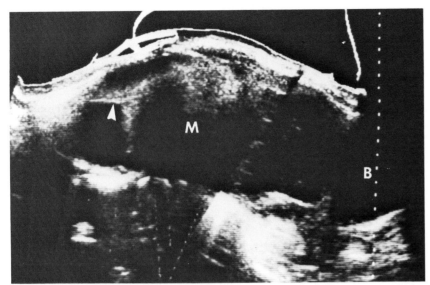

Arrowhead = Fluid level
B = Bladder
M = Dermoid

FIG 15–155.

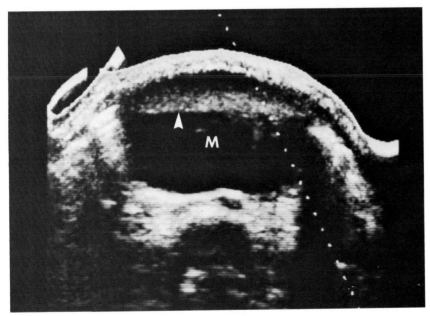

FIG 15–156.

## Ruptured Dermoid

Figures 15–157 through 15–159 are scans of a middle-aged woman who noticed a slight increase in abdominal girth 5 years previously. There was progressive increase in abdominal size with a sudden increase approximately 1 year before the examination. Four months before admission, she experienced pain and a further increase in abdominal size. When she finally entered the hospital, ultrasound examination revealed an extremely confusing picture. A longitudinal scan (Fig 15–157) demonstrates a solid component to a mass adherent to the anterior abdominal wall. This almost looks like placental tissue, and the mass could be confused wth an intra-abdominal pregnancy. The abdomen is filled with fluid in which the uterus and bowel loops appear to float. Figure 15–158 is a transverse scan through the midabdomen. Numerous solid and fluid components can be identified. Figure 15–159 is a transverse scan over the pelvis in which the uterus is seen surrounded by fluid. This was initially felt to be a neoplastic tumor because of the solid component and evidence of ascitic fluid. At operation a ruptured dermoid was found. Pathologic study disclosed that it was a benign cystic teratoma, with no evidence of malignancy.

Figure 15–160 is the scan of another patient with an extremely confusing ultrasound picture. A large abdominal mass is identified filling the pelvis and abdomen. The patient was pregnant, but much less so than the size of the abdomen indicated. The pregnancy is identified in the lower portion of the scan in Figure 15–160. Cephalad to the uterus was a large mass (D), which turned out to be a dermoid chiefly filled with keratin. The solid component of the dermoid has an appearance similar to that of placenta. Fetal echoes (Fe) are noted within the uterus lower in the pelvis.

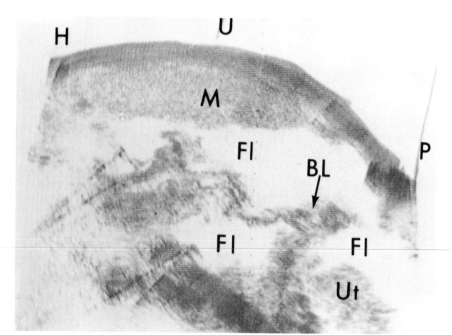

FIG 15–157.

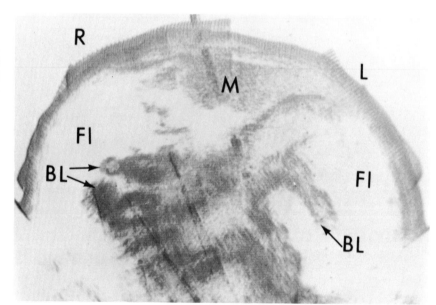

FIG 15–158.

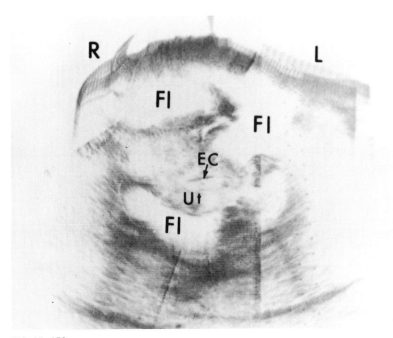

**FIG 15–159.**

| | | |
|---|---|---|
| **BL** | = | Bowel loops |
| **D** | = | Dermoid |
| **EC** | = | Endometrial cavity |
| **Fe** | = | Fetus |
| **FI** | = | Fluid in the abdomen |
| **H** | = | Head |
| **L** | = | Left |
| **M** | = | Solid component to ruptured dermoid |
| **P** | = | Symphysis |
| **R** | = | Right |
| **U** | = | Umbilicus |
| **Ut** | = | Uterus |

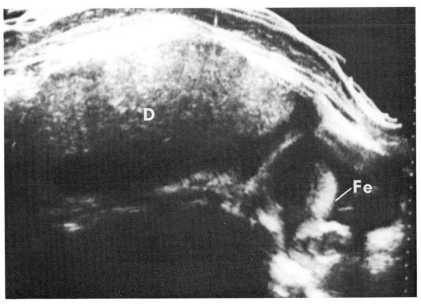

**FIG 15–160.**

## Pelvic Inflammatory Disease

Pelvic inflammatory disease presents an ultrasound spectrum that depends on the stage of infection. In the acute phase, masses within the pelvis may have a sonolucent appearance compatible with fluid. Also, tissue planes are difficult to delineate in the presence of inflammation. In the chronic phase, the fibrotic changes often yield solid-appearing masses within the pelvis that may be difficult to distinguish from neoplasm.

Figures 15–161 and 15–162 are longitudinal and transverse scans of a 17-year-old girl who experienced the onset of pain several weeks earlier. Fluid is seen in the cul-de-sac which could be from a recently ruptured ovarian cyst. However, the clinical findings suggested acute pelvic inflammatory disease. A culdocentesis was performed which yielded suppurative material in the cul-de-sac. A regimen of antibiotics was started and the patient showed clinical improvement. Pelvic inflammatory disease usually manifests on ultrasound as fluid in the peritoneal space in the acute phase.

Figures 15–163 and 15–164 are transverse and longitudinal scans of a 27-year-old woman who had recently experienced vomiting and right-sided abdominal pain. Figure 15–163 is a transverse scan in which both adnexal regions (arrowheads) are enlarged. Numerous small cystic areas are identified bilaterally. These areas may represent a small ovarian cyst. However, the patient had pelvic inflammatory disease and the findings are most consistent with small areas of abscess formation. The longitudinal scan in Figure 15–164 shows a large amount of fluid in the cul-de-sac. The patient was placed on antibiotics with dramatic improvement in symptoms and in the size of the adnexal area.

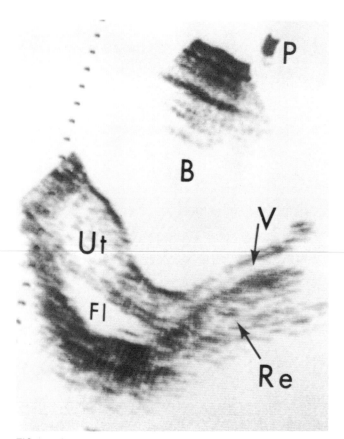

**FIG 15–161.**

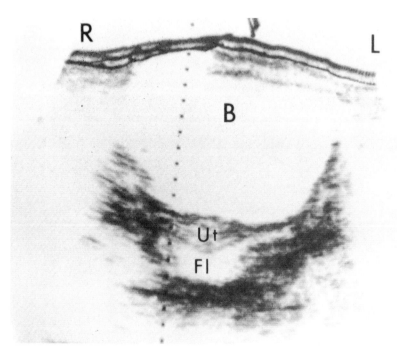

**FIG 15–162.**

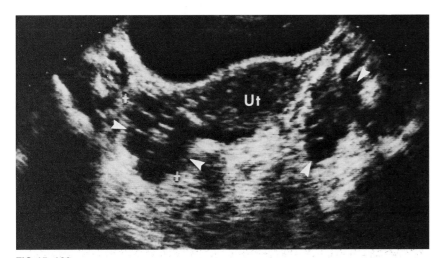

**FIG 15–163.**

| Arrowheads | = | Bilateral ovarian enlargement |
|---|---|---|
| B | = | Urinary bladder |
| Fl | = | Peritoneal fluid |
| L | = | Left |
| P | = | Symphysis |
| R | = | Right |
| Re | = | Rectum |
| Ut | = | Uterus |

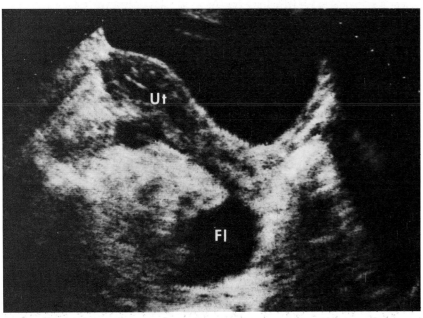

**FIG 15–164.**

## Progression of Pelvic Inflammatory Disease

Pelvic inflammatory disease may change dramatically over a short period of time. The following case is an excellent example. The patient was a 34-year-old woman who came to the emergency room with a 2-day history of fever and minimal abdominal pain. The initial ultrasound scans are shown in Figures 15–165 and 15–166. A small amount of fluid is noted in the cul-de-sac and adnexal region. The patient was started on antibiotic therapy and discharged home. She returned 2 weeks later complaining of increasing pelvic pain and fever. An ultrasound examination at that time demonstrated a dramatic increase in the amount of fluid in the cul-de-sac. Figure 15–167 is a longitudinal scan in which a multiloculated fluid collection is now present in the cul-de-sac region, displacing the uterus anteriorly. Figure 15–168 is a transverse scan demonstrating marked extension of the fluid into the adnexal region. Note the dramatic change in the size and contents of the fluid in the 2-week interim. The antibiotic therapy was changed, with marked clinical improvement. This case is an excellent example of the rapidity of development of pelvic fluid in the presence of acute pelvic inflammatory disease.

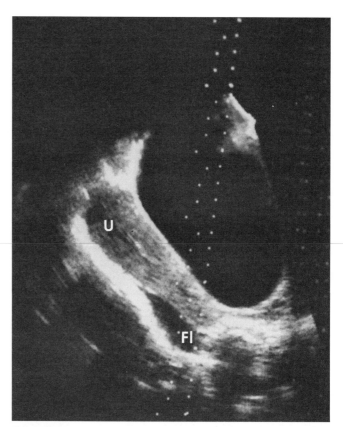

FIG 15–165.

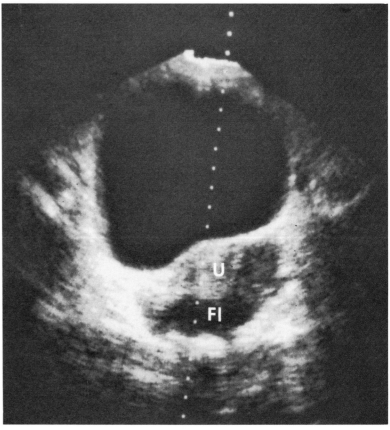

FIG 15–166.

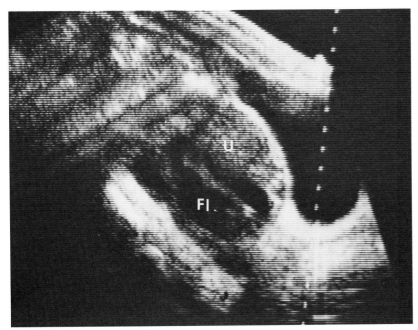

FI  = Pelvic inflammatory disease
U   = Uterus

**FIG 15–167.**

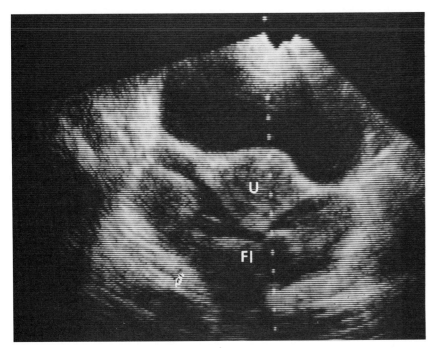

**FIG 15–168.**

## Tubo-Ovarian Abscess

Figures 15–169 and 15–170 are transverse and longitudinal scans of a 19-year-old woman with the recent onset of pelvic pain. She was found clinically to have pelvic inflammatory disease and an ultrasound examination was ordered. The ultrasound scans showed several fluid-filled areas in the right adnexal region. Examination suggested the presence of tubular lucencies throughout the right adnexa. The right adnexa was enlarged, as is noted by impression on the right side of the urinary bladder. Culture yielded *Gonococcus;* the infection responded well to antibiotic therapy.

Figures 15–171 and 15–172 are transverse and longitudinal scans of a 21-year-old patient with a 2-week history of abdominal pain and low-grade fever. Pelvic examination revealed a right-sided mass. Laboratory data indicated an elevated WBC count and sedimentation rate. Figure 15–171 is a transverse scan of the pelvis in which a cystic region is noted indenting the posterior aspect of the urinary bladder on the right side (arrowhead). This transverse scan would suggest a simple ovarian cyst. However, the longitudinal scan (Fig 15–172) indicated that the cystic region was a tubular structure, a tubo-ovarian abscess. The patient had a positive gonococcal culture and was placed on antibiotic therapy. The findings indicate fuid in the right fallopian tube. A portion of the fundus of the uterus is noted cephalad to the right tube.

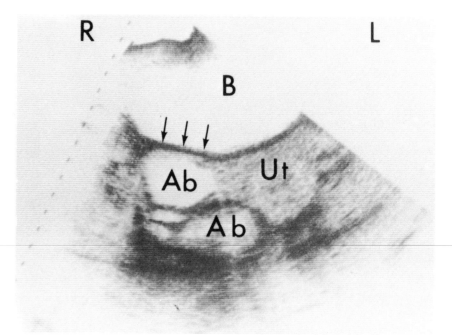

**FIG 15–169.**

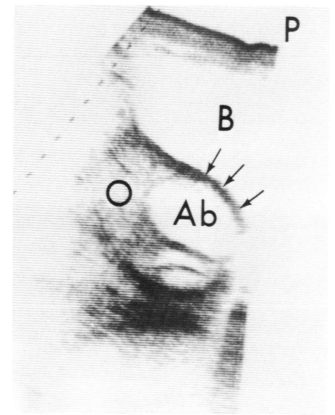

**FIG 15–170.**

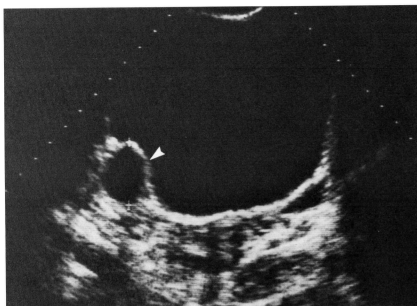

FIG 15–171.

| Arrows | = Indention on the urinary bladder |
|---|---|
| **Arrowhead** | = Tubo-ovarian abscess |
| **Ab** | = Tubo-ovarian abscess |
| **B** | = Urinary bladder |
| **L** | = Left |
| **O** | = Ovary |
| **P** | = Symphysis |
| **R** | = Right |

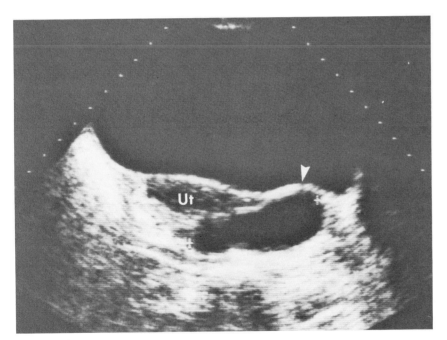

FIG 15–172.

## Pelvic Inflammatory Disease

Pelvic inflammatory disease frequently is associated with an intrauterine device. Figure 15–173 is a longitudinal scan with a strong echo within the uterus, indicating an intrauterine device. This has a fairly characteristic appearance of a Copper 7 or a Copper T intrauterine device. Posterior to the uterus is a large sonolucent mass that is secondary to a cul-de-sac abscess. The mass has a somewhat irregular border, highly consistent with an abscess. The possibility of a hematoma could not be ruled out. Clinically, however, the finding was consistent with pelvic inflammatory disease.

Often, long-standing pelvic inflammatory disease leads to hydrosalpinx. This entity is actually a sterile collection that has been scarred and blocked within the fallopian tube. The sonolucent collection in the fallopian tube often gives a picture similar to an ovarian cyst.

Figure 15–174 is an example of a moderately sized hydrosalpinx in the right fallopian tube. Again we see indentation on the posterior bladder wall characteristic of a right adnexal lesion. The hydrosalpinx is extremely lucent, indicating its fluid-filled nature. The walls are fairly sharp, although not quite as sharp as we might see in a simple ovarian cyst.

Figures 15–175 and 15–176 show a hydrosalpinx somewhat larger than the one in Figure 15–174. The walls of this hydrosalpinx are slightly sharper than in the previous case. This one could be confused with an ovarian cyst, or possibly a cystadenoma.

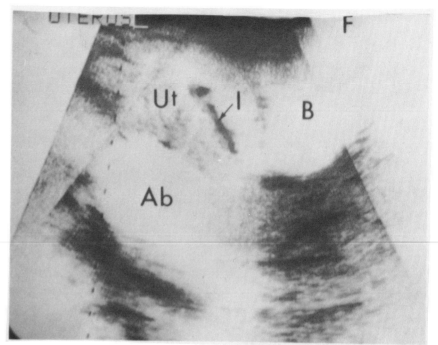

**FIG 15–173.**

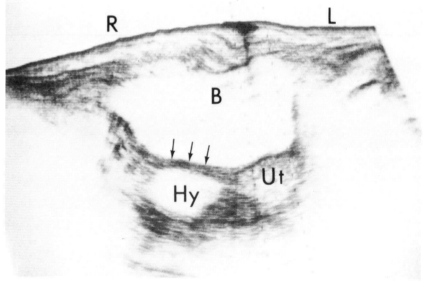

**FIG 15–174.**

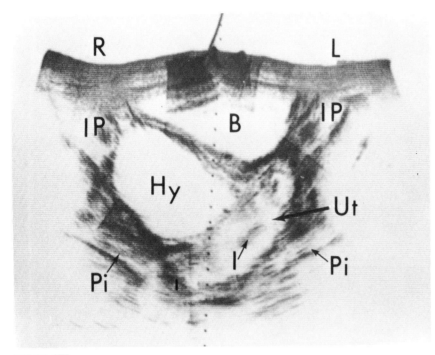

**FIG 15–175.**

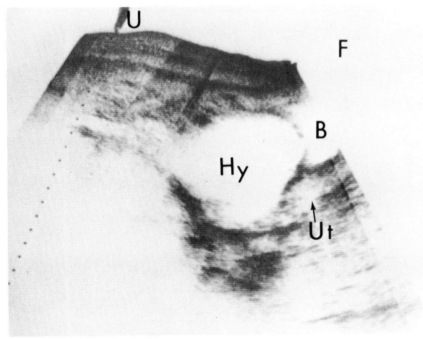

**FIG 15–176.**

Ab = Cul-de-sac abscess
Arrows = Indentation on the bladder
wall
B = Urinary bladder
F = Foot
Hy = Hydrosalpinx
I = Intrauterine device
IP = Iliopsoas muscle
L = Left
Pi = Piriform muscle
R = Right
U = Umbilical level
Ut = Uterus

## Pelvic Inflammatory Disease

Pelvic inflammatory disease also can appear to have a mixed echo pattern, rather than just sonolucent. Usually, when a mixed echo pattern of solid and cystic lesions is present, it is more characteristic of an abscess, as is found elsewhere in the body. When a mixed echo pattern is present, the diagnosis of pelvic inflammatory disease with ultrasound is usually easier.

Figures 15–177 and 15–178 are scans of a patient with severe pelvic inflammatory disease associated with an abscess anterior to the uterus and thickening of the urinary bladder wall. There also is evidence of debris (arrows) within the urinary bladder itself. The relatively sonolucent collection between the uterus and bladder wall has an appearance more characteristic of an abscess. Irregular borders are demonstrated. The internal echoes arising from the abscess also have an appearance of debris rather than a solid nature. There is evidence of some through-transmission through the abscess; again, this is somewhat characteristic.

Figures 15–179 and 15–180 are scans of a 21-year-old woman who had an intrauterine device removed 1 day previously because of pelvic pain. An ultrasound examination demonstrated two relatively lucent areas in the pelvis. It was difficult to visualize the uterus. Figure 15–179 is a transverse scan demonstrating the uterus in the midpelvis. The borders of the uterus (arrows), however, are quite difficult to see because of the adherent adnexal masses. Bilateral abscesses are present. Because of the inflammatory reaction, the interface between the abscesses and the uterus may be quite difficult to see. The abscesses present with a mixed echo pattern in which a portion is relatively sonolucent, indicating suppurative material, and a portion is echogenic, indicating fibrosis and debris. Figure 15–180 is a longitudinal scan of the patient showing the abscess collection posterior to the uterus.

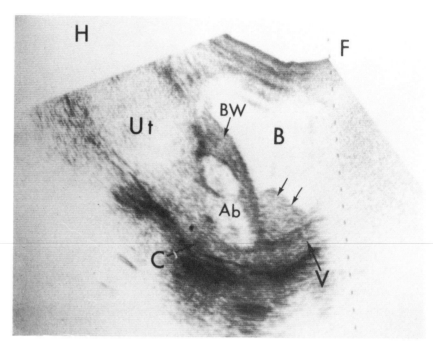

**FIG 15–177.**

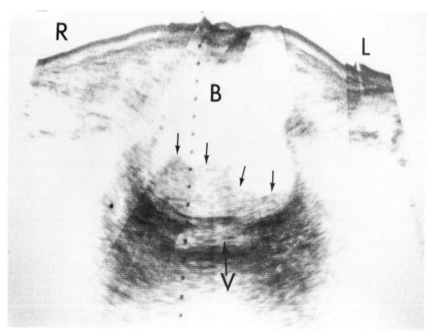

**FIG 15–178.**

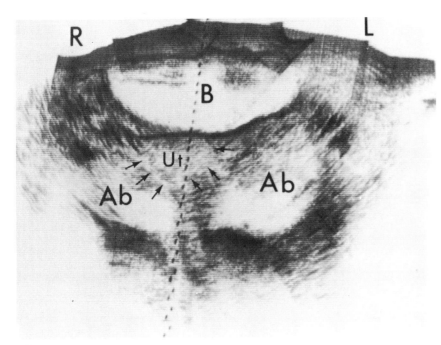

| Ab | = Pelvic abscess |
| Arrows | = Debris in the urinary bladder wall |
| B | = Urinary bladder wall |
| BW | = Thickened urinary bladder wall |
| C | = Cervix |
| F | = Foot |
| H | = Head |
| L | = Left |
| R | = Right |
| Ut | = Uterus |
| Ut and arrows | = Uterus that is difficult to see because of surrounding abscess |
| V | = Vagina |

FIG 15–179.

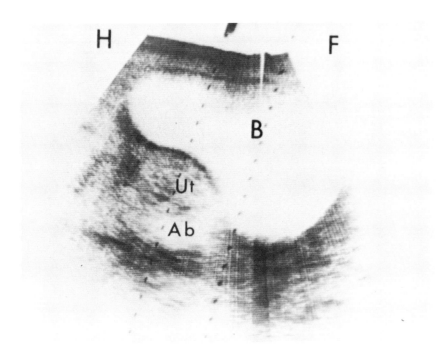

FIG 15–180.

## Other Entities Simulating Pelvic Inflammatory Disease

Other entities may have ultrasound appearances similar to that seen in pelvic inflammatory disease. These entities include endometriosis, infections from other etiologies, chronic ectopic pregnancies, necrotic tumors from pelvic organs, and tumors from other organs. Figures 15–181 and 15–182 are transverse and longitudinal scans of the pelvis that show a large, relatively lucent mass in the cul-de-sac region. This mass is displacing the uterus anteriorly and compressing it against the urinary bladder. The findings would be consistent with a large chronic abscess and pelvic inflammatory disease. However, the patient had a chronic ectopic pregnancy. Ectopic pregnancies can become quite large and walled off, as in this case. There is a large hemorrhagic region in the cul-de-sac, similar to what would be seen with an abscess.

Figure 15–183 is a longitudinal scan of the pelvis in a patient with a sonolucent mass posterior to the uterus. Through-transmission is noted deep to the mass, indicating its fluid-filled nature. This could easily be a pelvic abscess from pelvic inflammatory disease. The patient had diverticulitis. An abscess was arising in the pelvis secondary to the diverticular disease. There is no way to distinguish on ultrasound examination between the various entities causing the inflammation. They will all have similar appearances.

Figure 15–184 is a transverse scan of the pelvis of a 21-year-old woman with ulcerative colitis. Two months before the ultrasound examination she underwent a total colectomy. She was admitted to the hospital because of abdominal and pelvic pain. Figure 15–184 indicates a large mass in the cul-de-sac and adnexal region displacing the uterus anteriorly. This mass meets all of the ultrasound criteria of an abscess. The mass is relatively sonolucent, with a few internal echoes. The predominant feature is prominent through-transmission deep to the

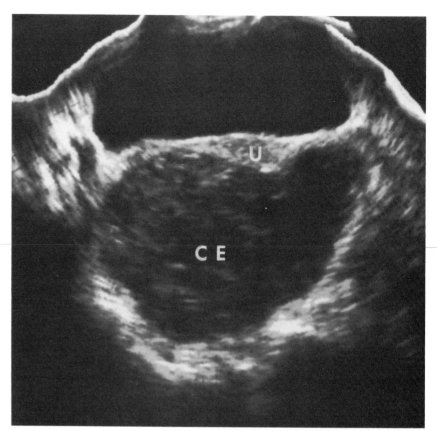

FIG 15–181.

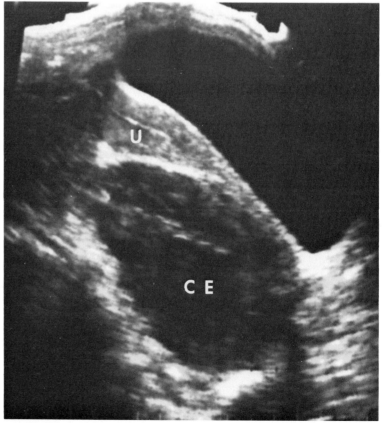

FIG 15–182.

mass, indicating its fluid-filled nature. Because of pelvic pain, an elevated white blood cell count, and appropriate clinical history, the diagnosis of a pelvic abscess was made. At operation a large pelvic abscess was drained.

As can be seen from the above cases, several entities may appear similar to pelvic inflammatory disease on ultrasound examination. It is necessary to correlate the clinical history and laboratory findings with the scan appearance to establish the correct diagnosis.

**Ab** = Pelvic abscess
**CE** = Chronic ectopic pregnancy
**U** = Uterus

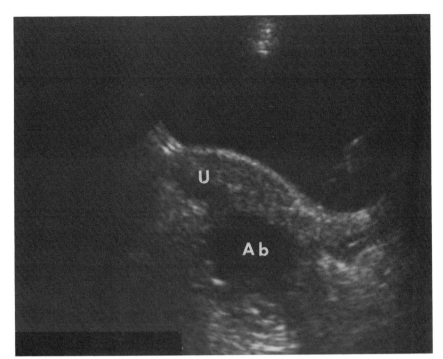

**FIG 15–183.**

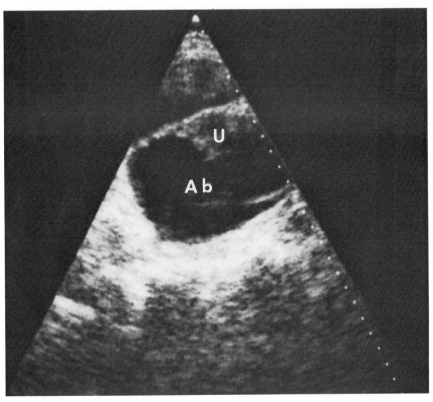

**FIG 15–184.**

## Endometriosis

Endometriosis has a varied ultrasound appearance, from cystic to solid-appearing lesions. The ultrasound findings are often similar in appearance to those seen in pelvic inflammatory disease. In fact, it is difficult to distinguish between these two entities on the basis of ultrasound findings alone. Clinical history and laboratory data will help distinguish them.

Figure 15–185 is a transverse scan of the pelvis of a 27-year-old woman with a 7-year history of endometriosis. Seven years earlier a large endometrioma had been surgically removed. The patient experienced increasing pain during menses. The ultrasound examination demonstrates a large sonolucent mass in the right adnexa compatible with an endometrioma. This is the usual appearance of the typical "chocolate cyst." Relatively few internal echoes are identified, with prominent through-transmission. The left adnexa is also slightly lucent. However, soft internal echoes are noted within the left adnexa. This finding is suggestive of an area of hemorrhage and clot in an endometrioma.

Figure 15–186 is a transverse pelvic scan of a 42-year-old woman with a long history of severe dysmenorrhea. The ultrasound examination demonstrates a large oval sonolucent mass on the left adnexa. Note the indentation on the posterior aspect of the urinary bladder, caused by the left adnexal mass. This is another typical appearance of endometrioma. In this instance, numerous soft internal echoes are present within the mass. These low-level echoes are suggestive of old blood.

Figures 15–187 and 15–188 are longitudinal and transverse scans of the pelvis in another patient with endometriosis. In this instance, a large cystic lesion is present cephalad to the uterus. Through-transmission is noted deep to the sonolucent area, indicating its fluid-filled nature. Very subtle low-level echoes are present within the cystic mass. These findings are typical of the "chocolate cyst" endometrioma found at surgery.

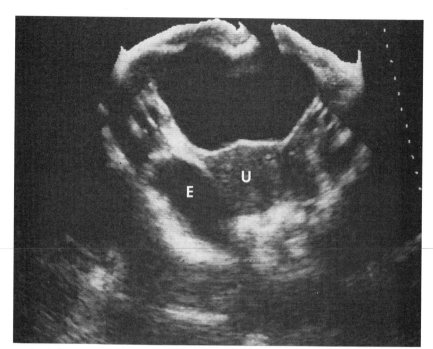

**FIG 15–185.**

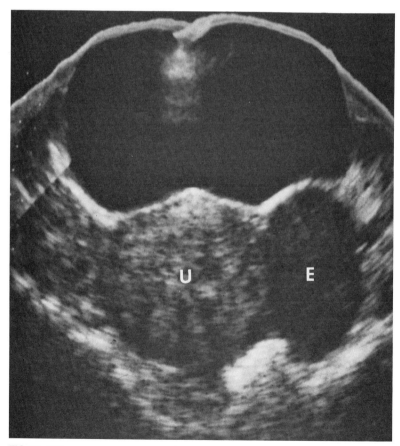

**FIG 15–186.**

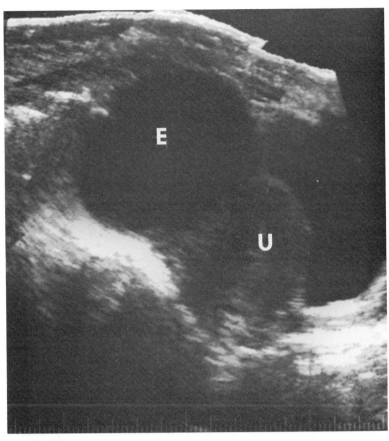

**FIG 15–187.**

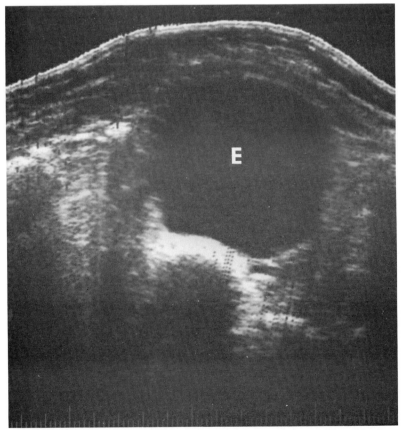

**FIG 15–188.**

E  =  Endometriosis
U  =  Uterus

## Endometriosis

Endometriosis can be the great mimicker in pelvic ultrasound evaluation, similar to pelvic inflammatory disease. Just as in pelvic inflammatory disease, endometriosis can give a spectrum of ultrasonic appearances, ranging from a nearly completely sonolucent mass all the way to a highy echogenic solid. Figures 15–189 through 15–191 are scans of a patient with a large pelvic mass secondary to endometriosis. The large cephalic sonolucent portion of the mass is a fluid-filled endometrioma. A solid component to the endometriosis, however, is posterior to the uterus. The greater echogenicity of this region in the cul-de-sac is most likely due to clotted blood or debris. A transverse scan of the same patient (Fig 15–191) shows the endometrioma with soft echoes within it, just posterior and to the left of the uterus.

Figure 15–192 is one scan of another patient with a large fuid-filled endometrioma in the left adnexa. The left adnexal mass is impinging on the posterior urinary bladder wall (arrows) as noted earlier. The endometrioma is displacing the left ovary away from the uterus. The ultrasound findings of this endometrioma are not specific for this entity. Other possibilities include an abscess, an ovarian cyst, or possibly cystadenoma.

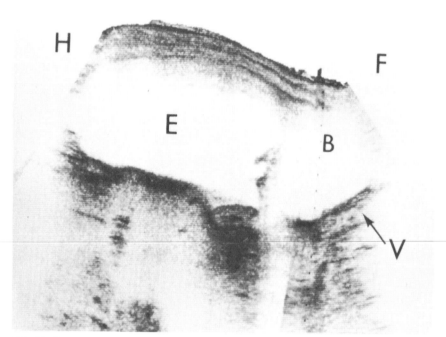

**FIG 15–189.**

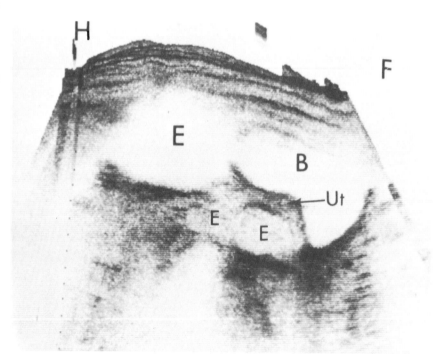

**FIG 15–190.**

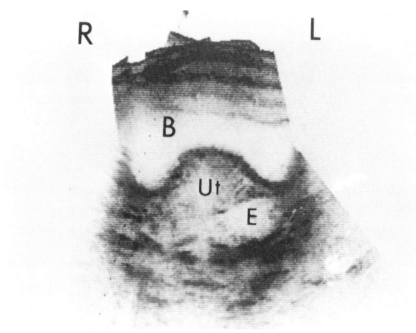

**FIG 15–191.**

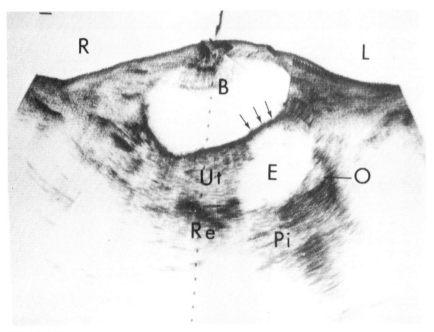

**FIG 15–192.**

| Arrows | = | Indentation of the endometrioma on the bladder wall |
|--------|---|-----|
| **B** | = | Urinary bladder |
| **E** | = | Endometriosis |
| **F** | = | Foot |
| **H** | = | Head |
| **L** | = | Left |
| **O** | = | Left ovary |
| **Pi** | = | Piriform muscle |
| **R** | = | Right |
| **Re** | = | Rectum |
| **Ut** | = | Uterus |
| **V** | = | Vagina |

## Endometriosis

Figures 15–193 and 15–194 are longitudinal and transverse scans of a 26-year-old woman who had a long history of chronic lower quadrant and pelvic pain that was most severe during menstruation. The longitudinal scan in Figure 15–193 shows a fluid collection posterior in the cul-de-sac. The extent of the disease is not appreciated until the transverse scan in Figure 15–194 is evaluated. This scan shows a large multiloculated sonolucent mass in the cul-de-sac in both adnexal regions. Septations are thickened and may represent some fluid-fluid levels. The ultrasound finding is highly suggestive of pelvic inflammatory disease. However, the patient's history was more compatible with endometriosis. At operation, resection of large bilateral endometriomas was performed.

Figures 15–195 and 15–196 are transverse and longitudinal scans of a young woman with long-standing pelvic pain and, recently, increasing discomfort. Ultrasound examination revealed two large sonolucent masses with through-transmission. Soft internal echoes were noted within the central portion of each mass. The findings were consistent with bilateral endometriomas, which were identified at operation. They had recently ruptured. Clotted blood was noted in the area, conforming to the findings on ultrasound. Note the indentation on the urinary bladder from the endometrioma in Figure 15–196.

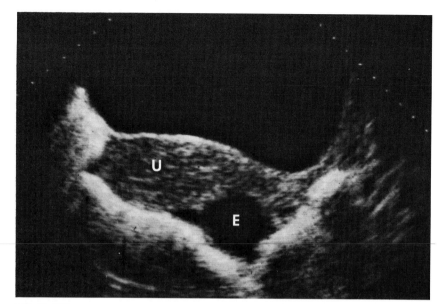

**FIG 15–193.**

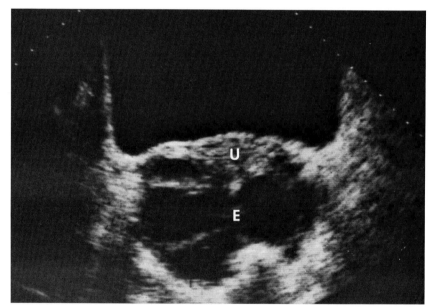

**FIG 15–194.**

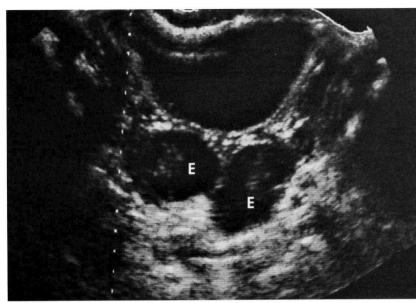

E  =  Endometrioma
U  =  Uterus

**FIG 15–195.**

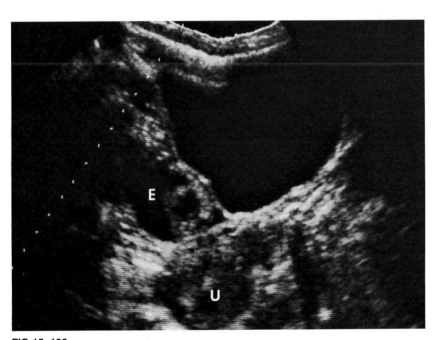

**FIG 15–196.**

## Endometriosis

Occasionally, endometriomas may have numerous internal echoes and be confused with solid ovarian lesions. Figure 15–197 is a transverse scan of the pelvis which demonstrates a solid-appearing endometrioma in the right adnexa. The urinary bladder wall is indented, indicating a right adnexal mass. This endometrioma appears solid in nature. There is evidence of a small amount of fluid in the cul-de-sac. At operation a large endometrioma involving the right ovary and posterior uterine wall was found.

Figure 15–198 is a transverse pelvic scan of another patient. The very solid-appearing mass in the right adnexa turned out to be an endometrioma. The findings are highly suggestive of a solid ovarian neoplasm or a pedunculated uterine fibroid. Chronic abscess and chronic ectopic pregnancy would also be included in the differential diagnosis. The mass was proved surgically to be an endometrioma.

Figures 15–199 and 15–200 are transverse and longitudinal scans of a 26-year-old woman who entered the hospital complaining of lower abdominal pain. Her abdominal pain had started at age 18 and was associated with dysmenorrhea. The symptoms disappeared when she was placed on oral contraceptives. In the preceding year, the symptoms became worse, and she finally entered the hospital because of increasing abdominal pain associated with menstruation. Figure 15–199 is a transverse scan demonstrating the uterus to be surrounded by a large echogenic mass. The mass penetrates the urinary bladder wall (arrows). A longitudinal scan (Fig 15–200) indicates that the uterus is retroverted. A large endometrioma is difficult to separate from the fundus of the uterus. Invasion of the urinary bladder wall is again seen on this scan. At operation, an endometrioma was found involving the fundal portion of the uterus and the posterosuperior aspect of the urinary bladder wall. This portion of the urinary bladder had to be resected.

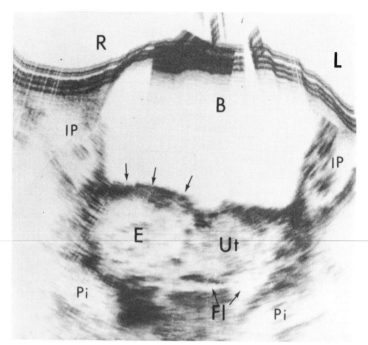

**FIG 15–197.**

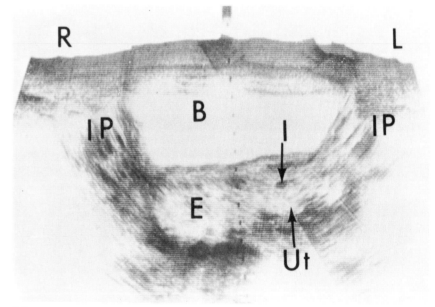

**FIG 15–198.**

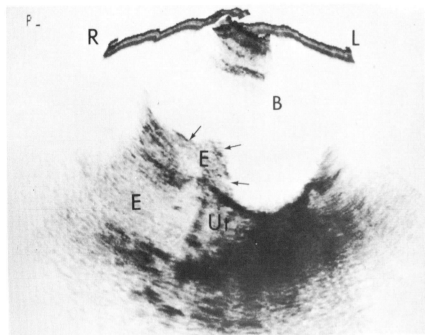

**Arrows** = Urinary bladder wall
**B** = Urinary bladder
**E** = Endometrioma
**F** = Foot
**Fl** = Fluid
**I** = Intrauterine device
**IP** = Iliopsoas muscle
**L** = Left
**Pi** = Piriform muscle
**R** = Right
**Ut** = Uterus

FIG 15–199.

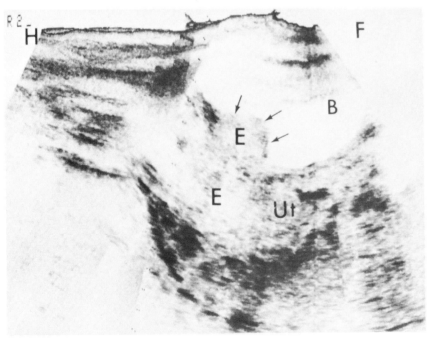

FIG 15–200.

## Pelvic Masses

Solid masses may arise from other tissue in the pelvis than the uterus and ovaries. These will be difficult to distinguish on ultrasound from gynecologic masses. Correlation with the clinical history is necessary to establish the correct diagnosis. Figure 15–201 is a transverse scan of the pelvis of a 5-year-old boy. He complained of abdominal pain and was noted to have a large pelvic mass on clinical examination. The transverse scan shows a solid pelvic mass posterior to the urinary bladder and indenting the posterior aspect of the bladder wall. A barium enema examination revealed narrowing of the rectum. The patient was found to have perirectal Burkitt's lymphoma.

Figure 15–202 is a longitudinal scan of the pelvis and lower abdomen in a 16-year-old boy who presented with a pelvic mass and urinary retention. The diagnosis of neuroblastoma was confirmed at open biopsy. The longitudinal scan shows the urinary bladder to be displaced anteriorly by a soft tissue mass with highly echogenic regions posteriorly. Acoustic shadowing is noted deep to the echogenic regions. The mass is dramatically impinging on the inferior aspect of the urinary bladder and causing urinary retention. An intravenous pyelogram demonstrated hydronephrosis on the left side. The ultrasound findings indicate a soft tissue mass with calcific components posteriorly. This correlated with the clinical diagnosis of neuroblastoma.

Figure 15–203 is a longitudinal scan of the pelvis and lower abdomen in a woman with diffuse metastatic colonic carcinoma. A large mass is seen posterior to the urinary bladder. A portion of the mass is highly echogenic (arrows). The patient had diffuse pelvic metastatic disease secondary to mucinous colonic carcinoma. Because of the mucin-containing material, high-amplitude echoes can be seen.

Figure 15–204 is a transverse scan of an elderly patient with recurrent liposarcoma. A large mass is noted posterior to the urinary bladder. There is no characteristic finding in this tu-

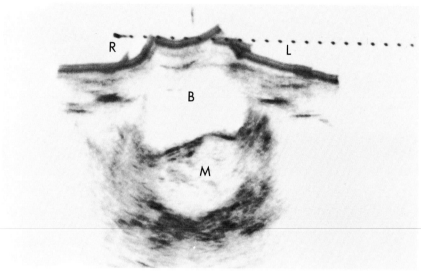

**FIG 15–201.**

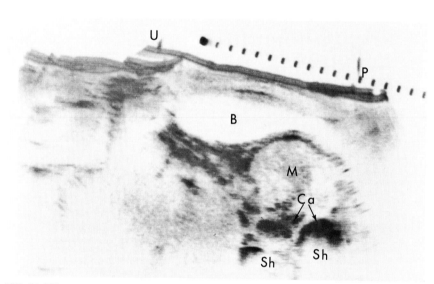

**FIG 15–202.**

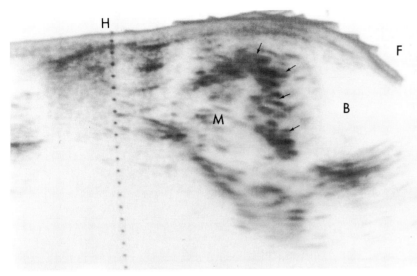

**FIG 15–203.**

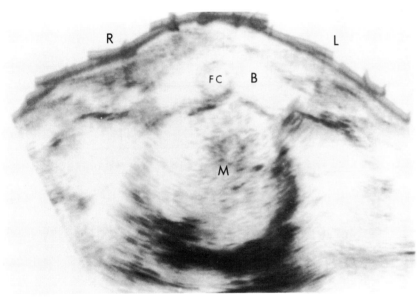

**FIG 15–204.**

mor to suggest its etiology. A Foley catheter is seen within the urinary bladder.

SOURCE: Figures 15–201 through 15–204 are provided through the courtesy of Barry Green, M.D.

| | | |
|---|---|---|
| **Arrows** | = | Highly echogenic region in mucinous adenocarcinoma of the colon |
| **B** | = | Urinary bladder |
| **Ca** | = | Calcification |
| **F** | = | Foot |
| **FC** | = | Foley catheter |
| **H** | = | Head |
| **L** | = | Left |
| **M** | = | Solid pelvic mass |
| **P** | = | Symphysis |
| **R** | = | Right |
| **Sh** | = | Acoustic shadowing |
| **U** | = | Umbilical level |

## Pelvic Masses

Large pelvic masses can be difficult to separate on ultrasound. Very often the pelvic enlargement may be secondary to the uterus. However, there may be other etiologies for the large masses noted in the pelvis on ultrasound. Figures 15–205 and 15–206 are longitudinal and transverse scans of a patient with uterine enlargement. A mass is definitely present within the uterus. To determine whether a mass is present in the uterus, it is most helpful to visualize the lower uterine segment and cervical region. If the uterus is noted to widen into the mass, then it most likely is uterine in origin. In Figures 15–205 and 15–206, there is a region in the central portion of the uterus with an unusual parenchymal texture that includes areas of increased and decreased echogenicity. The ultrasound findings would be consistent with degenerating fibroid, degenerating pregnancy, molar pregnancy, or hematocolpos. The patient had leiomyosarcoma of the uterus with degeneration in the central portion.

Figure 15–207 is a longitudinal scan in a 46-year-old woman who had a history of irregular menses and a large pelvic mass. The ultrasound examination demonstrates a large solid lesion cephalad to the region of the uterus. This lesion was initially thought to be a large pedunculated fibroid, as suggested by the texture of the mass and its smooth contour. At operation a large, 20-cm mass was removed. The mass was attached to the distal ileum and cecum. Pathology diagnosed a leiomyosarcoma of the distal ileum. The mass was cephalad to the uterus and had the ultrasound appearance of a pedunculated fibroid.

Figure 15–208 is a transverse scan of the pelvis in a 31-year-old man with a pelvic mass. A large mass (PS) is noted posterior to the urinary bladder (B). The bladder was recognizable because of the presence of a Foley catheter (FC). At operation, the mass was found to be a large pelvic sarcoma.

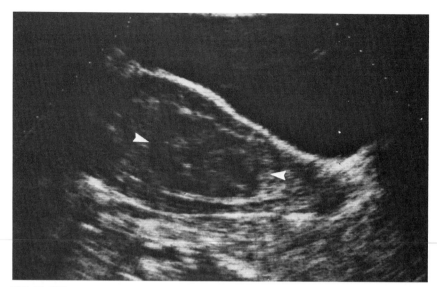

FIG 15–205.

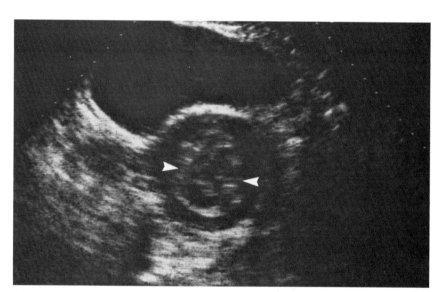

FIG 15–206.

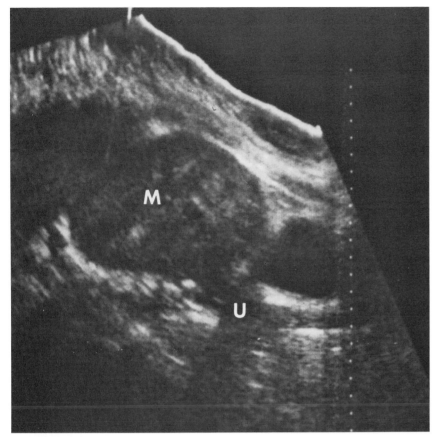

| Arrowheads | = Leiomyosarcoma of the uterus |
|---|---|
| **B** | = Urinary bladder |
| **FC** | = Foley catheter |
| **M** | = Leiomyosarcoma of the ileum |
| **PS** | = Pelvic sarcoma |

FIG 15–207.

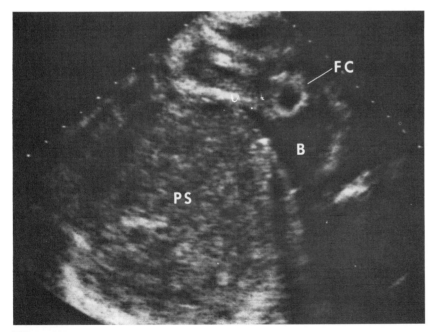

FIG 15–208.

## Pelvic Kidney

Examination of the pelvis may demonstrate a mass which has an unusual ultrasonic appearance. The bull's-eye appearance noted on these images is consistent with a pelvic kidney. However, other entities such as bowel lesions, dermoids, ovarian tumors, and degenerating fibroids may have a similar appearance. The possibilities of a pelvic kidney must be kept in mind when a bull's-eye lesion is noted in the pelvis.

Figures 15–209 and 15–210 are longitudinal and transverse scans of the abdomen and pelvis in a pregnant patient. The uterus is enlarged and the placenta is situated posteriorly. Posterior to the cervix (C) is a large mass that is elevating the cervix anteriorly. This could represent a rectal lesion or ovarian tumor. However, the appearance is that of a bull's-eye, especially on the transverse scan (Fig 15–210). The findings are consistent with a pelvic kidney. The position of this pelvic kidney would be slightly worrisome for a vaginal delivery because it is so low in the pelvis. However, the patient delivered a 9-lb infant vaginally without any difficulty.

Figure 15–211 is a transverse scan of the pelvis in a patient who had a clinical history consistent with endometriosis. She had increasing pelvic pain with menstruation. The pelvic ultrasound examination did not disclose any discrete masses suggestive of endometriosis. A bull's-eye area (arrowheads) was noted in the right adnexal region. The appearance was highly suggestive of a pelvic kidney. Both renal fossae were examined. The right kidney was in its normal position but no left kidney was identified. Therefore, the ultrasound diagnosis of a pelvic kidney was made. Because of the patient's clinical symptoms, surgery was performed to rule out endometriosis. Several small areas of endometriosis that were not visualized on ultrasound were found at surgery. The patient also had a right pelvic kidney.

Figure 15–212 is a transverse scan of the pelvis cephalad to the urinary bladder. The patient had a pelvic

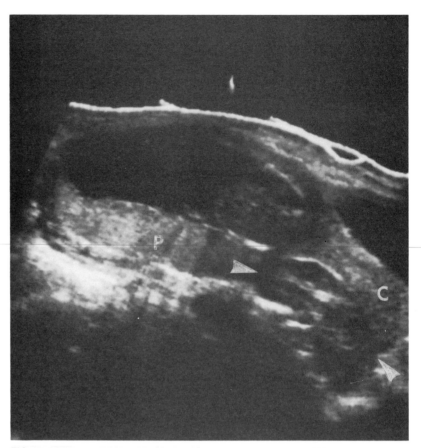

FIG 15–209.

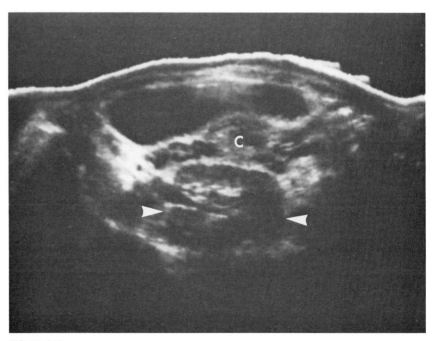

FIG 15–210.

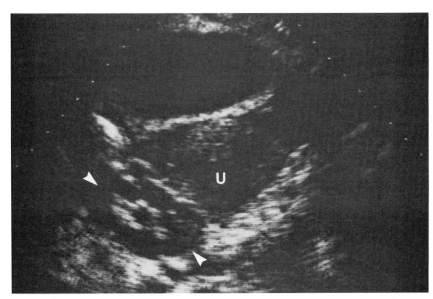

**FIG 15–211.**

mass and was referred by the gynecologist for ultrasonic evaluation. No discrete mass was noted posterior to the uterus or in the adnexal region. However, slightly cephalad to the urinary bladder was a bull's-eye lesion. The possibility of an intestinal mass versus a pelvic kidney was entertained. Examination of the renal fossae demonstrated absence of the right kidney. The bull's-eye (arrowheads) was the initial clue to the etiology of the pelvic mass, which turned out to be a pelvic kidney.

**Arrowheads** = Pelvic kidney
**C** = Cervix
**P** = Placenta
**U** = Uterus

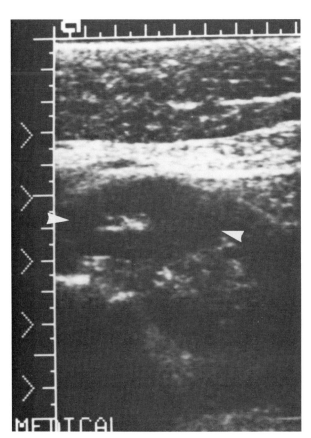

**FIG 15–212.**

## Pelvic Masses

Figure 15–213 is a longitudinal scan in a 16-year-old patient with a palpable pelvic mass. Ultrasound examination revealed a large soft-tissue mass cephalad to the uterus. Within the anterior portion of this mass is a sonolucent region. The possibility of a dermoid was initially considered. However, the appearance of the mass was slightly suggestive of a pelvic kidney. The renal fossae were examined and absence of the left kidney was identified. The mass in the pelvis turned out to be a pelvic kidney (K) with a peripelvic cyst (C). This is an unusual case because of the appearance of the peripelvic cyst in the kidney. However, the ultrasound findings were the initial clue to the etiology of the pelvic mass.

Figure 15–214 is a transverse scan of the pelvis in an 18-year-old girl. The uterus was slightly deviated to the left. There is a bull's-eye mass (arrowheads) in the right pelvis. Because of the appearance of the mass, the renal fossae were examined. Both kidneys were found in normal location and had a normal appearance. Therefore, other etiologies to the mass were sought. The patient had a small bowel follow-through in which an abnormality of the terminal ilium was identified, consistent with Crohn's disease, and documented. The bull's-eye mass in the right adnexa was secondary to an abnormal terminal ilium in Crohn's disease.

Figure 15–215 is a longitudinal scan of the pelvis in a 38-year-old woman who experienced discomfort after eating. The uterus (U) is well visualized. A bull's-eye mass (arrowheads) is situated cephalad to the uterus. It has the appearance of abnormal bowel rather than a pelvic kidney. The renal areas were examined to rule out a pelvic kidney. Both kidneys were normal in size and location.

Figure 15–216 is a transverse scan of the right lower quadrant in the same patient. In this instance, a tubular mass (arrowheads) is noted in the right lower quadrant. This represented a dilated abnormal terminal ilium. The cecum (Ce) is noted in the right lateral

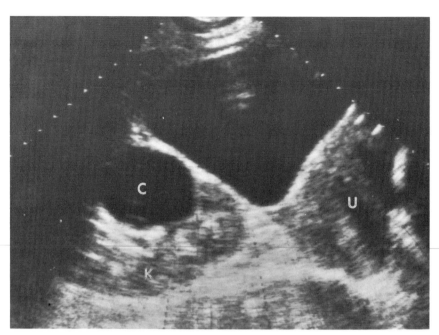

**FIG 15–213.**

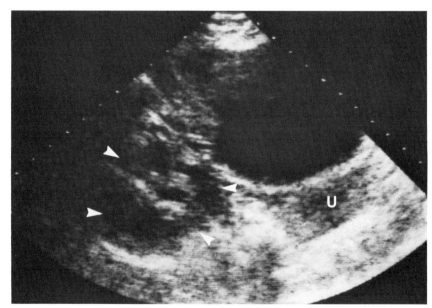

**FIG 15–214.**

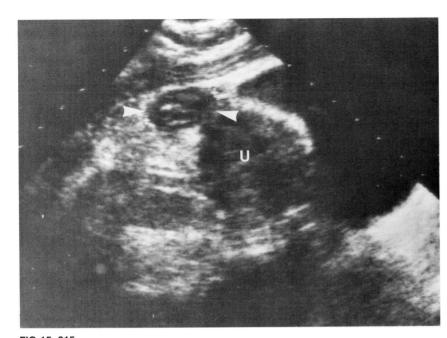

**FIG 15–215.**

quadrant with some fluid within it. The ultrasound findings were consistent with Crohn's disease.

| | | |
|---|---|---|
| **Arrowheads** | = | Crohn's disease |
| **C** | = | Renal cyst |
| **Ce** | = | Dilated cecum |
| **K** | = | Kidney |
| **R** | = | Right |
| **U** | = | Uterus |

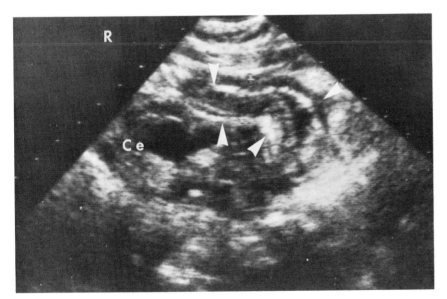

**FIG 15–216.**

## Urinary Bladder Diverticulum

A urinary bladder diverticulum may be visualized on pelvic ultrasound and present a confusing picture if the diagnosis is not considered. Urinary bladder diverticula usually present as sonolucent masses in the adnexal region. There is usually evidence of an interface between the bladder and the diverticulum over most of its border. However, close examination of bladder wall will often reveal an opening to the bladder diverticulum which leads to the correct diagnosis. Figure 15–217 is a longitudinal scan of the pelvis showing a sonolucent mass posterior to the urinary bladder. This may be considered an ovarian cyst or other fluid-filled structure. The interface between the bladder and the bladder diverticulum in Figure 15–217 is visualized in its entirety. The possibility of the bladder diverticulum should always be considered in such instances. In order to diagnose a urinary bladder diverticulum, the interface between the bladder and cystic mass should be scanned in its entirety. Figure 15–218 is a longitudinal scan of the same patient in which the opening between the bladder and bladder diverticulum is visualized. This leads to the correct diagnosis of a bladder diverticulum rather than a separate sonolucent mass posterior to the urinary bladder. The communication between the bladder and the bladder diverticulum in this case was approximately 6–7 mm in diameter. If this communication can be seen, the diagnosis and explanation of the sonolucent mass will be correctly determined.

Figure 15–219 is a longitudinal scan in a pregnant patient. A sonolucent mass (M) is noted posterior to the urinary bladder. In the presence of pregnancy, this was most likely a corpus luteum cyst. However, close examination of the urinary bladder revealed a communication between it and the sonolucent mass (Fig. 15–220). A large opening is present which leads to the correct diagnosis of a bladder diverticulum.

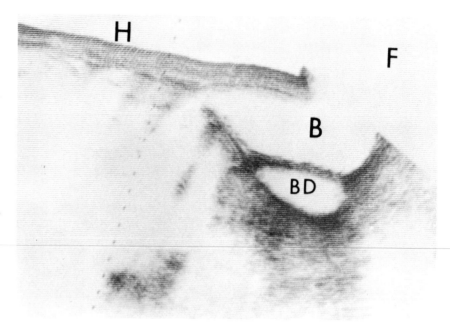

**FIG 15–217.**

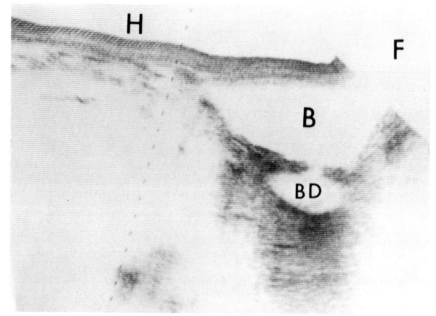

**FIG 15–218.**

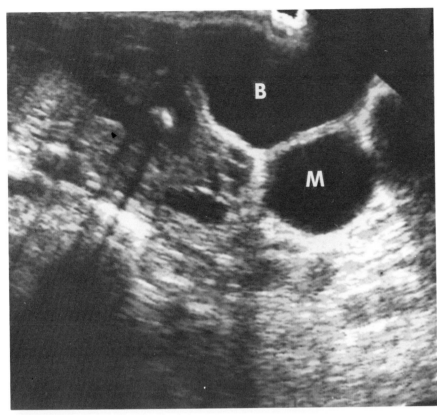

B   = Urinary bladder
BD  = Bladder diverticulum
F   = Foot
H   = Head
M   = Bladder diverticulum

FIG 15–219.

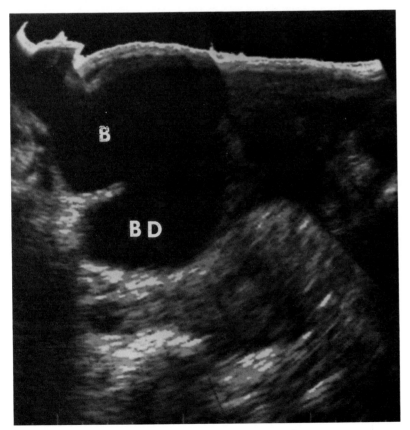

FIG 15–220.

## Cystic Urinary Masses

During the course of an ultrasound examination of the pelvis, the urinary bladder should be scrutinized for any masses. The urinary bladder is often forgotten during a pelvic ultrasound examination. However, masses within the urinary bladder are easily identified on ultrasound. Figures 15–221 and 15–222 are longitudinal scans in two different patients. Figure 15–221 is the scan of a male patient showing a circular and tubular mass at the base of the urinary bladder. Figure 15–222 is the scan of a female patient showing a similar mass. These characteristic echoes in the base of the bladder are easily identified as Foley catheters (FC). By lining up the long axis of the Foley catheter, the distal tube can be identified and will lead to the correct diagnosis. If only the balloon of the Foley catheter is visualized, then other entities must be considered.

Figures 15–223 and 15–224 are transverse and longitudinal scans in a male patient in which we see a circular sonolucent mass in the posterior aspect of the urinary bladder. Close scrutiny of the mass did not reveal the characteristic appearance of a Foley catheter. On real-time examination the mass filled and emptied with ureteral peristalsis. This confirmed the diagnosis of a simple ureterocele.

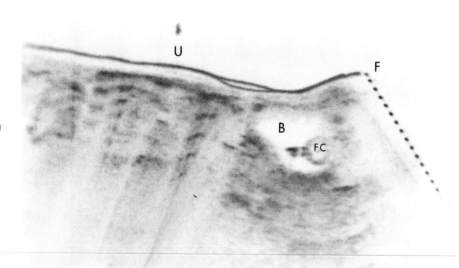

**FIG 15–221.**

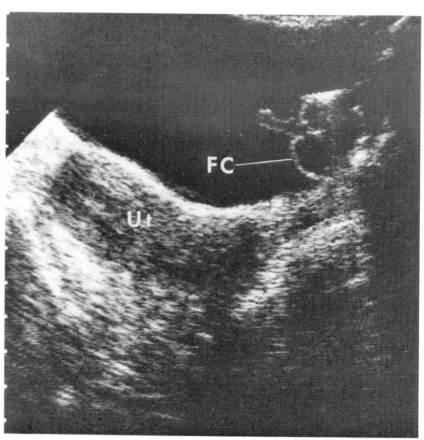

**FIG 15–222.**

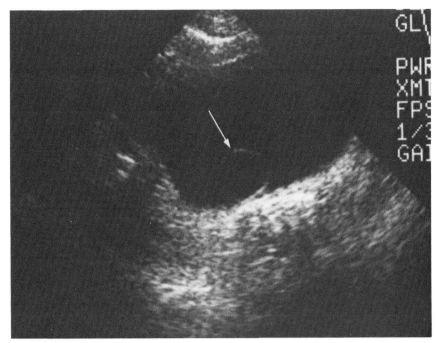

| Arrow | = | Ureterocele |
| B | = | Urinary bladder |
| F | = | Foot |
| FC | = | Foley catheter |
| U | = | Umbilicus |
| Ut | = | Uterus |

**FIG 15–223.**

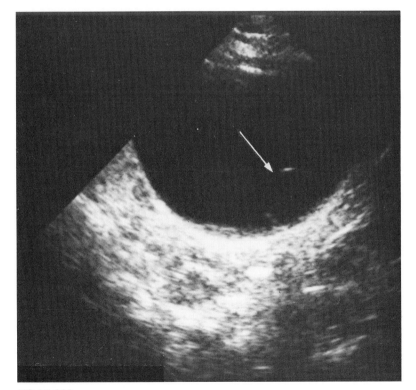

**FIG 15–224.**

## Urinary Bladder Masses

During examination of the pelvis, the urinary bladder walls should be examined to rule out any pathology. Figure 15–225 is a longitudinal scan in a 20-year-old patient that was obtained to rule out a possible right ovarian cyst. Examination of the pelvis did not reveal any pelvic masses in the adnexal region. However, during the course of the examination, a small, 1-cm irregularity was noted in the urinary bladder wall near its base (arrow). At operation a small polyp of the urinary bladder was removed. Pathologic study indicated that this was a papilloma of the urinary bladder wall.

Figure 15–226 is a transverse scan of the pelvis in which a solid-appearing mass is noted on the posterior urinary bladder wall. Although this could represent a bladder tumor, it is a blood clot which presented as an echogenic mass within the urinary bladder.

Figure 15–227 is a transverse scan of the pelvis of a middle-aged man with a suspected pelvic mass. A Foley catheter (FC) is noted in the urinary bladder. The left side of the urinary bladder has an irregular contour and a left pelvic mass was present. During the course of the examination, a high-amplitude echo (arrowhead) was noted in the posterior urinary bladder. Deep to this high-ampitude echo was an area of acoustic shadowing. The findings indicate a bladder calculus.

Figure 15–228 is a transverse scan in a man who was sent to ultrasound for a suspected pelvic mass. The urinary bladder is present in the midportion of the pelvis. Two sonolucent masses (BD) are identified lateral to the urinary bladder. Communication between these masses in the bladder was identified in each instance and the diagnosis of bilateral urinary bladder diverticula was made. The cystic mass on the right side contained a high-amplitude echo (arrowhead) with acoustic shadowing deep to the echo. The patient was found to have a urinary bladder stone in the bladder diverticulum on the right side.

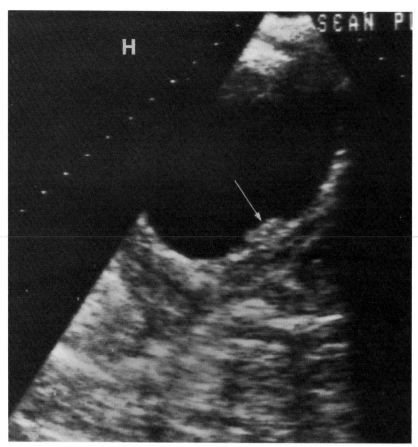

FIG 15–225.

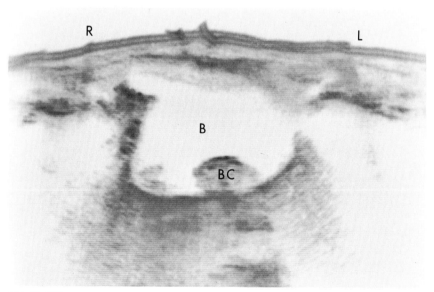

FIG 15–226.

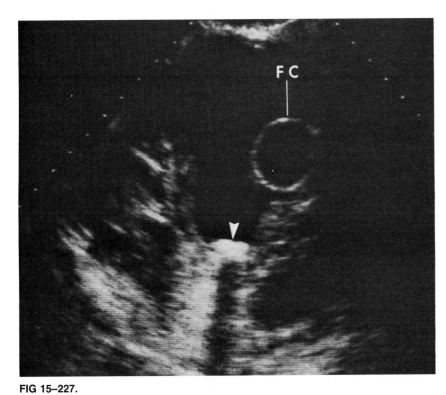

**FIG 15–227.**

SOURCE: Figure 15–226 is provided courtesy of Barry Green, M.D.

| | | |
|---|---|---|
| **Arrow** | = | Urinary bladder papilloma |
| **Arrowhead** | = | Urinary bladder stone |
| **B** | = | Urinary bladder |
| **BC** | = | Blood clot |
| **BD** | = | Bladder diverticulum |
| **FC** | = | Foley catheter |
| **H** | = | Head |
| **L** | = | Left |
| **R** | = | Right |

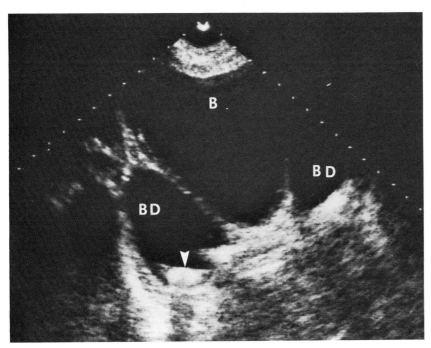

**FIG 15–228.**

## Bladder Tumors

Figures 15–229 and 15–230 are pelvic scans of a 42-year-old woman who had some difficulty on urination. The longitudinal scan (Fig 15–229) shows bladder wall thickening (arrows) on the posterior aspect. The bladder wall is approximately 1–1.5 cm in thickness, directly anterior to the vagina. Figure 15–230 is a transverse scan of the bladder wall thickening (arrows) on the posterior aspect of the bladder. The soft echoes, with no evidence of shadowing, indicate a soft-tissue tumor. This could represent either a blood clot or debris in the bladder. With the suggestion of wall thickening, however, a bladder tumor is most likely. At surgery, the patient was found to have urinary bladder carcinoma on the posterior left aspect of the bladder wall.

Another example of a urinary bladder wall carcinoma is seen in Figures 15–231 and 15–232. The bladder tumor is approximately 2 cm thick. We see a marked irregular surface to the bladder wall which is in contact with urine (arrows). Also noted on the transverse scan in Figure 15–231 is a circular structure secondary to a Foley catheter. When a soft-tissue density is noted within the urinary bladder or urinary bladder wall, the possibility of a urinary bladder carcinoma should be considered.

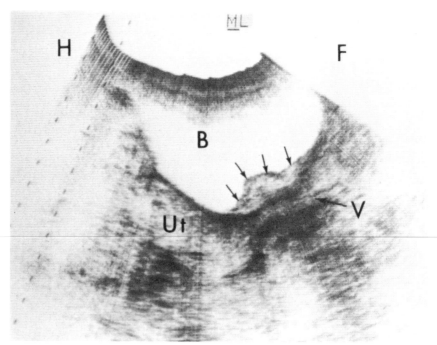

FIG 15–229.

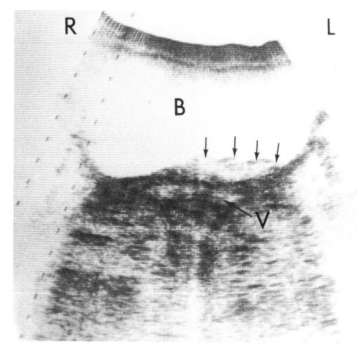

FIG 15–230.

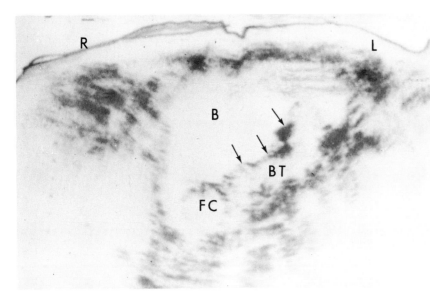

| **Arrows** | = | Urinary bladder wall carcinoma |
| **B** | = | Urinary bladder |
| **BT** | = | Urinary bladder wall tumor |
| **F** | = | Foot |
| **FC** | = | Foley catheter |
| **H** | = | Head |
| **L** | = | Left |
| **R** | = | Right |
| **Ut** | = | Uterus |
| **V** | = | Vagina |

**FIG 15–231.**

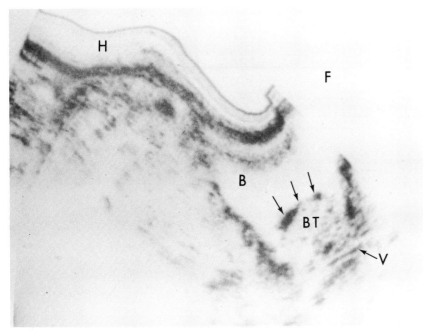

**FIG 15–232.**

## Pelvic Masses

Various masses in the pelvis may have confusing appearances on ultrasound. Figure 15–233 is an excellent example of a bladder duplication artifact. The urinary bladder may often appear as a sonolucent mass in the pelvis because of a duplication artifact. In this instance, there is a complete duplication artifact of the urinary bladder situated posterior to the vagina (B$^1$). What makes this scan interesting is the duplication artifact of the vagina (V$^1$). This artifact arises from the strong echo off the posterior urinary wall hitting the transducer skin interface and making a second trip. This yields a duplication artifact of the urinary bladder and the vagina. Duplication artifacts are discussed in greater detail in chapter 1.

Figure 15–234 is a longitudinal scan of a patient who had undergone a hysterectomy 15 years earlier. On ultrasound examination a mass was found posterior to the urinary bladder. The lucent anterior portion of the vagina is seen directly posterior to the urinary bladder. Deep to this, however, is an echogenic mass which turned out to be a vaginal tumor. This vaginal carcinoma could be somewhat difficult to separate from the rectum on ultrasound. We see the lucent anterior muscularis of the vagina separated from the vaginal tumor by a strong echogenic interface. The strong echogenic interface represents the vaginal mucosa.

Figure 15–235 is a longitudinal scan of the pelvis with a typically confusing ultrasound appearance. Very often, extremely large cystic masses may be mistaken for the urinary bladder. The cystic mass (M) in this case can be confused with the urinary bladder. There is a small triangular sonolucency inferior to the cystic mass (B) which represents a slightly filled urinary bladder. This is a very characteristic echo finding that must always be looked for on pelvic studies. This small triangular sonolucency is the only clue that the cystic mass does not represent the urinary bladder. Figure 15–236 is a longitudinal scan of the same patient who was told to

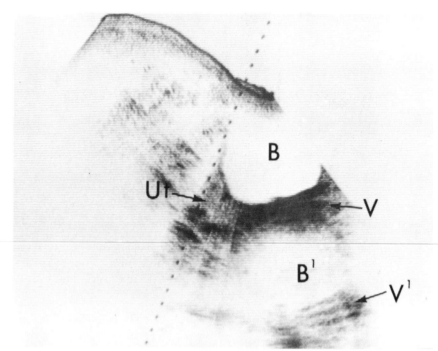

**FIG 15–233.**

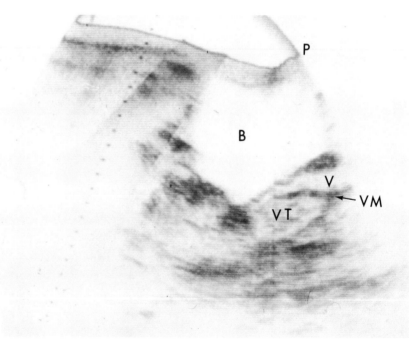

**FIG 15–234.**

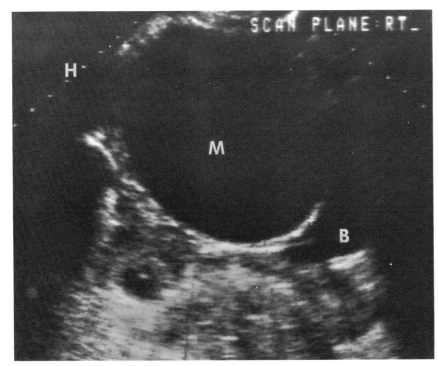

FIG 15–235.

completely void on urination. The triangular sonolucency is no longer identified. The bladder has been completely emptied and the cystic mass is now situated in the lower pelvis. In this instance, the cystic mass has the appearance of a typical urinary bladder. It would be almost impossible to diagnosis this rather large cystic mass on the scan in Figure 15–236 with the bladder completely empty. That is why the urinary bladder must be somewhat filled to make the correct diagnosis. The correct diagnosis was made from the scan shown in Figure 15–235 because of the small triangular lucency representing the filled urinary bladder.

| | | |
|---|---|---|
| **B** | = | Urinary bladder |
| **B**[1] | = | Bladder duplication artifact |
| **H** | = | Head |
| **M** | = | Ovarian cyst |
| **P** | = | Symphysis |
| **U** | = | Uterus |
| **Ut** | = | Uterus |
| **V** | = | Vagina |
| **V**[1] | = | Vaginal duplication |
| **VM** | = | Vaginal mucosa |
| **VT** | = | Vaginal tumor |

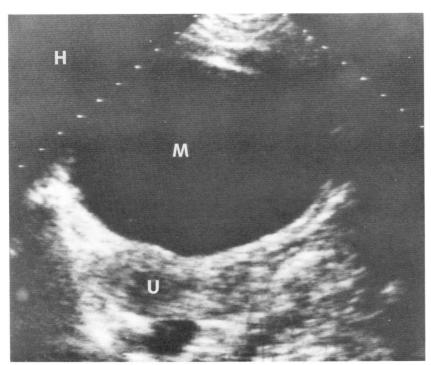

FIG 15–236.

## Normal Prepubescent Pelvis

When examining the prepubescent pelvis, it is important to visualize the uterus in its long axis. Normally, the cervical region of the prepubescent uterus is larger than the fundal region.

Figures 15–237 and 15–238 are longitudinal scans of a 4-year-old girl (Fig 15–237) and a 6-month-old girl (Fig 15–238). The cervical region is as large as or larger than the fundal region in both cases. Following puberty and hormonal stimulation, a reversal will occur, and the fundus of the uterus will become larger and more bulbous than the cervical region. Examination of the newborn and the pediatric pelvis can be quite difficult because the patients move about quite markedly during the course of a study. It is important, however, to attempt to visualize the uterus. Real-time examination can often facilitate the study and permit more rapid examination.

Finding the ovaries in a prepubescent child is also difficult. They are usually quite small, 1 cm or less. Again, the study can be quite difficult but usually does not require anesthesia.

Figure 15–239 is a transverse scan showing the ovaries bilaterally. The right ovary is approximately 1 cm in diameter; the left ovary is less than 1 cm in diameter. Here we see the ovaries cephalad to the uterus. The rectum is seen between the ovaries.

Figure 15–240 is a longitudinal scan of the right ovary, which appears as a relatively sonolucent oval-shaped structure in the adnexa. The marked difficulty encountered in visualizing the ovaries is due to their small size and poor patient cooperation.

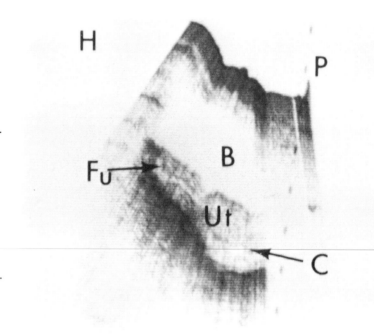

**FIG 15–237.**

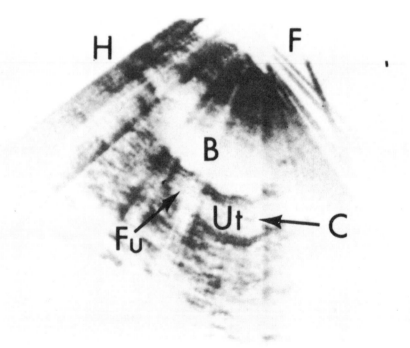

**FIG 15–238.**

B  =  Urinary bladder
C  =  Cervix
Fu =  Fundus of the uterus
H  =  Head
L  =  Left
O  =  Ovaries
P  =  Level of the symphysis pubis
R  =  Right
Re =  Rectum
Ut =  Uterus

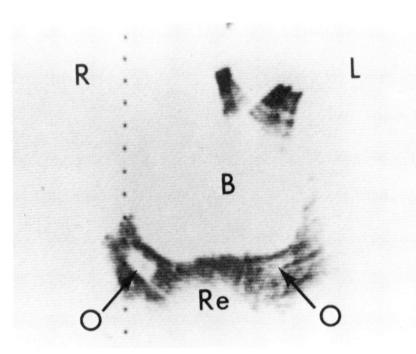

FIG 15–239.

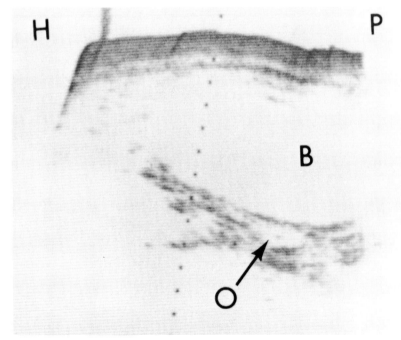

FIG 15–240.

## Precocious Puberty;
## Testicular Feminization

Figures 15–241 through 15–243 are scans of a 6-year-old child with precocious puberty. In precocious puberty, hormonal stimulation leads to changes in the uterus. The fundal size of the uterus is increased and becomes larger than the cervix. On a transverse scan (Fig 15–241) the uterus is visualized slightly to the left of midline. This uterus is much larger than normal in a 6-year-old. The ovaries are also quite large, measuring approximately 2 cm or greater in diameter in the transverse plane. Figure 15–242 is a longitudinal scan in which the uterus has a configuration more characteristic of the adult, or poststimulated, uterus. The fundus has a more bulky or bulbous appearance than the cervical region. Usually, in the unstimulated uterus the fundus is much smaller than the cervical region. In this 6-year-old girl with precocious puberty, however, the fundus was large compared with the cervical region. Figure 15–243 is a longitudinal scan of the right ovary. Again, the ovary appears much larger than expected in a 6-year-old. Normally, it should be 1 cm or less in diameter. This ovary is at least 2 cm in diameter and is impinging on the posterior aspect of the urinary bladder.

Figure 15–244 is a transverse scan of a 16-year-old patient who entered the hospital for an evaluation of primary amenorrhea. No pelvic organs can be seen. The uterus was not identified. Various pelvic muscles, such as the iliopsoas muscle, the obturator internus muscle, and the piriform muscles, can be seen, but we were never able to identify the ovaries during the course of the examination. The patient also underwent a pelvic examination, and the vagina was found to end in a blind pouch. The cervix was not identified. The findings are consistent with testicular feminization. For this entity, a pelvic ultrasound examination can be quite helpful. We were looking for a normal prepubescent uterus and ovaries but were unable to identify any such

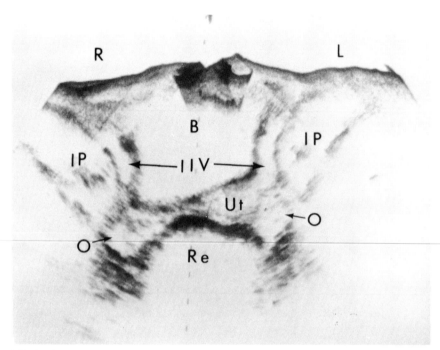

**FIG 15–241.**

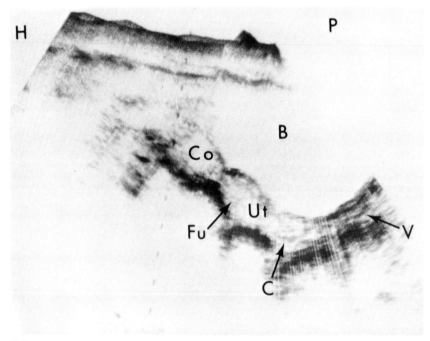

**FIG 15–242.**

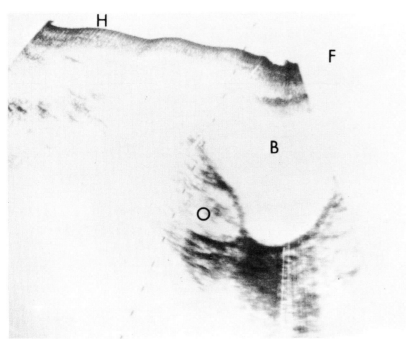

**FIG 15–243.**

structures during the course of pelvic sonography.

**B** = Urinary bladder
**C** = Cervix
**Co** = Colon
**F** = Foot
**Fu** = Fundus of the uterus
**H** = Head
**IIV** = Internal iliac vessels
**IP** = Iliopsoas muscles
**L** = Left
**O** = Ovaries
**OI** = Obturator internus muscle
**P** = Level of the symphysis pubis
**Pi** = Piriform muscle
**R** = Right
**Re** = Rectum
**Ut** = Uterus
**V** = Vagina

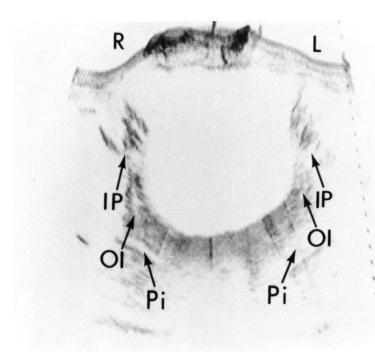

**FIG 15–244.**

## Normal Prostate; Benign Prostatic Hypertrophy

When the prostate is examined with ultrasound, the urinary bladder should be filled. The transducer must be angled more caudally for both longitudinal and transverse scans. The prostate is situated quite caudally, and if the transducer beam is perpendicular to the tabletop or slightly cephalad in angulation, the prostate gland cannot be visualized.

Figure 15–245 is a longitudinal scan in which the prostate appears as a soft echogenic region posterior to the urinary bladder and caudad to the seminal vesicles. Examination in the longitudinal planes best visualizes the prostate when the transducer beam is angled markedly caudally as in this case.

Figure 15–246 is a transverse scan with caudal angulation with the prostate indenting the posterior aspect of the urinary bladder. In the center of the prostate gland, a strong central echo represents the urethra and periurethral glands within the prostate.

Benign prostatic hypertrophy is suggested when a markedly enlarged prostate without disruption of the prostatic capsule is present on ultrasound. In Figure 15–247 we see marked indentation of the posteroinferior urinary bladder wall caused by the enlarged prostate. The circular appearance to the prostate in the longitudinal scan is indicative of prostatic enlargement. The transverse scan (Fig 15–248) demonstrates a nodularity to the prostate with two prominent curvilinear indentations on the posterior aspect of the bladder wall. A rectal ultrasound probe allows excellent visualization of the prostate. B-scan evaluation of the prostate does not determine volume quite as easily as the rectal probe scanner.

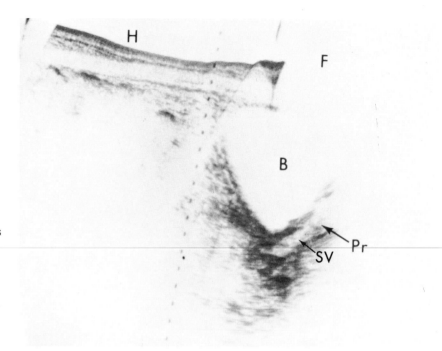

FIG 15–245.

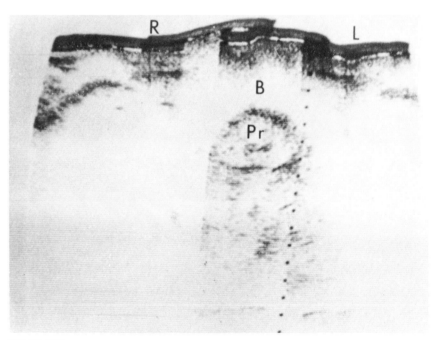

FIG 15–246.

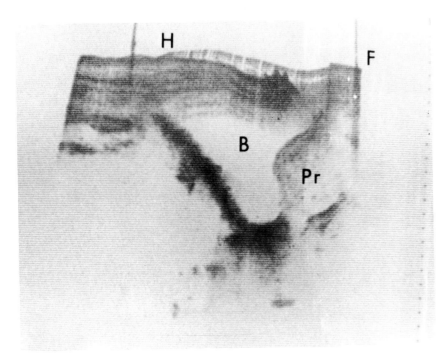

**B** = Urinary bladder
**F** = Foot
**H** = Head
**L** = Left
**Pr** = Prostate
**R** = Right
**SV** = Seminal vesicles

**FIG 15–247.**

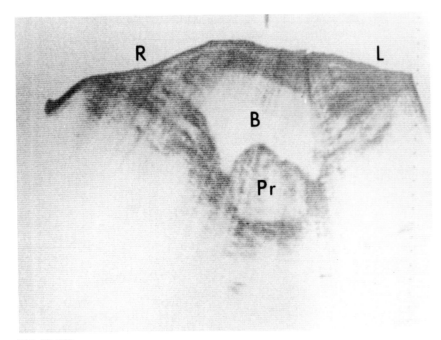

**FIG 15–248.**

## Prostatic Carcinoma; Prostatitis

Figures 15–249 and 15–250 are scans of a patient with prostatic carcinoma. The prostate is markedly enlarged and indenting the posterior aspect of the urinary bladder. It has a rather uneven echo pattern compared with that of the normal prostate. The irregular echogenicity is also accompanied by a somewhat irregular margin to the prostate wall. The interface between the urinary bladder and prostate is not as sharply seen as in a normal examination. The patient was found to have prostatic carcinoma. An uneven echo pattern and an irregular wall to the prostate are highly suggestive of prostatic carcinoma.

Figures 15–251 and 15–252 are scans of a patient with prostatitis. In Figure 15–251, the prostate has a fairly even echo pattern. The seminal vesicles, however, appear much more lucent than usual. The transverse scan (Fig 15–252) demonstrates fairly large seminal vesicles. They are not only more lucent, but they are increased in size, as compared with the normal findings.

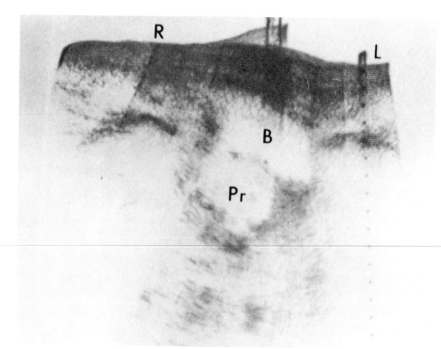

**FIG 15–249.**

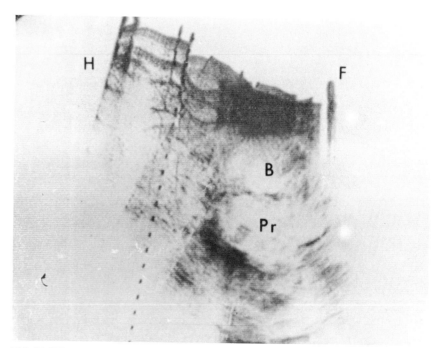

**FIG 15–250.**

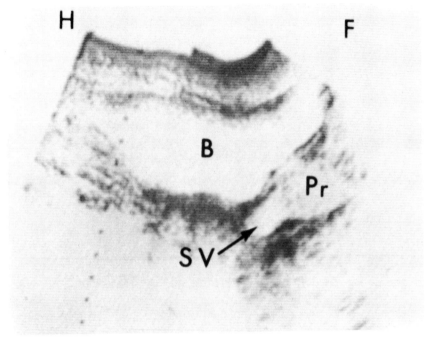

B  = Urinary bladder
F  = Foot
H  = Head
L  = Left
Pr = Prostate
R  = Right
SV = Seminal vesicles

**FIG 15–251.**

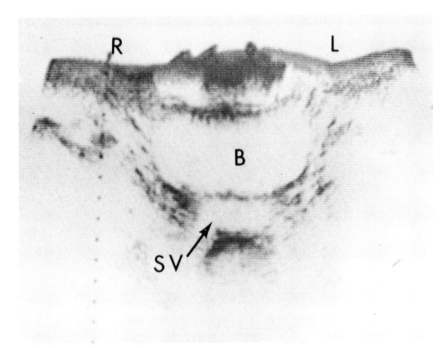

**FIG 15–252.**

# 16.
# Obstetrics

## 16a

## ULTRASONOGRAPHY OF FIRST-TRIMESTER PREGNANCY

David A. Nyberg, M.D.
Faye C. Laing, M.D.

Ultrasound provides a unique opportunity for monitoring human growth and development in utero. This diagnostic modality has had a major impact on the evaluation and clinical management of both normal and abnormal pregnancy during the first trimester. Because of its sensitivity in detecting and characterizing small fluid collections, ultrasound is extremely reliable for visualizing the changes associated with early intrauterine pregnancy.[1–3] The demonstration of cardiac and embryonic motion with real-time equipment permits direct and highly accurate assessment of gestational viability. The speed, flexibility, and ease of use of this modality permits accurate assessment of a variety of first-trimester complications. Finally, the lack of significant biologic hazard at diagnostic power levels is important throughout pregnancy and especially in early pregnancy, during the critical period of organogenesis.

The first section of this chapter will discuss ultrasound of normal gestation and will correlate sonographic findings of early gestation with normal embryologic development. The following section will discuss the role of ultrasound in evaluating complications of first-trimester pregnancy.

### Scanning Techniques

Sonographic examination of early pregnancy is performed with the patient supine and with a distended urinary bladder. A full bladder provides an acoustic window for examining uterine contents and displaces adjacent bowel loops. An overly distended bladder should be avoided, however, so as not to compress or distort the gestational sac. Real-time equipment using the highest possible transducer frequency is essential for accurate measurement of the crown-rump length and for assessing cardiac and fetal motion.

### Normal Embryologic Development

Early embryologic development is a dynamic sequence that includes ovulation, fertilization, implantation, and organogenesis. A brief review of this process is necessary in order to understand the sonographic findings of both normal and abnormal pregnancy.[4] Embryologic development will be discussed in terms of menstrual dating, in keeping with obstetric and sonographic methodology. Fetal age is approximately 2 weeks less than the menstrual age based on the "ideal" menstrual cycle. In actuality, individual variation in the time of ovulation causes inherent uncertainty in the gestational age.

Ovulation occurs 2 weeks after the last menstrual period when a mature graafian follicle releases an ovum. The graafian follicle subsequently becomes the corpus luteum, which helps maintain early pregnancy. Fertilization takes place within 24 hours in the distal fallopian tube. Following fertilization, the zygote undergoes rapid cell division to form a sphere of cells called the morula. The morula in turn develops a central cavity forming the blastocyst. The blastocyst consists of an outer cell layer called the trophoblast and an inner cell mass that subsequently forms the embryonic disk, the amniotic cavity, and the yolk sac.

The blastocyst implants in the secretory endometrium about 7–8 days after ovulation (3 weeks menstrual age). The invasive property of the trophoblast allows the blastocyst to burrow into the endometrial wall. During the fourth menstrual week, growth of the trophoblast forms a primitive uteroplacental circulation and primary chorionic villi. The chorionic villi rapidly proliferate into innumerable vascular fronds that cover the entire surface of the gestational sac. Concurrently, the endometrium undergoes adaptive changes (the decidual reaction) that provide nourishment to the developing blastocyst. Three layers of decidua are formed: the decidua basalis, deep to the blastocyst; the decidua capsularis, which covers the endometrial surface of the blastocyst; and the decidua vera or parietalis, which consists of the remaining endometrium.

Toward the end of the fourth week, the primary yolk sac regresses and a secondary yolk sac forms. The secondary yolk sac has important functions that include transfer of nutrients to the embryo, formation of hematopoietic cells, and development of the primitive embryonic gut and primary germ cells. Initially the yolk sac lies opposite the amniotic sac, immediately adjacent to the embryonic disk. As the amniotic sac grows, the yolk sac remains attached to the embryo by a yolk stalk and, together with the connecting stalk of the embryo, forms the umbilical cord. As the amniotic sac obliterates the chorionic cavity, the yolk sac becomes compressed between the amnion and chorion. At term it may be found under the amnion close to the umbilical cord attachment to the placenta.

The sixth to tenth menstrual weeks (the embryonic period) is a critical time of development during which virtually all major external and internal organs develop. The cardiovascular system is the first organ system to become functional. Fetal blood begins to circulate by the end of the fifth menstrual week in an ebb and flow pattern. By the end of the sixth menstrual week, coordinated contractions of the heart produce unidirectional flow. Most other organs have formed by the tenth week.

By 10 weeks, the chorionic villi associated with the decidua capsularis begin to degenerate and form the smooth chorion (chorion laeve). Concurrently, the chorionic villi in contact with the decidua basalis continue to proliferate and form the chorion frondosum, which represents the early placenta. By the end of the 12th week, the intestine, which had previously herniated into the umbilical cord, returns to the abdomen. The external genitalia are differentiated by the end of the 14th week.

## Sonographic Appearance of Normal First-Trimester Pregnancy

For the first 2 weeks after implantation (3–5 menstrual weeks) the blastocyst is too small to be resolved with ultrasound. The uterus becomes mildly enlarged and the central uterine cavity echo may become prominent, although this finding is not specific for pregnancy.[5] In addition, prominent arcuate vessels may be observed surrounding the uterus (unpublished data). This finding presumably reflects increased blood flow to the uterus following implantation.

The first reliable evidence of an intrauterine pregnancy is the appearance of the gestational sac, seen approximately 1 week after the missed menstrual period (5 menstrual weeks).[1–2] The normal sac appears as a rounded sonolucency (representing the blastocyst), surrounded by a prominent echogenic ring (representing chorionic villi and decidual reaction). When first seen, the gestational sac is about 5–8 mm in diameter, and its internal structures, including the embryo and yolk sac, are too small to be resolved. The gestational sac grows rapidly during the first trimester with its mean diameter increasing by 1–1.5 mm per day.[6–7] Concurrently, growth of the embryo (1.4 mm per day)[8, 9] results in its eventual detection between the sixth and seventh menstrual weeks.

It is important to recognize the sonographic appearance of a normal gestational sac prior to detecting an embryo, and to distinguish this appearance from that of an abnormal intrauterine pregnancy (IUP) or other intrauterine fluid collection.[10–12] The echo amplitude of a normal choriodecidual reaction is prominent (approaching that of the bladder-uterine interface) and demonstrates a smooth inner contour. The size of an "empty" gestational sac is normally less than 25 mm in mean diameter.[12] Its shape, which varies with the degree of bladder compression, should be round, oval, or crescentic, and its position should be in the middle or fundal portion of the uterus. Although the prognostic significance of a low-lying gestational sac has been debated, if a woman has vaginal bleeding, this appearance is probably due to an impending abortion.[10–12] Alternatively, if a woman is asymptomatic, a low-lying gestational sac may simply represent a low implantation, which is not associated with an increased risk of abortion.[13]

An important feature that can be used reliably to distinguish an IUP from other intrauterine fluid collections is the "double decidual sac" (DDS).[14–16] This finding, demonstrated in 98% of normal IUPs, is seen as two concentric echogenic lines surrounding a portion of the gestational sac. The inner line is thought to represent the chorionic villi and decidua capsularis surrounding the blastocyst, while the outer line is thought to represent the decidua parietalis.[14] Since the uterine cavity is normally collapsed, these two decidual layers remain closely opposed and create the paired echogenic lines seen on ultrasound. In contrast, other intrauterine fluid collections are located within the uterine cavity, causing separation of the endometrial walls. An ancillary observation that also relates to the DDS is a small triangular fluid collection within the uterine cavity adjacent to a portion of the gestational sac.[15] This fluid, which may be due to implantation bleeding, causes separation of the decidua capsularis from the decidua parietalis.[3]

The secondary yolk sac, seen between 6 and 7 gestational weeks, is the earliest structure visualized within the gestational sac.[12] It has a characteristic round, sac-like appearance that should not be confused with the embryo. Its presence may occasionally be helpful for confirming the presence of an IUP (before an embryo is detected). More importantly, as emphasized by Cadkin and McAlpin, the yolk sac is a useful landmark for locating a very small embryo.[17] Since the embryonic disk is contiguous with the yolk sac during early development, careful attention to the area adjacent to the yolk sac will frequently disclose a small embryo and/or embryonic cardiac motion.

An embryo is usually detected by the seventh week, when it is 5–10 mm in length.[18] In all cases it should be visible before the eighth week, at which time the gestational sac is about 25 mm in mean diameter. Using currently available electronically focused phased-array real-time equipment and careful scanning technique, it is possible to detect an embryo at 6 weeks or perhaps even a few days earlier.[17] Initially the embryo is seen as a thin linear structure adjacent to the yolk sac. Differentiation of the head from the trunk and recognition of the extremities are usually possible after 8 weeks. The umbilical cord and yolk stalk may also be observed at this time.

Embryonic viability is easily assessed with real-time ultrasound equipment by observing cardiac motion, seen as rhythmic pulsations emanating from the embryo. Cardiac motion is normally demonstrated as soon as embryonic echoes are detected. For very early gestations, cardiac motion may be more easily appreciated than the embryo itself. Rarely, a small (< 10 mm) embryo may be demonstrated in which cardiac motion cannot be confirmed on the initial sonogram. In these cases, a follow-up examination will be conclusive for determining embryonic viability.

The fetus continues to enlarge during the first trimester and reaches a length of about 5.5 cm by 12 weeks.[8] At that time the head has enlarged sufficiently that the biparietal diameter (BPD) can be measured. Occasionally, prior to 12 weeks, herniated fetal gut may be seen within the umbilical cord.[19] Because of their small size, a detailed examination of other fetal organs is not usually possible at this time.

The site of placental implantation can be seen at 8–9 weeks as a focal thickening of the choriodecidual reaction.[3] At the same time, the remaining choriodecidual reaction becomes less prominent, corresponding to degeneration of the chorionic villi with the formation of the chorion laeve. The amnion is seen as a very thin membrane that separates the embryo from the secondary yolk sac.[20] Visualization of the amnion may persist until 16 weeks when it normally fuses with the chorion.

## Gestational Age

Determining gestational age is more accurate during the first trimester than in later pregnancy, since fetal growth is less dependent on maternal and environmental factors at this stage.[9] Gestational age in early pregnancy can be determined by two methods: crown-rump length or gestational sac size. Crown-rump length is the most accurate sonographic indicator of gestational age with a range of 5 days between 6 and 12 weeks. It is obtained by measuring the maximal length of the embryo, excluding the extremities, in the neutral position. Accurate measurement depends on careful scanning with real-time equipment to ensure that a maximal length is obtained. This may be difficult in early pregnancy when the embryo is small and anatomic structures are not well defined. Care must be taken not to include the yolk sac when measuring the embryo.

Gestational age can also be determined during the first trimester by measuring gestational sac size. This method is particularly useful when an embryo is not detected or when it is too small to measure accurately. Gestational sac size may be expressed as either sac volume[21] or mean sac diameter.[9] Although sac volume more accurately reflects true sac size, because this is a difficult measurement to obtain, it is not routinely done. On the other hand, mean sac diameter (MSD) is easily calculated as an average of the longitudinal, anteroposterior, and transverse dimensions of the gestational sac (measured from inside the choriodecidual reaction). When properly performed, measurement of the MSD does not vary significantly with changes in bladder compression. Use of the MSD has the advantage that growth occurs at a nearly linear rate (1–1.5 mm in mean diameter per day) during the first trimester. As shown by Hellman et al., the mean sac size accurately predicts gestational age.[6] As a rule of thumb, menstrual age can be estimated as: MA (days) = MSD (mm) + 30.[15]

Gestational age is determined by the BPD beginning at about 12 weeks. The BPD and other parameters of fetal growth, including head circumference, abdominal circumference, and femur length, are subsequently utilized for the remainder of pregnancy.

## Use of Quantitative hCG Determinations

Following intrauterine implantation, the human chorionic gonadotropin (hCG) level normally increases in an exponential fashion, doubling about every 2–3 days.[22, 23] After 8 weeks, the hCG level plateaus and subsequently declines. During the first 8 weeks, a close relationship exists between quantitative hCG level and sonographic appearance for a normal pregnancy.[24, 25] Recent evidence indicates that an intrauterine gestational sac should always be visualized when the hCG level exceeds 1,800 mIU/ml.[25] Furthermore, there is a strong correlation between the quantitative serum level of hCG and the gestational sac size until 8 weeks, by which time an embryo is normally detected on ultrasound. Because the hCG level initially rises at a predictable rate, quantitative hCG determinations may be used to accurately determine menstrual age during the first 8 weeks.[26] Measuring the hCG level is also useful for diagnosing complications of early pregnancy, including threatened abortion, trophoblastic disease, and ectopic pregnancy. These entities will be discussed further in subsequent sections.

## Ultrasonography of First-Trimester Complications

The sequence of events that occurs during early gestational development represents a complex process that is frequently altered or interrupted by a variety of factors. Pelvic sonography has proved to be a valuable method that aids in the diagnosis and evaluation of these complications. The following section will discuss spontaneous and threatened abortion, hydatidiform degeneration, and concurrent uterine or adnexal masses. Because of the importance and complexity of ectopic pregnancy, this subject will be discussed separately in chapter 16B.

### Spontaneous Abortion

Spontaneous abortion is the natural termination of an IUP prior to 20 weeks.[27, 28] It is common and occurs in about 10%–20% of observed pregnancies. Occult abortions occur even more frequently, since it is estimated that up to 50% of conceptions terminate prior to implantation.[27] Clinically apparent spontaneous abortions occur after implantation, but usually before 12 gestational weeks. The majority of these early abortuses have chromosomal anomalies.[27] Other risk factors include a coexisting intrauterine contraceptive device, smoking, ingestion of toxins and drugs, pelvic irradiation, and some medical diseases, including diabetes mellitus.

Ultrasound's role in the evaluation of women with possible spontaneous abortion depends on the presenting clinical signs and symptoms. If the cervical os is dilated and/or products of conception are present within the cervical os or vagina, an incomplete abortion is diagnosed.[28] Under these circumstances, ultrasound is not usually indicated. Instead, uterine curettage should be performed to prevent further bleeding and infection. However, it is not always possible to determine clinically if a woman has recently passed gestational tissue, in which case ultrasound may be used in an effort to distinguish a complete or incomplete abortion from a potentially viable gestation (threatened abortion).

A recently completed spontaneous abortion appears on ultrasound as an empty uterus with a normal central cavity echo. The uterus may be mildly enlarged. An incomplete abortion may have a similar appearance if the retained tissue is scant. If sufficient gestational tissue is present, however, increased or irregular echoes will be evident within the central uterine cavity. It is important to realize that the sonographic appearance of a complete or incomplete abortion may be indistinguishable from that of an early normal pregnancy (between 3 to 5 menstrual weeks), or an ectopic pregnancy.[29] Correlation with the history and clinical findings is essential. If the diagnosis remains uncertain, serial hCG determinations may be useful since a spontaneous abortion will show a steady decline in the quantitative level.

### Threatened Abortion

The term threatened abortion applies to women during the first 20 weeks of pregnancy who have vaginal bleeding and who, on the basis of clinical evaluation, are considered to have a potentially viable gestation.[28] Approximately 20% of all women experience symptoms of threatened abortion. Of these threatened abortions, approximately one half terminate in spontaneous abortion and one half result in normal outcome.[27, 28] There is no known effective treatment for altering this outcome.

Ultrasound plays a major role in evaluating women with threatened abortion because it can frequently distinguish living from nonliving gestations.[30-33] A living conceptus may have one of three sonographic appearances, depending on the gestational age: (1) a gestational sac containing an embryo (> 7 weeks); (2) a gestational sac without a detectable embryo (5–7 weeks); (3) absence of a gestational sac (< 5

weeks). Ultrasonography is most accurate for assessing viability when an embryo is demonstrated, since cardiac activity may be evaluated. Cardiac motion not only proves the embryo is alive, but also indicates a favorable prognosis, since only 3%–8% of these fetuses subsequently abort.[30-32]

Most women who carry a living embryo do not have an apparent cause for their vaginal bleeding. Occasionally, however, there is sonographic evidence of placental abruption. Recent evidence suggests that this may be a more common cause of threatened abortion during the first trimester than has generally been recognized[34] and is the probable cause of the so-called live abortion. Large abruptions are frequently associated with a subchorionic fluid collection (representing blood) which may extend beneath the placenta.[20, 35, 36] Frequently a membrane is visible separating the hematoma from the amniotic fluid. This membrane, which represents the detached chorion, should be distinguished from the amnion, which is normally observed during early pregnancy (before chorioamniotic fusion). The detached chorion appears thick and echogenic and is relatively nonpliable, whereas the amnion is very thin and undulates when the fetus impresses upon it or the uterus is ballotted. Furthermore, the chorion is contiguous with the margin of the placenta, while the amnion can be traced to the base of the umbilical cord.[35] If an abruption is identified, the gestation should be monitored carefully since even large abruptions may have a favorable outcome with delivery of a normal fetus.

A missed abortion is diagnosed when an embryo is identified but cardiac motion is lacking. It is important to realize, however, that on rare occasions a very small normal embryo may be seen in which cardiac activity cannot be definitively confirmed on the initial sonogram.[37] Other sonographic findings seen with a missed abortion depend on the time interval between embryonic demise and the sonographic examination. Initially, the gestational sac and embryo can appear normal except that a nonliving embryo usually lies in a fixed and dependent position. Later the gestational sac becomes irregular in shape and/or position, the decidual reaction usually diminishes, and the amount of amniotic fluid frequently decreases. The appearance of the embryo also becomes distorted due to progressive maceration. Once embryonic demise is confirmed, the uterus should be promptly evacuated to circumvent clinical problems associated with prolonged vaginal bleeding, potential infection, and patient anxiety.

When the sonographic examination demonstrates a gestational sac but an embryo is lacking, it is more difficult to assess gestational viability.[10–12] If the gestational sac appears normal (see previous discussion of normal pregnancy), an early normal pregnancy (between 5 to 7 menstrual weeks) is likely. In these cases, however, the prognosis is not as favorable as when a living embryo is detected, because approximately 20% of patients with threatened abortion in whom the gestational sac appears sonographically normal subsequently abort.[12] These patients should be followed with serial ultrasound examinations to ascertain whether or not a living embryo develops.

Despite the absence of an embryo, a nonviable gestation may frequently be diagnosed on sonography on the basis of an abnormal-appearing gestational sac. Abnormal features of a gestational sac include a large sac size ($>$ 25 mm mean diameter); grossly aberrant shape; low position in the lower uterine segment; thin, weakly echogenic, irregular or incomplete choriodecidual reaction; and absent double decidual sac finding.[12] Although each of these findings strongly correlates with an abnormal outcome, interpreting a gestational sac as definitely abnormal should be done with caution to avoid terminating an early normal pregnancy. Confidence in reliably diagnosing a nonviable gestation increases as the number of abnormal features increases. Two features that have each been determined to have 100% specificity and predictive value for diagnosing an abnormal gestational sac are an abnormally large sac size and a grossly aberrant sac shape.[12] By using a combination of abnormal sonographic features, a recent study was able to detect 53% of all nonviable gestational sacs without any false positive diagnoses.[12] This accuracy approaches 100% when serial examinations are performed.

If the sonographic features are equivocal with regard to determining the status of a gestational sac, and if uterine evacuation is contemplated, supportive evidence of a nonviable gestation should be sought. Correlation with menstrual age may be helpful since a nonviable sac is usually small and immature when compared to the expected gestational age. Strict reliance on the menstrual history should be done with caution, however, since inaccurate dates can lead to termination of a potentially viable gestation.[31] Corre-

lating the sonographic findings with the hCG level is another useful method for confirming an abnormal gestational sac. A disproportionately low hCG level relative to the mean sac diameter supports the diagnosis of a nonviable gestation.[38] In any questionable case such as a gestational sac with minimally atypical sonographic features and/or a minimally depressed hCG level, follow-up sonography and/or serial hCG determinations are recommended. A normal gestational sac should grow approximately 1–1.5 mm per day and an embryo should become evident within 1–2 weeks following the appearance of the gestational sac.

The final sonographic appearance in patients with threatened abortion is an empty uterus without a gestational sac. As previously discussed, this finding may be observed during the first 5 weeks of a normal pregnancy. However, if a pregnant woman presents with vaginal bleeding, this appearance should suggest a recent spontaneous abortion, ectopic pregnancy, or even an early molar pregnancy. In this situation, clinical and laboratory correlation is essential for distinguishing the various diagnostic possibilities. Serial hCG determinations are useful because in normal pregnancy, hCG levels rise exponentially during the first 8 weeks.[23, 28] In comparison, patients with a recent abortion demonstrate a steady decline in hCG levels, while patients with an ectopic pregnancy usually demonstrate a plateau or subnormal rise in quantitative levels.[23]

*Trophoblastic Disease*

Trophoblastic disease represents a spectrum of proliferative diseases, throught to be initiated by persistence of chorionic villi from a blighted ovum. The clinical symptoms relate to the size and malignant behavior of the tumor. Symptoms of pregnancy, vaginal bleeding, and an enlarged uterus are frequently the presenting signs. Sonographically, the typical vesicular appearance of the uterus may not be present in first-trimester molar pregnancies.[40] The sonographic appearance of an early molar pregnancy may be indistinguishable from that of a missed abortion. In this situation, correlation of the sac size with quantitative serum hCG levels may be helpful. A molar pregnancy will be associated with disproportionately elevated hCG levels relative to the sac size, whereas a missed abortion will be associated with normal to low hCG levels.[38] As a molar pregnancy progresses, it will generally demonstrate the typical vesicular pattern, and theca lutein cysts may develop.

*Pelvic Masses*

Pelvic masses that are present during pregnancy may be discovered on routine physical examination or because they produce clinical symptoms. Potential complications of these masses include torsion, rupture or hemorrhage, pain, obstruction of vaginal delivery, and interference with effective labor.[41]

A corpus luteum cyst is the most commonly encountered "mass" during pregnancy. Although it normally is approximately 2 cm in size, it may attain a diameter of 10 cm prior to its regression by 16 weeks. Sonographically, a corpus luteum cyst becomes symptomatic by virtue of hemorrhage, rupture, or torsion. An uncomplicated corpus luteum cyst is a unilateral, simple unilocular cyst with a smooth, thin outer wall. When complications occur, it usually becomes more complex with the appearance of internal echoes and/or septations. If a corpus luteum cyst ruptures, it may produce acute pelvic pain and a hemoperitoneum which in every way mimics an ectopic pregnancy.[42] In this situation, laparoscopy or laparotomy is frequently necessary to establish the correct diagnosis.

Other cystic pelvic masses that may occur during pregnancy include abscesses and neoplasms. An ovarian cystadenoma, which is the most common pelvic mass to enlarge during pregnancy, should be considered when a cystic adnexal mass fails to regress after the first trimester. Occasionally a paraovarian cyst will become large enough to be detected by sonography.

A benign cystic teratoma, or dermoid cyst, is commonly discovered during pregnancy. Sonographically, most dermoid cysts appear as complex, extrauterine pelvic masses. Findings that suggest the diagnosis include cystic areas with fluid levels, echogenic masses with gradual acoustic shadowing, and changes that suggest the presence of calcification within a cystic mass. Predominantly cystic or solid masses may also be seen. Dermoid cysts may be difficult to identify on sonography since their echogenic texture may be confused with bowel. Because they are often pedun-

culated and mobile, they may be displaced out of the pelvis by an overly distended urinary bladder.

The most common solid pelvic mass associated with pregnancy is a uterine leiomyoma (fibroid). These tumors frequently enlarge and become more sonolucent during pregnancy due to estrogenic stimulation. Although frequently an incidental finding, they may cause clinical symptoms on the basis of size, degeneration, hemorrhage, or infarction. Fibroids are associated with an increased risk of spontaneous abortion. They may also inhibit effective labor, and, if large and in the lower uterine segment, they may mechanically obstruct vaginal delivery. Their sonographic appearance varies and depends on the presence of secondary changes which include degeneration, necrosis, hemorrhage, and calcification. The most common appearance is a hypoechoic solid mass that deforms the uterine contour. They should be distinguished from uterine contractions, which are more echogenic, are unlikely to alter the external contour of the uterus, and, most important, are transient.

## References

1. Ghorashi B, Gottesfeld KR: The gray scale appearance of the normal pregnancy from 4–16 weeks of gestation. *JCU* 1977; 5:195–201.
2. Chilcote WS, Asokan S: Evaluation of first-trimester pregnancy by ultrasound. *Clin Obstet Gynecol* 1977; 20:253–264.
3. Lyons EA, Levi CS: Ultrasound in the first trimester of pregnancy, in Callen PW (ed): *Ultrasonography in Obstetrics and Gynecology.* Philadelphia, WB Saunders Co, 1983, pp 1–19.
4. Moore KL: Formation of the bilaminar embryo, in Moore KL (ed): *The Developing Human:,* ed 3. Philadelphia, WB Saunders Co, 1982, pp 40–52.
5. Johnson MA, Graham MF, Cooperberg PL: Abnormal endometrial echoes: Sonographic spectrum of endometrial pathology. *J Ultrasound Med* 1982; 1:161–166.
6. Hellman LM, Kobayashi M, Fillisti L, Lavenhar M: Growth and development of the human fetus prior to the twentieth week of gestation. *Am J Obstet Gynecol* 1969; 103:789–798.
7. Bernard KG, Cooperberg PL: Sonographic differentiation between blighted ovum and early viable pregnancy. *AJR* 1985; 144:597–602.

8. Robinson HP: A critical evaluation of sonar crown rump length measurements. *Br J Obstet Gynaecol* 1975; 82:702–710.

9. Bowie JD, Andreotti RF: Gestational age in utero, in Callen PW (ed): *Ultrasonography in Obstetrics and Gynecology*. Philadelphia, WB Saunders Co, 1983, pp 21–39.

10. Donald I, Morley P, Barnett E: The diagnosis of blighted ovum by sonar. *Br J Obstet Gynaecol* 1979; 79:304–310.

11. Robinson HP: The diagnosis of early pregnancy failure by sonar. *Br J Obstet Gynaecol* 1975; 82:849–857.

12. Nyberg DA, Laing FC, Filly RA: Sonographic distinction of normal from abnormal gestational sacs in threatened abortion. *Radiology* (in press).

13. Smith C, Gregori C, Breen J: Ultrasonography in threatened abortion. *Obstet Gynecol* 1978; 51:173–177.

14. Bradley WG, Fiske CE, Filly RA: The double decidual sac sign of early pregnancy: Use in exclusion of ectopic pregnancy. *Radiology* 1982; 143:223–226.

15. Nyberg DA, Laing FC, Filly RA, et al: Ultrasonographic differentiation of the gestational sac of early intrauterine pregnancy from the pseudogestational sac of ectopic pregnancy. *Radiology* 1983; 146:755–759.

16. Nelson P, Bowie JA, Rosenberg ER: Early intrauterine pregnancy or decidual cast: An anatomic-sonographic approach. *J Ultrasound Med* 1983; 2:543–547.

17. Cadkin AV, McAlpin J: Detection of fetal cardiac activity between 41 and 43 days of gestation. *J Ultrasound Med* 1984; 3:499–503.

18. Shaub MS: Obstetrical ultrasonography, in Sarti DA, Sample WF (eds): *Diagnostic Ultrasound*. Boston, GK Hall, 1980, pp 590–607.

19. Cyr DR, Mack LA, Schoenecker SA, et al: Pitfalls in the diagnosis of abdominal wall abnormalities: Sonographic detection of normal bowel migration. Presented at the Seventy-first Annual Meeting of the Radiological Society of North America.

20. Burrows PE, Lyons EA, Phillips HJ, et al: Intrauterine membranes: Sonographic findings and clinical significance. *JCU* 1982; 10:1–8.

21. Robinson HP: Gestation sac volumes as determined by sonar in the first trimester of pregnancy. *Br J Obstet Gynaecol* 1975; 82:100–107.

22. Braunstein GD, Grodin JM, Vaitukaitis, et al: Secretory rates of human chorionic gonadotropin by normal trophoblast. *Am J Obstet Gynecol* 1973; 115:447–450.

23. Kadar N, Caldwell BV, Romero R: A method of screening for ectopic pregnancy and its indications. *Obstet Gynecol* 1981; 58:162–165.

24. Batzer FR, Weiner S, Corson SL, et al: Landmarks during the first forty-two days of gestation demonstrated by the β-subunit of human chorionic gonadotropin and ultrasound. *Am J Obstet Gynecol* 1983; 146:973–979.

25. Nyberg DA, Filly RA, Mahoney BS, et al: Early gestation: Correlation of HCG levels and sonographic identification. *AJR* 1985; 144:951–954.

26. Lagrew DC, Wilson EA, Fried AM: Accuracy of serum human chorionic gonadotropin concentrations and ultrasonic fetal measurements in determining gestational age. *Am J Obstet Gynecol* 1984; 149(2):165–168.

27. Fantel AG, Shepard TH: Basic aspects of early (first trimester) abortion, in Iffy L, Kaminetzky HA (eds): *Principles and Practice of Obstetrics and Perinatology*, vol 1. New York, John Wiley, 1981, pp 553–563.

28. Cavanagh D, Comas MR: Spontaneous abortion, in Danforth DN, (ed): *Obstetrics and Gynecology*. Philadelphia, Harper & Row, Publishers, 1982, pp 378–392.

29. Marks WM, Filly RA, Callen PW, et al: The decidual cast of ectopic pregnancy: A confusing ultrasonographic appearance. *Radiology* 1979; 133:451–454.

30. Hertz JB: Diagnostic procedures in threatened abortion. *Obstet Gynecol* 1984; 64:223–229.

31. Anderson SG: Management of threatened abortion with real-time sonography. *Obstet Gynecol* 1980; 55:259–264.

32. Ericksen PS, Philipsen T: Prognosis in threatened abortion evaluated by hormone assays and ultrasound scanning. *Obstet Gynecol* 1980; 55:434–438.

33. Duff GB: Prognosis in threatened abortion: A comparison between predictions made by sonar, urinary hormone assays and clinical judgment. *Br J Obstet Gynaecol* 1975; 82:858–862.

34. Goldstein *AJR* 1983; 141:975.

35. Kaufman AJ, Fleischer AC, Thieme GA, et al: Separated chorioamnion and elevated chorion: Sonographic features and clinical significance. *J Ultrasound Med* 1985; 4:119–125.

36. Mantoni M, Pedersen JF: Intrauterine hematoma: An ultrasonic study of threatened abortion. *Br J Obstet Gynaecol* 1981; 88:47–5.

37. Mahoney BS, Filly RA, Nyberg RA, et al: Sonographic evaluation of ectopic pregnancy. *J Ultrasound Med* 1985; 4:221–228.

38. Nyberg DA, Filly RA, Duarte Filho DL, et al: Correlation of sonography and quantitative serum hCG levels in diagnosing abnormal intrauterine pregnancy. *Radiology* (in press).

39. Braunstein GD, Karow WG, Gentry WC, et al: First-trimester chorionic gonadotropin measurements as an aid in the diagnosis of early pregnancy disorders. *Am J Obstet Gynecol* 1978; 131:25–32.

40. Callen PW: Ultrasonography in evaluation of gestational trophoblastic disease, in Callen PW (ed): *Ultrasonography in Obstetrics and Gynecology*. Philadelphia, WB Saunders Co, 1983, pp 259–270.

41. Fleischner AC, Boehm FH, James AE Jr: Sonography and radiology of pelvic masses and other maternal disorders. *Semin Roentgenol* 1982; 17:172–181.

42. Hallat JG, Steele CH, Snyder M: Ruptured corpus luteum with hemoperitoneum: A study of 173 surgical cases. *Am J Obstet Gynecol* 1984; 149:5–8.

# 16b
# ECTOPIC PREGNANCY

David A. Nyberg, M.D.
Faye C. Laing, M.D.

Ectopic pregnancy is a common complication of early pregnancy, estimated to occur in 1 of every 200 gestations in this country.[1] Because it is a leading cause of maternal morbidity and mortality, it is of critical importance to establish the correct diagnosis at the earliest possible time.[2] Nevertheless, clinical recognition of ectopic pregnancy is difficult, and until recently, the delay in making the correct diagnosis averaged 10 days following initial patient presentation. Undoubtedly this delay contributed to over one half of the 86 maternal deaths observed in this country from 1979 to 1980.[3] This chapter discusses recent laboratory and sonographic advances that permit an earlier and more reliable diagnosis of ectopic gestation to be made. It is hoped that increased awareness coupled with the use of improved diagnostic modalities will diminish the maternal morbidity and mortality associated with ectopic pregnancy.

Ectopic pregnancy results from extrauterine implantation of the blastocyst. In 95% of cases the ectopic site is the fallopian tube.[4] Predisposing factors for extrauterine implantation include pelvic adhesions, preexisting pelvic inflammatory disease, and intrauterine contraceptive devices. Initially, the blastocyst attempts to develop normally in spite of its aberrant location. Soon the ectopic gestation outgrows its vascular supply, producing poor trophoblastic growth. Eventually the invasive nature of the trophoblast and chorionic villi in combination with the thin supporting structures of the fallopian tube lead to leakage or rupture of the ectopic gestation. Concurrently, the endometrial lining of the uterus undergoes decidual changes in response to hormonal stimulation.

The presenting signs and symptoms of ectopic pregnancy are variable and depend on the size, location, and supporting vascularity of the developing blastocyst. The classic symptom-sign complex (amenorrhea with or without pelvic pain, irregular vaginal bleeding, and an adnexal mass) is often absent.[5] Pelvic pain is common but is variable in intensity and duration, and may be situated on the side opposite the ectopic gestation due to a contralateral corpus luteum cyst. Typically, the pain is suddenly exacerbated by tubal rupture, which occurs in 80%–90% of cases. Shock, secondary to intra-abdominal hemorrhage, occurs in less than 15% of cases.[6]

Because the clinical symptoms of ectopic pregnancy are nonspecific, a reliable laboratory test is necessary to identify those women who are pregnant from the patient group considered at risk. Virtually all currently used pregnancy tests screen for circulating levels of human chorionic gonadotropin (hCG) in maternal urine or serum. Although the role of hCG in early pregnancy is still incompletely understood, this glycoprotein appears to help maintain the corpus luteum and may contribute to fetal sex differentiation.[7] Because it is produced by trophoblastic cells within days after implantation, hCG is a sensitive marker for early gestation. Traditional urine pregnancy tests, which are performed in a test tube or on a slide, detect hCG by indirect agglutination. Although this test is easily performed and is readily available, it lacks the necessary sensitivity and specificity to make it a reliable screening procedure.[8] False negative results are frequent because this test requires hCG concentrations of more than 1,000 mIU/ml. Unfortunately, many patients with ectopic pregnancy have significantly lower hCG levels, probably due to poor trophoblastic growth.[9] False positive results are also common and are secondary to a variety of factors, including the use of various pharmaceuticals, proteinuria, hematuria, and pelvic inflammatory disease.

Dramatic improvement in the laboratory diagnosis of ectopic pregnancy occurred with the introduction of a sensitive radioimmunoassay able to detect as little as 5 mIU/ml of hCG in the serum.[10, 11] This sensitivity permits detection of virtually any gestational event, whether intrauterine or extrauterine. In addition, this method lacks false positive results since it is specific for the β-subunit of hCG. Another important advantage is that this test can quantitate the precise amount of circulating hCG within the serum. As will be discussed, this has important applications in the evaluation of ectopic pregnancy. Disadvantages of this test are that it utilizes specialized laboratory equipment and typically requires 24 hours for completion. Recently, a qualitative urinary pregnancy test has been developed that is specific for the β-subunit of hCG, can detect as little as 50 mIU/ml of hCG, and can be performed rapidly.[12]

Over the past few years ultrasound has evolved as a primary diagnostic modality for evaluating patients with suspected ectopic pregnancy. Although early reports suggested that sonography was accurate for detecting the ectopic gestation,[13, 14] subsequent experience revealed that the ultrasonographic findings were highly variable.[15–19] Unfortunately, demonstrating a living extrauterine embryo, although diagnostic, is un-

common, and is observed in approximately 10% of cases.[18] Other adnexal and extrauterine findings, while more common, are less specific. Even a sac-like structure surrounded by an echogenic ring, while highly suggestive of an extrauterine gestational sac, is not diagnostic.[16] Furthermore, it is well known that a normal sonogram does not exclude an ectopic pregnancy. A recent prospective study found that 20% of all ectopic pregnancies were associated with completely normal sonograms.[18]

The sensitivity and accuracy of ultrasound in the diagnosis of ectopic pregnancy can be significantly improved if high-resolution ultrasound is combined with the results of the radioimmunoassay pregnancy test. An elevated serum hCG level confirms a gestational event but does not distinguish an intrauterine from an extrauterine location. On the other hand, although sonography is relatively insensitive for demonstrating the ectopic gestation, it is highly accurate for detecting an intrauterine pregnancy (IUP) after 5 menstrual weeks.[20–21] Demonstrating an intrauterine gestation is very useful since most women suspected of having an ectopic pregnancy have an early IUP,[15, 16, 18] and this finding effectively excludes an ectopic gestation (since their coexistence is rare).[22] Absence of a detectable intrauterine gestation, on the other hand, places the patient in a high-risk group for ectopic pregnancy regardless of the extrauterine findings. The presence of free pelvic fluid, echogenic blood clot, or a complex adnexal mass proportionately increases that risk.[18, 23]

Since ultrasound's primary role in evaluating patients with suspected ectopic pregnancy is to identify patients with an IUP and to exclude them from the group at risk, careful scanning of the uterus and its contents is essential. The majority of patients with ectopic pregnancy have an empty uterus with normal or increased central uterine cavity echoes. Although this appearance suggests ectopic pregnancy, it may also be present with an early IUP (between 3 and 5 weeks) or a recent spontaneous abortion. Sonography is not usually able to distinguish between these entities, although the presence of an adnexal mass or free pelvic fluid favors an ectopic pregnancy.[18] Other diagnostic procedures that may be required for differentiation include uterine curettage, culdocentesis, and laparoscopy.

From a practical point of view, there are several ways to evaluate patients suspected of ectopic pregnancy. One common approach, which uses serial quantitative serum hCG determinations, relies on the fact that with a normal IUP the hCG level should double every 2–3 days. A subnormal rise or plateau in the hCG level suggests either an ectopic pregnancy or an abnormal intrauterine pregnancy.[24, 25] Another method used to identify patients with an ectopic pregnancy is to correlate a single hCG level with the sonographic appearance of the uterus.[26] Since an intrauterine gestational sac should always be visible when the hCG level exceeds 1,800 mIU/ml,[27] if it is absent when the hCG level is greater than 1,800 mIU/ml, an ectopic pregnancy is likely. This combination of findings, however, may also occur with a recent spontaneous abortion, in which case serial hCG determinations will show a steady decline or plateau in quantitative levels.[28] Absence of an intrauterine gestational sac at hCG levels less than 1,800 mIU/ml is nondiagnostic and may be due to an ectopic pregnancy, an early IUP, or a recent abortion. In this situation, serial hCG determinations may also be useful for distinguishing among these possibilities.

Occasionally, in patients with ectopic pregnancy, the uterine cavity is not empty but contains an intrauterine fluid collection.[19] If the fluid collection is not surrounded by an echogenic ring, it is clearly abnormal and uterine curettage should be recommended. If, however, the fluid collection is surrounded by an echogenic ring, it may be due to a "pseudogestational sac," which may simulate a true gestational sac. This sonographic appearance, seen in about 10% of patients with ectopic pregnancy,[18, 26, 28] is probably due to decidual changes within the endometrium secondary to hormonal stimulation. Sonographic demonstration of increased central uterine echoes ("decidual reaction"), seen in 20%–40% of patients with ectopic pregnancy, are also probably due to decidual changes.[29, 30] Pathologically, decidual changes are found in approximately 50% of patients with ectopic pregnancy.

Because a pseudogestational sac of ectopic pregnancy may simulate a true gestational sac, caution should be exercised when diagnosing an early IUP prior to detecting an embryo. Recent evidence indicates that a specific morphological feature, namely, the presence of a double decidual sac (DDS), may be reliably used to distinguish a true gestational sac from a pseudogestational sac.[29, 31, 32] Pathologically the two concentric lines, which on sonography account for the DDS, are thought to represent the chorion and the decidua capsularis in close apposition to the decidua parietalis.[31] Since the gestational sac develops within the uterine wall, the central uterine cavity remains collapsed and these two decidual layers remain closely apposed. In contrast, the fluid in a pseudogestational sac is within the uterine cavity. This causes separation of the endometrial walls and produces a single echogenic ring surrounding a fluid collection.

The presence of a DDS permits identification of a greater number of intrauterine pregnancies than is possible by detection of an embryo alone.[18, 29] In a prospective study of patients referred for possible ectopic pregnancy, 86% of intrauterine pregnancies were correctly identified by visualizing either an embryo (54%) or a gestational sac with a DDS (32%). Of the remaining patients with an IUP, only 2% had gestational sacs which lacked a DDS, and 12% were scanned before a gestational sac was detected.[18]

Any patient with an intrauterine fluid collection that lacks a DDS should be considered at risk for an ectopic pregnancy. Absence of a DDS has also been reported in 37% of patients with abnormal (nonviable) gestational sacs, probably secondary to decidual degeneration.[29, 33] Occasionally, in patients with normal gestational sacs whose diameter is less than 10 mm, a DDS finding may be lacking. Since approximately 2%–5% of normal gestational sacs fail to demonstrate a DDS finding, its absence should not be judged as definitely abnormal but should be interpreted in conjunction with other sonographic findings.[33]

In addition to a DDS, sonographic features of a normal gestational sac include a normal size, shape, and position of the sac, as well as a prominent surrounding choriodecidual reaction (see discussion of normal pregnancy in chapter 16A). These features are useful for identifying a normal IUP since, rarely, a pseudogestational sac may have findings that mimic a DDS but may lack other normal criteria.[29] In many cases the appearance of a pseudogestational sac is indistinguishable from that of a nonviable gestational sac. In these situations, uterine curettage is recommended. The recovery of chorionic villi confirms an IUP, whereas the recovery of decidual tissue without chorionic villi suggests the presence of an extrauterine pregnancy and requires further evaluation.

In the evaluation of patients with suspected ectopic pregnancy, the extrauterine findings are clearly secondary to the intrauterine findings but are often helpful for supporting the diagnosis.[18, 19] In their recent report, Mahony et al. assigned probability risks to pregnant women who were at risk for ectopic pregnancy and whose uteri lacked an IUP. When neither an adnexal mass nor pelvic fluid was present, the probability of an ectopic pregnancy was 20%, whereas the presence of either finding increased this risk to 71%.[18] The presence of either a noncystic adnexal mass or a moderate to large amount of pelvic fluid was associated with ectopic pregnancy in 85% and 91% of cases, respectively. In approximately 10% of cases, a living extrauterine embryo was demonstrated, which is, of course, diagnostic of ectopic pregnancy.[18]

Once an IUP is demonstrated, the extrauterine findings become statistically less helpful for diagnosing an ectopic pregnancy. In this situation, the combination of an adnexal mass and pelvic fluid is most likely due to a ruptured or hemorrhagic corpus luteum cyst, although the remote possibility of a coexisting ectopic gestation must be considered. An adnexal mass may also be present but unrelated to the pregnancy, as in patients with a dermoid cyst, endometrioma, or ovarian neoplasm.

Although more than 80% of ectopic gestations are in the isthmic and ampullary portions of the fallopian tubes, extrauterine implantation may occur in other sites.[4] An interstitial ectopic pregnancy develops in the medial third of the fallopian tube, within the uterine wall. Because the myometrium can support the developing blastocyst for a longer time period, this form of ectopic implantation tends to rupture when the gestation is relatively more mature, and is frequently associated with life-threatening hemorrhage.[19, 34]

Sonographically, an interstitial ectopic pregnancy may appear either extrauterine or intrauterine in location. Its interstitial location may be suggested if the gestational sac appears clearly extrauterine but contiguous with the uterus. An apparently intrauterine location is a more difficult diagnostic problem but may be suggested if the gestation is eccentrically positioned or lacks a complete myometrial mantle around the gestational sac.[34] Similar findings may be seen, however, if a gestation occupies one horn of a bicornuate uterus, or if a myoma is present. This appearance may also be artifactually produced by an overly distended urinary bladder displacing the gestational sac.[35]

An intra-abdominal ectopic pregnancy often persists until relatively late in pregnancy.[36] Establishing the correct diagnosis is important since life-threatening hemorrhage is a frequent complication. The sonographic findings, which may be subtle, include absence of myometrium between the fetus and urinary bladder or between the fetus and the anterior abdominal wall, as well as an indication that the uterus is separate from the fetus.

## Summary

Ectopic pregnancy is a common and life-threatening complication of early pregnancy. To make earlier diagnoses and diminish maternal morbidity and mortality, a high index of clinical suspicion is required. Recently, dramatic improvements have been made for detecting ectopic pregnancies by screening symptomatic patients with a combination of high-resolution ultrasound and a sensitive serum radioimmunoassay pregnancy test.

It is important to recognize that ultrasound's primary role is to evaluate the uterus. Identifying an intrauterine gestation effectively excludes an ectopic pregnancy, since their coexistence is rare. Absence of a detectable IUP, on the other hand, places the patient at risk for an ectopic gestation. Extrauterine findings of an adnexal mass and/or free pelvic fluid increase the likelihood that the pregnancy is ectopic. Occasionally the ectopic gestation itself is visualized, permitting a specific diagnosis to be made.

Further diagnostic evaluation of patients in the high-risk group depends on the specific sonographic findings, the availability of other diagnostic tests, and the particular clinical situation. Noninvasive diagnostic tests include repeated ultrasound examination, correlation of the sonographic findings with a simultaneous hCG determination, and serial hCG determinations. In selected cases, more invasive diagnostic procedures may be required, including uterine curettage, culdocentesis, and laparoscopy. A single approach cannot be recommended for every patient, so that familiarity with the advantages and limitations of each test and procedure is suggested.

## References

1. Dodson MG: Bleeding in pregnancy, in Aladjem S (ed): *Obstetrical Practice.* St Louis, CV Mosby Co, 1980, pp 451–472.
2. Dorfman SF: Deaths from ectopic pregnancy,

United States, 1979, to 1980. *Obstet Gynecol* 1983; 62:334–338.

3. Dorfman SF, Grimes DA, Cates W Jr, et al: Ectopic pregnancy mortality, United States, 1979 to 1980. *Clinic Aspects Obstet Gynecol* 1984; 64:386–389.

4. Iffy L: Ectopic pregnancy, in Iffy L, Kaminetzky HA (eds): *Principles and Practice of Obstetrics and Perinatology.* New York, John Wiley & Sons, Inc, 1981, pp 609–633.

5. McElin TW: Ectopic pregnancy, in Danforth PN (ed): *Obstetrics and Gynecology.* Hargerstown, Md, Harper & Row, Publishers, 1977, pp 336–357.

6. Tancer ML, Delke I, Veridiano NP: A fifteen year experience with ectopic pregnancy. *Surg Gynecol Obstet* 1981; 152:179–190.

7. Pritchard JA, MacDonald PC, Gant GF: The placental hormones, in Williams (ed): *Obstetrics.* Norwalk, Appleton-Century-Crofts, 1985, pp 119–137.

8. Derman R, Edelman DA, Berger GS: Current status of immunologic pregnancy tests. *Int J Gynaecol Obstet* 1979; 17:190–193.

9. Braunstein GD, Karow WG, Gentry WC, et al: First-trimester chorionic gonadotropin measurements as an aid in the diagnosis of early pregnancy disorders. *Am J Obstet Gynecol* 1978; 131:25–32.

10. Rasor JL, Braunstein GD: A rapid modification of the beta-hCG radioimmunoassay. Use as an aid in the diagnosis of ectopic pregnancy. *Obstet Gynecol* 1977; 50:553–558.

11. Schwartz RWO, Di Pietro DL: Beta-hCG as a diagnostic aid for suspected ectopic pregnancy. *Obstet Gynecol* 1980; 56:197–203.

12. Strubel JL, Rinke ML, Hussa RO: "Tandem Icon hCG" urine pregnancy test evaluated. *Clin Chem* 1985; 31:492–493.

13. Kobayashi M, Hellman L, Fillisti L: Ultrasound: An aid in the diagnosis of ectopic pregnancy. *Am J Obstet Gynecol* 1969; 103:1131–1140.

14. Maklad NF, Wright CH: Grey scale ultrasonography in the diagnosis of ectopic pregnancy. *Radiology* 1918; 126:221–225.

15. Lawson TL: Ectopic pregnancy: Criteria and accuracy of ultrasonic diagnosis. *AJR* 1978; 131:153–156.

16. Brown TW, Filly RA, Laing FC, et al: Analysis of

17. Pederson JF: Ultrasonic scanning in suspected ectopic pregnancy. *Br J Radiol* 1980; 53:1–4.

18. Mahony BS, Filly RA, Nyberg DA, Callen PW: Sonographic evaluation of ectopic pregnancy. *J Ultrasound Med* 1985; 4:221–228.

19. Laing FC, Jeffrey RB: Ultrasound evaluation of ectopic pregnancy, in Callen PW (ed): *Ultrasonography in Obstetrics and Gynecology.* Philadelphia, WB Saunders Co, 1983, pp 291–304.

20. Ghorashi B, Gottesfeld KR: The gray scale appearance of the normal pregnancy from 4–16 weeks of gestation. *JCU* 1977; 5:195–201.

21. Lyons EA, Levi CS: Ultrasound in the first trimester of pregnancy, in Callen PW (ed): *Ultrasonography in Obstetrics and Gynecology.* Philadelphia, WB Saunders Co, 1983, pp 1–19.

22. Berger MJ, Taymor ML: Simultaneous intrauterine and tubal pregnancies following ovulation induction. *Am J Obstet Gynecol* 1972; 113:812–813.

23. Jeffrey RB Jr, Laing FC: Echogenic clot: A useful sign of pelvic hemoperitoneum. *Radiology* 1982; 145:139–141.

24. Braunstein GD, Grodin JM, Vaitukaitis, et al: Secretory rates of human chorionic gonadotropin by normal trophoblast. *Am J Obstet Gynecol* 1973; 115:447–450.

25. Kadar N, Caldwell BV, Romero R: A method of screening for ectopic pregnancy and its indications. *Obstet Gynecol* 1981; 58:162–166.

26. Kadar N, DeVore G, Romero R: Discriminatory HCG zone: Its use in the sonographic evaluation for ectopic pregnancy. *Obstet Gynecol* 1981; 58:156–161.

27. Nyberg DA, Filly RA, Mahony BS, et al: Early gestation: Correlation of HCG levels and sonographic identification. *AJR* 1985; 144:951–954.

28. Steier JA, Bergsjo P, Myking OL: Human chorionic gonadotropin in maternal plasma after induced abortion, spontaneous abortion, and ectopic pregnancy. *Obstet Gynecol* 1984; 64:391–394.

29. Nyberg DA, Laing FC, Filly RA, et al: Ultrasonographic differentiation of the gestational sac of early intrauterine pregnancy from the pseudo-gestational sac of ectopic pregnancy. *Radiology* 1983; 146:755–759.

30. Marks WM, Filly RA, Callen PW, et al: The de-

cidual cast of ectopic pregnancy: A confusing ultrasonographic appearance. *Radiology* 1979; 133:451–454.

31. Bradley WG, Fiske CE, Filly RA: The double decidual sac sign of early pregnancy: Use in exclusion of ectopic pregnancy. *Radiology* 1982; 143:223–226.

32. Nelson P, Bowie JA, Rosenberg ER: Early intrauterine pregnancy or decidual cast: An anatomic-sonographic approach. *J Ultrasound Med* 1983; 2:543–547.

33. Nyberg DA, Laing FC, Filly RA: Sonographic distinction of normal from abnormal gestational sacs in threatened abortion. Radiology (in press).

34. Graham M, Cooperberg PL: Ultrasound diagnosis of interstitial pregnancy: Findings and pitfalls *JCU* 1979; 7:433–437.

35. Laing FC: Letter to the editor. *JCU* 1980; 8:287.

36. Allibone GW, Fagan CJ, Porter SC: The sonographic features of intra-abdominal pregnancy. *JCU* 1981; 9:383–387.

# 16c
# THE PLACENTA

Seymour Zemlyn, M.D.

Diagnostic ultrasound imaging is the first modality that allows easy and direct visualization of the placenta in situ. These images therefore have few preceding models other than pathologic material. It is important that the normal development and basic anatomy of the placenta be well understood by the sonographer. The placenta is a short-lived, highly vascular organ that derives from the interaction of the implanted ovum and the maternal uterine wall. Pathologic processes in the placenta are generally vascular events and are sometimes heralded by vaginal bleeding.

## Placental Development

According to Fox the placenta begins to form about the 21st day after conception and is anatomically complete by the end of the fourth month.[1] In prior events the villi of the chorion frondosum oriented to the endometrium proliferate and the mass of cells underlying the growing cytotrophoblast, called the syncytiotrophoblast, forms lacunae (fluid-filled spaces) by eroding small areas of the maternal tissue it contacts. About the 11th day maternal capillaries are pierced and maternal blood enters the lacunae to form the intervillous spaces. A few of the primary villi extend across these spaces and attach directly to the decidua basalis, serving to anchor the placenta. These anchoring villi are composed predominantly of connective tissue. The majority of the villi become increasingly vascularized, form secondary and tertiary buds, and continue to proliferate within these spaces, creating a vast surface area bathed in maternal blood.

When the maternal capillaries are reached at about the 10th or 11th day, human chorionic gonadotropin (hCG) arising from the trophoblast may be introduced directly into the maternal circulation, maintaining the corpus luteum and converting it to the corpus luteum of pregnancy. This results in the continuing progesterone secretion required to preserve the endometrium, prevent menses, and allow the pregnancy to continue. The earliest detection of pregnancy is based on radioimmunoassay or receptor techniques of maternal serum for the $\beta$-subunit of hCG. These tests are sensitive enough to be positive by the 10th or 11th day after conception. The rising titer may be quantitated for dates and for normal development of the pregnancy. By the sixth or seventh gestational week the placenta produces enough steroids to maintain pregnancy. The corpus luteum usually declines after about the 12th week, but occasionally it persists, sometimes throughout the pregnancy.

The first maternal vessels entered must be low-pressure capillaries, for if an arteriole is entered, hemorrhage is likely to destroy the pregnancy without the would-be mother knowing she had been pregnant.[2] On the other hand, delay in penetrating a suitable maternal vessel might result in low maternal levels of hCG and limit the nutrient and gas exchange of the growing trophoblast. In a clinical investigation elective hysterectomies were scheduled within 14 days of ovulation. A vigorous search for ova in these uteri revealed that more than 40% of preimplanted and implanted ova had major disorders of the germinal disks, including underlying hematomas, and are probably shed with the next menses.[3] A study of serial hCG determinations confirmed the surprisingly high rate of silent early abortion and indicated that only about 43% of implanted embryos become clinical pregnancies.[4]

By about the 18th day, capillaries have developed in the tertiary villi in the intervillous spaces, and the primitive embryonic heart and islands of hematopoiesis are forming the fetal side of the placental circulation. The embryonic heart will become responsible for pumping not only the blood volume of the small fetus, but also the vast fetal placental circulation through the cord. The embryonic heart is therefore relatively large early in embryologic development, and ultrasound detection of embryonic heart motion may be possible as early as the fifth conceptual or seventh gestational week.[5] It is estimated that ultimately the fetal heart pumps about 500 cc/min through the umbilical cord to the placenta.

It is critical that the maternal-placental circulation be a low-pressure, low-velocity unit. The maternal vascular system must deliver circulating blood at reduced pressure if it is not to overwhelm the relatively low intravascular pressure of the fetal circulation at their placental junction. High-volume, low-velocity flow bathing the villi allows optimal exchange of nutrients and waste. These goals are accomplished by means of changes in the vessels and tissue initiated by the invading syncytiotrophoblast. The tissue it contacts undergoes fibrinoid degeneration. The capillaries and arterioles of the maternal spiral arteries are disrupted and dilated, and become incorporated into the enlarging intervillous spaces. This results in an unusual circulatory system in which the diameter of the vessels increases in the direction of flow. In keeping with the laws of hydrodynamics, peripheral resistance and arterial pressure are progressively reduced and flow velocity slowed as the maternal-placental vessels expand, with dramatic change at the abruptly dilated intervillous spaces. The voluminous, quiet intervillous spaces are fed by arterial spurts, and drained by venules without an intervening capillary bed and with a small pressure gradient. Pulsations of maternal blood enter these smaller units centrally, each from a single coiled artery at the base of the intervillous space, and are propelled toward the chorionic surface.[6] The flow slows and reverses and venous drainage of blood introduced earlier occurs at the base. The unusual flow pattern through the jungle of villi is not uniform and produces eddy currents, stagnation, and streaming effects. As the intervillous space enlarges in radius during the course of the pregnancy, flow must become progressively slower within it. It is theorized that a critical volume may be reached at which the velocity becomes so slow as to invite thrombosis. These factors may play a role in the frequency with which thromboses and infarcts are routinely found post partum in the normal placenta. The stress of isolating maternal arterial pressures from the fetal circulation of 30–60 mm Hg systolic pressure or less also encourages vascular accidents and perhaps the changes we regard as "maturation" of the placenta. As these placental changes in calcification, thrombosis, and fibrin proliferation are also provoked in vascular systems by hypertension, it is not surprising that they occur prematurely in the setting of maternal hypertension.

Uterine contractions have been thought to temporarily reduce flow by compressing veins and arterioles and increasing intraluminal pressures, but Bleker et al., using ultrasound measurements, concluded that the intervillous spaces actually increase during contractions.[7] This work was performed with bistable equipment and a 1.5-MHz transducer. It may be that the measured increased thickness during contraction ascribed to the intervillous space was partially due to the thickened myometrium, because distinguishing muscle from placenta was not always possible within the technological limitations of equipment then available. These data await confirmation with modern equipment.

About the fourth month the placenta is about the same size as the fetus, but it does not keep up in growth with the fetus or the uterus for the rest of the pregnancy. It is estimated that about half the uterine surface is covered by the placenta in the fourth month, but at term the placenta occupies only about one fifth or one sixth of that surface, and weighs about one sixth as much as the fetus. The maternal surface of the term placenta is made up of 12–20 flat tufts called cotyledons. These do not totally correspond to the functional units of the villous spaces demonstrated by angiography, nor do the fetal and maternal units precisely match.[6] There are about 50 such functional units in the human placenta.

While there is great variability, the placenta at term is about 15 cm in diameter. According to sonographic measurements the normal placenta grows to a maximum thickness of 4 cm.[8] The placenta associated with intrauterine fetal growth retardation tends to be smaller in width, thickness, and area. Placentas over 5 cm thick are sometimes associated with maternal-fetal immunologic incompatibility, maternal diabetes mellitus or prediabetes, syphilis and other infections, maternal congestive heart failure, maternal anemia, edema and hydropic degeneration of the placenta accompanying an ill fetus, molar pregnancies, chorioangiomas, or intraplacental bleeding. Hyperplacentosis, an increase in trophoblastic activity with increased maternal serum hCG level, theca lutein cysts, pre-eclampsia, nausea, or pruritus may be present, but hyperplacentosis may also occur without apparent enlargement of the placenta.[9]

Fetal growth and maintenance depend on an adequate amount of functioning placental tissue to provide nutrition and exchange. Placental dysfunction may result from decreased perfusion or permeability, or decreased placental surface area.[10] Vascular insufficiency of the placenta is thought to be one of the causes of intrauterine growth retardation, usually manifested after 30 weeks' gestation, and of the post-maturity syndrome, manifested after 42 weeks' gestation. These neonates appear to be starved and are sometimes called dysmature. Several studies have demonstrated a relationship between maternal hypertension and growth retardation. Placental perfusion in fetuses with growth retardation may be one-fourth that of controls.[11] Diminished functioning placental tissue in pregnancies yielding dysmature infants may be reflected in decreased maternal blood levels of placental secretions such as human placental lactogen or schwangerschaftsprotein 1.[12] Diagnostic ultrasound

has a definite role in the detection of intrauterine growth retardation but is limited by its insensitivity to physiologic derangement that has not provoked anatomical changes beyond the normal range.

## Developmental Abnormalities of the Placenta

In 0.7%–6.6% of cases the placenta will have an accessory or succenturiate lobe. An undetected retained lobe can result in prolonged postpartum bleeding or infection, and, rarely, the connecting vessels of the two lobes may rupture during delivery. For these reasons physically separate accessory lobes should be reported when seen on sonography.[13] An even more rare pathologic condition (about 1 in 3,300 deliveries) occurs when the entire chorion frondosum continues into placentation. The circumferential placenta that forms is called placenta membranacea, and, because it is in part a placenta previa, it is associated with recurrent bleeding in the second and third trimesters that often ends in abortion or premature labor. The circumferential extent of the placenta may allow this condition to be detected by diagnostic ultrasound imaging.[14]

An anechoic subplacental space is normally seen on sonography and corresponds to the dilated endometrial veins of the decidua basalis.[15] This clear space varies between 0.5 and 2 cm in thickness and may be multiseptated. It is best seen when the placenta is posterior or fundal. The fundal clear space often lacks detail, in part because of refraction at the curved interface of placenta and wall. The septa are unlikely to be well seen here as the orientation of their reflecting surfaces is predominantly parallel to the ultrasound beam. Anterior infraplacental spaces are best visualized with high-frequency, short-focus transducers, with an intervening water-bath, or with the patient prone or upright. Real-time and Doppler studies indicate that venous flow in these areas is affected by position, the hydrostatic effect making anterior spaces less prominent than the posterior spaces when the patient is supine and more prominent when the patient is imaged upright [16] or prone.[17]

Invasion of the uterine wall by the placenta through the decidua basalis is termed placenta accreta. This condition may be further defined as placenta accreta vera (adherent to the myometrium), placenta increta (extending into the myometrium), or placenta percreta (extending through the myometrium onto the serosa). Placenta accreta vera, which accounts for up to 60% of cases, has not beenn detected ultrasonographically, but absence of the retroplacental clear space under optimal imaging techniques has been reported in placenta increta.[18, 19] Placenta accreta occurs more often in older and in multigravid women and is more likely in those who have had previous uterine curettages, especially if followed by prolonged amenorrhea and treatment for synechiae formation to achieve pregnancy.[20] An association with previous cesarean sections and with placentas implanted in the lower uterus has also been reported.[21] In those with placenta previa, the likelihood of concurrent placenta accreta rises dramatically in relation to the number of prior cesarean sections, reaching 67% in those with four previous cesarean sections.[22] The condition is thought to be due to a deficiency in the formation of the decidua basalis. These rare pathologic conditions are otherwise suggested by prepartum bleeding, uterine rupture, uterine inversion, or, most commonly, inability to extract the placenta at delivery. Hysterectomy may be required if the patient is to survive. Placenta accreta is the second most common reason, after uterine atony, for emergency hysterectomy due to obstetric hemorrhage.[23] The fetal and maternal mortality are each about 10%.

Chorioangiomas, also called placental hemangiomas, are regarded by some as hemangiomatous hamartomas and by others as benign neoplasms of the placenta. On microscopic examination they can be found in about 1% of examined placentas, but only large tumors are clinically significant, and these occur once in several thousand cases. This vascular tumor may act as an arteriovenous shunt, bypassing the normal placental tissue. Tumors 4 cm in diameter or larger have been associated with hydramnios (30%), antepartum hemorrhage (15%–20%), premature labor (10%), and also fetal anomalies, fetal demise, anemia, fetal hydrops, fetal heart failure, low birth weight, and toxemia.[24] The vascular pool created in these tumors may trap platelets and red blood cells. It has been suggested that these fetuses be stress-tested frequently,[25] and that care be taken at delivery that the baby receive a maximum amount of placental blood before the cord is clamped.[26] Chorioangioma can be detected ultrasonographically when it presents as a tumor on the fetal surface of the placenta or extending within the amniotic fluid.[27] An intra-amniotic clot may resemble this tumor.[28] In some cases a large placenta may be the only manifestation. Chorioangioma should be considered, especially when the combination of hydramnios, fetal edema, and a large placenta is present and immunologic causes have been excluded. The appearance of a thickened placenta should be readily distinguishable from hydatidiform mole or inwardly protruding uterine myomas.[29]

## Membranes and Umbilical Cord

The chorion is the limiting membrane of the fetus and its fluid environment. This shiny membrane is seen on sonograms as a well-defined, echo-dense line containing the amniotic fluid and, before it is resorbed, the chorionic fluid. In the early gestational sac it is seen sonographically as a thick, irregular density due to the chorion frondosum and decidual reaction, but thins rapidly as pregnancy continues. Once the conceptus fills the potential uterine lumen, the capsular chorion abuts the opposing uterine wall. When fluid is present within the uterine lumen, it displaces the chorion from the wall and forms a slit-like or crescentric sonolucent extrachorionic space. In early pregnancy this accounts for the pseudosac,[30] "double sac sign,"[31] "crescent,"[32] "double decidual sac,"[33] or deciduachorionic sac[34] that makes possible the ultrasonic distinction of a true intrauterine gestational sac. The hypoechoic slit, corresponding to the location of the uterine lumen, is sandwiched between the echogenic decidua vera and the echogenic chorion frondosum. Such a slit-like space is not present in the false sac of a pure decidual reaction, where only a single-thickness echogenic ring is present, as the chorion frondosum is not present. Larger intraluminal fluid collections are usually blood. If large enough they become almost spherical and resemble a second gestational sac. Each "sac" visualized should be analyzed for the tell-tale double sac sign to exclude a false twin gestational sac.[35] When blood collects here beyond the gestational sac stage, the chorion is indented or displaced centrally by the extrachorionic hematoma. Extrachorionic hematomas may extend laterally and superiorly, but are most often seen in the lower uterine cavity overlying the internal cervical os in patients who present with vaginal bleeding. These bleeding events need not be associated with fetal or maternal compromise.

The amnion initially forms a small sac about the embryo. With the accumulation of amniotic fluid and growth of the embryo, this sac expands within the chorionic sac until the amnion comes to lie against the chorion. These two membranes do not fuse, but only potential space remains between them, trapping the vestigial yolk sac. Once this occurs they are seen as a single membrane on sonograms, and the fetal surface of the placenta, called the chorionic plate, is composed of these two indistinguishable layers. Before this the amnion may be seen ultrasonically with difficulty as it is a much less reflective surface than the chorion.[36] Small segments of amnion may occasionally be seen slightly displaced from the chorion throughout pregnancy. The appearance may mimic that of the chorion displaced by an extrachorionic hematoma. Either is seen on a sonogram as a membrane suspended in fluid. The described sonographic characteristics are unproved, as it is not possible to verify pathologically that the membrane seen by the sonographer is the amnion. The difference in reflectivity of the amnion and chorion, and the fact that patients with a hematoma usually have been bleeding through the vagina, may aid in differentiating chorion from amnion. When the outer fluid collection contains either random echoes or septations, characteristics of hematomas, the membrane is the chorion. The continuity of the displaced chorion with the peripheral membrane is always clearly seen, whereas the amnion contacting the chorion is often obscure. The chorion is usually firm and fixed in its appearance, while the amnion may occasionally waver with fetal or maternal motion. The relationship of the membrane to the chorionic plate of the placenta may be helpful. Continuity at the margin of the placenta indicates that the membrane is the chorion. The amnion may be displaced from the chorion over a large arc and tends to run parallel to the chorionic wall. The external fluid collection of a hematoma tends to be crescentric, whereas that contour in chorioamniotic separation may be more of a wide ring or ribbon shape, tending to reflect its sac-within-a-sac origin. Theoretically, if the separated amnion can be followed to the base of the umbilical cord, it can be distinguished from the chorion. A large meningocele, lymphoceles, or extensive subcutaneous edema may give the confusing appearance of a membrane within the fluid medium of the pregnancy. Tracing the origin of the membrane to the fetus will facilitate the proper diagnosis. Substan-

tial chorioamniotic separation is uncommon in the third trimester and is sometimes associated with previous amniocentesis or hydramnios and congenital anomalies[30] or chorioangioma.[37] It is thought that rupture of the amnion and entanglement of the fetus in the floating membrane are the cause of the rare amniotic band syndrome, which results in degrees of constriction, vascular strangulation, or garroting amputation. A variety of congenital malformations, usually limb defects or amputations, may occur and may result in fetal death. It is possible to detect this syndrome ultrasonically if fetal parts straddle an intrauterine membrane and are associated with fetal edema, which is often asymmetric.[38]

Echogenic particles in the range of 1–5 mm long that are seen within the amniotic fluid on sonographic examinations were initially thought to represent vernix caseosa.[39] Such particles must be distinguished from acoustic noise. Gain settings should be below a level that would produce echoes within the urinary bladder. The particles should be seen to swirl with fetal or maternal movement or with external compression. Vernix usually does not appear before 36 weeks' gestation, and is not found prior to 32 weeks' gestation. The presence of these particles on the sonogram has therefore been taken as an indication that the pregnancy is near term and the fetal lungs are mature, and is reported to have some association with mature lecithin/sphingomyelin ratios.[40, 41] Such particles are also seen in the second trimester and are assumed to be due to meconium, possibly representing fetal distress,[42] but they have been reportedly seen as early as the 15th week of gestation with increasing frequency to term in normal pregnancies.[43] If they can be detected in early pregnancy the visualized particles cannot be presumed to be due to vernix, nor does their presence guarantee fetal pulmonary maturity.

The amnion forms the external surface of the umbilical cord and its interior is composed predominantly of a myxomatous material called Wharton's jelly, through which two arteries and a vein normally course. About 1% have a single artery, which may be noted on sonography,[44] and have a high fetal mortality due to an increased incidence of associated fetal anomalies. The ultrasound detection of echogenic thrombotic material within the cord has allowed the intrauterine diagnosis of umbilical vein thrombosis to be made.[45] The umbilical cord is normally about 1–2 cm in diameter but may be enlarged as a normal variant[46] or in association with erythroblastosis fetalis, maternal diabetes, abruptio placentae, patent urachus, hematoma, or umbilical cord tumor (angioma or myxosarcoma).[20, 47, 48] The small-for-gestational-age fetus often has a thin umbilical cord or a marginal insertion.[49]

## Intraplacental Sonolucent Spaces

Placental sonolucent spaces may contain serous or proteinaceous material, fibrin, or blood, and it is not possible to determine the nature of the material by sonography. Small subchorionic cystic areas are seen in 10%–15% of sonograms of placentas.[50] These represent areas of subchorionic fibrin deposition, septal cysts, or blood, and, especially near the umbilical cord insertion, umbilical vessels within the placenta. The umbilical vessels may be detected ultrasonographically by virtue of their pulsatile flow.[51]

Vascular accidents within the placenta are common. In placentas of full-term, normal pregnancies, Fox found 36% to have intervillous thromboses, 25% to have infarcts, and many more to have fibrin deposition, mostly in prerivillous and subchorionic areas.[20] The placenta does not form granulation tissue and organize clots in the usual fashion, but clotted blood is replaced by fibrin deposition which may, in turn, undergo cystic degeneration.[52] While the pathologist may distinguish red lesions (which are fresher and contain red blood cells and fibrin) from white (made up of bands of fibrin), and thromboses (with no contained villi) from infarcts (with contained necrotic villi), the sonographer is likely to see these only as sonolucent spaces. This creates no great clinical loss as they are common and are not individually significant. They rarely result in loss of enough functioning placenta to compromise the gas exchange or the nutrition of the fetus. However, the number and size of such lesions increase with the duration of the pregnancy, and in some pathologic situations, including Rh isoimmunization, severe toxemia, and maternal hypertension. An increased number of placental sonolucent spaces has been reported in the second trimester in cases of elevated maternal serum α-fetoprotein levels, with no identifiable cause.[53] An increase in fetal RBCs recovered in maternal blood is associated with intervillous thrombi.[20] The thrombi may contain nucleated (fetal) RBCs and may be the site of transmigration of fetal cells and elevated α-fetoprotein levels. Current interest has focused on the relationship of sonolucent areas to "aging" of the placenta and to intrauterine growth retardation.

## Placental Aging

Calcifications in the placenta occur microscopically in relation to the maternal surface of the villi, maternal vessels, and along the intercondylar septa and other areas.[54] Calcification may be laid down in larger amounts throughout the placenta, especially near term. The number and size of calcifications increase as pregnancy advances. Placental calcifications have been reported by some as more prevalent in young mothers and primigravidas, and they more readily detected by the radiologist and ultrasonographer than by the pathologist. When bistable equipment gave way to gray-scale ultrasonography, increasing detail of the previous formless interior of the placenta revealed sonolucent spaces and cotyledons related to the duration of pregnancy. Winsberg described increasing "transsonic" areas within the placentas of 36 weeks' gestation and later, and suggested this appearance might be useful in determining maturity.[55] Fisher's group described the appearance of intercotyledonary septa formation and readily detectable central sonolucencies within the cotyledons at about 36 weeks' gestation in normal pregnancies, but earlier in abnormal pregnancies associated with growth retardation.[56] The echo-free spaces correlated pathologically with circumscribed areas containing blood and fibrin, but virtually free of villi, except perhaps compressed at the periphery. These circumscribed sonolucent spaces seen in relation to cotyledon formation in late pregnancy have been variously identified as central avillous spaces,[56] maternal lakes,[57] calcified cotyledons,[58] or intervillous thromboses.[59]

Grannum et al. classified placental changes as grades 0–3 and correlated them with amniotic fluid lecithin/sphingomyelin (L/S) ratios.[60] The classification depends on changes in the linearity of the chorionic plate, the homogeneity of the placental substance, progressive calcification, especially of the basilar area, and the formation of cotyledons and their central sonolucent areas. Initially the placenta has a homogeneous echo pattern bounded on the interior by the distinct unwavering line of the chorionic plate. This pattern Grannum called grade 0. The chorionic plate in a grade 1 placenta is undulating and the parenchymal echo pattern is more uneven. Basilar and other placental calcifications are present in grade 2 placentas, and indentations of the chorion extend into the placenta, but not to the basilar plate. A grade 3 placenta is characterized by more calcifications, septations extending to the basilar levels forming cotyledons, and the appearance and enlargement of central clear areas within the cotyledons. When the placental changes are not uniform, grading is based on the appearance of the highest grading seen. Grading represent a general chronological progression, but the placenta may not pass through these grades and may not advance beyond grade 0 or 1 at the time of delivery. In Grannum's original series of 129 pregnancies, the 23 with grade 3 placentas had an amniotic fluid L/S ratio over 2, the accepted marker of fetal lung maturity. Mature L/S ratios were also present in 88% of the 32 patients with grade 2 placentas. Other slightly different classifications have also been proposed, but Grannum's remains commonly used in this country.

Based on Grannum's findings it was hoped that the presence of a grade 3 placenta predicting mature fetal lungs could be used as a substitute for amniocentesis, but the method has definite limitations. Roughly 20%–25% of near-term pregnancies achieve a grade 3 appearance, so the method does not apply to 75%–80% of those at term, and omits even more in the preterm ages. Posterior placentas are often obscured by the overlying fetus and cannot be accurately graded. Furthermore, instances of hyaline membrane disease have been reported after the placenta has been designated grade 3.[61-63] Other studies correlating grade 3 placentas with amniotic fluid L/S ratios, phosphatidylglycerol (PG) levels, or occurrences of hyaline membrane disease (HMD) were more qualified. In about 5%–23% of pregnancies with grade 3 placentas, amniotic fluid L/S ratios are "immature,"[63-67] and about 20%–25% of grade 3 placentas in uncomplicated cases are associated with negative PG levels[63, 64] indicative of fetal lung immaturity.

The few clinical cases of HMD in those with grade 3 placentas occurred between 29 and 37 weeks' gestation, conforming to the known fact that HMD is rare at 38 weeks' gestation or beyond.[63, 66] When the study group is limited to those of 37 weeks' gestation or older, no cases of HMD are seen, no matter what the placental grade.[65] This observation is sufficient to

explain the clinical success of using a grade 3 placenta to confirm fetal lung maturity in planning repeat cesarean sections in those with reliable dates of 38 weeks' gestation or more.[63, 66] If this is so, then evaluating the placental grade in that group is of dubious value, and ultrasound effort may be better directed toward confirming gestational age.[68]

Ultrasound parameters that place the pregnancy near term correlate with fetal lung maturity. Even though there is poor direct correlation between placental grading and fetal biparietal diameter (BPD), the fetal BPD in nondiabetics has been used for assessing timing of elective cesarean sections.[69] No instances of HMD, and few instances of borderline L/S ratios, were reported with a BPD of 9.3 cm or greater.[70] In another study the number of amniocentesis performed for maturity determination was markedly reduced by using either a BPD of at least 9.2 cm or a grade 3 placenta.[71] The BPD was useful more often than the less common grade 3 placenta.

The ultrasound demonstration of the epiphyseal centers of the femur and tibia has been related to L/S ratios.[72] Either a proximal tibial epiphysis of at least 3 mm or a distal femoral epiphysis of 5 mm or more is associated with mature L/S ratios in approximately 95% of cases. When the proximal tibial epiphysis is 5 mm or greater, 100% maturity has been found so far.

A more direct means of evaluating fetal lung maturity would be useful. Preliminary work in ultrasound tissue characterization suggests a future possibility of assessing placental maturity,[73] as well as evaluating fetal lung maturity directly in this fashion,[74] but has not been demonstrated to be effective with current equipment and techniques.[75, 76]

It seems a matter of fortuitous timing of codeveloping, independent factors that grade 3 placentas normally occur when the fetal lungs are likely to be mature.[65, 68] Certain complications may cause earlier "maturation" of the placenta without a similar effect on fetal pulmonary maturity. It has often been found that placental changes occur earlier in pregnancies complicated by chronic hypertension, growth retardation, and preeclampsia between 29 and 37 gestational weeks.[58, 66-68, 77-79] Those in this high-risk group are more likely to have immature L/S ratios or to develop HMD despite grade 3 placentas.[66, 68] A grade 3 placenta does not guarantee fetal lung maturity in this group and must be viewed with some caution.

Since the causes of early changes of placental maturation include intrauterine growth retardation, the prospect that such cases might be identified through placental grading in high-risk, preterm pregnancies has also been evaluated. Kazzi et al. selected newborns with birth weights of 2,700 gm or less to evaluate sonographic placental grading performed shortly before delivery.[78] Grade 3 placentas were associated with newborns judged to be growth retarded (SGA) over four times more often than they were with infants that were simply small and healthy (non-SGA), especially before 35 weeks' gestation. However, in those in the lower 10th percentile of birth weight, over 40% of those with grade 3 placentas were not growth retarded, and about 40% of the SGA infants did not have grade 3 placentas. A similar correlation was noted in preterm pregnancies associated with maternal disease.[80] Some 53% of growth-retarded fetuses were associated with a grade 3 placenta, and 56% of fetuses associated with a grade 3 placenta before 37 weeks' gestation were growth retarded. These two studies surveyed pregnancies of high suspicion for intrauterine growth retardation. In a retrospective study that did not select a high-risk group, grade 3 placentas before 34 weeks' gestation yielded four times the normal incidence of SGA infants (16% vs. 4%).[81] Still, this means that 84% of women seen in a random ultrasound practice with grade 3 placentas this early in pregnancy might be expected not to bear SGA infants, a rather weak diagnostic correlation. It is reported that a grade 3 placenta associated with a fetal BPD of 8.7 cm or less correlates with an 8.5 times increase in the likelihood of intrauterine growth retardation, and 59% of fetuses with intrauterine growth retardation may be detected by these criteria.[7] Hopper et al. analyzed over 1,000 sonograms and derived frequency graphs for all placental grades.[82] The early appearance of any placental grade above 0 was associated with a high incidence of preeclampsia and growth retardation. They recommend that grade 1 placentas seen prior to 27 weeks, grade 2 placentas seen prior to 32 weeks, and grade 3 placentas seen prior to 34 weeks be regarded with suspicion and followed for complications.

Several assessments have failed to demonstrate a clinically useful correlation of placental maturity and fetal postmaturity. Placentas tend to complete the changes we call maturity rapidly after 40 weeks, and the placenta is usually grade 3 in postmaturity,[83] but grade 2 and occasionally grade 1 placentas have also been noted.[84, 85] The placental grade, therefore, is not useful in identifying the fetus suffering from postmaturity syndrome, but the presence of a grade 0 or 1 placenta after 42 weeks is so rare as to call into question the validity of the historical dates of that pregnancy. Placental changes may be delayed in cases of diabetes mellitus and Rh sensitization.[80] There is microscopic evidence that the placenta is less mature when anencephaly is present, but this has not received ultrasonic attention as yet.[86]

In summary, the presence of a grade 3 placenta in a normal pregnancy has a different meaning when the pregnancy is at term (37–38 weeks or more) than it does in earlier or abnormal pregnancies. At term the fetal lungs are normally mature, no matter what the placental grade, and clinical HMD is absent. If a grade 3 placenta is found earlier in the pregnancy it is not a 100% reliable marker of fetal pulmonary maturity, and it may reflect the possibility of intrauterine growth retardation or the complications of hypertension or toxemia. The early appearance of any grade placenta has the same significance. A BPD of 9.2 cm or more correlates with fetal lung maturity, possibly because it tends to exclude early gestational ages, and it may be useful more often than placental grading. The grade of the placenta plays no part in evaluating postmaturity, with the exception that a grade 0 or 1 placenta in a supposed post-term pregnancy casts doubt upon the accuracy of the clinical dates. Placental changes may be delayed in diabetes mellitus and Rh sensitization, and perhaps with anencephaly.

## Placental Location

Since its initial description,[87] diagnostic ultrasound has become the method of choice for placental localization because it is safe, easy to perform and repeat, and provides information about the fetus and its environs. Often placenta location is a byproduct of obstetric sonography performed for many other reasons. The major clinical interest in the location of the placenta for possible placenta previa has been expanded, and ultrasound localization is commonly used to select an optimal amniocentesis site, and prior to cesarean sections. Gray-scale diagnostic ultrasonography is intrinsically the most accurate imaging technique as it is the only method that directly displays the placenta, the cervix, and the internal cervical os. As placenta previa is defined by the relationship of the placental attachment to the internal cervical os, the latter is a necessary landmark in accurate diagnosis. It would seem to be a simple matter for any sonographer to accurately locate and describe the location of the placenta. In fact, there has been great difficulty in both describing the position of the placenta and identifying placenta previa. This tarnished the early reputation of diagnostic ultrasound and its practitioners. Results are improving along with increased understanding and improved techniques of examination.

## Describing Placental Position

The placenta itself is easily noted on sonography. The inner surface of the placenta is the echodense line of the chorionic plate. The echogenicity of the placenta parenchyma is more intense than that of the uterine wall. Early in pregnancy the pattern is homogeneous and of uniform echo intensity. Late in pregnancy calcifications occur along the basilar plate and elsewhere, cotyledons are formed, and sonolucent areas appear. The retroplacental clear space may be useful in defining the deep and lateral limits of the placenta.[88] Even when the placenta can be precisely defined, the routine description of the placental position is not always a simple task. The uterus is a mobile, muscular structure, tethered to the pelvic walls by ligaments, connective tissue, and muscle. The uterus can rotate,[89] tilt, flex and extend,[90] and contract.[91, 92] The activity of the uterus may cause the apparent placental location to change, making a concise, accurate description impossible for the sonographer, and has contributed to an exaggerated sense of the mobillity of the placenta. The placenta seen on the mother's right (or anterior) at one moment may be on the left (or posterior) shortly thereafter, or on a later examination. These effects are most prominent in the second trimester when the amniotic fluid volume and placental size are great compared to the small fetus, and the pregnant uterus is quite malleable. The maternal urinary bladder volume often used in sonography may equal or exceed the size of such a uterus, and displace and contort it. Sandler et al. found that over 50% of 13–21-week and almost 25% of 24–34-week gestations seen for amniocentesis had a different placental position after the mother voided.[93] This underscores the importance of performing sonography at the time and place of second-trimester amniocentesis with the same urinary bladder volume for both procedures. As a rule this is best done with an empty bladder, which is also a more physiologic state for a meaningful description of placental position. The converse may also be useful, when a difficult placental position can be improved by performing the amniocentesis with the bladder filled to an optimal degree. Uterine contractions and the selection of diagnostic scan planes also affect the perception of placental position in the second trimester.

## Placenta Previa

The major value of ultrasonic placental localization is in the recognition of placenta previa. Placenta previa and premature separation of the placenta account for most cases of third-trimester bleeding. Maternal complications, in addition to those due to blood loss, include an increased incidence of placenta accreta, and unrelenting postpartum bleeding from other causes. In a prospective collaborative study of 53,518 pregnancies, the perinatal mortality for placenta previa of about 10% was due to blood loss, premature placental separation, or complications of early delivery.[94] An increased incidence of growth retardation was present, but the surviving children on later examination were normal in growth and development, indicating that their hardship was due to the intrauterine condition. Early detection is desirable as there is an initial peak of fetal death and bleeding due to placenta previa between 20 and 30 weeks' gestation. The incidence of placenta previa increases with maternal age, multiparity, and prior cesarean sections.[22]

Complete (or total or central) placenta previa is present when the thick midportion of the placenta overlies the internal cervical os. This sonographic diagnosis is more reliable than partial placenta previa (the peripheral portion of the placenta inserted upon the internal os), or marginal previa (the placenta extending to or very near the internal cervical os).[95] It is important to distinguish the degree of placenta previa when the corresponding obstetric approach differs, but it is not possible reliably to subclassify placenta previa unless the internal os is precisely identified. "Low-lying placenta" is a vague expression that has widely different limits in popular use, and sometimes its use includes placenta previa. Its use should be limited to those placentas which are not previa, but are close enough to the internal os to have some possible physiologic significance. As this level is not established, it would be well if an arbitrary limit were agreed upon, such as within 2 cm of the internal cervical os.[96] These definitions are often less precise in clinical practice than on the printed page, both by necessity and by neglect. As will be seen, there is probably no area of diagnostic ultrasound with more conflicting reports, diverse clinical results, and unusual concepts than second-trimester placenta previa. Definitions, criteria, and techniques of examination vary widely, and the conclusions of one group frequently disagree with those of another. It may be difficult to derive a clear physiologic understanding of events or a reasonable clinical approach from these offerings. Bowie's group, among others, devotes great attention to this problem, has reported outstanding results, and has unique techniques that are therefore worthy of emulation.[96-98]

There is an urge to err in the direction of overdiagnosis of placenta previa, as false negative examinations can lead to catastrophe.[99] Fortunately, false negative reports of placenta previa are rare. Accurate resolution of this issue on the first obstetric ultrasound examination is desirable and usually possible.[96] The number of unnecessary examinations can thereby be reduced and needless cost, confusion, and anxiety avoided.

### Anatomy of the Lower Uterus

A firm grasp of the anatomy of the lower uterus is needed to avoid pitfalls and allow the correct identification of the internal cervical os, a necessity in evaluating placenta previa. There are few reliable anatomical landmarks of the pregnant uterus in diagnostic ultrasound imaging. The vagina, cervical tip, endocervical canal, external isthmus, and placenta are often easier to identify than the internal cervical os. The cervix is the most fixed point of the uterus, being bound to the bony pelvis by the uterosacral ligaments posteriorly, the pubocervical fascia anteriorly, and the cardinal ligaments laterally. It undergoes the least change in size and shape during pregnancy. An echodense line attributed to vaginal mucus extends from the direction of the introitus and ends in the midvaginal axis at the cervix. Laterally this line may continue alongside the cervix into the lateral fornices. The external cervical os is at the intravaginal tip of the cervix. The superior limit of the anatomical cervix is the external isthmus, an alteration in the external contour of the uterus that identifies the lower uterine segment. The collar-like narrowing that gives the isthmus its name may sometimes be seen, but often only the tapering walls of the muscular uterine body meeting the parallel walls of the cervix mark its location. The maternal bladder may compress this area and cause the isthmus to appear to be more superiorly located than it actually is. In early pregnancy the conceptus does not normally extend into or expand the lower uterine segment. When the bladder is large or the lower segment is not opened, one must not be tempted to use the junction of the anterior and posterior uterine walls or the inferior limits of the amniotic fluid to identify the internal cervical os, as this is simply not accurate. At some time, usually in early or middle second trimester, the conceptus will become large enough to fill and expand the lower segment. Still later the lower segment will efface, thin out, and dilate.

The internal cervical os is located just inferior to the external isthmus. The endocervical canal is usually seen on sonograms as a line of increased or decreased echogenicity. The punctate superior termination of that line is the internal cervical os and is about the size of a nail head prior to dilatation. The nonpregnant cervix averages about 2.5 cm in length, and enlarges during pregnancy until effacement begins. The cervix probably never exceeds 6 cm in length.[100] Cervical effacement usually occurs late in pregnancy and begins superiorly,[101] moving the apparent internal os inferiorly. In the absence of placenta previa the placenta will appear to move away from the "os," even though physiologically the opposite is occurring, i.e., the "os" is moving away from the placenta. A placenta that had been immediately adjacent to the cervix may appear to be several centimeters from the "os" at full effacement. Dilation increases this distance even further.

### First Trimester

The location of the placenta may first be anticipated sonographically at about 6 weeks' gestation if a double sac sign is noted.[30] One side of the gestational sac has a sonolucent stripe within the echodense rim. This identifies the uterine lumen between the decidua vera of the endometrium and the decidua capsularis or chorion frondosum. The opposite surface of the conceptus, where the double ring is not present, is the decidua basalis, from which the placenta arises. The placenta may be predicted as anterior, posterior, fundal, or caudal. The implantation may then also be judged as high or low within the uterus. Low implantation has been assumed to be the forerunner of placenta previa, though interpretations of sonograms have challenged this understanding. The conceptus, in a normal high implantation, is confined to the uterine body, and the lower uterine segment is not expanded. Even if the placenta is in a caudal position in that situation, it is doubtful that it should be designated a placenta previa as, by definition, the pregnancy and the placenta do not extend to the internal cervical os. This is best called simply a caudally located placenta. The pregnancy, as it grows, will dilate and fill the lower segment and extend inferiorly beyond the placental implantation. Then the placenta will no longer be in the caudal position. This transition may be marked by some maternal bleeding from the disrupted margin of the placenta. The bleeding is usually limited and benign and is unlikely to adversely affect the outcome of the pregnancy.

As the uterus grows during pregnancy, the placenta will appear to recede from the cervix, a process called "placental migration" by King.[89, 102] This has been likened to the phenomenon of the imprinted decal on a balloon moving away from the orifice as the balloon is inflated.[103] In this analogy it can be seen that simply generalized enlargement of the balloon or uterus may cause this retreat. In the pregnant uterus there is also differential growth. The placenta does not continue to keep up with the growth of the fetus, or with the uterus, which must expand to house its growing contents. The relative surface area the placenta covers diminishes in proportion to the difference in growth. The expansion of the lower uterine segment and effacement of the cervix also contribute to the effect of the placenta increasing its distance from the uterine orifice. For this reason, ultrasound examinations are recommended late in pregnancy when placenta previa has been diagnosed earlier. The inferior edge of a marginal or partial placenta previa may separate enough after effacement and dilatation of the cervix to allow fetal passage per vagina. If the internal os can be visualized at that time, the obstetric judgment regarding vaginal delivery or cesarean section may be assisted.

### Second Trimester

In the second trimester the reasonable expectation of increased accuracy of diagnostic ultrasound imaging in the diagnosis of placenta previa was initially stunningly disappointing. Using bistable technology and pioneering techniques of that day, Wexler and Gottesfeld initially diagnosed placenta previa or low-lying placentas in almost half of the second-trimester pregnancies examined.[104] Compared to the known term incidence of placenta previa of about 0.5%, this is a predictive error of about 10,000%! As technical and interpretative skills improved, fewer and fewer second-trimester placenta previas were reported. Among other factors, it is evident that the most midtrimester placenta previas were reported when the mother was imaged with a full urinary bladder; the incidence was less in women who partially emptied the bladder before imaging,[105] and almost nil in those examined with an empty bladder.[96] Because the later in pregnancy the diagnosis is made, the more reliable it is likely to be, all second-trimester diagnoses of placenta previa should be confirmed on a late third-trimester examination.

False diagnoses of placenta previa have been related to large maternal urinary bladder volumes, myometrial contractions, use of erroneous scan planes, and extrachorionic hematomas. The distended maternal bladder[90, 97] or a myometrial contraction[91] may squeeze the lower uterine walls together. This constriction of the lower uterus in midpregnancy displaces the fetus and amniotic fluid superiorly, creating an apparent inferior location of the anchored placenta. If the junction of the compressed anterior and posterior uterine walls is regarded as the internal cervical os, its perceived location will be related to the degree of bladder filling and the presence or absence of uterine contractions. So, too, will be the likelihood of erroneously diagnosing placenta previa. Useful approximations used in the past included assuming that the internal cervical os was always in the midline, at the junction of the anterior and posterior uterine walls, at the lower margin of the amniotic fluid; was unaffected by maternal urinary bladder volume; was on a tangential line from the anterior uterine wall; could be seen on transverse scans; or that its sonographic location could be accurately related to physical examination. These criteria are no longer needed and should not be considered reliable substitutes for anatomical identification of this critical landmark.

A myometrial contraction often results in distortion of the lower uterus and the contained pregnancy. It is seen as a thickening of the uterine wall, usually an inwardly convex local expansion.[92] Its persistence may make it difficult to distinguish from a myoma, which may be more sonolucent than the remainder of the myometrium. A myoma is more likely than a contraction to distort the external uterine contour. In the lower uterus where the diameter is relatively small, the contraction may be circumferential, corresponding to circumferential muscle fibers. Uterine contractions are frequently seen in pregnancy (71% of Wilson's examinations), tend to be single, occur about equally anteriorly or posteriorly, and are usually seen under or close to the placenta, especially in the first trimester. It is possible that contractions are more common and prolonged during sonographic examinations because of the direct stimulation of the uterine musculature by the oppressive bladder volume. The chorionic surface of the placenta should be a flat to concave plane, but may be caused to bulge centally by an underlying uterine contraction or by a mass, including myoma, retroplacental hematoma, or a large maternal bladder. Occasionally the bulging chorionic surface of the lower margin of the placenta may innocently come to overlie the internal os and opposite uterine wall. This should not be mistaken for implantation over the os and wrongly called previa.

Hematomas in the distal uterine lumen may simulate placenta previa.[106] Hematomas may be echofree, septated, or have random echogenicity. The latter most resembles the placenta, and if the evolution through sonolucency or septation is not witnessed ultrasonically, only subtle echo quality distinction from the true placenta may allow recognition on a single examination. Because such cases always present with bleeding there is great temptation for the sonographer to confirm the clinical suspicion of placenta previa.

An association between transverse fetal lie and false placenta previa has been observed.[107] As with the previa diagnosis, few of these are actually transverse lies at term.[108] Placenta previa and pelvic tumors detour the usual vertical fetal attitude and are known to be associated with transverse lie. The large maternal bladder volume or uterine contraction responsible for a false previa diagnosis during sonography has the same mass effect as a pelvic tumor or placenta previa, producing a transverse lie. The fetus is displaced superiorly and the long axis of the uterus is shortened sagitally and increased transversely. The fetus probably accommodates passively to these dimensions by assuming a transverse attitude.

### Third Trimester

In third-trimester examinations in which women were imaged with full bladders and without postvoiding

studies, and in which the internal os was defined as the junction of the anterior and posterior walls, 82% (9/11) of women diagnosed as having placenta previa did not at delivery (false positives).[109] The impact of maternal urinary bladder volume cannot be overemphasized. Bowie et al. reported that nine of ten false positive diagnoses of placenta previa in late second and third trimester were recognized retrospectively as observer error due to large maternal bladder size.[9] Gorodeski et al., apparently using postvoiding examinations, reported no false positives in 56 diagnoses of placenta previa in a group of 159 third-trimester patients referred for vaginal bleeding.[110] Kurjak and Barsic reported no false positives in their four cases diagnosed in the third trimester by reexamining as close to delivery as possible.[111]

### Technique of Examination

If the internal cervical os is not covered by the overlying placenta, placenta previa is excluded. Placenta previa must be evaluated on a longitudinal scan which includes and demonstrates the internal cervical os, and preferably the inferior limits of the placenta as well. Transverse scans simply show the relationship of the placenta to the junction of the anterior and posterior uterine walls and do not allow identification of the internal os. Midsagittal scans are not necessarily appropriate, as the long axis of the uterus often does not coincide with that of the mother.

The level of the internal cervical os along the endocervical canal may be identified in relation to the external isthmus. When it cannot be otherwise identified the internal os may be assumed to be no further than 6 cm from the external cervical os, the maximum length of the cervix in pregnancy.[100] It follows that, if the placenta is more than 6 cm from the cervical tip, it cannot overlie the internal cervical os, and therefore does not fulfill the textbook definition of placenta previa. It is unclear whether a caudally located placenta may bridge across the lower segment and represent a physiologic placenta previa even though it does not adhere to the anatomicaly internal os. If placenta previa is not excluded by this examination, the patient should be reexamined after partially emptying her bladder. One may need to wait for the subsidence of a myometrial contraction, if present. Bowie et al. were able to visualize the cervix with an empty maternal urinary bladder in most patients at less than 30 weeks' gestation, but rarely in later pregnancy.[98] When successfully visualized, the cervix appeared significantly shorter (3.25 vs. 4.6 cm) than when the bladder was moderately filled. False locations of the internal os result in misplacing it superiorly, closer to the placenta. This is why false positive results are much more common than false negative results. Positive and doubtful cases are routinely reexamined in late pregnancy to reevaluate the diagnosis of placenta previa.

The placenta is generally easily identified except when a posterior placenta is obscured in late pregnancy by the overlying fetus. Placenta previa is unlikely when the space between the presenting fetal head and the maternal sacrum is 1.5 cm or less, according to King.[89] The apparent distance may be decreased by the extrinsic pressure of the transducer by a heavy-handed sonographer. The presenting fetal head often may be displaced superiorly by careful external manipulation,[112] which may be facilitated by the Trendelenburg position,[113] to permit visualization of the internal cervical os and accurately determine if the lower limits of the placenta extend to it. As a last resort, a skilled obstetrician may elect to manually displace the head per vagina. It is more difficult to elevate a breech.

The recognition of the common false diagnoses of second-trimester placenta previas and the present understanding of uniform growth, differential growth, expansion of the lower segment, and effacement of the cervix offer an explanation of placental migration. Placental migration may be simply the result of false positive early diagnoses of placenta previa. If rigid diagnostic techniques are used, few early placenta previas are detected, eliminating the basis for these concepts.[96]

## Abruptio Placentae and Retroplacental Hemorrhage

Abruptio placentae appears in the second half of pregnancy. The clinical picture may include vaginal bleeding, abdominal pain, hypertonic uterus, and fetal death. Blood loss may progress to shock, renal failure, coagulopathy, and maternal death. Abruptio placentae may complicate preeclampsia, but often there is no associated prior abnormality. The underlying pathology is premature separation of the placenta and retroplacental hemorrhage, but these events are more likely to occur without any such symptoms and without significant clinical sequelae. These three terms,

abruptio placentae, premature separation of the placenta, and retroplacental hemorrhage, are sometimes used interchangeably. They are probably best regarded as a spectrum, with silent small retroplacental hemorrhage the mildest form and symptomatic abruption the most severe. The diagnosis, in any case, has always been difficult to confirm. Detection is based in large part on the presence of an underlying hematoma, but a loculated hematoma may not form or it may not remain confined in the retroplacental area. Perhaps some fresh clots pass unnoticed during delivery, and some may organize and resorb, but pathologic confirmation is generally found in only 30% of clinical diagnoses.[20]

The ultrasonic sine qua non of abruptio placentae is the depiction of the retroplacental hematoma, and therefore only a small minority of cases are detected clinically. Such cases may have no associated vaginal bleeding. The hematoma is most often seen as a biconvex well-marginated, echo-free area. Like hematomas located elsewhere, retroplacental hematomas may be echo free, septated, or partially or fully echogenic. To be detected ultrasonically, a retroplacenta hematoma must be distinguishable from the sonolucency of the vessels normally visualized retroplacentally. The use of appropriate transducer frequency and focal length may be technically important to demonstrate such areas, especially for contact scanning of smaller anterior hematomas. In the case of large hematomas the mass effect of the hematoma may cause the placenta and chorionic plate to bulge inwardly, resembling a myometrial contraction or retroplacental myoma,[114] but the increased ultrasound transmission of hematomas is usually distinct from the attenuation of solid tissue.

More often nonspecific sonographic findings are present. When the hemorrhage does not remain localized in the retroplacental area the blood flows into the uterine lumen where it may be seen sonographically between the chorion and the uterine wall. These patients usually present with vaginal bleeding. This is most likely when the hemorrhage occurs from a peripheral area of the placenta, sometimes called marginal abruption. The extrachorionic hematoma appears as a membrane flanked by fluid on both sides, a picture that may be confused with chorioamniotic separation or an intra-amniotic septum dividing the imaged amniotic pool.[36, 37] It is useful to attempt to identify this "floating" membrane, as there is a different significance whether it is chorion with external blood, amnion with peripheral chorionic or amniotic fluid, or an intrauterine septation. (Differentiation was discussed in the section on Membranes and Umbilical Cord.) In the case of an intra-amniotic septation, fetal parts may often be seen to enter the outer fluid collection, which cannot occur with either a hematoma or chorioamniotic separation.[114] In amniotic band syndrome, the membrane is fixed to the fetus, which may be edematous or deformed.

Blood may dissect into the myometrium or placenta, creating sonolucent strips and sometimes expanding the thickness of the respective structure. Bleeding into the uterine wall is the cause of the hypertonic, rigid uterus in the symptomatic complex. Jaffe et al. found the placentas in a small group of controls to be no more than 5 cm thick, but some placentas of the group with abruptio placentae had thicknesses of up to 9 cm.[115] The placental margin was rounded in appearance more often in the study group than in controls, and other abnormal findings were usually present as well. Placental thrombus or infarct may rarely be distinguishable as a demarcated sonolucent or echogenic area within the placenta in association with retroplacental bleeding, but such findings also occur without associated bleeding. Occasionally blood that has dissected into the amniotic fluid may also be seen as random echoes, as a blood-fluid horizontal interface, or as a mass-like clot that may resemble a placental tumor.[28]

The foremost danger of this condition to the fetus is not the hematoma per se but the resulting loss of functioning tissue upon which its sustenance depends. Fox states than an otherwise healthy fetus may survive the loss of 30%–40% of the functioning placenta, but a lesser loss might doom an unhealthy fetus or high-risk pregnancy.[20] Nonstress testing and ultrasound imaging may play a role in following such cases, as the bleeding at the placenta-maternal interface may continue after the initial episode. It has been suggested that when a retroplacental hematoma can be seen on sonography, monitoring its size and growth may be useful in managing these patients,[116] but the size of the residual clot may not reflect the amount of placenta that may infarct in response to the vascular impairment. At this time clinical experience is too limited for firm conclusions to be drawn.

Fox described marginal hematomas in about 2% of term placentas. These hematomas nestle against the lateral margin of the placenta extending along the external surface of the membranes. They have been thought to be due to bleeding at the inferior margin of low-lying placentas, a minimal form of retroplacental bleeding. Such hematomas should be highly visible to the sonographer. In fact, a marginal extrachorionic sonolucency is occasionally seen at this site in the late first or early second trimester, associated with vaginal bleeding.[117, 118] In the collective data reported, 8 of 43 (18.6%) went on to fetal death or spontaneous abortion. Goldstein et al. reported on 40 prospective mothers with vaginal bleeding who did not have an extrachorionic hematoma detected on sonography. They continued to term and produced healthy babies. If the presence of a detectable hematoma seems to increase the risk, the size of the collection may offer little predictive value. Such fluid collections are sometimes interpreted by sonographers as second gestational sacs and called blighted twin ova.

Abruptio placentae is not always spontaneous. An isolated instance has been reported following amniocentesis.[119] About 2% of cases of retroplacental hemorrhage are due to trauma, most commonly an automobile accident. The shearing forces of deceleration are thought to disrupt one or more of the placenta-uterine interface vessels. Retroplacental hemorrhage is the most common cause of fetal death when the mother survives following trauma. It usually occurs within 48 hours after the trauma, but has been delayed as long as 5 days.[120] As a normal sonogram does not exclude retroplacental hemorrhage, continuous fetal monitoring for 48 hours or more after trauma may be important in evaluating that possible complication.

## References

1. Fox H: Placental structure, in MacDonald RR (ed): *Scientific Basis of Obstetrics and Gynecology.* New York, Churchill Livingstone, 1978, pp 30–35.
2. Kaiser IH: Fertilization and the physiology and development of fetus and placenta, in Danforth DN (ed): *Obstetrics and Gynecology,* ed 3. Hagerstown, Md, Harper & Row, 1977.
3. Hertig AT, Rock J, Adams EC, et al: On preimplantation stages of the human ovum. *Contrib Embryol* 1954; 35:199.
4. Edmonds DK, Lindsay KS, Miller JF, et al: Early

embryonic mortality in women. *Fertil Steril* 1982; 38:447.

5.  Robinson HP, Shaw-Dunn J: Fetal heart rates as determined by sonar in early pregnancy. *Br J Obstet Gynaecol* 1973; 80:805.

6.  Ramsey EM, Martin CR Jr, Donner MW: Fetal and maternal placental circulations: Simultaneous visualization in monkeys by radiography. *Am J Obstet Gynecol* 1967; 98:419.

7.  Bleker OP, Kloosterman GJ, Mieras DJ, et al: Intervillous space during uterine contractions in human subjects: An ultrasound study. *Am J Obstet Gynecol* 1975; 123:697.

8.  Hoddick WK, Mahony BS, Callen PW, et al: Placental thickness. *J Ultrasound Med* 1985; 4:479.

9.  Goodlin RC, Anderson JC, Skiles TL: Pruritis and hyperplacentosis. *Obstet Gynecol* 1985; 66:36s.

10. Seeds JW: Impaired fetal growth: Definition and clinical diagnosis. *Obstet Gynecol* 1984; 64:303.

11. Lunell NO, Sarby B, Lewander R, et al: Comparison of uteroplacental blood flow in normal and in intrauterine growth-retarded pregnancy. *Gynecol Obstet Invest* 1979; 10:106.

12. Westergaard JG, Teisner B, Hau J, et al: Placental function studies in low birth weight infants with and without dysmaturity. *Obstet Gynecol* 1985; 65:316.

13. Jeanty P, Kirkpatrick C, Verhoogen C, et al: The succenturiate placenta. *J Ultrasound Med* 1983; 2:9.

14. Molloy CE, McDowell W, Armour T, et al: Ultrasonic diagnosis of placenta membranacea in utero. *J Ultrasound Med* 1983; 2:377.

15. McGahan JP, Phillips HE, Reid MH: The anechoic retroplacental area. *Radiology* 1980; 134:475.

16. Smith DF, Foley WD: Real-time ultrasound and pulsed Doppler evaluation of the retroplacental clear area. *JCU* 1982; 10:215.

17. Marx M, Casola G, Scheible W, et al: The subplacental complex. *J Ultrasound Med* 1985; 4:459.

18. Tabsh KMA, Brinkman CR, King W: Ultrasound diagnosis of placenta increta. *JCU* 1982; 10:288.

19. Pasto ME, Kurtz AB, Rifkin MD, et al: Ultrasonographic findings in placenta increta. *J Ultrasound Med* 1983; 2:155.

20. Fox H: Pathology of the placenta, in Bennington L (ed): *Major Problems in Pathology.* Philadelphia, WB Saunders Co, 1978, vol 7.

21. Read J, Cotton DB, Miller F: Placenta accreta: Changing clinical aspects and outcome. *Obstet Gynecol* 1980; 56:31.

22. Clark SL, Koonings PP, Phelan JP: Placenta previa/accreta and prior cesarean section. *Obstet Gynecol* 1985; 66:89.

23. Clark SL, Yeh S, Phelan JP, et al: Emergency hysterectomy for obstetric hemorrhage. *Obstet Gynecol* 1984; 64:376.

24. Rodan BA, Bean WJ: Chorioangioma of the placenta causing intrauterine fetal demise. *J Ultrasound Med* 1983; 2:95.

25. Hurwitz A, Milwidsky A, Yarkoni S: Severe fetal distress with hydramnios due to chorioangioma. *Acta Obstet Gynecol Scand* 1983; 62:633.

26. Tonkin IL, Setzer Es, Brmocilla R: Placental chorioangioma: A rare cause of congestive heart failure and hydrops fetalis in the newborn. *AJR* 1980; 134:181.

27. Spirt BA, Gordon L, Cohen WN, et al: Antenatal diagnosis of chorioangioma of the placenta. *AJR* 1980; 135:1278.

28. McGahan JP, Phillips HE, Reid MH, et al: Sonographic spectrum of retroplacenta hemorrhage. *Radiology* 1982; 142:481.

29. O'Malley BP, Toi A, deSa DJ, et al: Ultrasound appearance of placental chorioangioma. *Radiology* 1981; 138:159.

30. Burrows PE, Lyons EA, Philips J, et al: Intrauterine membranes: Sonographic findings and clinical significance. *JCU* 1982; 10:1.

31. Bradley WG, Fiske CE, Filly RA: The double sac sign of early intrauterine pregnancy: Use in exclusion of ectopic pregnancy. *Radiology* 1982; 143:223.

32. Nelson P, Bowie, JD, Rosenberg ER: Early intrauterine pregnancy or decidual cast: An anatomic-sonographic approach. *J Ultrasound Med* 1983; 2:543.

33. Nyberg DA, Laing FC, Filly RA, et al: Ultrasonographic differentiation of the gestational sac of early intrauterine pregnancy from the pseudogestational sac of ectopic pregnancy. *Radiology* 1983; 146:755.

34. Cadkin AV, McAlpin J: The decidua-chorionic sac: A reliable sonographic indicator of intra-uterine pregnancy prior to detection of a fetal pole. *J Ultrasound Med* 1984; 3:539.

35. Baker MD, Mahony BS, Bowie JD: Adverse effect of an overdistended bladder on first trimester sonography. *AJR* 1985; 145:597.

36. Jeanty P, Renov P, Van Kerkem J, et al: Ultrasonic demonstration of the amnion. *J Ultrasound Med* 1982; 1:243.

37. Kaufman AJ, Fleischer AC, Thieme GA, et al: Separated chorioamnion and elevated chorion: Sonographic features and clinical significance. *J Ultrasound Med* 1985; 4:119.

38. Fiske CE, Filly RA, Golbus MS: Prenatal ultrasound diagnosis of amniotic band syndrome. *J Ultrasound Med* 1982; 1:45.

39. Bree RL: Sonographic identification of fetal vernix in amniotic fluid. *JCU* 1978; 6:269.

40. Gross TL, Wolfson RN, Kuhnert PM, et al: Sonographically detected free-floating particles in amniotic fluid predict a mature lecithin-sphingomyelin ratio. *JCU* 1985; 13:405.

41. Mullin TJ, Gross TL, Wolfson RN: Ultrasound screening for free-floating particles and fetal lung maturity. *Obstet Gynecol* 1985; 66:50.

42. Khaleghian R: Echogenic amniotic fluid in the second trimester: A new sign of fetal distress. *JCU* 1983; 11:498.

43. Paruleker SG: Ultrasonographic demonstration of floating particles in amniotic fluid. *J Ultrasound Med* 1983; 2:107.

44. Jasseni MN, Brennan JN, Merkatz IR: Prenatal diagnosis of single umbilical artery by ultrasound. *JCU* 1980; 8:447.

45. Abrams SL, Callen PW, Filly RA: Umbilical vein thrombosis: Sonographic detection in utero. *J Ultrasound Med* 1985; 4:283.

46. Casola G, Scheible W, Leopold GR: Large umbilical cord: A normal finding in some fetuses. *Radiology* 1985; 156:181.

47. Sutro WE, Tuck SM, Loesevitz A, et al: Prenatal observation of umbilical cord hematoma. *AJR* 1984; 142:801.

48. Seifer DB, Ferguson JE II, Behrens CM, et al: Nonimmune hydrops fetalis in association with hemangioma of the umbilical cord. *Obstet Gynecol* 1985; 66:283.

49. Davies BR, Casanueva E, Arrovo P: Placentas of small-for-dates infants: A small controlled series from Mexico City, Mexico. *Am J Obstet Gynecol* 1984; 149:731.

50. Spirt BA, Kagan EH, Rozanski RM: Sonolucent areas in the placenta: A sonographic and pathologic correlation. *AJR* 1978; 131:961.

51. Morin F, Winsberg F: Real-time identification of blood flow in the placenta and umbilical cord. *JCU* 1982; 10:21.

52. Fox H: White infarcts of the placenta. *Br J Obstet Gynaecol* 1963; 70:980.

53. Perkes EA, Baim RS, Goodman KJ, et al: Second trimester placental changes associated with increased maternal serum alpha-fetoprotein. *Am J Obstet Gynecol* 1982; 144:935.

54. Spirt BA, Cohen WN, Weinstein HM: The incidence of placental calcification in normal pregnancies. *Radiology* 1982; 142:707.

55. Winsberg F: Echogenic changes with placental aging. *JCU* 1973; 1:52.

56. Fisher CC, Garrett W, Kossoff G: Placental aging monitored by gray scale echography. *Am J Obstet Gynecol* 1976; 124:483.

57. Cooperberg PL, Wright VJ, Carpenter CW: Ultrasonic demonstration of a placental maternal lake. *JCU* 1979; 7:62.

58. Haney AF, Trought WS: The sonolucent placenta in high risk obstetrics. *Obstet Gynecol* 1980; 55:38.

59. Spirt BA, Gordon LP, Kagan EH: Intervillous thrombosis: Sonographic and pathologic correlation. *Radiology* 1983; 147:197.

60. Grannum P, Berkowitz RL, Hobbins JC: The ultrasonic changes in the maturing placenta and their relation to fetal pulmonic maturity. *Am J Obstet Gynecol* 1979; 133:915.

61. Kollitz J, Dattel BJ, Key TC, et al: Acute respiratory distress syndrome in an infant with grade III placental changes. *J Ultrasound Med* 1982; 1:205.

62. Gast MJ, Ott W: Failure of ultrasonic placental grading to predict severe respiratory distress in a neonate. *Am J Obstet Gynecol* 1983; 146:464.

63. Kazzi GM, Gross TL, Rosen MG, et al: The relationship of placental grade, fetal lung maturity, and neonatal outcome in normal and complicated pregnancies. *Am J Obstet Gynecol* 1984; 148:54.

64. Harman CR, Manning FA, Stearns E, et al: The correlation of ultrasonic placental grading and fetal pulmonary maturity. *Am J Obstet Gynecol* 1982; 145:941.

65. Raggozino MW, Hill LM, Breckle R, et al: The relationship of placental grading by ultrasound to markers of fetal lung maturity. *Radiology* 1983; 148:805.

66. Tabsh KMW: Correlation of real-time ultrasonic placental grading with amniotic fluid lecithin-sphingomyelin ratio. *Am J Obstet Gynecol* 1983; 145:504.

67. Clair ME, Rosenberg B, Tempkin D, et al: Placental grading in the complicated or high risk pregnancy. *J Ultrasound Med* 1983; 2:297.

68. Hadlock FP, Irwin JF, Roecker E, et al: Ultrasound prediction of fetal lung maturity. *Radiology* 1985; 155:469.

69. Ashton SA, Russo MP, Simon NV, et al: Relationship between grade III placentas and biparietal diameter determinations. *J Ultrasound Med* 1983; 2:127.

70. Havashi RH, Berry JL, Castillo MS: Use of ultrasound biparietal diameter in timing of repeat Cesarean section. *Obstet Gynecol* 1981; 57:325.

71. Petrucha RA, Golde SH, Platt LD: The use of ultrasound in the prediction of fetal pulmonary maturity. *Am J Obstet Gynecol* 1982; 144:931.

72. Tabsh KMA: Correlation of ultrasonic epiphyseal centers and the lecithin:sphingomyelin ratio. *Obstet Gynecol* 1985; 64:92.

73. Crawford DC, Fenton DW, Brice WI: Ultrasonic tissue characterization of the placenta: Is it of clinical value? *JCU* 1985; 13:533.

74. Benson DM, Waldrop LD, Kurtz AB, et al: Ultrasonic tissue characterization of fetal lung, liver, and placenta for the purpose of assessing fetal maturity. *J Ultrasound Med* 1983; 2:489.

75. Fried AM, Loh GK, Umer MA, et al: Echogenicity of fetal lung: Relation to fetal age and maturity. *AJR* 1985; 145:591.

76. Cayea PD, Grant DC, Doubilet PM, et al: Prediction of fetal lung maturity: Inaccuracy of study using conventional ultrasound instruments. *Radiology* 1985; 155:473.

77. Quinlan RW, Cruz AC, Buhi WC, et al: Changes in placental ultrasonic appearance: II. Pathologic significance of grade III placental changes. *Am J Obstet Gynecol* 1982; 144:471.

78. Kazzi GM, Gross TL, Sokol RJ, et al: Detection of intrauterine growth retardation: A new use for sonographic placental grading. *Am J Obstet Gynecol* 1983; 145:733.

79. Patterson RM, Hayashi RH, Cavazos D: Ultrasonically observed early placental maturation and perinatal outcome. *Am J Obstet Gynecol* 1983; 147:773.

80. Hills D, Irwin GAL, Tuck S, et al: Distribution of placental grade in high-risk gravidas. *AJR* 1984; 143:1011.

81. Kazzi GM, Gross TL, Sokol RJ: Fetal biparietal diameter and placental grade: Predictors of intrauterine growth retardation. *Obstet Gynecol* 1984; 62:755.

82. Hopper KD, Komppa GH, Bice P, et al: A reevaluation of placental grading and its clinical significance. *J Ultrasound Med* 1984; 3:261.

83. Rayburn W, et al: Antepartum prediction of the postmature infant. *Obstet Gynecol* 1982; 60:148.

84. Moya F, et al: Ultrasound assessment of the postmature pregnancy. *Obstet Gynecol* 1985; 65:319–332.

85. Yeh S, Petrucha R, Platt LD: Possible role of ultrasonic placental grading in predicting fetal dysmaturity in postterm pregnancies, in *Proceedings of the Society of Perinatal Obstetricians,* 1982, p 139.

86. Batson JL, Winn K, Dubin NH, et al: Placental immaturity associated with anencephaly. *Obstet Gynecol* 1985; 65:846.

87. Gottesfeld KR, Thompson HE, Holmes JH, et al: Ultrasonic placentography—a new method for placental localization. *Am J Obstet Gynecol* 1966; 96:538.

88. Callen PW, Filly RA: The placental-subplacental complex: A specific indicator of placental position on ultrasound. *JCU* 1980; 8:21.

89. King DL: Placental ultrasonography. *JCU* 1973; 1:21.

90. Zemlyn S: The effect of the urinary bladder in obstetrical sonography. *Radiology* 1978; 128:169.

91. Buttery B, Davison G: The dynamic uterus revealed by time-lapse echography. *JCU* 1978; 6:19.

92. Wilson RL, Worthen NJ: Ultrasonic demonstra-

tion of myometrial contractions in intrauterine pregnancy. *AJR* 1978; 132:243.

93. Sandler MA, Sznewajs SM, Bitvk LL: The effect of the distended urinary bladder on placental position and its importance in amniocentesis. *Radiology* 1979; 130:195–199.

94. Naeve RL: Placenta previa: Predisposing factors and effects on the fetus and surviving infants. *Obstet Gynecol* 1978; 52:521.

95. Gillieson MS, Winer-Muram HT, Muram D: Low-lying placenta. *Radiology* 1982; 144:577.

96. Artis AA, Bowie JD, Rosenberg ER, et al: The fallacy of placental migration: Effect of sonographic techniques. *AJR* 1985; 144:79.

97. Bowie JD, Rochester D, Cadkin AV, et al: Accuracy of placental localization by ultrasound. *Radiology* 1978; 128:177.

98. Bowie JD, Andreotti RF, Rosenberg ER: Sonographic appearance of the uterine cervix in pregnancy: The vertical cervix. *AJR* 1983; 140:737.

99. Laing FC: Placenta previa: Avoiding false-negative diagnoses. *JCU* 1981; 9:109.

100. Zemlyn S: The length of the uterine cervix and its significance. *JCU* 1981; 9:267.

101. Danforth DN: The morphology of the human cervix. *Clin Obstet Gynecol* 1983; 26:7.

102. King DL: Placental migration demonstrated by ultrasonography. *Radiology* 1973; 109:167.

103. Shaub MS, Sarti DA: Obstetrical ultrasonography, in Sarti DA, Sample WF (eds): *Diagnostic Ultrasound: Text and Cases.* Boston, GK Hall, 1980, p 596.

104. Wexler P, Gottesfeld KR: Second trimester placenta previa: An apparently normal placentation. *Obstet Gynecol* 1977; 50:706.

105. Rizos N, Duran TA, Miskin M, et al: Natural history of placenta previa ascertained by diagnostic ultrasound. *Am J Obstet Gynecol* 1979; 138:287.

106. Williams CH, VanBergen WS, Prentice RL: Extra-amniotic blood clot simulating placenta previa on ultrasound scan. *JCU* 1976; 5:45.

107. Lees RF, Teates CD: False placenta previa: A clinical observation. *JCU* 1978; 6:44.

108. Fried AW, Cloutier M, Woodring JH, et al: Sonography of the transverse fetal lie. *AJR* 1984; 142:421.

109. Mittelstaedt CA, Partain CL, Boyce IL, et al: Placenta praevia: Significance in the second trimester. *Radiology* 1979; 131:465.

110. Gorodeski IG, Neri A, Haimovich L, et al: Placenta previa: The ultrasonographic placental localization and its influence on the mode of delivery. *J Reprod Med* 1982; 27:655.

111. Kurjak A, Barsio B: Changes of placental site diagnosed by repeated ultrasonic examination. *Acta Obstet Gynecol Scand* 1977; 56:161.

112. Lee TG, Knochel JQ, Melendez MG, et al: Fetal elevation: A new technique for placental localization in the diagnosis of previa. *JCU* 1981; 9:467.

113. Jeffrey RB, Laing PC: Sonography of the low-lying placenta: Value of Trendelenburg and traction scans. *AJR* 1981; 137:547.

114. Spirt BA, Kagan EH, Rozanski RM: Abruptio placentae: Sonographic and pathologic correlation. *AJR* 1979; 133:877.

115. Jaffe MH, Schoen WC, Silver TM, et al: Sonography of abruptio placentae. *AJR* 1981; 137:1049.

116. Rivera-Alsina ME, Saldana IR, Maklad N, et al: The use of ultrasound in the expectant management of abruptio placentae. *Am J Obstet Gynecol* 1983; 143:924.

117. Goldstein SR, Subramanyam BR, Raghavendra BN, et al: Subchorionic bleeding in threatened abortion: Sonographic findings and significance. *AJR* 1983; 141:975.

118. Joupilla P: Clinical consequences after ultrasonic diagnosis of intrauterine hematoma in threatened abortion. *JCU* 1985; 13:107.

119. Zakut H, Lotan M, Ashiron R: Umbilical cord damage and placental abruption during amniocentesis. *Acta Obstet Gynecol Scand* 1984; 63:279.

120. Higgins SD, Garite T: Late abruptio placentae in trauma patients: Implications for monitoring. *Obstet Gynecol* 1984; 63:10s.

# 16d
# FETAL DATING

Lawrence D. Platt, M.D.
Greggory R. DeVore, M.D.
Janet Horenstein, M.D.

Accurate determination of gestational age is essential in the care and management of the pregnant patient. Information on gestational age allows one both to date the pregnancy and to distinguish normal from abnormal growth patterns. Traditional methods of determining pregnancy dates have relied on the patient's recollection of her last menstrual period and on the fundal height as assessed either by manual examination or by using a tape measure. Although fetal age in actuality begins with conception, the obstetric community dates pregnancy from the first day of the last menstrual period, thereby deriving a mean duration of pregnancy of 288 days. The ultrasound literature has proved to be somewhat confusing in that menstrual dating, fetal age, and gestational age have been used as reference points in establishing patterns of fetal development. In this chapter, pregnancy age is considered to date the last menstrual period.

Because of irregular menstrual cycles, a significant number of patients will not recall the time of their last menstrual period. In one study, Hertz et al.[1] reported that only 18% of patients were able to reliably give the dates of their last menstrual period. Wenner and Young[2] suggested the figure may be as high as 33%. The figure varies, depending on the population served. At Los Angeles County/USC Medical Center, which serves a large indigent population, approximately 40% of patients fail to provide an accurate gestational age assessment. In attempts to reduce the significant method-related variance in pregnancy dating, ultrasound morphometric measurements of fetal parts have been used to assess gestational age of the fetus, with improved accuracy. The following discussion addresses various ultrasonographic methods used in establishing gestational age.

At the outset it is imperative to understand that no single ultrasound measurements will precisely determine gestational age in every case. Even the best-prepared studies have reported a range of error in the predictive ability of one method or another to determine fetal age. It has generally been thought that the earlier the examination is performed, the more reliable the findings are. As a result of biologic variation, determination of fetal age after the first or second trimester will increase the error in these measurements.

## The Gravid Uterus

Studies on patients undergoing ovulation induction and in vitro fertilization have reported the changing appearance of the endometrial lining during different phases of the menstrual cycle.[4] These subtle changes can be clearly demonstrated on ultrasound examinations, but no studies have yet been carried out that describe a specific appearance of an endometrial lining corresponding to the first days of pregnancy. The first evidence of an intrauterine pregnancy is an anechoic area within the endometrial lining, seen 4½–5 weeks after the last menstrual period. This gestational sac is seen before a fetus is seen. Some authors have suggested that linear measurements of the gestational sac be utilized as a sign of gestational age.[5] However, a number of other investigators have stated that for patients with a reliable menstrual history, this method is no more accurate than the menstrual history. Measurements of the sac area and volume have proved to be more time-consuming with no improved accuracy. Therefore, it seems that dating of pregnancy prior to 6½ weeks' gestation is ineffective in improving pregnancy outcome. The benefits of dating pregnancy at this time seem negligible, and such examinations should be deferred until the second trimester, at which time accurate dating can be combined with a fetal anatomical survey. Occasionally some examiners have confused the yolk sac with a second, young fetus. Others have included the yolk sac in the crown-rump measurements. Both of these determinations may result in incorrect diagnoses.

Beginning at 6½–7 weeks' gestation, measurements of the fetal crown-rump length can be made and pregnancy can be dated to within 4–5 days. This single determination is one of the most accurate ways to assess pregnancy. The crown-rump length is measured along the long axis of the fetus and can be identified until 14 weeks' gestation. To improve accuracy the examiner should obtain multiple measurements and average them. Numerous tables have been published, but most rely on the data derived by Robinson and Fleming (Table 16D–1).[6] This particular work has stood the test of time and is most reliable. The use of real-time ultrasound simplifies this technique.[7]

It is our belief that this is the method of choice for early obstetric scanning. Whereas a sector linear-array or curved linear transducer can be used to measure crown-rump length, recent developments in transvaginal scanning are yielding remarkable images and may simplify the process.

Bovicelli et al.[8] have recently demonstrated the efficacy of measuring the biparietal diameter (BPD) in the first trimester for gestational age assessment. These investigators have also suggested that by combining the measurement of crown-rump length and BPD, one can narrow down the gestational age by an additional ½ to 1 day. Because of its minimal improvement, the additional steps, and the irregular shape of the fetal head, this technique has not gained wide acceptance.

## Second-Trimester Dating

The most commonly measured index of fetal size is the BPD. This measure was the most readily identified and apparently most reproducible in early studies. Un-

**TABLE 16D–1.**

**Fetal Crown-Rump Measurements vs. Fetal Age***

| MENSTRUAL MATURITY (WK + DAYS) | CORRECTED REGRESSIONAL ANALYSIS (CM); MEAN VALUES | MENSTRUAL MATURITY (WK + DAYS) | CORRECTED REGRESSIONAL ANALYSIS (CM); MEAN VALUES |
|---|---|---|---|
| 6 + 2 | 0.55 | 10 + 2 | 3.32 |
| 6 + 3 | 0.61 | 10 + 3 | 3.46 |
| 6 + 4 | 0.68 | 10 + 4 | 3.60 |
| 6 + 5 | 0.75 | 10 + 5 | 3.74 |
| 6 + 6 | 0.81 | 10 + 6 | 3.89 |
| 7 + 0 | 0.89 | 11 + 0 | 4.04 |
| 7 + 1 | 0.96 | 11 + 1 | 4.19 |
| 7 + 2 | 1.04 | 11 + 2 | 4.35 |
| 7 + 3 | 1.12 | 11 + 3 | 4.51 |
| 7 + 4 | 1.20 | 11 + 4 | 4.67 |
| 7 + 5 | 1.29 | 11 + 5 | 4.83 |
| 7 + 6 | 1.38 | 11 + 6 | 5.00 |
| 8 + 0 | 1.47 | 12 + 0 | 5.17 |
| 8 + 1 | 1.57 | 12 + 1 | 5.34 |
| 8 + 2 | 1.66 | 12 + 2 | 5.52 |
| 8 + 3 | 1.76 | 12 + 3 | 5.70 |
| 8 + 4 | 1.87 | 12 + 4 | 5.88 |
| 8 + 5 | 1.97 | 12 + 5 | 6.06 |
| 8 + 6 | 2.08 | 12 + 6 | 6.25 |
| 9 + 0 | 2.19 | 13 + 0 | 6.43 |
| 9 + 1 | 2.31 | 13 + 1 | 6.63 |
| 9 + 2 | 2.42 | 13 + 2 | 6.82 |
| 9 + 3 | 2.54 | 13 + 3 | 7.01 |
| 9 + 4 | 2.67 | 13 + 4 | 7.22 |
| 9 + 5 | 2.79 | 13 + 5 | 7.42 |
| 9 + 6 | 2.92 | 13 + 6 | 7.63 |
| 10 + 0 | 3.05 | 14 + 0 | 7.83 |
| 10 + 1 | 3.18 | | |

*From Robinson HP, Fleming JEE: A critical evaluation of sonar crown-rump length measurements. *Br J Obstet Gynaecol* 1975; 82:702.

fortunately, while easy to identify, the round structure with its midline falx was often mismeasured, which subsequently led to false assessments of gestational age and occasional untoward outcomes in the clinical management of the patients.

Early studies of the BPD were limited by the poor resolution of the equipment and differences in scanning and imaging techniques, as well as by assumptions about different tissue velocities. Recent advances in imaging have permitted guidelines to be established for imaging and measuring the BPD in a more consistent fashion.

### Establishing Guidelines for Measuring Techniques

Until recently many instruments utilized different assumptions for the speed of sound. It is generally thought however, that the velocity of ultrasound in human tissue averages 1,540 m/sec. Early work in the United Kingdom had assumed velocity of 1,600 m/sec.[9] The discrepancy between these instrumental measurements increases with increasing gestational age.

### Imaging Plane

The BPD is ideally measured when the fetus is in an occipital transverse position.[10] Using a series of scans made through the fetal brain, Hadlock et al. have shown that the midline structures can be seen in all planes.[10] However, the one that should be used to measure the BPD is a plane that demonstrates the cavum septum pellucidum, the thalamus, and the sylvian fissure.

### Other Factors Affecting Biparietal Diameter

Fetal position occasionally affects BPD measurement. A number of studies have shown that the fetus in breech presentation appears to have a smaller BPD and an elongated occipital frontal diameter (dolichocephaly).[11] The same findings have been observed in cases of premature rupture of membranes. These facts are important when attempting to determine gestational age in these patients. Hadlock has described something called the cephalic index, which entails measurement of the BPD and the occipital frontal di-

ameter. The cephalic index appears to be constant in the third trimester (i.e., 79% ± 7%). When these outer limits are reached, clinical pathology must be considered. In a study of 200 consecutive patients Hohler determined that the cephalic index was abnormal in approximately 14%. In these situations use of the BPD for determining gestational age is not advocated. When the cephalic index is abnormal, the fetus should be evaluated for possible congenital malformations. In addition, some other means of assessing gestational age should be used.

### Use of Single Versus Multiple Measurements

A number of investigators have questioned whether a single determination is adequate to assess gestational age. Most investigators agree that the benefits of the single determination are greatest in the second trimester. After this time, the use of multiple parameters has been shown to increase efficacy. In a recent study of timed pregnancies Kopta and Crane[12] found that the BPD is no less reliable than the crown-rump length measured in the first trimester. Coupled with the more optimal time to examine fetal anatomical structures, this suggests that the BPD can be adequately used to date pregnancies, and thus primary pregnancy dating in the first trimester becomes less valuable.

Some investigators have suggested that serial BPD measurements will improve the accuracy of dating techniques.[13] In a small study of 50 patients, O'Brien et al. demonstrated that the combination of a BPD measured early in pregnancy and a second measurement obtained between 18 and 30 weeks' gestation did not improve the ultimate accuracy. This appears to be at odds with both the method of growth-adjusted sonographic age (GASA), developed by Sabbagha et al.,[14] and the mean projected gestational age (HPGA), developed by Crane et al.[15]. Both these methods require that the BPD be measured before the 26th week of gestation and again between the 18th and 30th week of gestation. In Sabbagha's method the second examination is preferably performed at approximately 33 weeks' gestation. On the basis of evaluation of the head growth and the interval between the scans, one adjusts the original assigned gestational age if the head growth is greater or less than expected. For example, if head growth is above the 50th percentile on the second examination, the original gestational age is recalculated; the age is adjusted backward to make the first examination correspond to an earlier period of gestation. If, on the other hand, the fetus is found to be smaller than the 50th percentile on the second examination, the age is advanced to make the fetus older on the first examination. Crane uses a similar approach but reaches opposite conclusions. If on the second examination the head is larger than expected he will move the total curve toward the mean, making the fetus older. If the head is smaller than expected on the second examination, it is assumed that the fetus was in fact younger with a slower rate of growth based on those findings.

Although these methods are theoretically appealing, numerous limitations make them impractical for clinical use. (1) At a time when cost effectiveness is a major question in modern medicine, no studies have demonstrated the cost effectiveness of one, yet alone two, examinations. (2) The exact methods used by these two researchers have not been reproduced in other laboratories. In fact, Smazal et al.[16] found that the GASA was not beneficial in their studies. (3) Neither of the two methods takes into consideration the potential for head shape variances shown by the cephalic index concept as presented by Hadlock.

Nonetheless, the BPD remains a commonly measured parameter, for the following reasons: (1) improved resolution now allows defined end points of measurements and observations of intracranial landmarks, (2) a large database exists for correlating BPD with gestational age, and (3) the technique is easy to apply and can be performed in most patients.

## Head Circumference

The use of head circumference for fetal age assessment has gained wide acceptance in recent years. The head circumference can be measured in several ways. The initial use of map measure traced around the photograph of the fetal head. This tedious and often difficult technique gained little acceptance. Electronic calipers and software now provide the means for readily acquiring measurements. Furthermore, use of the average diameter can give an approximation of head circumference. The formula of an ellipse or a circle can be used for all practical purposes. In the case of the formula for a circle, the head circumference equaling BPD plus occipital frontal diameter divided by 2, the result multiplied by 3.14, has been shown to be clinically effective.[18]

Recently several authors have shown that the head circumference is a good index of menstrual age.[19, 20] Dating by head circumference is unaffected by head shape. In the last weeks of pregnancy, the head circumference is actually a better predictor of menstrual age than the BPD alone.[19] Theoretically one could use the formula for an ellipse, which involves a calculation of the square root. Unfortunately, some investigators have had great difficulty with this technique. One can simply use the formula for calculating the circumference of a circle. In a separate study we found that in most clinical situations, measurement abnormalities are unlikely when the simpler formula is used.[18]

## Abdominal Circumference

Abdominal circumference is readily measured by imaging a transverse section of the fetus at a right angle to the spine. Since the umbilical vein enters the fetal abdomen and traverses the liver obliquely in a cephalad and posterior direction, a scan that shows the umbilical vein extending to the anterior abdominal wall is likely an oblique rather than a true transverse scan. Therefore, the best measurement is obtained at the level of the portal umbilical venous complex with part of the fetal stomach showing in the scan. In identifying this plane one can also depict the long axis of the fetus and with an examining finger below a linear-array transducer identify that plane just below the fetal heart. Turning the transducer 90° will place the transducer within millimeters of the ideal plane of section.

Like the head circumference, the abdominal circumference can be measured by tracing the parameter with a map reader or electronic digitizer, or from two diameters obtained at right angles to each other. Unlike the head circumference, for which the formula for an ellipse should be used, the formula for the circle is most accurately used with measurement of the abdominal circumference: $(D_1 + D_2) \times 1.57$.

Because of occasional rapid growth of the abdominal circumference late in pregnancy, the relationship of the abdominal circumference to gestational age is less reliable than the BPD. Nonetheless, this measurement has been shown to be useful in midgestation as a single component of age assessment. Recently Selbing[21] reported that the use of mean abdominal diameters was as reliable as fetal femur length in gestational age assessment. The mean diameter has frequently been used in gestational age assessment.

Of all the fetal measurements discussed thus far, abdominal circumference is most susceptible to measurement error. Such errors occur as a result of an improper imaging plane, either too high or too low, which typically results in underestimation of the size and thereby underestimation of fetal age, or as a result of growth abnormalities. Particularly with regard to intrauterine growth retardation and macrosomia, the use of the abdominal circumference will either falsely reduce or raise the gestational age, respectively. Despite these concerns, Hadlock et al. believe that the abdominal circumference allows a more accurate assessment of age in the third trimester than any other measurement.[22]

## Femur Length

The fetal femur is best measured with a linear-array transducer. Although concern has been raised about images obtained from sector scanners, a number of studies have failed to demonstrate reproducibly the inadequacy of this technique. (For example, the angle of the femur to the ultrasound path does not appear to alter the measurements significantly.) As for all other measurements, multiple measurements should be made and the mean length used for dating purposes. In 1981 O'Brien, Queenan, and Campbell[23] first introduced the concept of using the fetal femur as an alternative means of gestational age assessment (Table 16D–2). Subsequently other investigators have evaluated the fetal femur as a alternative measurement of fetal age.[24–26] In general, these studies have demonstrated that measurement of the fetal femur length is quite reproducible. Table 16D–2 gives the relationship of fetal femur to gestational age and the variability of these measurements.

## Avoiding Sources of Error in Femur Length Measurements

To avoid erroneous measurements of the femur, sonographers should make sure they have not foreshor-

**TABLE 16D–2.**
**Fetal Age Measured by Femur Length***

| GESTATION (WK) | NO. OF MEASUREMENTS | FEMUR LENGTH: ARITHMETIC MEAN (MM) | ± 2 SD (MM) |
|---|---|---|---|
| 14 | 31 | 16.6 | 2.5 |
| 15 | 28 | 19.9 | 2.3 |
| 16 | 28 | 22.0 | 3.0 |
| 17 | 35 | 25.2 | 2.9 |
| 18 | 30 | 29.6 | 3.1 |
| 19 | 32 | 32.4 | 3.1 |
| 20 | 27 | 34.8 | 2.5 |
| 21 | 29 | 37.5 | 4.1 |
| 22 | 23 | 40.9 | 3.9 |
| 23 | 33 | 43.5 | 3.6 |
| 24 | 38 | 46.4 | 3.5 |
| 25 | 33 | 48.0 | 4.6 |
| 26 | 39 | 51.1 | 5.0 |
| 27 | 37 | 53.0 | 3.2 |
| 28 | 39 | 54.4 | 4.1 |
| 29 | 28 | 57.3 | 4.3 |
| 30 | 48 | 58.7 | 3.8 |
| 31 | 50 | 61.5 | 4.5 |
| 32 | 52 | 62.8 | 4.2 |
| 33 | 41 | 64.9 | 4.6 |
| 34 | 41 | 65.7 | 4.4 |
| 35 | 59 | 67.7 | 4.8 |
| 36 | 56 | 69.5 | 4.6 |
| 37 | 51 | 70.8 | 4.3 |
| 38 | 46 | 71.8 | 5.6 |
| 39 | 34 | 74.2 | 5.1 |
| 40 | 28 | 75.4 | 5.6 |

*From O'Brien GD, Queenan JT: Am J Obstet Gynecol 1981; 141:835. Reproduced by permission.

tened the measurement by obtaining oblique sections through the femur. In addition, novices often incorporate portions of the bony pelvis into the femur and thus overestimate gestational age. Additional errors have been introduced by attempting to measure the shadow produced by the femur bone, but this too will underestimate fetal age.

Most studies have demonstrated that the fetal femur length will provide equivalent age assessments as those obtained using head or abdominal circumference measurements. Because an ideal BPD cannot always be obtained, the alternative measurement of the fetal femur will provide the clinician with useful information. When a femur appears too short, careful analysis of all the long bones, including the humerus, radius, ulna, tibia, and fibula, must be undertaken as the fetus may be affected by a skeletal dysplasia, biochemical disorder, osteogenesis imperfecta, or possibly hypophosphatasia.

## The Ratio Game

These four parameters—BPD, head circumference, abdominal circumference, and femur length—can be used individually or in combination to identify the fetus with abnormal growth (Table 16D–3). Although this chapter is concerned primarily with dating, a number of authors have introduced checks and balances into the assessment of morphometric measurements. Hadlock et al.[27] have demonstrated the constant relationship of femur length to abdominal circumference throughout gestation. Abnormal findings should lead the examiner to consider abnormal fetal growth. Normal findings increase the reliability of the determinations. Hohler and Guetel[25] report that the femur/BPD ratio is also a constant late in pregnancy (79% ± 7%). This simple ratio, when abnormal, is helpful in identifying cases of skeletal dysplasia, hydrocephaly, and the like.

**TABLE 16D–3.**

**BPD, Head Circumference, and Abdominal Circumference as Functions of Gestational Age***

| GESTATIONAL AGE (WK) | BPD (CM) | HEAD CIRCUM. (CM) (1 SD = 0.96 CM) | ABDOMINAL CIRCUM. (CM) (1 SD = 1.14 CM) |
|---|---|---|---|
| 12.0 | 2.0 | 6.7 | 5.7 |
| 12.5 | 2.1 | 7.4 | 6.2 |
| 13.0 | 2.3 | 8.2 | 6.9 |
| 13.5 | 2.5 | 8.9 | 7.5 |
| 14.0 | 2.7 | 9.6 | 8.1 |
| 14.5 | 2.8 | 10.3 | 8.7 |
| 15.0 | 3.0 | 11.0 | 9.3 |
| 15.5 | 3.2 | 11.7 | 9.9 |
| 16.0 | 3.4 | 12.4 | 10.5 |
| 16.5 | 3.5 | 13.0 | 11.1 |
| 17.0 | 3.7 | 13.7 | 11.6 |
| 17.5 | 3.8 | 14.3 | 12.2 |
| 18.0 | 4.0 | 15.0 | 12.8 |
| 18.5 | 4.2 | 15.6 | 13.4 |
| 19.0 | 4.3 | 16.2 | 14.0 |
| 19.5 | 4.5 | 16.8 | 14.5 |
| 20.0 | 4.6 | 17.4 | 15.1 |
| 20.5 | 4.8 | 18.0 | 15.7 |
| 21.0 | 4.9 | 18.6 | 16.2 |
| 21.5 | 5.1 | 19.2 | 16.8 |
| 22.0 | 5.2 | 19.8 | 17.3 |
| 22.5 | 5.4 | 20.3 | 17.9 |
| 23.0 | 5.5 | 20.9 | 18.4 |
| 23.5 | 5.7 | 21.4 | 19.0 |
| 24.0 | 5.8 | 22.0 | 19.5 |
| 24.5 | 6.0 | 22.5 | 20.0 |
| 25.0 | 6.1 | 23.0 | 20.6 |
| 25.5 | 6.2 | 23.5 | 21.1 |
| 26.0 | 6.4 | 24.0 | 21.6 |
| 26.5 | 6.5 | 24.5 | 22.2 |
| 27.0 | 6.6 | 25.0 | 22.7 |
| 27.5 | 6.8 | 25.5 | 23.2 |
| 28.0 | 6.9 | 25.9 | 23.7 |
| 28.5 | 7.0 | 26.4 | 24.3 |
| 29.0 | 7.2 | 26.8 | 24.8 |
| 29.5 | 7.3 | 27.3 | 25.3 |
| 30.0 | 7.4 | 27.7 | 25.8 |
| 30.5 | 7.5 | 28.1 | 26.3 |
| 31.0 | 7.7 | 28.6 | 26.8 |
| 31.5 | 7.8 | 29.0 | 27.3 |
| 32.0 | 7.9 | 29.4 | 27.8 |
| 32.5 | 8.0 | 29.7 | 28.3 |
| 33.0 | 8.1 | 30.1 | 28.7 |
| 33.5 | 8.2 | 30.5 | 29.2 |
| 34.0 | 8.4 | 30.9 | 29.7 |
| 34.5 | 8.5 | 31.2 | 30.2 |
| 35.0 | 8.6 | 31.5 | 30.7 |
| 35.5 | 8.7 | 31.9 | 31.1 |
| 36.0 | 8.8 | 32.2 | 31.6 |
| 37.0 | 9.0 | 32.8 | 32.5 |
| 37.5 | 9.1 | 33.1 | 33.0 |
| 38.0 | 9.2 | 33.4 | 33.4 |
| 38.5 | 9.3 | 33.7 | 33.9 |
| 39.0 | 9.4 | 34.0 | 34.4 |
| 39.5 | 9.5 | 34.2 | 34.8 |
| 40.0 | 9.6 | 34.5 | 35.2 |
| 40.5 | 9.7 | 34.8 | 35.7 |
| 41.0 | 9.8 | 35.0 | 36.1 |
| 41.5 | 9.9 | 35.2 | 36.6 |
| 42.0 | 10.0 | 35.4 | 37.0 |

*From Hadlock FP: *Ultrasound Obstet Gynecol* 1981; 1:31. Reproduced by permission.

## Alternative Dating Methods

Gestational ages have been correlated with measurements of the interorbital and intraorbital distances.[28, 29] The assumed benefit of this technique occurs when fetuses are in the abnormal position and the orbital distances are more readily identified. In our experience this measurement is of limited value for gestational age assessment, and we do not use it for dating. However, we have used it on the rare occasions when hypotelorism or hypertelorism is present.

Jeanty et al.[26] and others have measured all the long bones in the fetus and demonstrated a relationship of bone length to gestational age. There are large variations, however, in the third trimester.

Yarkoni et al.[30] recently reported that the fetal clavicle can serve as an alternative means of fetal age assessment. The actual measurement in millimeters should correspond to the weeks of gestation.

In unpublished data, we have demonstrated the usefulness of obtaining the chest circumference as a predictor of gestational age. This measurement has become important in the assessment of skeletal dys-

# SEQUENTIAL ANALYSIS OF ULTRASONIC FETAL GROWTH PARAMETERS

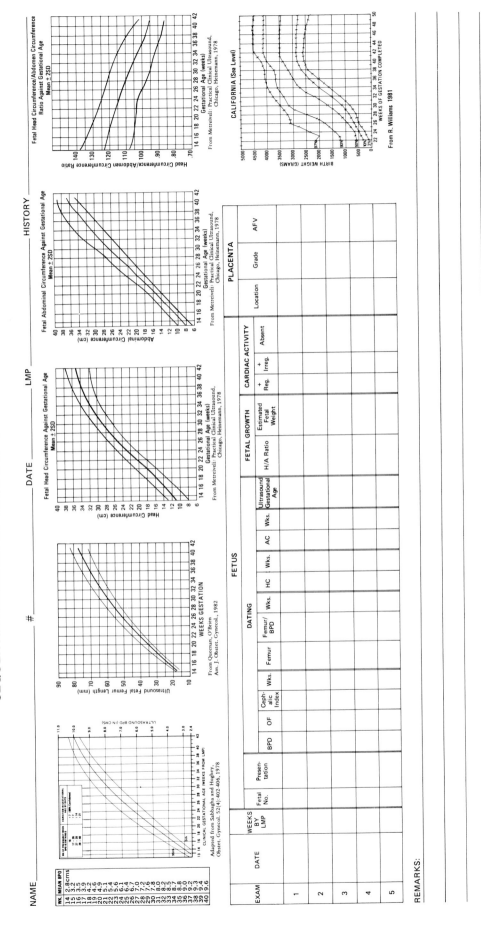

**FIG 16D–1.**
*Graphic reporting form developed by the authors.*

plasias and particularly in identifying those fetuses with small chests, which are therefore likely to have thoracic dystrophy. We have also published nomograms for the relationship of fetal heart structures to gestational age. Most of these nomograms, however, have been used for evaluation of fetal anatomy as it relates to congenital heart disease, and not specifically to gestational age.

A number of authors have described a relationship between specific anatomical features and gestational age. For example, McLeary and Kuhns[31] and Chinn et al.[32] have shown that the distal femoral epiphysis appears at a specific time in gestation. McLeary and Kuhns believe this can be detected at approximately 30 weeks' gestation, whereas Chin and co-workers believe it does not occur until 32 weeks. Regardless of the time of appearance, this observation offers little clinical help. Birnholz[33] has reported that the morphology of the fetal ear can be correlated with a specific gestational age. This technique has not gained wide acceptance for fetal age assessment.

## Clinical Use of the Mean Ultrasound Age

For a number of years we have been using a mean age as determined from multiple ultrasound parameters for the gestational age. Although our laboratory arbitrarily accepted the use of the mean ultrasound age, Hadlock et al.[34] have shown that the variability in predicting age from fetal measurements can indeed be reduced when two or more measurements are used in combination. This "composite age" has gained wide acceptance. Thus, after one measures the BPD, head and abdominal circumferences, and femur length, the average age of all these measurements is used for age assessment. One must recognize, however, that occasionally there is an abnormality and the value may represent a pathologic condition of the fetus. Every measurement deserves an adequate explanation. Therefore, when evaluating mean gestational age, one should average only those measurements that are reasonably close to each other.

Instead of using simple numerical dating for our report we have chosen to graphically display all of this data (Fig 16D–1).

Each ultrasound laboratory should develop a reporting form that adequately describes the examination. We have chosen to emphasize the graphic display of ultrasound data, particularly as they relate to fetal age. By plotting the values for fetal age at intervals between examinations the clinician not only will understand fetal age but will be provided with a clear picture of fetal growth.

## References

1. Hertz RH, Sokol RJ, Knoke JD, et al: Clinical estimation of gestational age: Rules for avoiding preterm delivery. *Am J Obstet Gynecol* 1978; 131:395.
2. Wenner WM, Young EB: Nonspecific date of last menstrual period: An indication of poor reproductive outcome. *Am J Obstet Gynecol* 1974; 120:1071.
3. Hadlock EP, et al: Fetal biparietal diameter: A critical reevaluation of the relation to menstrual age by means of realtime ultrasound. *J Ultrasound Med* 1982; 1:97.
4. Thickman D, Arger P, Tureck R: Sonographic assessment of endometrius in patients undergoing in vitro fertilization. *J Ultrasound Med* 1986; 5:197.
5. Hellman IM, et al: Growth and development of the human fetus prior to the twentieth week of gestation. *Am J Obstet Gynecol* 1969; 103:789.
6. Robinson HP, Fleming JEE: A critical evaluation of sonar crown-rump length measurements. *Br J Obstet Gynaecol* 1975; 82:702.
7. Nelson LH: Comparison of methods for determining crown-rump measurement by real-time ultrasound. *JCU* 1981; 9:67.
8. Bovicelli L, et al: Estimation of gestational age during the first trimester by realtime measurement of fetal crown-rump length and biparietal diameter. *JCU* 1981; 9:71.
9. Campbell S: Growth of the fetal biparietal diameter during normal pregnancy. *Br J Obstet Gynaecol* 1971; 78:513.
10. Hadlock FP, Deter RL, Harrist RB, et al: Fetal biparietal diameter: Rational choice of plane of section for sonographic measurement. *AJR* 1982; 138:871.
11. Hadlock FP, Deter RL, Carpenter RJ, et al: Estimating fetal age: Effect on head shape on BPD. *AJR* 1981; 137:83.

12. Kopta M, Crane JP, in *Proceedings of the Society of Gynecology Investigation,* 1985.

13. O'Brien WF, Coddington CC, Cefalo RC: Serial ultrasonographic biparietal diameters for prediction of estimated date of confinement. *Am J Obstet Gynecol* 1980; 138:467.

14. Sabbagha RE, Hughey M, Depp R: Growth-adjusted sonographic age: A simplified method. *Obstet Gynecol* 1978; 51:383.

15. Crane JP, Tomich PG, and Kopta M: Ultrasonic growth patterns in normal and discordant twins. *Obstet Gynecol* 1980; 55:678.

16. Smazal SF, et al: Comparative analysis of ultrasonographic methods of gestational age assessment. *J Ultrasound Med* 1983; 2:147.

17. Hohler CW: Cross checking pregnancy landmarks by ultrasound. *Contemp Obstet Gynecol* 1982; 20:169.

18. DeVore GR, Platt LD: Choosing the correct equation for computing the head circumference from two diameters: The effect of head shape. *Am J Obstet Gynecol* 1984; 148:221.

19. Hadlock FP, Deter RL, Harrist RB, et al: Fetal head circumference: Relation to menstrual age. *AJR* 1982; 138:649.

20. Law RG, McRae KD: Head circumference as an index of fetal age. *J Ultrasound Med* 1982; 1:281.

21. Selbing A: Conceptual dating using ultrasonically measured fetal femur length and abdominal diameters in early pregnancy. *Br J Obstet Gynecol* 1986; 93:116.

22. Hadlock FP, Deter RL, Harris RB, et al: Fetal abdominal circumference as a predictor of gestational age. *AJR* 1982; 139:367.

23. O'Brien GD, Queenan JT, Campbell S: Assessment of gestational age in the second trimester by realtime ultrasound measurement of the femur length. *Am J Obstet Gynecol* 1981; 140:165.

24. Hadlock FP, Harrist RB, Deter RL, et al: Fetal femur length as a predictor of menstrual age: Sonographically measured. *AJR* 1982; 138:875.

25. Hohler CW, Quetel TA: Fetal femur length: Equations for computer calculation of gestational age from ultrasound measurements. *Am J Obstet Gynecol* 1982; 143:479.

26. Jeanty P, Kirkpatrick C, Dramaix-Wilmet MS, et al: Ultrasonic evaluation of fetal limb growth. *Radiology* 1981; 140:165.

27. Hadlock FP, et al: A date-independent predictor of intrauterine growth retardation: femur length/abdominal circumference ratio. *AJR* 1983; 141:979.

28. Mayden KL, Tortora M, Berkowitz RL, et al: Orbital diameters: A new parameter for prenatal diagnosis and dating. *Am J Obstet Gynecol* 1982; 144:289.

29. Jeanty P, Dramaix-Wilmet M, VanGansebke D, et al: Fetal ocular biometry by ultrasound. *Radiology* 1982; 143:513.

30. Yarkorni S, Schmidt W, Jeanty P, et al: Clavicular measurement: A new biometric parameter for fetal evaluation. *J Ultrasound Med* 1985; 4:467.

31. McLeary RD, Kuhns LR: Sonographic evaluation of the distal femoral epiphyseal ossification center. *J Ultrasound Med* 1983; 2:437.

32. Chinn DH, et al: Ultrasonographic identification of fetal lower extremity epiphyseal ossification centers. *Radiology* 1983; 147:815.

33. Birnholz JC: The fetal external ear. *Radiology* 1983; 147:819.

34. Hadlock FP, Deter RL, Harrist RB, et al: Computer assisted analysis of fetal age in the third trimester using multiple fetal growth parameters. *JCU* 1983; 11:313.

## 16e

## ULTRASOUND DETECTION OF FETAL INTRAUTERINE GROWTH RETARDATION

Frank P. Hadlock, M.D.

The use of diagnostic ultrasound has made it possible to observe fetal growth in utero, and the development of normative biometric data for fetal growth parameters (Table 16E-1) allows us to evaluate objectively the growth process.[1, 2] A complete evaluation of the fetus can be achieved by the use of a sonographic fetal growth profile, which consists of measurements of head size, trunk size, femur length, estimated fetal weight, and body proportionality.[1, 2] This chapter addresses the use of the sonographic growth profile in the detection of fetal intrauterine growth retardation (IUGR).

### Definition and Classification

The most commonly used clinical criterion for defining IUGR is a fetal weight below the 10th percentile for age.[1] There are problems with this definition, however, in terms of both sensitivity and specificity. First, because of the statistical distribution of fetal weights in a general population, at least 7% of normal babies will be classified as growth-retarded when the 10th percentile line is used a a cutoff between normal and abnormal fetuses.[1, 2] Second, this definition does not take into account growth-retarded fetuses whose weights fall above the 10th percentile line—for example, a 3,000-gm term fetus that would have been a 4,000-gm fetus under proper nutritional circumstances. It is now known that fetuses affected by IUGR are not a homogeneous population and that varying degrees of compromise in height, weight, and soft tissue mass may be observed.[1, 2] The growth profile was designed to take into account these differences.

To make the matter more complex, the severity of retarded fetal growth depends on the etiology, duration, and degree of the IUGR process.[2] If a severe insult begins early in the first trimester of pregnancy, the fetus is proportionately small in all parameters, and the case is therefore referred to a symmetric IUGR.[3] The typical causes of this form of IUGR include a low genetic growth potential, intrauterine infection, severe maternal malnutrition, chromosomal aberrations, and severe congenital anomalies.[1-3] If the IUGR process begins in the late second or early third trimester, typically there is relative sparing of the fetal head size and body length in comparison with fetal soft tissue mass and weight.[3] This form of IUGR,

**TABLE 16E–1.**
**Predicted Normal Values for Measurements of the Fetus in Utero***

| MENSTRUAL AGE (WK) | HEAD CIRCUMFERENCE (HC) | | | ABDOMINAL CIRCUMFERENCE (AC) | | | FEMUR LENGTH | | | HC/AC RATIO | | | ESTIMATED WEIGHT PERCENTILES | | |
|---|---|---|---|---|---|---|---|---|---|---|---|---|---|---|---|
| | −2SD (CM) | MEAN (CM) | +2SD (CM) | −2SD (CM) | MEAN (CM) | +2SD (CM) | −2SD (CM) | MEAN (CM) | +2SD (CM) | −2SD | MEAN | +2SD | 10TH (KG) | 50TH (KG) | 90TH (KG) |
| 12 | 5.1 | 7.0 | 8.9 | 3.1 | 5.6 | 8.1 | 0.2 | 0.8 | 1.4 | 1.12 | 1.22 | 1.31 | | | |
| 13 | 6.5 | 8.9 | 10.3 | 4.4 | 6.9 | 9.4 | 0.5 | 1.1 | 1.7 | 1.11 | 1.21 | 1.30 | | | |
| 14 | 7.9 | 9.8 | 11.7 | 5.6 | 8.1 | 10.6 | 0.9 | 1.5 | 2.1 | 1.11 | 1.20 | 1.30 | | | |
| 15 | 9.2 | 11.1 | 13.0 | 6.8 | 9.3 | 11.8 | 1.2 | 1.8 | 2.4 | 1.10 | 1.19 | 1.29 | | | |
| 16 | 10.5 | 12.4 | 14.3 | 8.0 | 10.5 | 13.0 | 1.5 | 2.1 | 2.7 | 1.09 | 1.18 | 1.28 | | | |
| 17 | 11.8 | 13.7 | 15.6 | 9.2 | 11.7 | 14.2 | 1.8 | 2.4 | 3.0 | 1.08 | 1.18 | 1.27 | | | |
| 18 | 13.1 | 15.0 | 16.9 | 10.4 | 12.9 | 15.4 | 2.1 | 2.7 | 3.3 | 1.07 | 1.17 | 1.26 | | | |
| 19 | 14.4 | 16.3 | 18.2 | 11.6 | 14.1 | 16.6 | 2.3 | 3.0 | 3.6 | 1.06 | 1.16 | 1.25 | | | |
| 20 | 15.6 | 17.5 | 19.4 | 12.7 | 15.2 | 17.7 | 2.7 | 3.3 | 3.9 | 1.06 | 1.15 | 1.24 | 0.28 | 0.41 | 0.86 |
| 21 | 16.8 | 18.7 | 20.6 | 13.9 | 16.4 | 18.9 | 3.0 | 3.6 | 4.2 | 1.05 | 1.14 | 1.24 | 0.32 | 0.48 | 0.92 |
| 22 | 18.0 | 19.9 | 21.8 | 15.0 | 17.5 | 20.0 | 3.3 | 3.9 | 4.5 | 1.04 | 1.13 | 1.23 | 0.37 | 0.55 | 0.99 |
| 23 | 19.1 | 21.0 | 22.9 | 16.1 | 18.6 | 21.1 | 3.6 | 4.2 | 4.8 | 1.03 | 1.12 | 1.22 | 0.42 | 0.64 | 1.08 |
| 24 | 20.2 | 22.1 | 24.0 | 17.2 | 19.7 | 22.0 | 3.8 | 4.4 | 5.0 | 1.02 | 1.12 | 1.21 | 0.49 | 0.74 | 1.18 |
| 25 | 21.3 | 23.2 | 25.1 | 18.3 | 20.8 | 23.3 | 4.1 | 4.7 | 5.3 | 1.01 | 1.11 | 1.20 | 0.57 | 0.86 | 1.32 |
| 26 | 22.3 | 24.2 | 26.1 | 19.4 | 21.9 | 24.4 | 4.3 | 4.9 | 5.5 | 1.00 | 1.10 | 1.19 | 0.66 | 0.99 | 1.47 |
| 27 | 23.3 | 25.2 | 27.1 | 20.4 | 22.9 | 25.4 | 4.6 | 5.2 | 5.8 | 1.00 | 1.09 | 1.18 | 0.77 | 1.15 | 1.66 |
| 28 | 24.3 | 26.2 | 28.1 | 21.5 | 24.0 | 26.5 | 4.8 | 5.4 | 6.0 | 0.99 | 1.08 | 1.18 | 0.89 | 1.31 | 1.89 |
| 29 | 25.2 | 27.1 | 29.0 | 22.5 | 25.0 | 27.5 | 5.0 | 5.6 | 6.2 | 0.98 | 1.07 | 1.17 | 1.03 | 1.46 | 2.10 |
| 30 | 26.1 | 28.0 | 29.9 | 23.5 | 26.0 | 28.5 | 5.2 | 5.8 | 6.4 | 0.97 | 1.07 | 1.16 | 1.18 | 1.63 | 2.29 |
| 31 | 27.0 | 28.9 | 30.8 | 24.5 | 27.0 | 29.5 | 5.5 | 6.1 | 6.7 | 0.96 | 1.06 | 1.15 | 1.31 | 1.81 | 2.50 |
| 32 | 27.8 | 29.7 | 31.6 | 25.5 | 28.0 | 30.5 | 5.7 | 6.3 | 6.9 | 0.95 | 1.05 | 1.14 | 1.48 | 2.01 | 2.69 |
| 33 | 28.5 | 30.4 | 32.3 | 26.5 | 29.0 | 31.5 | 5.9 | 6.5 | 7.1 | 0.95 | 1.04 | 1.13 | 1.67 | 2.22 | 2.88 |
| 34 | 29.3 | 31.2 | 33.1 | 27.5 | 30.0 | 32.5 | 6.0 | 6.6 | 7.2 | 0.94 | 1.03 | 1.13 | 1.87 | 2.43 | 3.09 |
| 35 | 29.9 | 31.8 | 33.7 | 28.4 | 30.9 | 33.4 | 6.2 | 6.8 | 7.4 | 0.93 | 1.02 | 1.12 | 2.19 | 2.65 | 3.29 |
| 36 | 30.6 | 32.5 | 34.4 | 29.3 | 31.8 | 34.3 | 6.4 | 7.0 | 7.6 | 0.92 | 1.01 | 1.11 | 2.31 | 2.87 | 3.47 |
| 37 | 31.1 | 33.0 | 34.9 | 30.2 | 32.7 | 35.2 | 6.6 | 7.2 | 7.8 | 0.91 | 1.01 | 1.10 | 2.51 | 3.03 | 3.61 |
| 38 | 31.9 | 33.6 | 35.5 | 31.1 | 33.6 | 36.1 | 6.7 | 7.3 | 7.9 | 0.90 | 1.00 | 1.09 | 2.68 | 3.17 | 3.75 |
| 39 | 32.2 | 34.1 | 36.0 | 32.0 | 34.5 | 37.0 | 6.9 | 7.5 | 8.1 | 0.89 | 0.99 | 1.08 | 2.75 | 3.28 | 3.87 |
| 40 | 32.6 | 34.5 | 36.4 | 32.9 | 35.4 | 37.9 | 7.0 | 7.6 | 8.2 | 0.89 | 0.98 | 1.08 | | | |

*From Hadlock FP, Deter RL, Harriet RB, et al: Sonographic detection of fetal intrauterine growth retardation. *Perinatal Neonatol* 1983; 7:21–58. Reproduced by permission.

referred to as asymmetric IUGR, is usually the result of placental insufficiency. If this process is undetected and goes untreated to term, the fetal head size and body length will ultimately be affected, and the fetus will become more symmetrically growth retarded.[2] In our experience approximately 80% of growth-retarded fetuses are of the asymmetric type; only approximately 20% are in the symmetric IUGR category.

## Clinical Prospectives

One of the most important components in any strategy for detecting IUGR in utero is the identification of women who are at high risk for delivery of a growth-retarded fetus, since a majority of IUGR fetuses will come from this population of patients.[2] In our experience, the most important characteristics of this population are a history of a previous growth-retarded fetus, chronic hypertension, severe insulin-dependent diabetes mellitus, extremely poor weight gain, alcohol and/or drug abuse, and heavy cigarette smoking. One must also keep in mind, however, that at least one third of all IUGR fetuses will be born to patients with no high-risk factor for IUGR; for this reason, one should analyze the fetus for evidence of IUGR on all obstetric sonograms, regardless of the reason for the study.

Because the normal values for fetal measurements used to detect IUGR change with advancing menstrual age, it is imperative, particularly in high-risk patients, to establish menstrual age unequivocally early in pregnancy.[2] Ideally this should be done in the first trimester by use of the crown-rump length, which is accurate in dating to within 3–5 days (2 SD); however, successful dating (2 SD = ±1 week) can also be done prior to 20 weeks by use of the biparietal diameter (BPD) and/or femur length measurements.[4]

Finally, one must realize that the timing of the sonogram relative to the duration and degree of the IUGR process will have an impact on the detection rate of IUGR using sonography. For example, many of the growth parameters used to detect IUGR will not become abnormal until after 30 weeks, particularly in case of asymmetric IUGR. Thus, a normal examination in a high-risk patient at 28 weeks does not preclude the possibility of IUGR at 32 weeks, and in high-risk patients we prefer to examine the patient every 4 weeks until delivery. If evidence of IUGR is found, the interval between scans is reduced to 1–2 weeks.

## Sonographic Fetal Growth Profile

### Head Size

The fetal BPD was the first sonographic measurement used for detection of IUGR in utero.[1] The detection rates with this measurement, either at a single visit or by multiple examinations, were unsatisfactory, which is not surprising, for two reasons.[1] First, in the majority of fetuses affected by IUGR, fetal head size is spared until the third trimester of pregnancy and does not usually fall outside the normal range until very near term.[3] Thus, the use of this measurement alone would result in a very low sensitivity, with a high number of false negative results.[1] Second, variations in fetal head shape due to molding,[5] particularly the dolichocephaly which is observed in cases of fetal crowding (e.g., ruptured membranes, twins, breech fetuses), will result in abnormally low values in normal fetuses, which will lead to a high number of false positive diagnoses of IUGR.

It is well known that head circumference is a more shape-independent measurement of fetal head size than the BPD,[5] and its use in the growth profile will eliminate the high number of false positive diagnoses of IUGR when the BPD is used in cases of dolichocephaly. Head circumference is also known to be highly correlated with true fetal head volume and thus will allow one more accurately to monitor true fetal head growth. The head circumference is also an integral part of the head-to-body ratio used in evaluating body proportionality[3] (see later in this section), and is important in estimating fetal weight.

As with the BPD, proper plane selection and proper measurement techniques are important in ensuring that the largest head circumference measurement has been obtained. This measurement should be made from the same image used to measure the BPD.[1–4] The measurement can be made with the use of a map measurer or electronic digitizer for tracing the outer margins of the skull. Alternatively, head circumference may be determined more simply by measuring the largest transverse and longitudinal dimensions of the head profile (from outer boundary to outer boundary)[7] and calculating the head circumference based on the formula $(D_1 + D_2) \times 1.57.$* It cannot be overemphasized that the fetal head is typically the last fetal measurement adversely affected by the IUGR process.

## Trunk Size

The abdominal girth has been shown to be affected early in cases of IUGR, and this is thought to be due to the depletion of glycogen stores in the liver and subcutaneous fat in the soft tissues of the abdomen.[3] Measurement of the abdominal circumference at the level of the portal umbilical vein complex is known to be closely related to both fetal age and weight, and it is also known to be affected early in the IUGR process.[1-3] In our experience[2] and that of Campbell and Thomas,[3] this measurement has been affected earliest in IUGR in comparison with other fetal measurements, and ultimately it has been abnormal in all of the growth-retarded fetuses that we have studied. Measurements of this parameter can also be made with a map measurer or electronic digitizer, or it can be calculated from two diameter measurements, as described for the head circumference.[7]

## Length

The crown-heel length measurement obtained in the neonatal period is a difficult measurement to make prenatally because of fetal size and position. The femur length, however, is known to have a linear relationship to fetal crown-heel length.[8] It is this role as a substitute variable for crown-heel length that warrants the use of the femur length in the fetal growth profile. The femur length measurement is easy to obtain with real-time ultrasound and is typically made along the central shaft of the femur from the proximal greater trochanter region to the distal metaphysis.[1, 2] One should keep in mind that as with the fetal head, the femur length is affected late in cases of asymmetric IUGR.[2, 9]

---

*In dolichocephalic fetuses, head circumference =

$$4.443 \sqrt{\left(\frac{D1}{2}\right)^2 + \left(\frac{D2}{2}\right)^2}.$$

## Fetal Weight

A fetal weight below the 10th percentile for age is the traditional standard for defining IUGR,[1] and while there are certainly limitations to this definition, it has proved to be a useful standard in clinical practice. In our laboratory the most consistent in utero estimates of fetal weight using ultrasound techniques have come from the model using head circumference, abdominal circumference, and femur length.[6] One should be aware, however, that the variability of the weight estimate (2 SD = 16%) is quite large, and the use of this measurement alone would falsely classify some growth-retarded fetuses and some normal fetuses. In our laboratory we avoid using the BPD in estimating fetal weight because weight is underestimated in dolichocephaly and overestimted in brachycephaly.

## Body Proportionality

As indicated previously, approximately 80% of IUGR fetuses are asymmetrically growth retarded. The first sonographic measure of body proportionality used to detect IUGR was the head circumference/abdominal circumference ratio.[3] Although this measurement will fail to detect symmetric IUGR, sensitivity rates of approximately 70% have been reported with this technique for detecting asymmetric IUGR.[1-3] Unfortunately, this method has resulted in high false positive rates in screening a general population[1] and has the further limitation of requiring knowledge of menstrual age, since the normal range values change with time.[1-3]

We have recently evaluated the relation between femur length and abdominal circumference in detecting IUGR.[10] This ratio, which is analogous to the postnatal ponderal index, will not detect symmetric IUGR cases, but in our experience it has been abnormal in all cases of asymmetric IUGR.[10] This ratio has the further advantage of having normal range values that do not change with time after 22 weeks. The normal value for this ratio ($\pm 2$ SD), expressed as FL/AC $\times$ 100, is $22 \pm 2$. In our experience, a value greater than 24 indicates IUGR until proved otherwise.

## Other Sonographic Signs of IUGR

In 1977, Gohari and associates developed a method for determining total intrauterine volume (TIUV) using ultrasound.[11] Gohari et al. reasoned that this measurement should be of value in detecting IUGR fetuses because the TIUV is composed of fetal volume, placental volume, and amniotic fluid volume, all of which are known to be reduced in size in pregnancies affected by IUGR. Initial results using this technique were promising, but subsequent reports have demonstrated that this measurement is affected both by technique and by degrees of bladder filling, and most authors have concluded that it is not an ideal tool for detecting IUGR.[2] This is especially true in view of the normal fetal biometric data that have been gathered since 1977.[1, 2] The TIUV technique is also limited in that it requires a static-image scanner for uterine measurements, and it requires knowledge of menstrual age for proper use.

Oligohydramnios, a reduction in amniotic fluid volume, is a common finding in pregnancies affected by IUGR, and Manning and associates[12] initially advocated using a rough estimate of amniotic fluid volume as a screening tool for IUGR. They observed that when the largest pocket of amniotic fluid is less than 1 cm in its greatest axis, there is a high probability that the fetus is growth retarded. Good results were obtained when this method was used for the evaluation of fetuses that were small for gestational age clinically, but its efficacy in screening a general population for IUGR was not known. A more recent report, using less stringent criteria for defining oligohydramnios, suggests that oligohydramnios would result in detection of only 16% of IUGR fetuses.[13] Because oligohydramnios is also common in post-dates pregnancies, it obviously cannot be specific for the detection of IUGR. Nevertheless, whenever one suspects oligohydramnios in patients with intact membranes (either subjectively or by quantitative methods), the possibility of IUGR is increased, and follow-up studies are always recommended for monitoring fetal growth.

In 1977, a placental grading system was developed by Grannum et al. based on the distribution of calcium within the placenta substance and the basal plate, and it was the grade 3 placenta which was thought to represent placental maturity.[14] Petrucha and Platt[15] demonstrated that the incidence of various placental grades changes as a function of time and that only approximately 20% of normal patients will have a grade 3 placenta at term. They also noted that it was rare to find a grade 3 placenta prior to 36 weeks. Recently, Kazzi and associates[16] have demonstrated that when a grade 3 placenta is identified in the setting of a fetal weight estimate below 2,700 gm there is a fourfold increase in the incidence of IUGR, in comparison with fetuses of the same size with placental grades less than 3. While this study has not yet been confirmed in other laboratories, it is our impression that this observation has some validity, and certainly a high index of suspicion for IUGR is warranted when a grade 3 placenta is identified and the fetus weighs less than 2,700 gm or is less than 36 menstrual weeks in age.

## Recommendations

Symmetric IUGR is easy to detect if the dates are known, since all parameters in the growth profile are abnormal (Fig 16E–1). If the dates are not known, the diagnosis can be difficult to make, even with serial studies, since the growth parameters usually follow a pattern that is roughly parallel to the 10th percentile line; thus, one is never quite sure whether the fetal growth is abnormal or whether the dates are simply wrong. Prenatal diagnosis is not as critical in this form of IUGR, because in general, the causes (infection, chromosomal aberration, congenital anomalies) are not readily treatable or correctable.

Depending on the degree of the process, asymmetric IUGR is also relatively easy to diagnose if the dates are known (Fig 16E–2). In general, the fetal abdominal circumference is the most sensitive parameter, and in our experience a measurement more than 2 SD below the mean for age is unequivocal evidence of IUGR.[2] In addition, we believe that an abdominal circumference measurement below the 25th percentile warrants serial scans so that one can be certain that growth is not slowing or ceasing. If the dates are not known, one should pay particular attention to the femur length/abdominal circumference ratio, because the normal range values are independent of age. If an abnormal value (> 24) is encountered serial scans should be done at 2 to 3-week intervals to monitor growth of the abdominal circumference.

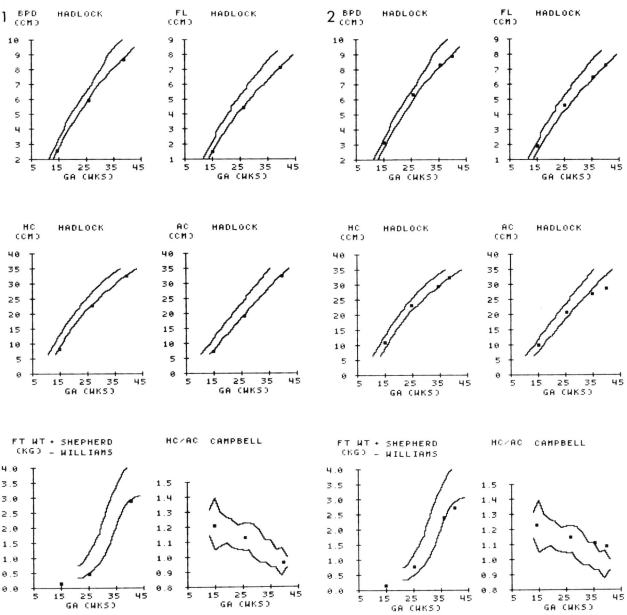

**FIG 16E–1.**
*Computer plot of growth profile data in a case of symmetric IUGR. (From Hadlock FP, Deter RL, Harrist RB, et al: Sonographic detection of fetal intrauterine growth retardation. Perinatol Neonatol 1983; 7:21–58. Reproduced by permission.)*

**FIG 16E–2.**
*Computer plot of growth profile data in a case of asymmetric IUGR. Note that the abdominal circumference is the first parameter to become abnormal. (From Hadlock FP, Deter RL, Harrist RB, et al: Sonographic detection of fetal intrauterine growth retardation. Perinatol Neonatol 1983; 7:21–58. Reproduced by permission.)*

## Conclusions

When evaluating fetal growth against objective standards such as the fetal biometric data listed in Table 16E–1, several important points should be kept in mind: (1) establish menstrual age early in pregnancy (preferably in the first trimester), especially in high-risk patients; (2) when using biometric data developed in another center, make sure that the population characteristics and the equipment and measuring techniques are appropriate for your institution; (3) recognize that a normal sonogram only indicates normal growth to that point and does not preclude the possibility of IUGR later in pregnancy, particularly in patients at high risk; (4) the abdominal circumference is the most sensitive measurement for detecting IUGR if dates are known, and the femur length/abdominal circumference ratio is the most sensitive if dates are not known; (5) the growth profile should be evaluated in serial scans at 3- to 4-week intervals in patients at high risk for IUGR; (6) because of the clinical difficulty in detecting IUGR, all patients referred for sonography for any reason should be evaluated for evidence of IUGR; and (7) when IUGR is identified in utero, early delivery should be considered, especially if fetal lung maturity can be demonstrated (L/S ratio > 2, PG +), since the rate of mortality and long-term morbidity is increased when such pregnancies are allowed to go to term.

Undoubtedly, new developments in this rapidly growing field will eventually increase our diagnostic accuracy for IUGR. The most notable examples to date are the biophysical profile, and Doppler evaluation of umbilical blood flow. Additional data will be required to define the role of these newer concepts.

## References

1. Deter RL, Hadlock FP, Harrist RB: Evaluation of normal fetal growth and the detection of intrauterine growth retardation, in Callen PW (ed): *Ultrasonography in Obstetrics and Gynecology.* Philadelphia, WB Saunders Co, 1983, pp 113–40.

2. Hadlock FP, Deter RL, Harrist RB, Park SK: Sonographic detection of fetal intrauterine growth retardation. *Perinatol Neonatol* 1983; 7:21–58.

3. Campbell S, Thomas A: Ultrasound measurement of the fetal head to abdomen circumference ratio in the assessment of growth retardation. *Br J Obstet Gynaecol* 1977; 84:165.

4. Hadlock FP, Deter RL, Harrist RB, Park SK: The use of ultrasound to determine fetal age: A review. *Med Ultrasound* 1983; 7:95.

5. Hadlock FP, Deter RL, Carpenter RJ, et al: Estimating fetal age: Effect of head shape on BPD. *AJR* 1981; 137:83.

6. Hadlock FP, Harrist RB, Carpenter RJ, et al: Sonographic estimation of fetal weight. *Radiology* 1984; 150:535–540.

7. Hadlock FP, Kent WR, Loyd J, et al: An evaluation of two methods for measuring fetal head and body circumferences. *J Ultrasound Med* 1982; 1(9):359.

8. Hadlock FP, Deter RL, Roecker E, et al: Relation of fetal femur length to neonatal crown-heel length. *J Ultrasound Med* 1984; 3:1–3.

9. O'Brien GD, Queenan JT: Ultrasound fetal femur length in relation to intrauterine growth retardation. *Am J Obstet Gynecol* 1982; 144:33.

10. Hadlock FP, Deter RL, Harrist RB, et al: A date-independent predictor of intrauterine growth retardation: Femur length/abdominal circumference ratio. *AJR* 1983; 141:979.

11. Gohari P, Berkowitz RL, Hobbins JC: Prediction of intrauterine growth retardation by determination of total intrauterine volume. *Am J Obstet Gynecol* 1977; 127:255.

12. Manning FA, Hill LM, Platt LD: Qualitative amniotic fluid volume determination by ultrasound: Antepartum detection of intrauterine growth retardation. *Am J Obstet Gynecol* 1981; 139:254.

13. Philipson EH, Sokol RJ, Williams T: Oligohydramnios: Clinical associations and predictive value for intrauterine growth retardation. *Am J Obstet Gynecol* 1983; 146:271.

14. Grannum PA, Berkowitz RL, Hobbins JC: The ultrasonic changes in the maturing placenta and their relation to fetal pulmonic maturity. *Am J Obstet Gynecol* 1979; 133:915.

15. Petrucha RA, Platt LD: Relationship of placental grade to gestational age. *Am J Obstet Gynecol* 1982; 144:733.

16. Kazzi GM, Gross TL, Sokol RJ, et al: Detection of intrauterine growth retardation: A new use for sonographic placental grading. *Am J Obstet Gynecol* 1983; 145:733.

## 16f

## ULTRASOUND EVALUATION OF NORMAL AND ABNORMAL FETAL ANATOMY

Dennis A. Sarti, M.D.

Ultrasound evaluation of the fetus has changed dramatically over the years with the development of newer high-resolution equipment. Initially an obstetric ultrasound examination consisted of identifying a fetus, placental position, and fetal viability. Initial evaluation of the fetus began with measurements of the biparietal diameter. For many years in early obstetric ultrasound, this was considered an adequate examination. With the development of higher resolution equipment, evaluation of the fetus has taken on greater significance. The fetus is now regarded as a patient, and the ultrasound examination as its first physical examination. In competent, highly skilled hands, specific information can be obtained from an obstetric ultrasound study that will yield accurate anatomical diagnoses.

Over the years normal ultrasound fetal anatomy has been described.[1-3] With study of the normal fetus, numerous criteria for recognizing an abnormal fetus have been developed.[4, 5] Prenatal diagnosis of numerous congenital anomalies is now commonplace in most medical centers.[6-9] It is difficult to visualize anomalies early in pregnancy. From approximately 6 to 14 weeks, the fetus is so small that only major abnormalities such as anencephaly can be detected. Usually in this early part of pregnancy fetal viability, amniotic fluid volume, and placental position are the major concerns of the ultrasonographer. After 14 to 16 weeks, anatomical structures become large enough that a systematic evaluation of the fetus can be undertaken, with surprising results. Many high-quality and sophisticated ultrasound examinations are performed from 14 to 20 weeks' gestation in conjunction with amniocentesis. The competency and experience of the ultrasonographer are major considerations in evaluating the adequacy of an ultrasound study. When an individual with little experience attempts a high-level fetal scan, numerous diagnostic errors are likely. Even in experienced hands these studies are quite difficult. Therefore, when there is a high index of suspicion of congenital anomalies, it is essential that the study be performed by an individual with adequate training and competence.

When doing a high-level fetal ultrasound study, it is most helpful to have a three-dimensional concept of the fetus. In the initial part of the examination, fetal position is identified. The right and left sides of the fetus must be continually evaluated since fetal movement is often present during the study. Maintaining this three-dimension concept of fetal position contributes to an increased level of diagnostic accuracy. A simple example is situs inversus, in which the stomach is on the right side. This entity will never be recognized unless the fetus is treated as a patient during the examination.

Before the fetus is evaluated, the uterus must be examined to rule out any masses or uterine anomalies. The placenta must be examined for areas of hemorrhage or increased maturation. An assessment of amniotic fluid volume is also important in evaluating fetal well-being. Amniotic fluid abnormalities will often be the initial clue that a fetal anomaly is present. Evaluation of amniotic fluid volume is quite difficult and requires years of experience. Amniotic fluid volume increases in linear fashion until late in pregnancy. However, the relative amount of fluid compared to the fetus changes during the course of pregnancy. In the second trimester the amniotic fluid volume appears quite large compared to the fetal volume. Often at 24–26 weeks the novice ultrasonographer will misinterpret this normal variation as polyhydramnios. Later in pregnancy the opposite is true. After 34–35 weeks, the amniotic fluid volume appears decreased compared to the fetal volume. Again, the novice will often misinterpret this normal finding as oligohydramnios. Although numerous attempts have been made to quantify amniotic fluid volume on ultrasound, these have been unsuccessful. To date the most adequate means of evaluating amniotic fluid volume is the experienced eye and rapid scanning. It is most helpful to scan the uterus with real time and in a rapid fashion to get an appropriate three-dimensional feel for the amount of amniotic fluid. If one scans continually over the same area and attempts to interpret amniotic fluid volume, diagnostic errors are made. If the area visualized contains a large amount of fluid, then polyhydramnios will be incorrectly diagnosed. If the opposite is true, then incorrect diagnosis of oligohydramnios will be made.

In order to present the ultrasound findings of a normal and abnormal fetus, I have chosen to discuss each anatomical location separately. The normal findings will be presented first, followed by the various fetal anomalies that may be diagnosed on ultrasound.

## Cranium

Anatomical study of the fetus begins with examination of the fetal cranium. The fetal skull can be visualized as early as 7–8 menstrual weeks when the crown-rump length is measured. Early ultrasound studies concentrated on obtaining a biparietal diameter (BDD). The midline structures of the cerebral peduncles, thalami, third ventricle, and falx cerebri are easily identified when one is measuring the BPD.[10] The cerebral hemispheres should appear symmetric. The near hemisphere is always more difficult to evaluate than the far hemisphere, because of reverberations off the portion of the fetal skull nearest the transducer. These reverberations are thrown into the near cerebral hemisphere, obscuring visualization of this area. If there is concern about the near hemisphere, the scan plane should be altered so that one views the fetal skull from either an anterior or posterior approach. To obtain the appropriate scan plane for measuring the BPD, it is often necessary to visualize the base of the skull and orbits. When both orbits are on the image, the appropriate scan plane is present for an adequate BPD and visualization of the midline structures. The lateral ventricles are identified by the presence of the highly echogenic choroid plexus.[11] The choroid plexus fills the region of the trigone of the lateral ventricles. The medial and lateral walls of the ventricles appear as sharp, highly reflective echoes on each side of the choroid plexus. When the midline echoes of the thalamic region are seen, slightly more caudad scans in the level of the midbrain will reveal pulsations of the basilar artery.[1]

A highly echogenic line is often seen near the skull echoes of the far table. This line is secondary to the subarachnoid space.[12] The subarachnoid space will have an echogenic region indenting into the cerebral echoes. This represents the sylvian fissure. Scanning the posterior fossa will reveal the cerebellar hemispheres and the cisterna magna, which is most pronounced from 20 to 26 weeks' gestation.

Systematic evaluation of the fetal cranium will lead to the correct diagnosis of any abnormalities if they exist. If the fetal skull is evaluated for size, contour deformity, hydrocephalus, intracranial cysts, intracranial hemorrhages, intracranial masses, or protrusions, the appropriate congenital anomaly may be identified.[13–15]

## Anencephaly

Anencephaly is a severe abnormality that belongs to the spectrum of neural tube defects (NTDs).[16] It is one of the more common CNS problems and occurs in approximately 1 in 1,000 births. Anencephaly results from failure of the neural tube to close completely near its cephalic end. This usually occurs in the second to third week of development. The cerebral hemispheres are completely absent, but a portion of the brain stem is still present. The cranial defect is not covered by bone or skin. This lack of covering results in an increased $\alpha$-fetoprotein (AFP) level in amniotic fluid and maternal serum. Most cases of anencephaly are presently discovered during an initial ultrasound examination or through maternal serum AFP screening programs. The initial ultrasound study if usually performed to determine gestational age. The diagnosis of anencephaly is made when attempts to measure the BPD are unsuccessful. The diagnosis of anencephaly can be made as early as 10 to 12 weeks.[15] An initial clue to the diagnosis is the presence of polyhydramnios, which is seen in approximately 50% of cases. It is usually not difficult to make the diagnosis of anencephaly on ultrasound in early and mid-pregnancy. The BPD is easily identifiable and seldom difficult to measure. Problems may arise in an obese patient or in cases of marked fetal activity. These problems are usually overcome with close scrutiny of the fetus. If the fetal cranium is not identified after 10–12 weeks, the possibility of anencephaly is immediately considered. The diagnosis of anencephaly later in pregnancy can be more difficult because of the low position of the fetal head in some patients. Very often the fetal head will not be well seen because of its position deep in the maternal pelvis. It will initially be thought that the BPD is not obtainable because of technical factors.[9] However, if the fetus is elevated out of the maternal pelvis, the correct diagnosis of anencephaly can be made.

As mentioned earlier, anencephaly is secondary to failure of the neural tube to completely close early in pregnancy. There are reports of anencephaly occurring secondary to amniotic bands within the uterus.[17] Acrania can be difficult to distinguish from anencephaly on ultrasound.[18] Acrania is the partial or complete absence of the cranium with the abnormal development of brain tissue. Brain tissue is present but markedly less than normal. The defect often occurs near the time of neural tube closure. The diagnosis can be distinguished from anencephaly by recognizing the presence of soft tissue brain substance cephalad to the high-amplitude echoes at the base of the fetal skull.[18]

## Microcephaly

Microcephaly is an uncommon fetal anomaly.[6] Various etiologic factors have been found to lead to microcephaly. Inherited traits such as Meckel's syndrome are involved. Meckel's syndrome includes microcephaly, polycystic kidneys, encephalocele, and polydactyly. Other causes such as chromosomal abnormalities and trisomies and environmental factors such as prenatal irradiation, infection, and maternal alcoholism or malnutrition have been found to cause microcephaly.[8, 15] Ultrasound diagnosis of microcephaly has been reported in maternal phenylketonuria.[19] The diagnosis of microcephaly can be quite difficult to make on ultrasound. Evidence of a disproportion in the craniofacial ratio may be the initial clue.[4] Mild forms of microcephaly are difficult to diagnose, whereas the more severe forms may be easy to diagnose.[19, 20] In the mild forms of microcephaly, it is important to compare the BPD and head circumference to other body parameters such as femur length and abdominal measurements. Microcephaly is very difficult to detect in early pregnancy, and comparison of the fetal head-body ratio has proved useful.[21]

## Skull Contour Deformity

The fetal skull usually has a sharp marginated, oval appearance on ultrasound. The skull yields high-amplitude echoes with fairly sharp borders. One normally sees a break in the fetal skull contour at the cranial sutures. Overlapping of the fetal skull echoes can be seen during labor with fetal molding or in fetal death.[8] Thanatophoric dwarfism is associated with a fetal skull deformity that has been described as cloverleaf in appearance. Because of premature suture closure, the skull contour has a trilobed appearance with prominence of the vertex and both temporal regions. This deformity resembles a cloverleaf on ultrasound examination.[22, 23] When this abnormality is visualized, close examination of the fetal long bones and thorax will often yield other abnormalities consistent with thanatophoric dwafism. Other craniofacial abnormalities have been reported such as orbits that cannot be visualized, hypoplasia of the mandible, and poor definition of the fetal cranium in otocephaly.[24]

### Hydrocephalus

Hydrocephalus may be an isolated finding or associated with other anomalies such as spina bifida, meningomyelocele, and encephalocele.[25] Hydrocephalus occurs in 0.5 to 1.8 in 1,000 births. There is also an increased incidence in the offspring of mothers who have previously borne children with hydrocephalus or spinal abnormalities.[26] Early in pregnancy, prior to 26 weeks' gestation, the lateral ventricles are normally quite large. This can easily lead to a false positive diagnosis of hydrocephalus.[27] When the novice begins looking at the cerebral ventricles in early pregnancy, he or she is initially concerned with the large size of the ventricles relative to that expected in the neonate or adult. A great deal of experience is needed to diagnose hydrocephalus in the second trimester. The lateral ventricles are large because they form earlier than the cerebral cortex. Measurements have been recorded in the normal population which compare the size of the lateral ventricle to the overall size of the hemisphere. Normal ratios have been determined which indicate that the ventricles make up 56% of the hemisphere at 15 weeks and 33% at 25 weeks.[28] This demonstrates the large size of the ventricles early in pregnancy and also indicates the rather rapid decrease in size of the ventricles relative to the cerebral cortex. This is an important finding when the diagnosis of hydrocephalus is entertained. Follow-up examinations in several weeks should show a relative decrease in the size of the ventricles in the normal case. If an increase occurs, the diagnosis of hydrocephalus is quite likely.

Because of the large size of the lateral ventricles early in pregnancy, it is often difficult to diagnose hydrocephalus prior to 20 weeks.[14] However, close examination of the normal anatomical structures of the ventricles will yield important information concerning the diagnosis of hydrocephalus. The choroid plexus

appear as highly echogenic regions in the trigone area of the lateral ventricles and should be in contact with the medial and lateral walls of the ventricle in this region. The occipital and frontal horns appear quite large in early pregnancy. However, the choroid plexus fills the lateral ventricles in the region of the trigone. Often the lateral wall of the lateral ventricles will not be visualized because it is a specular reflector. If the lateral wall of the ventricle is not visualized, structures such as the sylvian fissure and subarachnoid space can be mistaken for the lateral wall of the ventricle.[6] In these instances, the choroid will appear much smaller than the supposed lateral ventricle, and a mistaken diagnosis of hydrocephalus will be made. I have found it most helpful to scan the fetus in a plane which will allow the ultrasound beam to be perpendicular to the lateral wall of the ventricle. This is best done by scanning through the region of the near fetal ear and angling toward the far cranial echoes so that you are perpendicular to the cranium. This will also place the transducer beam perpendicular to the lateral wall of the deep ventricle. The lateral wall will then come into view adjacent to choroid plexus.

Hydrocephalus is usually easy to diagnose late in pregnancy because of the large size of the ventricles. The fetal head will often be increased in size secondary to ventricular dilatation in the third trimester. In the second trimester, ventricular dilatation occurs prior to an increase in head size. In fact, the fetal head is usually not increased in size in early hydrocephalus.[29, 30] Measuring the fetal head is not the best way to attempt to diagnose hydrocephalus. Instead, the ventricles and choroid plexus should be evaluated. The choroid plexus is compressed and small in hydrocephalus since it is under increased pressure. This is an important initial finding in the diagnosis of hydrocephalus.[15] Because of reverberations off the near skull, only the dilated deep ventricle may be visualized. The reverberations off the near skull will hide the dilated ventricle in the near hemisphere. A mistaken diagnosis of an intracranial cyst or unilateral hydrocephalus will be made. Unilateral hydrocephalus does occur but much less frequently than bilateral hydrocephalus.[31] Ultrasound has been used to assist in catheter placement in utero.[32] Under ultrasonic guidance, catheters have been placed in the dilated cerebral ventricles so that they may drain into amniotic fluid by a one-way valve.

## Holoprosencephaly and Hydranencephaly

Holoprosencephaly and hydranencephaly have a similar ultrasound appearance. The two entities can be distinguished on close examination. Holoprosencephaly results from incomplete division of the embryonic forebrain. Holoprosencephaly is divided into alobar, semilobar, and lobar categories, depending on the severity of the degree of separation of cerebral hemispheres. Alobar holoprosencephaly denotes a single common ventricle with fused thalami and no division of the cerebral hemispheres. In semilobar holoprosencephaly there is incomplete division of the cerebral hemispheres.[33] Holoprosencephaly appears on ultrasound has a large cystic space in the midline without evidence of a midline dividing structure. This midline cystic region represents a single common central ventricle.[15] A cortical mantle will be present in holoprosencephaly, which distinguishes it from hydranencephaly. The incomplete cleavage of the midline structures can have a varying degree of severity, which will affect the ultrasound presentation.[33–35]

Hydranencephaly appears as a large cranial vault that is completely filled with fluid. There is absence of a cerebral mantle.[14] The lack of a cerebral mantle permits the ultrasonographer to distinguish between hydranencephaly and holoprosencephaly. Theories explaining the development of hydranencephaly include occlusion of the internal carotid artery or intrauterine infections which lead to the failure of development of the cerebral hemispheres.

Agenesis of the corpus collosum can yield an ultrasound picture that may be confused with holoprosencephaly. Agenesis of the corpus callosum causes dilatation of the third ventricle, which is higher in position than usual.[36] The occipital horns are often dilated, and there is increased separation in the distance of the frontal horns. This often yields a large central ventricle, but the appearance is different from that seen in holoprosencephaly.

## Cystic Masses

Sonolucent fluid-filled regions within the cranium represent a variety of cystic masses. The sonographer must first attempt to visualize the ventricular system and see if the cystic regions are separate from the ventricles. A normal cystic region that can be quite pronounced in the second trimester is the cisterna magna. The cisterna magna is most prominent from 20 to 26 weeks' gestation. A prominent cisterna magna raises the possibility of pathologic cystic masses such as Dandy-Walker syndrome or a subarachnoid cyst.[37] Dandy-Walker syndrome is secondary to cystic dilatation of the fourth ventricle. This often leads to a dramatic increase in the size of the posterior fossa. Dandy-Walker syndrome is very difficult to distinguish from an arachnoid cyst.[38] Cysts may also arise in the choroid plexus. Usually they are of no consequence. There has been a case reported in which multiple cysts in the choroid plexus disappeared later in pregnancy.[39]

## Hemorrhage

Intraventricular and intracranial hemorrhage in the fetus have a similar ultrasound appearance as in the neonate. Such fetal hemorrhages usually appear as echogenic masses within the ventricle in the cerebral hemispheres. Intraventricular hemorrhage is diagnosed by identifying increased echogenicity of the ventricular system. Increased echogenicity in the lateral and third ventricles has led to the correct diagnosis.[40, 41] An echogenic region with a fluid level has been identified in the dependent hemisphere of the fetus.[42] It can be difficult to distinguish intraventricular hemorrhage from a large choroid plexus.[41] The choroid plexus is normally highly echogenic. Hemorrhage also results in increased echogenicity and may be difficult to distinguish from the normal variant. The etiology of hemorrhage is varied and includes preeclampsia, abruption, and isoimmune neonatal thrombocytopenia.[43]

Areas of increased echogenicity may be identified within the cerebral hemisphere. Such a finding is compatible with intracranial hemorrhage rather than intraventricular hemorrhage. An intracranial mass was found in a 26-week-old fetus in a mother who was suffering from abruptio placentae.[44] Autopsy confirmed the presence of an intracranial hemorrhage. A complex mass was identified in a 32-week-old fetus in the cerebral hemispheres. The mass had a mixed lucent and echogenic appearance secondary to intracranial hemorrhage.[45] An intraventricular and intracranial hemorrhage was identified in a 32-week-old fetus examined in utero after a maternal seizure. A large echogenic mass was demonstrated in the fetus, which had recently died, supposedly from the maternal seizure.[46]

### Intracranial Tumors

Fetal intracranial tumors are rare. They are usually secondary to intracranial teratomas. In children less than 2 months of age, intracranial teratomas account for 50% of brain tumors.[47] Therefore, it is not surprising that intracranial fetal teratomas have been diagnosed.[47, 48] The initial detection of this tumor may be secondary to an extremely large fetal head size.[6] Another presenting feature has been the unusual, sudden onset of rapid fetal head growth.[47] Evaluation of intracranial anatomy will disclose abnormal architecture and loss of the normal anatomical landmarks.[48] When a large fetal head is present without evidence of a cystic mass, the possibility of an intracranial fetal teratoma should be considered.

### Encephalocele

Encephaloceles are rare lesions that occur in approximately 1 to 4 in 10,000 live births.[49] They can be detected by elevated AFP levels in the maternal serum or amniotic fluid. Encephaloceles are defects within the calvarium with herniation of the meninges or of meninges and brain protruding through the defect. If the encephalocele is large, the size of the fetal head may be reduced.[8] Encephaloceles are usually located in the midline, with the majority situated posteriorly.[14, 49, 50] They occur because of failure of the neural tube to close in early embryonic development. Frontal encephaloceles are much less common.[51] Posterior encephaloceles may often be mistaken for other abnormalities such as cervical meningoceles and cystic hygromas. The important differential finding on ultrasound is the presence of a skull defect in an encephalocele. A potential for a false ear in the context of polyhydramnios.[52]

Midline encephaloceles arise from failure of the neural tube to close. Lateral encephaloceles may result from disruption of fetal skull growth secondary to amniotic bands which have been indicated in limb and other abnormalities. They are also thought to cause encephaloceles, especially those away from the midline.[50]

## Fetal Spine

Examination of the fetal spine has become extremely important because of the availability of other laboratory examinations that assist in the diagnosis of NTDs. AFP and acetylcholinesterase assays are laboratory tests that indicate the presence of NTDs. Ultrasound examination is often ordered in conjunction with these tests.

Evaluation of the fetal spine is extremely difficult. The fetal position is often not optimum. Fetal activity also makes the examination quite difficult. I have found it easiest to examine the fetal spine in segments. The cervical, thoracic, and lumbosacral segments should be examined separately. Fetal position will dictate which area is examined first. I attempt to examine the fetal spine in both transverse and longitudinal planes. The cervical spine is studied from the level of the occiput to the clavicles. By scanning back and forth numerous times, every vertebral body can be identified separately. The thoracic spine is then examined from the level of the clavicle to the level of the stomach. The same procedure is performed in transverse and longitudinal planes. Finally, the most difficult area, from the stomach to the distal sacrum, is examined. The lumbosacral region is where most of the pathology occurs. It is important that longitudinal scans of the spine be made from the posterior direction. Not only will the spinal defects be identified posteriorly, but many times the protruding masses will also be evident. If longitudinal scans are made only in a coronal plane, diagnostic errors will occur. Examination of the fetal spine is often quite tedious. However, it is important that each area be thoroughly scrutinized and no region inadvertently skipped. If all levels are scanned systemically, this can be avoided.

### Spinal Abnormalities

Spinal dysraphism denotes abnormal or incomplete fusion of the midline dorsal region of the spine during embryogenesis. The open forms of spinal dysraphism include meningocele and myelomeningocele.[53] These open forms can be identified on ultrasound. Occult forms of spinal dysraphism include intracanalicular lipoma and tethered cord, seen in neonates and infants. Spinal NTDs occur in 1.4–1.5 in 1,000 live births.[54] There are numberous causes of spinal NTDs, ranging from genetic to environmental. Valproic acid has been indicated as a causative agent and ultrasound diagnosis of a meningomyelocele has recently been reported.[55]

AFP can be detected in maternal serum and amniotic fluid. An elevated AFP level is highly suggestive of an NTD.[56, 57] When the AFP level is more than 5 SD above normal, a neural tube or other defect is usually present.[56] When the AFP level is 3 to 5 SD above normal, the fetus is most often normal, although abnormalities are occasionally identified. Ultrasound plays an important role in such cases. Ultrasound examination of the fetus is undertaken to confirm the presence of a fetal abnormality.

A second laboratory test used in conjunction with AFP assay is acetylcholinesterase assay.[54] When the acetylcholinesterase and AFP assays are both positive, the findings are highly consistent with NTD. If the AFP assay is positive and the acetylcholinesterase assay is negative, other abnormalities should be looked for, such as omphalocele, GI tract abnormalities, or GU tract abnormalities.

Ultrasound findings in spinal NTDs demonstrate widening of the lateral ossification centers. The posterior elements may be completely missing and a mass may be protruding from the site. Transverse scans will often show a U-shaped appearance to the spinal elements.[15] These findings or any combination of the above may be present in spinal NTDs. Prenatal diagnosis by ultrasound greatly assists the obstetrician in the management of such patients.[58] Attempts have been made to assess the severity of the neurologic deficits by evaluating fetal lower extremity motion. Most of these attempts have been unsuccessful. Fetal lower limb movement can occur passively rather than actively. This distinction is very difficult to assess on ultrasound.

Other spinal tumors may also be visualized on ultrasound. Diastematomyelia has been diagnosed in utero.[53] This entity results in equal or unequal division of the spinal cord. A bright echo in the midportion of the cord at the level of the defect can be identified. Lipomas can also cause widening of the spinal cord.

Sacrococcygeal teratomas have been visualized in the lumbosacral region. These present as solid masses in the lower spine.[48]

## Normal Fetal Neck and Thorax

Evaluation of the fetal neck and thorax reveals numerous anatomical structures. The ribs appear as high-amplitude echoes, often with acoustic shadowing obscuring visualization within the thoracic cage. The clavicles can be easily seen, along with the scapula. The fetal thorax is surrounded by spine and ribs. To evaluate the intrathoracic region, it is often necessary to scan between ribs. The fetal heart is easily recognized in the central to left side of the thoracic cavity. Fetal cardiac rate and anatomy should be noticed. These will be discussed in more detail later. The four chambers of the heart are usually easily visible with the apex of the heart, toward the left side of the thorax. It is important to maintain a three-dimensional mental image of how the fetus is lying so that the heart can be found on the correct side of the thorax. The aortic arch is visualized, with several neck vessels extending into the soft tissues of the neck. The descending thoracic aorta is present adjacent to the anterior aspect of the thoracic spine and slightly to the left. It is important to recognize the relationship of the aorta and inferior vena cava. The inferior vena cava should be to the right of the aorta. Following the neck vessels off the aortic arch, the soft tissues of the neck come into view. Very often, a fluid-filled trachea will be identified.[59] Besides cardiac activity, fetal breathing can be noticed on real-time examination.[60] Fetal breathing can be recognized by expansion of the fetal thorax and movement of the hemidiaphragms bilaterally. The hemidiaphragm on the right side is easy to visualize since it is adjacent to the liver. The hemidiaphragm on the left is slightly more difficult to visualize, although the fetal stomach acts as an anatomical landmark.

## Abnormal Fetal Neck and Thorax

Masses in the region of the neck can be easily identified. Masses such as encephaloceles and cervical meningomyeloceles were discussed earlier. Soft tissue masses that have been described in the region of the neck include cervical teratomas, which present as echogenic masses extending anteriorly.[61, 62] An intrauterine diagnosis of fetal goiter has also been made on ultrasound.[63] It appeared as a soft tissue mass in the anterior portion of the neck, which also resulted in polyhydramnios.

Fetal thoracic abnormalities that have been previously described include pleural effusions, diaphragmatic hernias, cystadenomatoid malformation of the lung, and enteric cysts.[6, 7] The contour of the thorax should be initially evaluated to determine whether it is proportional to the fetal abdomen and BPD. Cases of thanatophoric dwarfism have been diagnosed in utero. A small fetal thorax relative to the fetal abdomen led to the correct diagnosis.[64] Cystic masses within the lungs should suggest the diagnosis of adenomatoid malformations.[65] These can reach extremely large size, causing the mediastinum and cardiac structures to shift. Echogenic masses within the thorax have been reported in extralobar pulmonary sequestration.[66] Large fluid collections in the lung which appear within the pleural space have been diagnosed in fetal hydrothorax.[67] It is usually easy to differentiate hydrothorax from cystic adenomatoid malformation of the lung. In fetal hydrothorax the collapsed lung parenchyma appears to float within the fluid. Masses protruding from the thorax have been seen in sarcomatous lesions of the fetal body wall. Other protruding thoracic masses have been diagnosed in fetal ectopia cordis.[68–70] In this entity, fetal cardiac activity is identified outside the expected confines of the fetal thorax.

## Normal Fetal Abdomen

Numerous anatomical structures are easily identifiable in the fetal abdomen. Initially it is most important to evaluate the fetal abdominal contour. The abdominal wall is a sharp reflector in contact with amniotic fluid. Any disruption in the abdominal wall contour can be easily identified. The umbilical vessels are seen entering the abdominal wall at the umbilical level. The number of vessels can be determined at the site.

The various organs of the abdomen are easily identifiable on ultrasound.[71] The liver is the largest abdominal organ and is situated in the right upper quadrant. Vascular anatomy of the liver has been well delineated on ultrasound.[3, 72] The umbilical vein can be followed as it courses to the right side of the fetal abdomen and enters the liver. Within the liver the portal venous system and hepatic venous system can be identified. The hepatic veins are noted to empty into the inferior vena cava, which drains into the right atrium of the heart. It is important to maintain a right-left orientation of the fetus so that you are sure the liver is on the right side of the abdomen. The size of the liver is difficult to ascertain because of adjacent echogenic bowel. However, fetal liver ultrasound measurements have been determined during normal pregnancy.[73] A lucency is often seen lateral to the umbilical vein. This represents the fetal gallbladder. It is variable in size and may not always be seen. Cephalad to the liver is a curved lucency that represents the right hemidiaphragm. An echo texture difference is identified between the liver and the right lung. Fetal respirations can be checked by watching the right hemidiaphragm move with each respiration. The fetal stomach is usually seen on routine examination. It is a fluid-filled structure in the left upper quadrant of the fetal abdomen. If the fetal stomach is not visualized, the patient can be asked to wait for 20 or 30 minutes and then be reexamined. This will usually allow visualization of the fetal stomach in the left upper quadrant. The fetal spleen is slightly more difficult to demonstrate but can be visualized if fetal position permits. The left hemidiaphragm is more difficult to visualize than the right. However, it also presents as a curved lucency between the fetal stomach and the left lung and heart. The kidneys present a typical bull's-eye appearance on each side of the fetal spine. Occasionally the renal collecting systems are readily evident. The fetal stomach is usually the only fluid-filled bowel loop seen, especially early in pregnancy. The bowel and mesentery are present as echogenic regions in the middle and lower abdomen. The other fluid structure present in the lower abdomen represents the fetal urinary bladder, which is extremely variable in size. As with the fetal stomach, if the fetal bladder is not seen, the patient is asked to return in 20–30 minutes, after which time it should be readily visible.

### Polyhydramnios

GI tract abnormalities are often associated with polyhydramnios. Increased amniotic fluid volume is difficult to ascertain if it is present only to a minor degree.

Severe cases of polyhydramnios are readily evident on scanning the uterus. However, mild cases of polyhydramnios are difficult to diagnose because of variation in the ratio of amniotic fluid to fetus throughout pregnancy. Amniotic fluid appears quite prominent in the mid trimester compared to the fetus. It is less prominent in the third trimester. Therefore, a diagnosis of polyhydramnios should be made with caution in the second trimester. Polyhydramnios occurs in approximately 0.7%–1.4% of pregnancies. However, polyhydramnios is associated with a serious congenital fetal abnormality in approximately 20% of cases.[74] If polyhydramnios is identified, close examination of the fetal GI tract is necessary. GI tract abnormalities are usually associated with polyhydramnios. GU tract abnormalities are usually associated with oligohydramnios. Amniotic fluid volume often is an important clue as to which area of the fetus should be examined closely.

## Esophageal Atresia

Esophageal atresia very often has no characteristic appearance on ultrasound. Approximately 90% of cases of esophageal atresia are associated with tracheoesophageal fistula. This fistulous tract permits passage of fluid into the fetal stomach. Therefore, the fetal stomach will be identified on ultrasound, and no polyhydramnios will be present. However, approximately 10% of esophageal atresias do not have an associated tracheoesophageal fistula. In these cases, no fluid will be present in the fetal stomach, and polyhydramnios will often be present.[71] When polyhydramnios is identified, the fetal abdomen should be closely examined to determine whether or not the fetal stomach is present. Absence of the fetal stomach confirms the diagnosis of esophageal atresia.[75] Occasionally there may be a disparity in the ratio of the fetal abdominal diameter to the head diameter. The fetal abdominal diameter will be smaller than anticipated because of the empty fetal stomach.[76] If the fetal stomach is not identified, the patient should be examined over a 30-minute period to be sure that the fetal stomach is never present. Occasionally the sonographer may examine a normal fetus that has just emptied its stomach. Precaution dictates that a follow-up scan be obtained to confirm the absence of the fetal stomach.

## Duodenal Atresia

The "double bubble" seen on fetal abdominal x-ray films may also be seen on ultrasound examination of the abdomen in a fetus with duodenal atresia. Fluid-filled stomach and distended duodenum present as two large cystic masses in the upper abdomen of the fetus. Duodenal atresia usually has an easily recognizable ultrasound appearance. Later in pregnancy it is often associated with polyhydramnios. The fetal stomach is usually the larger of the two circular structures. It is important to recognize this entity before birth so that surgical treatment can be immediately instituted. If this entity is not recognized, neonatal problems secondary to emesis, aspiration, and electrolyte imbalance will occur.[77] Early ultrasound diagnosis forewarns the obstetrician and pediatrician of this correctable lesion.

## Meconium Peritonitis

Meconium peritonitis is often a complication of bowel perforation. Meconium may appear as an area of increased echogenicity within the fetal abdomen.[78, 79] In some instances this increased echogenicity may be transient in nature. On serial examinations of several patients, these areas of increased echogenicity disappeared over several weeks' time. However, some areas of increased echogenicity persist and increase. If perforation occurs, meconium peritonitis will result and lead to areas of fibrosis and calcification.[80, 81] This results in high-amplitude regions in the fetal abdomen which may demonstrate acoustic shadowing secondary to calcification. If meconium perforation occurs, an area of encapsulation may result in a large sonolucent cystic mass within the fetal abdomen.[82–85] The resulting fluid collections become localized and form a meconium cyst.

## Hepatobiliary System

Examination of the right upper quadrant may reveal abnormalities in the region of the liver and gallbladder. The fetal liver has an even parenchymal texture. The vascular anatomy of the liver has already been described. Abnormal echo texture in a portion of the liver along with distortion of vascular anatomy may lead to the diagnosis of an intrahepatic mass. If this mass is echo free with through-transmission, a liver cyst can be suspected. Liver hemangioma has been detected in utero.[86] It appeared as a region of abnormal liver parenchymal texture in the left lobe. Mesenchymal hamartoma has been visualized in utero as a hypoechoic liver mass.[87] This lesion is seen exclusively in childhood and has also been identified in the fetus.

Choledochal cysts present as fluid-filled masses in the right upper quadrant.[88, 89] Choledochal cysts result from dilatation of the distal common bile duct. These cysts can be difficult to diagnose correctly. It is necessary to recognize two fluid-filled structures in the right upper quadrant. A normal gallbladder must be demonstrated before the diagnosis of choledochal cyst can be considered, unless the choledochal cyst is massively enlarged. In the case of massive enlargement, duodenal atresia may be mistakenly diagnosed. Fetal gallstones have also been identified on ultrasound.[71, 90] These are extremely rare and usually associated with hemolytic anemia. Fetal gallstones have a similar ultrasonic appearance as gallstones found in the adult. A highly echogenic area in the right upper quadrant with deep acoustic shadowing in the fetal gallbladder bed confirms the diagnosis of fetal cholelithiasis.

## Diaphragmatic Hernia

Diaphragmatic hernia is a rare anomaly that occurs in approximately 1 in 4,000 births.[71] The diaphragm is usually visualized as a curvilinear lucent line between the liver and right lung or between the stomach and left lung and heart. Several findings can suggest the possibility of a diaphragmatic hernia. A shaft of the heart and mediastinum to the right or the left side should always raise the possibility of a diaphragmatic hernia. When a mediastinal shift is noted, close examination of the fetal stomach and liver should follow. If the fetal stomach and liver are in normal position, an intrathoracic mass is the most likely diagnosis. If the fetal liver and stomach are not identified in their usual location, a diaphragmatic hernia is quite likely.[91] When the diagnosis of a diaphragmatic hernia is made, the obstetrician and pediatrician should be notified so that surgery may be undertaken immediately after delivery. The difficulty with a diaphragmatic hernia is the problem that arises from hypoplasia of the lungs. If the lungs are severely hypoplastic, this will endanger the fetus at the time of delivery.

## Abdominal Wall Deformities

Examination of the fetal abdomen may reveal a deformity of the abdominal wall. A mass protruding from the fetal abdomen should raise the possibility of an omphalocele or gastroschisis. It is important to differentiate omphalocele from gastroschisis since omphalocele has a high association with other fetal anomalies. Omphalocele is a protrusion of abdominal contents through a midline defect. It has a covering membrane, and the umbilical cord is situated at the top of the omphalocele.[91, 92–95] Omphaloceles vary greatly in size. They may be quite small and contain a minimal amount of bowel, or they may be extremely large and contain the entire bowel, liver, spleen and even the heart. The umbilical cord inserts into the top of the herniated sac. An elevated AFP level is associated with omphalocele. This is one of the reasons for ultrasound examination of a pregnancy with an elevated AFP level. Close examination of the abdominal wall is necessary to rule out omphalocele and gastroschisis which is also associated with elevated AFP level.

Gastroschisis is herniation of bowel and abdominal contents lateral to the insertion of the umbilical cord. The umbilical cord enters the abdomen in its usual location. The abdominal contents herniate through a thin portion of the abdominal wall in a paraumbilical location. There is no covering membrane over gastroschisis. This is another way to determine whether or not we are dealing with gastroschisis or omphalocele. An omphalocele will contain a sharp, thin, reflective covering membrane that can often be identified over the area of protrusion. Gastroschisis does not have such a membrane. Therefore, the fetal bowel loops appear to float freely within the amniotic fluid without evidence of a covering membrane.[96] Gastroschisis also has a very low association with fetal anomalies.

## Normal Fetal Genitourinary System

The fetal kidneys are difficult to see in the first trimester and are often not visualized until 15 weeks at the earliest.[97] They present as circular, lucent regions on each side of the fetal spine in transverse plane. They are bean-shaped in coronal or sagittal views.[98] From 15 to 26 weeks, they are difficult to distinguish from surrounding tissue but can be seen in numerous instances. By the early third trimester, an echogenic border and central echoes are usually seen. This appearance is thought to be secondary to fatty deposition in the perirenal space and central collecting region.[97] The kidneys grow throughout pregnancy in proportion to fetal growth. However, there is a wide variation in the range of normal renal growth.[99] This may be due to factors which make it difficult to identify the borders in many fetal kidneys. Most of the time the central echoes are highly echogenic without evidence of fluid. Occasionally fluid may be identified in the renal collecting system. This is a normal anatomical variant and should not be misdiagnosed as hydronephrosis. When a kidney is absent in the renal fossa, the possibility of a congenital anomaly such as crossed fused ectopia should be considered.[100] If the kidneys are not visualized in normal position, the remainder of the fetal abdomen should be examined to determine whether or not an ectopic kidney is identified.

The fetal urinary bladder is usually always seen during the course of an ultrasound examination. It is very important to visualize the fetal urinary bladder because it indicates adequate urine production. If the bladder is not seen on the initial study, the patient should be asked to return for reexamination in 30–45 minutes to determine whether or not the fetal bladder has distended. If the fetal bladder has not distended, a genitourinary abnormality should be considered. The fetal urinary bladder has a wide variety of appearance, mainly depending on its size. It is circular to oval in the transverse plane. On longitudinal or coronal views the urinary bladder has an elongated, rectangular appearance. It can appear quite large and disturbing when initially seen in its maximally distended state. If the possibility of urinary bladder outlet obstruction is raised, the patient should be imaged at 15-minute intervals to determine whether or not bladder emptying occurs.

The fetal adrenal glands often present diagnostic problems on evaluation of the kidneys. The fetal adrenal glands are quite large, especially early in pregnancy. A typical sonographic appearance to the adrenals consists of a central echogenic line surrounded by two lucent limbs. The adrenal appears oval on cross-sectional view and triangular on coronal or sagittal views.[101, 102] Renal measurements may be difficult to obtain because of the indistinct border between the renal and adrenal gland. Close examination of this area usually separates these two organs.

## Oligohydramnios and Elevated AFP Levels

Severe bilateral renal disease is usually accompanied by oligohydramnios.[98] Evaluation of amniotic fluid is always difficult unless the ultrasonographer has a great deal of experience. However, in the setting of severe oligohydramnios, very little fluid is noted around the fetus. This is most definite in the second trimester, when a large amount of amniotic fluid should be present. Oligohydramnios poses diagnostic difficulty because of the poor quality of ultrasound images created in the absence of amniotic fluid. It is very difficult to obtain adequate fetal detail when oligohydramnios is present. Often the fetal kidneys cannot be visualized even though they are present. In such instances it is most important to evaluate the size and appearance of the fetal bladder. If the fetal bladder is present and adequate in size, then fetal urine production is occurring. If one can document emptying and refilling of the fetal bladder, a renal cause of oligohyramnios is less likely. However, if the urinary bladder is never seen or always appears extremely small, severe renal disease is the most likely cause of the oligohyramnios. One may or may not see renal masses in the renal fossa in the setting of severe renal disease. This is unimportant since the urinary bladder has yielded the most diagnostic information with regard to urine production.

A secondary consideration in the presence of severe oligohydramnios is the effects on the fetal lung. The lack of adequate amniotic fluid will often lead to hypoplasia of the fetal lungs. This becomes a serious consideration if the oligohydramnios persists for a long time.

Increased amniotic fluid and serum AFP levels have been found in GU tract abnormalities such as polycystic kidney disease and obstructive uropathy.[103] When a fetus is examined because of an elevated AFP level, the GU system should be studied closely. Again, the fetal bladder is an important diagnostic anatomical landmark and should be visualized. It will usually indicate whether or not urine production is adequate.

## Renal Agenesis

Bilateral renal agenesis is not compatible with extrauterine life. Severe oligohydramnios is usually present in pregnancy. By 20 weeks very little amniotic fluid will be visualized in the uterus. Most often examination of the renal fossa will reveal absence of the kidneys and nonvisualization of the fetal urinary bladder.[98] Occasionally, paraspinous sonolucencies may be seen. These areas are most likely secondary to prominent adrenal glands, which can be mistaken for the kidneys.[104] Evaluation of the fetal urinary bladder becomes extremely important in these cases. In bilateral renal agenesis the fetal urinary bladder will not be visualized. The fetal urinary bladder usually fills and empties in a cycle over a 1–1½-hour period.[7]

Unilateral renal agenesis is compatible with life. Often it will not be detected in utero. Since there is a normal and functioning kidney and urine production is adequate, oligohydramnios is not present. The urinary bladder will be well filled and emptied periodically.[105]

## Multicystic Kidney

Multicystic kidney is usually unilateral. On ultrasound it appears as a large multiloculated cystic mass in the upper abdomen in a paraspinous location.[106, 107] Numerous large cysts may be present. If the cystic region is quite large, it will increase the abdominal diameter and circumference. The contralateral kidney and urinary bladder are normal. There is no evidence of oligohyramnios since the normal kidney is producing adequate urine. These cystic masses may be difficult to distinguish from hydronephrosis. Usually coronal scans of the involved side will permit a distinction to be made between hydronephrosis and multicystic kidney. In hydronephrosis the typical finger-like projections of the dilated calyces as they extend from the renal pelvis will be visualized. In multicystic kidney the fluid masses have a random appearance rather than following anatomical planes. Multicystic kidney is rarely bilateral. When it is, severe oligohyramnios and nonvisualization of the fetal urinary bladder will be present. An interesting case has been reported of multicystic kidney disease in identical twins. Each twin had evidence of multicystic kidney on the same side.[108]

## Infantile Polycystic Kidneys

Infantile polycystic renal disease is bilateral. The kidneys present as large, homogeneous areas with increased echogenicity bilaterally.[109] The kidneys become so large that the abdominal diameter and circumference will be increased. Oligohydramnios is present, and the fetal urinary bladder cannnot be visualized because of inadequate urine production. The cause for the increased echogenicity of the kidneys is the small size of the cysts. The cysts are too small to image on ultrasound and create diffuse increased echogenicity throughout the renal fossa. These renal masses have been reported as early as 14 weeks, with oligohydramnios present at 18 weeks.[110] A word of caution is in order, however. A case has been reported which appeared normal at 19 weeks. The kidneys were not increased in size, and amniotic fluid was considered normal. However, reexamination at 25 weeks revealed oligohydramnios and increased size of, and echogenicity in, the renal fossa, consistent with infantile polycystic kidney disease.[111] This entity can also be seen as part of a spectrum of Meckel's syndrome. This syndrome includes occipital encephalocele, infantile polycystic kidney, and polydactyly.

## Urinary Tract Obstruction

Fetal urinary tract obstruction will have a varying appearance on ultrasound, depending on the level of obstruction. Obstruction may occur at the ureteropelvic junction. It may be unilateral or bilateral. When unilateral obstruction is present, a characteristic ultrasound appearance of a dilated renal pelvis along with dilated calyces can be identified.[113] This may be difficult to distinguish from multicystic kidney. However, a coronal scan of the involved kidney will usually show a characteristic appearance of hydronephrosis, whereas multicystic kidney has a random cystic appearance. Bilateral hydronephrosis will present as bilateral dilated collecting systems in the paraspinous region. It is important to attempt to evaluate the amount of surrounding renal parenchymal tissue in such cases.

Obstruction at the ureterovesical junction is less common.[114] The renal pelvis will be dilated, and a distended tubular structure on the involved side will be visualized down to the level of the fetal bladder. The possibility of an ectopic ureterocele should be considered. When bilateral hydronephrosis is present, close examination of the fetal bladder is undertaken. Very often the renal pelvis, calyces, and ureters are dilated down to the bladder.[115] The urinary bladder may also be distended and enlarged. In cases of prune belly syndrome, the abdominal musculature is lax and distended. Markedly dilated fetal ureters and fetal urinary bladder will be seen in the fetal abdomen.[116] When hydronephrosis is suspected, serial examinations are mandatory. Reports have indicated that hydronephrosis may be transient in nature.[117] Several cases have been reported in which bilateral hydronephrosis was definitely identified. Follow-up examinations several weeks later showed resolution of the suspected obstructive problem. The findings were thought to be secondary to varying degrees of bladder filling. The fetal collecting system may be lax in nature and appear dilated when the urinary bladder is markedly filled. After bladder emptying, the fetal collecting system may decompress and have a normal ultrasonic appearance.

Primary megaureter is an important entity to recognize so that fetal intrauterine surgery is not attempted. In primary megaureter the renal collecting system is dilated at the level of the renal pelvis and ureters. The fetal bladder is not enlarged, and adequate renal parenchyma is present.[118, 119] The important distinction to be made ultrasonographically is the presence of adequate renal parenchyma without evidence of dilatation of the calyceal system. The urinary bladder is also noted to empty periodically with no evidence of bladder outlet obstruction. Amniotic fluid volume is usually within normal limits.

Intrauterine fetal surgery is performed to relieve urinary tract obstruction in the fetus.[120-122] One must be absolutely sure that a definite obstruction persists. Often these cases are accompanied by oligohydramnios, indicating the severity of the obstruction. However, dilatation of the fetal collecting system does not always indicate severe obstruction. As noted previously, transient fetal obstruction has been reported. If persistent obstruction is present on numerous examinations and the site of obstruction can be localized, then definite obstruction can be considered. Fetal surgery carries numerous risks. It should only be undertaken in the most severe situations.

## Renal Tumors

Fetal renal tumors are not commonly identified in utero. A fetal renal hamartoma or mesoblastic nephroma has been identified in utero.[123] This is the most common renal neoplasm in the first few months of life. It must be remembered that the fetal adrenal glands can be quite large. It is important to recognize the normal fetal adrenal gland and not diagnose a renal tumor.[101, 102] Adrenal tumors do occur. Neuroblastoma has been diagnosed in utero.[124] It appeared as a cystic mass in the renal fossa and was initially thought to be of renal rather than adrenal origin.

Evaluation of the fetal pelvis is usually confined to examining the urinary bladder. As mentioned previously, the urinary bladder fills and empties over a period of approximately 1 hour. However, other cystic masses may be identified in the pelvis which can present a confusing picture. Ovarian cysts have been noted in female fetuses.[125] On ultrasound these appear as cystic masses in the pelvis that do not empty and refill periodically, as does the urinary bladder. If these cysts are large, they can compress the urinary bladder and make visualization of this normal structure difficult. Hydrometrocolpos also manifests as a pelvic mass. It has been reported as both echo free and echogenic.[126, 127] This large mass also compresses the fetal urinary bladder.

Determination of fetal gender can play a helpful role in certain diagnoses. An example is bilateral hydronephrosis with possible bladder outlet obstruction. Since posterior urethral valves are a common cause of this entity, ascertaining that the fetus is male would be helpful. Fetal gender has been determined in utero.[128, 129] Fluid has been identified in the fetal scrotum consistent with hydrocele.[130] It is often difficult to determine fetal gender, especially if fetal position is not optimum. However, a recent case in which ambiguous genitalia were identified indicates the diagnostic accuracy that is possible in this area.[131]

## Fetal Hydrops

There are numerous ultrasound findings in fetal hydrops. Massive soft tissue edema along with pleural and pericardial effusions and ascites can be visualized. These findings often signify a grave prognosis for the fetus. They have been associated with Rh isoimmunization, α-thalassemia, congenital heart disease, other congenital anomalies, fetal anemia, and fetal tumors.[132] Ultrasound findings are usually characteristic of a fluid collection within the fetus. The ultrasound findings of fetal ascites and pleural effusion are similar to those seen in the neonate and adult. An entity termed pseudoascites has been described.[133, 134] It is important not to diagnose ascites when a small lucent rim is identified beneath the abdominal wall. This rim may represent a normal anatomical variant, most likely fetal abdominal wall musculature.[134] Recent reports have also noted the occurrence of transient fetal ascites.[135] Two cases were described in which fetal ascites was well documented in the second trimester but no longer present on follow-up examinations near term.

## Cystic Hygromas

Cystic hygromas are secondary to abnormal development of the lymphatic system. On ultrasound they usually appear as multiloculated cystic masses, most often in the posterior region of the fetal neck and head.[136] Approximately 80% of cystic hygromas are in this cervical location.[7] A recent report indicates that some cystic hygromas may have a solid component in addition to their multiloculated appearance.[137] Although cystic hygromas can be isolated anatomical abnormalities, there is an increased association with Turner's syndrome.[138] When cystic hygromas are identified, chromosome analysis is needed to determine whether or not Turner's syndrome is present. Cystic hygromas are one of the causes of increased AFP levels. The neck region is always examined to determine if a multiloculated mass is present. Cystic hygromas pose a diagnostic problem since occipital encephaloceles and meningomyeloceles of the cervical region may have a similar appearance on ultrasound.[8, 139] In order to distinguish an encephalocele and a meningomyelocele from a cystic hygroma, it is necessary to evaluate the bony structures in the region.[139] If an encephalocele is present, there will be a break in the occipital bone. If a cervical meningomyelocele is present, the osseous structures of the cervical spine will be widened and disrupted. If the osseous structures are intact, the diagnosis of a cystic hygroma can be made.

## Normal Fetal Skeleton

With improved equipment, evaluation of the fetal skeleton has become more sophisticated. The fetal cranium and spine have already been discussed. Most long bones can be visualized by mid-second trimester.[140] Even the phalanges and metatarsals are visible at this time. The hands and feet may be difficult to see because of fetal position. The long bones are usually readily visible, the only drawback being marked fetal activity. Numerous long bones have been measured on ultrasound. Ultrasound measurements are more accurate than radiographic measurements since no magnification is present. Femur length has been used to predict gestational age.[141] To measure the adequate femur length, it is necessary to scan the femur parallel to its long axis. Scanning off the long axis will yield falsely small measurements. Other long bones including the humerus, radius, ulna, tibia, and fibula have been measured in large series.[142, 143] Epiphyseal ossification centers are also noted to occur at various times in pregnancy. The distal femoral epiphysis is visible on ultrasound at approximately 34–36 weeks.[144, 145] All of the data in evaluation of the normal fetal skeleton now permits diagnosis of skeletal abnormalities.

## Fetal Skeletal Abnormalities

In pregnancies at risk for skeletal abnormalities, the fetal skeleton should be evaluated for bone brightness, deformity, fractures, and abnormal growth.[146] A comparison of the long bones with the BPD may be helpful in early detection of abnormalities.[147] This is not always the case if the fetal skull is not growing appropriately. Deformities of the fetal skull and thorax have been reported in thanatophoric dwarfism. Once these deformities are identified, the long bones may also demonstrate shortening.[22, 23, 64]

Achondroplasia has been diagnosed in utero by following the femur length in serial studies. In heterozygous achondroplasia the femur length is in the normal range early in pregnancy.[148, 149] However, the femur length falls below the range of normal at approximately 21 to 27 weeks' gestation. In the homozygous form of achondroplasia a short femur length appears much earlier in gestation.

Achondrogenesis will manifest with retarded growth of vertebral bodies and sacral ossification centers, along with shortened limbs.[150, 151] Decreased bone echogenicity in the region of the vertebrae and sacrum can suggest the correct diagnosis in the presence of shortened long bones. Osteogenesis imperfecta has been diagnosed at 17 weeks' gestation based on the ultrasound findings of numerous long bone fractures.[152] Isolated limb abnormalities may be seen in amniotic band syndrome. This can be identified on a routine ultrasound examination. Fusion of the lower extremities and congenital short femur have been diagnosed in utero.[153, 154] Abnormalities of the fetal hand and foot, including clubfoot, are also identifiable.[155–157] Evaluation of the fetal hands and feet is quite difficult because of fetal movement and fetal position. With increased awareness and attention to the fetal skeleton, improvement in the diagnosis of fetal skeletal abnormalities can be anticipated.

### Conjoined Twins

Conjoined twins is an extremely rare event that occurs in 1 in 50,000 live births.[158, 159] Whenever twins are present, it is necessary to visualize that they are completely separate by ultrasound. This may be difficult especially later in pregnancy when very little amniotic fluid is noted. The degree of conjunction is extremely variable. It may be minimal to highly severe.[158–162] The severity of conjunction will help the obstetrician and surgeon determine the best method of delivery. Fortunately this event is very rare. Scanning one of these cases is quite difficult, especially with both parents watching the TV monitor and asking questions.

## References

1. Johnson ML, Hattan RA, Rees GK: The normal fetus. *Semin Roentgenol* 1982; 17:182.
2. Hattan RA, Rees GK, Johnson ML: Normal fetal anatomy. *Radiol Clin North Am* 1982; 20: 271.
3. Jeanty P, Romero R, Hobbins JC: Vascular anatomy of the fetus. *J Ultrasound Med* 1984; 3:113.
4. Lyons EA, Levi CS, Greenberg CR: The abnormal fetus. *Semin Roentgenol* 1982; 17:198.
5. Bree RL, Mariona FG: The role of ultrasound in the evaluation of normal and abnormal fetal growth. *Semin Ultrasound* 1980; 1:264.
6. Hobbins JC, Venus I: Congenital anomalies. *Clin Diagn Ultrasound* 1979; 3:95.
7. Knochel JQ, Lee TG, Melendez MG, et al: Fetal anomalies involving the thorax and abdomen. *Radiol Clin North Am* 1982; 20:297.
8. Miskin M, Rothberg R: Prenatal detection of congenital anomalies on ultrasound. *Semin Ultrasound* 1980; 1:278.
9. Hobbins JC, Grannum PAT, Berkowitz RL, et al: Ultrasound diagnosis of congenital abnormalities. *Am J Obstet Gynecol* 1979; 134:331.
10. Johnson ML, Dunne MG, Mack LA, et al: Evaluation of fetal intercranial anatomy by static and renal time ultrasound. *JCU* 1980; 8:311.
11. McGahan JP, Phillips HE: Ultrasound evaluation of the size of the trigone of the fetal ventricle. *J Ultrasound Med* 1983; 2:315.
12. Laing FC, Stamler CE, Jeffrey RB: Ultrasonography of the fetal subarachnoid space. *J Ultrasound Med* 1983; 2:29.
13. Carrasco CR, Stierman ED, Harnsberger HR, et al: An algorithm for prenatal ultrasound diagnosis of congenital CNS abnormalities. *J Ultrasound Med* 1985; 4:163.
14. Hidalgo H, Bowie J, Rosenberg ER, et al: In utero sonographic diagnosis of fetal cerebral anomalies. *AJR* 1982; 139:143.
15. Fiske CE, Filly RA: Ultrasound evaluation of the normal and abnormal fetal neural axis. *Radiol Clin North* 1982; 20:285.
16. Robinson HP, Hood VD, Adam AH, e al: Diagnostic ultrasound: Early detection of fetal neural tube defects. *Obstet Gynecol* 1980; 56:705.
17. Worthen NJ, Lawrence D, Bustillo M: Amniotic band syndrome: Antepartum ultrasonic diagnosis of discordant anencephaly. *JCU* 1980; 8:453.
18. Mannes EJ, Crelin ES, Hobbins JS, et al: Sonographic demonstration of fetal acrania. *AJR* 1982; 139:181.
19. Lenke RR, Platt LD, Koch R: Ultrasonographic failure of early detection of fetal microcephaly in maternal phenylketonuria. *J Ultrasound* 1983; 2:177.
20. Kurtz AB, Wagner RJ, Rubin CS, et al: Ultrasound criteria for in utero diagnosis of microcephaly. *JCU* 1980; 8:11.

21. Sarti DA, Crandall BF, Winter J, et al: Correlation of biparietal and fetal body diameters: 12–26 weeks gestation. *AJR* 1981; 137:87.

22. Burrows PE, Stannard MW, Pearrow J, et al: Early antenatal sonographic recognition of thanatophoric displasia with cloverleaf skull deformity. *AJR* 1984; 143:841.

23. Mahony BS, Filly RA, Callen PW, et al: Thanatophoric dwarfism with the cloverleaf skull: A specific antenatal sonographic diagnosis. *J Ultrasound Med* 1985; 4:151.

24. Cayea PD, Bieber FR, Ross MJ, et al: Sonographic findings in otocephaly (synotia). *J Ultrasound Med* 1985; 4:377.

25. Chervenak FA, Berkowitz RL, Romero R, et al: The diagnosis of fetal hydrocephalus. *Am J Obstet Gynecol* 1983; 147:703.

26. Robertson RD, Sarti DA, Brown WJ, et al: Congenital hydrocephalus in two pregnancies following the birth of a child with neural tube defect: Aetiology and management. *J Med Genet* 1981; 18:105.

27. Chinn DH, Callen PW, Filly RA: The lateral cerebral ventricle in early second trimester. *Radiology* 1983; 148:529.

28. Pretorius DH, Drose JA, Manco-Johnson ML: Fetal lateral ventricular ratio determination during the second trimester. *J Ultrasound Med* 1986; 5:121.

29. Callen PW, Choolijian D: The effect of ventricular dilatation upon biometry of the fetal head. *J Ultrasound Med* 1986; 5:17.

30. Gillieson MS, Hickey NM: Prenatal diagnosis of fetal hydrocephalus associated with a normal biparietal diameter. *J Ultrasound Med* 1984; 3:227.

31. Hartung RW, Yiu-Chiu V: Demonstration of unilateral hydrocephalus in utero. *J Ultrasound Med* 1983; 2:369.

32. Bernholz JC, Frigoletto FD: Antenatal treatment of hydrocephalus. *N Engl J Med* 1981; 304:1021.

33. Chervenak FA, Isaacson G, Hobbins JC, et al: Diagnosis and management of fetal holoprosencephaly. *Obstet Gynecol* 1985; 66:322.

34. Chervenak FA, Isaacson G, Mahoney MJ, et al: The obstetric significance of holoprosencephaly. *Obstet Gynecol* 1984; 63:115.

35. Chervenak FA, Isaacson G, Hobbins JC, et al: Diagnosis and management of fetal holoprosencephaly. *Obstet Gynecol* 1985; 66:322.

36. Comstock CH, Culp D, Gonzalez J, et al: Agenesis of the corpus callosum in the fetus: Its evolution and significance. *J Ultrasound Med* 1985; 4:613.

37. Comstock CH, Boal DB: Enlarged fetal cisterna magna: Appearance and significance. *Obstet Gynecol* 1985; 66:25S.

38. Kirkinen P., Jouppila P, Valkeakari T, et al: Ultrasonic evaluation of the Dandy-Walker syndrome. *Obstet Gynecol* 1982; 59:18S.

39. Friday RO, Schwartz DB, Tuffli GA: Spontaneous intrauterine resolution of intraventricular cystic masses. *J Ultrasound Med* 1985; 4: 385.

40. McGahan JP, Haesslein HC, Meyers M, et al: Sonographic recognition of in utero intraventricular hemorrhage. *AJR* 1984; 142:171.

41. Kim MS, Elyaderani MK: Sonographic diagnosis of cerebroventricular hemorrhage. *Radiology* 1982; 142:479.

42. Mintz MC, Arger PH, Coleman BG: In utero sonographic diagnosis of intracerebral hemorrhage. *J Ultrasound Med* 1985; 4:375.

43. Morales WJ, Stroup M: Intracranial hemorrhage in utero due to isoimmune neonatal thrombocytopenia. *Obstet Gynecol* 1985; 65:20S.

44. Bondurant S, Boehm FH, Fleischer AC, et al: Antepartum diagnosis of fetal intracranial hemorrhage by ultrasound. *Obstet Gynecol* 1984; 63:25S.

45. Donn SM, Barr M, McLeary RD: Massive intracerebral hemorrhage in utero: Sonographic appearance and pathologic correlation. *Obstet Gynecol* 1984; 63:28S.

46. Minkoff H, Schaffer RM, Delke I, et al: Diagnosis of intracranial hemorrhage in utero after a maternal seizure. *Obstet Gynecol* 1985; 65:22S.

47. Lipman SP, Pretorius DH, Rumack CM, et al: Fetal intracranial teratoma: US diagnosis of three cases and a review of the literature. *Radiology* 1985; 157:491.

48. Chervenak FA, Isaacson G, Touloukian R, et al: Diagnosis and management of fetal teratomas. *Obstet Gynecol* 1985; 66:666.

49. Graham D, Johnson RB, Winn K, et al: The role of sonography in the prenatal diagnosis

and management of encephalocele. *J Ultrasound Med* 1982; 1:111.

50. Chervenak FA, Isaacson G, Mahoney MJ, et al: Diagnosis and management of fetal cephalocele. *Obstet Gynecol* 1984; 64:86.

51. Chervenak GA, Isaacson G, Rosenberg JC, et al: Antenatal diagnosis of frontal cephalocele in a fetus with atelosteogenesis. *J Ultrasound Med* 1986; 5:111.

52. Fink IJ, Chinn DH, Callen PW: A potential pitfall in the ultrasonographic diagnosis of fetal encephalocele. *J Ultrasound Med* 1983; 2:313.

53. Williams RA, Barth RA: In utero sonographic recognition of diastematomyelia. *AJR* 1985; 144:87.

54. Main DM, Mennuti MT: Neural tube defects: Issues in prenatal diagnosis and counselling. *Obstet Gynecol* 1986; 67:1.

55. Weinbaum PJ, Cassidy SB, Vintzileos AM, et al: Prenatal detection of a neural tube defect after fetal exposure to valproic acid. *Obstet Gynecol* 1986; 67:31S.

56. Slotnick N, Filly RA, Callen PW, et al: Sonography as a procedure complementary to alpha-fetoprotein testing for neural tube defects. *J Ultrasound Med* 1982; 1:319.

57. Hashimoto BE, Mahony BS, Filly RA, et al: Sonography, a complimentary examination to alpha-fetoprotein testing for fetal neural tube defects. *J Ultrasound Med* 1985; 4:307.

58. Chervenak FA, Duncan C, Ment LR, et al: Perinatal management of meningomyelocele *Obstet Gynecol* 1984; 63:376.

59. Cooper C, Mahony BS, Bowie JD, et al: Ultrasound evaluation of the normal fetal upper airway and esophagus. *J Ultrasound Med* 1985; 4:343.

60. Boylan P, O'Donovan P, Owens OJ: Fetal breathing movements and the diagnosis of labor: A prospective analysis of 100 cases. *Obstet Gynecol* 1985; 66:517.

61. Patel RB, Gibson JY, D'Cruz CA, et al: Sonographic diagnosis of cervical teratoma in utero. *AJR* 1982; 139:1220.

62. Chervenak FA, Tortora M, Moya FR, et al: Antenatal sonographic diagnosis of epignathus. *J Ultrasound Med* 1984; 3:235.

63. Barone CM, Van Natta FC, Kourides IA, et al: Sonographic detection of fetal goiter, an unu-

sual cause of hydramnios. *J Ultrasound Med* 1985; 4:625.

64. Fink IJ, Filly RA, Callen PW, et al: Sonographic diagnosis of thanatophoric dwarfism in utero. *J Ultrasound Med* 1982; 1:337.

65. Graham D, Winn K, Dex W, et al: Prenatal diagnosis of cystic adenomatoid malformation of the lung. *J Ultrasound Med* 1982; 1:9.

66. Romero R, Chervenak FA, Kotzen J, et al: Antenatal sonographic findings of extralobar pulmonary sequestration. *J Ultrasound Med* 1982; 1:131.

67. Bovicelli L, Rizzo N, Orsini LF: Ultrasonic real time diagnosis of fetal hydrothorax and lung hypoplasia. *JCU* 1981; 9:253.

68. Wicks JD, Levine MD, Mettler FA: Intrauterine sonography of thoracic ectopia cordis. *AJR* 1981; 137:619.

69. Haynor DR, Shuman WP, Brewer DK, et al: Imaging of fetal ectopia cordis: roles of sonography and computed tomography. *J Ultrasound Med* 1984; 3:25.

70. Todros T, Presbitero P, Montemurro D, et al: Prenatal diagnosis of ectopia cordis. *J Ultrasound Med* 1984; 3:429.

71. Mukuno DH, Lee TG, Harnsberger HR, et al: Sonography of the fetal gastrointestinal system. *Semin Ultrasound CT MR* 1984; 5:194.

72. Chinn DH, Filly RA, Callen PW: Ultrasonic evaluation of fetal umbilical and hepatic vascular anatomy. *Radiology* 1982; 144:153.

73. Vintzileos AM, Neckles S, Campbell WA, et al: Fetal liver ultrasound measurements during normal pregnancy. *Obstet Gynecol* 1985; 66:477.

74. Alexander ES, Spitz HB, Clark RA: Sonography of polyhydramnios. *AJR* 1982; 138:343.

75. Zemlyn S: Prenatal detection of esophageal atresia. *JCU* 1981; 9:453.

76. Pretorius DH, Meier PR, Johnson ML: Diagnosis of esophageal atresia in utero. *J Ultrasound Med* 1983; 2:475.

77. Nelson LH, Clark CE, Fishburne JI, et al: Value of serial sonography in the in utero detection of duodenal atresia. *Obstet Gynecol* 1982; 59:657.

78. Lince DM, Pretorius DH, Manco-Johnson ML, et al: The clinical significance of increased echogenicity of the fetal abdomen. *AJR* 1985; 145:683.

79. Denholm TA, Crow HC, Edwards WH, et al: Prenatal sonographic appearance of meconium ileus in twins. *AJR* 1984; 143:371.

80. Nancarrow PA, Mattrey RF, Edwards DK, et al: Fibroadhesive meconium peritonitis: In utero sonographic diagnosis. *J Ultrasound Med* 1985; 4:213.

81. Blumenthal DH, Rushovich AM, Williams RK, et al: Prenatal sonographic findings of meconium peritonitis with pathologic correlation. *JCU* 1982; 10:350.

82. Silverbach S: Antenatal real time identification of meconium cyst. *JCU* 1983; 11:455.

83. Lauer JD, Cradock TV: Meconium pseudocyst: Prenatal sonographic and antenatal radiologic correlation. *J Ultrasound Med* 1982; 1:333.

84. Hartung RW, Kilcheski TS, Greaney RB, et al: Antenatal diagnosis of cystic meconium peritonitis. *J Ultrasound Med* 1983; 2:49.

85. Williams III J, Nathan RO, Worthen NJ: Sonographic demonstration of the progression of meconium peritonitis. *Obstet Gynecol* 1984; 64:822.

86. Platt LD, Devore GR, Benner P, et al: Antenatal diagnosis of a fetal liver mass. *J Ultrasound Med* 1983; 2:521.

87. Foucar E, Williamson RA, Yiu-Chiu V, et al: Mesenchymal hamartoma of the liver identified by fetal sonography. *AJR* 1983; 140:970.

88. Elrad HE, Mayden KL, Ahart S, et al: Prenatal ultrasound diagnosis of choledochal cyst. *J Ultrasound Med* 1985; 4:553.

89. Frank JL, Hill MC, Chirathivat S, et al: Antenatal observation of a choledochal cyst by sonography. *AJR* 1981; 137:166.

90. Beretsky I, Lankin DH: Diagnosis of fetal cholelithiasis using real time high resolution imaging employing digital detection. *J Ultrasound Med* 1983; 2:381.

91. Chinn DH, Filly RA, Callen PW, et al: Congenital diaphragmatic hernia diagnosed prenatally by ultrasound. *Radiology* 1983; 148:119.

92. Schaffer RM, Barone C, Friedman AP: The ultrasonographic spectrum of fetal omphalocele. *J Ultrasound Med* 1983; 2:219.

93. Nelson PA, Bowie JD, Filston HC, et al: Sonographic diagnosis of omphalocele in utero. *AJR* 1982; 138:1178.

94. Fried AM, Woodring JH, Shier RW, et al: Omphalocele in limb/body wall deficiency syndrome: Atypical sonographic appearance. *JCU* 1982; 10:400.

95. Fink IJ, Filly RA: Omphalocele associated with umbilical cord allantoic cyst: Sonographic evaluation in utero. *Radiology* 1983; 149:473.

96. Lenke RR, Hatch EI: Fetal gastroschisis: A preliminary report advocating the use of cesarean section. *Obstet Gynecol* 1986; 67:395.

97. Bowie JD, Rosenberg ER, Andreotti RF, et al: The changing sonographic appearance of fetal kidneys during pregnancy. *J Ultrasound Med* 1983; 2:505.

98. Hadlock FP, Deter RL, Carpenter R, et al: Sonography of fetal urinary tract anomalies. *AJR* 1981; 137:261.

99. Jeanty P, Dramaix-Wilmet M, Elkhazen N, et al: Measurement of fetal kidney growth on ultrasound. *Radiology* 1982; 144:159.

100. Greenblatt AM, Beretsky I, Lankin DH, et al: In utero diagnosis of crossed renal ectopia using high resolution real time ultrasound. *J Ultrasound Med* 1985; 4:105.

101. Rosenberg ER, Bowie JD, Andreotti RF, et al: Sonographic evaluation of fetal adrenal glands. *AJR* 1982; 139:1145.

102. Lewis E, Kurtz AB, Dubbins PA, et al: Real time ultrasonographic evaluation of normal fetal adrenal glands. *J Ultrasound Med* 1982; 1:265.

103. Dean WM, Bourdreau EJ: Amniotic fluid alpha-fetoprotein in fetal obstructive uropathy. *Pediatrics* 1980; 66:537.

104. Dubbins PA, Kurtz AB, Wapner RJ, et al: Renal agenesis: Spectrum of in utero findings. *JCU* 1981; 9:189.

105. Austin CW, Brown JM, Friday RO: Unilateral renal agenesis presenting as a pseudomass in utero. *J Ultrasound Med* 1984; 3:177.

106. Friedberg JE, Mitnick JS, Davis DA: Antepartum ultrasonic detection of multicystic kidney. *Radiology* 1979; 131:198.

107. Older RA, Hinnan CG, Crane LM, et al: In utero diagnosis of multicystic kidney by gray scale ultrasonography. *AJR* 1979; 133:130.

108. Fillon R, Grignon A, Boisvert J: Antenatal diagnosis of ipsilateral multicystic kidney in identical twins. *J Ultrasound Med* 1985; 4:211.

109. Habif DV, Berdon WE, Yeh MN: Infantile polycystic kidney disease: In utero sonographic diagnosis. *Radiology* 1982; 142:475.

110. Shenkar L, Anderson C: Intrauterine diagnosis and management of fetal polycystic kidney disease. *Obstet Gynecol* 1982; 59:385.

111. Mahony BS, Callen PW, Filly RA, et al: Progression of infantile polycystic kidney disease in early pregnancy. *J Ultrasound Med* 1984; 3:277.

112. Pardes JG, Engel IA, Blomquist K, et al: Ultrasonography of intrauterine Meckel's syndrome. *J Ultrasound Med* 1984; 3:33.

113. Blane CE, Koff SA, Bowerman RA, et al: Non-obstructive fetal hydronephrosis: Sonographic recognition and therapeutic implications. *Radiology* 1983; 147:95.

114. Montana M, Cyr DRK, Lenke RR, et al: Sonographic detection of fetal ureteral obstruction. *AJR* 1985; 145:595.

115. Glazer GM, Filly RA, Callen PW: The varied sonographic appearance of the urinary tract in the retus and newborn with urethral obstruction. *Radiology* 1982; 144:563.

116. Christopher CR, Spinelli A, Severt D: Ultrasonic diagnosis of prune-belly syndrome. *Obstet Gynecol* 1982; 59:391.

117. Sanders R, Graham D: Twelve cases of hydronephrosis in utero diagnosed by ultrasonography. *J Ultrasound Med* 1982; 1:131.

118. Dunn V, Glasier CM: Ultrasonographic antenatal demonstration of primary megaureter. *J Ultrasound Med* 1985; 4:101.

119. Deter RL, Hadlock FP, Gonzales ET, et al: Prenatal detection of primary megaureter using dynamic image ultrasonography. *Obstet Gynecol* 1980; 56:759.

120. Golbus MS, Harrison MF, Filly RA, et al: In utero treatment of urinary tract obstruction. *Am J Obstet Gynecol* 1982; 142:383.

121. Gore RM, Callen PW, Filly RA, et al: Prenatal percutaneous antegrade pyelography in posterior urethral valves: Sonographic guidance. *AJR* 1982; 139:994.

122. Vallancien G, Dumez Y, Aubrey MC, et al: Percutaneous nephrostomy in utero. *Urology* 1982; 20:647.

123. Ehman RL, Nicholson SF, Machin GA: Prenatal sonographic detection of congenital mesoblastic nephroma in a monozygotic twin pregnancy. *J Ultrasound Med* 1983; 2:555.

124. Newton ER, Louis F, Dalton ME, et al: Fetal neuroblastoma and catecholamine-induced maternal hypertension. *Obstet Gynecol* 1985; 65:49S.

125. Tabsh K: Antenatal sonographic appearance of a fetal ovarian cyst. *J Ultrasound Med* 1982; 1:329.

126. Hill SJ, Hirsh JH: Sonographic detection of fetal hydrometocolpos. *J Ultrasound Med* 1985; 4:323.

127. Davis GH, Wapner RJ, Kurtz AB, et al: Antenatal diagnosis of hydrometrocolpos by ultrasound examination. *J Ultrasound Med* 1984; 3:371.

128. Dunne MG, Cunat JS: Sonographic determination of fetal gender before 25 weeks gestation. *AJR* 1983; 140:741.

129. Scholly TA, Sutphen JH, Hitchcock DA, et al: Sonograpic determination of fetal gender. *AJR* 1980; 135:1161.

130. Meizner I, Katz M, Zamora E, et al: In utero diagnosis of congenital hydrocele. *JCU* 1983; 11:449.

131. Cooper C, Mahony BS, Bowie JD, et al: Prenatal ultrasound diagnosis of ambiguous genitalia. *J Ultrasound Med* 1985; 4:433.

132. Fleischer AC, Killam AP, Boehm FH, et al: Hydrops fetalis: Sonographic evaluation and clinical implications. *Radiology* 1981; 141:163.

133. Rosenthal SJ, Filly RA, Callen PW, et al: Fetal pseudoascites. *Radiology* 1979; 131:195.

134. Hashimoto BE, Filly RA, Callen PW: Fetal pseudoascites: Further anatomic observations. *J Ultrasound Med* 1986; 5:151.

135. Mueller-Heubach E, Mazer J: Sonographically documented disappearance of fetal ascites. *Obstet Gynecol* 1981; 61:253.

136. Phillips HE, McGahan JP: Intrauterine fetal cystic hygromas: sonographic detection. *AJR* 1981; 136:799.

137. Rahmani MR, Fong KW, Connor TP, et al: The varied sonographic appearance of cystic hygromas in utero. *J Ultrasound Med* 1986; 5:165.

138. Robinow M, Spisso K, Buschi AJ, et al: Turner syndrome: Sonography showing fetal hydrops simulating hydramnios. *AJR* 1980; 135:846.

139. Pearce JM, Griffin D, Campbell S: The differential prenatal diagnosis of cystic hygromata and encephalocele by ultrasound examination. *JCU* 1985; 13:317.

140. Filly RA, Golbus MS: Ultrasonography of the normal and pathologic fetal skeleton. *Radiol Clin North Am* 1982; 20:311.

141. Hadlock FP, Harrist RB, Deter RL, et al: Fetal femur length as a predictor of menstrual age: Sonographically measured. *AJR* 1982; 138:875.

142. Jeanty P, Kirkpatrick C, Dramaix-Wilmet M, et al: Ultrasonic evaluation of fetal limb growth. *Radiology* 1981; 140:165.

143. Jeanty P, Dramaix-Wilmet M, van Kerkem J, et al: Ultrasonic evaluation of fetal limb growth: Part II. *Radiology* 1982; 143:751.

144. Chinn DH, Bolding DB, Callen PW, et al: Ultrasonographic identification of fetal lower extremity epiphyseal ossification centers. *Radiology* 1983; 147:815.

145. McLeary RD, Kuhns LR: Sonographic evaluation of the distal femoral epiphyseal ossification center. *J Ultrasound Med* 1983; 2:437.

146. Kurtz AB, Wapner RJ: Ultrasonographic diagnosis of second trimester skeletal dysplasias: A prospective analysis in a high risk population. *J Ultrasound Med* 1983; 2:99.

147. Wladimiroff JW, Niermeijer MF, Laar J, et al: Prenatal diagnosis of skeletal dysplasia by real time ultrasound. *Obstet Gynecol* 1984; 63:360.

148. Filly RA, Golbus MS, Carey JC, et al: Short limbed dwarfism: Ultrasonographic diagnosis by mensuration of femoral length. *Radiology* 1981; 138:653.

149. Kurtz AB, Filly RA, Wapner RJ, et al: In utero analysis of heterozygous achondroplasia: Variable time of onset as detected by femur length measurements. *J Ultrasound Med* 1986; 5:137.

150. Mahony BS, Filly RA, Cooperberg PL: Antenatal sonographic diagnosis of achondrogenesis. *J Ultrasound Med* 1984; 3:333.

151. Johnson VP, Yiu-Chiu VS, Wierda DR, et al: Midtrimester prenatal diagnosis of achondrogenesis. *J Ultrasound Med* 1984; 3:223.

152. Shapiro JE, Phillips JA, Byers P, et al: Prenatal diagnosis of lethal perinatal osteogenesis imperfecta. *J Pediatr* 1982; 100:127.

153. Roabe RD, Harnsberger HR, Lee TG, et al: Ultrasonographic antenatal diagnosis of "mermaid's syndrome": Fusion of fetal lower extremities. *J Ultrasound Med* 1983; 2:463.

154. Grahan M: Congenital short femur: Prenatal sonographic diagnosis. *J Ultrasound Med* 1985; 4:361.

155. Jeanty P, Romero R, d'Alton M, et al: In utero sonographic detection of hand and foot deformities. *J Ultrasound Med* 1985; 4:595.

156. Hashimoto BE, Filly RA, Callen PW: Sonographic diagnosis of clubfoot in utero. *J Ultrasound Med* 1986; 5:81.

157. Chervenak FA, Tortora M, Hobbins JC, et al: Antenatal sonographic diagnosis of clubfoot. *J Ultrasound Med* 1985; 4:49.

158. Sakala EP: Obstetric management of conjoined twins. *Obstet Gynecol* 1986; 67:21S.

159. Wood MJ, Thompson HE, Roberson FM: Real time ultrasound diagnosis of conjoined twins. *JCU* 1981; 9:195.

160. Abrams SL, Callen PW, Anderson RL, et al: Anencephaly with encephalocele in craniopagus twins: Prenatal diagnosis by ultrasonography and computed tomography. *J Ultrasound Med* 1985; 4:485.

161. Wilson DA, Young GZ, Crumley CS: Antepartum ultrasonographic diagnosis of ischiopagus: A rare variety of conjoined twins. *J Ultrasound Med* 1983; 2:281.

162. Gore RM, Filly RA, Parer JT: Sonographic antepartum diagnosis of conjoined twins. *JAMA* 1982; 247:3351.

# 16g

# FETAL CARDIAC ULTRASOUND

Greggory R. DeVore, M.D.

As the result of improved ultrasound technology and training, a number of structural malformations of the fetus have been diagnosed prenatally.[1-4] Of the organ systems evaluated, the heart and great vessels can pose some difficulty for the fetal sonographer. However, the importance of antenatal diagnosis of congenital heart disease is emphasized by the fact that of the 1 million fetuses sonographically examined each year in the United States by radiologists, obstetricians, or their assistants, 8,000 are born with some form of cardiovascular defect.[5-6] Although most clinicians believe that antenatal detection of structural anomalies of the heart should be undertaken in those patients at risk (Table 16G–1), the majority of affected newborns have no antecedent risk factors.[7-8] Therefore, a diagnostic approach that could be applied during the course of a "routine" fetal ultrasound examination would be advantageous so that the sonographer could *screen* for congenital anomalies of the cardiovascular system in an efficient, logical manner.

This chapter reviews an approach that allows major malformations of the heart to be identified during the course of fetal sonography. To accomplish this, the sonographer must understand the following: (1) the fetal circulation, (2) the screening echocardiogram, and (3) the consulative examination.

## Fetal Circulation

Unlike the pediatric or adult patient, in whom blood is delivered to the body and head by the left ventricle, the fetus requires both ventricles to meet its systemic needs. Initially oxygenated blood flowing from the inferior vena cava enters the right atrium where most of it crosses through the foramen ovale to the lower-pressure left atrium. During ventricular diastole blood from the left atrium enters the left ventricle where, during ventricular systole, it is ejected through the aortic valve into the ascending aorta. The greatest volume of blood from the left ventricle is distributed to the fetal heart, head, and upper extremities.

Blood from the right atrium flows through the tricuspid valve into the right ventricle. During ventricular systole it is ejected through the pulmonary valve into the pulmonary outflow tract where the major portion flows through the ductus arteriosus into the descending aorta. From here it is distributed to the fetal trunk

**TABLE 16G–1.**

**Prenatal Risk Factors Congenital Heart Disease[8]**

FETAL RISK FACTORS
　Intrauterine growth retardation
　Fetal cardiac dysrhythmia
　Abnormal karyotype (trisomy 13, 18, 21 Turner's syndrome)
　Noncardiovascular structural anomalies
MATERNAL RISK FACTORS
　Heart disease
　　Congenital
　　Acquired
　Drug ingestions
　　Alcohol
　　Aspirin
　　Narcotics
　　Amphetamines
　　Anticonvulsants
　　Lithium
　　Birth control pills
　　Other sex hormones
　Polyhydramnios
　Oligohydramnios
　Rh sensitization
　Diabetes mellitus
　Preeclampsia
　Collagen vascular disease
FAMILIAL RISK FACTORS
　Congenital heart disease
　Genetic syndrome

and placenta. Therefore, as a result of fetal circulation, the right and left ventricles function as a parallel system—that is, the left ventricle pumps blood to the heart, head, and upper extremities, and the right ventricle supplies blood to the body and placenta.[9–11]

An important point to remember is that this parallel system is dependent on the patency of the foramen ovale and ductus arteriosus. A partial or complete obstruction to blood flow at the level of the inflow (mitral and tricuspid valves) or outflow (aortic and pulmonic valves) tracts will result in redistribution of blood within the cardiac chambers which is manifested in the fetal and immediate newborn period as disproportion between the right and left atrial and ventricular chambers.[12–15] This important observation is the basis for the screening fetal echocardiographic examination, which can be easily performed by sonographers who routinely evaluate the fetus from the 16th to the 40th week of gestation.

## Screening Echocardiographic Evaluation

*Real-Time Examination of the Four-Chamber View*

EXAMINATION OF NONCARDIAC STRUCTURES

Before the heart is examined, the fetal head, abdomen, and extremities should be imaged and the biparietal diameter, cephalic index, head circumference, abdominal circumference, and femur length measured, as described elsewhere.[16–19] Once gross anomalies of these organ systems have been screened for, identification of the fetal stomach on the left side of the abdominal cavity should be confirmed.

THE FOUR-CHAMBER VIEW

Because of fetal circulation, it is important to be able to identify both the right and left ventricles and the atria in the same view. The four-chamber view at the level of the inflow tracts is ideal since it allows examination of the right and left atrial and ventricular chambers, walls, interatrial and interventricular septa, foramen ovale, and the tricuspid and mitral valves. Besides containing these structures, the four-chamber view at this level is easiest to image for the noncardiologist involved with fetal sonography.[20–22]

**Identification of the Right and Left Ventricular and Atrial Chambers.**—To obtain the four-chamber view the transducer is directed parallel to the long axis of the fetal spine or aorta. After either of these structures has been identified, the ultrasound beam is rotated 90° at the level of the thorax, and the four chambers are imaged. The easiest way to identify atrial and ventricular anatomy on a transverse image of the thorax is first to locate the fetal spine and mentally draw a line to the opposite anterior chest wall. The ventricle lying beneath the intersection of this line and the anterior chest wall should be the right ventricle. The left ventricle is inferior to the right ventricle and is on the same side of the fetal trunk as the stomach. Table 16G–2 lists the differences in shape and location between the right and left ventricles in the normal fetus.

**TABLE 16G–2.**

**Identification of Right and Left Ventricles From the Four-Chamber View**

| GEOMETRIC FEATURE | RIGHT VENTRICLE | LEFT VENTRICLE |
|---|---|---|
| Position within thorax | Beneath anterior chest wall | Left side of thorax, above spine, same side of trunk a stomach |
| Geometric shape | Conical | Ellipsoid |
| Flap of foramen ovale | | Present within le atrium |
| Insertion of AV valve leaflets on interventricular septum | Tricuspid valve inserts lower than mitral valve | Mitral valve inserts higher than tricuspid valve |

Once the ventricles have been identified, movement of the flap of the foramen ovale within the left atrium should be confirmed to occur on the same side of the trunk as the fetal stomach.

**Examination of the Mitral and Tricuspid Valves.**—In the four-chamber view the mitral and tricuspid valves can be seen to open and close. Normally the tricuspid valve inserts lower on the interventricular septum than the mitral valve. Occasionally one can see prominent papillary muscles within the right ventricular chamber.

**Examination of the Interventricular and Interatrial Septa.**—The interventricular septum separates the ventricular chambers and has an elongated V-shaped appearance. At the apex of the heart the interventricular septum is thickest and narrows as it approaches the base where the mitral and tricuspid valves insert. During ventricular systole the septum shortens in length and thickens in width.

The interatrial septum is a thin, membrane-like structure that can be seen as a continuation of the interventricular septum. Approximately one-half the distance from the interventricular-interatrial junction an interruption of the interatrial septum occurs. This is the foramen ovale.

*The Abnormal Four-Chamber View*

ABNORMAL ANATOMY

Congenital anomalies that grossly distort normal anatomy of the four-chamber view can be readily identified. The four-chamber view has been used to diagnose a rhabdomyoma of the interventricular septum that infiltrated the right ventricle and compressed the left ventricular chamber. It can demonstrate a large ventricular and atrial septal defect in a fetus with an atrioventricular canal defect.

VENTRICULAR DISPROPORTION

As a consequence of fetal circulation, abnormalities of the inflow or outflow of blood to the ventricles result in ventricular disproportion, that is, one ventricle appearing larger than the other. Ventricular disproportion can best be screened for by carefully examining the four-chamber view. Once it is suspected, the following questions must be answered: (1) Is the larger of the two ventricles normal or increased in size? (2) Is the smaller of the two ventricles normal or decreased in size? (3) Is the overall diameter of the heart normal,

large, or small? (4) What is the severity of the disproportion? (5) Are the aortic and pulmonic outflow tracts properly related? (6) Are the aortic and pulmonic outflow tracts normal, decreased, or increased in size? Table 16G–3 lists anomalies reported in the literature and from our own experience in which abnormal anatomy and/or ventricular disproportion would be noted in the four-chamber view of the heart.

*Further Evaluation*

Once abnormal anatomy or ventricular disproportion is noted during the screening examination, further evaluation of ventricular dimensions, the aortic and pulmonic outflow tracts, the arch of the aorta, and the ductus arteriosus should be carried out. These examinations, which should be performed by an experienced fetal cardiovascular sonologist, constitute the consultative evaluation.

## Consultative Echocardiographic Evaluation

*Real-Time-Directed M-Mode Examination*

Following assessment of the structural anatomy seen on the four-chamber view, it is important to quantify accurately contractility of the ventricles, their chamber size, the thickness of the ventricular walls and inter-

**TABLE 16G–3.**

**Congenital Anomalies Detected in Utero With an Abnormal Four-Chamber View[12]**

ANATOMIC ABNORMALITY
  Septal rhabdomyoma
  Endocardial cushion defect
  Ventricular septal defect
  Simple
    Tetralogy of Fallot
    Truncus arteriosus
    Double-outlet right ventricle
  Single ventricle
  Epsteins' anomaly
VENTRICULAR DISPROPORTION
  Hypoplastic left ventricle
  Hypoplastic right ventricle
  Hypoplastic aortic arch
  Aortic stenosis
  Coarctation of the aorta (simple)
  Coarctation of the aorta (complex)
  Subaortic stenosis
  Ostium primum defect with gooseneck deformity

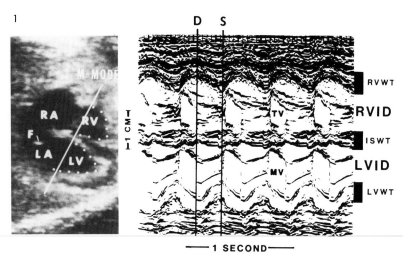

**FIG 16G–1.**
*Real-time-directed M-mode echocardiogram. The M-mode cursor is directed perpendicular to the interventricular septum at the level of the atrioventricular valves, and the M-mode recorded. RA = right atrium; RV = right ventricle; LA = left atrium; LV = left ventricle; F = foramen ovale; D = diastole; S = systole; RVWT = right ventricular wall thickness; RVID = right ventricular internal dimension; ISWT = interventricular septal wall thickness; LVID = ventricular internal dimension; LVWT = left ventricular wall thickness.*

ventricular septum, and the opening excursion of the tricuspid and mitral valves.[23–26] To achieve this, M-mode echocardiography is used.

## METHODOLOGY

Using a real-time-directed system, the sonographer directs the M-mode cursor perpendicular to the interventricular septum at the level of the mitral and tricuspid valves (Fig 16G–1). Once the M-mode cursor is properly positioned, the M-mode view can be recorded.

## MEASUREMENTS

Although there are a number of measurements and calculated values derived from computer analysis of the M-mode image, the following can be obtained without the assistance of the computer program.

### Ventricular Chamber Dimensions

1. Biventricular outer dimension (diastole). This measures the outer dimension of the heart from the epicardium of the right ventricle to the epicardium of the left ventricle (Fig 16G–2, points 1–6).

2. Biventricular inner dimension (diastole). This measures the overall dimension of the heart, including the right and left ventricular chambers and interventricular septum (Fig 16G–2, points 2–5).

3. Right ventricular internal dimension (diastole).

This measurement is obtained at the point where the tricuspid valve leaflets close. It reflects the size of the right ventricle at end diastole (Fig 16G–2, points 2–3).

4. Right ventricular internal dimension (systole). This measurement is obtained at the point of maximal inward excursion of the right ventricular wall and reflects end systole (Fig 16G–2, points 8–9).

5. Left ventricular internal dimension (diastole). This measurement is obtained at the point where the mitral valve leaflets close. It reflects the end-diastolic dimension of the left ventricle (Fig 16G–2, points 4, 5).

6. Left ventricular internal dimension (systole). This measurement is obtained at the point of maximal inward excursion of the right ventricular wall (Fig 16G–2, points 10, 11).

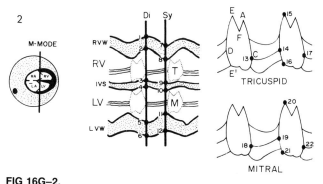

**FIG 16G–2.**
*Schematic of the M-mode tracing identifying points used for quantitative assessment of ventricular size and function.*

## Ventricular Wall Thickness

1. Left ventricular wall thickness (diastole). This measurement is obtained between the epicardium and endocardium (Fig 16G–2, points 5, 6).

2. Right ventricular wall thickness (diastole). This measurement is obtained between the epicardium and endocardium (Fig 16G–2, points 1,2).

3. Interventricular septal wall thickness (diastole). This measurement is obtained at the level of the septum between the right and left ventricular endocardium (Fig 16G–2, points 3, 4).

## Atrioventricular Valve Excursion

1. Tricuspid valve opening excursion. This measures the separation of the valve leaflets during diastole (Fig 16G–2, points 15, 16).

2. Mitral valve opening excursion. This measures the separation of the valve leaflets during diastole (Fig 16G–2, points 20, 21).

### M-MODE COMPUTATIONS

**Right and left ventricular fractional shortening.**—To evaluate how well the ventricles are contracting, the fractional shortening can be computed from their respective end-diastolic and end-systolic measurements using the formulas in Table 16G–4.[23]

**Ratios.**—Table 16G–5 lists the mean, 5%, and 95% confidence limits for the following ratios between 18 to 40 weeks of gestation: right/left ventricular internal dimension, right/left ventricular wall thickness, and tricuspid/mitral valve opening excursion.

### ASSESSMENT OF VENTRICULAR DIMENSIONS AS A FUNCTION OF FETAL GROWTH

Because the fetus is growing at a rapid rate, it is imperative to correlate the relationship of ventricular chamber dimensions with noncardiac growth parameters. Unlike previously published studies, in which M-mode measurements were related to gestational age (derived from regression analysis of the biparietal diameter of the fetal head), we have chosen to compare M-mode measurements against direct fetal growth measurements (biparietal diameter, head circumference, abdominal circumference, and femur length) (Table 16G–6).[23–29] This allows versatility, especially when evaluating a fetus with a nonlethal anomaly of

**TABLE 16G–4.**

**Computation of Right and Left Ventricular Fractional Shortening[23]**

*Right ventricle:*
$$\frac{(RVID\text{-}D) - (RVID\text{-}S)}{RVID\text{-}D} \times 100 = \quad (Normal = 24.7\text{–}39.5)$$

*Left ventricle:*
$$\frac{(LVID\text{-}D) - (LVID\text{-}S)}{LVID\text{-}D} \times 100 = \quad (Normal = 25.7\text{–}33.1)$$

RIVD-D = *Right ventricular internal dimension (diastole)*
RVID-S = *Right ventricular internal dimension (systole)*
LVID-D = *Left ventricular internal dimension (diastole)*
LVID-S = *Left ventricular internal dimension (systole)*

**TABLE 16G–5.**

**Mean, 5%, and 95% Confidence Limits for M-Mode Computations (N = 82)[23]**

| RIGHT/LEFT RATIOS | 5% | MEAN | 95% | SD |
|---|---|---|---|---|
| Internal dimension (diastole) | 0.80 | 0.98 | 1.15 | 0.08 |
| Fractional shortening | 0.74 | 0.98 | 1.21 | 0.12 |
| Tricuspid/mitral excursion | 0.83 | 0.99 | 1.15 | 0.08 |
| Wall thickness (diastole) | 0.58 | 1.12 | 1.65 | 0.27 |

one of the above organ systems, for example, hydrocephaly, in which the gestational age cannot be determined from the biparietal diameter because it can be abnormally increased in size.

## The Outflow Tracts

### REAL-TIME EXAMINATION

In the normal fetus the aortic outflow tract is perpendicular to the pulmonic outflow tract. This relationship can be identified in one of two ways. The first approach involves rotating the transducer approximately 30° from the plane of the four-chamber view until the characteristic "left parasternal image" is seen. This view contains a portion of the right ventricle, left atrium, left ventricle, mitral valve, aortic valve, and aortic outflow tract and reveals anatomical continuity of the internal anatomy of the left ventricle with its corresponding outflow tract. The left ventricular outflow tract, however, must be examined further to confirm that the brachiocephalic, common carotid, and left subclavian arteries originate from the arch of the aorta.

In the second approach the heart is imaged in the short axis. In this view the sonographer can identify

**TABLE 16G–6.**
**Ventricular End-Diastolic and Aortic Dimensions[23–27]\***

| VENTRICULAR END-DIASTOLIC ($N$ = 82) | $r$ | $R^2$ | SEE |
|---|---|---|---|
| Biventricular outer | | | |
| BPD | 0.958 | 0.918 | 0.238 |
| FL | 0.943 | 0.889 | 0.279 |
| AC | 0.951 | 0.904 | 0.259 |
| HC | 0.937 | 0.877 | 0.290 |
| Biventricular inner | | | |
| BPD | 0.957 | 0.917 | 0.197 |
| FL | 0.944 | 0.892 | 0.227 |
| AC | 0.948 | 0.899 | 0.218 |
| HC | 0.937 | 0.877 | 0.239 |
| RV internal | | | |
| BPD | 0.945 | 0.893 | 0.109 |
| FL | 0.930 | 0.867 | 0.123 |
| AC | 0.942 | 0.887 | 0.112 |
| HC | 0.919 | 0.844 | 0.132 |
| LV internal | | | |
| BPD | 0.940 | 0.884 | 0.103 |
| FL | 0.923 | 0.852 | 0.112 |
| AC | 0.925 | 0.856 | 0.114 |
| HC | 0.921 | 0.848 | 0.118 |
| Tricuspid valve excursion | | | |
| BPD | 0.933 | 0.871 | 0.082 |
| FL | 0.926 | 0.857 | 0.087 |
| AC | 0.916 | 0.839 | 0.092 |
| HC | 0.910 | 0.828 | 0.094 |
| Mitral valve excursion | | | |
| BPD | 0.922 | 0.851 | 0.084 |
| FL | 0.919 | 0.845 | 0.086 |
| AC | 0.900 | 0.810 | 0.098 |
| HC | 0.900 | 0.810 | 0.099 |
| RV wall thickness | | | |
| BPD | 0.778 | 0.606 | 0.062 |
| FL | 0.762 | 0.580 | 0.064 |
| AC | 0.774 | 0.598 | 0.062 |
| HC | 0.769 | 0.591 | 0.063 |
| LV wall thickness | | | |
| BPD | 0.727 | 0.526 | 0.061 |
| FL | 0.700 | 0.490 | 0.064 |
| AC | 0.731 | 0.534 | 0.060 |
| HC | 0.697 | 0.485 | 0.064 |
| Interventricular septal wall thickness | | | |
| BPD | 0.767 | 0.588 | 0.046 |
| FL | 0.745 | 0.558 | 0.048 |
| AC | 0.753 | 0.568 | 0.047 |
| HC | 0.771 | 0.594 | 0.045 |
| Aortic dimensions ($N$ = 43) | | | |
| Aortic root dimension | | | |
| BPD | 0.915 | 0.837 | 0.087 |
| FL | 0.937 | 0.878 | 0.077 |
| AC | 0.945 | 0.894 | 0.077 |
| HC | 0.921 | 0.848 | 0.085 |
| Aortic valve excursion | | | |
| BPD | 0.845 | 0.713 | 0.083 |
| FL | 0.869 | 0.756 | 0.077 |
| AC | 0.867 | 0.757 | 0.077 |
| HC | 0.852 | 0.725 | 0.082 |

\*BPD = biparietal diameter; FL = femur length; AC = abdominal circumference; HC = head circumference; SEE = standard error of the estimate.

the normal relationship of the aorta and pulmonary outflow tract. The transducer beam is directed parallel to the long axis (spine, aorta) of the fetal trunk. As the ultrasound beam is directed laterally through the proper plane, the circular left and right ventricular chambers are seen, with the pulmonic valve opening and closing off to the side of the right ventricle. By rocking the transducer medially, the sonographer can identify the short axis of the outflow tract. In this view the aorta is circular and in the center of the image, with the pulmonic outflow tract draping over it. Once this view has been obtained, the right ventricular outflow tract should be examined carefully to confirm the bifurcated pulmonary arteries medially, and the ductus arteriosus laterally.

Once the anatomical relationships of the outflow tracts have been examined with real-time imaging, it is important to quantify their dimensions. For this purpose, we have again chosen to use the M-mode view.

### M-Mode Examination of the Aortic Root and Valve

Although real-time measurements of the aortic and pulmonic roots have been reported for the fetus, the correlation coefficients and the coefficient of determination are much lower than for M-mode measurements.[27–29] In a recently completed study, we found that evaluation of the aortic root with M-mode imaging was easy to accomplish (see Table 16G–6).[27] We chose to measure the aortic root dimension and aortic valve opening excursion because of the ease of accessibility from either the left parasternal or short axis views. As with ventricular disproportion, the sonographer must ascertain whether the outflow tracts are of equal size or if one is larger than the other. By quantifying the aortic root and valve dimensions, one can establish that the aortic valve is normal, increased, or decreased in size. Ventricular disproportion has been demonstrated in which the left ventricle was smaller than the right. The M-mode measurement of the aortic root and valve demonstrated it to be smaller than normal, thus confirming a hypoplastic left ventricle. In another case a ventricular septal defect was noted in the four-chamber and left parasternal views. Evaluation of the aortic and pulmonic outflow tracts revealed disproportion, with the aortic root dimension increased in size, as determined from the M-mode measurement. This fetus had tetralogy of Fallot.

## Conclusion

Using the approach outlined in this chapter, the fetal sonographer can begin to examine the fetal heart and identify fetuses with major malformations of the cardiovascular system. It is important to emphasize that the screening examination requires a subsequent comprehensive study to completely define anatomical abnormalities.

## References

1. Stephensen SR, Weaver DD: Prenatal diagnosis: A compilation of diagnosed conditions. *Am J Obstet Gynecol* 1981; 141:319.
2. DeVore GR, Hobbins JC: Ultrasound diagnosis of congenital birth defects, in Sciarra JW (ed): *Gynecology and Obstetrics.* New York, Harper & Row, 1982, chap 72.
3. DeVore GR, Hobbins JC: The use of ultrasound in the diagnosis and management of fetal congenital anomalies: The challenge of the 1980's, in Warshaw JB (ed): *The Biological Basis of Reproductive and Developmental Medicine.* New York, Elsevier Biomedical, 1983, p 391.
4. DeVore GR, Hobbins JC: Antenatal diagnosis of congenital structural anomalies with ultrasound, in Beard RW, Nathanielsz PW (eds): *Fetal Physiology and Medicine: The Basis of Perinatology.* New York, Marcel Dekker, Inc, 1984, pp 1–56.
5. *Diagnostic Ultrasound Imaging in Pregnancy.* Washington, DC, National Institutes of Health, 1984.
6. Taussig HB: World survey of common cardiac malformations: Developmental error or genetic variant? in Engle MA, Perloff J (eds): *Congenital Heart Disease After Surgery.* New York, Yorke Medical Publications, 1983, pp 1–42.
7. Rowe RD, Freedom RM, Mehrizi A, et al: *The Neonate with Congenital Heart Disease.* Philadelphia, WB Saunders Co, 1981.
8. Kleinman CS: Fetal echocardiography, in Sanders R (ed): *Ultrasound Annual.* New York, Raven Press, 1982, pp 321–346.
9. Goodwin JW: The fetal circulation, in Goodwin JW, Gooden JV, and Chance GW (eds): *Perinatal Medicine.* Baltimore, Williams & Wilkins Co, 1976, p 143.
10. Gootman N, Gootman P: *Perinatal Cardiovascular Function.* New York, Marcel Dekker, Inc, 1983.
11. Rudolph AM: *Congenital Disease of the Heart.* Chicago, Year Book Medical Publishers, Inc, 1974.
12. DeVore GR: The prenatal diagnosis of congenital heart disease: A practical approach for the fetal sonographer. *JCU* 1985; 13:229–245.
13. Goldberg SJ, Allen HD, Sahn DJ: *Pediatric and Adolescent Echocardiography.* Chicago, Year Book Medical Publishers, Inc, 1980.
14. Silverman NH, Snider AR: *Two-Dimensional Echocardiography in Congenital Heart Disease.* Norwalk, Appleton-Century Crofts, 1982.
15. DeVore GR: The prenatal diagnosis of congenital heart disease: A practical approach for the fetal sonographer. *JCU* 1985; 13:229–245.
16. Hadlock FP, Deter RL, Harrist RB, et al: Fetal biparietal diameter: A critical re-evaluation of the relation to menstrual age by means of real-time ultrasound. *J Ultrasound Med* 1982; 1:97.
17. Hadlock FP, Deter RL, Harrist RB, et al: Fetal abdominal circumference as a predictor of menstrual age. *AJR* 1982; 138:367–370.
18. O'Brien GD, Queenan JT: Growth of the ultrasound fetal femur length during normal pregnancy: Part I. *Am J Obstet Gynecol* 1981; 141:833–837.
19. DeVore GR, Platt LD: Choosing the correct equation for computing the head circumference: The effect of head shape. *Am J Obstet Gynecol* 1984; 148:221–222.
20. DeVore GR, Kleinman CS, Donnerstein RL, et al: Fetal echocardiography: I. Normal anatomy as determined by real-time directed M-mode ultrasound. *Am J Obstet Gynecol* 1982; 144:249–260.
21. DeVore GR, Donnerstein RI, Kleinman CS, et al: Fetal echocardiography: II. The diagnosis and significance of a pericardial effusion in the fetus using real-time-directed M-mode ultrasound. *Am J Obstet Gynecol* 1982; 144:693–701.
22. Kleinman CS, Hobbins JC, Jaffe CC, et al: Echocardiographic studies of the human fetus: Prenatal diagnosis of congenital heart disease and cardiac dysrhythmias. *Pediatrics* 1980; 65:1059–1067.
23. DeVore GR, Siassi B, Platt LD: Fetal echocar-

diography: IV. M-mode assessment of ventricular size and contractility during the second and third trimesters of pregnancy in the normal fetus. *Am J Obstet Gynecol* 1984; 150:981–988.

24. DeVore GR, Siassi B, Platt LD: The use of the abdominal circumference as a means of assessing M-mode ventricular dimensions during the second and third trimesters of pregnancy in the normal fetus. *J Ultrasound Med* 1985; 4:175–182.

25. DeVore GR, Siassi B, Platt LD: The use of the femur length as a means of assessing M-Mode ventricular dimensions during the second and third trimesters of pregnancy in the normal fetus. *JCU* (in press).

26. DeVore GR, Siassi B, Platt LD: The use of the head circumference as a means of assessing M-

mode ventricular dimensions during the second and third trimesters of pregnancy in the normal fetus. (in press).

27. DeVore GR, Siassi B, Platt LD: Fetal echocardiography: V. M-mode measurements of the aortic root dimension and aortic valve excursion in the second and third trimester in the normal human fetus. *Am J Obstet Gynecol* 1985; 152:543–550.

28. Sahn DJ, Lange LW, Allen HD, et al: Quantitative real-time cross-sectional echocardiography in the developing normal human fetus and newborn. *Circulation* 1980; 62:588–597.

29. Allan LD, Joseph MC, Boyd EC, et al: M-mode echocardiography in the developing human fetus. *Br Heart J* 1982; 47:573.

# ULTRASOUND AND BIOCHEMICAL TESTS FOR THE PRENATAL DETECTION OF NEURAL TUBE DEFECTS AND OTHER ABNORMALITIES

Barbara F. Crandall, M.D.
Myles Matsumoto, M.D.

Over the past 10 years we have performed routine amniotic fluid α-fetoprotein (AFP) assays on about 53,000 pregnancies monitored by second-trimester amniocentesis. The fluids were from patients seen at ten different centers in California. We analyzed the results in 50,000 pregnancies for which consecutive fluids were sent to us to assay, excluding those submitted to confirm an abnormal AFP. Pregnancy outcomes are known in 96%. The indications for amniocentesis are listed in Table 16H–1. Amniocentesis was usually recommended when either a parent or a maternal first cousin had a neural tube defect (NTD); these are listed under "Other" in Table 16H–1.

AFP levels were measured by radioimmunoassay in the first 30,000 cases; in the last 20,000 an enzyme-linked immunosorbent assay was used instead. All samples were assayed in duplicate.[1] Interassay variation was less than 10% (4.2%–9.6%). Our normal range was established from clear amniotic fluid samples from pregnancies in which the outcome was known to be normal. Gestational dates were confirmed by ultrasonography. At least 100 samples were assayed for each week of gestation from 14 to 22 weeks, and the means and standard deviations were established. An SD of +3 above the mean is about 2 times the median, and of +5 above the mean is between 2.5 and 3 times the median. Bloody samples were tested by the Betke-Kleihauer test or by immunoelectrophoresis for the presence of fetal blood.

Acetylcholinesterase (AChE) gel electrophoresis was performed using the disk technique.[2] This test was performed when the AFP level was more than +2 SD above the mean or when there was a higher risk for an NTD, such as a positive family history or two elevated maternal serum AFP levels. It was not in use for the first 5,000 amniocenteses, although many of the samples showing elevated amniotic fluid AFP levels were tested retrospectively. AFP levels 3 SD or more above the mean were an indication for a repeat amniocentesis unless the AChE test was negative and the sample contained fetal blood. AFP levels 5 SD or more above the mean were always an indication for a repeat amniocentesis whether the AChE test was positive or negative.

The first amniotic fluid AFP value was 3 SD or more above the mean in 426 individuals (0.8%): the fetus was normal (did not have an NTD or certain other abnormalities) in 201 (47%) and abnormal or dead in 225 (53%) (Table 16H–2). This does not include pre-

**TABLE 16H–1.**

**Indications for Amniocentesis**

| INDICATION | % |
|---|---|
| Maternal age | 84.5 |
| Previous NTD | 2.5 |
| Previous chromosome abnormality | 1.9 |
| Elevated maternal serum AFP | 0.4 |
| Other* | 10.8 |

*Includes relative with NTD previous pregnancy(ies) with multiple malformations, spontaneous abortions or stillbirths, radiation, drugs, parent carriers of a genetic disorder, intrauterine growth retardation, anxiety.

maturity, growth retardation, congenital heart defect, cleft lip and palate, hip dislocation, club feet, inguinal hernia, or polydactyly.

The initial levels were between +3 SD and +5 SD above the mean in 204 individuals (0.4%); the fetus was normal in 169 (83%) and abnormal in 35 (17%) cases. If bloody fluids were excluded, 135 of 167 (82%) had a normal outcome and 32 (18%) had an abnormal outcome. In 43 of the 73 (59%) normal cases, the amniotic fluid AFP level measured at or just above +3 SD. The AChE test was weakly positive in one normal case, but both the AFP and AChE results were normal on repeat amniocentesis. A second sonogram gave slightly earlier gestational dates, usually confirmed by last menstrual period dating, in a number of cases, so the amniotic fluid AFP was corrected to <+3 SD. A number of patients underwent repeat amniocentesis, particularly in the earlier part of the series; all but one had a normal second amniotic fluid level and the outcomes were normal. There were four sets of twins in this group and in each set the level was elevated in one twin or both; all had a normal outcome.

In 222 (0.4%) cases the initial amniotic fluid AFP level was ≥+5 SD: the outcome was normal in 32 (14%) and abnormal in 190 (86%). Seventeen of the former and 9 of the latter patients had bloody amniotic fluid. When these were excluded, 15 of 196 (8%) were normal and 181 of 195 (92%) were abnormal.

There was one set of normal twins in which one had an AFP level of ≥+5 SD and the other, ≥+3 but <+5 SD. The parents elected not to repeat the amniocentesis; one twin died 8 weeks later and the other was normal. A second amniocentesis was performed in the rest of the normal cases; in five cases amniotic fluid AFP levels remained ≥+5 SD. In the others it decreased but remained between +3 and +5 SD above the mean in 22 women; in 5 it was <+3 SD.

## Abnormalities Detected

With the use of the protocol specified, 231 abnormal or dead fetuses were identified: 107 had open NTDs, and 124 had other abnormalities. Three open NTDs, one cystic hygroma, and two omphaloceles had AFP levels of 2 SD; the NTDs and cystic hygroma had positive AChEs, the two omphaloceles had negative AChEs but were identified by sonograms. In addition, two closed encephaloceles (one first seen at 38 weeks), three cystic hygromas, and one closed cervical spina bifida were identified by sonography and had normal AFP levels and AChE tests.

No NTD was missed (Table 16H–3). All open NTDs were associated with clearly positive AChE tests. However, eight anencephalies and two encephaloceles occurred prior to AChE tests. All anencephalies had AFP levels above +5 SD. Of the 47 open spina bifidas in 36 the AFP level was >+5 SD, but in 10 it was between >+3 and +5, and in one it was +2 SD (hence, 23% it was <+5 SD). Of the nine open encephaloceles, in four the AFP level was >+5 SD, in three it was between +3 and +5 SD, and in two it was at +2 SD (or approximately 50% measured >+5).

Fetal demise was the most common of the non-NTD abnormalities detected, followed by omphalocele (Table 16H–4). In the earlier part of the study, some of the omphaloceles were not distinguished from gas-

**TABLE 16H–2.**

**Pregnancy Outcomes With Amniotic Fluid AFP 3SD or More Above Mean (%)***

| OUTCOME | AF ≥ +3 | AFP ≥ +3, < +5 | | | AFP ≥ +5 | | |
|---|---|---|---|---|---|---|---|
| | | TOTAL | BLOODY | CLEAR | TOTAL | BLOODY | CLEAR |
| Normal | 201 (47) | 169 (83) | 34 | 135 | 32 (14) | 17 | 15 |
| Abnormal | 225 (53) | 35 (17) | 3 | 32 | 190 (86) | 9 | 181 |
| Total | 426 | 204 | 37 | 167 | 222 | 26 | 196 |

*Parentheses enclose percentages.

**TABLE 16H–3.**
**Open NTDs Detected (AChE Test Positive)**

| CATEGORY | NO. | +2 | ≥+3, <+5 | ≥+5 |
|---|---|---|---|---|
| | | AFP LEVEL | | |
| Spina bifida | 47 | 1 (1) | 10 (10) | 36 (36) |
| Anencephaly | 51 | | | 51 (43)* |
| Encephalocele | 9 | 2 (2) | 3 (3) | 4 (2)† |
| Total | 107 | 3 | 13 | 91 (81) |

*Eight cases prior to AChE test.
†Two cases prior to AChE test.

troschises: all the gastroschises were identified in the past 2 years. Prior to the last 5 years, an elevated AFP level was usually the first indication of a problem. Lately, two thirds of the omphaloceles and most of the cystic hygromas and hydrops were first identified on sonography. Fetal hydrops resulted from severe Kell sensitization in one case, Turner's syndrome in two cases, trisomy 21 in one case, and an unknown cause in the other five cases. Two of the latter occurred in succeeding pregnancies in one woman. Cystic hygroma was mainly associated with Turner's syndrome, and with trisomy 21 and trisomy 18 (one case each). The "other" category included 2 cases each of duodenal atresia and sacral teratoma and trisomy 13 and 18 and one case each of Dandy-Walker cyst,

acardia, "severe brain and renal" anomalies, complete atresia of the colon, congenital nephrosis, amniotic band syndrome and facial teratoma.

## AChE

The specific band associated with an open NTD was usually quite clear and unequivocal and all open NTDs tested positive. This was true even in the presence of fetal blood, when a fainter, broad, blurred characteristic band may be present, which partially disappears with the inhibitor. There were 14 false positive AChE tests on clear fluid; the specific band was faint, and all were normal on a repeat amniocentesis. In 6 of these 14 cases, the placenta was anterior. Six were associated with AFPs measuring <+3 SD, five between +3 and +5 SD, and three ≥+5 SD above the mean.

## Outcomes of Pregnancies Combining US With AFP and AChE Tests of First Amniocentesis (Table 16H–5)

AFP LEVELS ≥+3 AND <+5 SD ABOVE THE MEAN
If the AChE test was negative, the risk of an open NTD was practically zero, but the incidence of other

**TABLE 16H–4.**
**Other Abnormalities Detected (AChE Test Positive)***

| CATEGORY | NO. | +2 SD | ≥+3, <+5 SD | ≥+5 SD |
|---|---|---|---|---|
| | | AFP LEVEL | | |
| Fetal demise† | 38 (25) | | 8 (1) | 30 (24)** |
| Omphalocele‡ | 32 (18) | 2 (0) | 4 (2) | 26 (16) |
| Gastroschisis§ | 4 (4) | | | 4 (4) |
| Hydrops/ascites†‖ | 9 (4) | | | 9 (4) |
| Cystic hygroma† | 22 (17) | 1 (1) | 4 (1) | 17 (15) |
| Urinary obstruct | 4 (2) | | | 4 (2) |
| Other | 15 (4) | | 6 (0)¶ | 9 (4)†† |
| Totals | 124 (74) | 3 (1) | 22 (4) | 99 (69) |

*Parentheses enclose percentages.
†AFP <+2 SD in one additional case.
‡Trisomy 18 (two cases).
§Some earlier cases not separated from omphalocele.
‖Trisomy 21 (one case)
¶Trisomy 13 (two cases, one with hydrocephalus), trisomy 18 (one case), Dandy-Walker cyst (one), acardia (one), severe "brain and renal anomalies" (one)
**Twins. One twin was dead. In the other, AFP and AChE continued to be abnormal 3 weeks later.
††Duodenal atresia (two cases, AChE positive in one), sacral teratoma (two, in both AChE was positive), complete atresia of the colon (one, AChE negative), trisomy 18 (one, AChE positive), congenital nephrosis (one, AChE negative), amniotic band syndrome (one, AChE negative), facial teratoma (one, AChE negative).

**TABLE 16H–5.**

Number of Abnormalities Identified by Ultrasound, First Amniocentesis AFP > +3 SD, AChE Positive or Negative

| AFP | NO. ABNORMAL | AChE NEG. | US POS. | AChE POS. | US POS. |
|---|---|---|---|---|---|
| ≥ +3, < +5 | 35 | 18† | 13† | 17¶ | 15†† |
| ≥ +5 | 190* | 30‡ | 27‡ | 150** | 147‡‡ |

*Ten open NTDs not tested by AChE.
†Demise (seven), omphalocele (two), cystic hygroma (three, one with trisomy 18, one with trisomy 21, one with XO), trisomy 13 (two), trisomy 18 (one), brain and kidney abnormalities (one), Dandy-Walker cyst (one), and acardia (one).
‡Omphalocele (ten), hydrops (five), demise (six), cystic hygroma (two), bladder obstruction (two), other (five).
§US normal in chromosome abnormality (three), omphalocele (two).
‖US normal in congenital nephrosis (one), duodenal atresia (one), and atresia of colon (one).
¶SB (ten), encephalocele (three), cystic hygroma (one), omphalocele (two), demise (one).
**Anencephaly (43), SB (36), encephalocele (two), demise (24), omphalocele (16), gastroschisis (four), hydrops (four), cystic hygroma (15), bladder obstruction (two), other (four).
††US normal in SB (two).
‡‡US normal in SB (two), omphalocele (one), trisomy 18 (one).

abnormalities was 9.9%. These were usually identified on a second ultrasound examination, but two small omphaloceles were missed (excluding three chromosome abnormalities identified by amniocentesis). Ultrasound failed to detect 2 of 18 abnormalities (11%). If the AChE test was positive, there was a 77% risk of abnormality, including open NTDs. Repeat ultrasound and amniocentesis are recommended, unless the abnormality is identified unequivocally. Two cases of open spina bifida were not detected on ultrasound; both were low-lying and both occurred more than 3 years ago. Ultrasound failed to detect 2 of 17 abnormalities (12%) (excluding chromosome abnormalities).

AFP LEVELS > +5 SD ABOVE THE MEAN

If the AChE test was normal, there was a 51% risk of demise or abnormality, but not an open NTD. Repeat ultrasound and amniocentesis was recommended, unless the presence of an abnormality was unequivocal. One case of congenital nephrosis was associated with consistently and markedly elevated AFP levels, and in this case and one case each of duodenal atresia and complete atresia of the colon, ultrasound scans were normal. Ultrasound failed to detect 3 of 30 abnormalities (10%).

If the AChE test was positive, there was a high risk of abnormality (98%). Two cases of spina bifida and one omphalocele were not detected on ultrasound (1.9%); all three occurred more than 3 years ago.

There were two pregnancies with a dead twin (one with anencephaly) in which the amniotic fluid AFP level remained above +5 SD and the AChE test was positive on the second amniocentesis 3 weeks later. We believe that perfusion of the liver of the dead twin may have accounted for this. One triplet pregnancy in which one fetus had spina bifida led to amniotic fluid AFP levels above +5 SD. The AChE test was positive in one normal triplet and between 3 and 5 SD above normal in the second normal triplet. The sonogram correctly delineated all three. Selective termination was attempted, but both normal triplets were spontaneously aborted later.

## Results of Second Amniocentesis

A second amniocentesis was usually performed if the first AFP level was more than +3 SD above the mean unless the AChE test and the sonogram were normal and the elevation appeared to result fromm FB contamination. A second amniocentesis was always done if the AFP level was more than +5 SD unless an abnormality or demise was clearly visualized on the sonogram. Of 169 normal pregnancies in which the initial AFP level was between +3 and +5 SD, only one normal showed an elevated second AFP level, and this was explained by FB contamination. Of 32 normal pregnancies with an initial AFP level at or above +5 SD, five normal fetuses remained above +5 SD on restudy. In 22 the AFP level was +3 to +5 SD and in 5 it was below +3 SD in the second amniotic fluid sample. All had normal AChE values, but two were tested retrospectively. The risk of an abnormality was therefore 60% if the second AFP level was +3 to +5 SD, and 97% for AFP levels at or above +5 SD.

These results are combined with the ultrasound findings in Table 16H–6. Excluding chromosome abnormalities, 10 of 225 abnormalities (4%) were missed on ultrasound.

## False Positives and Negatives

There were four true false positives, defined as the termination of the pregnancy of a normal fetus. In one, the initial amniotic fluid-AFP level measured +4 SD, and the sample contained fetal blood; a second amniocentesis resulted in an AFP of about the same level. In the second case, both amniotic fluid samples

**TABLE 16H–6.**

**Risk of Abnormality With Normal Ultrasound Findings and Elevated Second AFP Level**

| 2d AFP | TOTAL ABNORM. | AChE NEG. | | AChE POS. | |
|---|---|---|---|---|---|
| | | NO. | NO. MISSED BY US (%)* | NO. | NO. MISSED BY US (%)* |
| >+3, <+5 | 35 | 18 | 2 (11.5)‡ | 17 | 2 (12)‖ |
| >+5 | 190† | 30 | 3 (10.0)§ | 150 | 3 (2.0)¶ |

*Chromosome abnormalities excluded.
†Ten open NTDs not tested by AChE, all identified by US.
‡Two small omphaloceles.
§Congenital nephrosis (one), duodenal atresia (one), complete atresia of colon (one).
‖Two cases of spina bifida.
¶Two cases of spina bifida, one omphalocele.

were clear; the first AFP measured above +9 SD and the second between +6 and +7 SD above the mean. Spina bifida occulta of the lower vertebrae and the entire sacrum were noted at autopsy: the kidneys were not examined. In the third case, the amniotic fluid sample was clear and the AFP measured >+9 SD and remained >+5 SD in the second amniocentesis. The AChE test was consistently negative. The pregnancy was terminated, and no abnormalities were detected at autopsy, although the kidneys were not examined microscopically. The identical findings recurred in a succeeding pregnancy, which was continued with a normal outcome. AFP levels in the mother and child were normal. Exactly the same situation occurred in another woman: The first pregnancy was terminated and the kidneys were not studied. The second resulted in a normal baby. These two families with "normal" elevated AFP levels are being studied further. The incidence of true false positives in this series was 1/12,500. AChE gel electrophoresis, which was added after the first two false positives, would have excluded an open NTD in both. It correctly predicted that the other case was not an open NTD. There were no false negatives for open NTDs. Congenital nephrosis, although a rare genetic disorder, usually results in AFP levels >+5 SD, negative AChE tests, and normal US. It is inherited as an autosomal recessive trait and is usually fatal within the first 2 months of life.

## Recurrence Risk for NTDs

Some 2.5% of the amniocenteses were performed because of a previous open NTD. The recurrence risk was 1.8%. One case of encephalocele was probably due to Meckel's syndrome. Another woman had a fetus with anencephaly, followed by one with an encephalocele, and then two with hydrocephalus. Two cases of simple hydrocephaly occurred in pregnancies of women with a previous anencephaly; both were detected by ultrasound.

## NTDs and Maternal Age

Eighty-five percent of the amniocenteses were done for maternal age only, and the incidence of open NTD in this group was 1.5/1,000. This compares to 1.1/1,000 in a group of women identified in our maternal age AFP pilot program.[1]

## Discussion

In our experience, AFP assay was the best test for the detection of NTDs, particularly if a large number of samples were being tested. However, the AFP level was more sensitive to fetal blood contamination and changes in gestational age than AChE. AChE can be measured quantitatively or examined qualitatively. Most reports suggest that the former fails to discriminate clearly between normals and abnormals.[3, 4] The qualitative test may be included routinely for all amniotic fluid samples if a slab gel technique is used. Nevertheless, we have found the bands to be less equivocal with disk electrophoresis, although this has a more limited application for a large number of cases. As a compromise, we included the test when AFP levels measured >+2 SD or when there was an increased risk for NTDs. Our experience suggests that it would be very unlikely to miss an open NTD with this protocol.

There have been several other large series of amniotic fluid AFPs reported. The United Kingdom collaborative report collected data on 13,490 pregnancies, of which 385 had an open NTD.[5] They used different cut-off levels at different gestational ages, and 90% of open NTDs were identified. Milunsky published data on 20,000 second-trimester amniotic fluid AFP assays; no open NTDs were missed.[6] Our previously published studies are included in this series.[7, 8]

The identification of NTDs and certain other fetal abnormalities on ultrasound is usually highly accurate in expert hands. However, low-lying or "flat" SBs such as myeloscheses may prove particularly difficult to identify, and sonography is best used in conjunction with biochemical studies. Four SBs were not detected on sonography, even after abnormal AFP and AChE levels suggested their presence. All occurred in the earlier part of the study, and none have been missed in the last 3 years. More than 50% of the abnormalities were detected on the initial ulltrasound examination (this figure is now 75%).

We believe AFP should be measured routinely in all amniotic fluid samples. With the addition of AChE, the false positive rate as defined, will be extremely low, and very few open NTDs will be missed. We have tried to avoid a second amniocentesis when possible, and, providing the AChE test and sonogram are normal, it was sometimes avoidable when fetal blood contamination appeared to be responsible for an AFP level of +3 to +5 SD. However, this decision is dependent on uniformally high caliber equipment, expertise, and good sonographic visualization on more than one examination, and only if the AChE is unequivocally negative. Accurate diagnosis of fetal abnormalities is best achieved by combining ultrasound with both AFP assay and AChE electrophoresis.

## Summary

Of 50,000 initial amniotic fluid samples, 0–8% had an AFP level $\geq +3$ SD above the mean. The risk of an open NTD or other serious fetal abnormality was 53% if AFP levels measured $\geq +3$ SD, 17% for levels between $\geq +3$ and $+5$, and 86% for levels $\geq +5$. If the AChE test was positive, the risk for an abnormality was 77%, for AFP levels between $+3$ and $+5$ and 98% for AFP levels $\geq +5$. If the second AFP was $\geq +3$ SD, the risk of an abnormality was 89% and 97% for levels $\geq +5$ SD. No abnormal fetus had a normal repeat AFP. In this series, there were 107 open NTDs and all were identified. The true false positive rate was 1 per 12,500 of the cases screened. Ultrasound performed at ten different amniocentesis centers identified 96% of the abnormalities, excluding chromosomal ones. We conclude that the identification of NTDs and other serious abnormalities prenatally is best done by combining ultrasound with biochemical studies of amniotic fluid.

## Acknowledgments

This research was supported in part by grant HD-00345 for Research Training in Mental Retardation, grant HD-05616 for Developmental Biology in Mental Retardation, and grant 83-00043 from the Genetic Disease Section of the California State Department of Health Services.

The authors thank the following physicians and their staff for supplying amniotic fluid samples and follow-up data: Mitchell Golbus (UCSF Medical Center), John Mann (Permanente Hospital, San Jose), Howard Cann (Stanford Medical Center), Michael Kaback (Harbor-UCLA Medical Center, Torrance), Sanford Sherman (Oakland Children's Hospital), Miriam Wilson (County-USC Medical Center), Cindy Curry (Valley Children's Hospital, Fresno), Kenneth Dumars (UC-Irvine), William Conte (Prenatal Diagnostics, Inc.) Drs. T. Lebherz, Lidia Rubinstein, K. Tabsh, A. Ketupanya, and Dennis Sarti, and Ms. K. Yamazaki, R.N.

## References

1. Crandall BF, Robertson RD, Lebherz TB, et al: Maternal serum AFP screening for the detection of NTDs. *West J Med* 1983; 138:524–530.
2. Crandall BF, Kasha W, Matsumoto M: Prenatal diagnosis of NTDs: Experience with AChE. *Am J Med Genet* 1982; 12:361–366.
3. Chubb IW, Pilowsky PM, Springell HJ, et al: AChE in human amniotic fluid: An index of fetal neural development? *Lancet* 1979; 1:688–690.
4. Smith AD, Wald NJ, Cuckle HS, et al: Amniotic

fluid acetylcholinesterase as a possible diagnostic test for NTD in early pregnancy. *Lancet* 1979; 1:684–688.

5. Second Report of the UK Collaborative Study on AFP in relation to NTDs: Amniotic fluid AFP measurement in antenatal diagnosis of anencephaly and open spina bifida in early pregnancy. *Lancet* 1979; 11:651–661.

6. Milunsky A: Prenatal detection of neural tube defects: VI. Experience with 20,000 pregnancies. *JAMA* 1980; 244:2731–2735.

7. Crandall BF, Matsumoto M: Routine amniotic fluid alpha-fetoprotein measurement in 34,000 pregnancies. *Am J Obstet Gynecol* 1984; 149:744–747.

8. Crandall BF, Matsumoto M: Routine amniotic fluid alphafetoprotein assay: Experience with 40,000 pregnancies. *Am J Med Genet* 1986; 24:143–149.

## 16i

# FETAL DEATH EVALUATED BY ULTRASONOGRAPHY

Seymour Zemlyn, M.D.

There is evidence that far fewer conceptions result in a fruitful pregnancy than is commonly believed. Hertig et al., after carefully searching the uterus and tubes following hysterectomy performed late in the menstrual cycle, found that 40% of very early embryos were anatomically abnormal.[1] They concluded that many pregnancies are shed before or just after implantation. Hormonal studies confirm a high early embryonic mortality.[2] Urinary human chorionic gonadotropin (hCG) levels indicated an implanted pregnancy in about 60% of the ovulatory cycles in a group of 198 women trying to conceive. More than half of these implantations did not result in a clinical pregnancy. These women never missed a menstrual period and would be unaware of their close brush with motherhood. An additional 5% or more of implantations were lost before the 12th gestational week.

There is some dispute as to whether spontaneous abortion predisposes to additional abortions. These unhappy events are likely to recur.[3] Following a spontaneous abortion about one third of pregnancies result in another abortion. In contrast, more than 92% of normal pregnancies are followed by a normal pregnancy. After a stillbirth the subsequent pregnancy results in abortion in about 15% of cases and in stillbirth in about 20% of cases.

The generally accepted rate of combined abortion and fetal death in clinical pregnancy is 15%–20%. In the second and third trimesters of pregnancy fetal death is clinically suspected when heart tones cannot be heard and fetal motion is not felt after 20 weeks' gestation. Some of these cases will be found to be molar pregnancies. Suspicion of fetal death may be aroused when the fundal height of the uterus does not change or decreases, or when biochemical or hormonal values associated with pregnancy decline or are at nonpregnancy levels. Vaginal bleeding may or may not be present. Ultrasound is the best method of resolving clinical suspicions and has made previous techniques obsolete.

Fetal death can be excluded when fetal heart motion or definite fetal activity is detected. Conversely, the absence of fetal heart motion once a fetus can be visualized is indicative of fetal death. If uncertainty exists it is prudent to reexamine in 1–2 weeks, as there is no leeway in pronouncing a fetus dead. This is more likely to be a problem in the 7- to 10-week gestational age pregnancy, and the absence of detectable fetal heart motion on real-time sonographic examination should be reliable in the second or third trimester.[4] Secondary criteria may also be noted. In general order of earliest to latest appearance after fetal death, these include absence of fetal activity, echogenic blood[5, 6] or gas[7] in the heart and vessels, absence of internal fetal fluids, angulation of the fetal position, overriding of the skull bones, derangement of the fetal skeleton, and loss of normal morphology. There may be subcutaneous edema, pleural and pericardial effusions, ascites, and hydropic degeneration of the placenta, findings also seen in the live fetus with severe fetal hydrops. Oligohydramnios may be present and may be severe. Rarely, a long-standing missed abortion may present as a calcified fetus, a lithopedion.

Passive motion may be imparted to a small dead fetus by uterine contractions, maternal aortic pulsation, or a change in maternal position. Manipulation of the uterus may be useful in provoking reflex tonic movement by the live fetus, which, according to Platt et al., is easily distinguished from the flaccid, passive motion of the dead fetus. The absence of fetal movement over a 5-minute observation period with real-time ultrasound is said to be 100% reliable in diagnosing fetal death in pregnancies of 20 weeks' gestation or more. A refraction artifact as the transducer is passed across the rectus muscle in the midline may cause the image to appear to "jump," simulating fetal movement.

In the final analysis, absence of fetal cardiac activity on real-time examination is the method for diagnosis of fetal demise.

## References

1. Hertig AT, Rock J, Adams EC: A description of 34 human ova within 17 days of development. *Am J Anat* 1936; 98:435.
2. Edmonds DK, Lindsay KS, Miller JF, et al: Early embryonic mortality in women. *Fertil Steril* 1982; 38:447–453.
3. Hathout H, Kasrawi R, Moussa MA, et al: Influence of pregnancy outcome on subsequent pregnancy. *Int J Gynaecol Obstet* 1982; 20:145–147.
4. Platt LD, Manning FA, Murata Y, et al: Diagnosis of fetal death in utero by real-time ultrasound. *Obstet Gynecol* 1980; 55:191.
5. McLeary RD: An early sign of fetal demise: Ultrasonic demonstration of clotted blood within the fetal heart. *Radiology* 142:712.
6. Abrams SL, Callen PW, Filly RA: Umbilical vein thrombosis: Sonographic detection in utero. *J Ultrasound Med* 1985; 4:283.
7. Weinstein BJ, Platt LD: The ultrasonic appearance of intravascular gas in fetal death. *J Ultrasound Med* 1983; 2:451.

## 16j

## A BIOPHYSICAL PROFILE OF THE HUMAN FETUS

Harbinder S. Brar, M.D.
Lawrence D. Platt, M.D.

In obstetrics and gynecology, ultrasound imaging is used to assess events that change over relatively long periods of time, including growth, biparietal diameter (BPD), fetal weight, and congenital anomalies. The accurate assessment of biophysical indices of fetal condition based on short-term constants such as fetal breathing movements, fetal movements, and fetal heart rate has only recently been possible. We are entering an era of physical diagnosis of the human fetus. Before this era, the development and perfection of specific and accurate diagnostic tests for identification of the fetus at risk for death or damage in utero had been a major challenge and elusive goal for obstetricians and perinatologists. With the advent of high-resolution real-time ultrasound and the development of Doppler ultrasound, fetal medicine has shifted away from reliance on nonspecific maternal clinical markers of potential fetal disease, such as fundal height measurement, to more specific and direct examination of the fetus.

### Need for Assessment of Fetal Condition and Risk

The improvement in medical management of high-risk pregnancy factors like diabetes and hypertension and better understanding of the effect of maternal disease on the fetus have resulted in a need for better assessment of fetal well-being and for the correct identification of the fetus at risk. This has been further necessitated by the following factors: (1) advances in neonatal care over the last two decades have lowered the minimal gestational age at which neonatal survival occurs. Also, there has been a reduction in neonatal mortality and morbidity. Since perinatal asphyxia dramatically effects neonatal survival (especially in the premature fetus), there is a great need for accurate assessment of fetus at risk. (2) Medicolegal, societal, and consumer pressures and demands for a perfect outcome of a pregnancy have added impetus to the development of accurate diagnostic tests.

### Evolution of the Biophysical Profile

*Era of Biochemical Markers*

Historically, initial attempts to assess fetal well-being relied heavily on measurement of various biochemical markers in maternal serum or urine. These tests focused primarily on the integrity of the "fetoplacental unit" as an indirect measure of fetal condition. A variety of tests were used or described, such as determinations of placental alkaline phosphatase, human placental lactogen, leucine amino peptidase (oxytoninase), and steroids such as progesterone, estriol, estrone, estetrol, and total estrogen. Later, "placental function tests" were described, such as the metabolic clearance rate of DHEAS and the DHEAS loading tests. These tests fall into disrepute because of difficulties encountered in measurement and interpretation. Furthermore, they had a low specificity and sensitivity for predicting fetal well-being.

### Era of Antepartum Fetal Heart Rate Testing

With the introduction of the non-stress test, the contraction stress test, and improved neonatal care, perinatal mortality has fallen drastically to less than 12 in 1,000 live births. The ratio of stillbirth to neonatal death has changed from 1:2 in 1970 to 2:1 in 1980.[1] Thus, prevention of stillbirth has become a major challenge in modern perinatal medicine. The non-stress test and the contraction stress test predict normal outcome reasonably well; however, they are much less accurate in predicting poor outcome. The non-stress test has a low false negative rate (1% or less) and a high false positive rate (more than 75%).[2, 3] The contraction stress test has a somewhat higher false negative rate (2%–2.7%),[2, 3] and a false positive rate ranging from 50% to more than 75%.[4–6] Moreover, use of the contraction stress test presents both practical and theoretical difficulties, inasmuch as it is lengthy and cumbersome, and it also has failed to identify the dying fetus in certain terminal instances.[7]

### Era of the Biophysical Profile

The antepartum stillbirth rate in an untested population is about 8 per 1,000 and accounts for about 66% of all perinatal morbidity. The causes of stillbirths falls into four major groups: chronic intrauterine asphyxia (60%–70%), congenital anomalies (20%–25%), acute complications (e.g., placental abruption and infection) (5%–10%), and idiopathic (5%–10%).

Clearly, then, specific, accurate methods for detection of developing fetal asphyxia can result in early appropriate intervention and hence reduce fetal loss. Elimination of sustained fetal asphyxia is also likely to reduce neonatal loss from complications of prematurity.[8] An ideal antepartum fetal test must have a high specificity, sensitivity, and positive and negative predictive values, and low false negative and false positive rates. Formulas for statistical evaluations are shown below.

| | Outcome | |
| --- | --- | --- |
| | Normal | Abnormal |
| *Test result:* Normal | TN | FN |
| Abnormal | FP | TP |

*Predictive values:*

$$\text{Negative} = \frac{TN}{TN + FN} \qquad \text{Positive} = \frac{TP}{TP + TP}$$

$$\text{Sensitivity} = \frac{TP}{TP + FN} \qquad \text{Specificity} = \frac{TN}{TN + FP}$$

True negatives refer to unaffected patients with a negative (normal) test result. Test positives refer to affected patients with a positive (abnormal) test result. False negatives refer to affected patients with a negative test result. False positives refer to unaffected patients with a positive test result.[9, 10] An ideal antepartum test should be (1) highly sensitive and specific, since low sensitivity can result in asphyxial fetal death (false negative result) and low specificity can result in inappropriate intervention for the normal fetus (false positive result), leading in turn to iatrogenic neonatal mortality and morbidity as well as iatrogenic maternal morbidity, and (2) capable of identifying the fetus with major anomalies incompatible with extrauterine life, thus avoiding unnecessary surgical intervention in the mother. This is further underscored by the fact that a high incidence of abnormal antepartum and intrapartum fetal heart rate patterns are reported in infants with major anomalies, and surgical intervention is more likely in this group. Conversely, a high incidence of anomalies (up to 30%) is seen in selected populations, with abnormal antepartum fetal heart rate testing.[11, 12]

With the appropriate use of fetal biophysical variable monitoring and particularly with the use of the composite biophysical profile, nearly all fetuses with chronic asphyxia can be detected, the majority of congenital anomalies can be detected, and a lesser proportion of fetuses at risk for acute asphyxia can be detected.[13] The advantage of high-resolution dynamic ultrasound imaging is the ability to visualize the fetus and its activities, allowing application of the time-honored principle of physical examination, albeit indirectly to the fetus. This is creating the emerging concept of the fetus as a patient.[14] It allows one to assess fetal responses to detrimental maternal fetal risk accurately and as different from maternal risk. This also enables the physician to selectively intervene when fetuses are at risk (for example, by initiating delivery in preterm patients with oligohydramnios),[15, 16] thus reducing iatrogenic maternal and fetal disease.

## Fetal Biophysical Activities and Their Scope

The number of biophysical activities that can be studied by real-time B-mode ultrasound are numerous. They include: (1) generalized biophysical activities such as gross body movements, breathing movements, and fetal tone;[17–19] (2) specific activities such as sucking, swallowing, micturition, and reflex activities;[20] (3) recognizing sleep states by monitoring lens motion of the fetal eye;[21] (4) recording fetal heart rates;[22] (5) complex measurements of flow in umbilical vessels;[23] (6) assessing intrauterine environment, including quantitative amniotic fluid volume determination,[16, 24, 25] placental architecture, grade, and pathology,[26, 27] and cord position;[26] (7) assessing peristaltic patterns, purposeful movements, and evoked fetal reflex responses, like the fetal startle response evoked using an artificial larynx.[29]

The extent of fetal biophysical activities that may be incorporated in the profile is not limited by technical ability but by practicalities of time constraints. These biophysical activities vary with sleep cycles in humans as well as in experiment animals.[30, 31]

### Effects of Asphyxia

The response of these areas to hypoxemia is unknown but it has been speculated that variation may exist.[32] During fetal neural development a higher oxygen level is required for newly developing CNS centers. The biophysical activities that become active first in fetal development are the last to disappear under the influence of progressive asphyxia, which, when severe, arrests all biophysical activities.[33] For example, the fetal tone center (cortex-subcortical area), which is the earliest to function (7.5–8.5 weeks),[33, 34] is the last to disappear during progressively worsening asphyxia. The presence of poor fetal tone was indeed found to be associated with the highest perinatal death rate (42.8%) because it signifies hypoxemia of a highly significant degree. On the other hand, the fetal heart rate reactivity starts operating at about 28 weeks and therefore is more sensitive to asphyxia; it is the first biophysical activity to be affected by progressively worsening asphyxia (Table 16J–1). The temporal and functional characteristics of fetal CNS function during recovery from asphyxia are unclear. Animal studies seem to indicate that recovery of CNS function (return to normal of the biophysical profile) occurs before the restoration of blood gas values to normal.[35–43]

### Effects of Drugs

Drugs that depress CNS activity, such as sedatives (barbiturates, diazepam), analgesics (morphine, meperidine), and anesthetics (halothane), usually abolish

**TABLE 16J–1.**

**Fetal CNS Centers***

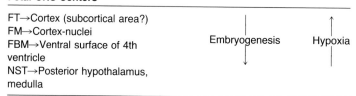

FT→Cortex (subcortical area?)
FM→Cortex-nuclei
FBM→Ventral surface of 4th ventricle
NST→Posterior hypothalamus, medulla

*FT = fetal tone; FM = fetal movements; FBM = fetal breathing movements; NST = non-stress test.

fetal biophysical activities.[44] In contrast, CNS stimulants such as amphetamines and hyperglycemia can result in increased fetal biophysical activities. A knowledge of maternal drug use prior to clinical testing thus is essential.

## Single Biophysical Variable Testing

### Antepartum Fetal Heart Rate Testing

#### Non-stress Test

The combination of fetal heart rate acceleration and fetal body movements has been associated with a high probability of a favorable perinatal outcome.[45] Movement precedes the onset of most acceleration, thus indicating some kind of reflex feedback mediated through the neurophysiologic pathways initiating the acceleration.[46] Lavery has reviewed 11 reported series (total of 7,884 patients) in which the non-stress test was used.[47] The false negative rate (uncorrected for lethal anomalies) was 6.80 per 1,000. Among the group with abnormal tests the perinatal death rate was 12%. Major advantages of the non-stress test include ease of testing. Major disadvantages of any single test (including the non-stress test) are: (1) the frequency of an abnormal test result is relatively high (9%–10%);[48] (2) the true positive predictive accuracy of the abnormal test result is low (12%–13%),[47] although it may be improved by extending the duration of the test[49] (to allow for sleep cycles) or by combining the test with other tests like the FBM[50] or the contraction stress test;[54] and (3) the false negative rate is relatively high (4–6 per 1000).[47]

In a prospective randomized clinical study comparing the non-stress test to fetal biophysical profile (FBP), the frequency of abnormal tests was significantly higher with the non-stress test and the positive predictive accuracy was lower,[51] although the negative predictive accuracy did not vary.

#### Contraction stress test

The contraction stress test entails the observation of periodic heart rate changes in relation to contractions. The false negative rate is about 0.4 per 1,000;[52] however, fetal death during a negative test has been reported.[53] The reported false positive rate varies from 25% to 100%.[54, 55] In a blinded clinical study, fetal death rate with a positive test was 327 per 1,000.[56]

Combining the contraction stress test with other biophysical variables may reduce the false positive rate.[57]

### Fetal Breathing Movements

The occurrence of rhythmic episodes of breathing movements in utero as part of normal fetal development has been documented in chronically catheterized fetal rats and monkeys[35, 36] and in the human fetus.[58, 59] In the normal fetus, breathing movements are episodic, with bursts of fetal breathing interspersed with periods of apnea. The proportion of time the human fetus spends breathing varies with the time of the day, reaching a zenith in late evening and a nadir in early morning.[59] Boddy and Dawes[60] found that fetuses that spent at least 50% of the time breathing had a good outcome and ones that spent less than 50% of the time breathing had a poor outcome. Prolonged apnea associated with fetal gasping was invariably associated with severe fetal compromise or death. In another prospective study,[61] the presence of fetal breathing movements before delivery was a strong predictor of a normal nonasphyxiated fetus (90%), whereas only 50% of fetuses with absent breathing were asphyxic or depressed at birth. These results are similar to those of the non-stress test in that when abnormal they are poor predictors of outcome, but the predictive accuracy improves markedly when both tests are combined.[32]

### Fetal Movement

Clinical studies of subjective (maternal) reporting of decreased fetal movement have confirmed that decreased fetal movement is associated with adverse outcome.[62, 63] These movements can be monitored by real-time ultrasound[64, 65] and they occur in episodes of 30 minutes (with 10–16 discrete movements) in each 90-minute period[66] and appear to be related to sleep-wake cycles.[67] Unlike breathing movements, gross body movements have little circadian activity and do not fluctuate with glucose concentrations.[68] There are two ways of recording fetal movement, subjectively and objectively. Subjective recording refers to the mother's perception of fetal movement. Women who perceive decreased fetal movement are at higher risk of bearing abnormal infants.[62] Objective monitoring is performed with real-time ultrasound. In a prospective, blinded study of 216 high-risk pregnancies,[32] the incidences of low 5-minute Apgar score, fetal distress in labor, and perinatal mortality were all significantly increased in inactive fetuses as compared to active fetuses. As with all other single tests, the predictive accuracy was greatest with the normal test. A high false positive rate[64] was explained as due to fetal quiescence during a sleep cycle.

*Fetal Tone*

Hypotonia, characterized by limb deflexion, loss of fist formation, and a "frog-like" posture, is the usual finding in an asphyxiated newborn.[69] Fetal tone has not been studied in animals, but in the human fetus normal tone is defined as active flexion-deflexion of a fetal limb or opening and closing of the fetal hand. Fetal tone is considered abnormal if there is no return to a position of complete flexion after fetal movement or if the fetus is in a deflexed position (partial or complete) in the absence of fetal movement. In the previously mentioned prospective, blinded study of 216 high-risk pregnancies,[32] absent fetal tone was associated with a high incidence of fetal distress in labor, low 5-minute Apgar score, and perinatal morbidity, as compared to fetuses having normal tone on the last test before delivery.

A better objective method of detecting fetal tone is to evoke a fetal startle response using the artificial larynx. By doing this one may actually visualize forearm motion, which allows one to evaluate fetal tone.[29]

## Evolution of Composite Fetal Biophysical Variable Monitoring

We have used different biophysical variables singly to predict fetal outcome. The common denominator of use of any single variable is that a normal test result is a much more powerful predictor of normal fetal condition than the abnormal test is a predictor of fetal compromise. All variables individually continue to have false negative results (rate of 4–6 per 1,000 for the non-stress test)[47] and unacceptably high (30%–70%) false positive rates because of sleep-wake cycles.

Since an abnormal variable could be explained because of asphyxia or a sleep-wake cycle, a test is required that could differentiate these two entities. This diagnostic dilemma may be resolved by observing multiple biophysical profiles in combination and by extending the period of observation beyond a sleep-wake cycle. This brought about the development of a combined biophysical profile of the fetus.

## Biophysical Profile Scoring as a Clinical Test

There are two different kinds of scoring systems reported in the literature. The first is the one described by Manning et al.[32] in which each variable is either normal (score = 2) or abnormal (score = 0) (Table 16J–2). The second is the one described by Vintzileos et al.[70] in which each variable is scored of 0, 1, or 2 (Table 16J–3). They also include placenta grading in the biophysical profile scoring.

## Fetal Biophysical Profile for Antepartum Fetal Assessment: Clinical Studies

Variables may be divided into two types, acute and chronic. Acute variables reflect immediate fetal condition (e.g., FM, FBM, FT, and NST). Chronic variables reflect chronic progressive intrauterine asphyxia (e.g., amniotic fluid volume).

Table 16J–4 summarizes several published studies. The details of the studies are as follows.

1. In an initial study, 216 patients were studied, and with the exception of the non-stress test, the score was not used for management purposes.[18] There was a high correlation between abnormal score and low 5-minute Apgar scores, fetal distress in labor, and antepartum and perinatal death rate. The lower the score the greater the correlation.

A combination of test results always resulted in improved positive predictive accuracy for both normal and abnormal test results. The maximal positive predictive accuracy for the normal test was achieved when all variables were abnormal. The perinatal death rate when all variables were normal (combined score = 10) was 0, as compared with 400 per 1,000 when all variables were abnormal (score = 0).

**TABLE 16J–2.**

**Biophysical Profile Scoring: Techniques and Interpretation***

| BIOPHYSICAL VARIABLE | NORMAL (SCORE = 2) | ABNORMAL (SCORE = 0) |
|---|---|---|
| Fetal breathing movements | At least 1 episode of FBM of at least 30 sec duration in 30 min observation | Absent FBM or no episode of ≥ 30 sec in 30 minutes |
| Gross body movement | At least 3 discrete body/limb movements in 30 min (episodes of active continuous movement considered as single movement) | Two or fewer episodes of body/limb movements in 30 min |
| Fetal tone | At least 1 episode of active extension with return to flexion of fetal limb(s) or trunk; opening and closing of hand considered normal tone | Either slow extension with return to partial flexion or movement of limb in full extension or absent fetal movement |
| Reactive FHR | At least 2 episodes of FHR acceleration of ≥ 15 beats/min and of at least 15 sec duration associated with fetal movement in 30 min | Less than 2 episodes of acceleration of FHR or acceleration of >15 beats/min in 30 min |
| Qualitative AFV | At least 1 pocket of AF that measures at least 1 cm in two perpendicular planes | Either no AF pockets or a pocket <1 cm in two perpendicular planes |

*FBM = fetal breathing movement; FHR = fetal heart rate; AFV = amniotic fluid volume; AF = amniotic fluid.

2. In a follow-up study of 5,182 pregnancies, fetal biophysical profile scores were obtained in 1,184 consecutive high-risk pregnancies.[70] Score results were used to guide clinical management as per the protocol in Table 16J–5.

Although the above protocol was used for management in the study it is probably better to individualize management schemes. For example, intervention in a fetus with oligohydramnios would depend on the etiology of the condition and the duration of gestation.

**TABLE 16J–3.**

**Criteria for Scoring Biophysical Variables***

NON-STRESS TEST:
   *Score 2 (NST 2):* Five or more FHR accelerations of at least 15 bpm in amplitude and at least 15 sec duration associated with fetal movements in a 20-minute period.
   *Score 1 (NST 1):* Two to four accelerations of at least 15 bpm in amplitude and at least 15 sec duration associated with fetal movements in a 20-minute period.
   *Score 0 (NST 0):* One or no acceleration in a 20-minute period.
FETAL MOVEMENTS
   *Score 2 (FM 2):* At least three gross (trunk and limbs) episodes of fetal movements within 30 minutes. Simultaneous limb and trunk movements were counted as a single movement.
   *Score 1 (FM 1):* One or two fetal movements within 30 minutes.
   *Score 0 (FM 0):* Absence of fetal movements within 30 minutes.
FETAL BREATHING MOVEMENTS:
   *Score 2 (FBM 2):* At least one episode of fetal breathing of at least 60-sec duration within a 30-minute observation period.
   *Score 1 (FBM 1):* At least one episode of fetal breathing lasting 30–60 sec within 30 minutes.
   *Score 0 (FBM 0):* Absence of fetal breathing or breathing lasting less than 30 sec within 30 minutes.
FETAL TONE:
   *Score 2 (FT 2):* At least one episode of extension of extremities with return to position of flexion, and also one episode of extension of spine with return to position of flexion.
   *Score 1 (FT 1):* At least one episode of extension of extremities with return to position of flexion, or one episode of extension of spine with return to position of flexion.
   *Score 0 (FT 0):* Extremities in extension; fetal movements not followed by return to flexion; open hand.
AMNIOTIC FLUID VOLUME:
   *Score 2 (AF 2):* Fluid evident throughout the uterine cavity; a pocket that measures 2 cm or more in vertical diameter.
   *Score 1 (AF 1):* A pocket that measures less than 2 cm but more than 1 cm in vertical diameter.
   *Score 0 (AF 0):* Crowding of fetal small parts. Largest pocket less than 1 cm in vertical diameter.
PLACENTAL GRADING:
   *Score 2 (PL 2):* Placental grading 0, 1, or 2.
   *Score 1 (PL 1):* Placenta posterior, difficult to evaluate.
   *Score 0 (PL 0):* Placental grading 3.

*NST = nonstress test; FHR = fetal heart rate, bpm = beats/minute, FM = fetal movements; FBM = fetal breathing movements; FT = fetal tone; AF = amniotic fluid; PL = placental grading. Maximal score = 12; minimal score = 0.

Performing a contraction stress test in these patients might be a reasonable way to obtain more information about the status of the fetus.

Only one fetus suffered unpredictable and unpre-

**TABLE 16J–4.**

**Cumulative Results of Fetal Biophysical Profile for Antepartum Fetal Assessment**

| STUDY POPULATION | NO. OF PATIENTS | NO. OF TESTS | | | | | CRUDE PNM | | CORRECTED PNM* | | FALSE NEGATIVE RATE | |
| | | HIGH-RISK | TOTAL | NORMAL | EQUIVOCAL | ABNORMAL | NO. | RATE | NO. | RATE | NO. | RATE |
|---|---|---|---|---|---|---|---|---|---|---|---|---|
| Manitoba, general population, 1979–1982 | 65,979 | 20 | . . . | . . . | . . . | . . . | 943 | 14.1 | 586 | 8.81 | . . . | . . . |
| Manitoba, prospective study | 12,620 | 100 | 26,257 | 97.52% | 1.72% | 0.76% | 93 | 7.37 | 24 | 1.90 | 8 | 0.643 |
| Baskett et al. | 2,400 | 100 | 5,618 | 97.1% | 1.70% | 1.2% | 23 | 9.20 | 11 | 4.40 | 1 | 0.500 |
| Platt et al.† | 286 | 100 | 1,112 | 94% | 3.5% | 2.4% | 4 | 14.00 | 2 | 7.00 | 2 | 7.40 |
| Schifrin et al.† | 158 | "Most" | 240 | . . . | . . . | . . . | 7 | 44.00 | 2 | 12.60 | 1 | 6.300 |
| Vintziles et al. | 150 | 100 | 342 | 94.9% | 2% | 3.1% | 5 | 33.30 | 4‡ | 26.60 | 0 | 0 |
| Total | 15,614 | >90 | 33,569 | >95% | 2% | 1% | 132 | 8.40 | 43 | 2.70 | 12 | 0.770 |

*Corrected to exclude death due to lethal anomaly or Rh disease.
†Modified use of biophysical profile scoring.
‡All neonatal deaths.

**TABLE 16J–5.**

**Biophysical Profile Scoring: Management Protocol**

| SCORE | INTERPRETATION | MANAGEMENT |
|---|---|---|
| 10 | Normal infant, low risk for chronic asphyxia | Repeat testing at weekly intervals; repeat twice weekly in diabetics and patients ≥42 wk gestation |
| 8 | Normal infant, low risk for chronic asphyxia | Repeat testing at weekly intervals; repeat testing twice weekly in diabetics and patients ≥42 wk Oligohydramnios an indication for delivery |
| 6 | Suspect chronic asphyxia | Repeat testing in 4–6 hr Deliver if oligohydramnios present |
| 4 | Suspect chronic asphyxia | If ≥36 wk and favorable, then deliver; if <36 wk and L/S* 2.0, repeat test in 24 hr; if repeat score ≤4, deliver |
| 0–2 | Strong suspicion of chronic asphyxia | Extend testing time to 120 min; if persistent score ≤4, deliver regardless of gestational age |

*L/S, amniotic fluid lecithin/spingomyelin ratio.

ventable death (true false negative rate, 0.8/1,000). Six perinatal deaths occurred, for a corrected perinatal mortality rate of 5.06/1,000, lower than the rate expected even in a low-risk population. In addition, 13 fetuses with major congenital anomalies (8 lethal) were detected.

3. Baskett et al.[71] reported on a similar prospective study conducted on 2,400 high-risk pregnancies. The perinatal death rates ranged from 0.3 per 1,000 when the score was 10 (false negative rate) to 292 per 1,000 when the score was 0. The corrected perinatal morbidity rate was 2.8 per 1,000.

4. The largest experience has been recently reported by Manning et al.[72] in 12,620 referred high-risk pregnancies. A total of 26,257 tests were performed. Ninety-three perinatal deaths occurred (gross perinatal mortality rate, 7.37/1,000), of which only 24 occurred among structurally normal nonisoimmunized fetuses and were presumed to be asphyxial in origin (corrected perinatal mortality, 1.9/1,000). Eight structurally normal fetuses died within 1 week of a normal test result (corrected false negative rate, 0.634/1,000), 97.52% of tests were normal, and only 0.75% were scored 4 or less.

5. Vintzileos et al.[70] reported their experience with 150 high-risk pregnancies in which 342 examinations were performed. There was a high correlation of an abnormal score with abnormal intrapartum fetal heart rate patterns, meconium during labor, fetal distress, and perinatal mortality rate, but the predictive value increased when variables were combined (Figs 16J–1 through 16J–4). The predictive value of biophysical scoring with a nonreactive non-stress test in 33 patients is shown in Table 16J–6. Seven patients had a

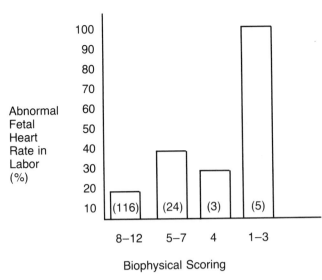

FIG 16J–1.

*The relationship of fetal biophysical scoring to incidence of abnormal fetal heart rate patterns in labor. Number of patients is given in parentheses.*

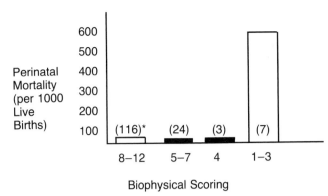

FIG 16J–3.

*Relationship of fetal biophysical score to perinatal mortality. Number of patients is given in parentheses. \*One case of Potter's syndrome.*

score of 1 to 3 and accounted for 57.1% of neonatal deaths. They recommended an antepartum fetal evaluation protocol as shown in Figure 16J–5.

The results confirm the high predictive value of negative test results for a good neonatal outcome. In contrast, each abnormal variable was associated with a high false positive rate. The absence of fetal movements was the best predictor of abnormal heart rate patterns in labor (80%), the nonreactive non-stress test was the best predictor of meconium (33.3%), decreased amniotic fluid was the best predictor of fetal

distress (37.5%), and poor fetal tone was the best predictor of perinatal death rate.

6. Platt and co-workers[72] in a study of 286 fetuses reported a corrected perinatal mortality rate of 7.0/1,000, compared to 22.6/1,000 for all patients in their institution. They confirmed the predictive values of the abnormal score but challenged whether the predictive value of the normal score exceeds that of the non-stress test. In this regard it is interesting to note that the combined studies of fetal biophysical profile scoring have consistently yielded a false negative rate of less than 1 in 1,000, whereas cumulative studies of the non-stress test alone yield a false negative rate of 4–6 per 1,000.[77] In another study by Platt et al.,[73] 279 patients were randomly assigned to a biophysical pro-

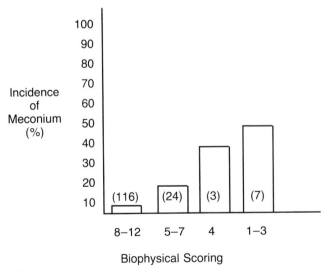

FIG 16J–2.

*The relationship of fetal biophysical scoring to incidence of meconium in labor. Number of patients is given in parentheses.*

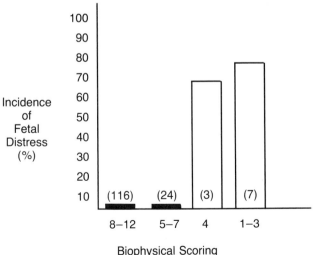

FIG 16J–4.

*Relationship of fetal biophysical scoring to incidence of fetal distress. Number of patients is given in parentheses.*

**TABLE 16J–6.**

**Predictive Value of Biophysical Scoring With Nonreactive Non-Stress Test***

| NO. OF BIOPHYSICAL SCORES | % | SCORE | OUTCOME |
|---|---|---|---|
| 13/33 | 39.3 | 8–12 | Good (100%) |
| 10/33 | 30.3 | 6–7 | Good (80%) Fetal distress (20%) |
| 3/33 | 9.0 | 4 | Fetal distress (100%), no neonatal deaths |
| 7/33 | 21.2 | 1–3 | Good (14%), fetal distress (28.5%), neonatal deaths (57.1%) |

*Zero to one accelerations every 20 minutes. As the biophysical score decreases, the incidence of good outcomes decreases while fetal distress increases ($P < .00005$).

file group and 261 to the non-stress test group; and there was no significant difference in the negative predictive value, the sensitivity, or the specificity of the two tests in identifying overall abnormal outcome as measured by perinatal mortality, fetal distress in labor, low 5-minute Apgar score, and infants small for gestational age. The corrected perinatal mortality in the biophysical profile group was 5 per 1,000, compared

to 7 per 1,000 in the non-stress test group. A statistically significant difference was found between biophysical profile and the non-stress test for a positive predictive value in determing abnormal outcome.

## Fetal Biophysical Profile as an Early Predictor of Fetal Infection

Vintzileos et al.[74] serially assessed the modified fetal biophysical profile in 73 patients with ruptured membranes and who were not in labor. A score of 8 or higher was associated with an infection rate of 2.7% and a score of 7 or lower was associated with an infection rate of 93.7%. They suggested that rupture of membranes by itself does not alter the biophysical activity of the healthy fetus. A low score ($\leq$7) was a good predictor of impending fetal infection, and the biophysical activities were altered in this group in a manner similar to uteroplacental insufficiency. The first manifestations of impending fetal infection were a nonreactive non-stress test and absent fetal breathing movements. Loss of fetal motion and poor fetal tone

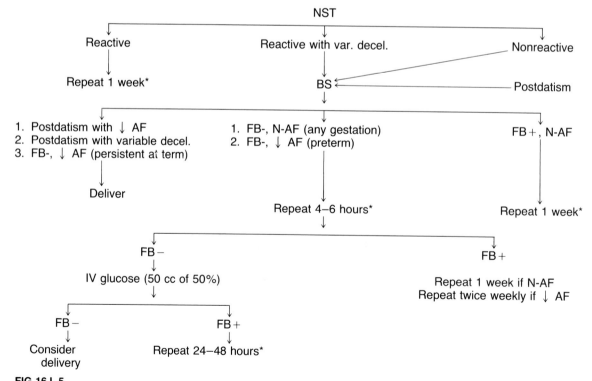

**FIG 16J–5.**

*Protocol for antepartum fetal evaluation. *Repeat fetal evaluation beginning with NST. $\downarrow$ AF = decreased amniotic fluid volume; N-AF = normal amniotic fluid volume; Fb– = fetal breathing absent; FB+ = fetal breathing present; BS = biophysical scoring.*

were late signs. The presence of fetal breathing movements had the highest specificity in predicting absence of fetal infection, with no cases of fetal infection seen when breathing was present 24 hours before delivery. The mechanism by which fetal infection diminishes fetal biophysical activities seems to occur by increasing fetal oxygen demands and causing local tissue hypoxia and thereby malfunction of CNS centers that control reflex biophysical activities.[70] With these observations, Vintzileos et al. have recommended a protocol as outlined in Figure 16J–6.

In a follow-up study by the same authors, a prospective comparison between the daily fetal biophysical profile and amniocentesis in predicting infection was undertaken in 58 patients with preterm premature rupture of the membranes.[75] The biophysical profile had a sensitivity, specificity, positive predictive value, and negative predictive value of 80%, 97.6%, 92.3%, and 93.2%, respectively, in predicting infection outcome, as compared to 60%, 81.3%, 52.9%, and 85.3%, respectively, of Gram stain.

## Advantages of Biophysical Profile Scoring

Fetal assessment based on biophysical profile scoring offers several advantages in clinical practice.

1. The test can be done by specially trained personnel with the average time to complete the test about 20 minutes.

2. It results in a substantial fall in false positive results and has false negative results comparable with those of OCT.

3. It also provides other useful information with regard to fetal position and number, the risk of IUGR, and placental location and grade. The impact of this information cannot be measured but is likely to be great.

4. It may identify major congenital anomalies not detected earlier in pregnancy in which obstetric management may be altered.

5. It can be widely applied.

6. Assurance of fetal well-being in at-risk pregnancies has allowed conservative therapy and prevented early intervention and the associated risks of failed induction, iatrogenic prematurity, and increased operative delivery.

7. The test potentially helps monitor patients with preterm premature rupture of the membranes for impending infection, thus preventing neonatal and maternal sepsis.

## Limitations of the Biophysical Profile

1. Long-term developmental sequelae of fetuses with low scores is still unknown.

2. The different CNS centers responsible for the biophysical activities have a varying degree of sensitivity. The duration and frequency of hypoxemia and their effect on the fetus are as yet unknown.

## Summary

Based on the cumulative experience of more than 15,000 patients in several centers, fetal biophysical profile scoring holds promise as an improved methd of fetal risk detection. Antepartum detection, classification, determination of severity, and ultimately treat-

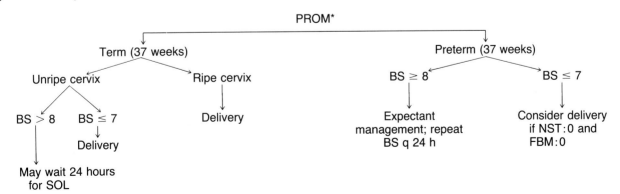

**FIG 16J–6.**
*Proposed protocol for management of premature rupture of the membranes. *Premature rupture of the membranes. BS = biophysical score, NST 0 = nonreactive non-stress test, FBM 0 = fetal breathing movements absent, SOL = spontaneous onset of labor.*

ment of the fetus at risk for death and damage in utero form the basis of modern perinatal medicine. It remains to be determined whether the addition of more variables or refinement of existing variables will improve accuracy still further. The assessment of multiple biophysical variables and responses to intrinsic and extrinsic stimuli is most helpful in differentiating a normal sleeping fetus from an asphyxiated fetus.

## References

1. Morrison I: Perinatal morbidity. *Semin Perinatol* 1985; 9(4).
2. Schifrin BS: The rationale of antepartum fetal heart rate monitoring. *J Reprod Med* 1979; 23:213.
3. Evertson LR, Gauthier RJ, Schifrin BS et al: Antepartum fetal heart rate testing: I. Evaluation of the nonstress test. *Am J Obstet Gynecol* 1979; 133:29.
4. Christie CB, Cudmore W: The oxytocin challenge tests. *Am J Obstet Gynecol* 1979; 1118:327.
5. Gauthier RJ, Evertson LR, Paul RH: Antepartum fetal heart rate testing: II. Intrapartum fetal heart rate testing and neonatal outcome following a positive contraction stress test. *Am J Obstet Gynecol* 1979; 133:34.
6. Ray M, Freeman R, Pine S, et al: Clinical experiences with the oxytocin challenge test. *Am J Obstet Gynecol* 1972; 114:1.
7. Evertson LR, Gauthier RJ, Collea JV: Fetal demise following negative contraction stress tests. *Obstet Gynecol* 1978; 51:671.
8. Martin CB, Schifrin BS, in Aladjem S, Brown A (eds): *Perinatal Fetal Monitoring.* St Louis, CV Mosby Co, 1976.
9. Schifrin BS, Guntes V, Gergely RC, et al: The role of real time scanning in antenatal fetal surveillance. *Am J Obstet Gynecol* 1981; 140:525.
10. Manning FA, Baskett TF, Morrison I, et al: Fetal biophysical profile scoring: A prospective study in 1,184 high risk patients. *Am J Obstet Gynecol* 1981; 140:289.
11. Druzin M, Gratacos J, Keegan K, et al: Antepartum fetal heart rate testing: The significance of fetal bradycardia. *Am J Obstet Gynecol* 1981; 139:194.
12. Powell-Phillips WD, Towell ME: Abnormal fetal heart rate associated with congenital anomalies. *Br J Obstet Gynaecol* 1980; 87:270.
13. Manning FA, Morrison I, Lange IR, et al: Antepartum determination of fetal health composite biophysical profile scoring, in *Symposium on Fetal Monitoring. Clin Perinatol* 1982; 9(2).
14. Manning FA: Assessment of fetal condition and risk: Analysis of single and combined biophysical variable monitoring. *Semin Perinatol* 1985; 9(4):168–183.
15. Johnson J, Harman CR, Lange IR, et al: Fetal biophysical profile scoring in the management of the post-date pregnancy: A prospective study. *Am J Obstet Gynecol* (in press).
16. Phelan JP, Platt LD, Yeh S: The role of ultrasound assessment of amniotic fluid volume in the management of the post-date pregnancy. *Am J Obstet Gynecol* 1985; 151:304.
17. Chamberlain PF, Manning FA: Ultrasound: Fetal movements and fetal condition, in *Principles and Practice in Obstetrics and Gynecology,* ed 3. New York, Appleton-Century-Crofts, 1984, pp 175–188.
18. Platt LD, Manning FA: Fetal breathing movements: An update. *Clin Perinatol* 1980; 7:425.
19. Patrick JE, Challis JRG: Measurement of human fetal breathing in healthy pregnancies using real time ultrasound. *Semin Perinatol* 1980; 4:275.
20. Chamberlain PF, Manning FA, Morrison I, et al: Circadian rhythm in bladder volume in the term human fetus. *Obstet Gynecol* 1984; 674:657.
21. Martin CB Jr: On behavioral states in human fetus. *J Reprod Med* 1981; 26:425.
22. DeVore GR, Donnelstein RL, Kleinman CS, et al: Fetal echocardiography: I. Normal anatomy using realtime directed M-mode ultrasound. *Am J Obstet Gynecol* 1982; 144:249–260.
23. Campbell S, Griffin DR, Pearce JM, et al: New doppler technique for assessing utero placental blood flow. *Lancet* 1983; 1:675.
24. Chamberlain PFC, Manning FA, Morrison I, et al: Ultrasound evaluation of amniotic fluid volumes: I. The relationship of marginal and decreased amniotic fluid volumes to perinatal outcome. *Am J Obstet Gynecol* 1984; 150:245.
25. Chamberlain PFC, Manning FA, Morrison I, et al: Ultrasound evaluation of amniotic fluid: II. The

relationship of increased amniotic fluid to perinatal outcome. *Am J Obstet Gynecol* 1984; 150:250.

26. Grannum PAT, Berkowitz RL, Hobbins JC: The ultrasonic changes in the maturing placenta and their relationship to fetal pulmonic maturity. *Am J Obstet Gynecol* 1979; 133:915.

27. Kaufman AJ, Fleischer AC, Thieme G, et al: Separated chorioamnion and elevated chorion: Sonographic features and clinical significance. *J Ultrasound Med* 1985; 4:119.

28. Lange IR, Manning FA, Morrison I, et al: Prenatal diagnosis of cord prolapse. *Am J Obstet Gynecol.*

29. Divon MY, Platt LD, Cantrell CJ, et al: Evoked fetal startle response: A possible intrauterine neurological examination. *Am J Obstet Gynecol* 1985; 153:454.

30. Dawes GS, Fox HE, Leduc BM, et al: Respiratory movements and rapid eye movement sleep in the foetal lamb. *J Physiol* (London) 1972; 220:119.

31. Ruckebusch L, Gaujoux M, Eghbali B: Sleep cycles and kinesis in the fetal lamb. *Electroencephalogr Clin Neurophysiol* 1977; 42:226.

32. Manning FA, Platt LD, Sipos L: Antepartum fetal evaluation: Development of a fetal biophysical profile score. *Am J Obstet Gynecol* 1980; 136:787.

33. Humphrey T: Function of the nervous system during prenatal life, in Uwe S (ed): *Perinatal Physiology.* New York, Plenum, 1978, p 651.

34. Ianniruberto A, Tejani E: Ultrasonographic study of fetal movements. *Semin Perinatol* 1981; 5:175.

35. Boddy K, Dawes GS, Fisher R, et al: Fetal respiratory movements, electrocortical and cardiovascular responses to hypoxemia and hypercapnia in sheep. *J Physiol (London)* 1974; 243:599.

36. Manning FA, Platt LD: Maternal hypoxemia and fetal breathing movements. *Obstet Gynecol* 1979; 53:758.

37. Manning FA, Wyn-Pugh E, Boddy K: Effect of cigarette smoking on fetal breathing movements in normal pregnancies. *Br Med J* 1975; 1:552.

38. Gennsar Y, Marsand K, Brantmark B: Maternal smoking and fetal breathing movements. *Am J Obstet Gynecol* 1975; 123:861.

39. Thalar I, Goodman JD, Dawes GS: Effect of cigarette smoking on fetal breathing movements. *Am J Obstet Gynecol* 1980; 138:282.

40. Socol ML, Manning FA, Murata Y, et al: Maternal smoking causes fetal hypoxia: Experimental evidence. *Am J Obstet Gynecol* 1982; 142:214.

41. Natale R, Clewlow F, Dawes GS: Measurement of fetal forelimb movements in the lamb in utero. *Am J Obstet Gynecol* 1981; 140:545.

42. Dalton KJ, Dawes GS, Patrick JE: Diurnal, respiratory and other rhythm of fetal heart rate in lambs. *Am J Obstet Gynecol* 1977; 127:414.

43. Murata Y, Martin CB, Ikenoue IT: Fetal heart rate accelerations and late deceleration during the course of intrauterine death in chronically catheterized fetal monkeys. Proc. SGI No. 253, 1981 (Abstract).

44. Boddy K, Dawes GR: Fetal breathing. *Br Med Bull* 1976; 31:3.

45. Rochard F, Schiffrin BS, Goupil F, et al: Nonstressed fetal heart rate monitoring in the antepartum period. *Am J Obstet Gynecol* 1976; 126:699.

46. Timor-Tritsch TE, Dierker LJ, Sador I, et al: Fetal movement associated with fetal heart rate acceleration and deceleration. *Am J Obstet Gynecol* 1978; 131:276.

47. Lavery JP: Non-stress fetal heart rate testing. *Clin Obstet Gynecol* 1982; 25:689.

48. Schiffrin BS, Foye G, Amato J, et al: Routine fetal heart rate monitoring in the antepartum period. *Obstet Gynecol* 1981; 57:320.

49. Brown R, Patrick JE: The non-stress test: How long is enough? *Am J Obstet Gynecol* 1981; 141:645.

50. Manning FA, Platt LD, Sipos L, et al: Fetal breathing movements and the non-stress test in high risk pregnancies. *Am J Obstet Gynecol* 1979; 135:511.

51. Manning FA, Lange IR, Morrison I, et al: Fetal biophysical profile score and the NST: A comparative trial. *Obstet Gynecol* 1984; 64:326–331.

52. Freeman RK, Anderson G, Dorchester W, et al: A prospective multi-institutional study of antepartum fetal heart rate monitoring: Risk of perinatal mortality and morbidity according to AFHR test results. *Am J Obstet Gynecol* 1982; 143:771.

53. Flood B, Lee J: Fetal death during a negative

contraction stress test. *Obstet Gynecol* 1978; 52(suppl):41.

54. Christie CB, Cudmore DW: The oxytocin challenge test. *Am J Obstet Gynecol* 1974; 118:327.

55. Collea JV, Holls WM: The contraction stress test. *Obstet Gynecol* 1982; 25:707.

56. Staisch KJ, Westlake JR, Bashore RA: Blind oxytocin challenge test and perinatal outcome. *Am J Obstet Gynecol* 1980; 138:399.

57. Manning FA, Platt LD: Human fetal breathing movements and the abnormal contraction stress test. *Am J Obstet Gynecol* 1980; 133:590.

58. Manning FA, Platt LD: Human fetal breathing monitoring—Clinical considerations. *Semin Perinatol* 1980; 4:311.

59. Patrick JE, Campbell K, Carmichael L, et al: A definition of human fetal apnea and the distribution of fetal apneic intervals during the last 10 weeks of pregnancy. *Am J Obstet Gynecol* 1980; 136:471.

60. Boddy K, Dawes GS: Fetal breathing. *Br Med Bull* 1975; 31:1.

61. Platt LD, Manning FA, LeMay M: Fetal breathing movements: The relationship to fetal condition. *Am J Obstet Gynecol* 1978; 132:542.

62. Sadovsky E, Polishuk WZ: Fetal movements in utero. *Obstet Gynecol* 1977; 50:49.

63. Rayburn WF: Antepartum fetal assessment: Monitoring fetal activity. *Clin Perinatol* 1982; 9:231.

64. Patrick J, Fetherston W, Vick H, et al: Human fetal breathing movements and gross body movements at weeks 34–35 of gestation. *Am J Obstet Gynecol* 1978; 130:693.

65. Manning FA, Platt LD, Sipos L: Fetal movements in human pregnancies in the third trimester. *Am J Obstet Gynecol* 1979; 54:699.

66. Manning FA, Morrison I, Lange IR: Fetal biophysical profile scoring: A prospective study in 1,184 high risk patients. *Am J Obstet Gynecol* 1981; 140:289.

67. Campbell K: Ultradian rhythms in the human fetus during the last 10 weeks of gestation: A review. *Semin Perinatol* 1980; 4:301.

68. Patrick JE, Campbell K, Carmichael L, et al: Patterns of gross fetal body movements over 24 hour observation intervals during the last 10 weeks of pregnancy measured with a real time scanner. *Am J Obstet Gynecol* 1982; 142:363.

69. Freeman JM, Brann AW Jr: Central nervous system disturbances, in Behrman RE (ed): *Neonatal-Perinatal Medicine: Disease of the Fetus and Infant.* St Louis, CV Mosby Co, 1977, p 799.

70. Vintzileos AM, Campbell WA, Ingardia CJ, et al: The fetal biophysical profile and its predictive value. *Obstet Gynecol* 1983; 62(3):271–278.

71. Baskett TG, Gray JH, Prewett SJ, et al: Antepartum fetal assessment using a fetal biophysical profile score. *Am J Obstet Gynecol* 1984; 148:630.

72. Platt LD, Eglington GS, Sipos L, et al: Further experience with the fetal biophysical profile score. *Obstet Gynecol* 1983; 61:480.

73. Platt LD, Walla CA, Paul RH, et al: A prospective trial of fetal biophysical profile versus the nonstress test in the management of high risk pregnancies. *Am J Obstet Gynecol* 1985; 153:624.

74. Vintzileos AM, Campbell WA, Nochimson DJ, et al: The fetal biophysical profile in patients with premature rupture of membranes: An early predictor of fetal infection. *Am J Obstet Gynecol* 1985; 152:510–516.

75. Vintzileos AM, Campbell WA, Nochimson DJ, et al: Fetal biophysical profile vs. amniocentesis in predicting infection in preterm premature rupture of the membrane. Personal communication.

## 16k
## ULTRASOUND FINDINGS IN INCOMPETENT CERVIX

Dennis A. Sarti, M.D.

Incompetent cervix manifests in the second trimester as a painless, bloodless abortion with minimal warning. It is frequently secondary to previous trauma, such as a difficult delivery or a previous dilation and curettage procedure. Besides trauma, other etiologies, such as functional or congenital ones, have been entertained.[1]

Ultrasound examination of the lower uterine segment and endocervical canal can confirm the clinical impression of an incompetent cervix.[2–6] When the clinical history suggests an incompetent cervix, ultrasound can be performed to confirm the diagnosis. Most often these patients present with two or three previous second-trimester abortions. If such a patient is encountered, an ultrasound examination of the endocervical canal should be undertaken. Occasionally an incompetent cervix will be visualized in a patient without any previous history. This is an extremely important finding since it would not normally be detected prior to the spontaneous abortion.

The technique for ultrasound examination of the endocervical canal is extremely important. The cervix and endocervical canal can usually be seen early in pregnancy, prior to 28 weeks. Later on in pregnancy visualization of these areas becomes more difficult because the low position of the fetus obstructs visualization of the lower uterine segment. Evaluation of the endocervical canal is usually performed utilizing the full urinary bladder technique. The urinary bladder can alter the anatomy by rotating the uterus and flattening the endocervical canal and cervix.[7] When the urinary bladder is full, the length of the cervix varies from 2.6 to 6 cm.[8] Some advocate visualization of the endocervical canal with an empty urinary bladder.[9] This can be quite difficult since the cervix will appear in a vertical direction which is not parallel to the ultrasound beam.

It is most important to determine the axis of the cervix on transverse scans. If the cervix and lower uterine segment are scanned in a transverse plane, the cervix will be noted to be midline, deviated to the right or left. Once the axis is determined, longitudinal scans paralleling the long axis of the cervix are obtained. The cervix has an echo pattern similar to that of the remainder of the uterine musculature. Scans along the long axis of the endocervical canal are obtained at several-millimeter intervals until the endocervical canal comes into view. The endocervical canal most often appears as a single linear high-amplitude echo in the cervical myometrial echoes.[2] The endocervical canal may also appear as multiple echogenic columns and occasionally is surrounded by a lucent zone.[9] Rarely, the endocervical canal appears as a slightly lucent region throughout. This is thought to be secondary to a mucous plug.[9] If the longitudinal scan plane is slightly off the endocervical canal, only the musculature of the cervix will be visualized. In such cases an incompetent cervix can be missed. It is important to scan completely across the cervix at small increments so that the linear high-amplitude echo of the endocervical canal comes into view.

When incompetent cervix is present, sonolucency secondary to amniotic fluid will be noted in the endocervical canal. The sonolocency may extend nearly the entire length of the endocervical canal to the external os. An early clue may be that the cervix appears shorter than expected. Some authors advocate measuring the region of the internal os in a transverse plane. They have found that the diameter of the cervix at this site is greater than the diameter in the normal patient.[1, 4]

The degree of bladder filling plays an important role in the diagnosis of incompetent cervix. Overdistention of the urinary bladder can lead to collapse of an incompetent cervix from increased pressure in the urinary bladder.[2] Therefore, if on initial examination the urinary bladder appears overdistended, the patient should partially void and then be reexamined to determine if the lower uterine segment distends and fluid is noted in the endocervical canal.

It is extremely difficult and unusual to visualize an incompetent cervix with ultrasound prior to the 14th or 15th week. At this early stage of pregnancy, the volume of fluid and fetus within the uterus is not adequate to cause distention of the lower uterine segment and cervix. By the 17th or 18th week of pregnancy, however, an incompetent cervix can be visualized on ultrasound. In any patient clinically suspected of having incompetent cervix, ultrasound examinations of the lower uterine segment should be performed serially at 1-week intervals until approximately the 24th week. By this stage of pregnancy, if fluid is not identified in the endocervical canal on ultrasound, it is extremely unlikely that an incompetent cervix is present. Usually the serial examinations will reveal the presence of incompetent cervix. Very often the first finding is shortening of the endocervical canal. There has been a report of a case in which very rapid dilatation of the endocervical canal occurred 20 minutes after a normal ultrasound examination.[10] However, this has been disputed as an incorrect interpretation of the intitial ultrasound findings.[11]

If an incompetent cervix is diagnosed or suspected, cerclage is performed using the Shirodkar or McDonald procedures. Ultrasound has been used to visualize the position of the sutures in these procedures.[12] Often the sutures can be seen, to determine their location and if adequate therapy is present. Since the internal structures of the uterus can be visualized on ultrasound, this modality is extremely helpful to the clinician in confirming or ruling out the diagnosis of incompetent cervix.

## References

1. Comparetto G, Gullo D, Venezia R: Ultrasonographic diagnosis of cervico-isthmic incompetence during pregnancy. *Acta Eur Fertil* 1981; 12:323.
2. Sarti DA, Sample WF, Hobel CJ, et al: Ultrasonic visualization of a dilated cervix during pregnancy. *Radiology* 1979; 130:417.
3. Bernstine RL, Lee SH, Crawford WL, et al: Sonographic evaluation of the incompetent cervix. *JCU* 1981; 9:417.
4. Brook I, Feingold M, Schwartz A, et al: Ultrasonography in the diagnosis of cervical incompetence in pregnancy: A new diagnostic approach. *Br J Obstet Gynaecol* 1981; 88:640.
5. Vaalamo P, Kwikoski A: The incompetent cervix during pregnancy diagnosed by ultrasound. *Acta Obstet Gynecol Scand* 1983; 62:19.
6. Feingold M, Brook I, Zakut H: Detection of cervical incompetence by ultrasound. *Acta Obstet Gynecol Scand* 1984; 63:407.
7. Zemlyn S: The effect of the urinary bladder in obstetrical sonography. *Radiology* 1978; 128:169.
8. Zemlyn S: The length of the uterine cervix and its significance. *JCU* 1981; 9:267.
9. Bowie JD, Andreotti RF, Rosenberg ER: Sonographic appearance of the uterine cervix in pregnancy: The vertical cervix. *AJR* 1983; 140:737.

10. Witter FP: Negative sonographic findings followed by rapid cervical dilatation due to cervical incompetence. *Obstet Gynecol* 1984; 64: 136.

11. Vintzileos AM, Campbell WA, Nochimson DJ: Letter to the editor. *Obstet Gynecol* 1985; 65:600.

12. Parulekar SG, Kiwi R: Ultrasound evaluation of sutures following cervical cerclage for incompetent cervix uteri. *J Ultrasound Med* 1982; 1:223.

# 16I
# ULTRASONOGRAPHIC EVALUATION OF THE LARGE-FOR-DATES UTERUS

Seymour Zemlyn, M.D.

The assessment of a pregnancy that appears too large for the historical dates is a common reason for performing obstetric sonography. In some cases the clinical impression will not be verified, and normal fetal measurements and a normal amount of amniotic fluid for gestational age will be found on the sonogram. The sonogram is usually more reliable than clinical measurement of the fundal height as the latter is affected by body build, fetal position, and urinary bladder volume.[1] Apparent enlargement is often simply due to an error in dating, possibly due to irregular menses, poor recollection of the last menses, or post-conceptual bleeding viewed as the last menstrual period. In these instances sonographic dating is usually more advanced by 4 weeks and is appropriate for the fundal measurement.

Enlargement, when present, may be due to an increase in size of one or more elements of the pregnancy. Proliferation of abnormal trophoblastic tissue causes increased size in molar pregnancy, excessive amniotic fluid in hydramnios, oversized fetus in macrosomia, enlargement of the uterus itself due to leiomyoma(s), or apparent enlargement due to an adjacent pelvic mass. Of course, all elements are involved in erroneous dating or multiple pregnancy. Enlargement in the first trimester is often due to an error in dating, molar pregnancy, leiomyoma(s), or adjacent mass(es) contributing to the perceived size of the pregnancy. In the second or third trimester, multiple gestations or hydramnios are likely to be detected, and fetal macrosomia is usually manifest in very late pregnancy.

## Uterine Myomas and Pelvic Masses

Uterine myomas and pelvic masses that are not palpably separate from the uterus may cause the uterus to seem large for dates. This is most likely to occur in early pregnancy with a sizeable myoma that constitutes a significant volume of the overall structure. This becomes a crucial matter in timing when a therapeutic abortion is refused because the size of the uterus is larger than the menstrual history indicates. Clinically detected uterine myomas are said to accompany about 1% of pregnancies. Myomas seldom affect the outcome of the pregnancy. The treatment, myomectomy, is more hazardous than the myoma and is rarely performed during pregnancy. Complications of pregnancies that have been reported in association with myomas include abortion, premature rupture of membranes, excessive growth or carneous degeneration of the myoma, and dystocia due to a cervical myoma. Ectopic pregnancy, disseminated intravascular coagulation, hemoperitoneum, extrusion of the myoma, and inversion of the uterus have also been reported.

Clinically a myoma may go unnoticed, cause the pregnancy to seem larger and therefore more advanced, or present as an unknown pelvic mass. Ultrasound is capable of clarifying about 95% of these clinical confusions. Myomas, especially small ones, may be easier to identify by ultrasound imaging than by clinical palpation, but those under 2 cm are unlikely to be detected by any technique.[2] Sonographically, a myoma is best recognized as a spherical thickening of the myometrial wall that expands the uterine contour. It may be difficult to distinguish from the frequently seen myometrial contraction. If the mass disappears during the course of a sonographic examination, it clearly is a contraction. Its persistence is not always indicative of a myoma, as a contraction may endure for a long interval. The diagnosis is more reliable when the myoma disturbs the external contour, but it may predominantly encroach upon the conceptus.

Myomas typically are echo-poor structures compared to the myometrium or the placenta, and transmit ultrasound as though they were a solid. However, degenerating myomas may have increased echogenicity and enhanced through-transmission. When the area of degeneration is large compared to the pregnancy, the "snowstorm" echogenicity may be mistaken for a molar pregnancy.[3, 4] Occasionally the myoma may become painful and tender due to degeneration and hemolysis. This is called carneous or red degeneration, because of the color and appearance of the myoma. The pain may be severe and resemble the pain of an acute abdomen. Once the diagnosis is established, treatment is generally directed to relieving the pain.

The chance of a myoma affecting a pregnancy is thought to be greater if the myoma is large. Muram et al., based on a small series, felt that the relation of the placenta to the myoma may be an important factor.[5] While there was no increase in the overall complication rate in their group, most of the complications occurred in the 10 of 13 patients whose placenta was

located adjacent to the myoma. The complications included premature rupture of membranes and postpartum hemorrhage with no adverse consequences, and bleeding during pregnancy, including three first-trimester abortions and one 16-week abortion. It has often been said that myomas tend to increase in size during pregnancy due to hormonal stimulation. The size of the myoma as determined by serial ultrasonography, however, did not change throughout the pregnancy in 82 of 89 patients.[6] Those myomas followed after the pregnancy all diminished in size post partum, often dramatically. A myoma followed during pregnancy may not always appear at the same location, owing to the ability of the uterus to rotate.

The physiologic corpus luteum cyst usually declines after the first trimester but may occasionally persist. The most common pelvic mass to enlarge during pregnancy is an ovarian cystadenoma.[7] Ovarian neoplasms, including cystic teratomas, parovarian cysts, endometriomas, and hydrosalpinx, are other cystic configurations seen in pregnancy. One horn of a bicornuate uterus may expand with a decidual reaction or part of the amniotic sac when the pregnancy is in the other horn.[8, 9] This may be very confusing if the congenital anomaly has been unknown to the patient or her obstetrician. The nonpregnant side of a double uterus may resemble a solid mass, especially a myoma, when seen by the sonographer.[10] Real-time imaging allows visualization of peristalsis, enabling the identification of confusing fluid-filled bowel loops. Teratomas may have associated solid components, hair, calcifications, and lipid. Pelvic abscesses may arise from appendicitis, ileitis, or other inflammatory conditions. They are especially dangerous as a source of maternal septicemia. Ectopic pelvic kidney is regarded as an indication for cesarean section.

### Hydatidiform Mole

Hydatidiform mole occurs in about 1 of 2,000 pregnancies in the United States. It is more common in Asians and in those under 15 or over 40 years of age.[11] Hydatidiform mole (molar pregnancy) is a proliferation of abnormal vesicular trophoblastic tissue within the uterus. Microscopically these small grape-like vesicles are seen to be hydropic, enlarged villi. Such vesicles proliferate readily, and, as they are trophoblastic in nature, are responsible for the remarkably high levels of serum human chorionic gonadotropin (hCG) that often mark this disorder. The absence of a fetal circulation has been thought to be responsible for the edematous, degenerated appearance of the villi and was cited in support of the once popular theory that moles are the result of a pregnancy in which the fetus died. In recent years forms of hydatidiform molar pregnancy with unusual features, including a fetus and/or fetal circulation, have been increasingly described. A maternal circulation is always present, and bleeding and hematomas are common among the abnormal villi. Internal areas of necrosis may be present, possibly as a result of the mole outgrowing its blood supply, and secondary infection may ensue. Invasive mole or choriocarcinoma, more malignant forms of gestational trophoblastic disease, may follow this relatively benign disorder, or may occur after a normal pregnancy.

Szulman and Surti describe two forms of this entity, complete or classic mole and partial mole.[12] In complete or classic molar pregnancy, the entire placenta is abnormal and a fetus is not present. About 90% of cases of molar pregnancy are this form, and usually present clinically with vaginal bleeding and a uterus too large for dates in the first or second trimester of pregnancy. Bleeding may be severe, and anemia may be present. Diagnostic vesicular tissue may be passed. In association with excessive hormonal secretion, the symptoms of early pregnancy, especially nausea, may be unusually severe. Hydatidiform mole is the only cause of true toxemia in the first trimester of pregnancy.

The sonographic appearance of classic molar pregnancy was first described in 1963 by MacVicar and Donald as a homogeneous speckled echogenic pattern caused by the surfaces of the innumerable vesicles filling an enlarged uterus, interrupted by sonolucent areas representing clots or necrosis.[13] The vesicles may vary in size, and the high fluid content allows enhanced transmission of the ultrasound beam. Multiseptated ovarian theca lutein cysts are commonly present in the pelvis and frequently are over 5 cm in diameter. The usual "snowstorm" appearance of the intrauterine molar tissue is so distinctive that series were reported without false positive diagnoses even during the days of bistable technology.[14] Variations of the pattern also occur, which are less likely to be so precisely diagnostic.[15] A degenerating uterine myoma[16] or an ovarian malignancy

with[17] or without necrosis[18] could resemble a mole, but the cystic spaces are not as regular and uniform as the vesicles of molar tissue. The serum hCG level may be helpful in the differential diagnosis as it is not elevated with myomas or ovarian tumors in the absence of associated pregnancy. Evaluating the vesicular spaces, especially in the anterior aspect of the uterus, requires properly focused transducers of the highest appropriate frequency. Incomplete abortion with hydropic degeneration of the placenta[15, 19] or retained products of conception[16] also may resemble complete molar pregnancy. Incomplete abortion should be suspected if a history of recent decline in uterine size is present. As evacuation of the uterus is the treatment for any of these conditions, the differential diagnosis may not be clinically important, but prostaglandin probably should not be used if a mole is suspected.

Rarely, a complete hydatidiform mole may coexist with a normal fetus and a seperate normal placenta. This is generally regarded as a form of twinning, one twin being the molar pregnancy. It is distinguished on sonographic examination from other forms of hydatidiform mole when a placenta with the classic vesicular pattern of hydatidiform mole is seen separately from a placenta with a normal appearance and a coexisting fetus.[20] Such pregnancies rarely survive, and are sacrificed in the need to evacuate the uterus of its menacing contents. The molar pregnancy may present as a placenta previa, and may proceed to invasive mole or choriocarcinoma.[21] Complete mole in an ectopic ovarian pregnancy has been reported.[22]

In partial molar pregnancy, only a variable portion of the placenta is abnormal, and an abnormal fetus may be coexist. Jones and Lauersen reported eight cases of hydatidiform mole and a coexisting fetus and described the value of sonography in the diagnosis.[23] This condition occurred in about 1 in 22,000 pregnancies. While coexisting fetus and mole may be a useful descriptive grouping, it lacks correlation with pathologic classification, as it may be the result of either complete or partial hydatiform mole. The fetus in partial molar pregnancy is said to usually have a triploid karyotype, but many normal karyotypes have been reported. The fetus, if still present, is often growth retarded or dead early in the pregnancy.[20] Unlike the classic mole, the uterus may be small for dates, and these patients are much less likely to have symptoms.

Ultrasound examination of partial hydatidiform mole

may reveal one of three patterns, according to Woo et al.[24] The placenta has the typical vesicular pattern of a complete mole in type A, which occurred in five of their 15 cases. Pattern B, present in two cases, is characterized by irregular heterogeneous areas of echogenicity within the enlarged uterus, with or without a deformed gestational sac. The ultrasonographer is likely to diagnose this as a missed or incomplete abortion.[15, 25] Pattern C, which Woo et al. regarded as diagnostic, occurred in over half of their patients. A greatly enlarged placenta and a large gestational sac, which may be empty or contain a small, dead fetus, are seen. The sac is thin-walled, and the usual echogenic rim of missed abortion or blighted ovum, for which these are often mistaken, is notably absent.

The size of the vesicles of molar pregnancy increases with the duration of the pregnancy.[12] In early pregnancy the vesicles may be small and difficult to identify. The typical cystic spaces of a mole may be few or absent,[26] but their detection may be significantly improved by the use of technically optimal transducers.[16] Hydropic degeneration of the placenta[19] or hypervascularity of the uterine wall during pregnancy[27] may resemble hydatidiform mole with coexistent fetus. In hypervascularity of the uterine wall, the large vascular spaces are confined to the myometrium, and may be present in area of the wall remote from the placenta. If seen very early a mole may look like an ordinary gestational sac.[28] Conversely, a coexisting true gestational sac may be mistaken for an area of hemorrhage or necrosis in the hydatidiform mole, and a small embryo may be overlooked,[15] especially if the bulky tissue pushes it anterior or posterior to the optimal transducer focal zone.

The recurrence of symptoms or persistence of an elevated hCG level after a molar pregnancy has been evacuated indicates an invasive mole. About 20% of complete molar pregnancies are followed by invasive mole. The figure is slightly higher in women over 50.[11] The diagnosis is often greatly delayed in this older group, as pregnancy is often not considered initially as a cause of amenorrhea or of irregular bleeding in 50-year-old women. In invasive mole, molar tissue is present within the myometrium and sometimes creates echogenic areas within the uterine wall that can be seen on sonography.[15] It was thought that partial moles never resulted in invasion, but a few such cases have now been reported.[29, 30] After therapy, persistence or recurrence of theca lutein cysts is presumptive evidence that the treatment is ineffective,[31] but serial hCG determinations are more sensitive for evaluating the course of the disease.[32]

Metastatic disease beyond the myometrium, including choriocarcinoma, may be detected sonographically as nonspecific pelvic masses or hepatic metastases.[33] The metastases tend to be echogenic and undergo cystic degeneration. Pulmonary metastases are not uncommon, but pulmonary dysfunction may occur with benign disease and may be severe, even leading to death.[34] The latter, it has been theorized, may be due to occult pulmonary emboli of trophoblastic cells.

**Multiple Gestation**

Twins occur in about 1% of pregnancies. They are slightly more common in blacks, the difference being due to dizygotic or fraternal twins. Triplets occur in about 1 in 10,000 births. Drugs that stimulate ovulation, such as clomiphene, increase the likelihood of dizygotic multiple pregnancies, with the number of fetuses related to the drug dosage. Because twins are much more common than other multiple pregnancies, most of the data and comments will be derived from and directed to twinning. Abnormalities found in twins will occur in triplets and other multiple pregnancies. Two thirds of twins are dizygotic. Monozygotic twins are always of the same sex and are nearly identical to one another. Any anomaly found in one monozygotic twin is likely to be present in the other. The degree of duplication of extrafetal gestational elements in monozygotic twins depends on the timing of division of the conceptus and may result in separate sacs and membranes, partial duplication, or, least likely, a single placenta and sac. Dizygotic twins have separate sacs, but the two placentas may fuse and appear as one. In most cases it is not possible to distinguish the zygotic nature of the twinning on ultrasonic examination, but if twins are recognized as of opposite sex they must be dizygotic, and a single sac identifies monozygotic twins.

A single sac is not proved simply because a dividing membrane is not seen on ultrasound, as one may be present and difficult to visualize, but should be based on an intertwining of sibling fetal parts or umbilical cords. Limitation of the sphere of travel of one or both twins suggests that an unseen dividing membrane is present.[135] Even though a membrane defining the sacs is not visualized, the sac size may be inferred from the range of movement of the twins. If the confined area of one fetus is greatly restricted relative to its twin, oligohydramnios of the "stuck" twin should be suspected. The prognosis for such a fetus is very poor, as in each of six instances reported by Mahony et al. fetal or neonatal death resulted. When hydramnios is present the proportional participation of each sac may be assessed in a similar fashion when the separating membrane is not clearly evident. About 30% of monozygotic twins, as well as all dizygotic twins, have dichorionic placentation. The presence of two separate placentas is indicative of a dichorionic pregnancy. If there is only one placenta, a dividing membrane within the sac should be sought. A thick membrane indicates the chorion and a dichorionic-diamniotic pregnancy. If the membrane is thin, reflecting ultrasound poorly, it is probably the amnion and is indicative of a diamniotic monochorionic pregnancy. Monochorionic twins are at risk and should be followed more closely for twin transfusion syndrome due to intraplacental vascular shunts.[36]

Multiple pregnancy may be suspected when growth is excessive, multiple fetal parts are palpated, more than one fetal heart is heard, or the family history suggests the possibility. Ultrasound imaging is the diagnostic method of choice. Multiple pregnancy is regarded as high risk, and early diagnosis is much more than convenience. Complications are related to the increased size of the pregnancy, an increased incidence of fetal anomalies, and interrelationship of fetuses sharing the uterus. Hydramnios is said to be common, adding to the enlargement of the uterus. The most common complication of twins is premature labor and resultant small babies, with increased morbidity and mortality. Some 10%–12% of perinatal deaths and 17% of growth-related infants are the result of multiple pregnancies.[37] In addition to an increased fetal mortality, a French study concluded that infants born of a twin pregnancy average 8.3 patient-days in the neonatal intensive care unit and are almost seven times more likely to be handicapped than are infants born of a single pregnancy.[38]

The diagnosis of multiple pregnancy may be suspected early in the first trimester when more than one gestational sac is seen on sonography. The false appearance of two intrauterine sacs may be created by uterine contractions, technical artifacts, or fluid (blood)

within the uterine lumen. A single sac centrally squeezed by a myometrial contraction may resemble two sacs. A search for the connecting fluid isthmus will uncover the potential error. Artifactual double or even triple sac appearances may occur on transverse scans, due to refraction at interfaces of fat, muscle, and urine. This is more frequent when the acoustic path through the bladder is long and the rectus muscles or the extraperitoneal fat are well developed. Such a mechanism may also create false duplication of embryos, or apparent fetal movement as the transducer is moved. It occurs when the transducer is in or near the midline, and is ascribed to ultrasound beam refraction caused by the lenticular-shaped margins of the rectus muscles[39] or the interface between the abdominal muscles and the extraperitoneal fat collection.[40] Though this artifact is said to be quite common, it is not seen in longitudinal scan planes, or in transverse scans performed with the transducer just lateral to the midline. The lateral margin of the rectus must also be avoided as it is possible for duplication to occur at this refractive contour by the same mechanism, according to Buttery and Davison. An excessively large maternal urinary bladder volume may distort the twin sacs and obscure the embryonic pole or yolk sac contents, leading to erroneous diagnoses of blighted ovum or missed abortion. Partially emptying the bladder allows the sacs to expand to their normal spherical configurations.[41]

In early pregnancy, especially in cases of threatened abortion, blood within the uterine lumen adjacent to the gestational sac creates a second intrauterine fluid collection. In the first trimester the fluid will be outlined by an echogenic rim, composed of the decidua parietalis and decidua capsularis or chorion frondosum, usually forming a crescentic shape about the conceptus. Burrows et al. termed this collection a pseudosac.[42] When the shape is more oval or round, the resemblance to a second gestational sac increases, and is analogous to the pseudogestational sac outlined by decidua in ectopic pregnancy. Under these circumstances the second sac never contains an embryo or fetus, but echoes derived from contained blood may simulate an embryonic pole,[43] and a shed decidual cast may mimic a macerated fetus.[44] The true sac contains the singleton embryo or fetus, unless the bleeding is due to blighted ovum or abortion, when a viable fetus will not be present.

Several authors have described the transient ultrasound appearance of two intrauterine fluid collections in early pregnancy which they suggest may be gestational sacs, and therefore interpreted these as complete abortions of one (or both) of twin pregnancies.[45–47] In the pregnancies that went to term only a single fetus was present. Despite the fact that these are called failed twins or vanishing twins, a second embryo or fetus was never seen or recovered. One possible exception is one of Finberg and Birnholz's 22 cases, in which some contained echoes were interpreted as a macerated second fetus. In fact the only pathologic material that might support this concept is a flattened empty sac present on the fetal surface of the placenta at the time of delivery in one of Robinson and Caines' 30 cases. These sonographic interpretations may be especially arbitrary in the setting of maternal bleeding, as any bleeding single pregnancy is likely to have a second intrauterine thick-rimmed fluid collection (of blood) in early pregnancy. When two intrauterine fluid collections are identified they should each be put to the test of the "double ring" sign to distinguish a false sac due to hematoma from a true gestational sac.[48] In a singleton pregnancy with bleeding, the hematoma supplants the sonolucent crescent marking the uterine lumen, and no additional evidence of a "double ring" will be present. In true twin sacs there should be an additional sonolucent stripe for one or both sacs. Unfortunately, none of the illustrated cases of so-called blighted twin ovum satisfy that criterion. Finberg and Birnholz were unable to find a single such case in a review of more than 1,000 reported cases of threatened abortion.

The normal growth curve for biparietal diameters of twins has not been completely established. Many reports are based on a limited number of twin pregnancies. Some have found that concordant twins (biparietal diameter difference 4 mm or less), and the larger of discordant twins (difference in biparietal diameters greater than 4 mm), follow normal singleton biparietal growth curves.[49, 50] Many have found twin dimensions to fall below those of singletons in late pregnancy. Leveno et al., in a study of 123 normal twin pregnancies, found twin biparietal diameters to be slightly smaller than singleton measurements throughout pregnancy by an average of 3.5 mm, and more in late pregnancy, and constructed a table of twin biparietal diameters from their data.[51] A tendency for the abdominal circumference and the biparietal diameter to be less than in singletons in the third trimester has

been noted.[52, 53] So far, twin femur lengths have been found to be similar to singleton measurements,[53] but Iffy et al., reporting on 43 twin abortions between 8.5 and 21 weeks' gestation, found the average crown-rump length to be smaller than in singletons by 7 mm in early pregnancy.[54] Others found a marked decrease in average twin size after 30 weeks,[55–57] which may be predominantly due to severe compromise of the smaller discordant twin.[50]

There is some evidence that the fetal lungs of twins tend to mature earlier than in singletons.[58] Based on the lecithin/sphingomyelin (L/S) ratio of amniotic fluid collected at cesarean section of 42 twin pregnancies, it was found that twins usually had similar values, and that a mean L/S ratio of 2 was reached at 31–32 weeks in twins and at 36+ weeks in singletons. Instances of respiratory distress syndrome do occasionally occur in one neonate of a multiple pregnancy, and significant differences in L/S ratios in the two sacs of dizygotic twins have been reported.[59] Phosphatidyl glycerol (PG) levels or the combination of L/S and PG values appear to have better twin agreement than L/S alone. In twins of less than 36 weeks' gestation, sampling both sacs for these factors is prudent when possible. Respiratory distress is more common in male newborns. Female fetuses have chemical evidence of lung maturity 1–1.4 weeks earlier than males.[60] The contribution of fetal sex to discrepancies of lung maturity in dizygotic twins is not known, but it implies that, when only one sac is tapped in sexually unlike twins, the male's is more likely to be critical. Male-male twin pregnancies have a shorter gestation and are more likely to be premature.[61, 62]

Small differences in the size of twins are common, but large discrepancies (discordant twins) suggest growth retardation or fetofetal transfusion syndrome. The latter is the result of vascular shunting in the common placenta of monozygotic twins dividing the shared flow unequally. Growth retardation usually manifests after 30 weeks' gestation, but the discordancy of fetofetal transfusion may become evident much earlier.[63] Vascular shunts are present in about 80% of monochorionic placentas in live births, and about one third of these develop evidence of this syndrome.[64] The donor fetus is undernourished and anemic, and the larger recipient may have a vascular overload resulting in congestive heart failure.[65] At birth, one may require transfusion and the other phlebotomy. Extreme cases result in intrauterine death of one or both twins.

A bizarre product of multiple pregnancy and placental shunting is the rare acardiac monster. The monster may lack a head (acardia acephalus), or human shape (acardia amorphus). Extremities, when present, may be seen actively moving in utero. Even though it has no heart, the acardiac monster may survive and grow until the cord is occluded, as the heart of its monozygotic sibling acts as the pump to propel its own circulation via vascular shunting at the placenta. This vascular load may lead to heart failure of the otherwise healthy fetus. If the abnormal fetus dies the remaining twin is likely to survive. When acardia acephalus has been identified in utero at sonography, occlusion of the umbilical cord via amnioscope has been suggested as an appropriate treatment to allow salvage of the other fetus.[66] Fetus papyracea is a desiccated, compressed, parchment-like residuum of a dead fetus that may be seen sonographically[67] but is usually found by the pathologist trapped between membranes pressed against the uterine wall by the sac of the live remaining twin. It could result from total demise correlated with velamentous insertion of the umbilical cord.[68]

Conjoined twins is another rare (1:50,000 births) complication of monozygotic twinning. Since the description of the first antenatal sonographic detection in 1977,[69] many case reports have followed. Fusion between twins should be searched for when there appears to be a single (monoamniotic) sac.[70] The twins may be joined at any point of the head or body, but about 75% of conjoined twins are united at the thorax or anterior abdominal wall. They tend to be oriented in a face-to-face constant attitude, with opposing organs, which may be shared by the twins to any degree, at the same level. Even more rare are twins joined at the buttocks, ischia, or heads.[71] These latter groups are sometimes oriented with their spines aligned, and the two heads or tails forming the north and south poles. Forms that do not fit well into these brackets also occur.[72] At attempt at evaluating the degree of sharing of organs may be useful in determining the management of such cases.[73] When conjoined twins are suspected examination may be repeated until the sonographer is satisfied of the constancy of the relationship. Conjoined twins at term must be delivered by section.

Fetus in fetu, a rare, parasitic, malformed portion of a fetus included in the body of its twin, may be identified on sonography as a mass,[74] usually in the high retroperitoneal area. Unlike a teratoma, which is more likely to occur in the pelvis, there is no known potential for malignancy. Its morphology depends on the extent of development of the parasitic twin, but should contain elements of vertebral column and/or formed body parts.[75] It is fortunate that single sac twins are rare as they offer a myriad of peculiar complications, including conjoined twins, intermingling of fetal parts, and interlocking fetuses, which may preclude safe vaginal delivery, and intertwining of umbilical cords, which may be responsible for fetal death.[76, 77]

## Hydramnios

Hydramnios or polyhydramnios is the condition of an excessive amount of amniotic fluid, sometimes defined as more than 2 L at term. In clinical practice the quantity of this fluid is rarely accurately measured, and the diagnosis is based on a subjective evaluation on physical examination, at delivery, or by radiographic or sonographic imaging. Sonography is the diagnostic method of choice, as it alone identifies the excessive fluid as the source of the large palpable uterus. Total intrauterine volume measurements, which include the fetus and placenta, may be used to quantitatively define those with hydramnios,[78] but the correlative data for this determination have focused on low volumes and the detection of growth retardation, and its efficacy for detection of hydramnios is not clearly demonstrated. The reliability of this measurement has been questioned.[79–81] Volume determination of greater accuracy may be accomplished by totaling the multiple calculated areas of stepped interval cross sections,[82] a procedure unsuited to real-time scanners and tedious for common clinical use. Chamberlain et al., seeking usable criteria for real-time scanning, arbitrarily selected an amniotic fluid collection of 8 cm depth or more as representing hydramnios.[83] Their resulting data did not correlate with known statistics. In sonography, the diagnosis is usually made on eyeball judgment and probably improves with moderate experience. Advanced cases are readily recognized, but an objective means of distinguishing lesser degrees of hydramnios from normal is not available.

Hydramnios is usually detected in the third or late

second trimester when the large size of the uterus is noted. On sonography, the fetus in advanced hydramnios is seen lying on the dependent surface with a wide surrounding area of fluid over and about it, described as "at the bottom of the sea." The uterus may appear rounded and tense, and more circular than ovoid on transverse sections. On rare occasions, accumulated fluid contained in cystic hygromas or massive ascites where the fetal skin is pressed to the amnion may simulate hydramnios.[84] Judgments of hydramnios must be made in reference to the appropriate time frame of the pregnancy. There is normally more fluid than fetus in early midtrimester. Near term the uterus is almost totally occupied by the fetus and only a few small pockets of fluid may normally be seen.

Amniotic fluid is believed to be initially formed from transudate of maternal origin. As pregnancy proceeds, the fetus is an increasingly active participant in its formation, swallowing from and excreting into this pool. The fluid is not static, and an active interchange across fetal mucous membranes may amount to 450 cc/hour. Some interchange occurs across the umbilical cord. At term amniotic fluid is biochemically similar to fetal urine.[85] Much of the volume of amniotic fluid seems to be formed by fetal urinary excretion as oligohydramnios occurs with renal agenesis and with reduced fetal urinary output. However, increased urinary excretion is not found in cases of hydramnios in diabetic mothers.[86] The fetus swallows about 200 ml/day. Abnormalities that interfere with this function may result in hydramnios, but the measured swallowing rate is the same in normal or fetuses with hydramnios.[87] There is also believed to be an unmeasured interchange in the respiratory tree. Surprisingly little is known of the causes of hydramnios. The mechanisms postulated are often inferred from the associated abnormality. Hydramnios is associated with some maternal disorders, including diabetes mellitus, preeclampsia, anemia, and obesity. It is known to occur when the fetal hypothalamus is absent, and it is sometimes present in multiple pregnancies, hydrops fetalis, congenital anomalies, and placental hemangiomas (chorioangiomas).

The abnormally large uterine volume of hydramnios may create clinical problems due to the maternal burden and is more likely to result in rupture of membranes, premature labor, premature separation of the placenta, prolapsed umbilical cord, poor labor, and postpartum uterine atony. The perinatal mortality is said to be as high as 50%,[88] but if associated congenital anomalies are excluded, the corrected mortality is about twice normal, about 4 in 1,000 births.[83] The deaths are usually associated with prematurity, prolapsed cord, maternal diabetes, congenital anomalies, multiple pregnancies, or hydrops fetalis. These last three categories fall within the diagnostic province of the sonographer and should be the focus of that examination when hydramnios is present. One may also occasionally fortuitously observe a prolapsed cord in the endocervical canal during labor or in prolapsed "hourglass" membranes distal to the presenting fetal part.[89–91]

In about 60% of cases of hydramnios no underlying pathology is discovered. Nonetheless, the presence of hydramnios should stimulate careful scrutiny for congenital anomalies, as they are present in about 18%–26% of cases.[92, 93] Most anomalies associated with hydramnios are of the CNS or gastrointestinal tract. Others include cystic mass lesions, dilatation of the urinary tract, mesoblastic nephroma, neck masses, dwarfism, and transient fetal ascites. If elevated serum and amniotic fluid levels of $\alpha$-fetoprotein (AFP) are also present, abnormalities of open neural tubes, anencephaly, omphalocele, gastroschisis, or high intestinal obstruction should be expected. The elevated AFP concentrations in cases of open neural tubes, omphalocele, and gastroschisis are thought to be due to transudation across the exposed fetal membranes. In high gastrointestinal tract obstruction, such as duodenal atresia, it may be secondary to regurgitation of fetal bile, which normally has a high AFP concentration.[94] The AFP level is normal in esophageal atresia, but the amniotic fluid acetylcholinesterase level may be elevated.[95]

Anencephaly accounts for about 40% of all anomalies associated with hydramnios, and neural tube defects and hydrocephaly are present in an additional 10%.[93] Gastrointestinal anomalies include high obstructive lesions such as tracheoesophageal fistula, duodenal atresia, and annular pancreas; and nonobstructive lesions, including cleft palate, omphalocele, gastroschisis, and diaphragmatic hernia. This list includes the vast majority of all fetal gastrointestinal abnormalities. Obstructive lesions usually result in dilated fluid-filled bowel proximal to the lesion and an absence of fluid in the tract distally. If the obstruction is located in the esophagus, as in esophageal atresia or some cases of tracheoesphageal fistula, the sonographer may note hydramnios, an absence of fluid in the fetal stomach and intestine, and sometimes a dilated fluid-filled esophagus. The ultrasonic findings were thought initially to be the counterpart of the "gasless stomach" seen on radiographs with esophageal atresia without tracheoesophageal fistula.[96] The in utero examination for this anomaly may be more sensitive than examination of the newborn, as the fetal stomach may not contain fluid in several forms of tracheoesophageal fistula, even though air is seen in the stomach on the radiograph of the same neonate later.[97] The reason for this difference may be related to the ability of material within the amniotic fluid to plug the fistula, the lesser fetal muscular activity of the chest in the absence of respiration and crying, and the difference in viscosity between amniotic fluid and air. In duodenal atresia or annular pancreas, the dilated stomach and duodenum may be seen as separate fluid collections, creating a "double bubble" appearance.[98–100] This fairly specific finding may be mimicked by bilateral hydronephrosis.[101] Other patterns of dilated bowel may represent more unusual intestinal obstructions, which may be anticipated at the termination of the dilated segment.[102] A large upper abdominal cyst representing the entire infarcted small bowel and proximal colon in a case of midgut volvulus has been described.[103] Prenatal detection of high obstructing lesions averts feeding of the neonate and the attendant aspiration pneumonia, and allows early planning for optimal treatment. Amniocentesis may be desirable if duodenal atresia is detected, as there is about a 30% incidence of associated trisomy 21.[104]

Hydramnios in the presence of omphalocele was thought to be due to transudation across the membrane, but it has been suggested that it only occurs in those cases of omphalocele associated with other complicating factors.[105] About 50% of omphaloceles are accompanied by an additional anomaly, including anencephaly and neural tube defects, and cardiovascular or chromosomal abnormalities.[106] There is an increased incidence of midgut volvulus, which may cause intestinal obstruction. Genetic amniocentesis should be performed to detect chromosomal abnormalities, even if it is too late for elective abortion, as the results may be instrumental in determining if delivery should be by section.[107] The umbilical cord is centrally located in relation to the mass and abdominal wall in omphalocele but enters the fetal abdomen at

the periphery of the mass in gastroschisis.[108] Amniocentesis is not clearly indicated in gastroschisis because, unlike omphalocele, there is no associated increase in karyotype abnormalities.[109] There is about a 25% incidence of associated anomalies with gastroschisis, predominantly intestinal atresias and malrotation.

Intra-abdominal cysts associated with hydramnios are usually large, and the hydramnios is often acute. Hydramnios has been reported to resolve spontaneously[10] or with drainage of the cyst.[111, 112] One theory is that these intra-abdominal cystic masses, which are usually at least 8 cm in diameter, cause pressure on the intestine, leading to partial obstruction and diminished swallowing.[113] Some support for this view is a case report of hydramnios in which an amniogram performed because of a "cystic mass," the urinary bladder, which filled the fetal abdomen, failed to opacify the intestinal tract, ascribed to lack of fetal swallowing.[114] On the other hand, on amniography before delivery in a fetus with hydramnios and a large ovarian cyst, swallowing was normal and there was no evidence of intestinal obstruction.[115]

About 10% of fetal ovarian cysts reported in the literature are associated with hydramnios. These cysts are usually of graafian follicular origin and are under hormonal influence. They are more common in diabetics and in erythroblastosis fetalis.[116] When hydramnios is present the cyst is usually very large, filling the abdomen and making it difficult to be certain of its ovarian origin. Of course, it is wise to check the fetal sex to be sure it is female before suggesting this diagnosis.

Hydronephrosis is usually associated with normal or decreased amounts of amniotic fluid, but about 10% of cases have hydramnios. Hydramnios has been associated with bilateral ureteropelvic junction obstructions,[101] bilateral vesicoureteral reflux,[117] and unilateral hydronephrosis.[118] A flurry of individual case reports describe hydramnios accompanying congenital mesoblastic nephroma, a nonmetastasizing renal tumor.[119–121] All were detected as a solid mass in the fetal abdomen or flank on obstetric sonography. In these instances the left renal tumors each had a dimension of 7 or 8 cm, again suggesting that the hydramnios may be secondary to the mass effect and compression of adjacent structures. Hydramnios has been described in a male fetus that had a temporarily markedly distended urinary bladder (megacystis) not due to obstruction, and no other abnormalities.[114] Another unique case report involves hydramnios associated with a giant aneurysm of the intra-abdominal portion of the umbilical vein which resulted in fetal demise at 36 weeks' gestation.[122]

Cystic adenomatoid malformation of the lung may be associated with hydramnios, nonimmune fetal hydrops, pleural effusions, and ascites. The hydramnios accompanying cystic adenomatoid malformation of the lung may be acute, and may resolve spontaneously.[110] Theoretical etiologies of hydramnios include partial obstruction of the esophagus, decreased fetal swallowing, and abnormal interchange across the abnormal respiratory tree.[123, 124] Hydramnios may be part of nonimmune fetal hydrops with pleural effusion, and/or ascites accompanying cystic adenomatoid malformation. Cystic adenomatoid malformation is seen as a mass of one or more cysts within the fetal chest, which may resemble fluid-filled loops of bowel secondary to diaphragmatic hernia but lack peristalsis and are relatively constant in configuration.[125] Solid or type III lesions of cystic adenomatoid malformation may be more difficult to recognize but are associated with increased size of the affected lung and shift of the heart and midline chest structures.[126] Diaphragmatic hernia, also often associated with hydramnios, is accompanied by a scaphoid abdomen due to the displacement of the bowel which normally fills it. The umbilical cord may appear to enter the abdomen in a high location.[127] Other anomalies are present in about half of those with diaphragmatic hernia, and in 87% if growth retardation is also present. Enterogeneous and pericardial cysts and other fluid collections that may have to be theoretically considered in the differential diagnosis have not yet been reportedly identified in utero ultrasonically. Symptomatic newborns that survive with cystic adenomatoid malformation often benefit from resection of the abnormal lung,[128] but the survival rate is poor if hydrops is present.[129]

Fetal neck masses that have been associated with hydramnios include cervical teratomas, metastatic neuroblastoma, and goiter.[130–133] The hydramnios is assumed to be the result of obstruction of the esophagus and interference with swallowing. The postnatal period may be hazardous due to airway obstruction, and intubation and surgery may be required for survival. Cystic hygromas (fetal Turner's syndrome) have a distinctive septated cystic appearance on sonography and are sometimes associated with hydrops fe-

talis. Epignathus, a mass arising from the face, is associated with hydramnios, probably by a similar mechanism.[134]

Extremity measurements may be important in patients with hydramnios as dwarfism has been associated with hydramnios.[135, 136] In dealing with anomalies rarely associated with hydramnios, it must be remembered that hydramnios frequently occurs without a detectable underlying cause. The association of an anomaly may be a random event, and there may not be a cause-and-effect relationship. In addition, multiple factors may be present, such as multiple anomalies, or an anomaly and maternal diabetes or fetal hydrops, making it unclear which is the important instigating factor. Extralobar pulmonary sequestration seen in utero was accompanied by hydramnios and nonimmune hydrops fetalis and ended in interpartum death in a single reported case.[137] The sequestered lung was seen as a solid mass in the most typical location of the left lower chest and was thought to be a mediastinal tumor on sonographic examination. In a few instances hydramnios has been associated with temporary, benign fetal ascites which may resolve as late as 48 hours after birth.[138] The relationship of these findings remains a mystery.

Hydramnios is said to be associated with multiple pregnancies. Useful standards for the normal quantity of fluid in multiple pregnancies have not been established, and, theoretically, twins are entitled to twice as much amniotic fluid as a single pregnancy. Some confirmation of this by measured total intrauterine volumes of twice singleton standards has been reported through 35 weeks' gestation.[139] This fact must be taken into account in making the subjective diagnosis of hydramnios in multiple pregnancies. In addition to the maladies associated with hydramnios faced by any singleton, the fetus in a multiple pregnancy may suffer congestive heart failure due to transfusion syndrome.

## Hydrops Fetalis

Hydrops fetalis refers to generalized fetal anasarca and usually indicates a very sick fetus with a poor chance of survival. It may result from a variety of abnormal states, but often none is found. The specific outlook may depend on the underlying cause of hydrops fetalis, but predicting the outcome on the basis of the sonogram is difficult.[140] Hydrops fetalis may include fetal peripheral edema, ascites, pleural and pericardial effusions, hepatosplenomegaly, cardiomegaly, hydramnios, and a thick placenta. Peripheral edema is represented on sonograms by soft-tissue thickness greater than 5 mm, but subcutaneous fat deposition of a diabetic pregnancy, or soft tissue thickening not due to edema (see in some dwarfs), should not be mistaken for generalized edema. When only a single feature, such as ascites, is present it is questionable whether it is appropriate to call this hydrops fetalis.[140] Ascites unaccompanied by other evidence of fetal edema may be transient and benign,[141, 142] or it may be caused by an abnormality that does not produce the full-blown syndrome,[143] and it must be distinguished from pseudoascites.[144]

Hydrops fetalis is generally divided into isoimmune and nonimmune forms. In isoimmunization, maternal antibodies, provoked by prior direct exposure to the responsible antigen, destroy the fetal red blood cells (RBCs) and result in a hemolytic anemia in utero. Frantic erythropoiesis causes immature forms of RBCs (erythroblasts) to enter the fetal circulation and led to the designation of erythroblastosis fetalis. Elevated maternal antibody titers, as well as the obstetric history and family blood types, are important in identifying erythroblastosis. Secondary congestive heart failure and compensatory erythropoiesis may cause the anasarca, and enlargement of the liver, spleen, and placenta that mark the process. Other mechanisms implicated in the formation of fetal hydrops include hypoproteinemia, diminished osmolality, hepatic dysfunction, and obstruction of hepatic circulation.

Rh isoimmunization, the most common cause of hydrops fetalis in the past, has diminished with the clinical use of Rh immunoglobulin to suppress sensitization. Currently, about 76%–86% of sonographically identified cases are due to nonimmune causes.[145, 146] Isoimmunization may rarely be due to AB and more unusual blood group antigens present in the fetus and its father, but not in the mother. These result in a less severe form of reaction than Rh incompatibility, and the affected fetuses seldom require transfusions or terminate as stillbirths.

The role of diagnostic ultrasound in isoimmunization includes the diagnosis of hydrops fetalis and estimation of its severity. Ultrasound offers a safe, effective method of following the patient as frequently as desired. The amniotic fluid bilirubin content as assessed on spectrophotometry is another sensitive indicator of the severity of the process, but amniocentesis has an associated complication rate and is not always successful. Discoloration of the fluid gives inaccurate readings. If amniocentesis is to be performed, ultrasound monitoring for placental position is most important to avoid fetomaternal hemorrhage or bloody discoloration of the fluid. In suspect cases ultrasonic detection of disproportionate growth of the fetal abdomen compared to the biparietal diameter is an early indicator of hepatomegaly due to anemia.[147] Bilateral theca lutein cysts have been reported in a few instances in association with erythroblastosis fetalis and even more rarely with nonimmune hydrops fetalis.[148]

In nonimmune hydrops fetalis immunologic screening tests are negative. The condition is most likely to be discovered in utero when ultrasonography is performed because of the increased size of associated hydramnios. Hutchison et al. found that 75% of their cases of nonimmune hydrops fetalis were associated with hydramnios.[149] Almost half the cases are idiopathic, and a significant associated abnormality is not uncovered. Of the rest, many processes have been reported to be associated with nonimmune hydrops fetalis. Among these are congestive heart failure of any cause, including arrhythmias, congenital heart disease, myocarditis, fibroelastosis, twin transfusion, or parasitic twin; hematologic disorders, including α-thalassemia and fetal anemia; pulmonary disorders such as cystic adenomatoid malformation, pulmonary hypoplasia, pulmonary lymphangectasia, and extralobar pulmonary sequestration; renal abnormalities, including congenital nephrosis, renal dysplasia, and renal vein thrombosis; intrauterine infections such as syphilis, leptospirosis, congenital hepatitis, and Chagas disease; congenital anomalies including trisomies 18 and 21, Turner's syndrome, cystic hygromas, cervical cavernous hemangiomas, mosaicism, achondroplasia, tuberous sclerosis, storage disease, polycystic ovaries, and sacral teratoma; brain tumor; meconium peritonitis; neuroblastomatosis; idiopathic arterial calcification; disseminated intravascular coagulopathy; chorioangioma; umbilical vein thrombosis, chorionic vein thrombosis, umbilical vein aneurysm, and hemangioma of the umbilical cord; and dysmaturity.[137, 150–158] There is an association with maternal diabetes mellitus and toxemia.

Table 16L–1 lists important ultrasonic foci for evaluating the causes of hydrops fetalis (similar to those

**TABLE 16L–1.**

**Sonographic Survey for Abnormalities Associated With Hydrops Fetalis**

| LOCATION | SONOGRAPHIC FINDING | ABNORMALITY |
|---|---|---|
| FETUS | | |
| Head | Intracranial mass and: Congestive heart failure | Arteriovenous malformation, vein of Galen aneurysm |
| Microcephaly | Large BPD and midline shift | Cytomegalic inclusion virus, toxoplasmosis |
| | | Brain tumor |
| Neck | Cystic masses | Lymphatic dysplasia, Turner's syndrome, Cavernous hemangioma |
| Thorax | Poorly contracting heart, pericardial effusion | Congestive heart failure, myocarditis, fibroelastosis |
| | | ?Cardiac anomalies |
| | Arrhythmia | Mediastinal tumor, extralobar pulmonary sequestration |
| | Solid chest mass | |
| | Cystic chest mass(es) | Cystic adenomatoid malformation, diaphragmatic hernia |
| | Small thorax | Dwarfism |
| Abdomen | Hepatomegaly | Heart failure, anemia, extramedullary hematopoiesis, storage disease |
| | Masses | Neuroblastomatosis |
| | Densities | Meconium peritonitis |
| | Cyst | Umbilical vein aneurysm |
| Limbs | Short limbs | Dwarfism |
| | Fractures | Osteogenesis imperfecta |
| | Contractures | Arthrogryposis |
| Mass | Sacrum | Sacral teratoma |
| | External | Parasitic twin |
| TWINS | Discordant | Fetofetal transfusion |
| PLACENTA | Thick | Infection, extramedullary hematopoiesis, anemia, chorioangioma |
| | Mass | Chorioangioma |
| UMBILICAL CORD | | |
| Echogenic interior mass | | Umbilical vein thrombosis Hemangioma of umbilical cord |

reported by Fleischer et al.[146]). Complete recovery of a normal infant is possible in only a few conditions on this list if the intrauterine crisis is survived. These become very important issues for the sonographer. Drug therapy may correct a fetal tachyarrhythmia,[159–161] and early delivery may save the compromised fetus from the final effects of a threatening chorioangionma or umbilical cord hemangioma. It is thought that amnioscopic occlusion of the cord of an acardiac monster may save the donor twin.[162] Spontaneous remission of fetal hydrops has occurred in at least one instance.[163] Occasionally oligohydramnios is associated with hydrops fetalis. This is an ominous combination that may reflect renal failure, as reported cases of oligohydramnios with fetal hydrops have resulted in fetal death.

## Macrosomia

Macrosomia refers to an excessively large fetus. These large fetuses are difficult to deliver through the vagina. Shoulder dystocia may occur and may result in fractures of the clavicle or extremities, and brachial nerve injuries. Asphyxia may result in perinatal death. Cesarean section is often recommended in these patients, especially if labor is prolonged.[164] Macrosomia is associated with maternal diabetes or weight over 180 pounds, older mothers, higher parity, and postmaturity.[165] The newborn is more likely to be male, to have a low Apgar score, and to have increased perinatal mortality or morbidity. The frequency of macrosomia diminishes when the local altitude is high above sea level, assumedly the effect of lesser oxygenation. It is more unusual at 5,000 feet altitude (Denver), and almost never occurs above 9,000 feet.[166]

Macrosomia is often defined as a birth weight over 4,000 gm but personal definitions of over 4,100, 4,200, or 4,500 gm have been used in the literature. In any of these cases, it would be rare before the 37th week of gestation and more common in postdated pregnancy (42 weeks or greater).[167] "Mechanical macrosomia" has been suggested to describe the fetuses that are large relative to the maternal pelvis, and "metabolic macrosomia" for the generally overgrown fetus, the large-for-gestational-age (LGA) fetus.[168] Many of these definitions are not very useful for the sonographer, who is not capable at present of commenting on disproportion and would be very limited in trying to identify these fetuses weighing more than 4,000 gm. Sonographers screening for large fetuses in the last trimester prefer to identify those in the upper 10th percentile of fetal weight (LGA). These fetuses are assumed to be at risk for macrosomia.

Measurements used to estimate fetal weight include biparietal diameter, head circumference, head area, thoracic diameter, abdominal diameter, abdominal circumference, abdominal area, thigh circumference or area, and femoral length. The use of head measure-

ments alone might be expected to be a weak corollary as weight is more closely related to variance in body size. Body size is reflected in thoracic and abdominal dimensions. Circumferences have been preferred to diameters by some on the basis that they deviate less when head or body shapes are not average. Area calculations seem to suffer from compounding mensuration errors. The use of femoral length is an attempt to introduce the effect of the length of the fetus upon its weight. The above measurements have been used individually and in almost every combination. In addition, some have used multiplanar techniques and extensive calculations to compute surface area or fetal volume as determinants of fetal weight. Such exercises promise greater accuracy when properly done but are not suitable for real-time imaging, are easily derailed by fetal movement, and are too tedious to be readily accepted for routine studies. The originators and enthusiasts of a measurement technique often report results that are not commonly attained by others using those techniques. The multiplicity of formulas offered reflect the inability of one method to produce satisfactory results in all situations. The above methods produce 95% confidence limits (2 SD) of ±15% to 28%, and are often less accurate at the extreme portions of the curve, the ones of greatest clinical interest. Individual variance may be great.

Weight estimates are generally compared to Shepard's[169] modification of Warsoff's tables of average fetal weight, so the degree of deviation, if any, can be easily appreciated. This relative weight may remain constant to term if the growth rate remains constant, but diabetics' fetuses seem to undergo accelerated growth in late pregnancy.[170] Volume studies suggest that growth patterns in nondiabetics may normally be linear or nonlinear, the curves of the latter being either "convex" or "concave."[171] An excessive drop-off in growth rate may theoretically indicate an element of growth retardation in a potentially macrosomic fetus, even though it is not small for dates. When compared to birth weights, fetal weights estimated on the basis of biparietal diameter and abdominal diameter[172] or biparietal diameter and abdominal circumference[173] were found to have limited ability to identify LGA. A normal ultrasound scan was reliable in over 90%, about the same as chance in excluding the upper 10th percentile. The predictive power of a positive ultrasound examination was 18% and 63%, respectively, in the two studies. The ratio of femur length/abdominal circumference $\times$ 100 has been used in predicting macrosomia.[174] Macrosomic fetuses have values of 20.5 ± 2 compared to the normal ratio of 22 ± 2. In 156 fetuses the predictive power of a positive ratio was 68% and the sensitivity was 63%. It was more effective in screening diabetics, where its predictive power for macrosomia was 89%. A retrospective study of diabetic mothers indicated that 20 of 23 (87%) macrosomic fetuses could have been predicted by the fact that the difference between the average "thoracic" diameter (measured 1 cm below cardiac pulsation, actually the abdomen) and the biparietal diameter was 1.4 cm or more.[175]

Diabetics are at hight risk for bearing macrosomic infants as excessive fetal subcutaneous fat may accumulate in late pregnancy due to increased insulin and high blood sugar levels. Accelerated growth in some fetuses of diabetic mothers as early as the 28th to 32d weeks was demonstrated by serial studies of fetal abdominal circumstances.[170] This group also had higher amniotic fluid levels of insulin, more subcutaneous fat, and weighed more at birth. The increased subcutaneous fat may be seen on sonograms as a sonolucency separating the scalp from the skull by 4 mm or more in some diabetics and has been described as "diabetic halo."[176] Initially thought to reflect poor diabetic control, it has been correlated with LGA fetuses as determined by other ultrasound estimates. A halo effect unrelated to diabetes or macrosomia may also be created by edema and may be present due to hydrops fetalis, Turner's syndrome, lymphangectasia, trisomy 18, or dwarfism.

## References

1. Worthen N, Bustillo M: Effect of urinary bladder fullness on fundal height measurements. *Am J Obstet Gynecol* 1980; 138:759.
2. Gross BH, Silver TM, Jaffe MH: Sonographic features of uterine leiomyomas: Analysis of 41 proven cases. *J Ultrasound Med* 1983; 2: 401.
3. Levin S, Feingold M, Brook I, et al: False positive ultrasonography diagnosis of molar pregnancy. *Acta Obstet Gynecol Scand* 1981; 60:435.
4. Rinehart JS, Hernandez E, Rosenshein NB, et al: Degenerating leiomyomata uteri, an ultrasonic mimic of hydatidiform mole. *J Reprod Med* 1981; 26:142.
5. Muram D, Gillieson M, Walters JH: Myomas of the uterus in pregnancy: Ultrasonographic follow-up. *Am J Obstet Gynecol* 1980; 138:16.
6. Winer-Muram HT, Muram D, Gillieson MS, et al: Uterine myomas in pregnancy. *Can Med Assoc J* 1983; 128:949.
7. Fleischer AC, Boehm FH, James AE Jr: Sonography and radiology of pelvic masses and other maternal disorders. *Semin Roentgenol* 1982; 17:172.
8. Bezjian AA: Pelvic masses in pregnancy. *Clin Obstet Gynecol* 1984; 27:402.
9. Pennes DR, Bowerman RA, Silver TM: Congenital uterine anomalies and associated pregnancies: Findings and pitfalls of sonographic diagnosis. *J Ultrasound Med* 1985; 4:531.
10. Jones TB, Fleischer AC, Daniell JF, et al: Sonographic characteristics of congenital uterine abnormalities and associated pregnancy. *JCU* 1980; 8:435.
11. Bandy LC, Clarke-Pearson DL, Hammond CB: Malignant potential of gestational trophoblastic disease at the extreme ages of reproductive life. *Obstet Gynecol* 1984; 64:395.
12. Szulman AE, Surti U: The syndromes of hydatidiform mole: 1. Cytogenic and morphologic considerations. *Am J Obstet Gynecol* 1978; 132:20.
13. MacVicar J, Donald I: Sonar in the diagnosis of early pregnancy and its complications. *J Obstet Gynaecol Br Commonw* 1963; 70:387.
14. Gottesfeld KR, Taylor ES, Thompson HE, et al: Diagnosis of hydatidiform mole by ultrasound. *Obstet Gynecol* 1967; 30:163.
15. Fleisher AC, James AE Jr, Krause DA, et al: Sonographic patterns in trophoblastic diseases. *Radiology* 1978; 126:215.
16. Reid MH, McGahan JP, Oi R: Sonographic evaluation of hydatidiform mole and its look-alikes. *AJR* 1983; 140:307.
17. Kobayashi M: Use of diagnostic ultrasound in trophoblastic neoplasms and ovarian tumors. *Cancer* 1976; 33:441.
18. Nelson LH, Fry RJ, Homesley HD, et al: Malignant ovarian tumors simulating hydatidiform mole on ultrasound. *JCU* 1982; 10:249.
19. Buschi AJ, Brenbridge ANAG, Cochrane JA, et

al: Hydropic degeneration of the placenta simulating hydatidiform mole. *JCU* 1979; 7:60.

20. Sauerbrei EE, Salem S, Fayle B: Coexistent hydatidiform mole and live fetus in the second trimester: An ultrasound study. *Radiology* 1980; 135:415.

21. Yee B, Tu B, Platt LD: Coexisting hydatidiform mole with a live fetus presenting as a placenta previa on ultrasound. *Am J Obstet Gynecol* 1982; 144:726.

22. Switzer JM, Weckstein ML, Campbell LF, et al: Ovarian hydatidiform mole. *J Ultrasound Med* 1984; 3:471.

23. Jones WB, Lauersen NH: Hydatiform mole with coexistent fetus. *Am J Obstet Gynecol* 1975; 122:267.

24. Woo JSK, Wong LC, Hsu C, et al: Sonographic appearances of the partial hydatidiform mole. *J Ultrasound Med* 1983; 2:261.

25. Woodward RM, Filly RA, Callen PW: First trimester molar pregnancy: Nonspecific ultrasonographic appearance. *Obstet Gynecol* 1980; 55:31S.

26. Naumoff P, Szulman AE, Weinstein B, et al: Ultrasonography of partial hydatidiform mole. *Radiology* 1981; 140:467.

27. Hadlock FP, Deter RL, Carpenter R, et al: Hypervascularity of the uterine wall during pregnancy: Incidence, sonographic appearance, and obstetric implications. *JCU* 1980; 8:399.

28. Reuter K, Michiewitz H, Kahn PC: Early appearance of hydatidiform mole by ultrasound. *AJR* 1980; 134:588.

29. Szulman AE, Ma HK, Wong LS, et al: Residual trophoblastic disease in association with partial hydatidiform mole. *Obstet Gynecol* 1982; 57:392.

30. Looi LM, Silvanesaratnam V: Malignant evolution with fatal outcome in a patient with partial hydatidiform mole. *Aust NZ J Obstet Gynaecol* 1981; 21:51.

31. Scheer K, Goldstein DP: Use of ultrasonography to follow regression of theca lutein cysts. *Radiology* 1973; 108:673.

32. Requard CK, Mettler PA: The use of ultrasound in the evaluation of trophoblastic disease and its response to therapy. *Radiology* 1980; 135:419.

33. Munyer TP, Callen PW, Filly RA, et al: Further observations on the sonographic spectrum of gestational trophoblastic disease. *JCU* 1983; 9:349.

34. Huberman RP, Fon GT, Bein ME: Benign molar pregnancies: Pulmonary complications. *AJR* 1982; 138:71.

35. Mahony BS, Filly RA, Callen PW: Amnionicity and chorionicity in twin pregnancies: Prediction using ultrasound. *Radiology* 1985; 155:205.

36. Barss VA, Benacerraf BR, Frigoletto FD: Ultrasonographic determination of chorion type in twin gestation. *Obstet Gynecol* 1985; 66:779.

37. Manlan G, Scott KE: Contributions of twin pregnancy to perinatal mortality and fetal growth retardation: Reversal growth retardation after birth. *Can Med Assoc J* 1978; 118:365.

38. Papiernik E: Social cost of twin births. *Acta Genet Med Gemellol* 1983; 32:105.

39. Buttery B, Davison G: The ghost artifact. *J Ultrasound Med* 1984; 3:49.

40. Sauerbrei EE: The split image artifact in pelvic ultrasonography: The anatomy and physics. *J Ultrasound Med* 1985; 4:29.

41. Baker ME Mahony BS, Bowie JD: Adverse effect of an overdistended bladder on first trimester sonography. *AJR* 1985; 45:597.

42. Burrows PE, Lyons EA, Phillips HJ, et al: Intrauterine membranes: Sonographic findings and clinical significance. *JCU* 1982; 10:1.

43. Schafter RM, Stein K, Shih YH, et al: The echoic pseudogestational sac of ectopic pregnancy simulating early intrauterine pregnancy. *J Ultrasound Med* 1983; 2:215.

44. Dunne MG: Shed decidual cast simulating an intrauterine fetus. *AJR* 1982; 139:591.

45. Robinson HP, Caines JS: Sonar evidence of early pregnancy failure in patients with twin conceptions. *Br J Obstet Gynaecol* 1977; 84:22.

46. Finberg HJ, Birnholz JC: Ultrasound observations in multiple gestation with first trimester bleeding: The blighted twin. *Radiology* 1979; 132:137.

47. Landy HJ, Keith L, Keith D: The vanishing twin. *Acta Genet Med Gemellol* 1982; 31:179.

48. Cadkin AV, MacAlpin J: The decidua-chorionic sac: A reliable sonographic indicator of intrauterine pregnancy prior to detection of a fetal pole. *J Ultrasound Med* 1984; 3:539.

49. Scheer K: Ultrasound in twin gestation. *JCU* 1975; 2:197.

50. Crane JP, Tomich PG, Kopta M: Ultrasonic growth patterns in normal and discordant twins. *Obstet Gynecol* 1980; 55:678.

51. Leveno KJ, Santos-Ramos R, Duenhoelter JH, et al: Sonar cephalometry in twins: A table of biparietal diameters for normal twin fetuses and a comparison with singletons. *Am J Obstet Gynecol* 1979; 135:727.

52. Socol ML, Tamura RK, Sabbagha RE, et al: Diminished biparietal diameter and abdominal circumference growth in twins. *Obstet Gynecol* 1984; 64:235.

53. Grumbach K, Coleman BG, Arger PH, et al: Twin and singleton growth patterns cmpared using ultrasound. *Radiology* 1986; 158:237.

54. Iffy L, Lavenhar MA, Jakovits A, et al: The rate of early intrauterine growth in twin gestation. *Am J Obstet Gynecol* 1983; 146:970.

55. Bhargva V, Agarwal RD, Singh LI, et al: Intrauterine growth of twins. *Indian Pediatr* 1983; 20:401.

56. Leroy B, Lefort F, Neveu P et al.: Intrauterine growth charts for twin fetuses. *Acta Genet Med Gemellol* 1982; 31:199.

57. Secher NJ, Kaern J, Hansen PK: Intrauterine growth in twin pregnancies: Prediction of fetal growth retardation. *Obstet Gynecol* 1985; 66:63.

58. Leveno KJ, Quirk JG, Whalley PJ, et al: Fetal lung maturation in twin gestation. *Obstet Gynecol* 1984; 148:405.

59. Dobbie HG, Whittle MJ, Wilson AT, et al: Amniotic fluid phospholipid profile in multiple pregnancy and the effect of zygosity. *Br J Obstet Gynaecol* 1983; 90:1001.

60. Fleisher B, Kulovich MV, Hallman M, et al: Lung profile: Sex differences in normal pregnancy. *Obstet Gynecol* 1985; 66:327.

61. MacGillivray I: Determinants of birthweight of twins. *Acta Genet Med Gemellol* 1983; 32:151.

62. Newton W, Keith L, Keith D: The Northwestern University multihospital twin study: IV. Duration of gestation according to fetal sex. *Am J Obstet Gynecol* 1984; 149:655.

63. Elejalde BR, de Elejalde MM, Wagner AM, et al: Diagnosis of twin to twin transfusion syndrome at 18 weeks of gestation. *JCU* 1983; 11:442.

64. Galea P, Scott JM, Goel KM: Feto-fetal transfusion syndrome. *Arch Dis Child* 1982; 57:781.

65. Brennan JD, Diwan RV, Rosen MG, et al: Feto-fetal transfusion syndrome: Prenatal ultrasonographic diagnosis. *Radiology* 1982; 143:535.

66. Platt LD, DeVore GR, Bienarz A, et al: Antenatal diagnosis of acephalus acardia: A proposed management scheme. *Am J Obstet Gynecol* 1983; 146:857.

67. Hantman SS, Zara HD; In utero sonographic detection of abnormal twin pregnancy. *JCU* 1982; 10:282.

68. Livnat EJ, Burd L, Cadkin A, et al: Fetus papyraceus in twin pregnancy. *Obstet Gynecol* 1978; 51:41s.

69. Wilson RL, Shaub MS, Cetrulo CJ: The antepartum findings of conjoined twins. *JCU* 1977; 5:35

70. Apuzzio JJ, Ganesh V, Landau I, et al: Prenatal diagnosis of conjoined twins. *Am J Obstet Gynecol* 1984; 148:343.

71. Wilson DA, Young GZ, Crumley CS: Antepartum ultrasonographic diagnosis of ischiopagus: A rare variety of conjoined twins. *J Ultrasound Med* 1983; 2:281.

72. Weingast GR, Johnson ML, Pretorius DH, et al: Difficulty in sonographic diagnosis of cephalothoracopagus. *J Ultrasound Med* 1984; 3:421.

73. Gore RM, Filly RA, Parer JT: Sonographic antepartum diagnosis of conjoined twins. *JAMA* 1982; 247:3351.

74. Nicolini U, Dell'Agnola A, Ferrazzi E, et al: Ultrasonic prenatal diagnosis of fetus in fetu. *JCU* 1983; 11:321.

75. Nocera RM, Davis M, Hayden CK Jr, et al: Fetus-in-fetu. *AJR* 1982; 138:762.

76. Golan A, Amit A, Baram A, et al: Unusual cord intertwining in monoamniotic twins. *Aust NZ Obstet Gynaecol* 1982; 22:165.

77. Nyberg DA, Filly RA, Golbus MS, et al: Entangled umbilical cords: A sign of monoamniotic twins. *J Ultrasound Med* 1984; 3:29.

78. Gohari P, Berkowitz RL, Hobbins JC: Prediction of intrauterine growth retardation by total intrauterine volume. *Am J Obstet Gynecol* 1977; 127:255.

79. Grossman M, Flynn JJ, Aufrichtig D, et al: Pit-

falls in ultrasonic determination of total intrauterine volume. *JCU* 1982; 10:17.

80. Kurtz AB, Shaw WM, Kurtz RJ, et al: The inaccuracy of total uterine volume measurements: Sources of error and a proposed solution. *J Ultrasound Med* 1984; 3:289.

81. Giersson RT, Patel NB: Longitudinal and transverse uterine area measurements (LTUA) are not representative of intrauterine volume. *JCU* 1984; 3:353.

82. Kurtz AB, Kurtz RJ, Rifkin MD, et al: Total uterine volume: A new graph and its clinical applications. *J Ultrasound Med* 1984; 3:299.

83. Chamberlain PF, Manning FA, Morrison I, et al: Ultrasound evaluation of amniotic fluid volume: II. The relationship of increased amniotic fluid volume to perinatal outcome. *Am J Obstet Gynecol* 1984; 150:250.

84. Robinow M, Spisso K, Buschi AJ, et al: Turner syndrome: Sonography showing fetal hydrops simulating hydramnios. *AJR* 1980; 135:846.

85. Finnegan JK: Amniotic fluid and midtrimester amniocentesis: A review. *Br J Obstet Gynaecol* 1984; 91:745.

86. Van Otterloo LC, Wladmiroff JW, Wallenburg HCS: Relationship between fetal urine production and amniotic fluid volume in normal pregnancy and pregnancy complicated by diabetes. *Br J Obstet Gynaecol* 1977; 84:205.

87. Abramovich DR, Garden A, Jandial L, et al: Fetal swallowing and voiding in relation to hydramnios. *Obstet Gynecol* 1978; 54:15.

88. Stander RW: Abnormalities of the placenta, membranes, and fetus, in Danforth DN (ed): *Obstetrics and Gynecology,* ed 3. Hagerstown, Md, Harper & Row, 1977.

89. Donnelly PB, Rosenberg MA, Kay CJ, et al: Sonographic demonstration of occult umbilical cord prolapse. *AJR* 1980; 134:1060.

90. Hales ED, Westney LS: Sonography of occult cord prolapse. *JCU* 1984; 12:283.

91. Vintzileos AM, Nochimson DJ, Lillo NL, et al: Ultrasonic diagnosis of fundic presentation. *JCU* 1983; 11:510.

92. Hobbins JC, Grannum PAT, Berkowitz RL et al: Ultrasound in the diagnosis of congenital anomalies. *Am J Obstet Gynecol* 1979; 134:331.

93. Jacoby HE, Charles D: Clinical conditions associated with hydramnios. *Am J Obstet Gynecol* 1966; 94:910.

94. King CR, Prescott GH: Amniotic fluid alpha fetoprotein elevation with fetal omphalocele and a possible mechanism for its occurrence. *Am J Obstet Gynecol* 1978; 130:279.

95. Holzgreve W, Beller FK, Pawlowitzki IH: Amniotic fluid acetylcholinesterase as a marker in prenatal diagnosis of esophageal atresia. *Am J Obstet Gynecol* 1983; 145:641.

96. Zemlyn S: Prenatal detection of esophageal atresia: Case report. *JCU* 1981; 9:453.

97. Eyheremendy E, Pfister M: Case report: Antenatal real-time diagnosis of esophageal atresias. *JCU* 1983; 11:395.

98. Houlton MC, Sutton M, Aiken: Antenatal diagnosis of duodenal atresia. *J Obstet Gynaecol Br Common* 1974; 81:818.

99. Lees RF, Alford BA, Brenbridge ANAG, et al: Case Report: Sonographic appearance of duodenal atresia in utero. *AJR* 1978; 131:701.

100. Boomsma JHB, Weemhof RA, Polman HA: Sonographic appearance of annular pancreas in utero: A case report. *Diagn Imaging* 1982; 51:288.

101. Sanders R, Graham D: Twelve cases of hydronephrosis in utero diagnosed by ultrasonography. *J Ultrasound Med* 1982; 1:341.

102. Lee TG, Warren BH: Antenatal ultrasonic demonstration of fetal bowel. *Radiology* 1977; 124:471.

103. Cloutier MG, Fried AM, Selke AC: Antenatal observation of midgut volvulus by ultrasound. *JCU* 1983; 11:286.

104. Jassani MN, Gauderer SL, Fanaroff AA, et al: A perinatal approach to the diagnosis and management of gastrointestinal malformations. *Obstet Gynecol* 1982; 59:33.

105. Nelson PA, Bowie JD, Filston HC, et al: Sonographic diagnosis of omphalocele in utero. *AJR* 1982; 138:1178.

106. Baird PA, MacDonald EC: An epidemiological study of congenital malformations of the anterior abdominal wall in more than half a million congenital births. *Am J Hum Genet* 1981; 23:470.

107. Hauge M, Bugge M, Nielsen J: Early prenatal diagnosis of omphalocele constitutes indication for amniocentesis. *Lancet* 1983; 2:507.

108. Schaffer RM, Barone C, Friedman AP: The ultrasonographic spectrum of fetal omphalocele. *J Ultrasound Med* 1983; 2:219.

109. Giulian BB, Alvear DT: Prenatal ultrasonographic diagnosis of fetal gastroschisis. *Radiology* 1978; 29:473.

110. Glaves J, Baker JL: Spontaneous resolution of maternal hydramnios in congenital cystic adenomatoid malformation of the lung: Antenatal ultrasound features. A case report. *Br J Obstet Gynaecol* 1983; 90:1065.

111. Redwine FO, Petres RE, Cruikshank DP: Reversal of hydramnios by drainage of a fetal renal cyst: A case report. *J Reprod Med* 1983; 28:421.

112. Seeds JW, Cefalo RC, Hervert WNP, et al: Hydramnios and maternal renal failure: Relief with fetal therapy. *Obstet Gynecol* 1984; 64:26s.

113. Tabsh KMA: Antenatal sonographic appearance of a fetal ovarian cyst. *J Ultrasound Med* 1982; 1:329.

114. Hurwitz A, Yagel S, Rabinovitz R, et al: Hydramnios caused by pure megacystis. *JCU* 1984; 12:110.

115. Valenti C, Kassner EG, Yermakov V, et al: Antenatal diagnosis of a fetal ovarian cyst. *Am J Obstet Gynecol* 1975; 123:216.

116. Suita S, Ikeda K, Koyanagi R, et al: Neonatal ovarian cyst diagnosed antenatally: Report of two patients. *JCU* 1984; 12:517.

117. Philipson EH, Wolfson RN, Kedia KR: Fetal hydronephrosis and polyhydramnios associated with vesico-ureteral reflux. *JCU* 1984; 12:585.

118. Ray D, Berger N, Ensor R: Hydramnios in association with unilateral fetal hydronephrosis. *JCU* 1982; 10:82.

119. Geirsson RT, Ricketts NEM, Taylor DJ, et al: Prenatal appearance of a mesoblastic nephroma associated with polyhydramnios. *JCU* 1985; 13:488.

120. Howey DD, Farrell EE, Sholl J, et al: Congenital mesoblastic nephroma: Prenatal ultrasonic findings and surgical excision in a very-low-birth-weight infant. *JCU* 1985; 13:506.

121. Walter JP, McGahan JP: Mesoblatic nephroma: Prenatal sonographic detection. *JCU* 1985; 13:686.

122. Fuster JS, Benasco C, Saad I: Giant dilatation of the umbilical vein. *JCU* 1985; 13:363.

123. Kohler HF, Rymer BA: Congenital cystic adenomatoid malformation of the lung and its relation to hydramnios. *Br J Obstet Gynaecol* 1973; 80:130.

124. Ostor AG, Fortune DW: Congenital cystic adenomatoid malformation of the lung. *Am J Clin Pathol* 1978; 70:595.

125. Graham D, Winn K, Dex W, et al: Prenatal diagnosis of cystic adenomatoid malformation of the lung. *J Ultrasound Med* 1982; 1:9.

126. Diwan RV, Brennan JN, Philipson EH, et al: Ultrasonic prenatal diagnosis of type III congenital cystic adenomatoid malformation of lung. *JCU* 1983; 11:218.

127. Stiller RJ, Roberts NS, Weiner S, et al: Congenital diaphragmatic hernia: Antenatal diagnosis and obstetrical management. *JCU* 1985; 13:212.

128. Cohen FA, Moskowitz PS, McCallum WD: Sonographic diagnosis of cystic adenomatoid malformation in-utero. *Prenatal Diagn* 1983; 3:139.

129. Pezzuti RT, Isler RJ: Antenatal ultrasound detection of cystic adenomatoid malformation of lung: Report of a case and review of the recent literature. *JCU* 1983; 11:342.

130. Rosenfeld CR, Coin CD, Duenhoelter JH: Fetal cervical teratoma as a cause of polyhydramnios. *Pediatrics* 1979; 64:176.

131. Trecet JC, Claramunt V, Larraz J, et al: Prenatal ultrasound diagnosis of fetal teratoma of the neck. *JCU* 1984; 12:509.

132. Gadwood KA, Reynes CJ: Prenatal sonography of metastatic neuroblastoma. *JCU* 1983; 11:512.

133. Barone CM, Van Natta FC, Kourides IA, et al: Sonographic detection of fetal goiter, an unusual cause of hydramnios. *J Ultrasound Med* 1985; 4:625.

134. Kang K, Hissong S, Langer A: Prenatal ultrasonic diagnosis of epignathus. *JCU* 1978; 6:330.

135. Wong WS, Filly RA: Polyhydramnios associated with fetal limb abnormalities. *AJR* 1983; 140:1001.

136. Zimmerman EZ, Weinraub Z, Raijman A, et al: Antenatal diagnosis of a fetus with an extremely narrow thorax and short limb dwarfism. *JCU* 1984; 12:112.

137. Romero R, Chervanek FA, Kotzen J, et al: Antenatal sonographic findings of extralobal pulmonary sequestration. *J Ultrasound Med* 1982; 1:131–132.

138. Bryan EM: Benign fetal ascites associated with

maternal polyhydramnios. *Clin Pediatr* 1975; 14:88.

139. Redford DHA: Uterine growth in twin pregnancy by measurement of total intrauterine volume. *Acta Genet Med Gemellol* 1982; 31:145.

140. Mahony BS, Filly RA, Callen PW, et al: Severe nonimmune hydrops fetalis: Sonographic evaluation. *Radiology* 1984; 151:757.

141. Bryan EM: Benign fetal ascites associated with maternal polyhydramnios. *Clin Pediatr* 1975; 14:88.

142. Platt LD, Collea JV, Joseph DM: Transitory fetal ascites: An ultrasound diagnosis. *Am J Obstet Gynecol* 1978; 132:906.

143. Graif M, Shalev J, Mashiach S, et al: Free intra-abdominal fluid in the fetus: Ultrasonic assessment. *JCU* 1983; 11:458.

144. Rosenthal SJ, FIlly RA, Callen PW, et al: Fetal pseudoascites. *Radiology* 1979; 131:195.

145. Graves GR, Baskett TF: Nonimmune hydrops fetalis: Antenatal diagnosis and management. *Am J Obstet Gynecol* 1984; 148:563.

146. Fleischer AC, Killam AP, Boehm FJ, et al: Hydrops fetalis: Sonographic evaluation and clinical implications. *Radiology* 1981; 141:163.

147. Weiner S, Bolognese RJ, Librizzi RJ: Ultrasound in the evaluation and management of the isoimmunized pregnancy. *JCU* 1981; 9:315.

148. Fleming P, McLeary RD: Nonimmunological fetal hydrops with theca lutein cysts. *Radiology* 1981; 141:169.

149. Hutchison AA, Drew JH, Yu VYH, et al: Nonimmunologic hydrops fetalis: A review of 61 cases. *Obstet Gynecol* 1982; 59:347.

150. Davis CL: Diagnosis and management of nonimmune hydrops fetalis. *J Reprod Med* 1982; 27:594.

151. Etches PC, Lemons JA: Nonimmune hydrops fetalis: Report of 22 cases including three siblings. *Pediatrics* 1979; 64:326.

152. Jouppila P, Kirkinen P, Herva R, et al: Prenatal diagnosis of pleural effusions by ultrasound. *JCU* 1983; 11:516.

153. Gadwood KA, Reynes CJ: Prenatal sonography of metastatic neuroblastoma. *JCU* 1983; 11:512.

154. Jones DED, Pritchard KI, Gioanni CA, et al: Hydrops fetalis associated with idiopathic arterial calcification. *Obstet Gynecol* 1972; 39:435.

155. Riboni G, DeSimoni M, Leopardi O, et al: Ultrasound appearance of a glioblastoma in a 33 week fetus in utero. *JCU* 1985; 13:345.

156. Grundy H, Glasman A, Burlbaw J, et al: Hemangioma presenting as a cystic mass in the fetal neck. *J Ultrasound Med* 1985; 4:147.

157. Fuster JS, Benasco C, Saad I: Giant dilatation of the umbilical vein. *JCU* 1985; 13:363.

158. Seifer DB, Ferguson JE II, Behrens CM, et al: Nonimmune hydrops fetalis in association with hemangioma of the umbilical cord. *Obstet Gynecol* 1985; 66:283.

159. Harrigan JT, Kangos JJ, Sikka A, et al: Successful treatment of fetal congestive heart failure secondary to tachycardia. *N Engl J Med* 1981; 304:1527.

160. Silverman NH, Enderlein MA, Stanger P, et al: Recognition of fetal arrhythmias by echocardiography. *JCU* 1985; 13:255.

161. Kleinman CS, Copel JA, Weinstein EM, et al: Treatment of fetal supraventricular tachyarrhythmias. *JCU* 1985; 13:265.

162. Platt LD, DeVore GR, Bienvariz A, et al: Antenatal diagnosis of acephalus acardia: A proposed management scheme. *Am J Obstet Gynecol* 1983; 146:857–859.

163. Shapiro I, Sharf M: Spontaneous intrauterine remission of hydrops fetalis in one identical twin: Sonographic diagnosis. *JCU* 1985; 13:427.

164. Dor N, Mosberg H, Stern W, et al: Complications in fetal macrosomia. *NY State J Med* 1984; 84:302.

165. Spellacy WN, Miller S, Winegar A, et al: Macrosomia: Maternal characteristics and infant complications. *Obstet Gynecol* 1985; 66:158.

166. Lichty JA, Ting RY, Brunx PD, et al: Studies of babies born at high altitude. *Am J Dis Child* 1957; 93:666.

167. Boyd ME, Usher RH, McLean FH: Fetal macrosomia: Prediction, risks, proposed management. *Obstet Gynecol* 1983; 61:715.

168. Deter RL, Hadlock FP: Use of ultrasound in the detection of macrosomia: A review. *JCU* 1985; 13:519.

169. Shepard MT, Richards VM, Berkowitz RT, et al: An evaluation of two equations for the prediction of fetal weight by ultrasound. *Am J Obstet Gynecol* 1982; 136:45.

170. Ogata ES, Sabbagha R, Metzger BE, et al: Serial ultrasonography to assess evolving fetal macrosomia: Studies in 23 pregnant diabetic women. *JAMA* 1980; 243:2405.

171. Deter RL, Harrist RB, Hadlock FP, et al: Longitudinal studies of fetal growth using volume parameters determined with ultrasound. *JCU* 1984; 12:313.

172. Eik-Nes PH, Grottum P, Persson P, et al: Prediction of fetal growth deviation by ultrasonic biometry: II. Clinical application. *Acta Obstet Gynecol Scand* 1983; 62:117.

173. Ott WJ, Doyle S: Ultrasonic diagnosis of altered fetal growth by use of a normal ultrasonic fetal weight curve. *Obstet Gynecol* 1984; 63:201.

174. Hadlock FP, Harrist RB, Fearneyhough TC, et al: Use of femur length/abdominal circumference ratio in detection of the macrosomic fetus. *Radiology* 1985; 154:503.

175. Elliott JP, Garite TJ, Freeman RK, et al: Ultrasonic prediction of fetal macrosomia in diabetic patients. *Obstet Gynecol* 1982; 60:159.

176. Miller JM, Horger EO: Diabetic halo. *South Med J* 1983; 76:1484.

# CASES

## Dennis A. Sarti, M.D.

### Normal Early Pregnancy

In discussing gestational age in the case section, we will use menstrual dating, which is also used by the referring obstetrician. Therefore, 2 weeks after conception will be referred to as the fourth menstrual week.

Fertilization occurs in the distal end of the fallopian tube. The fertilized ovum takes 3 days to traverse the fallopian tube. The blastocyst then floats around the uterine cavity for approximately 3–4 days. By 7 days after conception, the blastocyst implants in the uterine wall. At 4 menstrual weeks, or 2 weeks after conception, the ultrasound findings are minimal. Some decidual reaction can be identified in the uterine cavity. Figures 16–1 and 16–2 are longitudinal scans of the uterus at approximately 4 menstrual weeks. Some increased echogenicity is noted in the fundal region of each uterus (arrow). This is secondary to decidual reaction in preparation for the developing pregnancy. These ultrasound findings cannot be distinguished from the findings in early menstruation, an abortion in progress, or decidual reaction in an ectopic pregnancy. There is no way to distinguish those three entities from a normal intrauterine pregnancy at this time.

Figure 16–3 is a longitudinal scan of the uterus at approximately 4½ menstrual weeks. There is the suggestion of a very early gestational sac with a small lucency identified centrally in the echogenic region. This is not a measurable gestational sac but only suggestive.

Finally, a gestational sac is identified in the fundal region of this uterus in Figure 16–4. This is a longitudinal scan in which a fluid-containing structure is noted in the fundal region. Highly echogenic areas are noted surrounding the fluid-containing structure, with a double ring appearance in the inferior border. This is at approximately 5 menstrual weeks when the gestational sac is 8–10 mm in diameter.

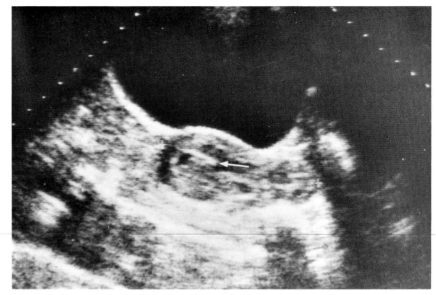

**FIG 16–1.**

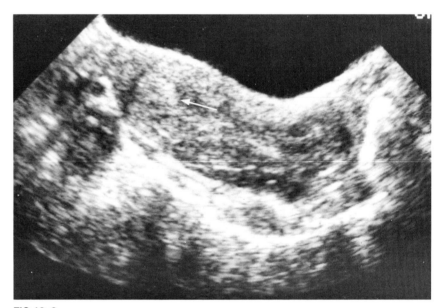

**FIG 16–2.**

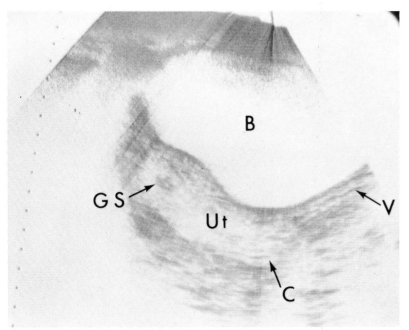

| Arrow | = | Decidual reaction |
|-------|---|-------------------|
| B     | = | Bladder           |
| C     | = | Cervix            |
| GS    | = | Gestational sac   |
| H     | = | Head              |
| Ut    | = | Uterus            |
| V     | = | Vagina            |

FIG 16–3.

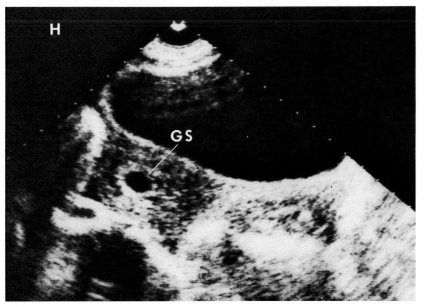

FIG 16–4.

## Normal Early Pregnancy

Implantation usually occurs in the fundus or miduterus. Rarely, it is identified in the lower uterine segment. It is very important to follow implantation in the lower uterine segment since it may indicate impending abortion. Most often implantation occurs in the fundal region. It initially begins with a highly echogenic region. Eventually a small gestational sac develops. Figure 16–5 is a longitudinal scan in the midline of the uterus which shows a small cystic region in the cervical area secondary to a nabothian cyst (C). The pregnancy is approximately 4–4½ weeks old by menstrual dating. An echogenic region is noted in the fundal area (arrows). This is the earliest ultrasound sign of an intrauterine pregnancy. There is nothing specific about this appearance to indicate that it represents a normal pregnancy. The only way to confirm that the pregnancy is normal is to scan the patient in approximately 7–10 days. Figure 16–6 is a longitudinal scan of the same patient made approximately 4 weeks after the scan in Figure 16–5. It demonstrates an early intrauterine pregnancy in the fundal and body region of the uterus. The placenta (P) is situated anteriorly and appears as a highly echogenic region. Amniotic fluid volume is identified, with embryonic echoes present within the midportion. The crown-rump length of the fetus was 2 cm, which corresponds to a gestational age of 8½ weeks.

The earliest suggestive evidence of an intrauterine pregnancy is the finding of a normal-appearing gestational sac in the fundal region. Figures 16–7 and 16–8 are longitudinal scans in which a gestational sac is well visualized. Note that the sac is usually oval to circular in appearance. It has a highly echogenic rim. There is also the suggestion of a double appearance to the gestational sac, which will be discussed later. The size and shape of the gestational sac must always be evaluated. The echogenic amplitude should equal that of the urinary bladder–uterus interface.

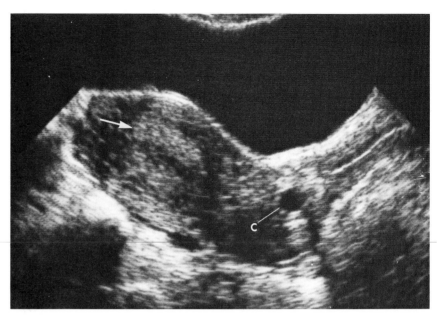

**FIG 16–5.**

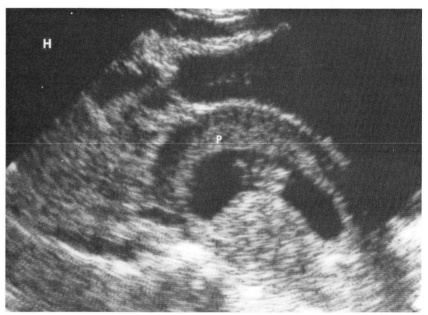

**FIG 16–6.**

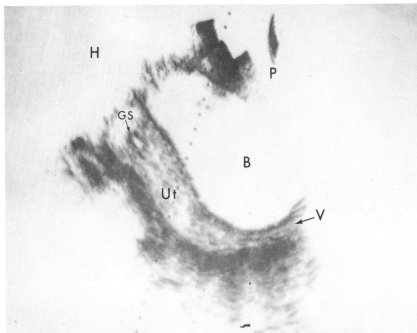

FIG 16–7.

| Arrow | = | Decidual reaction |
|---|---|---|
| B | = | Urinary bladder |
| C | = | Nabothian cyst |
| GS | = | Gestational sac |
| H | = | Head |
| P | | Placenta (Fig 16–6) |
| P | = | Symphysis pubis (Figs 16–7, 16–8) |
| U | = | Umbilical level |
| Ut | = | Uterus |
| V | = | Vagina |

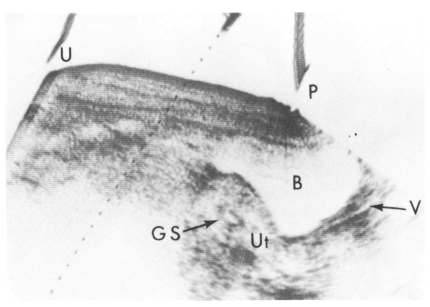

FIG 16–8.

## Human Chorionic Gonadotropin Levels and Gestational Sac

The size and appearance of the gestational sac indicate that there is a strong relationship with the serum human chorionic gonadotropin (hCG) level until approximately 8 weeks. Figure 16–9 shows data developed by Nyberg which correlate the hCG level with gestational sac size. There is a linear correlation from 5 to 8 menstrual weeks. The hCG level increases rapidly, doubling approximately every 2–3 days. The gestational sac size also grows quite rapidly during early pregnancy. Therefore, correlation of these two findings can be an important clue to the progression of early pregnancy.

Figure 16–10 (contributed by Dr. Nyberg) shows the development of the deciduae in early pregnancy. The decidua just deep to the blastocyst is termed the decidua basalis. The decidua covering the top of the blastocyst is termed the decidua capsularis. The remainder of the decidua over the cavity is called the decidua parietalis. Between the decidua parietalis and decidua capsularis lies the uterine cavity. This space is the reason we are able to see a double decidual gestational sac. The double decidual gestational sac can be identified in early pregnancy over part of the gestational sac. It will not be seen entirely around the gestational sac because of the region of the decidua basalis. Figures 16–11 and 16–12 are longitudinal scans of very early pregnancy in which the double decidual gestational sac can be seen. The echogenic area causing the double appearance (arrowheads) is secondary to the decidua parietalis lying outside the decidua capsularis.

Figure 16–11 is a longitudinal scan in which the mean diameter of the gestational sac is 6.8 mm. This corresponds to a gestation of 5 weeks 2 days since last menstrual period.

Figure 16–12 is a longitudinal scan in which the mean sac diameter measures 8 mm. This corresponds to a gestation of approximately 5 weeks 3 days. The hCG level was 3,460. The

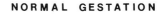

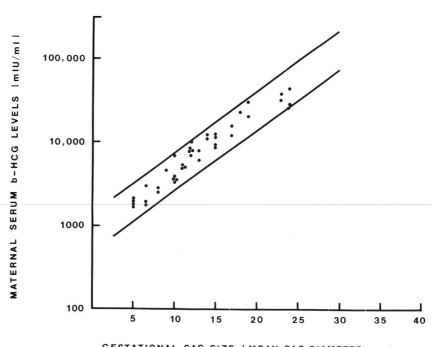

FIG 16–9.

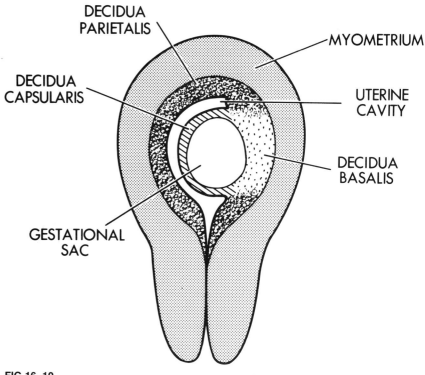

FIG 16–10.

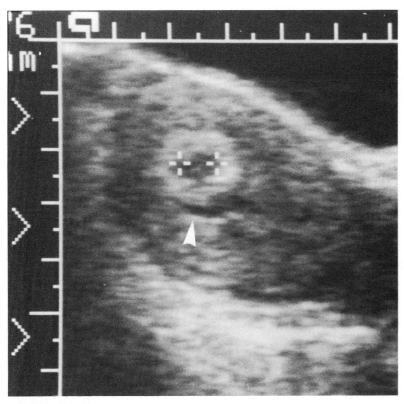

FIG 16–11.

mean diameter of the gestational sac is measured from the inside borders of the decidua capsularis and basalis. The sac diameter is measured in three planes, as will be illustrated later. The double ring appearance is extremely important, as it is the first sign that the pregnancy is truly intrauterine. Even though an embryo is not visualized, the double decidual sac appearance is highly indicative of an intrauterine pregnancy.

**Arrowhead** = Decidua parietalis representing a double decidual gestational sac

SOURCE: Figure 16–10 is reproduced with permission from Nyberg DA, Laing FC, Filly RA, et al: Ultrasonographic differentiation of the gestational sac of early intrauterine pregnancy from the pseudogestational sac of ectopic pregnancy. *Radiology* 1983; 146:755.

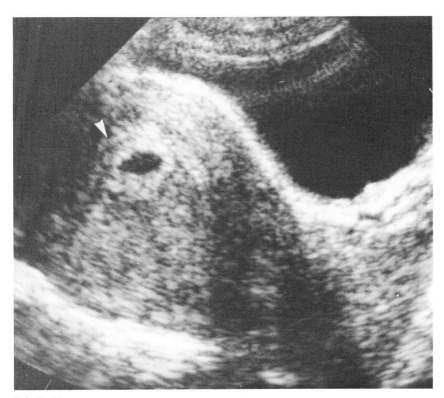

FIG 16–12.

## Normal Gestational Sac

The normal gestational sac has a double ring appearance that indicates an intrauterine pregnancy. Figure 16–13 is a longitudinal scan in which a large sonolucent mass is seen posterior to the cervical region. The mass represents a corpus luteum cyst. A gestational sac is present within the fundal portion of the uterus. It has a circular appearance with highly echogenic surrounding echoes. There is a double ring appearance (arrowhead) indicating an intrauterine pregnancy. A yolk sac and embryo are not identified at this time. The ultrasound findings indicate a pregnancy of about 5 menstrual weeks. The secondary yolk sac can be visualized at approximately 6 menstrual weeks. The ultrasound findings also are confirmatory evidence of an intrauterine pregnancy even though an embryo cannot be visualized. The secondary yolk sac is characteristically round and has a sharp interface. The transducer must be perpendicular to the interface to bring out the echoes of the secondary yolk sac. Figure 16–14 is a longitudinal scan of the uterus which has a gestational sac in the fundal region. The curvilinear echoes of the small yolk sac (Y) are seen in the inferior portion of the gestational sac. An embryo is not visualized at this time. However, the presence of the yolk sac indicates an intrauterine pregnancy.

When the yolk sac becomes visible, the embryonic pole is in close proximity. Often the embryo will not be visualized but cardiac activity can be identified adjacent to the yolk sac. This is secondary to the small size of the embryo. Close examination of the region of the yolk sac may reveal cardiac activity even when the embryo cannot be seen. Figure 16–15 is a longitudinal scan in a pregnancy of 6 menstrual weeks. The gestational sac has an oval appearance and a double ring, characteristic of an intrauterine pregnancy. Note the yolk sac within the gestational sac. Figure 16–16 is a longitudinal scan of the same patient, with magnification of the region of the gestational sac. Cephalad to the yolk sac is a slightly echogenic region that

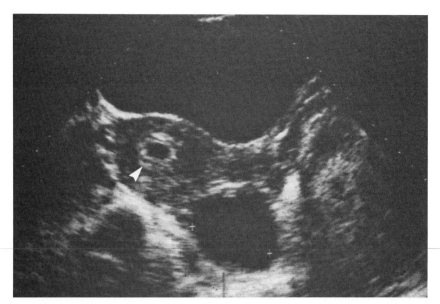

**FIG 16–13.**

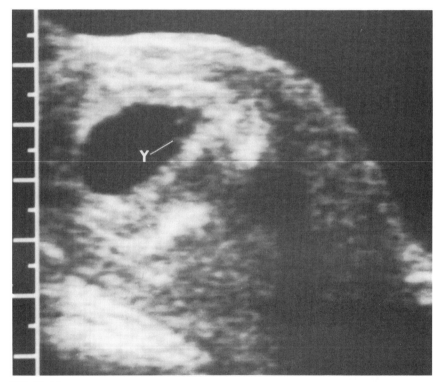

**FIG 16–14.**

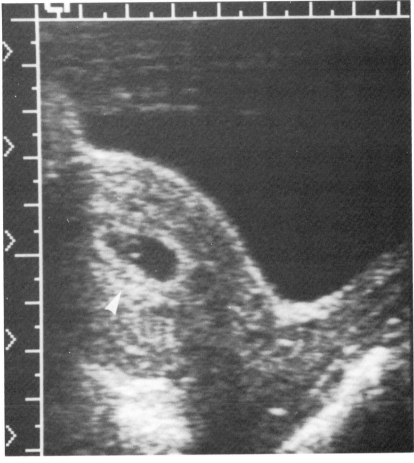

FIG 16–15.

represents the embryonic pole (E). With focused transducers, these small anatomic details can be well visualized. Cardiac activity was identified in the region of the embryonic pole. The findings indicated an intrauterine pregnancy and also viability with visualization of the cardiac activity. In very early pregnancy, close examination of the region of the yolk sac may yield evidence of an embryo with cardiac activity.

**Arrowhead** = Double decidual gestational sac
**E** = Embryonic pole with cardiac activity
**Y** = Yolk sac

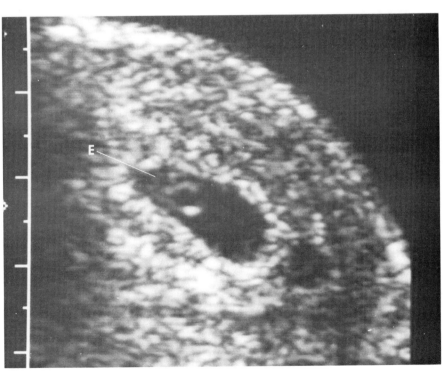

FIG 16–16.

## Normal Early Pregnancy

Figure 16–17 is a transverse scan of a pregnancy of 6 weeks by menstrual dating. There is a double decidual gestational sac sign (arrowheads). This double sac is slightly exaggerated compared to what was seen in previous cases. The lucent area between the echogenic regions represents the uterine cavity. The patient was experiencing some vaginal bleeding at the time of examination. The exaggerated double decidual gestational sac appearance is secondary to fluid within the endometrial cavity. The separation is between the decidual parietalis and the decidua capsularis. This appearance may be seen in patients with clinical symptoms of vaginal bleeding. Often these symptoms are inconsequential and a normal pregnancy ensues.

Figure 16–18 is a transverse scan showing the uterine cavity in magnified view. In vitro fertilization had been performed 35 days before the scan. The ultrasound findings correspond to a gestational age of 7 weeks by menstrual dating. The mean gestational sac diameter was 2.1 cm, corresponding a gestational age of 51 days by menstrual dating. The menstrual age can be roughly determined by adding 30 to the mean gestational sac diameter: 30 + 21 (mm) = 51 days, which corresponds closely to the patient's history of 49 days since fertilization. The yolk sac is well seen in this case (Y). Adjacent to the yolk sac are some linear echoes representing the embryo (E). In this magnified view, fetal cardiac activity was easily identified, indicating viability.

A corpus luteum cyst is often seen in association with pregnancy. These cysts can become quite large and are disturbing when initially seen. Figure 16–19 is a longitudinal scan in which a large oval sonolucency is seen posterior to the cervical region of the uterus. The sonolucency is secondary to a corpus luteum cyst. An embryo is identified within the gestational sac. The gestational sac has an elongated appearance secondary to overdistention of the urinary bladder. The gestational sac may appear deformed when

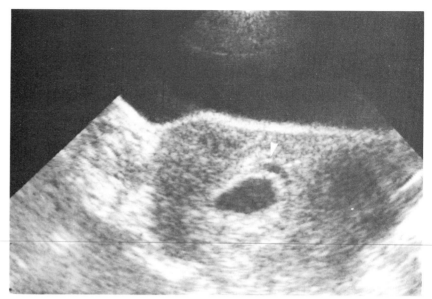

FIG 16–17.

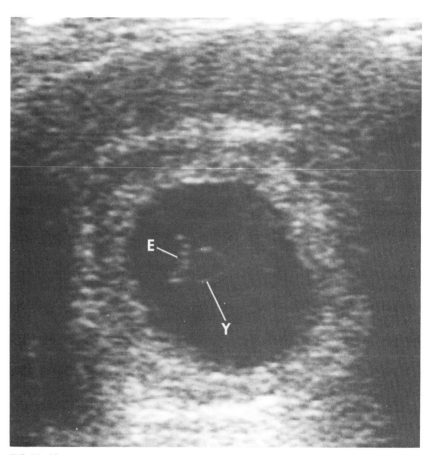

FIG 16–18.

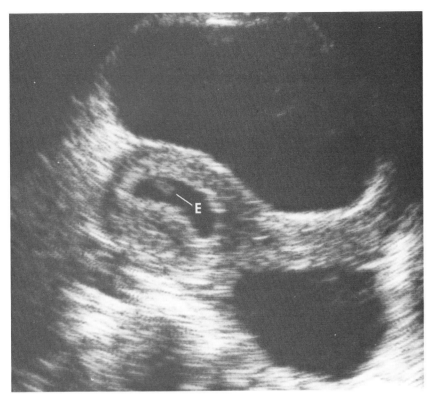

FIG 16–19.

the urinary bladder markedly compresses the uterine body and fundus. In this instance, both the embryonic pole and cardiac activity were well seen, indicating a normal intrauterine pregnancy.

Figure 16–20 is a longitudinal scan in which the gestational sac has a more oval appearance. An embryonic pole is again identified adjacent to the thickened echogenic region which will eventually develop into the placenta. A double sac appearance is noted anteriorly. Embryonic activity was identified in the region of the embryonic pole.

**Arrowhead** = Double decidual gestational sac
**E** = Embryonic pole with cardiac activity
**Y** = Yolk sac

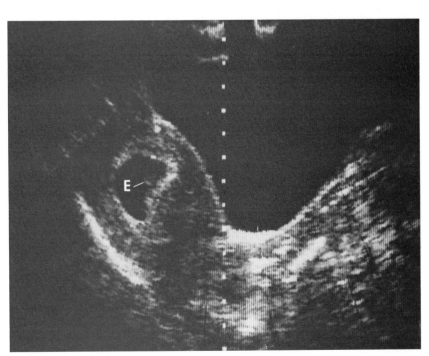

FIG 16–20.

## Normal Early Pregnancy

Occasionally, two fluid-filled areas are seen within the uterine cavity. Care must be taken to rule out the possibility of hemorrhage within the sac. The possibility of multiple pregnancies must also be considered. The earliest definite diagnosis of twin pregnancy will occur when two embryos are identifed, as in Figure 16–21. Note the curvilinear echo between the embryos, which represents the separate amniotic sacs (S). Fetal cardiac activity was identified within each fetal pole.

Crown-rump length is measured in early pregnancy. Figure 16–22 is a transverse scan of a pregnant uterus in which the embryo is seen adjacent to the yolk sac. The strong linear echo represents the midline echoes of the fetal head. Crown-rump length can be measured at this time. In this instance, the crown-rump length was 1.9 cm, corresponding to a gestational age of 8.4 weeks by menstrual dating.

Eventually the gestational sac disappears and the region of the decidua capsularis and decidua parietalis atrophies. The only region of chorionic villi that remains is in the area of the decidua basalis, which eventually develops into the placenta. Figure 16–23 is a scan made at approximately 10 menstrual weeks in which the echogenic region of the decidua capsularis and the decidua parietalis has disappeared (arrows). The echogenic region remaining in the area of the decidua basalis is the platental site (Pl).

The umbilical cord can be seen at approximately 8–10 menstrual weeks. Figure 16–24 is a scan in which the umbilical cord (arrowhead) is identified between the high-amplitude echoes of the placenta and the fetus. The crown-rump length was 2.3 cm, corresponding to a gestational age of 8.9 weeks by menstrual dating.

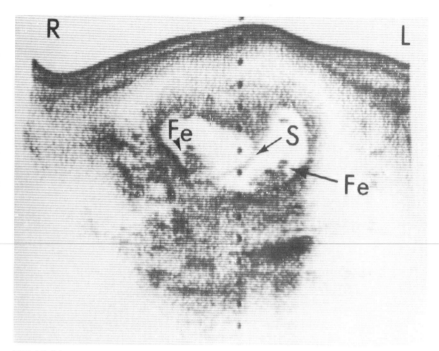

**FIG 16–21.**

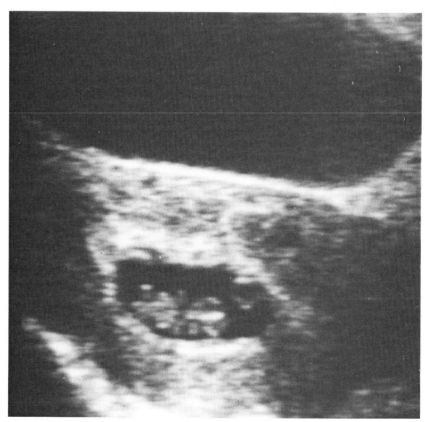

**FIG 16–22.**

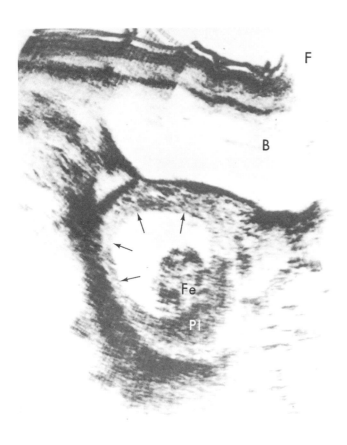

| | | |
|---|---|---|
| **Arrows** | = | Atrophy of the decidua capsularis and decidua parietalis |
| **Arrowhead** | = | Umbilical cord |
| **B** | = | Urinary bladder |
| **F** | = | Foot |
| **Fe** | = | Fetus |
| **L** | = | Left |
| **Pl** | = | Placenta |
| **R** | = | Right |
| **S** | = | Amniotic membrane separating the twin pregnancy |

**FIG 16–23.**

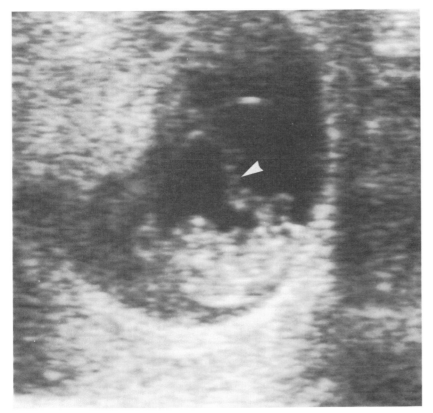

**FIG 16–24.**

## Abnormal Gestational Sac

Numerous ultrasonic signs can indicate an abnormal gestational sac. In Figure 16–25 a longitudinal scan demonstrates a gestational sac without the usual round or oval appearance. In the caudal portion of the gestational sac we see a pointed segment. A pointed segment is a strong indication that an abnormal sac is present. The same patient was scanned in the transverse plane (Fig 16–26). Here we see an uneven thickness and echogenicity to the surrounding echoes of the gestational sac. Areas of thinner echogenicity (arrows) are present on the anterior and posterior segments of the gestational sac (Fig 16–26). This is compatible with decreased vascular supply to an abnormal sac. The vascularity of a gestational sac can be evaluated from the thickness and strength of the surrounding echoes. Here we have evidence of an abnormal vascular supply.

The patient was brought back for examination 10 days later (Figs 16–27 and 16–28). Figure 16–27 is a longitudinal scan indicating marked decrease in the surrounding echoes (arrows). A transverse scan confirms the decreased echogenicity. Also of extreme importance is the fact that the gestational sac did not increase in size. If there is any question as to whether an abnormal sac is present, the patient should be studied 7–10 days later, during which time the mean diameter of the sac should increase by at least 1 cm. The main findings of this case are the pointed segment and decreased echogenicity, indicating an abnormal gestational sac.

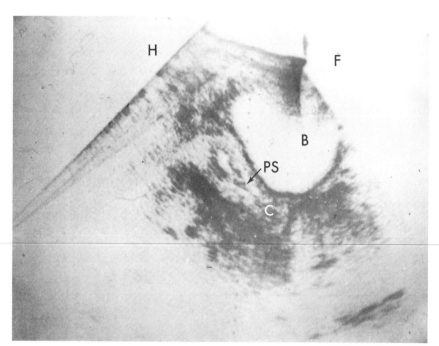

FIG 16–25.

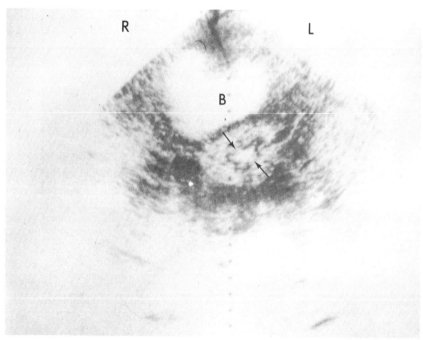

FIG 16–26.

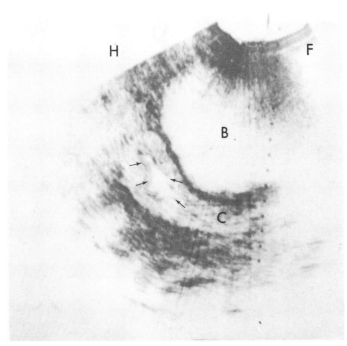

| Arrows | = | Decreased vascular supply to the gestational sac |
|---|---|---|
| B | = | Urinary bladder |
| C | = | Cervix |
| F | = | Foot |
| H | = | Head |
| L | = | Left |
| PS | = | Pointed segment |
| R | = | Right |

FIG 16–27.

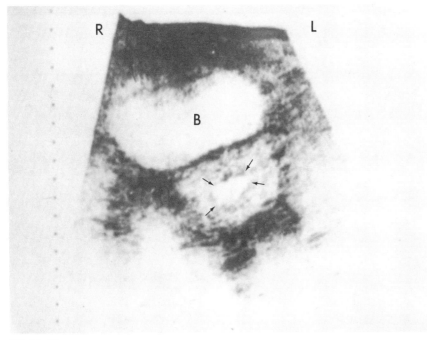

FIG 16–28.

## Abnormal Gestational Sac

The figures on these two pages show gestational sacs that have a typical round to oval appearance. The abnormality in these cases is the weak surrounding echogenicity. Decidual reaction and chorionic villi are highly echogenic. They are equal in echogenicity to the urinary bladder–uterus interface. In a healthy gestational sac, the surrounding echoes are also quite thick. These four cases are examples of normal-shaped gestational sacs with very weak surrounding echoes.

Figure 16–29 is a longitudinal scan of the uterus in a patient whose last menstrual period was 8 weeks earlier. The size of the sac is much smaller than expected for an 8-week gestation. Very weak surrounding echoes indicate an abnormal gestational sac (arrowhead). Figure 16–30 is a longitudinal scan of another patient whose last menstrual period was 11 weeks earlier. The size of the gestational sac is much smaller than expected. Because the menstual history may often be inaccurate, the appearance of the gestational sac is very important. In this case the gestational sac is seen in the miduterine body. That in itself is not abnormal. However, the surrounding echoes of the gestational sac are thin and weak (arrowhead), indicating a poor vascular supply to the gestational sac and an abnormal pregnancy.

Figure 16–31 is a transverse scan in a young woman whose last menstrual period was 10 weeks earlier. The mean gestational sac diameter was 2.7 cm. An embryo and yolk sac should be visualized by this time. The surrounding echoes are extremely thin and weak, confirming an abnormal pregnancy (arrowhead).

Figure 16–32 shows another blighted ovum; the surrounding gestational sac echoes are extremely weak and thin. The patient's last menstrual period was 12 weeks earlier. The mean sac diameter was 3.1 cm. With a sac diameter of that size, we should have no trouble visualizng an embryo.

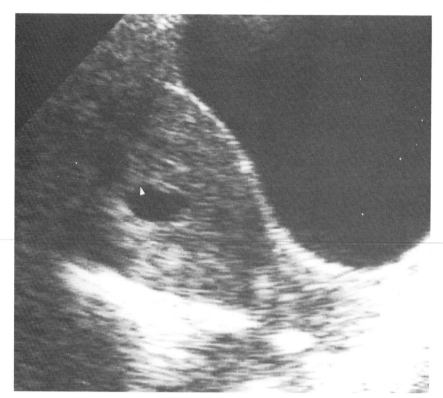

**FIG 16–29.**

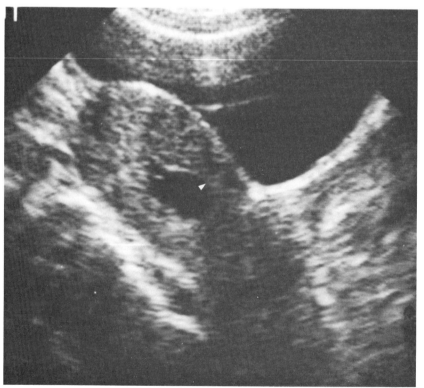

**FIG 16–30.**

**Arrowhead** = Weak surrounding echoes
of the gestational sac

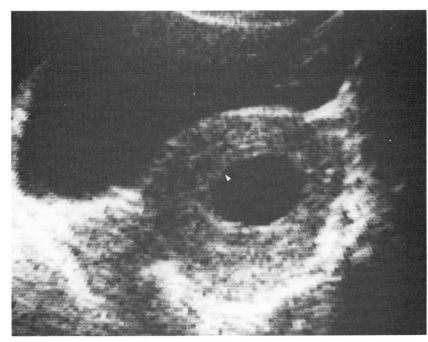

FIG 16–31.

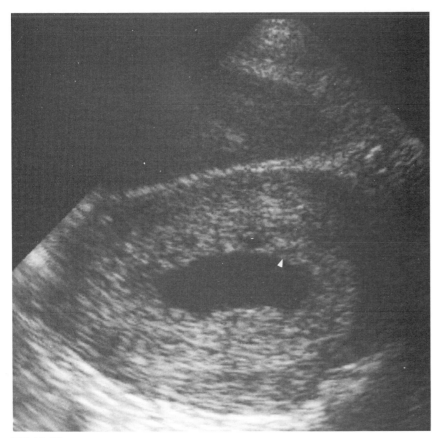

FIG 16–32.

## Abnormal Gestational Sac

Frequently a large amount of fluid is seen in the gestational sac, but without evidence of any fetal echoes. This has been termed an anembryonic pregnancy or a blighted ovum. A longitudinal scan of the uterus (Fig 16–33) demonstrates a large amount of fluid in the gestational sac. The surrounding echoes however, are quite thin and weak, indicating an abnormal pregnancy. A break in the gestational sac with some fragmentation of the surrounding echoes supports this interpretation. Figure 16–34 is a transverse scan of an anembryonic pregnancy with markedly weak surrounding echoes (arrows). This finding indicates a poor vascular supply to the gestational sac. There is no evidence of fetal echoes within this rather large gestational sac. Once a gestational sac reaches a size of approximately 2–3 cm, fetal echoes should be detectable. If fetal echoes are not present on a close and meticulous examination, an anembryonic pregnancy can be diagnosed.

Figures 16–35 and 16–36 are longitudinal and transverse scans of a patient with an anembryonic pregnancy. Here we see an empty gestational sac. Weak, thin surrounding echoes (arrows) indicate poor vascular supply to this pregnancy. When there is no evidence of a placental site with a gestational sac of this size, an anembryonic pregnancy can be diagnosed. This gestational sac is approximately 7–8 cm. By this time a markedly thick portion that will eventually be the placental site should be seen. The fetus should also be quite large by this time.

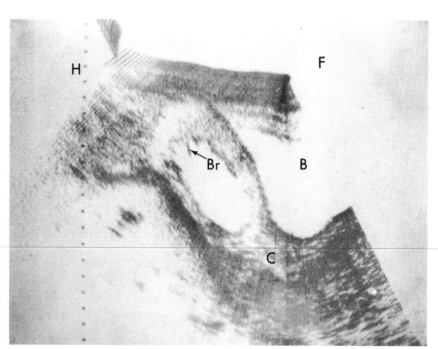

FIG 16–33.

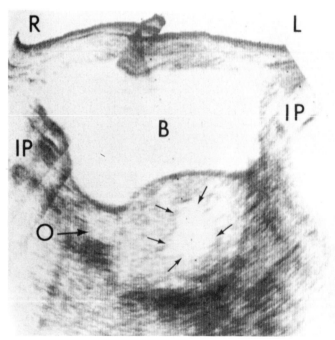

FIG 16–34.

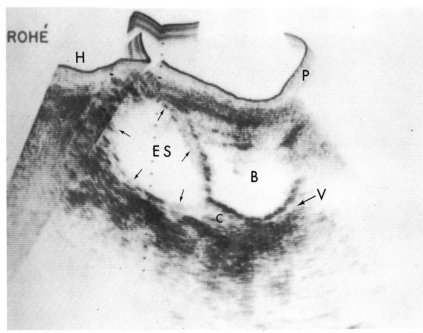

FIG 16–35.

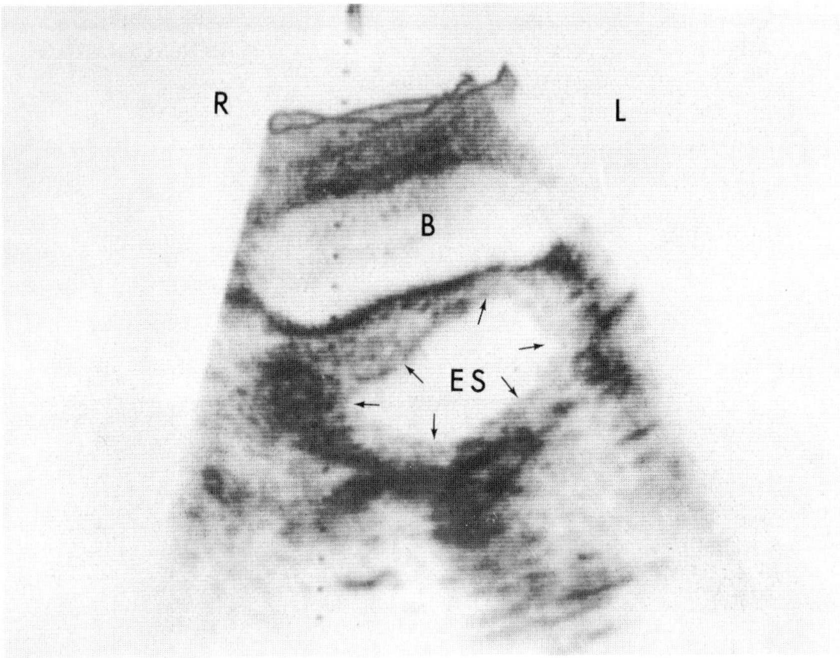

| Arrows | = | Weak and thin surrounding echoes, indicating an abnormal gestational sac |
|---|---|---|
| B | = | Urinary bladder |
| Br | = | Break in the gestational sac indicating fragmentation |
| C | = | Cervix |
| ES | = | Empty gestational sac |
| F | = | Foot |
| H | = | Head |
| IP | = | Iliopsoas muscle |
| L | = | Left |
| O | = | Right ovary |
| R | = | Right |

FIG 16–36.

## Sac-Embryo Size Disparity

The embryo, like the gestational sac, grows quite rapidly from 5 to 10 menstrual weeks. The gestational sac is first seen when it is 5–8 mm in diameter. It grows at a rate of 1–1.5 mm/day. The embryo is first visualized at approximately 6 menstrual weeks. The growth of the embryo is 1.4 mm/day. There is an expected relationship between the size of the embryo and the size of the gestational sac.

Figures 16–37 through 16–40 are ultrasound scans of four separate patients in whom there is a disparity between the size of the gestational sac and the size of the embryo. In all four cases the embryo is much smaller than would be expected from the size of the gestational sac. This is always a disturbing finding and mandates close examination of the embryonic pole to detect fetal cardiac activity. In all four cases the embryo (arrow) did not demonstrate any fetal cardiac activity. Note the large size of the gestational sacs relative to the embryos, compare the appearance with the previous cases of normal pregnancy. Another disturbing finding in these cases is the lack of high-amplitude echoes surrounding the gestational sac. The thickness of the surrounding echoes is much less than anticipated. In all four cases it would be difficult to determine the placenta site. In a normal pregnancy and with a sac of this size, the placenta is easily identified.

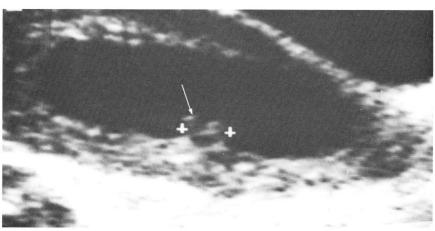

FIG 16–37.

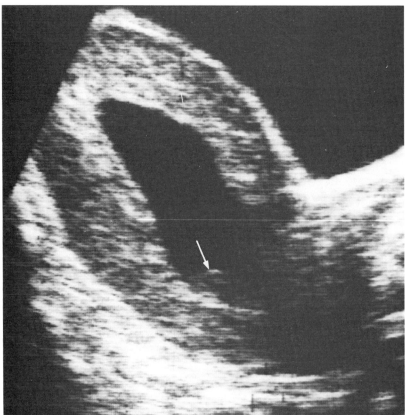

FIG 16–38.

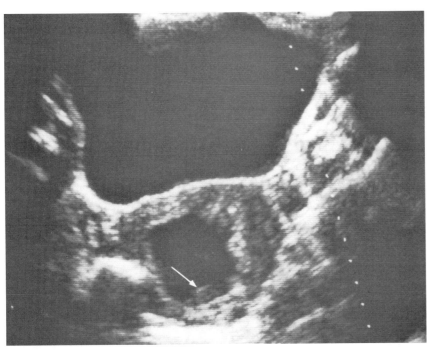

**Arrow** = Embryonic pole
**Cursors** = Embryonic pole

**FIG 16–39.**

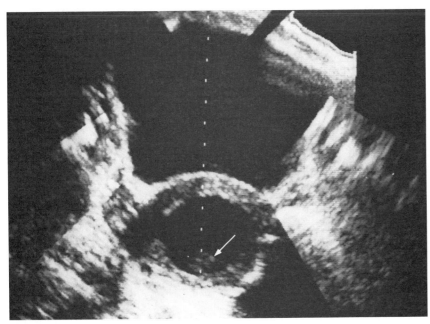

**FIG 16–40.**

## Abnormal Gestational Sac

Occasionally echoes are seen within the gestational sac that do not represent embryonic echoes. Figure 16–41 is a transverse scan in a patient whose last mentrual period was 9 weeks earlier. The gestational sac has a double ring sign, and a linear echo is noted within the gestational sac (arrow). This is secondary to layering of hemorrhage. An echo this sharp, linear, and well demarcated is most consistent with hemorrhage. There was no evidence of an embryonic pole in this case.

Figure 16–42 is a transverse scan in a patient with recent vaginal bleeding. The surrounding echoes of the decidua are less echogenic than anticipated. There is also evidence of increased sonolucency (arrowheads) to the surrounding decidual echoes. This is often an indication of hemorrhage in the decidual lining and may indicate an abortion in progress.

Figure 16–43 is a transverse scan in another patient with vaginal bleeding. Again, areas of hemorrhage are noted within the echogenic decidual reaction (arrowheads). This appearance indicates poor vascular supply to the pregnancy, as well as hemorrhage within the decidual region. Close examination of the fluid within the gestational sac reveals some soft echoes. This finding is abnormal and is most consistent with hemorrhage.

Figure 16–44 is the scan of another patient with vaginal bleeding and early pregnancy. The shape of the gestational sac is markedly abnormal (C-shaped). Also, the borders of the sac are slightly irregular. An important finding is the soft echo appearance to the fluid within the gestational sac, indicating hemorrhage. When such soft echoes are noted within the gestational sac, the pregnancy usually is nonviable. No embryo was identified in any of these cases.

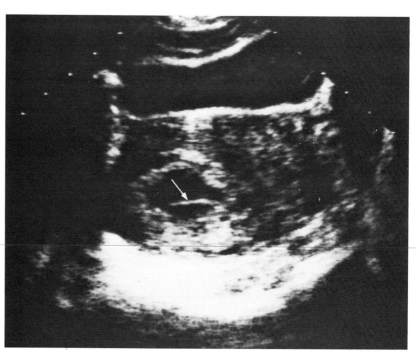

FIG 16–41.

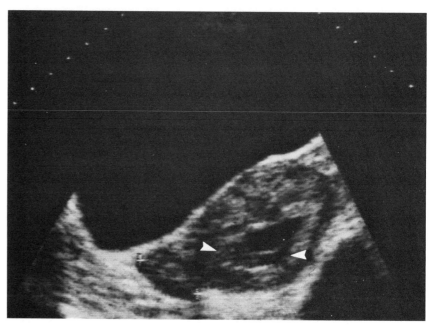

FIG 16–42.

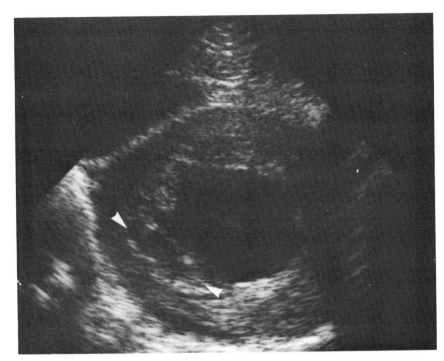

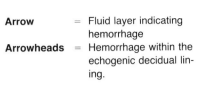

**Arrow**      = Fluid layer indicating hemorrhage

**Arrowheads** = Hemorrhage within the echogenic decidual lining.

FIG 16–43.

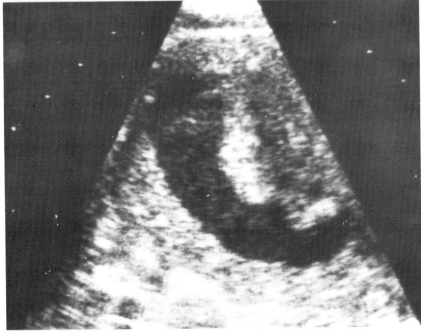

FIG 16–44.

## Low-Lying Gestational Sac

When the gestational sac is situated in the cervical region, it is an extremely worrisome finding. A follow-up examination performed several days later will often reveal that an abortion has occurred. Gestational sacs can be low-lying and normal. However, it is an unusual finding, since they are most commonly seen in the uterine body or fundal area. Figure 16–45 shows a gestational sac situation in the cervical region. No embryo was identified. The patient had a small amount of bleeding. A follow-up scan, obtained 1 week later, is shown in Figure 16–46. At this time the gestational sac had completely disappeared and a complete abortion had occurred.

Figure 16–47 is a longitudinal scan of the uterus in which the gestational sac is identified at the level of the cervical os (arrows). Although this finding could represent an ectopic cervical pregnancy, the patient was aborting at the time of examination. The gestational sac was being expelled from the uterus into the vagina.

Figure 16–48 is a longitudinal scan of another patient who was aborting during the ultrasound examination. A large amount of fluid is seen in the endocervical and lower uterine segment. The echogenic region above the fluid represents residual products of conception. During the examination the patient completely aborted, with expulsion of the fluid content into the vagina.

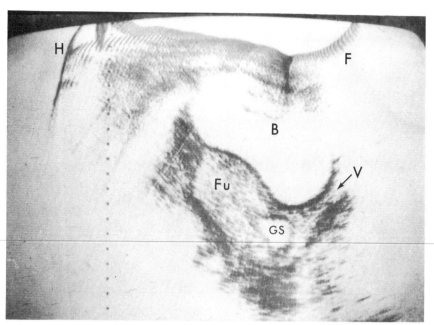

**FIG 16–45.**

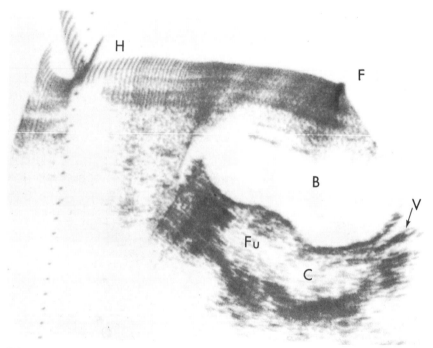

**FIG 16–46.**

Arrows = Aborting gestational sac
B = Bladder
C = Empty cervix
F = Foot
Fu = Uterine fundus
H = Head
GS = Gestational sac
V = Vagina

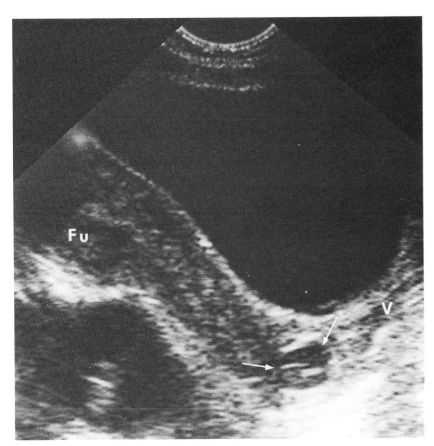

FIG 16–47.

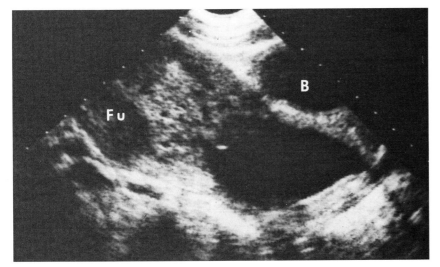

FIG 16–48.

## Incomplete Abortion

Figure 16–49 shows the retained products (arrows) of conception within the central point of the uterus. It almost appears to be an incomplete sac. However, the uterus was almost twice as large approximately 2 weeks earlier. Not only did the uterus contract down, but the central echoes of the uterus became smaller. These findings are compatible with incomplete, inevitable abortion.

Occasionally the uterus will reach a fairly large size. If abortion is taking place, the fetus and placenta degenerate. Often, such degeneration may be difficult to distinguish from a molar pregnancy. Figure 16–50 is a transverse scan of a patient with an incomplete abortion. The uterus is markedly enlarged. Diffuse, irregular echoes within it could be confused with a molar pregnancy. We can often distinguish an incomplete abortion from a molar pregnancy by the strong echoes present in an incomplete abortion.

Figure 16–51 is a longitudinal scan in which numerous strong echoes (arrows) are seen within the uterus. This uneven echo pattern is highly suggestive of an inevitable abortion, rather than a molar pregnancy. Figure 16–52 further confirms this diagnosis, since calcification is noted within the uterus. That this is a calcific density is confirmed by the shadow distal to it. If such strong calcific echoes can be identified, the diagnosis of an inevitable abortion, as opposed to a molar pregnancy, can be made.

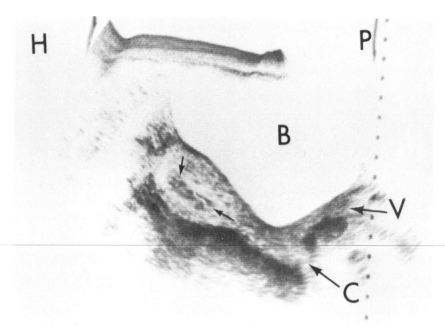

**FIG 16–49.**

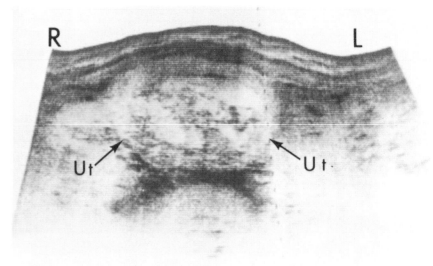

**FIG 16–50.**

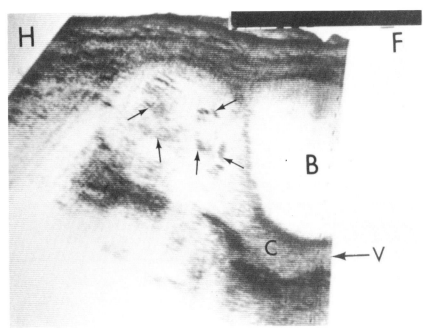

Arrows = Retained products of conception
B = Urinary bladder
C = Cervix
Ca = Calcification
H = Head
L = Left
P = Level of the symphysis pubis
R = Right
Sh = Shadowing
Ut = Uterus
V = Vagina

FIG 16–51.

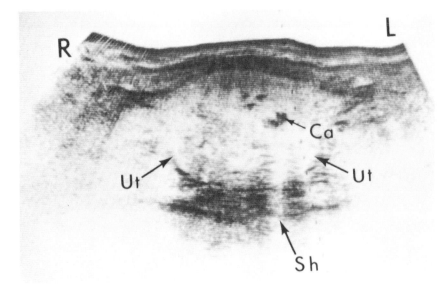

FIG 16–52.

## Incomplete Abortion

Often, a patient may undergo ultrasound examination to determine whether or not she has aborted completely. Clinically, she will be having some spotting and pain. It is not believed that the pregnancy is viable, but it must be determined whether or not the uterus has completely emptied.

Figures 16–53 and 16–54 are scans typical of a patient who has had an incomplete abortion. Strong echoes (arrows) are seen in the endometrial cavity, which is somewhat thicker than we usually see with normal menstruation. In the right clinical setting, however, the findings are compatible with an incomplete abortion. The patient can be followed up for several weeks to see whether or not the uterus empties completely. If central echoes are still present over a prolonged period of time, a dilatation and curettage should be performed.

Figures 16–55 and 16–56 are scans of an incomplete abortion which has gone on for more than 3 years. The patient had an abortion 3 years earlier without complete emptying of the uterus. Strong central echoes (arrows) are seen within the midportion of the uterus. In this instance, shadowing distal to the echoes indicates calcification within the midportion of the uterus. The retained products of conception actually contained bony structures from the fetus.

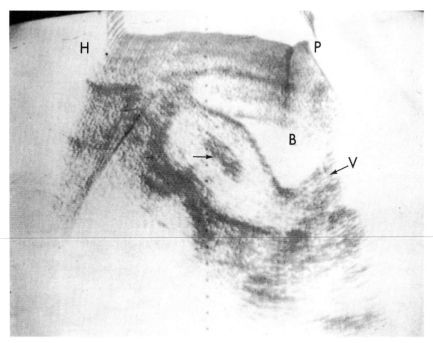

**FIG 16–53.**

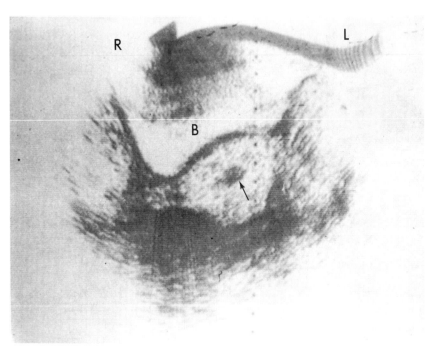

**FIG 16–54.**

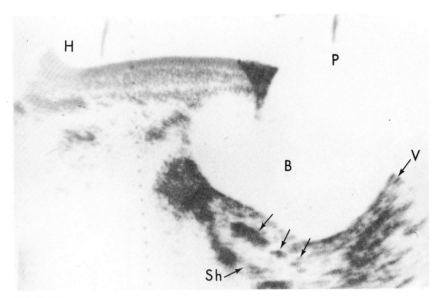

FIG 16–55.

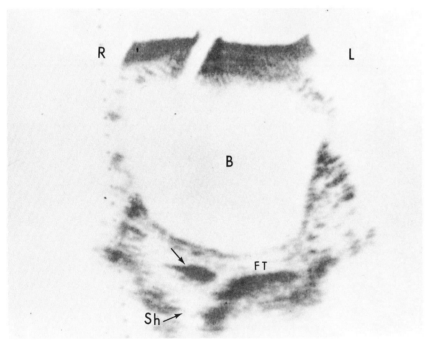

FIG 16–56.

## Ectopic Pregnancies

Ectopic pregnancies are pregnancies in which the blastocyst implants in an area other than the uterine cavity. Approximately 95% of ectopic pregnancies are located in the fallopian tube. The major role of the ultrasonographer is to ascertain whether or not a normal intrauterine pregnancy is present. If this diagnosis cannot be made with certainty, the possibility of an ectopic pregnancy is increased. The chance of finding a viable pregnancy in an ectopic location is less than 10%. Although a viable ectopic pregnancy has an impressive ultrasound picture, it is not routinely seen. The scans shown here are four different patients who had tubal ectopic pregnancies in which a viable embryo was identified outside the uterus.

Figure 16–57 is a transverse scan in a patient who had a right tubal ectopic pregnancy. The high-amplitude echoes of the chorio decidual reaction (arrow) are seen in the right adnexal area. Amniotic fluid is noted surrounding the echogenic region of an embryo. Cardiac activity was identified within the embryonic pole, indicating a viable ectopic pregnancy. The uterus (U) has an oval sonolucent region representing a pseudo-gestational sac (arrowhead).

Figure 16–58 is a transverse scan of a 24-year-old woman whose last menstrual period was 8 weeks earlier. She presented with vaginal spotting and pelvic pain. No gestational sac is identified within the uterus (U). A gestational sac is noted in the right adnexal region with the highly echogenic, surrounding chorio decidual reaction (arrow). Within the gestational sac is an embryonic pole, outlined by cursors. Cardiac activity was noted within the embryonic pole.

Figure 16–59 is a transverse scan in a 34-year-old woman whose last menstrual period was 8 weeks and 4 days earlier. She presented with a pelvic mass and pain on the left side. The clinical history does not fit the ultrasound findings. The left adnexal pain was secondary to a corpus luteum cyst, not seen on this scan. A right ectopic pregnancy is identified by

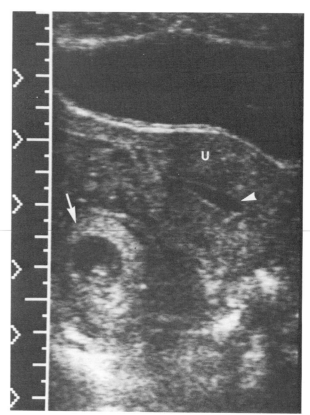

FIG 16–57.

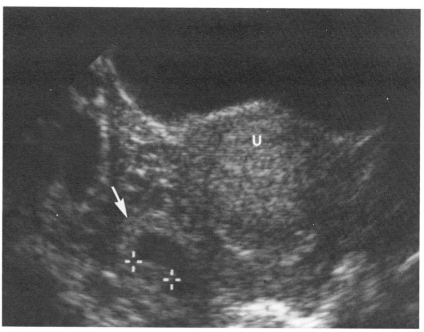

FIG 16–58.

the highly echogenic surrounding gestational sac (arrow). Within the gestational sac is an echogenic embryonic pole which demonstrated cardiac activity.

Figure 16–60 is a transverse scan of another patient who had an ectopic pregnancy on the right side. The conceptus was situated in the cornual region of the uterus. Notice the eccentric location of the pregnancy compared to uterine echoes (U). The gestational sac was situated in the right anterior region adjacent to the uterus (arrow). An embryonic pole is seen in the dependent portion. Cardiac activity was present within the embryonic pole.

All four of these cases are unusual in that the embryonic pole was identified with cardiac acitivity. Although they are impressive ultrasound scans, they are not commonly seen.

**Arrow** = Gestational sac
**Arrowhead** = Pseudo-gestational sac
**U** = Uterus

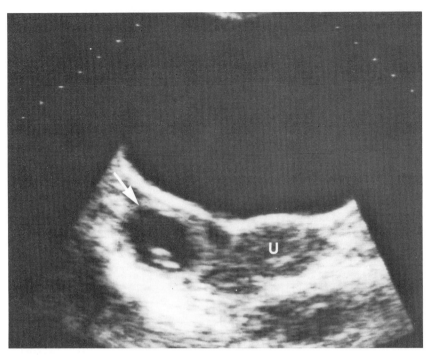

FIG 16–59.

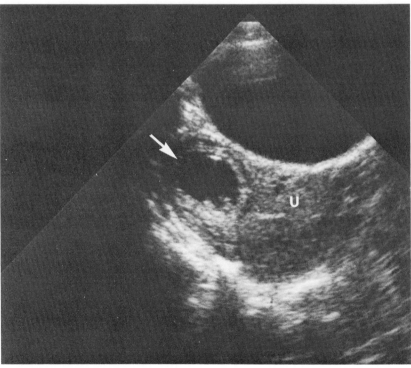

FIG 16–60.

## Ectopic Pregnancy With No Pelvic Mass

Very often an ectopic pregnancy will be present in which the ultrasound findings are normal. No mass will be identified in the pelvis or adnexal region. This is a common occurrence which has been identified in 20% of ectopic pregnancies. Therefore, *a negative pelvic ultrasound examination does NOT rule out an ectopic pregnancy.* Figures 16–61 and 16–62 are longitudinal and transverse scans in a 33-year-old woman whose last menstrual period was 6 weeks and 1 day earlier. The patient presented with mild pelvic pain. The ultrasound examination revealed no evidence of an intrauterine pregnancy. A single linear echo is noted in the uterine cavity in Figure 16–61. This could represent menstruation, very early pregnancy (< 5 weeks), or decidual reaction of an ectopic pregnancy. The left ovary was identified on a transverse scan (Fig 16–62). The left ovary is normal in size (arrowhead). No adnexal masses or free fluid were noted. At operation a right ectopic pregnancy was found.

Figure 16–63 is a longitudinal scan of the pelvis in a 25-year-old woman with pelvic pain and vaginal bleeding. Her menstrual history was uncertain. The uterus was clinically noted to be slightly enlarged. Ultrasound examination of the pelvis revealed an empty uterus without evidence of an intrauterine pregnancy. There was no free fluid and no adnexal mass noted on ultrasound examination. The hCG level was 4,000 IU, an abnormal combination of ultrasound finding and hCG level. The study was highly suspicious for ectopic pregnancy. At operation a left ectopic pregnancy was found.

Figure 16–64 is a transverse scan of another patient who was studied approximately 7 weeks after her last menstrual period. A pregnancy test was positive. The ultrasound scan shows an empty uterus and no evidence of a gestational sac or embryo. A cystic mass is seen on the right side. This cyst has through-transmission and very little internal echoes.

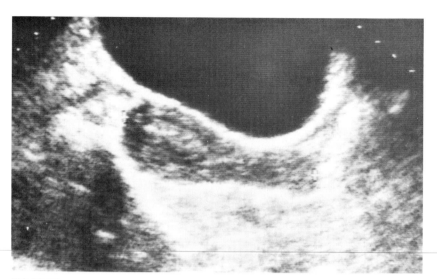

**FIG 16–61.**

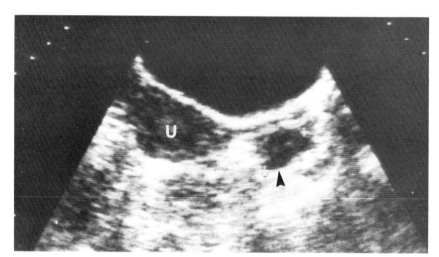

**FIG 16–62.**

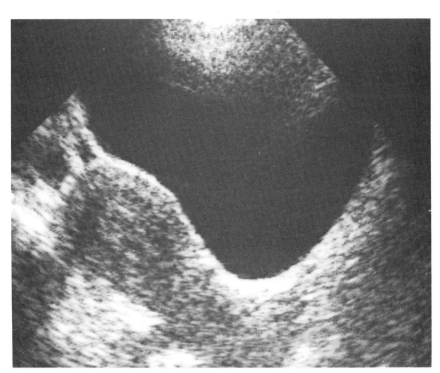

**FIG 16–63.**

The findings could represent an ectopic pregnancy, except that minimal echoes are noted. Corpus luteum cysts are usually seen early in pregnancy. This study indicates a normal right corpus luteum cyst. At operation a left ectopic pregnancy was found. No mass was deleted in the left adnexal region on ultrasound examination. The only finding was a cystic mass on the right side, which represented a normal corpus luteum cyst. A corpus luteum cyst should not be confused with an ectopic pregnancy. The important finding was that there was no evidence of an intrauterine pregnancy in all four patients, who were thought to be pregnant. No adnexal masses were found at ultrasound except for the corpus luteum cyst in Figure 16–64. In all four cases, an ectopic pregnancy was found at surgery.

**Arrowhead** = Normal left ovary
**C** = Right corpus luteum cyst
**U** = Uterus

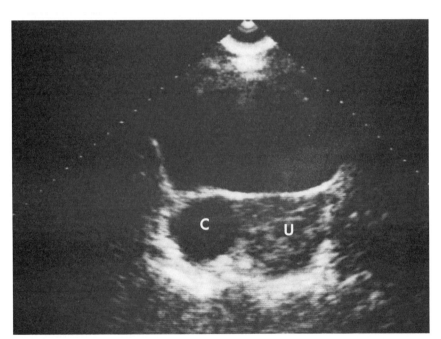

**FIG 16–64.**

## Pseudosac of an Ectopic Pregnancy

A confusing ultrasound finding is a pseudosac in an ectopic pregnancy. Figure 16–65 is an anatomic drawing contributed by Dr. Nyberg which explains the presence of a pseudosac. Decidual reaction occurs in the uterine cavity as the uterus prepares for implantation. If hemorrhage occurs, the central portion of the uterine cavity may be echo free. The surrounding decidual reaction will be echogenic. Therefore, the ultrasound findings will be those of an echogenic sac with central lucency. However, there will not be the double gestational sac appearance that is noted in a normal intrauterine pregnancy. Therefore, a sac within the uterus must be closely examined to ascertain whether or not it has a double or single ring appearance. If a single ring appearance is present, the possibility of a pseudosac should be considered. A single ring may also be seen in a very early normal pregnancy or in an abortion in progress. Unless a double sac can be seen, the possibility of an ectopic pregnancy must be considered. The pseudo-gestational sac is recently been reported to be present in approximately 10% of patients with ectopic pregnancy.

Figure 16–66 is a transverse scan in a patient whose last menstrual period was 7½ weeks earlier. A sac-like structure (arrowhead) is identified in the uterus. It has a single ring with some soft internal echoes. The findings are compatible with a pseudosac in an ectopic pregnancy. Other scans demonstrated an ectopic pregnancy in the left adnexal region. An embryo was identified by fetal cardiac activity was not seen.

Figure 16–67 is a transverse scan in a 20-year-old woman with vaginal bleeding and pelvic pain. The uterus is deviated to the left side. A pseudosac (arrowhead) is present within the uterine cavity. Some soft echoes are noted within the pseudosac, compatible with hemorrhage. A large mass is seen within the right adnexal region, along with some fluid in the cul-de-

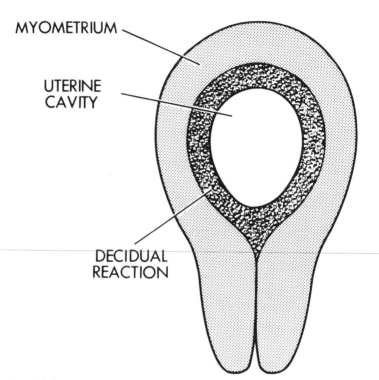

FIG 16–65.

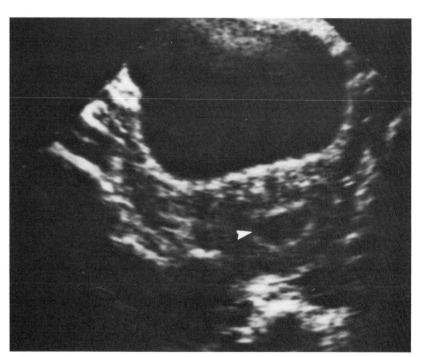

FIG 16–66.

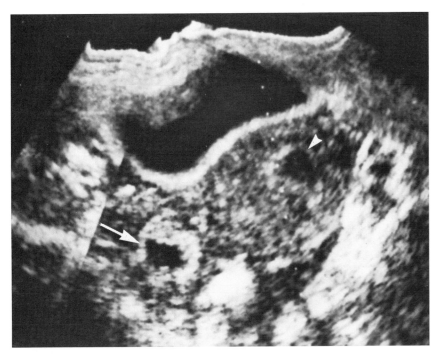

**FIG 16–67.**

sac. In the central portion of the mass are a decidual reaction and chorion villi secondary to an ectopic pregnancy (arrows). Fetal cardiac activity was visualized within the ectopic pregnancy in the right adnexa.

Figure 16–68 is a longitudinal scan of the uterine cavity in another patient with an ectopic pregnancy. A sac-like structure is seen within the uterine cavity (arrowhead). It only has a single echogenic ring. The sac is also abnormally formed and elongated. The findings indicate a pseudosac in the uterus secondary to an ectopic pregnancy.

SOURCE: Figure 16–65 is reproduced with permission from Nyberg DA, Laing FC, Filly RA, et al: Ultrasonographic differentiation of the gestational sac of early intrauterine pregnancy from the pseudogestational sac of ectopic pregnancy. *Radiology* 1983; 146:755.

**Arrow** = Right ectopic pregnancy
**Arrowhead** = Pseudosac within the uterus

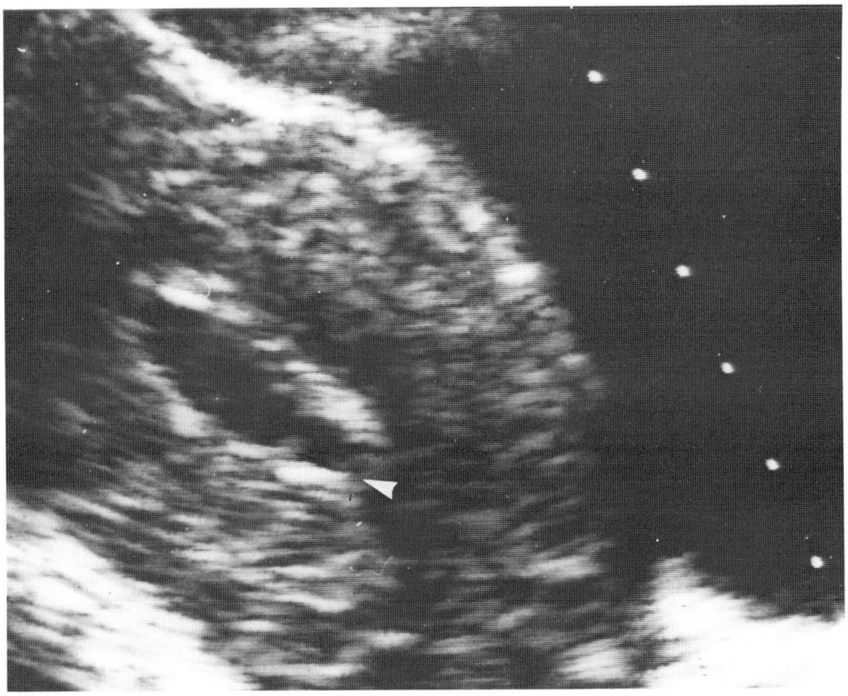

**FIG 16–68.**

## PSEUDOSAC OF AN ECTOPIC PREGNANCY

Usually the pseudosacs of an ectopic pregnancy are quite small in size. Occasionally larger sacs are identified that give an extremely confusing picture. These are most often confused with an abortion in progress. Figures 16–69 and 16–70 are transverse and longitudinal scans of a patient who had a pseudosac that measured 3 cm in greatest diameter. The patient was a 22-year-old woman who entered the emergency room for vaginal bleeding. The ultrasound examination suggested an abortion in progress. Figure 16–70 demonstrates a fluid-fluid level consistent with hemorrhage. The patient underwent dilatation and currettage, and no chorionic villi were found. At operation a left tubal ectopic pregnancy was found. The ultrasound findings in this case indicate that a pseudosac can reach fairly large size and present a confusing picture.

Figure 16–71 is a longitudinal scan in another patient who had an extremely large pseudosac in the uterine fundus and body (arrows). The pseudosac measured 3.5 cm in average diameter. It has the ultrasound appearance of a blighted ovum. However, the finding was secondary to a large decidual cast and pseudosac secondary to an ectopic pregnancy.

Occasionally, clotted blood may be present within a pseudosac and may be mistaken for an embryo. Figure 16–72 is a longitudinal scan of another patient who had an ectopic pregnancy. Within the uterine fundus is an echogenic ring suggesting a sac. This turned out to be a pseudosac (arrows). Within the pseudosac is an echogenic region (indicated by the cursors) that was thought to be a nonviable embryo. It turned out to be clotted blood within the false sac of an ectopic pregnancy.

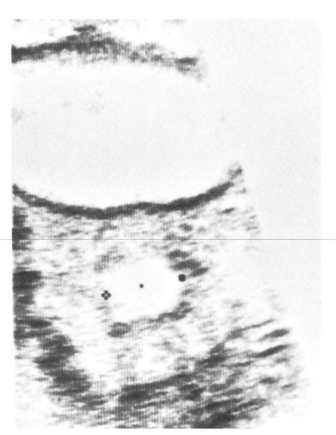

**FIG 16–69.**

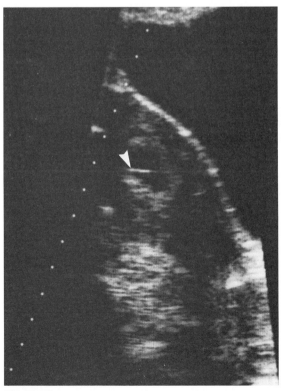

**FIG 16–70.**

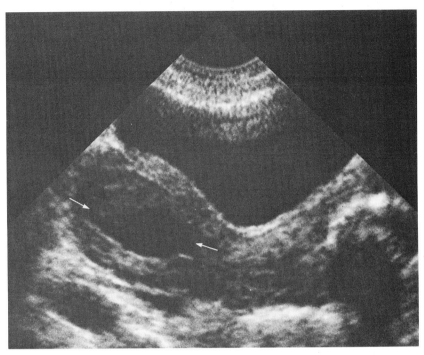

**Arrows** = Pseudosac
**Arrowhead** = Fluid layer compatible with hemorrhage

FIG 16–71.

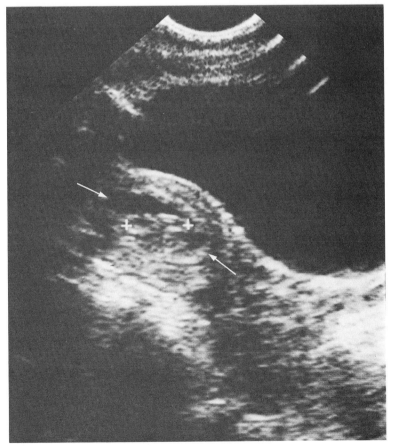

FIG 16–72.

## Ectopic Pregnancy With Pelvic Fluid

In an ectopic pregnancy, a mass may or may not be seen. Sometimes the only finding is fluid in the pelvis. This fluid could be secondary to a recently ruptured corpus luteum cyst. However, the possibility of hemorrhage within the pelvis must always be considered. On ultrasound, an ectopic pregnancy often appears as an ill-defined mass in the pelvis that is very adherent to the uterus. When the borders between the uterus and mass are lost, the appearance may be similar to that of chronic pelvic inflammatory disease or endometriosis. Figures 16–73 and 16–74 are transverse and longitudinal scans of a right ectopic pregnancy. Pelvic fluid is noted posterior to the uterus in both scans. The fluid is secondary to hemorrhage from the ectopic pregnancy.

Figure 16–75 is a longitudinal scan in the midline in which a moderate amount of fluid is noted posterior to the uterus. The fluid was the only ultrasound finding in this case of ectopic pregnancy. The uterus was completely empty, with no evidence of an intrauterine pregnancy. The fluid in the cul-de-sac could represent a recently ruptured cyst. However, in this instance it represented blood in the pelvis secondary to an ectopic pregnancy.

Figure 16–76 is a transverse scan of the pelvis of another patient with ectopic pregnancy. The patient's last menstrual period was 6 weeks earlier. A corpus luteum cyst is present in the left adnexal region. This cyst does not represent the ectopic pregnancy. The ectopic pregnancy was not visualized on this study. Instead, a false sac (arrowhead) is identified in the uterus. Posterior to the uterus is fluid consistent with hemorrhage within the pelvis. The cyst on the left side is a normal anatomic finding and should not be confused with an ectopic pregnancy.

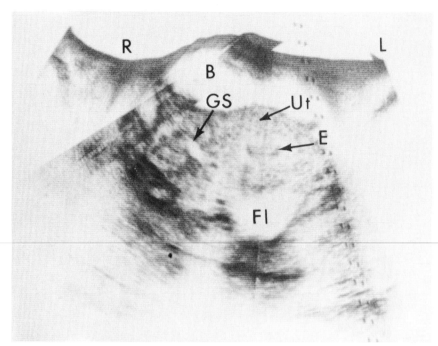

FIG 16–73.

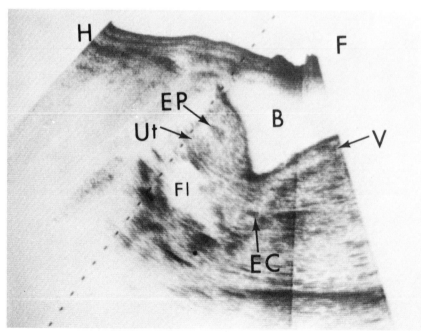

FIG 16–74.

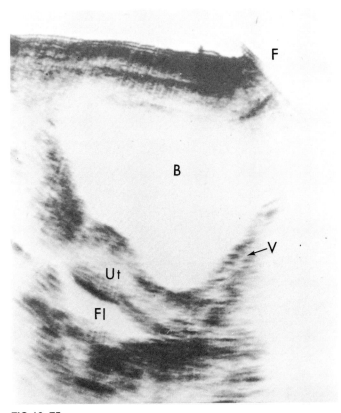

| Arrowhead | = Pseudosac |
|---|---|
| **B** | = Urinary bladder |
| **E** | = Endometrial cavity |
| **EC** | = Endocervical canal |
| **EP** | = Endometrial proliferation |
| **F** | = Foot |
| **FI** | = Hemorrhage in the pelvis |
| **GS** | = Gestational sac (ectopic) |
| **H** | = Head |
| **L** | = Left |
| **R** | = Right |
| **Ut** | = Uterus |
| **V** | = Vagina |

FIG 16–75.

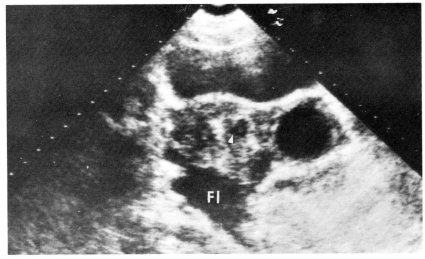

FIG 16–76.

## Ectopic Pregnancy With Hemorrhage

An ectopic pregnancy can be life-threatening. A large amount of hemorrhage may be identified in the pelvis and abdomen. It is extremely important that the ultrasonographer recognize the hemorrhage as a surgical emergency. Not only the pelvis but also the rest of the abdomen should be examined to determine if any abdominal fluid is present. Figures 16–77 and 16–78 are transverse and longitudinal scans of a patient with pelvic pain. The uterus (U) is difficult to visualize on both scans because of a large pelvic mass with numerous echoes. The mass does not have the appearance of free fluid, as was noted in the previous cases. However, it does have an echogenic appearance secondary to hemorrhage (He). The hemorrhage represents some clotted blood, which gives the numerous interfaces. It is often difficult to identify the uterus in such cases since it is lost in the hemorrhagic mass. This is a surgical emergency and life-threatening. A left ectopic was found at surgery.

Figure 16–79 is a longitudinal scan of a patient with pelvic pain. Her last menstrual period was approximately 7 weeks earlier. The uterus is empty, without evidence of an intrauterine pregnancy. The uterus is displaced anteriorly against the urinary bladder by a large echogenic oval mass with through-transmission. This mass has the characteristic appearance of hemorrhage. Because of the pelvic findings, the patient's abdomen was examined. Figure 16–80 is a transverse scan of the right upper quadrant in which fluid in the peritoneal cavity is seen displacing the liver away from the abdominal wall. The fluid was secondary to hemoperitoneum. At operation a large hemoperitoneum was identified. About 1½ L of blood was removed from the peritoneal cavity. The hemoperitoneum was caused by a right ectopic pregnancy.

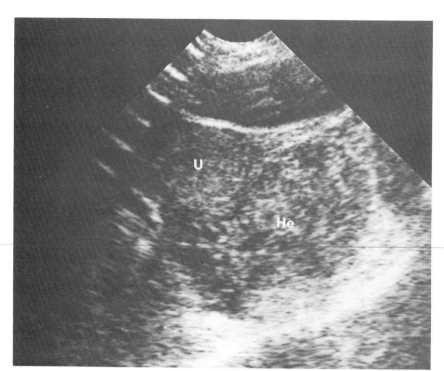

**FIG 16–77.**

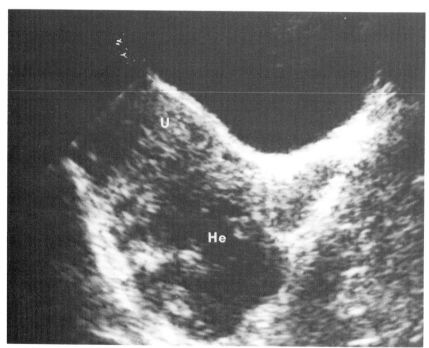

**FIG 16–78.**

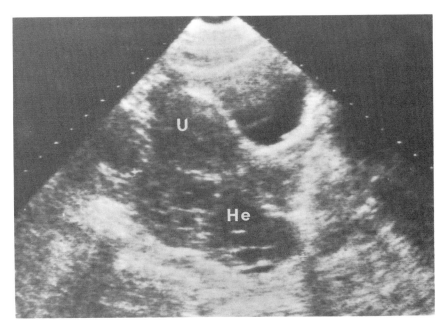

He = Hemorrhage
Li = Liver
U = Uterus

FIG 16–79.

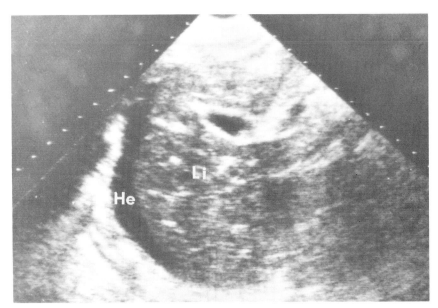

FIG 16–80.

## Chronic Ectopic Pregnancy

Occasionally an ectopic pregnancy presents as an adnexal or pelvic mass with numerous internal echoes suggesting a solid lesion. In such cases the pregnancy may be mistaken for an ovarian tumor, chronic pelvic inflammatory disease, endometriosis, or uterine myoma. Figure 16–81 is a transverse scan of a 37-year-old patient whose last normal menstrual period was 3 months previously. She had complained of some mild pelvic pain several weeks earlier. A questionably palpable mass was noted in the left adnexal region. On pelvic ultrasound a mildly enlarged left adnexal was identified (M). The findings were suggestive of chronic ectopic, endometriosis, or possibly solid ovarian tumor. At operation a chronic left ectopic pregnancy was found.

Figure 16–82 is a transverse scan of the pelvis in which a solid-appearing right adnexal mass is noted lateral to the uterus. A small linear echo is noted in the uterine cavity that may be secodary to menstrual blood or decidual reaction. No gestational sac was identified in the uterus. At operation an ectopic pregnancy of the right side was found.

Figures 16–83 and 16–84 are longitudinal and transverse scans of a patient who had a large pelvic mass posterior to the uterus. The uterus is displaced anteriorly against the urinary bladder. The pelvic mass has a mixed echo pattern with numerous internal linear echoes. Some through-transmission is identified. At operation a large chronic ectopic pregnancy was found in the cul-de-sac displacing the uterus anteriorly.

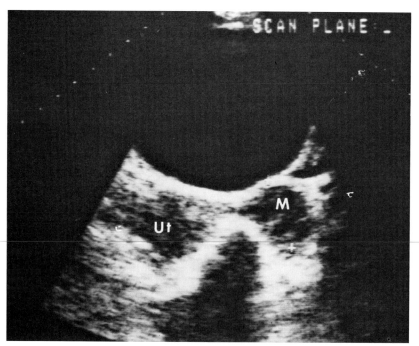

**FIG 16–81.**

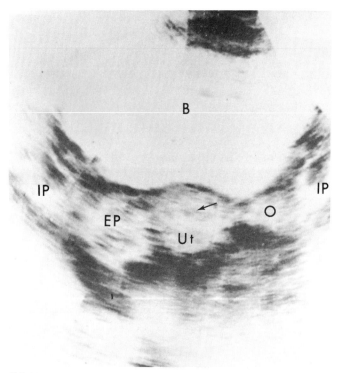

**FIG 16–82.**

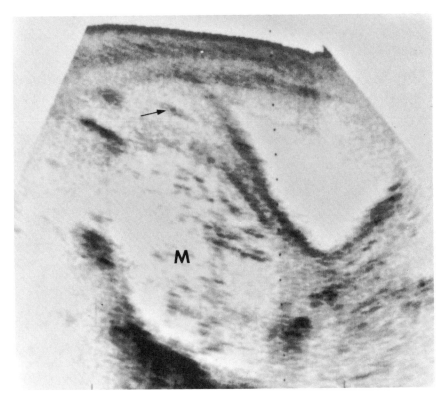

Arrow = Uterine cavity
B = Bladder
EP = Ectopic pregnancy
IP = Iliopsoas muscle
M = Ectopic pregnancy
O = Normal left ovary
Ut = Uterus

FIG 16–83.

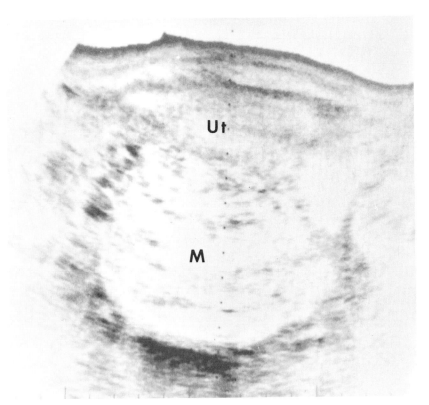

FIG 16–84.

## Abdominal Pregnancy

An intra-abdominal pregnancy is extremely rare. It often persists until relatively late in pregnancy, since the fetus has room to grow within the abdomen. Establishing a correct diagnosis by ultrasound is often quite difficult. The clue is absence of the myometrial echo between the fetus and urinary bladder or between the fetus and the anterior abdominal wall. This is often difficult to recognize because the myometrium thins out during the course of pregnancy. A second helpful clue is identification of an empty uterus low in the pelvis. Figures 16–85 and 16–86 are longitudinal and transverse scans of a 19-year-old woman who had an abdominal pregnancy that was not suspected initially. The patient elected to have a therapeutic abortion at 19 weeks. Several attempts at abortion were unsuccessful, and an ectopic pregnancy was finally suspected. At operation an abdominal pregnancy was found. Figure 16–85 is a longitudinal scan showing a small amount of fluid cephalad to the urinary bladder. The placenta is anterior to the fluid. The empty uterus is the only clue that this may be an ectopic pregnancy. The uterus (U) is inferior to the abdominal pregnancy. At the time of examination, the uterus was thought to be the lower uterine segment. the transverse scan in Figure 16–86 suggests oligohydramnios. The placenta is situated to the left side with the fetal head to the right side.

Figure 16–87 is a transverse scan of a 43-year-old woman who was approximately 30 weeks pregnant. The mass in the left side of the abdomen was thought to be a myomatous uterus. The abdominal pregnancy was not identified on ultrasound examination. At the time of delivery a cesarian section was undertaken. The patient had an abdominal pregnancy in the right side of the abdomen. She also had a 16- to 18-week-size fibroid uterus.

Figure 16–88 is another example of an abdominal pregnancy. In this instance, a moderate amount of amniotic fluid surrounds the fetus (F). Ab-

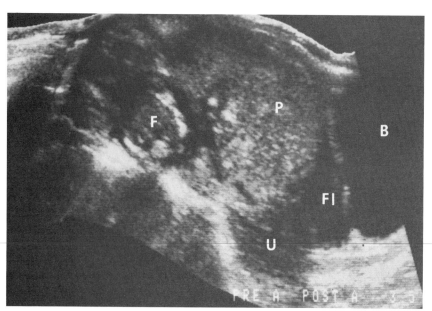

**FIG 16–85.**

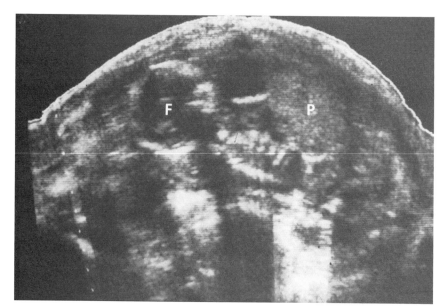

**FIG 16–86.**

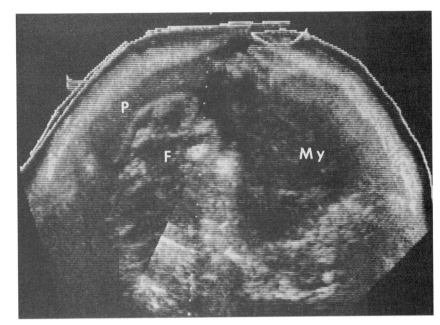

FIG 16–87.

dominal pregnancies usually are not associated with this much amniotic fluid.

**B** = Urinary bladder
**F** = Fetus
**Fl** = Abdominal fluid
**My** = Myomatous uterus
**P** = Placenta
**U** = Uterus

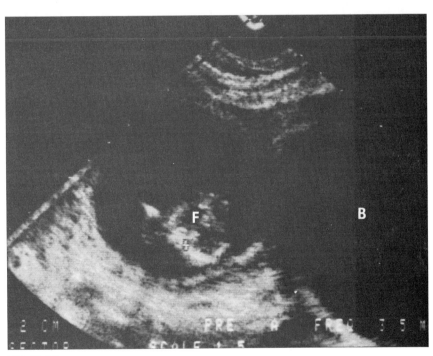

FIG 16–88.

## Gestational Age

Numerous anatomic structures are measured by ultrasound throughout the course of pregnancy. Ultrasound is a very accurate means of measuring anatomic structures because no magnification is present, as in roentgenography. In early pregnancy, the first measurable structure is the gestational sac. The gestational sac is measured from the internal diameter of the echogenic ring of the gestational sac. Figures 16–89 and 16–90 are width and height measurements of the gestational sac. The third measurement would be made in a plane perpendicular to the images shown in Figures 16–89 and 16–90. These three measurements are then averaged for a mean gestational sac diameter. The distance between the cursors is measured in a height, width, and length dimensions. Gestational sac measurements are used from 5 to 10 menstrual weeks.

The first measurable aspect of the embryo is the crown-rump length. This is measured from the top of the fetus to the rump, as is indicated by the cursors in Figure 16–91. Fetal crown-rump measurements can be obtained from approximately 6 to 12 menstrual weeks. This is probably the most accurate time for dating pregnancy. Fetal cardiac activity is easily documented at this time.

Fetal femur length measurements can be obtained from approximately 12 weeks until term. Fetal femur length is obtained by measuring the osseous structure of the femur, as shown in Figure 16–92. The high-amplitude linear echo represents the osseous structure of the femur; the cursors mark the end of the femur. The small arrow represents the femoral epiphysis.

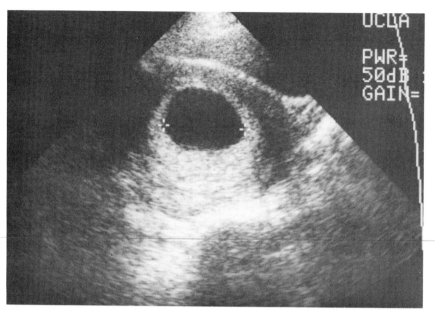

FIG 16–89.

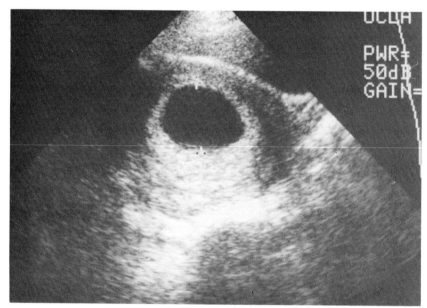

FIG 16–90.

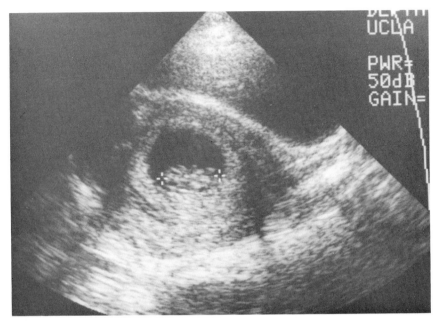

**FIG 16–91.**

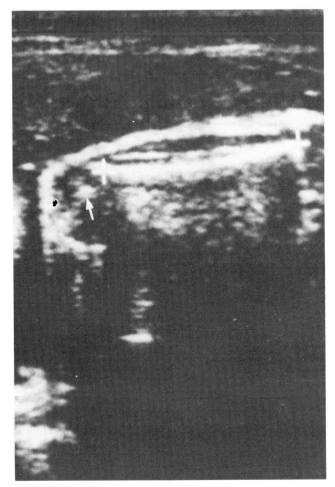

**FIG 16–92.**

## Gestational Age

Later in pregnancy, the biparietal diameter (BPD) is measured to determine gestational age. The BPD can be measured from 10 weeks until term. Measurement is done at the thalamic level. The cursors are then placed on the calvarial high-amplitude echoes. They can be placed at the beginning of each calvarial echo or in the central portion of it. It is important not to have too much gain because of gray scale widening of the fetal skull and soft tissue echoes. High-contrast, low-gain images are best when the BPD is to be measured. Figure 16–93 is an example of BPD measurement. The cursors are placed in the center of the calvarial echoes. The triangular sonolucencies in the central portion of the brain are at the thalamic level.

Fetal head circumference is also used to determine gestational age. In Figure 16–94, the circumference surrounds the outer border of the calvarial echoes.

Fetal abdominal measurements may be used to determine gestational age. Fetal abdominal diameters are measured at the level of the umbilical vein in its horizontal portion (small arrowhead). If the umbilical vein is seen in its entirety, an oblique scan of the fetal abdomen has been obtained and the measurement is not valid. Once abdominal portion of the umbilical vein has been located, the abdominal diameter is measured, as is shown in Figure 16–95. The larger sonolucent area represents the fetal stomach (large arrowhead). After the horizontal portion of the umbilical vein has been identified, the fetal abdominal circumference can be measured in a similar manner. Figure 16–96 shows the fetal abdominal circumference measured at the level of the umbilical vein.

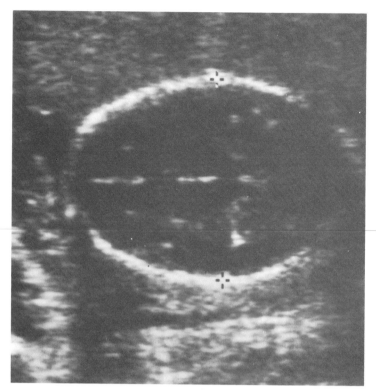

FIG 16–93.

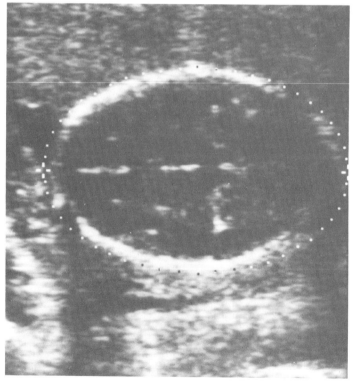

FIG 16–94.

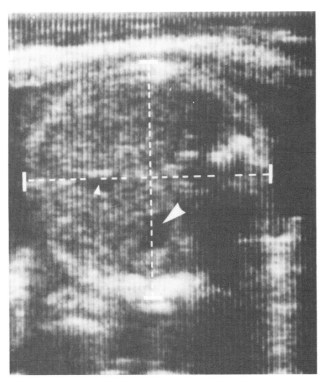

**FIG 16–95.**

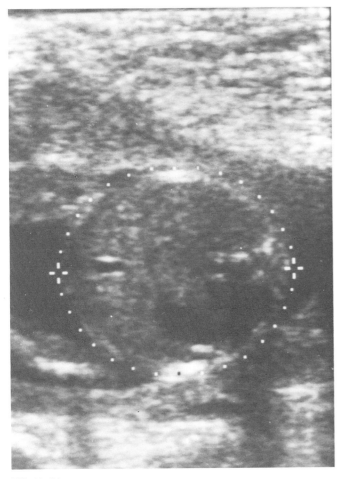

**FIG 16–96.**

## Normal Placenta

Placental tissue will appear either as an echogenic area or as a sonolucent area, depending on its position relative to the fetus and the ultrasound transducer. If an anterior placenta is present in which there is only uterine and abdominal wall between the placenta and the transducer, the placenta will appear as an evenly speckled echogenic structure. Figure 16–97 is a longitudinal scan showing an anterior placenta. Note the even parenchymal pattern through the placental texture. A strong linear echo is present between the placenta and amniotic fluid. This echo arises from the chorionic plate. Since the chorionic plate is a specular reflector, the transducer must be close to perpendicular to visualize it. It is not unusual to scan over an anterior placenta and be unable to see the chorionic plate because the transducer is not perpendicular to the interface. Figure 16–98 is another example of an anterior placenta. In this instance, several small sonolucencies are situated just beneath the chorionic plate. These sonolucencies may be secondary to choriol cysts or venous lakes. With real-time imaging, blood flow can be detected, which will aid in determining whether or not the sonolucencies represent venous lakes.

When a placenta is fundal, it has an evenly speckled appearance until it is posterior to the fetus. Figure 16–99 shows fundal posterior placenta. When the placenta has amniotic fluid or uterine wall anterior to it, it speckles in evenly as would be expected. Note the through-transmission of the placental tissue where it is deep to amniotic fluid. There is placental tissue inferior to this site which is very sonolucent. This is secondary to attenuation of the returning echoes by the fetus.

Figure 16–100 is a transverse scan of a posterior lateral placenta. Note the shadowing deep to the fetal body and fetal extremities. The left lateral portion of the placenta is well seen. It has an evenly speckled appearance as long as there is no attenuation by the fetus anteriorly. The placental

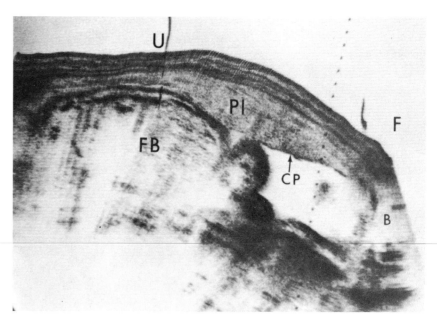

**FIG 16–97.**

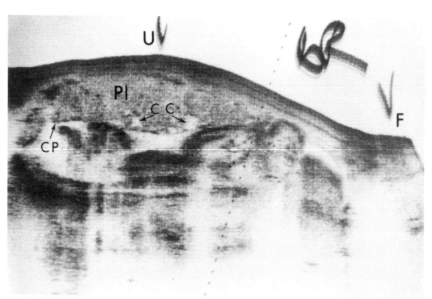

**FIG 16–98.**

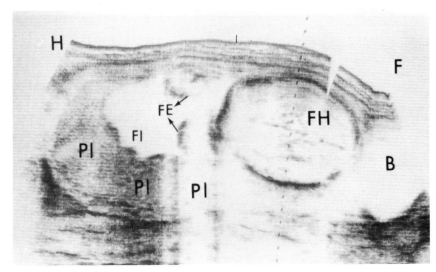

**FIG 16–99.**

myometrial interface on the lateral border (arrows) is seen. The placenta tissue is higher in amplitude than the adjacent myometrium.

| | | |
|---|---|---|
| **Arrows** | = | Placental myometrial interface |
| **B** | = | Urinary bladder |
| **C** | = | Choriol cysts |
| **CP** | = | Chorionic plate |
| **F** | = | Foot |
| **FB** | = | Fetal body |
| **FE** | = | Fetal extremities |
| **FH** | = | Fetal head |
| **FI** | = | Amniotic fluid |
| **FS** | = | Fetal spine |
| **H** | = | Head |
| **PI** | = | Placenta |
| **R** | = | Right |
| **Sh** | = | Acoustic shadow |
| **U** | = | Umbilical level |
| **UC** | = | Umbilical cord |

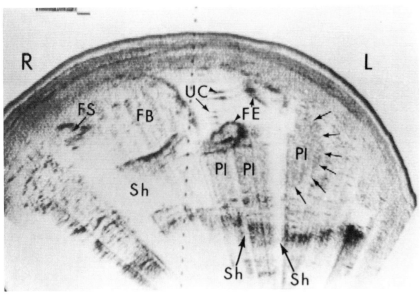

**FIG 16–100.**

## Normal Placenta

A posterior placenta is usually sonolucent because of attenuation by the fetus. It may be echogenic if it is posterior to amniotic fluid. The only way to
evaluate posterior placental texture is
by scanning through the amniotic fluid
or by scanning from the side of the
mother. Figure 16–101 is a transverse
scan of the gravid uterus in which we
see a posterior placenta. The placental tissue on the left side of the mother
has an even echo pattern, which can
be visualized because the placenta is
situated deep to amniotic fluid. The
placenta on the left side of the mother
was scanned from the anterior maternal abdominal wall. The placenta on
the right side of the mother is also
posterior. We are able to visualize the
gray level echo of the placenta. However, we did not scan from an anterior
approach since it would have been
obscured by the fetal body. Scanning
was carried out from the lateral aspect
of the mother. This may be necessary
when you are trying to determine the
placental grade.

Figure 16–102 is an excellent example of the varying appearances of a
placenta. In the fundal region, the placenta has an echogenic texture because it is situated posterior to amniotic fluid. There are then several
areas in which the placenta is completely echo free secondary to acoustic shadowing deep to fetal extremities. Between the two large areas of
acoustic shadowing is a small, thin,
echogenic region which has enhanced
through-transmission (TT). This represents placental tissue, which is visualized deep to a small area of amniotic
fluid. Further down the posterior segment is another area of shadowing
which is deep to the region of the fetal
neck. In the area deep to the fetal
head is another relatively sonolucent
region. The distance between the fetal
head (FH) and the maternal sacrum
(MS) is demarcated on the scan in
Figure 16–102. This becomes an important measurement to rule out the
possibility of placenta previa. If this
distance is greater than 2.5 cm, the
question of placenta previa should be
raised. If the fetal head is elevated out

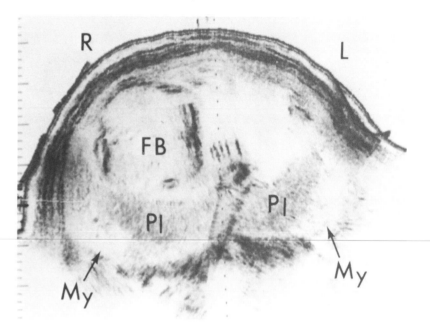

FIG 16–101.

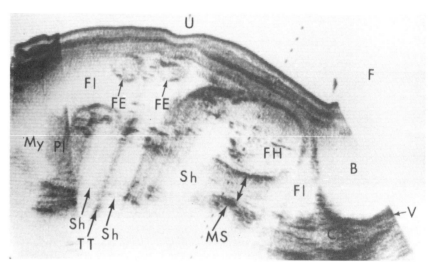

FIG 16–102.

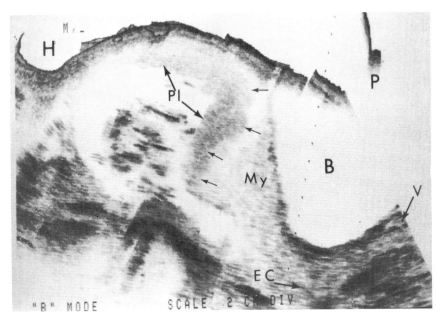

**FIG 16–103.**

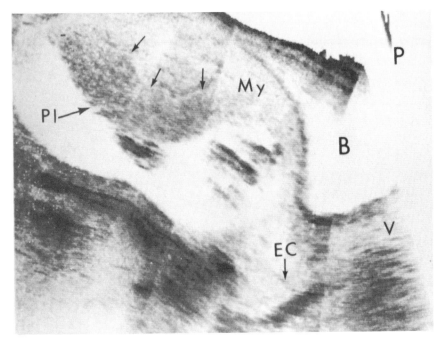

**FIG 16–104.**

of the pelvis, the region can be evaluated to determine whether or not placenta tissue is in this area or whether it represents myometrium.

Uterine contractions can present a confusing ultrasound picture. Figure 16–103 is a midline scan of a low-lying anterior placenta. Note the difference in echogenicity between the placenta and the myometrium. The arrows in Figure 16–103 indicate the placental myometrial interface. Note the low position of the placenta on this scan. Figure 16–104, a scan of the same patient, was made approximately 5 minutes later after partial emptying of the urinary bladder. The lower uterine segment is not as thick as in Figure 16–103. The patient had a uterine contraction in Figure 16–103 which had relaxed by the time she was rescanned in Figure 16–104. The placenta is now situated in an anterior location. With relaxation of the lower uterine contraction, the placenta has moved away from the internal os into a more anterior position. This becomes a problem in evaluating placenta previa.

| **Arrows** | = | Placenta-myometrium interface |
| **B** | = | Urinary bladder |
| **C** | = | Cervix |
| **EC** | = | Endocervical canal |
| **F** | = | Foot |
| **FB** | = | Fetal body |
| **FE** | = | Fetal extremities |
| **FH** | = | Fetal head |
| **FI** | = | Amniotic fluid |
| **H** | = | Head |
| **L** | = | Left |
| **MS** | = | Maternal sacrum |
| **My** | = | Myometrium |
| **P** | = | Symphysis |
| **PI** | = | Placenta |
| **R** | = | Right |
| **Sh** | = | Acoustic shadowing |
| **TT** | = | Through-transmission |
| **U** | = | Umbilicus |
| **V** | = | Vagina |

## Placental Maturation

During the course of pregnancy, the placenta undergoes changes that have been termed maturation. Ultrasound findings have permitted grading of these changes. Figure 16–105 is a longitudinal scan of an anterior placenta that is considered a grade 0. The placental texture is even. The chorionic plate is fairly sharp. A small choroidal cyst is noted just beneath the chorionic plate. The placental myometrial interface does not have any area of increased echogenicity.

Figure 16–106 is considered a grade 1 placenta. The placental texture is slightly uneven compared to a grade 0 placenta. There may be the beginning signs of undulation in the chorionic plate. The texture is slightly uneven, with one area of increased echogenicity (arrow) noted within the placental region.

Figure 16–107 shows a grade 2 placenta. The internal architecture of the placenta is more uneven than in a grade 0 or grade 1 placenta. A grade 2 placenta has increased echogenicity at the basilar region at the placenta-myometrium interface. There is also some evidence of calcification elsewhere with slight attenuation. The chorionic plate is more undulated than in the previous two cases.

Figure 16–108 shows a grade 3 placenta. In this instance, the cotyledons are identified. They are completely surrounded by high-amplitude echoes which represent fibrotic and calcific changes. The cotyledons often appear as sonolucent areas between these highly echogenic regions. The septations extend from the basilar plate to the chorionic plate.

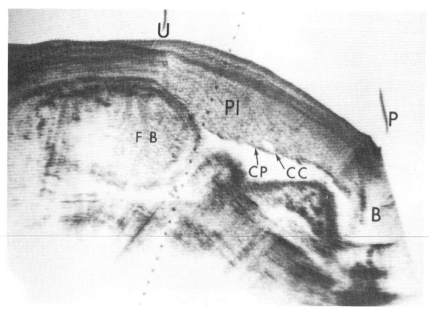

FIG 16–105.

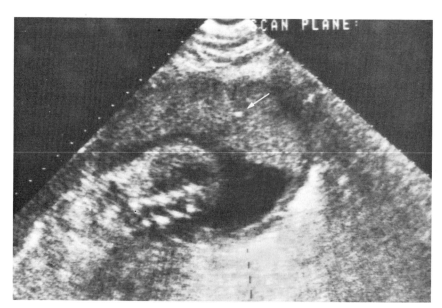

FIG 16–106.

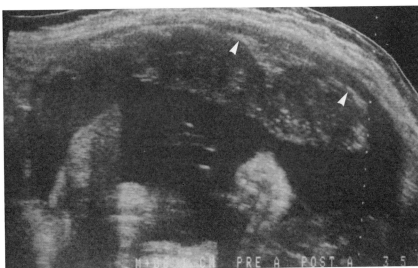

| Arrow | = Uneven placental texture (Fig 16–106) |
|---|---|
| Arrows | = Fibrous septations between the cotyledons (fig 16–108) |
| Arrowheads | = Increased basilar echogenicity at the placenta-myometrium interface |
| B | = Urinary bladder |
| CC | = Choroidal cyst |
| CP | = Chorionic plate |
| Co | = Cotyledons |
| F | = Foot |
| FB | = Fetal body |
| H | = Head |
| P | = Symphysis pubis |
| Pl | = Placenta |
| U | = Umbilicus |

FIG 16–107.

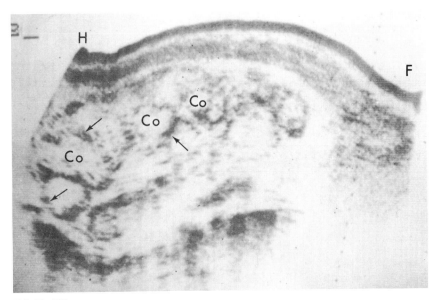

FIG 16–108.

## Placenta Previa

In examining a patient with third-trimester bleeding for placenta previa, it is extremely important to visualize not only the cervix but also the endo-cervical canal. Figure 16–109 is a longitudinal scan in which the strong linear echo of the endocervical canal can be seen within the myometrial echoes of the cervix. Since the cervix is quite wide, we can scan over a 4-cm area and just visualize the cervical myometrium without visualizing the endocervical canal. An important measurement in ruling out a posterior placenta previa is visualization of the distance between the fetal head and the maternal sacrum. In Figure 16–109 the distance between the fetal head and maternal sacrum (small arrows) is only about 1 cm. This is within normal limits, since anything less than 1.6–2 cm is considered within normal limits. Figure 16–110 is another longitudinal scan in which the distance between the fetal head and maternal sacrum is normal. Again, it is extremely important to visualize the linear echo of the endocervical canal, which is well seen in Figure 16–110.

Figure 16–111 is an example of an increased distance between the fetal head and maternal sacrum. In this instance it is approximately 3 cm. When the fetal head is elevated above the maternal sacrum, the possibility of a posterior placenta previa should be considered. Other causes for elevation of the fetal head include an extremity interposed between the fetal head and the maternal sacrum, or a fetal head that is off center, causing us to scan a lateral aspect that will appear to be elevated off the maternal sacrum. Whenever there is any question, it is important to have the patient continue filling her bladder and to make strong efforts to visualize the endocervical canal.

Figure 16–112 is an example of a bladder filled adequately enough to allow visualization of the endocervical canal. The placenta extends completely over the cervix on this scan. The placental-myometrial interface (arrows) is well seen on this study. When attempting to diagnose a poste-

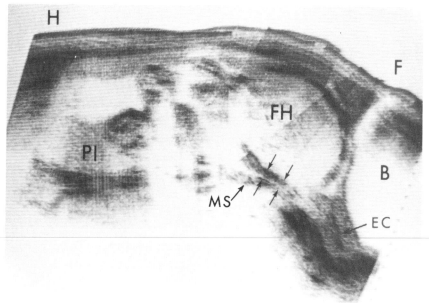

FIG 16–109.

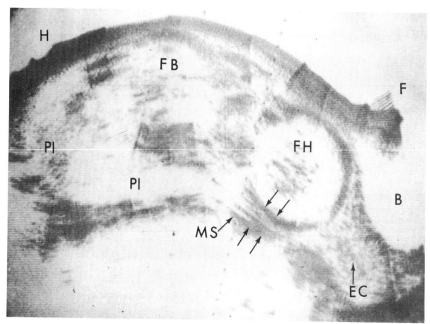

FIG 16–110.

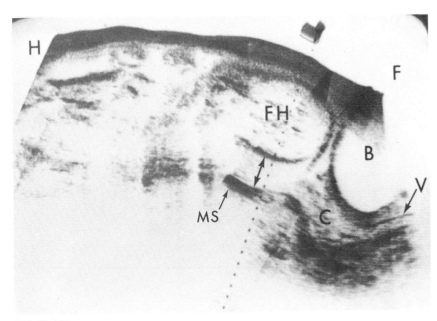

FIG 16–111.

rior placenta previa, it is extremely important to visualize not only the cervix but also the endocervical canal and the placental-myometrial interface, as is seen in Figure 16–112. If this placental-myometrial interface can be seen extending over the entire cervix, the diagnosis of posterior placenta previa can be made.

| | | |
|---|---|---|
| **Arrows** | = | Fetal head-maternal sacral distance |
| **Arrows** | = | Placental-myometrial interface (Fig 16–112) |
| **B** | = | Urinary bladder |
| **C** | = | Cervix |
| **EC** | = | Endocervical canal |
| **F** | = | Foot |
| **FB** | = | Fetal body |
| **FH** | = | Fetal head |
| **H** | = | Head |
| **MS** | = | Maternal sacrum |
| **PI** | = | Placenta |
| **V** | = | Vagina |

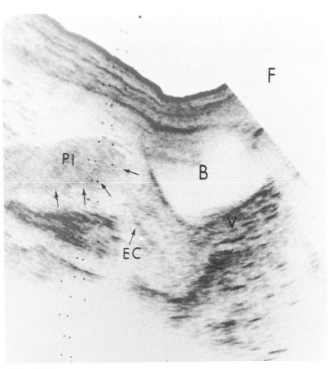

FIG 16–112.

## Placenta Previa

A central placenta previa exists when the midportion of the placenta is situated over the internal cervical os. There is usually evidence that equal portions of the placenta are situated over the anterior myometrium and over the posterior myometrium. Figure 16–113 shows a central placenta previa in which placental tissue is identified over the cervix. The placenta-myometrium interface (arrows) is well visualized as the relatively lucent band caudal to the placenta itself. This is consistent with a central placenta previa. Figure 16–114 is a longitudinal scan near the midline in another patient. A small amount of placenta tissue (Pl) can be seen over the cervix. The placenta-myometrium interface (arrows) is again identified between the placenta and the cervix. The strong linear echo within the cervix represents the endocervical canal. Visualizing the endocervical canal helps locate the region of the internal os. By looking just cephalad to this, visualization of placental tissue will indicate a placenta previa.

Figures 16–115 and 16–116 are examples of a placenta previa with sonolucent areas also visualized within the placenta and slightly inferior to the placenta. In Figure 16–115 a sonolucent area, secondary to hemorrhage, is seen just beneath the chorionic plate of the placenta. This is a complete posterior placenta previa since placental tissue is seen over the cervix and in the cervical canal. Figure 16–116 is a longitudinal scan of another patient demonstrating not only a posterior placenta previa but also hemorrhage slightly separating the placenta from the cervix.

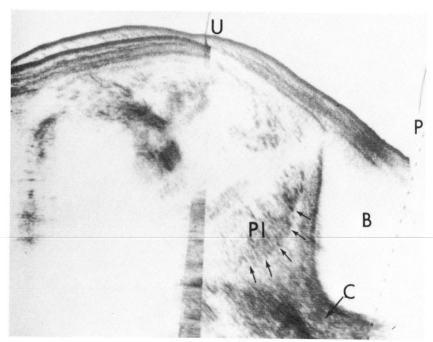

FIG 16–113.

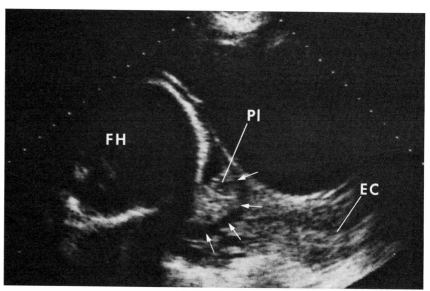

FIG 16–114.

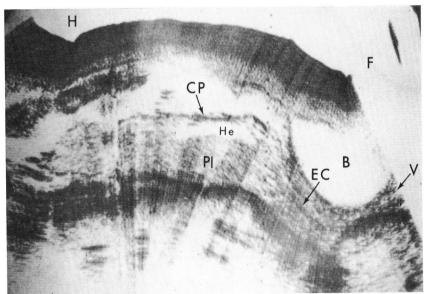

**FIG 16–115.**

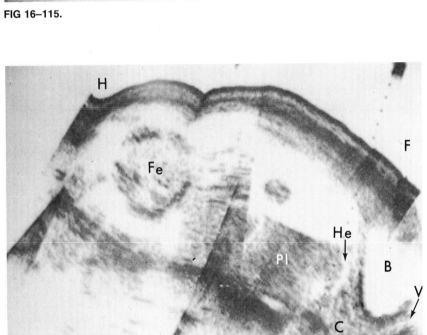

**FIG 16–116.**

| Arrows | = | Placenta-myometrium inter-face |
|---|---|---|
| **B** | = | Urinary bladder |
| **C** | = | Cervix |
| **CP** | = | Chorionic plate |
| **EC** | = | Endocervical canal |
| **F** | = | Foot |
| **Fe** | = | Fetus |
| **FH** | = | Fetal head |
| **H** | = | Head |
| **He** | = | Hemorrhage |
| **P** | = | Symphysis pubis |
| **PI** | = | Placenta |
| **U** | = | Umbilicus |
| **V** | = | Vagina |

## False Placenta Previa

Numerous situations can arise in which a placenta previa may falsely be visualized on ultrasound. The number of false positive diagnoses of placenta previas is quite high. Care should be taken to rule out a false positive diagnosis. If there is any question, a follow-up examination later in pregnancy is recommended. Placenta previa is greatly overdiagnosed in the midtrimester.

Figure 16–117 is a longitudinal scan of a patient thought to have a placenta previa. The endocervical canal (EC) is seen as a slightly lucent area in the cervical region. Note the echogenic placental tissue situated over what appears to be the internal os. An important finding on this scan is the thick myometrium posteriorly. Figure 16–118 is a longitudinal scan of the same patient obtained approximately 10 minutes later. The myometrium is much thinner than in the earlier study. In Figure 16–117, the patient was having uterine contractions of the posterior wall. When the contractions relaxed, the placenta moved into its normal position, which was more cephalad, as shown in Figure 16–118. The endocervical canal and the internal os are now visualized. The placenta is approximately 2 cm away from the internal os. Therefore, Figure 16–118 indicates that this is not a placenta previa. The findings are a good example of what uterine contraction can do to placental location.

Figure 16–119 is a longitudinal scan of the lower uterine segment. The placental tissue appears to be located entirely over the lower portion of the uterus. However, we are not over the cervix and the endocervical canal on this scan. We are off to the side of the cervix. Therefore, placental tissue over the lower uterine segment does not make a diagnosis of the placenta previa. This is another example of a false placenta previa secondary to technical factors. By scanning near the midline, we are able to visualize the endocervical canal in Figure 16–120. The endocervical canal is the highly echogenic line. The region of the internal os can be well seen. The

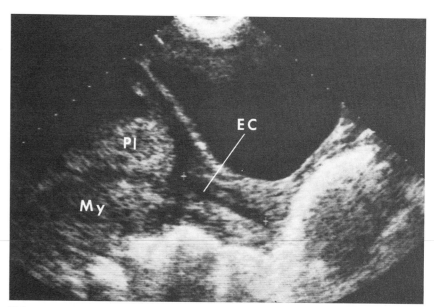

FIG 16–117.

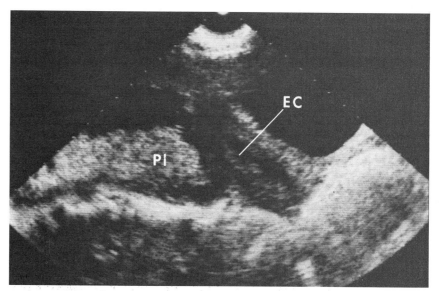

FIG 16–118.

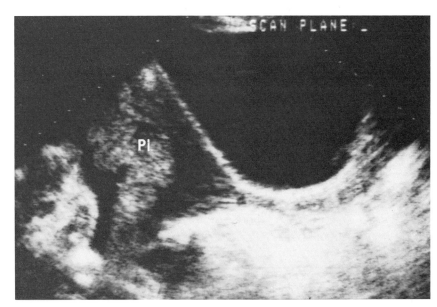

FIG 16–119.

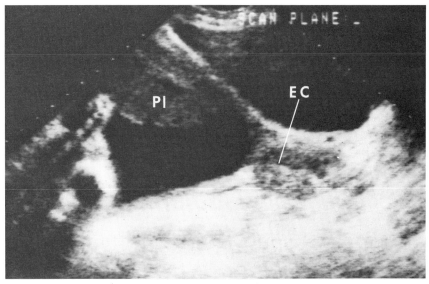

FIG 16–120.

placenta is situated anteriorly but no placenta previa is present. These two cases are excellent examples of how false placenta previas may be overdiagnosed.

**EC** = Endocervical canal
**My** = Myometrium
**Pl** = Placenta

## Subamnionic Hemorrhage

Many women undergo ultrasound examination in the second trimester for vaginal bleeding. Often an area of hemorrhage can be identified during an ultrasound examination. It is important to estimate the amount and location of the hemorrhage. Depending on the location, hemorrhage may have serious consequences. Before discussing hemorrhage, it is necessary to remind the reader that two membranes, the amnion and the chorion, are present surrounding the fetus. In the second trimester, the amnion can often be normally identified. Figure 16–121 is a transverse scan of an early pregnancy in which a sharp specular reflector (arrowhead) is identified within the amniotic fluid. This is secondary to the amnion, which is separate from the chorion. Eventually the amnion and chorion abut each other. The space between them is only a potential space later in pregnancy. One can determine that this is the amnion by watching the fetus move against it. The amnion will move easily in the amniotic fluid. Ballotting the uterus will also determine that this represents the amnion as it floats easily in the amniotic fluid.

Figure 16–122 is the scan of a patient who presented with first-trimester bleeding. A membrane is elevated off the surface of the placenta. It appears to be going anterior to the placenta. Deep to the membrane are some soft echoes indicating hemorrhage. In this instance, we have chorioamniotic separation. It is important to ascertain that the membrane is being elevated over the surface of the placenta rather than going behind it.

Figures 16–123 and 16–124 are longitudinal and transverse scans of another patient who presented with vaginal bleeding. The amnion is again noted to be elevated away from the chorion. There is no evidence of the membrane going behind the placenta in Figure 16–123. Soft echoes are present deep to the amnion, secondary to the large area of hemorrhage. It is difficult to ascertain whether or not these large areas of hemorrhage will result in an abortion. I have seen very

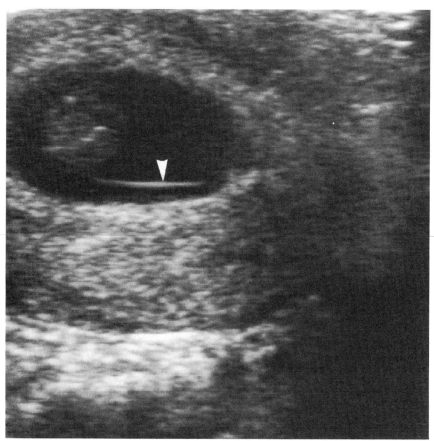

**FIG 16–121.**

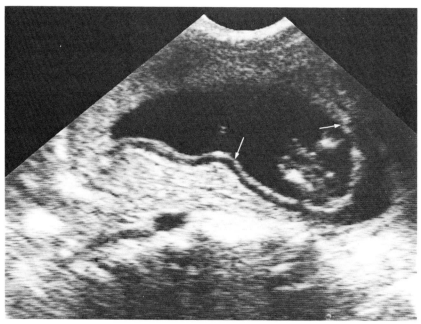

**FIG 16–122.**

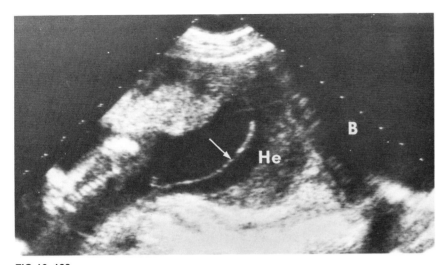

**FIG 16–123.**

large areas of hemorrhage that go on to term pregnancies. The ultrasonographer must try to distinguish whether or not the membrane being elevated is the amnion or the chorion. If it is the amnion, it will not go behind the placenta and may go over the surface of the placenta. If it is chorionic separation, the membrane will go behind the placenta.

| | |
|---|---|
| **Arrowhead** | = Normal amnion |
| **Arrows** | = Elevated amnion secondary to hemorrhage |
| **B** | = Bladder |
| **He** | = Hemorrhage |

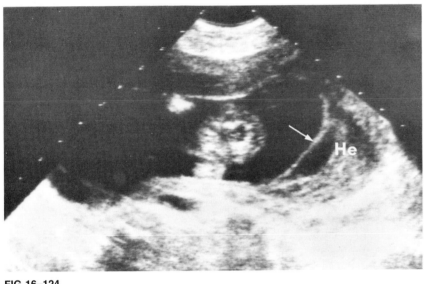

**FIG 16–124.**

## Subchorionic Hemorrhage

When membrane elevation is noted to go posterior to the placenta, it is secondary to subchorionic hemorrhage. Retroplacental hemorrhage has more serious implications than subamnionic hemorrhage. If the hemorrhage tamponades off and there is no further bleeding, then pregnancy may continue normally. However, if hemorrhage continues, the possibility of an abortion is increased. Figure 16–125 is the scan of a patient who presented at 14 weeks with bleeding and cramping of 2 days' duration. This transverse scan shows elevation of the chorion due to retrochorionic echogenic material secondary to hemorrhage (H). The hemorrhage is dissecting posterior to the lateral aspect of the placenta on the left side.

Figure 16–126 is the transverse scan of another patient experiencing first-trimester bleeding. A sonolucent area of hemorrhage (H) can be seen dissecting retroplacentally. This is another example of subchorionic hemorrhage. The important feature is the retroplacental location of the hemorrhage. Figure 16–127 is the transverse scan of a third patient who presented with vaginal bleeding and discomfort. The area of hemorrhage is quite large and is also dissecting posterior to the placenta. Figure 16–128 is a transverse scan in which we again see evidence of subchoronic hemorrhage. Note the thickness of the membrane. This is confirmatory evidence that it is subchoronic. Fetal viability was identified at the time of ultrasound examination. The patient returned approximately 4 days later with further bleeding and fetal demise.

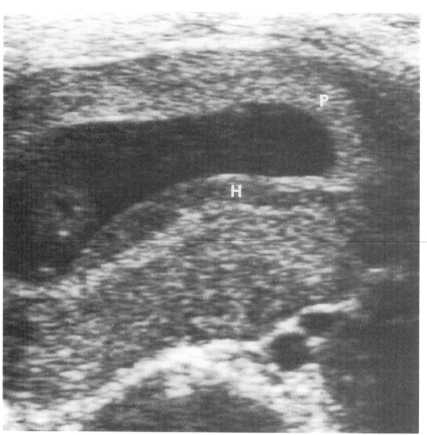

FIG 16–125.

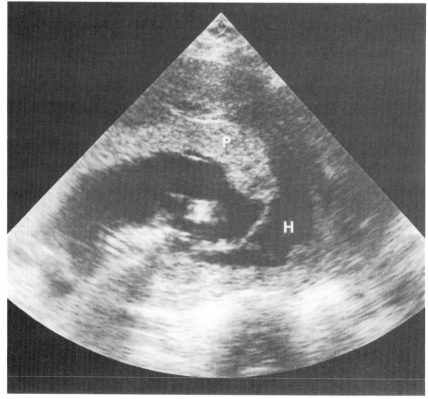

FIG 16–126.

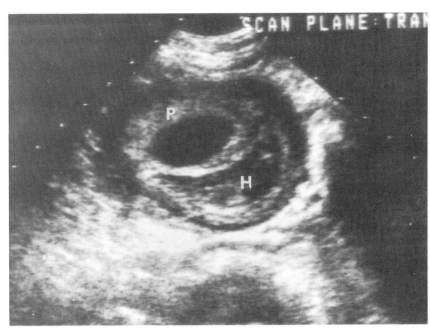

H = Subchorionic hematoma
P = Placenta

**FIG 16–127.**

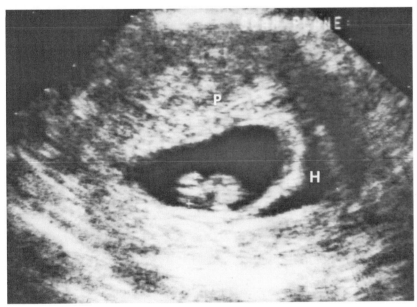

**FIG 16–128.**

## Abruptio Placentae

Abruptio placentae is often a surgical emergency. In severe cases of abruption, the patient enters the hospital with dramatic uterine contractions and bleeding. Because it is often a surgical emergency, ultrasound may be bypassed. However, we are seeing more cases of subclinical abruption that tamponade off.

Figure 16–129 is a longitudinal scan of the uterus in which a posterior placenta (P) is elevated off the fundal region of the uterus by a large sonolucent hematoma (H). The distance between the top of the uterus and the placenta is larger than anticipated. Note the abnormal contour of the placental interface. Also important is the through-transmission deep to the area of hematoma. This is not secondary to normal myometrium. It is too lucent, and too much transmission is occurring. This represents a large area of hemorrhage secondary to abruptio placentae.

Figure 16–130 is a transverse scan over the left upper quadrant of the uterus. The patient sought medical attention because of abdominal pain. Ultrasound examination revealed a viable pregnancy of approximately 32 weeks' gestation. Over the region of maximal tenderness was an area of sonolucency demonstrated on the scan in Figure 16–130 (arrowheads). The patient was extremely tender at this site. This sonolucent mass was secondary to a retroplacental area of hemorrhage. The patient was placed on bed rest, and her symptoms quickly subsided. There was no further progression of the area of hemorrhage.

Figures 16–131 and 16–132 are longitudinal and transverse scans of another patient who came to the emergency room with severe abdominal pain and uterine contraction. She was in the second trimester of pregnancy. A large sonolucent area is identified in the retroplacental regions separating the placenta from the myometrium. This large sonolucency was secondary to an area of hemorrhage from an abruptio placentae. The patient's symptoms continued, with re-

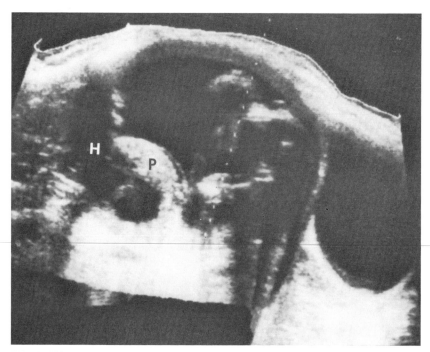

**FIG 16–129.**

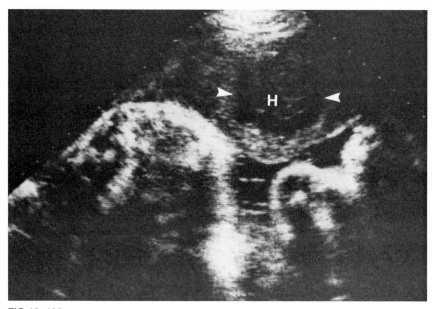

**FIG 16–130.**

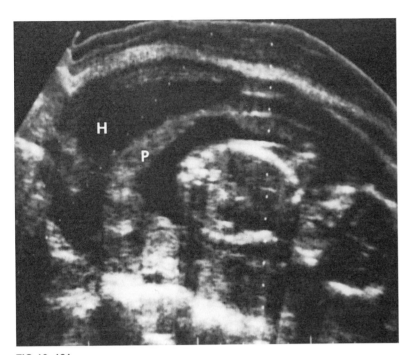

FIG 16–131.

sultant fetal demise and surgical intervention.

**Arrowheads** = Abruptio placentae
**H** = Hemorrhage in abruptio placentae
**P** = Placenta

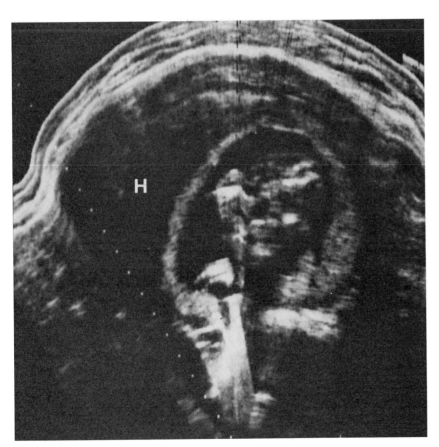

FIG 16–132.

## Abnormal Placenta

Five centimeters is considered the upper limit for normal placental thickness. It is important to measure placental thickness perpendicular to the chorionic plate. Tangential scans through the placenta can give falsely large measurements.

Several clinical entities can cause increased placental thickness. The entity most often seen in the recent past was Rh sensitization. This is decreasing with present treatment, however. Other entities such as infection, diabetes, and maternal congestive heart failure may also cause a thickened placenta. Figures 16–133 and 16–134 show an extremely thickened placenta in a patient who had Rh sensitization. The placenta is so large it occupies most of the uterine volume. Figure 16–133 is a longitudinal scan in which only a portion of the fetal head is visualized. A small amount of amniotic fluid is present. In Figure 16–134, a transverse scan, some amniotic fluid is identified along with fluid in the fetus. The fluid is secondary to ascites. Fetal bowel loops are noted floating within the ascites.

Placenta accreta is present when placental tissue invades through the decidua basalis. Placenta accreta may be suggested when there is absence of a clear space in the retroplacental region between the placenta and myometrium. Although it will not affect the viability of the fetus, placenta accreta does create problems at delivery. These problems include prepartum bleeding, uterine rupture, and the possibility of complete separation of the placenta from the myometrium at the time of delivery. Figures 16–135 and 16–136 are transverse and longitudinal scans of a patient with placenta accreta. The placental-myometrial interface is not well defined (arrowheads). In the region of the interface is a highly echogenic area with tubular lucencies suggesting placental invasion into the uterine wall.

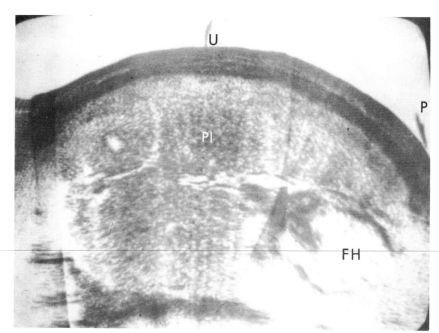

FIG 16–133.

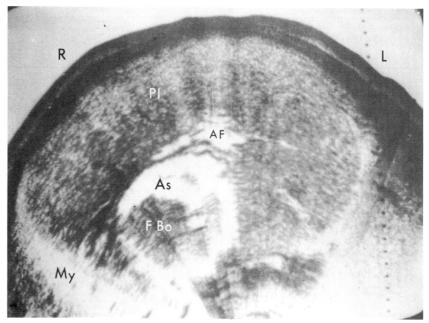

FIG 16–134.

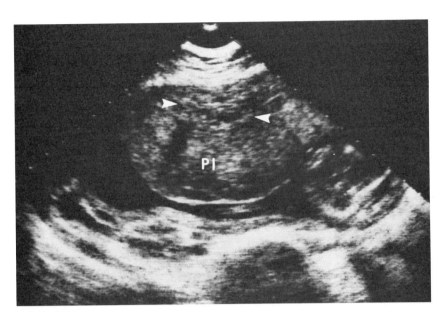

**FIG 16–135.**

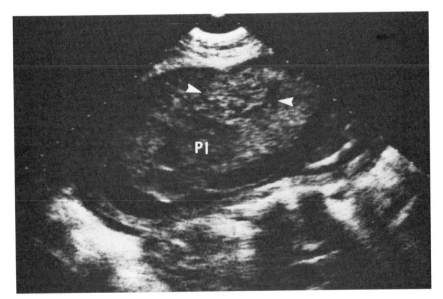

**FIG 16–136.**

| | | |
|---|---|---|
| **Arrowheads** | = | Poorly defined placental-myometrial interface secondary to placental accreta |
| **AF** | = | Amniotic fluid |
| **As** | = | Fetal ascites |
| **FBo** | = | Fetal bowel |
| **FH** | = | Fetal head |
| **L** | = | Left |
| **My** | = | Myometrium |
| **P** | = | Symphysis |
| **Pl** | = | Placenta |
| **R** | = | Right |
| **U** | = | Umbilicus |

## Hydatidiform Mole

Hydatidiform mole can present as large for dates. In this instance, the fetus is felt to be at 16 or 18 weeks' gestation, and no fetal heart tones are present. Usually the clinician will request an ultrasound study to rule out fetal death. A hydatidiform mole gives a fairly characteristic echo pattern on ultrasound. Figures 16–137 and 16–138 are longitudinal and transverse scans of a patient with a molar pregnancy. Here we see a fairly even echo pattern throughout the uterus. The mole looks like placental tissue. If, when scanning the uterus, we find echogenicity of placental tissue throughout, the diagnosis of a molar pregnancy can be made.

Figures 16–139 and 16–140 are scans of another molar pregnancy within the confines of the uterus. Here we see some lucent structures indicating the larger grapelike structures within a hydatidiform mole. This type of molar pregnancy can be confused with a degenerated placenta and fetus. Even when scanning the uterus in its entirety, however, we do not find any calcific echoes or shadows when dealing with a molar pregnancy.

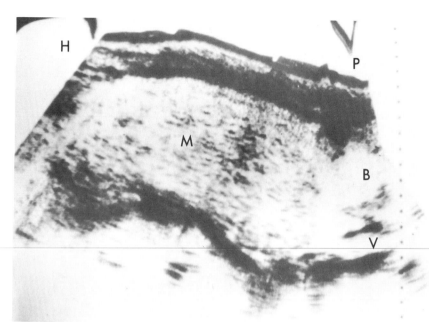

**FIG 16–137.**

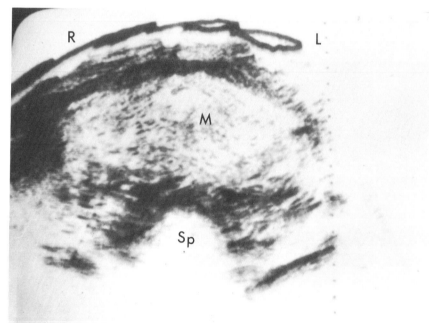

**FIG 16–138.**

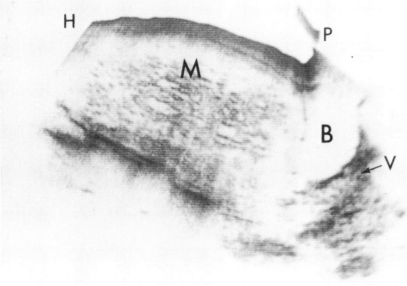

FIG 16–139.

B = Urinary bladder
H = Head
L = Left
M = Hydatidiform mole
P = Level of the symphysis pubis
R = Right
Sp = Spine
V = Vagina

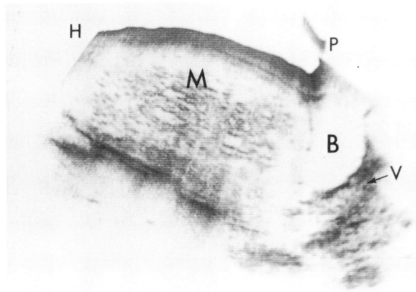

FIG 16–140.

## Early Molar Pregnancy

An early molar pregnancy is a difficult diagnosis to make. The entity could be confused with decidual reaction in an ectopic pregnancy or an abortion in progress. Figure 16–141 is a transverse scan of the pelvis in a 24-year-old woman with symptoms of hyperemesis. The uterus was much smaller than anticipated by hCG levels. Numerous small sonolucent areas are present within the uterine cavity (arrowheads). This appearance is compatible with an impending abortion. However, the high hCG levels suggested the possibility of a molar pregnancy. The patient underwent dilatation and curettage, and a molar pregnancy was confirmed.

Figure 16–142 is a transverse scan of another patient with a molar pregnancy. The uterine size was approximately 10–12 weeks. The central portion of the uterus was highly echogenic with numerous tubular lucencies throughout. These findings were secondary to hydatidiform mole (arrowhead). The possibility of a degenerating pregnancy could not be entirely excluded. However, in the presence of a degenerating pregnancy, there are usually regions of increased echogenicity suggesting some fetal degeneration. Such regions were not noted in this case.

Figure 16–143 is a longitudinal scan of the pelvis of a young woman who was thought to have an abortion in progress. Ultrasound revealed increased echoes in the uterine cavity, suggesting the possibility of an abortion. The patient did not return to the clinic and was lost to follow-up. She returned 10 weeks later with hyperemesis. Another ultrasound examination was ordered (Fig 16–144). The uterus was diffusely enlarged to approximately 16 weeks in size. An uneven echo pattern is present throughout the uterus with areas of increased echogenicity and numerous sonolucencies (arrowhead). The findings are compatible with a molar pregnancy, which she was found to have. The earlier scan (Fig 16–143) shows what a very early mole can look like. This is the same ultrasound appearance that

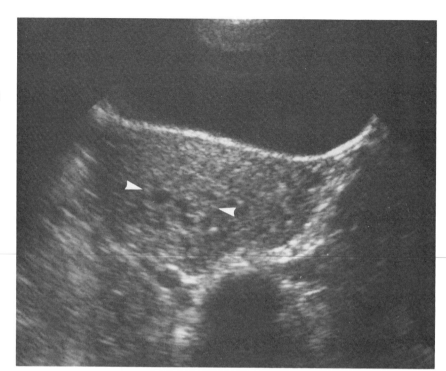

FIG 16–141.

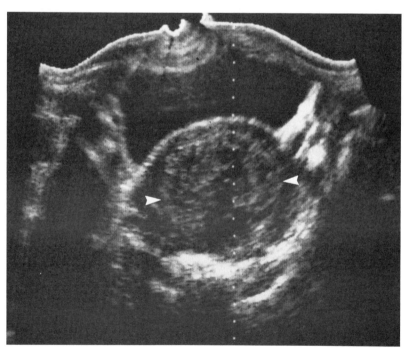

FIG 16–142.

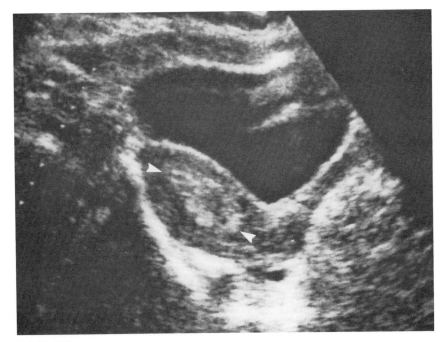

**FIG 16–143.**

may be seen in decidual reaction of an ectopic pregnancy, a nonviable pregnancy with an abortion in progress, or severe hemorrhage secondary to uterine carcinoma. There is no distinguishing feature on this scan to indicate a molar pregnancy. This did turn out to be a very early mole, which progressed to the size seen in Figure 16–144.

**Arrowheads** = Hydatiform mole

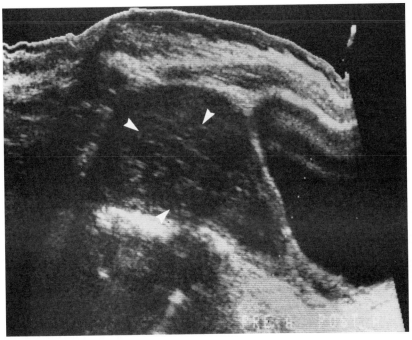

**FIG 16–144.**

## Multiple Gestation

A diagnosis of multiple gestation requires visualization of more than one embryo. The scans shown here are consistent with twin pregnancy. Occasionally a double gestational sac may be seen early in pregnancy that is secondary to a twin pregnancy. Until the embryos are identified, the diagnosis of a twin pregnancy cannot be made with certainty. One sac may be the normal gestational sac and the second sac an area of hemorrhage. Often the diagnosis of twin pregnancy in early gestation is made erroneously. Figure 16–145 is a transverse scan of the uterus in which two embryos (arrows) are identified. Cardiac activity was noted within each embryo, indicating viability. We do not see a membrane separating the embryos at this time. However, it is necessary that the transducer be perpendicular to the membrane for visualization of the membrane. The time of gestation in this case is approximately 7½ gestational weeks.

Figure 16–146 is a scan of a gravid uterus in another twin pregnancy of approximately 10 weeks' gestation. The membrane is not visible because the imager is not perpendicular to it. Fetal cardiac activity was noted within each embryo.

Figures 16–147 and 16–148 are transverse scans of the same patient. In Figure 16–147 fetal echoes are seen in each sac, and the membrane separating the two embryos can be identified. Fetal cardiac activity was detected in each embryonic pole. Figure 16–148 is a scan obtained slightly caudad. An embryo is visible on one side but not on the other side. In such an instance, the possibility of a bighted ovum could be considered. However, careful scanning would identify the presence of an individual embryo in each sac.

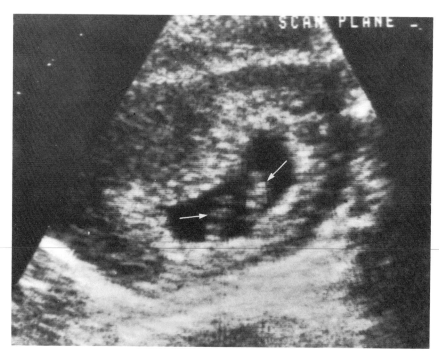

FIG 16–145.

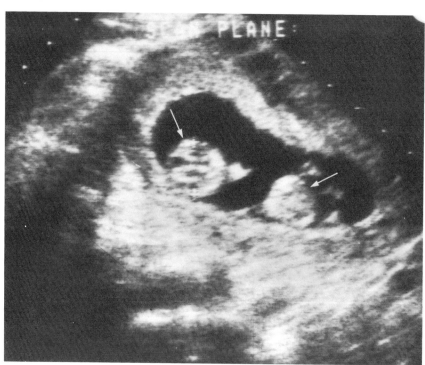

FIG 16–146.

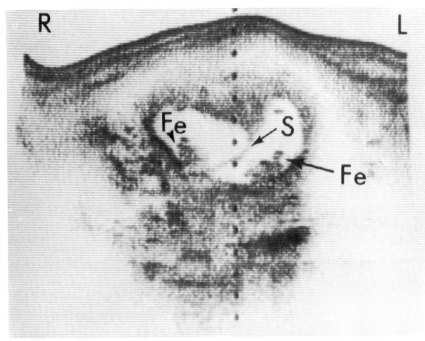

FIG 16–147.

**Arrows** = Embryos
**Fe** = Fetus
**L** = Left
**R** = Right
**S** = Membrane separating the amniotic cavities

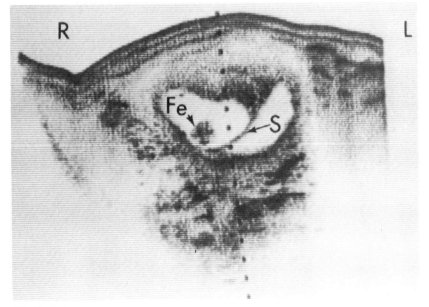

FIG 16–148.

## Twin Pregnancy With Demise

Occasionally a twin pregnancy is identified in which only one viable embryo is present. The second embryo may be visualized and found to have no fetal cardiac activity, or an empty second sac may be found. When there is an empty second sac, it is difficult to determine whether or not a twin pregnancy was ever present. The empty second sac may represent a blighted ovum of the second embryo, or what appears to be an empty second sac may be an area of hemorrhage within the uterine cavity. Unless an embryo is identified, the diagnosis of demise of a twin should always be made with caution. Figure 16–149 is a transverse scan of a 10-week pregnancy in which we see a single viable fetus (arrow). Cardiac activity was identified in the fetal echoes. An empty sac (S) is noted on the right side of the uterus. It is difficult to determine whether or not this sac represents the blighted ovum of a twin pregnancy or an area of hemorrhage within the uterine cavity.

Figure 16–150 shows another double gestational sac suggestive of a twin pregnancy. An embryonic pole is noted within the sac on the right side (arrow). Cardiac activity was identified in this embryonic pole. The pregnancy was at approximately 7 menstrual weeks. An empty sac is noted to the left (S). This most likely represents a blighted twin pregnancy because of the surrounding echogenicity. However, the possibility of hemorrhage into the uterine cavity must always be considered as the cause of such a finding.

Figure 16–151 shows a twin pregnancy in which there has been demise of one of the embryos. The embryo on the left is viable (arrow). It represents a normal 10-week pregnancy. The sac on the right (S) is much smaller than the one on the left. There is a nubbin of soft tissue (arrowhead) within the sac on the right side which is suggestive of a nonviable embryonic pole. When such findings are seen, they provide confirmatory evidence that a twin pregnancy did exist but that demise of one of the twins has occurred.

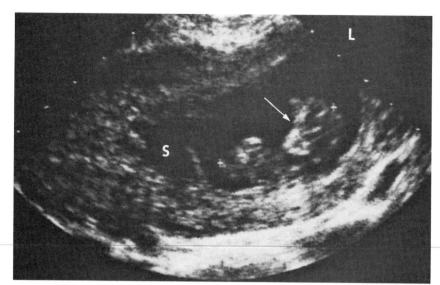

**FIG 16–149.**

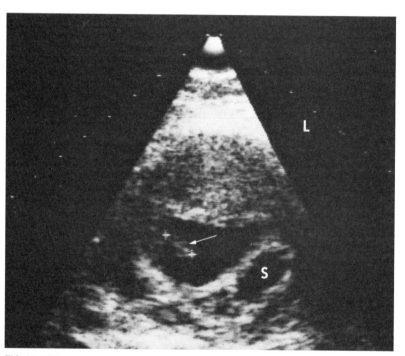

**FIG 16–150.**

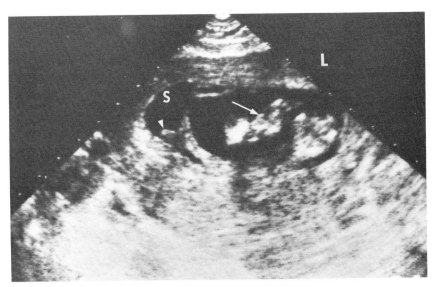

FIG 16–151.

In Figure 16–152 there is definite ultrasound evidence of a twin pregnancy. The gestational sac on the left side contains a viable embryo (arrow). The amniotic fluid in the sac on the left is quite clear. The sac on the right (S) has soft internal echoes and an area of markedly increased echogenicity (arrowhead). The area of increased echogenicity represents a macerated fetus. No cardiac activity was detected within these echoes. The soft echoes within the fluid represent the region of hemorrhage. This is definite evidence that a twin pregnancy was present but one of the embryos has died.

**Arrow** = Viable fetus
**Arrowhead** = Nonviable fetus
**L** = Left
**S** = Nonviable gestational sac

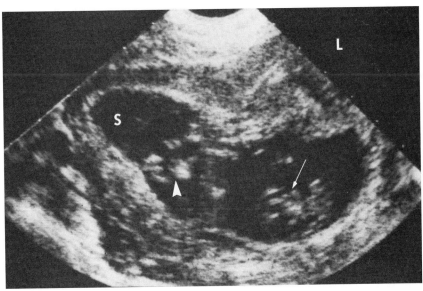

FIG 16–152.

## Multiple Gestation

Multiple gestation is usually easy to identify. If anything, there may be difficulty in ascertaining the correct number of fetuses. Triplets may be present when only twins are diagnosed. One must keep in mind that fetuses are quite active. They can move about dramatically during the course of an ultrasound examination. Therefore, it is most helpful to scan the uterus quickly to get a three-dimensional understanding of the uterine contents. By determining which fetus is attached to which body, the mistaken diagnosis of twins in the presence of triplets can be avoided. Figure 16–153 is a longitudinal scan in the midline of the uterus in which two fetuses are present in the vertex position. Figure 16–154 is a transverse scan of a different pregnancy in which we see the abdomen of the left fetus and the pelvis of the right fetus. The membrane (arrow) separating the two fetuses indicates that the fetuses are within their separate sacs. Occasionally scanning the uterus will reveal only the membrane separating the two fetuses (Fig 16–155). The amniotic membrane separating the two fetuses is quite pliable, especially in the midtrimester. It is amazing to visualize the membrane as both fetuses move about the uterine cavity. The resilience of this structure is quite impressive. Figure 16–156 is a transverse scan of a patient who was initially thought to have a twin pregnancy. However, the location of the second fetal head is actually in the myometrium. The first fetal head is within amniotic fluid and surrounded by placental tissue. The second fetal head represents a calcified myoma. It happened to be approximately the same size as the biparietal diameter of the fetus at the time of the scan. Scans made much later in pregnancy revealed that the fetus had grown while the calcified myoma stayed the same size.

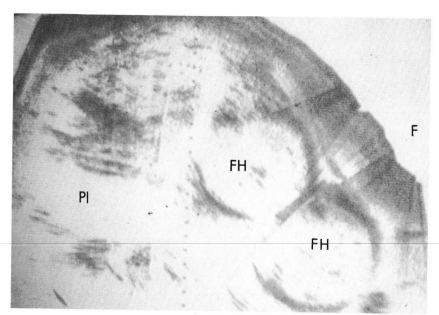

**FIG 16–153.**

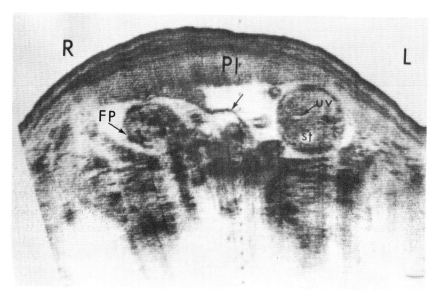

**FIG 16–154.**

A      = Aorta
Arrow  = Membrane separating the twin pregnancies
F      = Foot
FH     = Fetal head
? FH   = Calcifified myoma simulating fetal head
FP     = Fetal pelvis
H      = Head
L      = Left
PI     = Placenta
R      = Right
Sp     = Spine

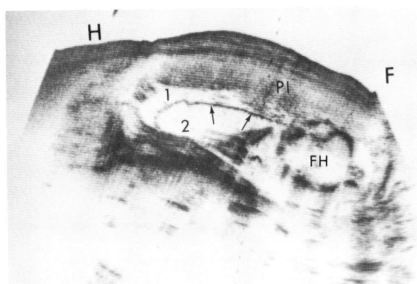

FIG 16–155.

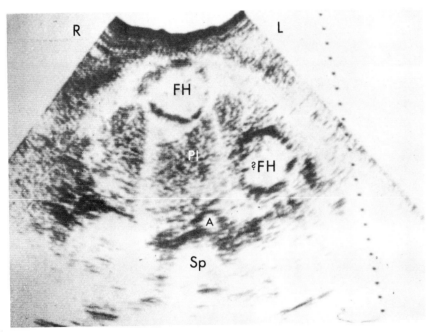

FIG 16–156.

## Multiple Gestation

When two fetuses are identified during the course of an ultrasound examination, care must be taken that additional fetuses have not been missed. By obtaining transverse and longitudinal scans quite rapidly, this error can be avoided. In Figure 16–157 three fetal heads are visualized in one scan. This patient had triplets at approximately 18 weeks' gestation. Figure 16–158 shows triplets later in the second trimester. Two fetal heads and the body of the third infant can be visualized.

Fertility drugs have increased the incidence of multiple gestations. Figures 16–159 and 16–160 are scans of the same patient in whom quintuplets were identified. The patient was taking fertility drugs, which resulted in multiple gestations. Figure 16–159 is a transverse scan in which three of the sacs are identified. Figure 16–160 is a longitudinal scan in which four of the five sacs are noted. It was impossible to obtain a scan in which all five sacs could be seen in a single image. All five fetuses were alive at the time of scanning. The time of gestation was approximately 12 menstrual weeks.

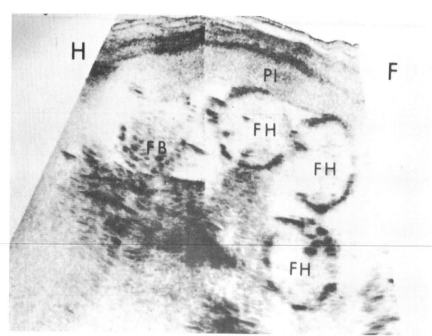

FIG 16–157.

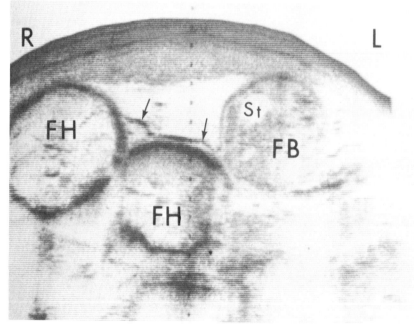

FIG 16–158.

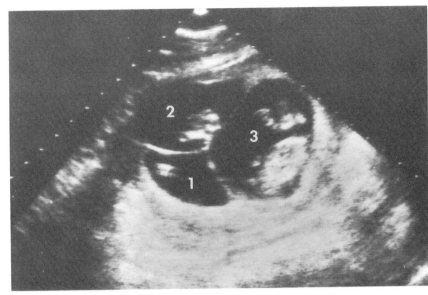

**FIG 16–159.**

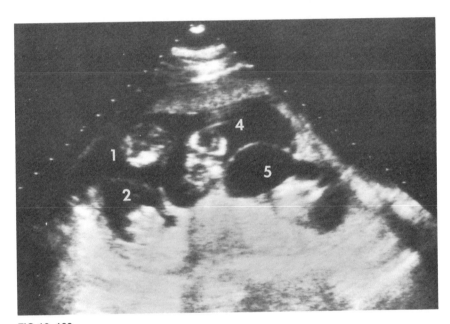

**FIG 16–160.**

## Abnormal Twin Pregnancy

A disproportion in the size of twins can be seen in cases of fetal demise. Figures 16–161 and 16–162 are scans of a twin pregnancy in which the second embryo (2) has died. In Figure 16–161, both fetal heads are identified. The normal fetal head (1) is much larger than the abnormal fetal head (2). There has been degeneration and a decrease in size of the second twin secondary to death. Figure 16–162 is a scan through the fetal abdomens of both twins. Again, the normal abdomen (1) is much larger than the abnormal fetal abdomen (2).

Occasionally the rare twin-twin transfusion syndrome may be identified. In these cases, there is an arteriovenous shunt between the twins. Often it leads to major abnormalities. A twin-twin transfusion syndrome is shown in Figure 16–163. Both twins are dramatically affected and small (arrowheads). Severe polyhydramnios was present and fetal demise was noted for each fetus. More commonly, a twin-twin transfusion syndrome causes an increase in size and edema to the twin receiving most of the blood. The twin yielding the majority of the blood because of the shunt is usually small. Figure 16–164 is an example of a twin-twin transfusion syndrome in which we see ascites (As) in the involved twin. There is also thickening of the fetal abdominal wall secondary to edema.

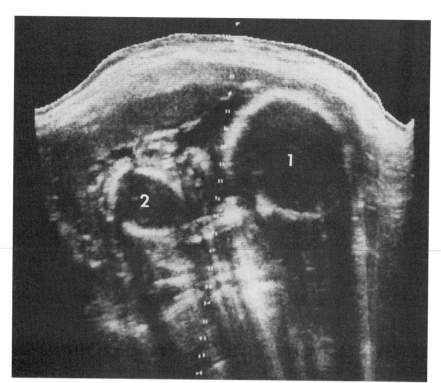

FIG 16–161.

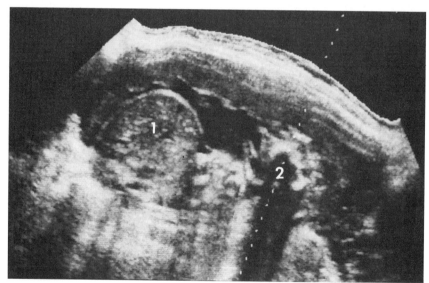

FIG 16–162.

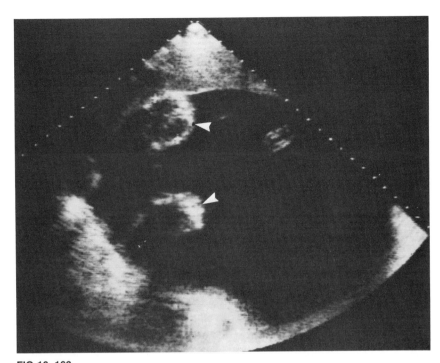

FIG 16–163.

**Arrowheads** = Twins with demise
**As** = Fetal ascites
**B** = Fetal urinary bladder
**1** = Viable twin
**2** = Twin with demise

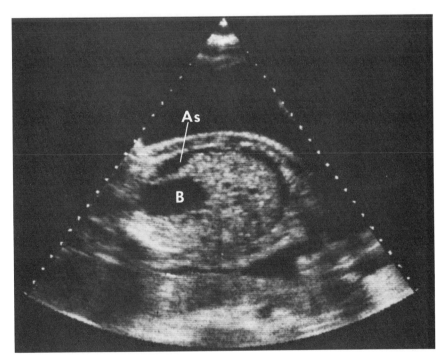

FIG 16–164.

## Conjoined Twins

Conjoined twins are an extremely rare event that occurs in approximately 1 in 50,000 live births. Whenever twin pregnancy is present, the fetuses must be examined to make sure they are completely separate. This is usually easy in the second trimester because of the amniotic fluid present. However, it can be much more difficult in the third trimester when relatively little fluid is present. Figure 16–165 is an example of conjoined twins fused at the abdomen and thorax. The fetal spines (arrows) are on opposite ends. This scan is a transverse scan through the fetal abdomen. The fetuses had a single heart. They were joined nearly the entire length of the thorax and abdomen.

Figures 16–166, 16–167, and 16–168 show another case of conjoined twins which were fused near the spine. Figure 16–166 is a transverse scan showing a single abdomen with two fetal spines present posteriorly (arrows). Figure 16–167 is a longitudinal coronal scan through the area of the fetal spines. Note the two complete sets of fetal spines (arrows) in close proximity to each other. From Figures 16–166 and 16–167, you can imagine the appearance of the fetal spine in two dimensions. Figure 16–168 is a scan of the fetuses in the region of the fetal head and neck. Two separate heads were identified (H). The fetal necks were separate. These fetuses were joined at the thorax and abdomen and had a single thorax and abdomen with duplication of the spine posteriorly.

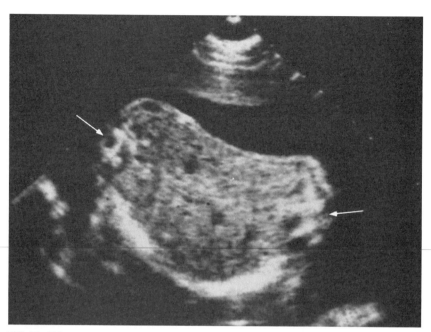

FIG 16–165.

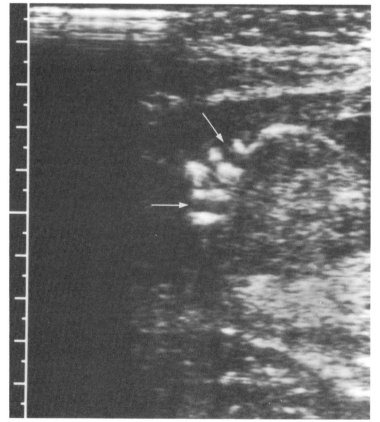

FIG 16–166.

**Arrows** = Fetal spine
**H** = Fetal heads

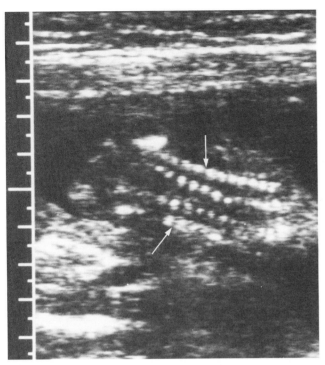

**FIG 16–167.**

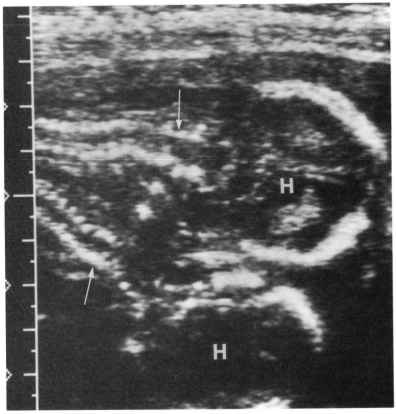

**FIG 16–168.**

## IUD and Pregnancy

Ultrasound examination is often requested to locate an intrauterine device (IUD). If the request is made during the first 10 weeks of pregnancy,
the examination can be successfull. In
early pregnancy the IUD will stand out
as a highly echogenic structure adjacent to the gestational sac. If the
pregnancy is past 10 or 12 weeks, visualization of the IUD is more difficult
because of the numerous strong
echoes arising from the fetus. In Figure 16–169, the gestational sac is
seen as a sonolucent region in the
midportion of the uterus. Lateral to the
gestational sac on the right side is a
highly echogenic circular structure
compatible with an intrauterine device.
This appearance is commonly seen in
a Copper 7 IUD. Figure 16–170
shows another Copper 7 IUD which is
seen to the left of the gestational sac.
A small amount of shadowing is noted
deep to the high-amplitude echo of
the IUD, confirming its nature.

Figure 16–171 is a longitudinal
scan of the pelvis showing a gestational sac in the fundal region of the
uterus. Three high-amplitude echoes
are noted anterior to the gestational
sac. These are the step-like echoes
characteristically seen when a Lippes
loop IUD is present. Figure 16–172 is
a transverse scan of the pelvis in
which we visualize an abnormal gestational sac. Instead of being round or
oval, the gestational sac has an irregular lobulated appearance. Anterior in
the uterine cavity is a highly echogenic region that is casting an acoustic shadow. This is secondary to a
Copper 7 IUD. In this instance an
abortion is present, as indicated by
the abnormal-appearing gestational
sac. Very often an IUD will be associated with an abortion in progress. This
is not an unusual finding. Note the
shadowing deep to the IUD which is
characteristic of these structures.

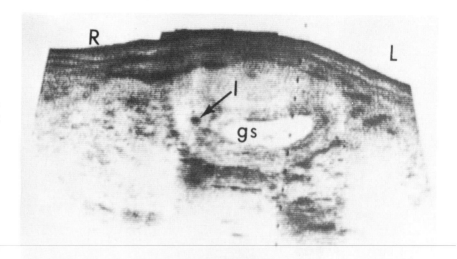

**FIG 16–169.**

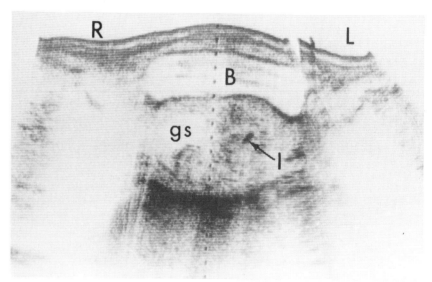

**FIG 16–170.**

B   = Urinary bladder
**gs** = Gestational sac
l   = Intrauterine device
L   = Left
R   = Right

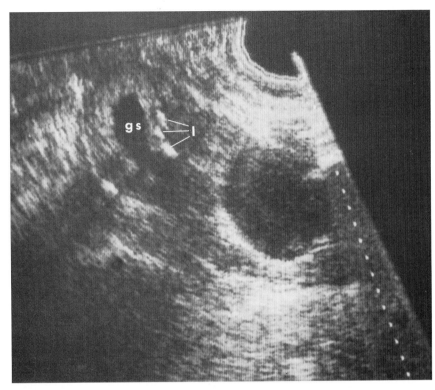

FIG 16–171.

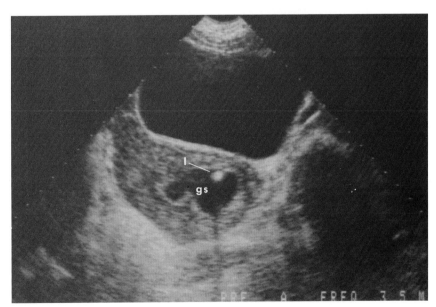

FIG 16–172.

## Mass Associated With Pregnancy

A common reason for ultrasound referral is a patient who is considered too large for dates. A common explanation for the large size is a pelvic mass found in association with pregnancy. Often a pelvic mass will elevate the uterus out of the pelvis. Under these circumstances, the patient will clinically be felt to be larger than expected for dates. A common mass seen during pregnancy is a corpus luteum cyst of pregnancy. This usually supports the pregnancy for the first 4 or 5 months. Corpus luteum cysts are usually only a few centimeters in size, but some have been reported to reach 10 cm. Figure 16–173 is a longitudinal scan in the midline of the pelvis in which we see a very early pregnancy with a small gestational sac. Posterior to the lower uterus is a sonolucent region representing a corpus luteum cyst. The cyst is elevating the uterus out of the pelvis, making the uterus appear longer under physical examination than would be expected from the patient's menstrual history.

Figure 16–174 is a longitudinal scan in a patient who has a nonfunctioning cyst. The cyst appears as a large sonolucent mass cephalad to the uterine fundus. A small gestational sac is present within the uterine cavity. The obstetrician palpated the top of the cyst mistakenly as the top of the uterus. Therefore, he thought she was approximately 6 weeks further along than her history indicated. Figure 16–175 is a transverse scan in a patient with a sonolucent mass in the right adnexal region. The mass has sharp borders and through-transmission. There is septation noted posteriorly. The mass turned out to be a large, multiloculated ovarian cyst.

Figure 16–176 is a longitudinal scan in a 23-year-old woman whose last menstrual period was 4½ weeks earlier. She was sent to ultrasound because of right pelvic pain. The possibility of an ectopic pregnancy was considered. The longitudinal scan shows an empty uterus without evidence of a gestational sac. A solid-appearing mass is present superior to

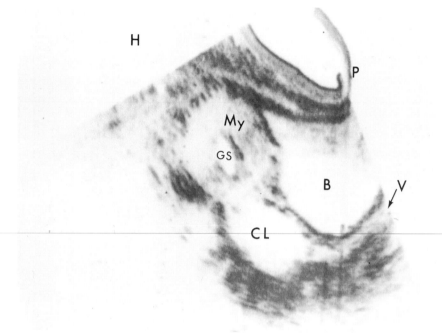

FIG 16–173.

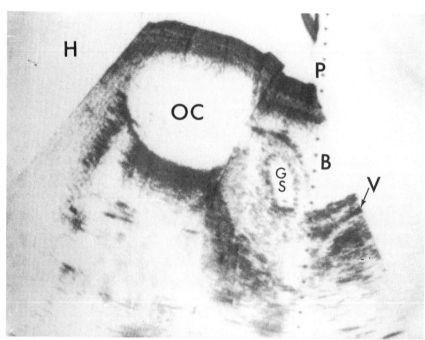

FIG 16–174.

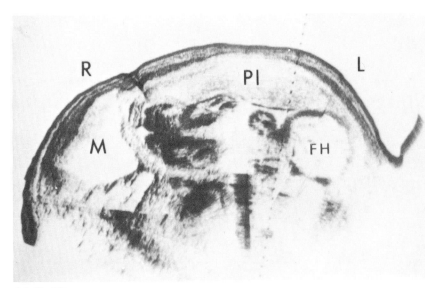

FIG 16–175.

the uterus. The patient was watched closely and a normal intrauterine pregnancy was identified. The ultrasound findings are consistent with a hemorrhagic corpus luteum cyst. This is not an uncommon event and can often be confused with an ectopic pregnancy.

**B** = Urinary bladder
**CL** = Corpus luteum cyst
**F** = Foot
**FH** = Fetal head
**GS** = Gestational sac
**H** = Head
**He** = Hemorrhagic corpus luteum cyst
**L** = Left
**M** = Multiloculated ovarian cyst
**My** = Myometrium
**OC** = Ovarian cyst
**P** = Symphysis pubis
**PI** = Placenta
**R** = Right
**U** = Uterus
**V** = Vagina

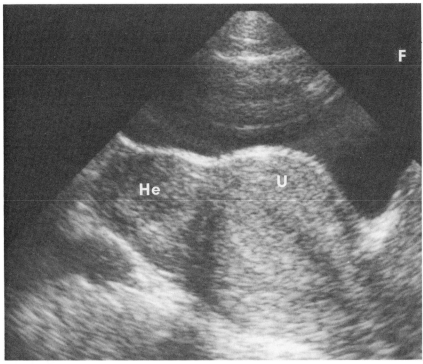

FIG 16–176.

## Mass Associated With Pregnancy

Very often a mass will be identified in assocation with pregnancy. Previous cases demonstrated several fluid-filled masses consistent with cystic structures. The following cases demonstrate solid masses in association with an intrauterine pregnancy. These masses often present as large-for-dates pregnancy. They can elevate the uterus out of the pelvis, as is shown in Figure 16–177. A large mass is noted posterior to the lower uterine segment (M). The mass has some soft internal echoes and lacks enhanced through-transmission. The findings indicate a solid lesion in the lower uterine segment. This turned out to be a large lower uterine fibroid.

Figure 16–178 is the scan of another patient with a large-for-dates pregnancy. A pregnancy is identified in the fundus of the uterus, along with the fetus (arrowhead). The size of the fetus indicates that the pregnancy is only about 9 menstrual weeks. However, the mass cephalad to the uterus is palpable above the umbilical level, suggesting a 20-week pregnancy. The obstetrician mistook the cephalad portion of this mass for the fundus of the uterus. The mass has internal echoes and lacks through-transmission. These ultrasound findings indicate that it is a solid lesion. The mass turned out to be a large fundal myoma.

Figure 16–179 is a scan of another fundal myomatous uterus in association with pregnancy. The uterus was thought on palpation to be large for dates because of the myoma. The gestational sac was approximately 9–10 weeks in size. The fundal myoma measured 10–12 cm in diameter and placed the time of pregnancy (by palpation) at approximately 20–22 weeks. This explained the large-for-dates finding. Note the numerous internal echoes and lack of through-transmission in association with this fundal mass. This indicates its solid nature.

Figure 16–180 is a transverse scan of a pregnant uterus. The fetus (arrowhead) can be seen within the fluid-

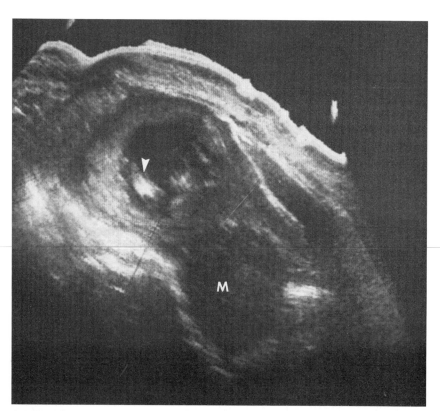

**FIG 16–177.**

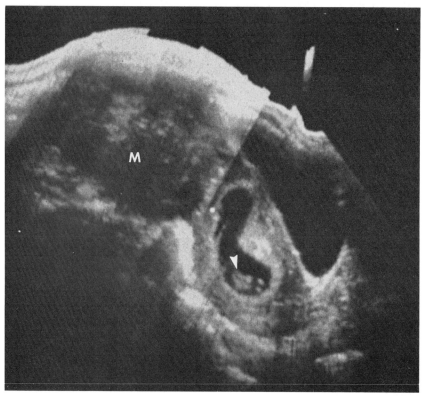

**FIG 16–178.**

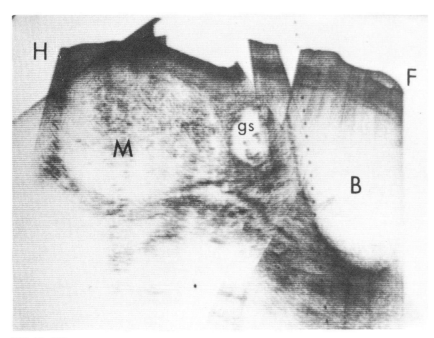

**FIG 16–179.**

filled gestational sac. However, very little internal fetal anatomy is identified. This has been called the empty thorax or empty abdomen sign of fetal demise and will be discussed later in the section on fetal demise. No fetal cardiac activity was identified, confirming fetal demise. Lateral to the gestational sac is a circular echogenic region with marked acoustic shadowing deep to it. This turned out to be a calcified myoma in association with pregnancy. The location of the myoma is within the uterine wall.

| **Arrowhead** | = Fetus |
| **B** | = Urinary bladder |
| **F** | = Foot |
| **gs** | = Gestational sac |
| **H** | = Head |
| **M** | = Uterine fibroid |

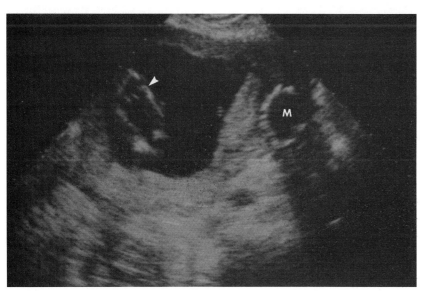

**FIG 16–180.**

## Mass Associated With Pregnancy

Figure 16–181 is a longitudinal scan of a 21-year-old woman with a 5-week intrauterine pregnancy. She reported pain on the left side, and an ectopic pregnancy was suspected. The gestational sac is within the uterus, which rules out an ectopic pregnancy. However, an oval mass is present in the left adnexal and cul-de-sac region. Through-transmission is present, indicating its fluid nature. There were some internal echoes especially on the posterior aspect. The mass increased in size during early pregnancy. At operation a cystadenoma of the left ovary was removed.

Figure 16–182 is a transverse scan of a patient who was sent for ultrasound because of a large-for-dates pregnancy. On palpation she was thought to be approximately 14 weeks' size but was only 7 weeks pregnant by menstrual history. In this scan the gestational sac is seen within the uterus. The sac would correspond to a pregnancy of approximately 7 weeks. Anterior and to the left of the uterus was an echogenic solid-appearing mass (M) which was quite worrisome because of its echo texture, and surgery was performed. This is an unusual case in which an ovarian neoplasm was found in association with a very early intrauterine pregnancy. The ultrasound findings of a soft tissue mass without evidence of attenuation suggesting a fibroid led to surgery because of a suspected solid ovarian lesion.

Figure 16–183 is a longitudinal scan of the lower pelvis in a 26-year-old woman. An intrauterine pregnancy is identified superior to the urinary bladder. Amniotic fluid (A) is present. Posterior to the cervix and endocervical region is a large mass which has an echogenic region superiorly and a sonolucent region inferiorly. This highly echogenic mass was consistent with a dermoid. At operation a dermoid was removed.

Figure 16–184 is a transverse scan of the pelvis in a patient with a 5-week pregnancy by menstrual dating. A

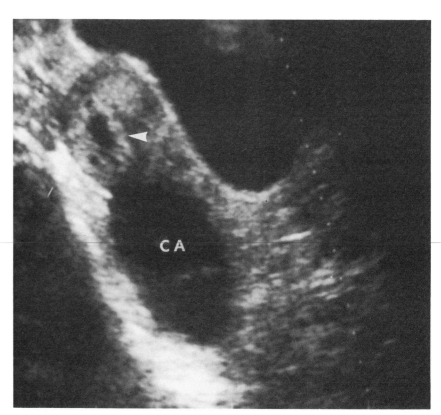

**FIG 16–181.**

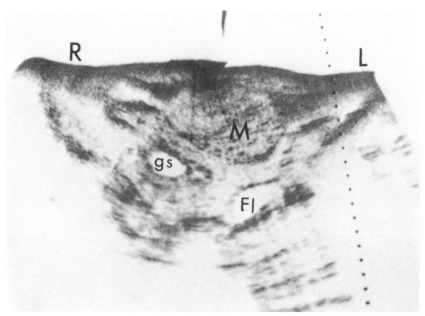

**FIG 16–182.**

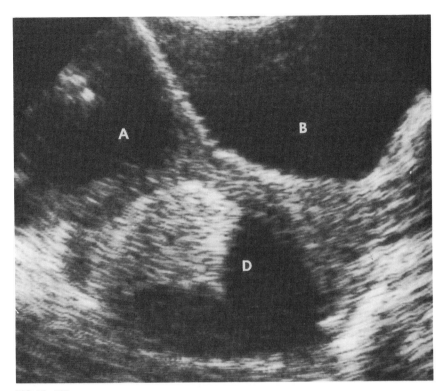

FIG 16–183.

double-ring gestational sac is identified in the uterine cavity (arrowhead). The size of the sac is appropriate for a 5-week pregnancy. The left ovary is normal. In the right adnexal region is an echogenic ring-like structure that is indenting the posterior aspect of the urinary bladder. The central portion in the echogenic region is sonolucent. Surrounding the echogenic area is a soft tissue region representing a capsule. The ultrasound findings were most consistent with a right dermoid. At operation a right dermoid was removed.

| Arrowhead | = | Gestational sac |
|-----------|---|-----------------|
| A | = | Amniotic fluid |
| B | = | Urinary bladder |
| CA | = | Cystadenoma |
| D | = | Dermoid |
| Fl | = | Pelvic fluid |
| gs | = | Gestational sac |
| L | = | Left |
| M | = | Ovarian neoplasm |
| O | = | Normal left ovary |
| R | = | Right |

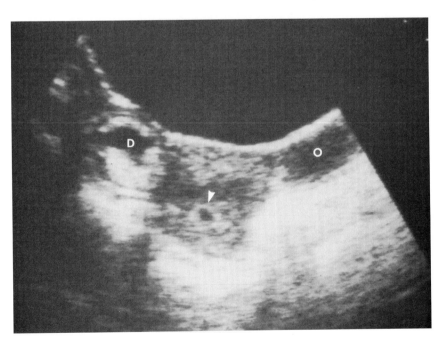

FIG 16–184.

## Masses Associated With Pregnancy

Figure 16–185 is a longitudinal scan of the midline in which we see a pregnancy within the uterus. Cephalad to the uterus is a soft tissue mass that has an echogenic central region. Figure 16–186 is a transverse scan of the same patient. The mass is secondary to an ectopic kidney in association with an intrauterine pregnancy. The "bull's-eye" appearance, especially noted in Figure 16–186, indicates the reniform appearance. Other entities that can give a bull's-eye appearance are gastrointestinal tract lesions. When such an appearance is noted in the pelvis, both renal fossae should be examined to rule out the possibility of an ectopic kidney.

Figure 16–187 is another example of a pelvic ectopic kidney. The patient's last menstrual period was 6 weeks earlier. The gestational sac (arrowhead) within the uterus is compatible with that menstrual history. Cephalad to the uterus is a pelvic kidney. Examination of the renal fossae revealed absence of the right kidney in that location.

Figure 16–188 is a transverse scan of the lower abdomen in a patient with a renal transplant in the right iliac fossa. The fetal head is situated in the midline. On the right side is the renal transplant with a small amount of fluid in the collecting system. This may be minimal hydronephrosis versus extrarenal pelvis.

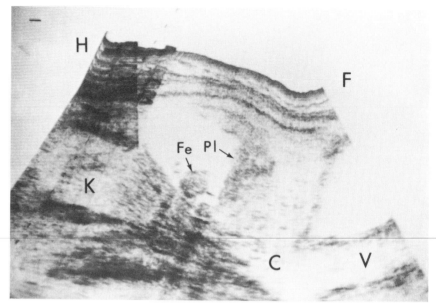

FIG 16–185.

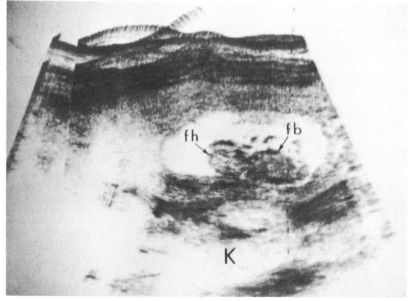

FIG 16–186.

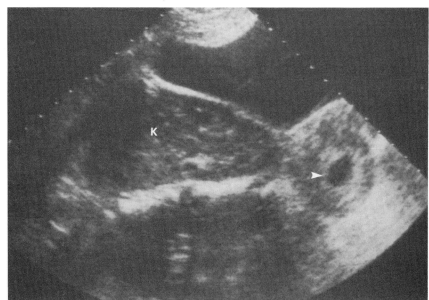

**FIG 16–187.**

| | | |
|---|---|---|
| **Arrowhead** | = | Gestational sac |
| **C** | = | Cervix |
| **F** | = | Foot |
| **fb** | = | Fetal |
| **Fe** | = | Fetus |
| **FH** | = | Fetal head |
| **fh** | = | Fetal head |
| **H** | = | Head |
| **Hy** | = | Minimal hydronephrosis |
| **K** | = | Kidney |
| **L** | = | Left |
| **Pl** | = | Placenta |
| **R** | = | Right |
| **V** | = | Vagina |

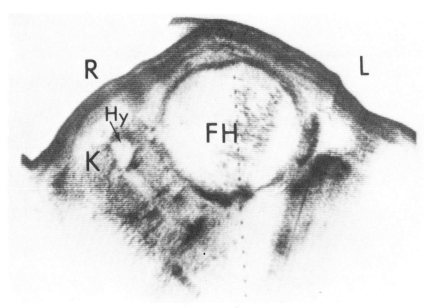

**FIG 16–188.**

## Bicornuate Uterus

The diagnosis of pregnancy in a bicornuate uterus is most easily made in the first 10 weeks of pregnancy. At that time, the gestational sac will often develop in one cornu. The nongravid cornu will demonstrate increased echogenicity secondary to decidual reaction. After 10 weeks, the gravid cornu increases in size dramatically and the nongravid cornu may only appear as a small nubbin of tissue laterally. As pregnancy progresses, the nongravid cornu becomes less and less evident. Figure 16–189 is a transverse scan of a first-trimester pregnancy. The pregnancy is present in the left horn of a bicornuate uterus where the embryo (E) is identified in the midportion of the nongravid cornu. This is secondary to decidual reaction in response to pregnancy. Later in pregnancy, the nongravid cornu would not be visible because of its small size relative to the overall size of the uterus.

Figure 16–190 is a transverse scan of a uterus in a 29-year-old woman whose last menstrual period was 8 weeks and 2 days previously. There is evidence of a bicornuate uterus with a pregnancy present in the left cornu. The gestational sac has increased echogenicity in the endometrial cavity of the right cornu (arrowhead). Figure 16–191 is a transverse scan of another patient with a bicornuate uterus and an early pregnancy. A gestational sac (S) is present in the gravid right cornu. Decidual reaction (arrowhead) is present in the nongravid left cornu. Figure 16–192 is a hysterosalpingogram of the same patient prior to pregnancy. The hysterosalpingogram confirms the presence of a bicornuate uterus.

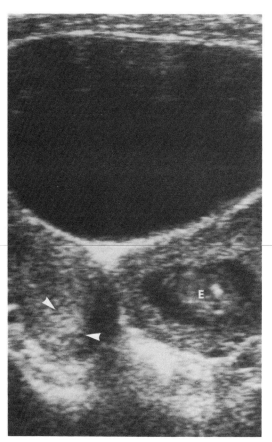

FIG 16–189.

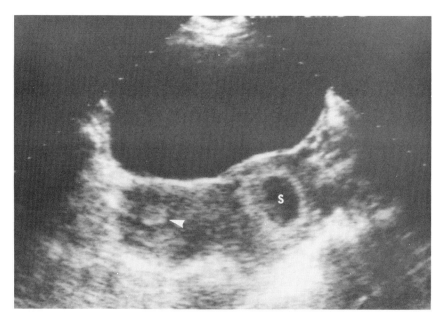

FIG 16–190.

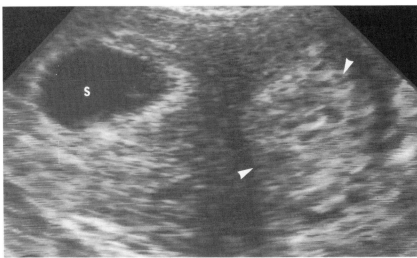

| Arrowhead | = | Decidual reaction in the nongravid cornu |
| E | = | Embryo |
| S | = | Gestational sac |

FIG 16–191.

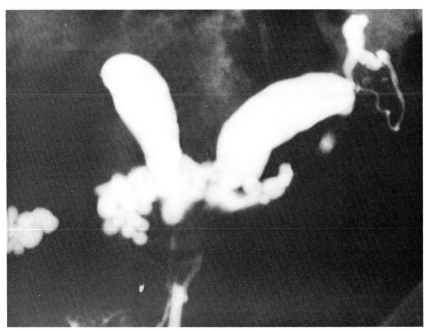

FIG 16–192.

## Bicornuate Uterus

Pregnancy in a bicornuate uterus can result in complications when the patient undergoes a therapeutic abortion. Often the therapeutic abortion will be unsuccessful because of this uterine anomaly. Figures 16–193 and 16–194 illustrate such a case. Figure 16–193 is a transverse scan obtained after an attempted therapeutic abortion. A gestational sac with fetal echoes is present in the right cornu. The left side of the uterus has a mixed echo pattern. In Figure 16–194, a longitudinal scan through the left side of the uterus, a small lucency is noted. The lucent area was secondary to hemorrhage following an unsuccessful therapeutic dilatation and curettage. During the procedure, the nongravid uterine cavity was entered rather than the gravid right cornu. Ultrasound can be extremely helpful in delineating the cause of the unsuccessful abortion.

Figure 16–195 is a transverse scan of a 22-year-old woman with a bicornuate uterus. The patient reported that 10 weeks and 3 days had passed since her last menstrual period. She underwent ultrasound examination because of vaginal bleeding. This is an example of an inevitable abortion. The right cornu demonstrates increased decidual reaction with a sonolucency centrally, compatible with hemorrhage. The left cornu demonstrates increased echogenicity compatible with decidual reaction. The right cornu contains a nonviable pregnancy; the left contains decidual reaction.

Figure 16–196 is a transverse scan through the uterus of a patient with a known bicornuate uterus. A twin pregnancy is present, one fetus in each cornu. Fetal echoes (arrows) are identified. Fetal cardiac activity was noted bilaterally.

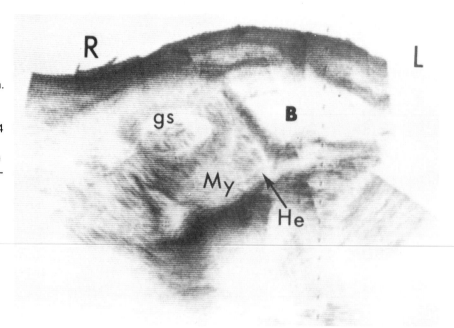

**FIG 16–193.**

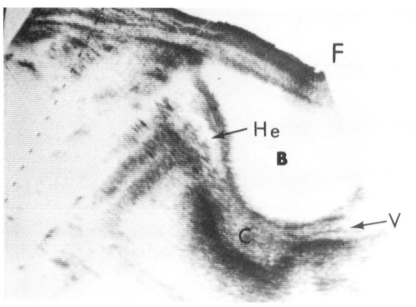

**FIG 16–194.**

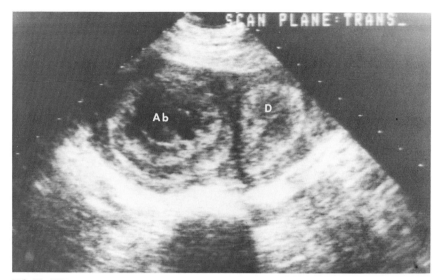

**FIG 16–195.**

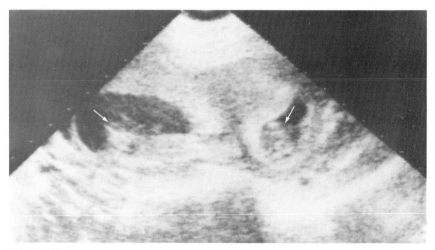

**FIG 16–196.**

| Arrows | = | Viable embryo |
|--------|---|---------------|
| **Ab** | = | Abortion |
| **B** | = | Urinary bladder |
| **C** | = | Cervix |
| **D** | = | Decidual reaction |
| **F** | = | Foot |
| **gs** | = | Gestational sac |
| **He** | = | Hemorrhage |
| **L** | = | Left |
| **My** | = | Myometrium |
| **R** | = | Right |
| **V** | = | Vagina |

## Uterine Anomalies

Figure 16–197 shows a pregnancy in a double uterus. It is often difficult to distinguish a double uterus from a bicornuate uterus on ultrasound. However, visualization of two cervices on scanning the lower pelvis can help one make this diagnosis. Figure 16–197 demonstrates a 7-week pregnancy in the left uterus. A gestational sac is identified on that side. The right uterus demonstrates increased echogenicity in the uterine cavity secondary to decidual reaction (arrows).

Figure 16–198 is another example of pregnancy in a double uterus. In this instance, the pregnancy is on the right side. A small amount of amniotic fluid is noted in the right uterus. The left uterus contains decidual reaction, manifested by increased echogenicity in the uterine cavity (arrows).

Figures 16–199 and 16–200 are longitudinal scans obtained in a 16-year-old girl who had a 15 week-sized uterus with no heart tones identified. A longitudinal scan in the midline revealed an empty uterus (Fig 16–199). A large mass in the left pelvis was thought to represent an ectopic pregnancy (Fig 16–200). At operation an unusual uterine anomaly was found. The nongravid uterus was seen in the midline, as shown in Figure 16–199. However, there was an atretic horn of a duplicated uterus present in the left pelvis. This atretic horn did not communicate with the cervix. The atretic horn contained a nonviable pregnancy with retained products of conception.

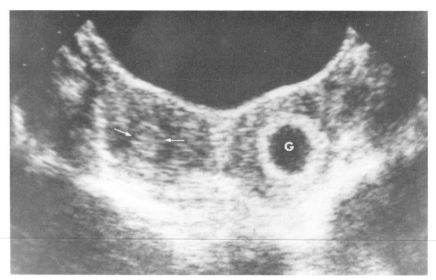

FIG 16–197.

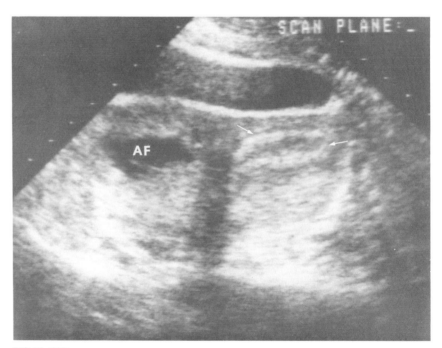

FIG 16–198.

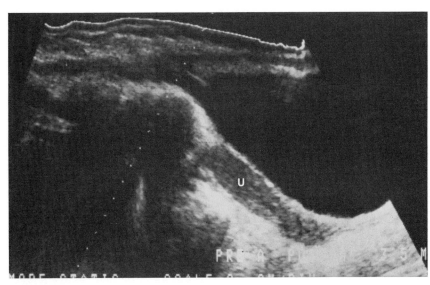

**Arrows** = Decidual reaction
**AF** = Amniotic fluid
**EP** = Ectopic pregnancy in atretic horn
**G** = Gestational sac
**U** = Nongravid uterus

**FIG 16–199.**

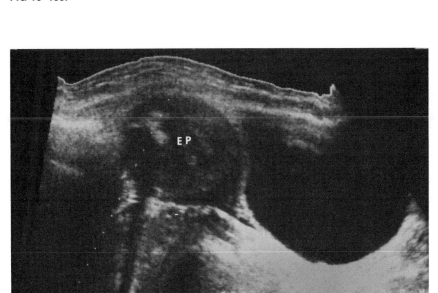

**FIG 16–200.**

## Uterine Septum

Occasionally a septum may be present in the uterus. This may affect the pregnancy by altering the lie of the fetus. When the fetus is in an unusual lie, the possibility of a uterine anomaly should be considered. Another concern in the presence of a uterine septum is that a fetal extremity may become trapped on one side of the septum, leading to limb abnormalities in serious cases. Figures 16–201 and 16–202 are longitudinal and transverse scans of the same patient. Uterine septation (arrow) is identified in the anterior half of the uterine cavity. The placenta is situated anteriorly. Deep to the placenta is some amniotic fluid. The tubular structure in the uterus is secondary to uterine septation. The fetal extremities are seen deep to the structure.

Figure 16–203 is a transverse scan near the fundus of the uterus in another patient. The fetal head (F) can be distinguished in the right fundal region. The thick echo in the midportion represents a uterine septation (arrow). On the left of the uterine septation is amniotic fluid, with no evidence of fetal echoes. The fetus was in a breech presentation and remained so until term because of the uterine septation.

Figure 16–204 shows another example of uterine septation. The placenta is situated anteriorly and is low-lying. The fetus is in a breech position. The septum extends only through a portion of the lower uterine segment. It is situated on the right side and is indicated by the echogenic structure in the lower uterine segment (arrow).

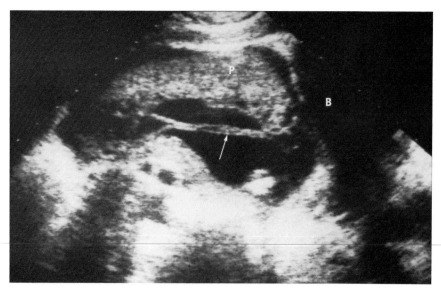

FIG 16–201.

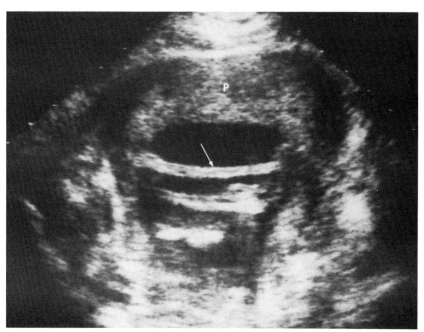

FIG 16–202.

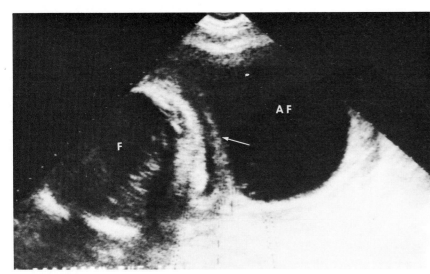

Arrow = Uterine septum
AF = Amniotic fluid
B = Bladder
F = Fetus
p = Placenta

FIG 16–203.

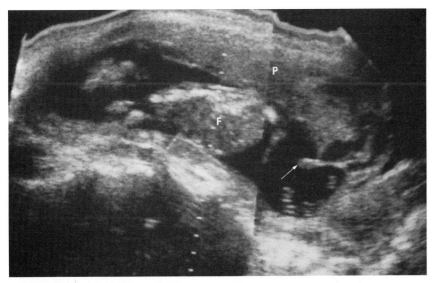

FIG 16–204.

## Normal Fetal Anatomy

With present-day equipment, ultrasound evaluation of the fetus has become extremely important. The fetus is regarded as a patient, and the ultrasound examination as its first physical examination. Before approximately 13–14 weeks' gestation, only major abnormalities can be identified. Fetal detail increases dramatically from 14 to 20 weeks. By 20 weeks, the fetus can be examined from head to toe for major abnormalities. With present-day equipment, which can be focused at different levels, excellent anatomical detail is possible. A large number of fetal anatomical scans are performed from 16 to 20 weeks' gestation because of amniocentesis. With the increased use of maternal serum α-fetoprotein studies and other screening procedures, the number of fetal anatomical studies will most likely increase. Examination of the fetus at this stage requires a great deal of experience and an understanding of normal anatomy.

Figure 16–205 is a transverse scan of the fetal cranium at the level of the lateral ventricles. This is cephalad to the level at which we usually measure the biparietal diameter. The choroid plexus (CP) appear as highly echogenic structures in the posterior aspect of the lateral ventricle. The choroid plexus should be in contact with the medial and lateral walls of the ventricle (arrows). This is a normal finding. The frontal and occipital horns are often fluid-filled. The choroid is present at the level of the trigone and should contact the walls of the lateral ventricle.

Occasionally a small sonolucency may be identified within the highly echogenic choroid plexus. This sonolucent area has been noted to be secondary to cysts (C) of the choroid plexus. Figure 16–206 is an example of a choroid plexus cyst. Usually the choroid plexus of the deep hemisphere is readily visible. The near hemisphere is not well seen on ultrasound because of reverberations off the near skull echo. Figure 16–207 is a magnified scan of the fetal brain near the midline. The triangular lu-

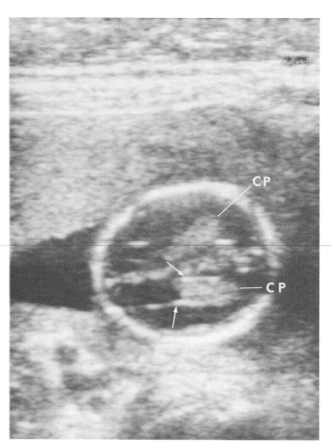

**FIG 16–205.**

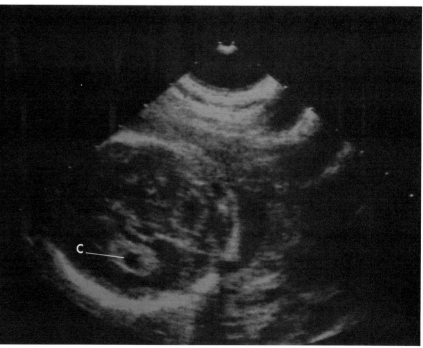

**FIG 16–206.**

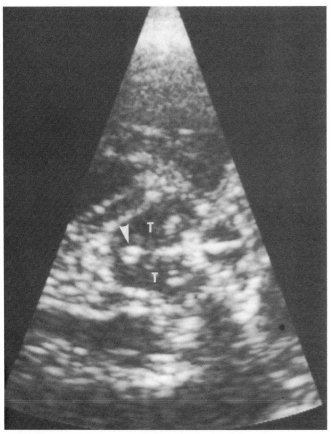

**FIG 16–207.**

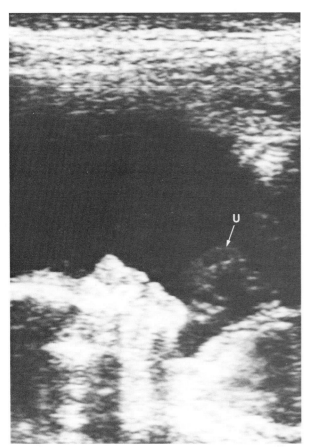

**FIG 16–208.**

cents areas of the thalami (T) are identified. The circular echogenic region posterior to the thalami is the cerebral aqueduct (arrowhead). Distinguishing the anatomical detail of the fetal brain can help the sonographer rule out major abnormalities. Figure 16–208 is a scan of the fetal profile. The umbilical cord is seen beneath the fetal chin. The fetal forehead, nose, lips, and chin are well visualized in this profile view.

| | | |
|---|---|---|
| **Arrows** | = | Walls of the lateral ventricle |
| **Arrowhead** | = | Cerebral aqueduct |
| **C** | = | Choroid plexus cyst |
| **CP** | = | Choroid plexus |
| **T** | = | Thalami |
| **U** | = | Umbilical cord |

## Normal Fetal Anatomy

The fetal spine examination is one of the most difficult intrauterine studies to perform. It is most often done at 16–18 weeks' gestation, in conjunction with amniocentesis. In the setting of elevated α-fetoprotein and acetylcholinesterase levels, the possibility of a neural tube defect is quite likely. Ultrasound evaluation of the fetal spine is performed to rule out a meningomyelocele or meningocele. It is best to examine the fetal spine in segments. The cervical, thoracic, and lumbar regions should be examined separately in both transverse and longitudinal planes. The osseous structures at each level can be identified. Any missing elements should be noted, along with protrusion of a multiloculated cystic mass posteriorly. Figure 16–209 is a longitudinal scan through the occipital and cervical region. The skin line is well seen because it is adjacent to amniotic fluid. It is most helpful to attempt to visualize the skin line. This is not always possible since the fetus may rest against the inside of the uterine cavity. Figure 16–210 is a longitudinal posterior scan through the cervical and thoracic region. Each osseous structure can be identified. There is no evidence of any missing elements posteriorly.

The most difficult area of the fetal spine to examine is the lumbosacral region. Since most meningomyeloceles occur in this area, it is necessary to examine this region closely. Often several studies are required before one yields an adequate view of the region. The osseous structures of the lumbosacral region taper as they approach the sacrum. Figure 16–211 shows the lumbosacral region with tapering.

Transverse scans should be obtained at all levels. Figure 16–212 is a transverse scan of the cervical region. The circular high-amplitude echoes represent the osseous structures of the cervical spine (arrow). The high-amplitude echoes are intact all the way around. If there were a major defect, a large U-shaped deformity would be present. The tubular structure around the soft tissues of the neck represents the umbilical cord.

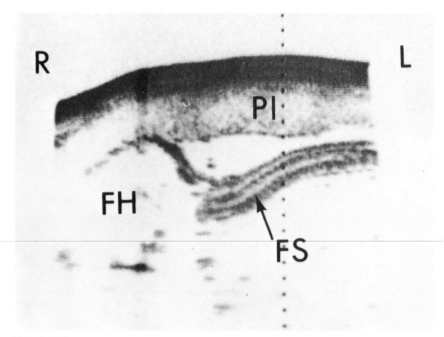

**FIG 16–209.**

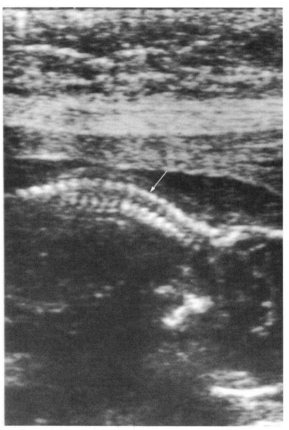

**FIG 16–210.**

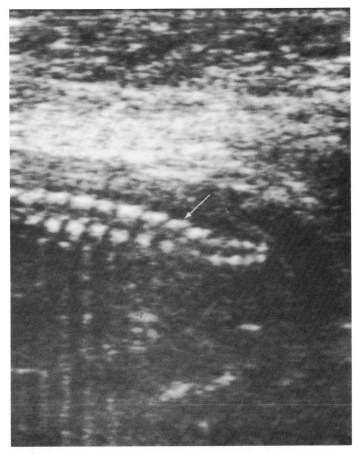

**Arrow** = Fetal spine
**FH** = Fetal head
**FS** = Fetal spine
**L** = Left
**PI** = Placenta
**R** = Right
**U** = Umbilical cord

**FIG 16–211.**

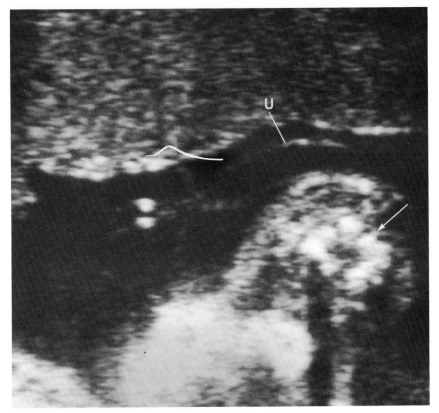

**FIG 16–212.**

## Normal Fetal Anatomy

Examination of the fetal thorax is somewhat difficult because of the overlying fetal ribs. The fetal ribs are represented by high-amplitude echoes surrounding the thoracic cage. Figure 16–213 is a coronal scan through the thorax. The ribs cast acoustic shadows (arrows). The thorax is evaluated by scanning through the fetal intercostal spaces. Ultrasound windows can usually be found with slight angling of the transducer. Figure 16–214 is a four-chamber view of the heart. The intraventricular septum and intraatrial septum are clearly depicted. Cardiac evaluation is becoming increasingly important in fetal ultrasound. This study is difficult to perform because fetal position plays a dramatic role in evaluation of the fetal heart.

Figure 16–215 is a longitudinal scan of the thorax and neck. The sonolucent area represents the right atrium. The superior vena cava is seen as a tubular structure extending cephalad to the right atrium. Just below the right atrium is a curved structure representing the right hemidiaphragm. The liver is situated inferior to this. The tubular structure in the neck is a fluid-filled trachea. We do not usually see a fluid-filled esophagus. Figure 16–216 is a longitudinal scan made slightly to the left of the scan in Figure 16–215. The "candycane" appearance of the aortic arch and descending thoracic aorta is evident. The aortic arch (AA) is definitely identified because neck vessels (arrows) are seen arising from the arch. This separates it from the pulmonary artery, which does not have neck vessels arising from it. The descending thoracic aorta and abdominal aorta (A) are seen anterior to the high-amplitude vertebral echoes.

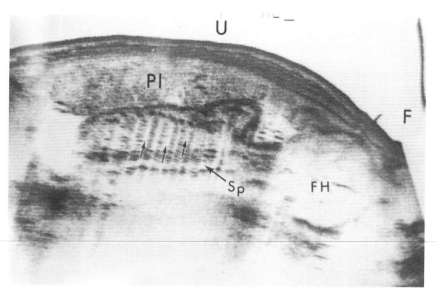

FIG 16–213.

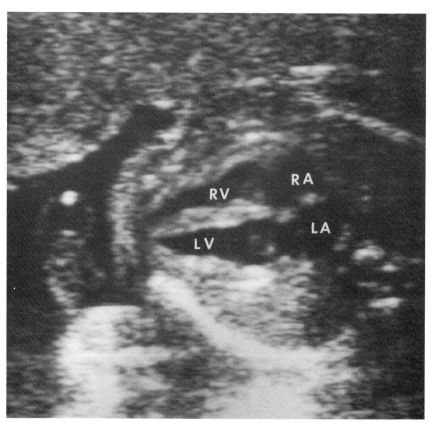

FIG 16–214.

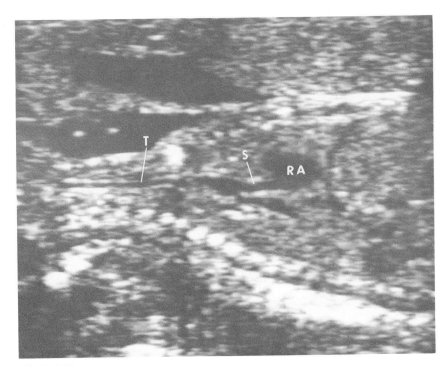

**FIG 16–215.**

| Arrows | = Acoustic shadowing from ribs (Fig 16–213) |
| --- | --- |
| **Arrows** | = Neck vessels arising from the aortic arch (Fig 16–216) |
| **A** | = Descending thoracic aorta |
| **AA** | = Aortic arch |
| **F** | = Foot |
| **FH** | = Fetal head |
| **LA** | = Left atrium |
| **LV** | = Left ventricle |
| **PI** | = Placenta |
| **RA** | = Right atrium |
| **RV** | = Right ventricle |
| **Sp** | = Fetal spine |
| **T** | = Trachea |
| **U** | = Umbilicus |

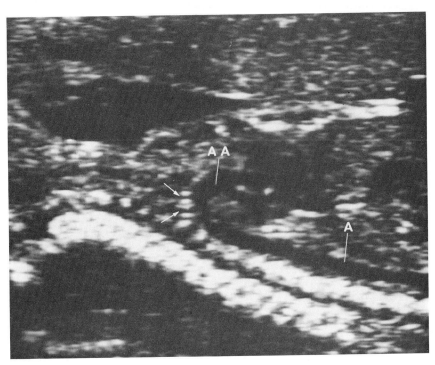

**FIG 16–216.**

## Normal Fetal Anatomy

Numerous anatomical structures are easily identified in the fetal abdomen. The fetal abdomen is well seen since no overlying ribs are obstructing its view. The umbilical vein can be seen entering the abdomen and appears as a tubular structure in the anterior abdomen, coursing to the right into the liver (Fig 16–217). Numerous fluid-filled structures are seen in the fetal abdomen. These should be recognized as normal anatomical findings and not mistaken for pathology. It is important to identify these anatomical structures so that fetal abnormalities will be detected when they are present. Figure 16–217 demonstrates the sonolucent stomach in the left abdomen. It is important to maintain a continuous three-dimensional concept of the fetus. When I begin scanning, the first thing I decide is which is the right and which the left side of the fetus. Once that is decided, one must continually be aware of fetal movement so that the right-to-left orientation of the fetus is always documented. The fetal stomach is on the left side of the fetal abdomen and any findings to the contrary become extremely important. The fetal spine is usually highly echogenic and often has acoustic shadowing.

Figure 16–218 is a coronal scan of the fetus. The coronal plane is very important, especially in the evaluation of fetal kidneys. The left kidney (K) is well seen on this scan. The fetal heart is present in the thorax, and fluid is seen in the stomach on the left side of the fetal abdomen.

The fluid-filled structures of the fetal abdomen are the fetal stomach and fetal urinary bladder. Figure 16–219 is a scan showing both the fluid-filled stomach and the fetal bladder. When the fetal bladder is first visualized on longitudinal scans, it can be extremely disturbing. The fetal bladder is larger than one expects when it is maximally distended. It has a rectangular appearance, as is seen in Figure 16–219. The fetal bladder is round on transverse scans, as is seen in Figure 16–220. The scans are of a male fetus, and the fetal urinary bladder is

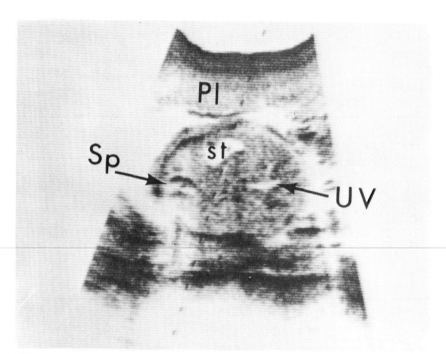

FIG 16–217.

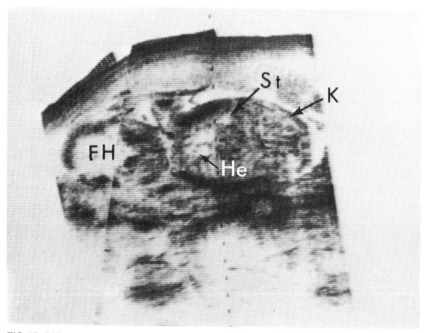

FIG 16–218.

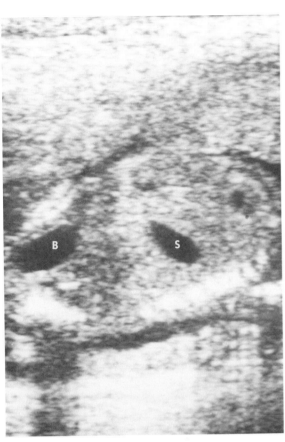

**FIG 16–219.**

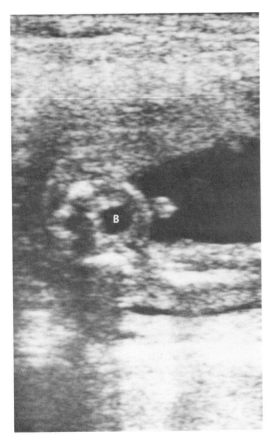

**FIG 16–220.**

shown normally distended. When evaluating fetal renal problems, it is important to examine the fetal urinary bladder. Usually the fetal urinary bladder will fill and empty within 1–1½ hours. This is the normal cycle for fetal urinary voiding. If there is suggestive evidence of renal disease, the fetal urinary bladder should be examined at 15-minute intervals for 45 minutes to 1 hour.

| | | |
|---|---|---|
| **B** | = | Fetal bladder |
| **FH** | = | Fetal head |
| **He** | = | Fetal heart |
| **K** | = | Fetal kidney |
| **Pl** | = | Placenta |
| **S** | = | Fetal stomach |
| **St** | = | Fetal stomach |
| **Sp** | = | Fetal spine |
| **UV** | = | Umbilical vein |

## Normal Fetal Anatomy

Currently available real-time equipment permits excellent evaluation of fetal anatomy. Figure 16–221 is a transverse scan through the fetal abdomen. In this enlarged view of the fetal abdomen the kidneys can be seen posteriorly. The aorta and inferior vena cava can be seen anterior to the spine. The small tubular sonolucency anterior to the inferior vena cava and aorta represents the splenic vein. Note the centimeter markers laterally. The splenic vein is less than 1 mm in size. The arrowheads outline the head of the pancreas. An echogenic region surrounds the splenic vein and portal junction. We are seeing the head of the pancreas and part of the uncinate process of the fetus. Figure 16–222 is a coronal scan of the fetal pelvis and lower abdomen. The curved tubular lucency in the fetal pelvis and lower abdomen represents the large intestine. The rectum (R), sigmoid (S), and descending colon (D) are well seen in this scan. The lucency just above the descending colon represents fluid in the stomach.

Examination of the fetal kidneys is important if oligohydramnios is present. The fetal kidneys are usually well seen by the 20th week. Before that time visualization is more difficult. As pregnancy progresses, fetal kidneys stand out better because of the position of fat in the fetus. Figure 16–223 is a transverse scan through the fetal kidney (arrowheads) in which we see the typical bull's-eye appearance of the kidney. Figure 16–224 is a longitudinal scan through the kidney. The central collecting systems are minimally separated, suggesting some fluid in the renal pelvis. There is a varying degree of fluid in the renal pelvis. Occasionally the fluid volume may appear quite large and suggest hydronephrosis. However, it is important not to overdiagnose hydronephrosis from a single study.

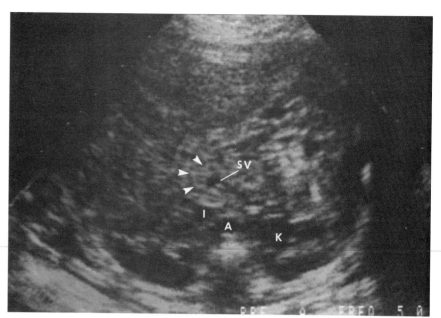

FIG 16–221.

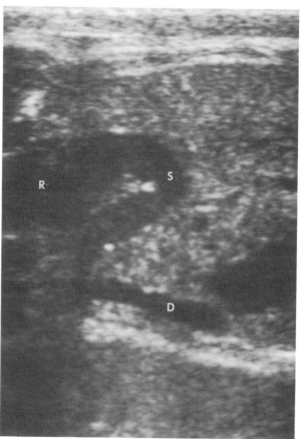

FIG 16–222.

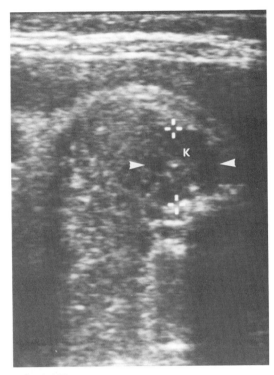

**FIG 16–223.**

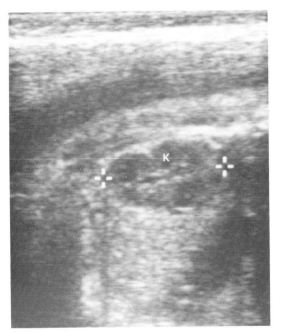

**FIG 16–224.**

| Arrowheads | = | Head of the pancreas (Fig 16–221) |
|---|---|---|
| Arrowheads | = | Kidney (Fig 16–223) |
| A | = | Aorta |
| D | = | Descending colon |
| I | = | Inferior vena cava |
| K | = | Kidney |
| R | = | Rectum |
| S | = | Sigmoid colon |
| SV | = | Splenic vein |

## Amniotic fluid

The amniotic fluid volume yields important information on the status of the pregnancy. Evaluation of amniotic fluid volume is quite difficult and still subjective. Years of experience are necessary to evaluate amniotic fluid adequately. The uterus must be scanned quickly so that one achieves a three-dimensional image of the amount of amniotic fluid present. The ratio of amniotic fluid volume to fetal volume changes during the course of pregnancy. In the second trimester the amniotic fluid volume is large relative to the fetal volume. This is a normal finding and should not be called polyhydramnios. Later in pregnancy the amniotic fluid volume decreases relative to the fetal volume. This is also a normal finding and should not be called oligohydramnios. With time the sonographer will develop a feeling for what is normal amniotic fluid volume.

Figures 16–225 and 16–226 are transverse and longitudinal scans of a patient with polyhydramnios. The tense appearance of the abdominal wall is the first important clue. The placenta appears compressed and flattened. Because of the increased pressure, placental thickness will often be less than anticipated. The fetal extremities will float in the amniotic fluid. Polyhydramnios is found in approximately 1% of pregnancies. In the great majority of cases there is no identifiable cause of the polyhydramnios. However, in about 20% of cases of polyhydramnios, there will be associated fetal anomalies. Anencephaly and gastrointestinal tract abnormalities are the most common causes.

Decreased amniotic fluid volume, or oligohydramnios, is of serious importance especially if it is present in the second trimester. When low amniotic fluid volume is identified in the second trimester, one must first ascertain whether rupture of the membranes has occurred. If the membranes have not ruptured, one must be immediately concerned about the fetus. Figures 16–227 and 16–228 are transverse and longitudinal scans of a fetus in the second trimester. There is practically no amniotic fluid volume present.

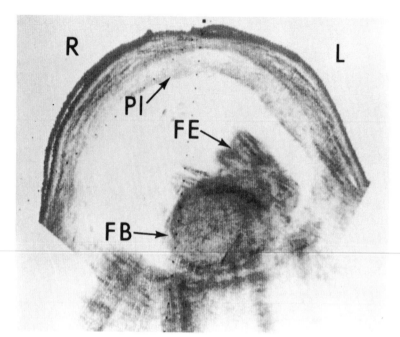

FIG 16–225.

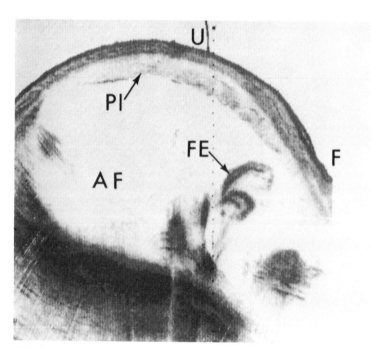

FIG 16–226.

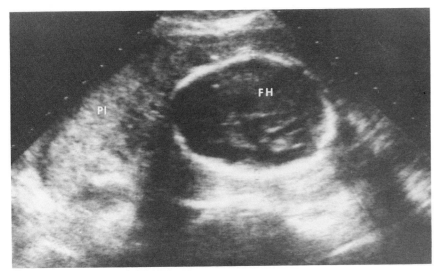

**FIG 16–227.**

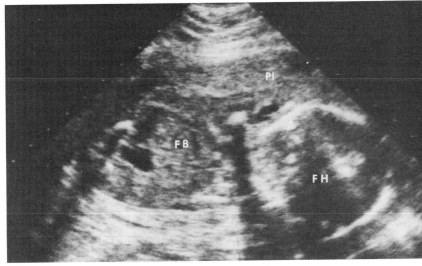

**FIG 16–228.**

The membranes had ruptured. If there had been no history of ruptured membranes, the major concern would have been a severe renal abnormality. Oligohydramnios is often associated with genitourinary tract abnormalities. The major concern in these cases is hypoplasia of the lungs. Lack of amniotic fluid during the second trimester inhibits the normal development of fetal lung tissue. Hypoplasia of the lungs will result in respiratory difficulty at birth. Later in pregnancy, the amount of amniotic fluid relative to the fetus appears quite small. It is a normal anatomical finding.

**AF** = Amniotic fluid
**F** = Foot
**FB** = Fetal body
**FE** = Fetal extremities
**FH** = Fetal head
**L** = Left
**Pl** = Placenta
**R** = Right
**U** = Umbilicus

# Anencephaly

An elevated α-fetoprotein (AFP) level in the maternal serum or amniotic fluid is often indicative of neural tube defect. A major cause of an extremely high AFP level is anencephaly. Anencephaly is lack of development of cerebral hemispheres. The base of the skull and primitive brain is present. There is a marked disproportion between the echoes of the fetal skull and those of the fetal body. It is extremely important to line up the fetal body with the presumed site of the fetal head when attempting to diagnose anencephaly. This diagnosis is easily made on ultrasound after 14 weeks. There is usually a cluster of echoes in the region of the base of the skull that is fairly characteristic of anencephaly.

Figure 16–229 is a longitudinal scan of the uterus in which ill-defined echoes are present in the region of the fetal head (FH). Several attempts at measuring the biparietal diameter were unsuccessful. This is usually the initial finding in the diagnosis of anencephaly. The discrepancy in size between the fetal head and the fetal body is quite apparent. Figure 16–230 is another example of anencephaly in which we see an inappropriate size relationship between the fetal head and fetal body. Often (50% of cases) anencephaly is accompanied by polyhydramnios.

When the fetal head is situated quite low in the pelvis, the diagnosis of anencephaly can be difficult to make. Figure 16–231 is a longitudinal scan in which the fetal head is situated quite inferiorly. The important finding is the cluster of echoes in the region of the fetal calvarium. There is no evidence of any strong echoes representing the normal fetal skull. Instead, numerous high-amplitude echoes are present in the region where the fetal head should be. No discrete calvarium was ever identified. Figure 16–232 is another example of anencephaly. The fetal body is appropriate in size for the menstrual history. In this case the few echoes at the base of the skull represent the only evidence of the fetal head.

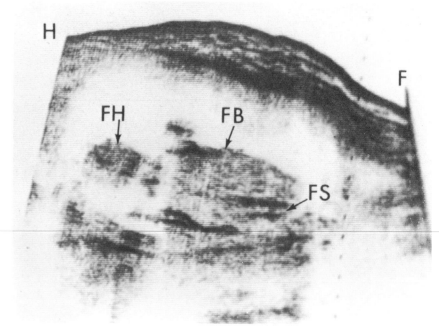

FIG 16–229.

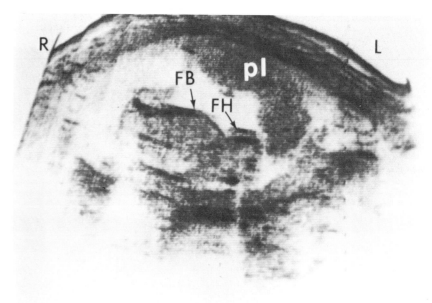

FIG 16–230.

F   = Foot
FB  = Fetal boddy
FH  = Fetal head
FS  = Fetal spine
H   = Head
L   = Left
PI  = Placenta
R   = Right

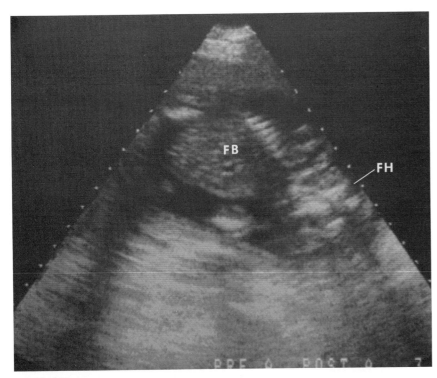

FIG 16–231.

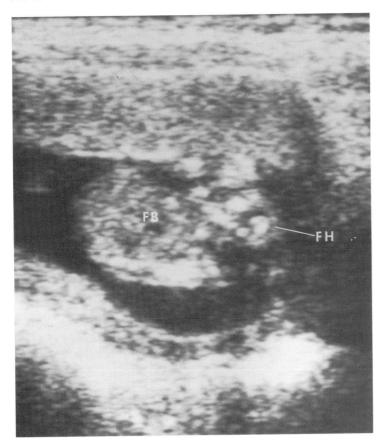

FIG 16–232.

## Hydrocephalus

Hydrocephalus can be detected before it causes an increase in head size. Detection of hydrocephalus is usually based on evaluation of the choroid plexus and the ventricles themselves. When the cerebral ventricles are first examined, at 14 to 24 weeks' gestation, they are quite large relative to the size of the cerebral hemisphere and decrease in relative size in later pregnancy. It is important to evaluate the relationship of the choroid plexus to the ventricular walls. The choroid is usually situated in the region of the trigone. It should be in contact ith the medial and lateral walls of the lateral ventricles. Often the frontal horn and occipital horn will not contain choroid and will appear fluid filled. However, the critical point is the relationship of the choroid to the walls of the ventricle in the region of the trigone. Since the lateral wall of the ventricle is a specular reflector, it will not be imaged unless it is scanned close to the perpendicular. Figure 16–233 was obtained by scanning the lateral wall of the far ventricle slightly off the perpendicular. The choroid (C) is visualized as an echogenic region. The lateral wall of the lateral ventricle is not seen, and the mistaken diagnosis of hydrocephalus could be made. This mistake can be avoided by scanning over the base of the skull on the near hemisphere and angling up toward the calvarium on the far hemisphere. This will place the ultrasound beam perpendicular to the lateral wall of the deep ventricle. In this instance (Fig 16–234), both the medial and the lateral walls of the deep ventricle are visualized (arrowheads). Note that the choroid plexus is in contact with both the medial and lateral wall. This rules out hydrocephalus.

Figure 16–235 is a scan of a patient with early hydrocephalus. The ventricle is slightly dilated (H). The echogenic choroid is present in the ventricle. Its borders are not in contact with either the medial wall or the lateral wall. Although in this case hydrocephalus is not causing any enlargement of the fetal skull, the diagnosis

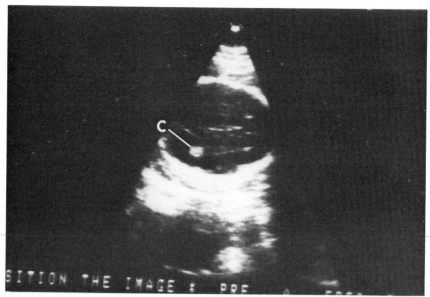

FIG 16–233.

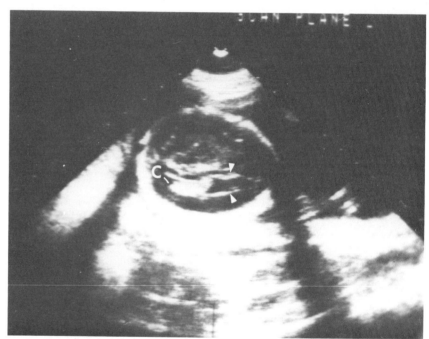

FIG 16–234.

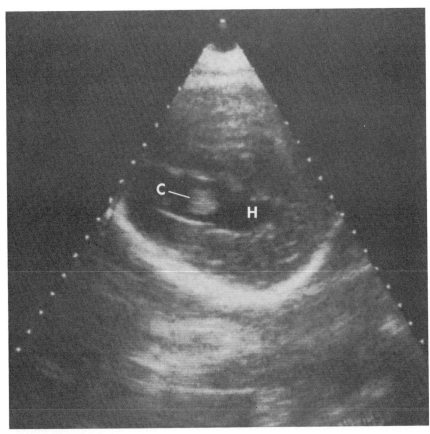

**FIG 16–235.**

can still be made because of the internal anatomy of the dilated ventricle.

Figure 16–236 is the scan of another patient with hydrocephalus (H). The dilatation of the lateral ventricle is more severe than in the previous case (Fig 16–235). The choroid plexus (C) in Figure 16–236 appears much smaller relative to the fluid-filled lateral ventricle. This is more severe hydrocephalus, with only a small rim of cortex present peripherally. The deep ventricles are better visualized than the near ventricle and hemisphere because of reverberation artifacts emanating from the near skull. It is often difficult to see the ventricle on the near hemisphere because of reverberation artifacts.

| | |
|---|---|
| **Arrowheads** | = Walls of the lateral ventricle |
| **C** | = Choroid plexus |
| **H** | = Hydrocephalus |

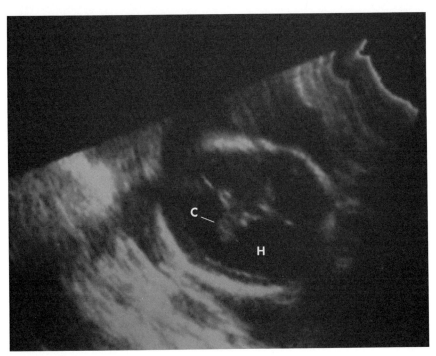

**FIG 16–236.**

## Hydrocephalus

Ventricular dilatation can reach dramatic size, even before an increase in the biparietal diameter. Figure 16–237 is an example of dramatic increase in the size of the ventricle with hydrocephalus present (H). The choroid plexus (C) is extremely small. It appears shrunken and tiny relative to the size of the dilated lateral ventricle. A helpful maneuver in confirming the diagnosis of hydrocephalus is ballotting the fetal head. If no hydrocephalus is present, the choroid plexus will move with the fetal head. If hydrocephalus is present, the choroid plexus will move in the opposite direction as the fetal head for the first few oscillations. The choroid plexus will appear to be a leaf floating in the breeze in the presence of a dilated ventricle.

Reverberation artifacts emanating from the near table present diagnostic difficulties. In Figure 16–238 several reverberation artifacts (R) are noted off the near skull echoes. These artifacts hide the dilated near ventricle. The dilated deep ventricle demonstrates hydrocephalus (H) and a small shrunken choroid plexus (C). The initial diagnosis may be that of a brain cyst rather than hydrocephalus because of lack of visualization of the dilated near ventricle.

Toxoplasmosis can cause hydrocephalus. Figure 16–239 is a scan of a fetal skull in which hydrocephalus (H) is identified in the deep hemisphere. There is also an area of increased echogenicity in the cortex lateral to the dilated ventricle (arrowhead). The same patient was scanned at a slightly different plane in the occipital region (Fig 16–240). Two more areas of increased echogenicity (arrowheads) were identified within the fetal cerebrum. These were areas of calcification secondary to toxoplasmosis.

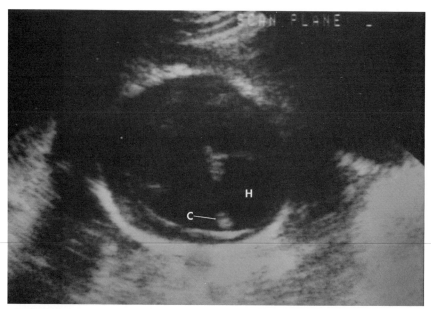

**FIG 16–237.**

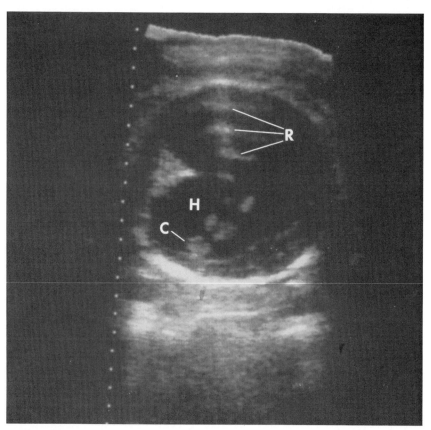

**FIG 16–238.**

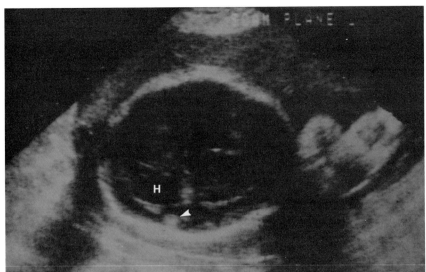

FIG 16–239.

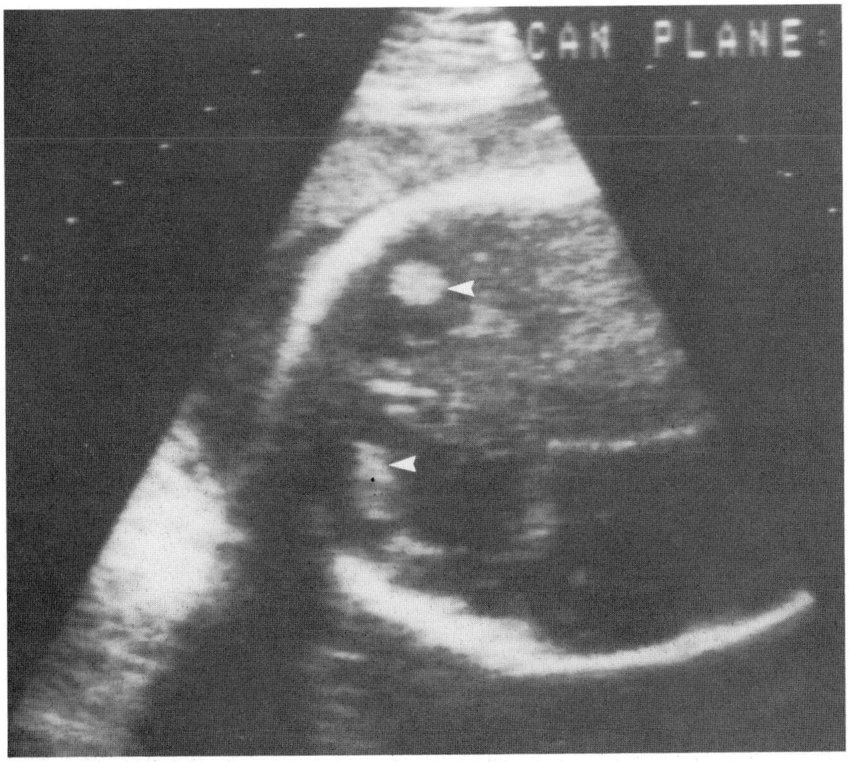

Arrowheads = Areas of calcification from toxoplasmosis
C = Compressed choroid plexus
H = Hydrocephalus
R = Reverberation artifacts

FIG 16–240.

## Intracranial Cystic Masses

Fluid-filled regions may be identified within the brain that do not correspond to dilated lateral ventricles. These may be cystic masses arising from various etiologies. If the cystic mass is secondary to a dilated fourth ventricle, the Dandy-Walker syndrome is present. Figure 16–241 is a scan through the fetus in which the fetal head (FH) appears much larger than the fetal body. The fetal head was enlarged because of a large cystic mass, which was found to be a dilated fourth ventricle (Dandy-Walker syndrome). Fourth ventricular dilatation can achieve massive size, as in this case.

The cisterna magna may be fairly prominent normally, especially from approximately 20 to 26 weeks' gestation. However, dilatation of the posterior fossa may indicate pathology. Figure 16–242 is an example of dilatation of the posterior fossa. The possibility of Dandy-Walker syndrome should be considered. However, the mass was secondary to an arachnoid cyst causing fluid accumulation in the posterior fossa region, which is a common site for arachnoid cyst formation.

Figure 16–243 is a scan through the fetal occipital region that shows dilatation of a lateral ventricle. In the midportion of the lateral ventricle is a cystic (Cy) mass. The intracranial cyst was causing obstruction of the foramen of Monro on that side, leading to unilateral hydrocephalus (H). Figure 16–243 demonstrates dilatation of the occipital and frontal horns. The cyst is seen centrally.

Figure 16–244 is the scan of a fetal cranium in which no cerebral tissue was identified. The fetal calvarium was filled with fluid. Numerous reverberation artifacts are identified. However, the study revealed a completely fluid-filled calvarium except for the remaining primitive brain noted at the base of the skull. This appearance was secondary to hydranencephaly. Hydranencephaly and holoprosencephaly can be difficult to distinguish. A mantel of cerebrum is present in holoprosencephaly but not in hydranencephaly. That is usually the major distinguishing factor between these two.

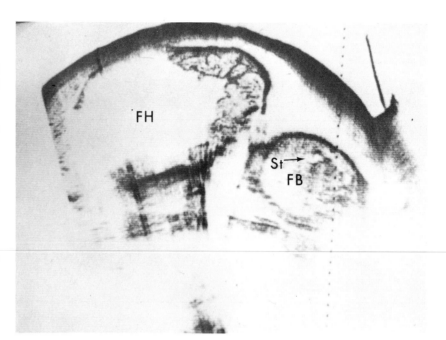

FIG 16–241.

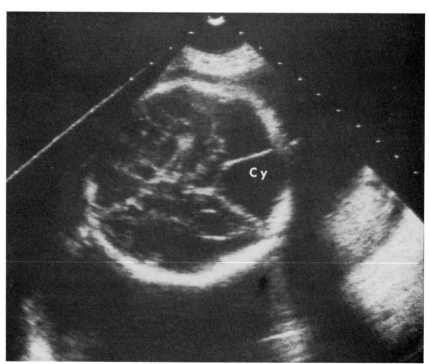

FIG 16–242.

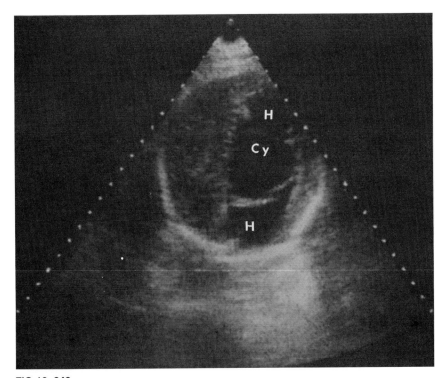

**FIG 16–243.**

Hydranencephaly is thought to be secondary to blockage or nondevelopment of the internal carotid cerebral arteries.

**Cy** = Intracranial cyst
**FB** = Fetal body
**FH** = Large fetal head secondary to dilated fourth ventricle
**H** = Unilateral hydrocephalus
**Hy** = Hydranencephaly
**St** = Fetal stomach

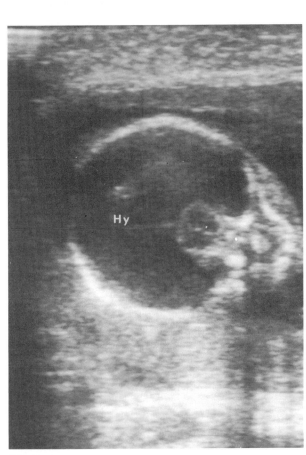

**FIG 16–244.**

## Encephalocele

Another cause for an elevated α-feto-protein (AFP) level in maternal serum or amniotic fluid is an encephalocele. An encephalocele is a protrusion or herniation of brain covering and brain substance through an opening in the fetal calvarium. When encephaloceles are large, they are easily detected. Small encephaloceles can be difficult to see, especially if they are flattened and pancaked against the fetal skull. When a fetal ultrasound examination is performed because of an elevated AFP level, an encephalocele should be looked for immediately after anencephaly has been ruled out. Encephaloceles necessitate close examination of the fetal calvarium. Figure 16–245 is a scan of the fetal calvarium in an 18-week fetus. The calvarial echoes are intact and no disruption of the fetal skull is identified. Initial quick examination of the fetal skull did not reveal any abnormalities. Closer examination of the fetal skull revealed an abnormality in the occipital region, shown in Figure 16–246. There is protrusion of brain substance secondary to a small encephalocele (arrowhead) in the occipital region. This was not easily seen. If the fetal skull had not been closely examined, the encephalocele would have been missed.

Figure 16–247 is a longitudinal scan of the posterior aspect of the fetus. Just inferior to the occipital bone is a large cranial defect (arrow) through which an encephalocele is protruding (arrowheads). The cervical spine is inferior to this protruding mass. Most encephaloceles are in the midline, and more are situated posteriorly than anteriorly.

Figure 16–248 is a transverse scan of the fetal skull in which there is a large encephalocele (arrowheads) protruding from the lateral aspect of the fetal skull. These are usually from amniotic bands and do not have genetic importance.

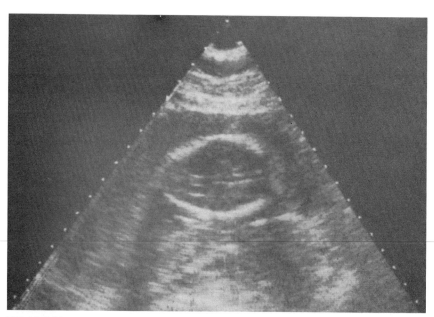

FIG 16–245.

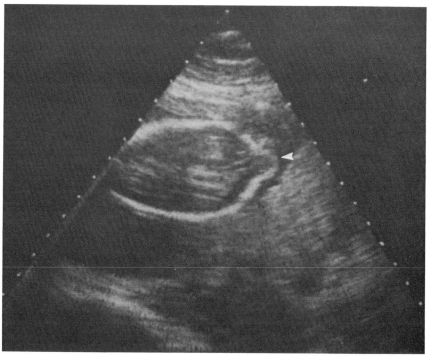

FIG 16–246.

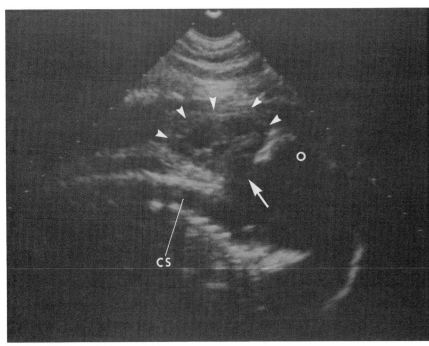

**Arrow** = Cranial defect
**Arrowheads** = Encephalocele
**CS** = Cervical spine
**FH** = Fetal head
**O** = Occiput

FIG 16–247.

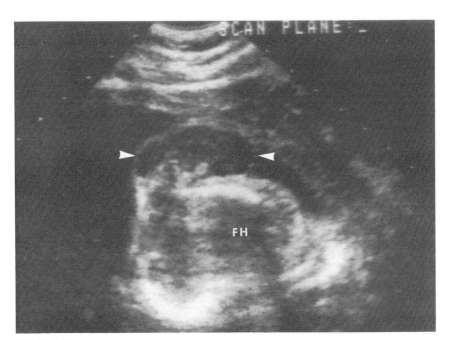

FIG 16–248.

## Meningocele

Because elevated AFP levels can be detected in the maternal serum and in the amniotic fluid, the number of ultrasound examinations performed to assess neural tube defects has increased. Often a fetus may be examined at 16 to 20 weeks' gestation because of an elevated serum or amniotic fluid AFP level. The initial part of the examination concentrates on the fetal skull to rule out anencephaly. The second part of the examination concentrates on evaluation of the fetal spine. This is often a difficult examination to do because of fetal position. In a thorough examination the cervical, thoracic, and lumbar segments of the spine are studied separately. It is important to evaluate the spine in both transverse and longitudinal views. In Figure 16–249 a meningomyelocele is visualized at the upper lumbar level. The posterior elements of the spine (S) are intact until the site of defect (arrow). There is absence of the high-amplitude echoes of the spinal elements at that site. A protruding mass (arrowheads) is present in association with the spinal defect.

Most spinal defects occur in the lumbosacral region. The lower lumbosacral area is difficult to examine because of fetal position. Figure 16–250 is another example of a meningocele diagnosed at approximately 16 weeks. The spinal elements (S) are indicated by high-amplitude echoes that appear intact until the very end of the spine. There is an opening with a protruding cystic mass (arrowhead) secondary to meningocele. This was a difficult examination to perform because of adipose tissue in the mother. Also, the back of the fetus was against the uterine wall. Only occasionally did the fetus bounce away, permitting visualization of fluid behind the lower fetal back.

The ultrasound appearance can suggest other causes of elevated AFP levels, including fetal demise, incorrect dates, abdominal abnormality, and twin or multiple gestations. Figures 16–251 and 16–252 are scans of a pregnancy in which the AFP level was elevated. A twin pregnancy was diag-

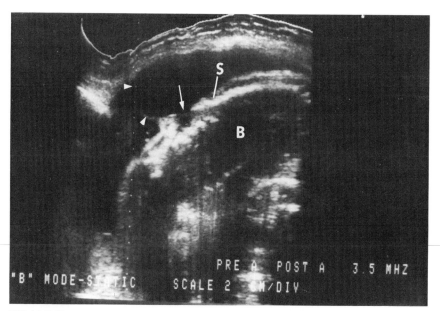

**FIG 16–249.**

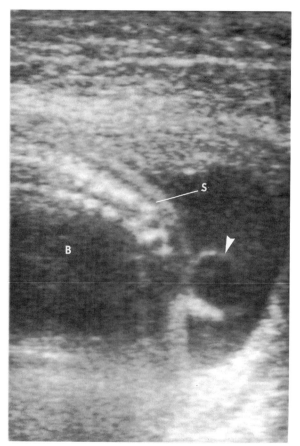

**FIG 16–250.**

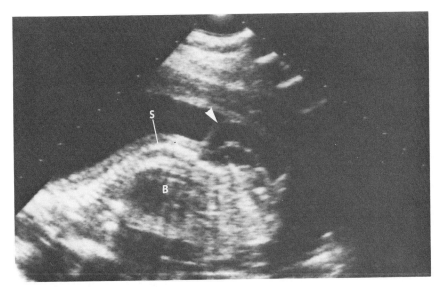

**FIG 16–251.**

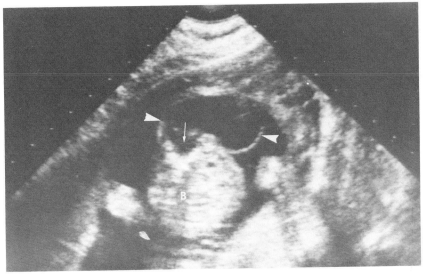

**FIG 16–252.**

nosed. This is a common cause of elevated serum AFP levels. However, it is important to examine each twin to rule out the possibility of any abnormalities. In this case, one of the twins was normal. Scans of the second twin are shown in Figures 16–251 and 16–252. A large mass protrudes from the posterior lower bacck of this fetus (arrowheads). The longitudinal scan in Figure 16–251 demonstrates an intact spine (S) until the lumbar region is encountered. At approximately L-2 there was loss of the posterior elements of the spine. A multiloculated mass is present posteriorly. The transverse scan in Figure 16–252 demonstrates the spinal defect. In this view, the spinal elements have a large U-shaped appearance, with loss of the posterior elements (arrow). This is a characteristic appearance of a defective spine. The mass protrudes posterior to the spinal defect (arrowheads).

| **Arrow** | = Spinal defect |
| **Arrowheads** | = Multiloculated cystic mass secondary to meningocele |
| **B** | = Fetal body |
| **S** | = Spinal elements |

## Meningocele

Evaluation of fetal spine on ultrasound examination is extremely difficult and requires a great deal of experience. Figure 16–253 is a transverse scan of the lower fetal body (B) in a patient with an elevated amniotic fluid AFP level. Ultrasound study did not initially demonstrate any spinal problem. Figure 16–253, a scan of the lower fetal spine and pelvic region, was the only view on the initial study which revealed an abnormality. The major finding in this view is the U-shaped deformity to these spinal elements (arrow). When this is found, the diagnosis of a spinal defect can be made. During the time of examination, the fetus was continually against the uterine wall. It is most helpful to visualize the fetal spine when amniotic fluid is situated behind the skin line, which was not possible during the initial study. The patient was reexamined the next day. Figure 16–254 is a longitudinal scan in which a small, 6-mm meningocele (arrowhead) is identified off the posterior lumbosacral region. Note the missing posterior elements, and the small mass. The initial study in Figure 16–253 was quite difficult to assess. However, the finding of an abnormally shaped fetal spine in the transverse view indicated the diagnosis.

Figure 16–255 is a longitudinal scan in which a multiloculated mass is seen over the posterior lower fetal back. This multiloculated mass is compatible with a meningocele or meningomyelocele. Typically these entities appear as sharply marginated, fluid-filled structures, often associated with some septations. If the mass is large, as it is in this case, it is usually detected. However, if the mass is small, as it is in Figure 16–256, it can often be missed. Figure 16–256 is a longitudinal scan in which the posterior spinal elements are distorted in the lower lumbosacral region. A small multiloculated cystic structure (arrowheads) is present in the posterior back. This is secondary to a meningomyelocele. When the lesions are this small, they are easily missed. One must strive to obtain both transverse and longitudinal views of the lower

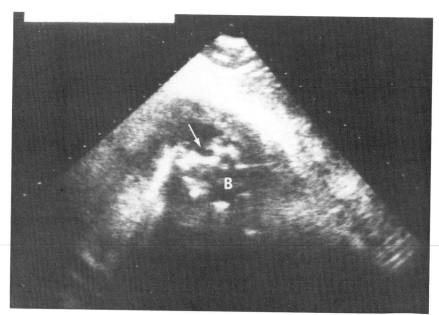

FIG 16–253.

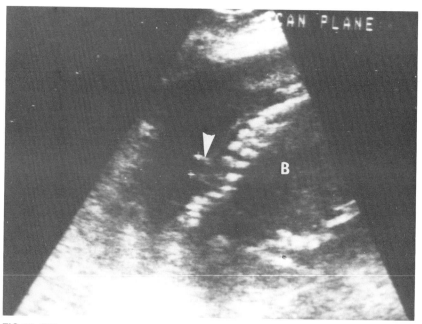

FIG 16–254.

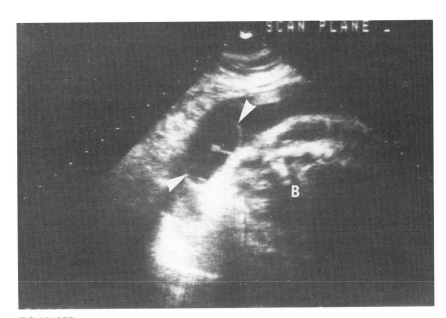

**FIG 16–255.**

lumbosacral region. If the sonographer waits until the fetus moves away from the uterine wall, amniotic fluid can be positioned posterior to the skin line. When the skin line is visualized and found to be normal, a spinal abnormality is usually unlikely. Until amniotic fluid is positioned posterior to the skin line, the diagnosis is always uncertain.

| **Arrow** | = U-shaped deformity of spinal abnormality |
| **Arrowheads** | = Meningomyelocele |
| **B** | = Fetal body |

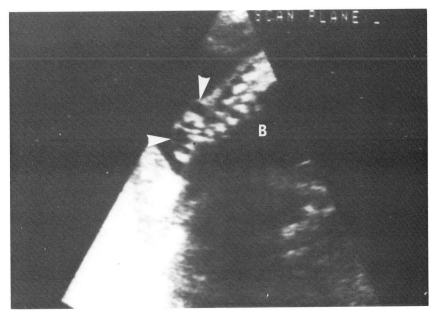

**FIG 16–256.**

## GI Tract Obstruction

During examination of the fetal abdomen, the fetal stomach and urinary bladder should always be seen. If they are not seen, follow-up examinations 15–20 minutes later are suggested. Figure 16–257 is a transverse scan of the fetal thorax and abdomen. Rib shadowing is noted through the fetal thorax. The oval sonolucent mass in the pelvis is the fetal urinary bladder. The fetal urinary bladder has a variable size, and this one is certainly within normal limits. During examination of the fetal abdomen, the fetal stomach was never identified. The patient was scanned at 15-minute intervals for 1 hour. During this time, the fetal stomach was never seen. Mild polyhydramnios was present. The findings indicate an esophageal atresia. The pediatricians were warned of this finding prior to delivery, and the patient was treated surgically. Since 90% of esophageal atresias are associated with a tracheal esophageal fistula, fluid will be seen in the stomach in 90% of esophageal atresias. However, in 10% of esophageal atresias there is no communication with the distal GI tract. Such was true in this case, as fluid was never identified in the fetal stomach.

Occasionally too many fluid-filled structures will be noted in the fetal abdomen. When this is encountered, as in Figure 16–258, the possibility of a GI tract obstruction or other cystic mass of the abdomen should be considered. The fetus had polyhydramnios. The two superior sonolucent structures represent the fetal stomach (S) and a dilated duodenal bulb (D) secondary to duodenal atresia. This is the typical "double bubble" sign seen on x-ray studies. The three sonolucent masses in the fetal abdomen are secondary to a dilated proximal stomach and duodenum and fluid in the urinary bladder.

Figures 16–259 and 16–260 illustrate another case of duodenal atresia. Polyhydramnios was present. Polyhydramnios is often seen in cases of high GI tract obstruction. Whenever polyhydramnios is detected on ultrasound, close examination of the fetal

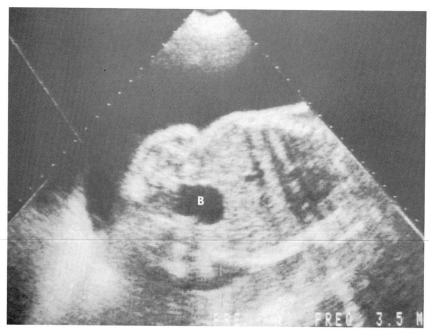

FIG 16–257.

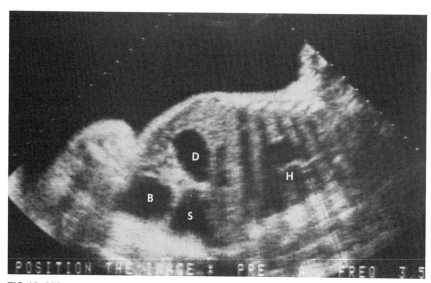

FIG 16–258.

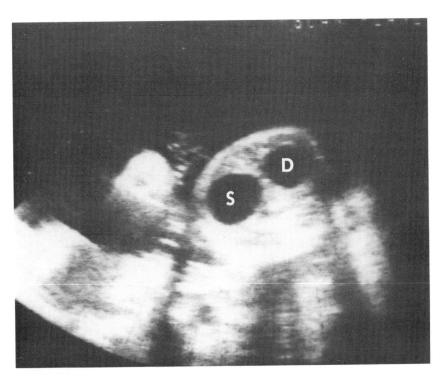

**FIG 16-259.**

abdomen is necessary. Figure 16-259 is a transverse scan of the fetus showing the classic "double bubble" sign. The stomach is on the left side of the fetal abdomen and a dilated duodenum (D) is on the right side. Figure 16-260 is a coronal scan of the fetus showing the dilated duodenum (D) in the right abdomen. The fetal stomach is well seen (S). Peristaltic waves were visible on real-time examination and are noted near the antral region. Note the pylorus, situated between the duodenum and the stomach. Near the fundus of the stomach is a tubular structure, secondary to a dilated distal esophagus.

**B** = Fetal urinary bladder
**D** = Dilated duodenum
**S** = Stomach
**H** = Heart

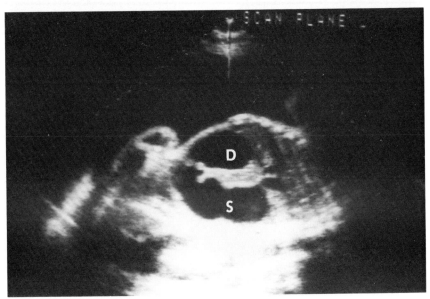

**FIG 16-260.**

## Omphalocele and Gastroschisis

Protrusion of the abdominal contents through the region of the fetal umbilical cord is secondary to an omphalocele. Omphalocele and gastroschisis are additional reasons for elevated maternal serum or amniotic fluid AFP levels. When such elevation is identified, examination of the fetal wall is necessary to rule out these abnormalities. Omphalocele is herniation of the abdominal contents through the midportion of the fetal abdomen. The umbilical cord will arise from the herniated mass. A surrounding membrane of peritoneum is present in omphalocele and is an important ultrasound finding. In gastroschisis, the abdominal wall defect is lateral to the umbilical cord. There is no evidence of a covering membrane in gastroschisis. Figure 16–261 is a longitudinal scan of a fetus that shows a soft tissue mass (arrowheads) protruding from the fetal body (FB). This scan is off to the side of the fetal head, which is seen on another view.

The size of omphaloceles can vary greatly. They may contain a small amount of intestine or nearly the entire abdominal contents. Figures 16–262 and 16–263 are transverse scans of the same fetus. Figure 16–263, a scan near the upper abdomen, shows a soft tissue mass protruding from the fetal body. The fetal body (FB) is much smaller than the size anticipated from the menstrual history. The reduced size is caused by protrusion of the liver (L) through a large omphalocele. Figure 16–263 is a scan through the lower pelvis. There is further evidence of protrusion of GT contents on this view. Note the covering membrane (arrowheads), which confirms the presence of an omphalocele. The fetal bladder (B) is noted on this scan between the iliac wings.

Gastroschisis is a herniation of abdominal contents to the side of the umbilical cord, which is seen to arise in its usual location. Protrusion of intestinal contents is noted. There is no covering peritoneal membrane in gastroschisis, as is present in omphalocele. It is important to make these dis-

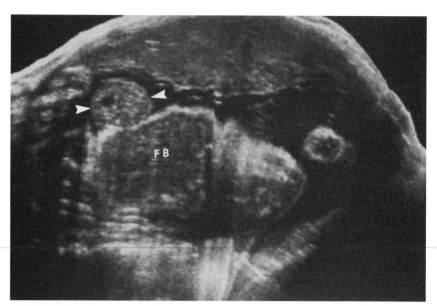

**FIG 16–261.**

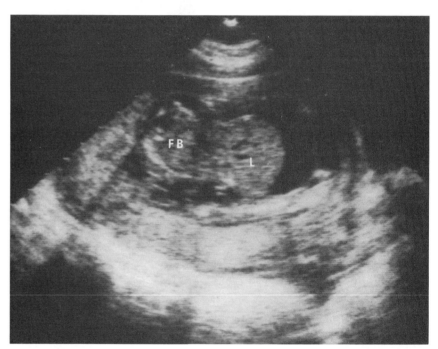

**FIG 16–262.**

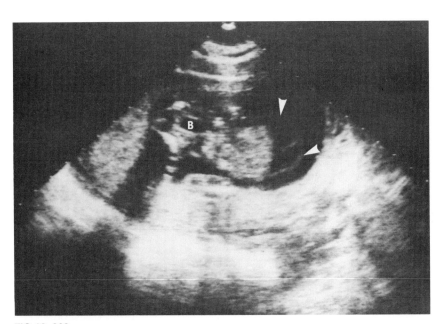

**FIG 16–263.**

tinctions since omphalocele has a high association with other congenital anomalies. Gastroschisis does not. Figure 16–264 is a transverse scan of the fetal abdomen (FB) in which an echogenic mass (M) is seen protruding from the right lower quadrant of the fetal abdomen. The umbilical cord (arrow) arises in its usual location. The mass contains numerous small bowel loops in which peristalsis was noted on real-time examination. No covering membrane was identified during the course of the examination.

| | | |
|---|---|---|
| **Arrow** | = | Umbilical cord |
| **Arrowheads** | = | Covering membrane of an omphalocele |
| **B** | = | Urinary bladder |
| **FB** | = | Fetal body |
| **L** | = | Liver |
| **M** | = | Small intestine |
| **S** | = | Fetal spine |

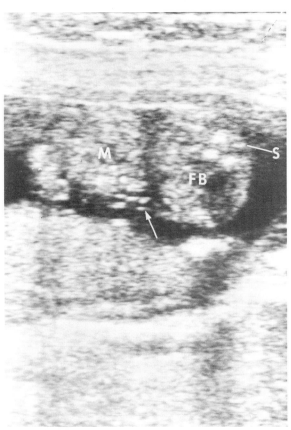

**FIG 16–264.**

## Fetal Renal Disease

Severe renal disease is accompanied by oligohydramnios. When oligohydramnios is seen in the second trimester, rupture of membranes should first be ruled out. If rupture of membranes is not present, then the most likely diagnosis is severe fetal renal disease. It is not always necessary to identify a mass in the renal bed. Severe oligohydramnios can be evaluated by visualizing the fetal urinary bladder. In the second trimester, the status of the fetal urinary bladder is more important in the diagnosis of severe renal disease than visualizing the kidneys themselves. The fetal urinary bladder increases in size over a period of 1–1½ hours and then empties. When severe oligohydramnios is present, the fetal urinary bladder must be closely examined. If it is not seen, the patient should be scanned at 15-minute intervals to see if the fetal bladder is visualized or changes in size. Figure 16–265 is the scan of a fetus in which severe oligohydramnios is present. Only a small amount of amniotic fluid (AF) was visualized on this study. The amount was dramatically decreased for the second trimester. The fetal urinary bladder was never visualized. The fetal body (arrowheads) is often difficult to see because of the oligohydramnios. No definite masses were identified in the renal fossa. The patient had a therapeutic abortion, and severe renal dysplasia was found in the fetus.

Figure 16–266 is a second-trimester scan showing severe oligohydramnios in another fetus. It is difficult to visualize the fetal body (arrowheads) because of the lack of amniotic fluid. The woman did not have rupture of membranes. The fetal urinary bladder was never visualized. There is a cystic mass present in the region of the renal fossa (arrow). This was the only tissue identified in what supposedly was the fetal renal beds. The important finding was lack of visualization of the fetal urinary bladder. The patient had a therapeutic abortion. At autopsy, the right kidney was absent and there was dysplastic disease of the left kidney.

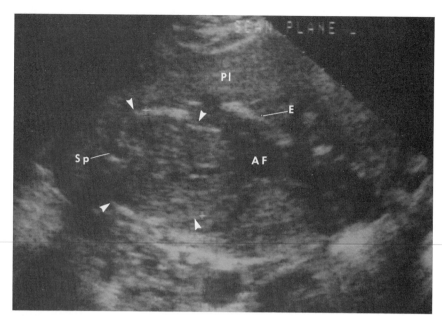

**FIG 16–265.**

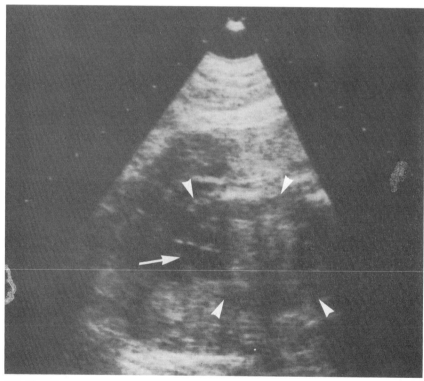

**FIG 16–266.**

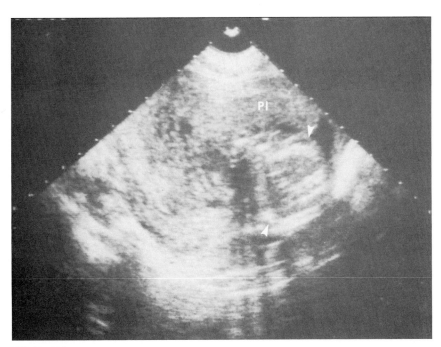

FIG 16–267.

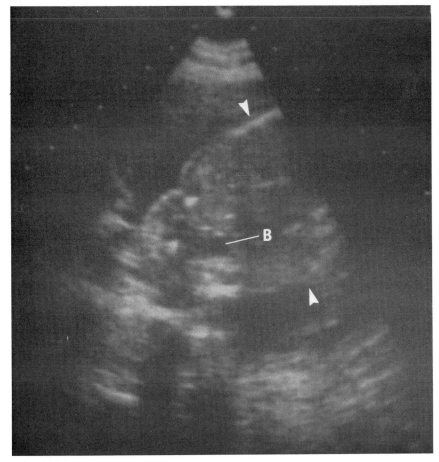

FIG 16–268.

Figure 16–267 also shows severe oligohydramnios in the second trimester. Little amniotic fluid is present. No masses were identified in the renal fossa and no normal kidneys were noted. The fetal bladder was examined and appears on the coronal scan shown in Figure 16–268. The fetal bladder was quite small. Additional scans were performed over a period of 1½ hours, with close examination of the fetal bladder at 15-minute intervals. The fetal bladder measured 6 mm in diameter and never increased in size. Some advocate giving diuretics to see if a fetal urinary bladder will change in size. We have not found this technique to be helpful. Because of the findings, the patient was asked to return in 1 week to determine whether or not the fetal urinary bladder findings were consistent. The entire procedure was again repeated 1 week later. No change in size and shape of the fetal urinary bladder was detected. Therefore, the diagnosis of severe renal disease was made. The patient had a therapeutic abortion. At autopsy, the left kidney was absent and the right kidney was severely hypoplastic.

| | |
|---|---|
| **Arrow** | = Dysplastic fetal kidney |
| **Arrowheads** | = Fetal body |
| **AF** | = Amnioticc fluid |
| **B** | = Fetal urinary bladder |
| **E** | = Extremity |
| **Pl** | = Placenta |
| **Sp** | = Spine |

## Fetal Renal Disease

When severe oligohydramnios is noted in the second trimester, the diagnosis of severe renal disease is quite likely. A major problem associated with low amniotic fluid volume is hypoplasia of the lungs. Even though the fetus may go to term, fetal breathing will be ccompromised because of lung hypoplasia. Figure 16–269 is the scan of a fetus examined in the second trimester. Severe oligohydramnios was present. As usual, it is difficult to identify the fetal body (arrowheads) because of the lack of surrounding amniotic fluid. Numerous cystic areas were present in the fetal renal fossa (arrows). This fetus was found to have bilateral dysplastic renal disease. Figure 16–270 is a longitudinal scan of another fetus with severe oligohydramnios in the second trimester. Practically no amniotic fluid is identified surrounding the fetus. The left kidney was visualized. A few small cystic aras were identified in the right kidney. This was an example of agenesis of the left kidney and dysplastic disease of the right kidney.

Figures 16–271 and 16–272 are transverse and coronal scans of a fetus in which a different entity is present. Oligohydramnios was noted in the second trimester. In this instance, both kidneys were visualized. They are unusual in appearance and are bilaterally enlarged and extremely echogenic. This appearance is seen in infantile polycystic disease. The reason for the increased echogenicity of the kidneys is the extremely small size of the abnormal cysts. They are too small to separate on ultrasound. Therefore, they appear as highly echogenic structures within the kidneys. The result is severe oligohydramnios and subsequent hypoplasia of the lungs due to lack of room for lung expansion.

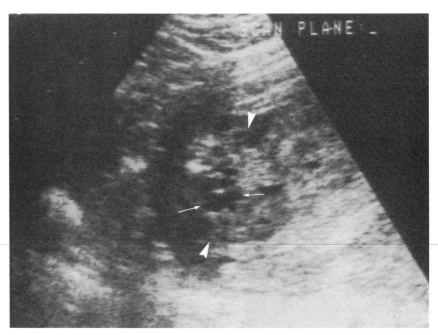

FIG 16–269.

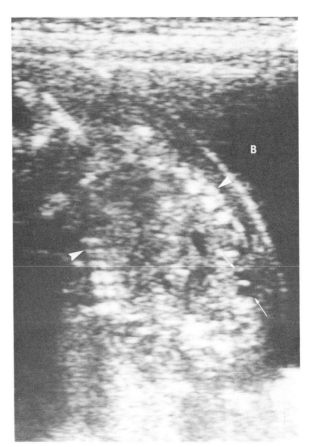

FIG 16–270.

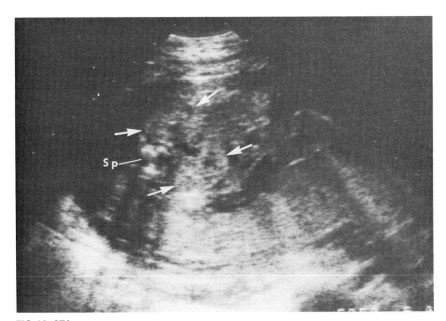

FIG 16–271.

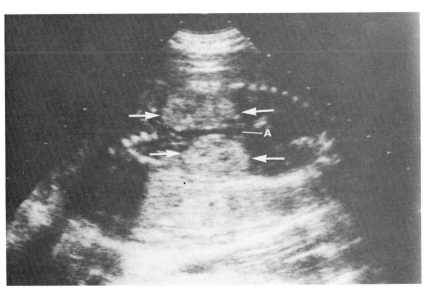

FIG 16–272.

| **Arrowheads** | = | Fetal body |
| **Small arrows** | = | Dysplastic kidneys |
| **Large arrows** | = | Infantile polycystic kidneys |
| **A** | = | Fetal aorta |
| **B** | = | Maternal urinary bladder |
| **Sp** | = | Fetal spine |

## Renal Obstruction

Renal obstruction in the fetus has a similar ultrasound appearance as that noted in the adult. It is important that several studies be performed since transient renal obstruction in utero has been described. Follow-up scans performed on a different day and with different maternal hydration would be helpful in determining whether or not the fetal renal obstruction persists.

Figures 16–273 and 16–274 are scans in which bilateral hydronephrosis (H) is present. Figure 16–273 is a coronal scan in which the renal pelves and calyces are dilated. There is also evidence of dilatation of the ureters. Figure 16–274 is a longitudinal scan of the pelvis in which the fetal bladder (B) is noted to be markedly distended. The tubular structure on the inferior aspect of the fetal bladder (arrow) represents a dilated ureter. This fetus was found to have posterior urethral valves leading to a bladder outlet obstruction. This in turn resulted in bilateral hydronephrosis, which was identified in Figure 16–273. Mild oligohydramnios was present.

Figure 16–275 is a scan through the fetal abdomen in which numerous large sonolucencies were identified. They corresponded bilaterally to the renal bed. The architecture and appearance suggested bilateral hydronephrosis. Very little parenchymal tissue was identified. Severe oligohydramnios was noted. The findings indicated bilateral fetal hydronephrosis.

Figure 16–276 is a longitudinal scan of the uterus in which the fetal abdomen is large and distended compared to the fetal head. Within the fetal abdomen are numerous fluid-filled tubular structures. These structures were secondary to hydroureter and hydronephrosis. The fetus had prune-belly syndrome. When we see large dilated ureters within the entire abdomen, the possibility of prune-belly syndrome should be considered. A cesarean section was performed because of the large size of the fetal abdomen.

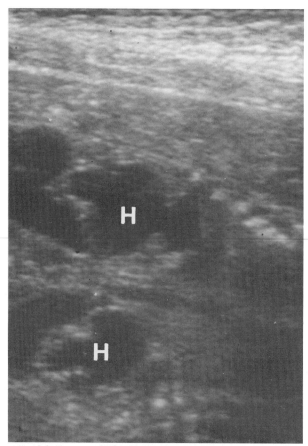

**FIG 16–273.**

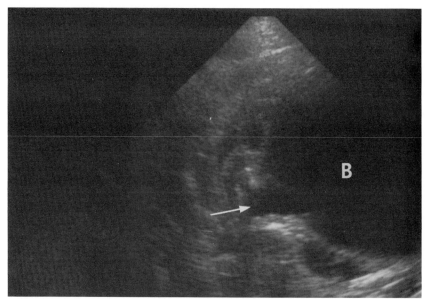

**FIG 16–274.**

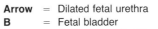

Arrow = Dilated fetal urethra
B     = Fetal bladder
H     = Hydronephrosis (Figs 16–273,
         16–275)
H     = Fetal head (Fig 16–276)
S     = Symphysis
Ur    = Dilated ureters

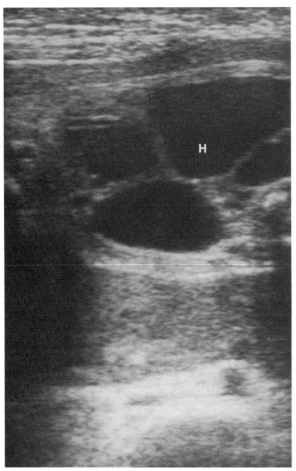

**FIG 16–275.**

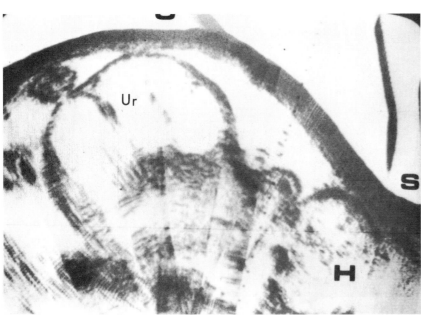

**FIG 16–276.**

## Hydronephrosis and Multicystic Kidney

Fetal hydronephrosis can be transient in nature. This must always be kept in mind. Figure 16–277 is the coronal scan of a fetal kidney at 37 weeks' gestation. The ultrasound findings are consistent with hydronephrosis. A ureter (U) and the renal pelvis (P) are dilated. The renal outline is well seen (arrowheads). Dilated calyces are also identified. The neonate was examined to determine whether or not hydronephrosis was present after birth, and the kidneys were found to be normal. This is an excellent example of the caution that must be exercised when intrauterine hydronephrosis is diagnosed.

Multicystic kidneys are a cause of cystic masses in the upper abdomen. Usually they are unilateral. The other kidney functions normally and the fetal urinary bladder is well seen. It is sometimes difficult to distinguish multicystic kidney from hydronephrosis. This can best be done on coronal scans showing the calyces, pelves, and ureters in the hydronephrotic kidney. In multicystic kidney, the cystic areas are random in appearance. Figure 16–278 is a coronal scan in a patient with multicystic kidney (C). One large cyst and numerous small ones are identified.

Figure 16–279 is a coronal scan in which a fluid-filled structure is noted in the left renal fossa (C). This was secondary to a multicystic kidney on that side. The possibility of hydronephrosis could be considered. However, a transverse scan of the area (Fig 16–280) demonstrates multiple cysts situated in a random fashion rather than in the expected anatomical location for hydronephrosis. Therefore, the diagnosis of multicystic kidney was more likely than hydronephrosis.

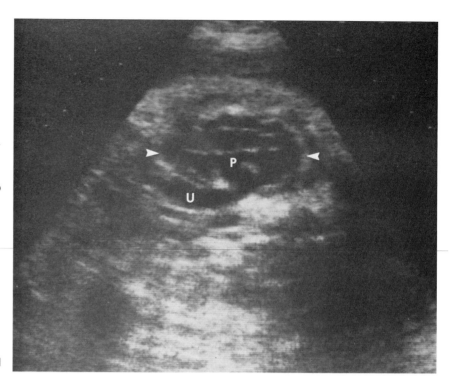

**FIG 16–277.**

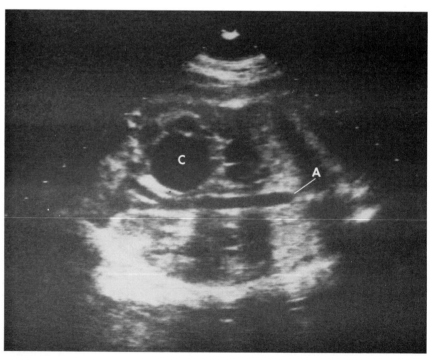

**FIG 16–278.**

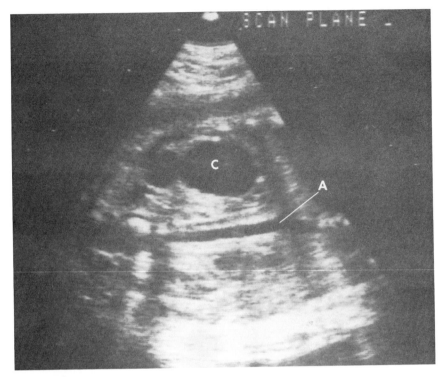

| **Arrowheads** | = | Renal outline |
| A | = | Aorta |
| C | = | Multicystic kidney |
| P | = | Renal pelvis in hydrone- |
|   |   | phrosis |
| Sp | = | Fetal spine |
| U | = | Hydroureter |

FIG 16–279.

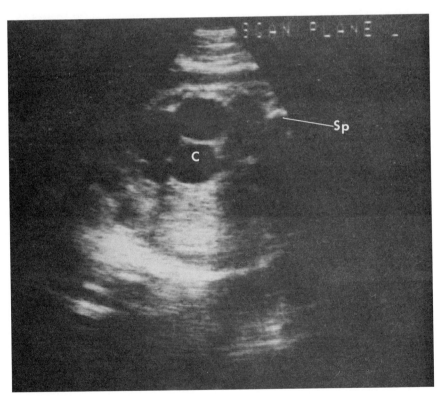

FIG 16–280.

## Abnormal Fetal Abdomen

Occasionally echogenic masses can be identified in the fetal abdomen. These are most often secondary to meconium. If meconium extravasates from the GI tract, it can create highly echogenic masses that may eventually calcify. However, we have seen cases of transient increased echogenicity that have disappeared in the course of the pregnancy. These are extremely important to identify and follow so that the mistaken diagnosis of a persistent abnormality is not made. Figure 16–281 is a scan through the fetal abdomen at approximately 17 weeks. A highly echogenic, well-marginated mass (arrowheads) was visualized in the fetal abdomen. This mass persisted in location and appearance throughout the entire study. The patient was rescanned at weekly intervals for 4 weeks. The first examination revealed very little change. However, some change in the appearance of the echogenic region was eventually detected. Figure 16–282 is a scan through the fetal abdomen made 4 weeks after the scan shown in Figure 16–281. The echogenic mass (arrowheads) is less discrete in appearance and less echogenic. The patient was rescanned periodically throughout pregnancy. The echogenic region disappeared and a normal infant was delivered. We feel these areas most certainly represent areas of meconium that are transient and eventually resolve.

Occasionally, fetal ascites can be identified in which a fluid lucency is present in the fetal abdomen. Figure 16–283 is a scan showing fluid in the fetal abdomen near the umbilical cord. The umbilical cord is actually seen entering the fetal abdomen and bifurcating.

It has been repeatedly emphasized that the fetus should be treated as a patient. Three-dimensional visualization of the fetus along with continual orientation while doing the ultrasound examination is a necessity. The scan in Figure 16–284 appears to be entirely normal. However, the fetal stomach (S) is situated on the right side of the fetal abdomen. There is no way to

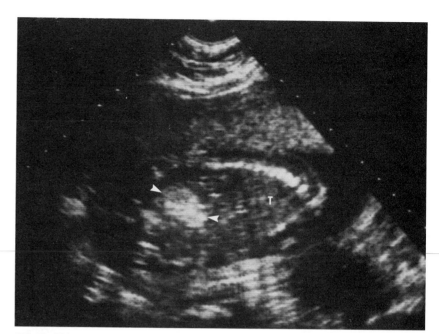

FIG 16–281.

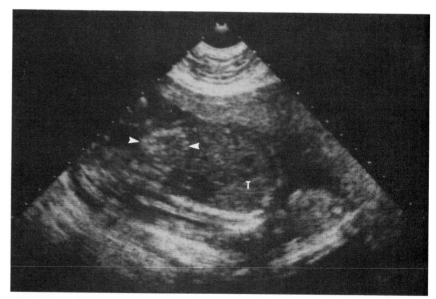

FIG 16–282.

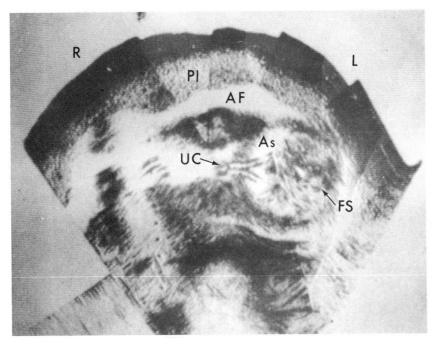

**FIG 16–283.**

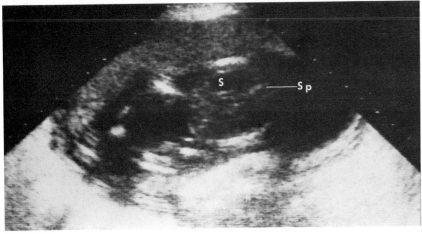

**FIG 16–284.**

determine its location on a single scan. However, by maintaining a three-dimensional mental image of the fetus, the sonographer was able to detect this anomaly, and a thorough examination of the remainder of the fetus was performed. The fetal heart was also on the right side. The aorta and inferior vena cava were completely reversed, with the aorta on the right side and inferior vena cava on the left side. These findings were secondary to a complete situs inversus. There are no congenital abnormalities associated with a complete situs inversus. If the heart and great vessels had been on the left side, numerous associated abnormalities would have been present. The parents decided to continue the pregnancy. A normal infant was born with complete situs inversus.

| Arrowheads | = Echogenic abdominal mass |
|---|---|
| AF | = Amniotic fluid |
| AS | = Ascites |
| FS | = Fetal spine |
| L | = Left |
| Pl | = Placenta |
| R | = Right |
| S | = Fetal stomach |
| Sp | = Fetal spine |
| T | = Fetal thorax |
| UC | = Umbilical cord |

## Fetal Ascites

The ultrasound findings of fetal ascites are similar to the findings in adult ascites. Fetal ascites can occur because of numerous problems such as Rh sensitization, infection, congenital anomalies and cardiac abnormalities. The term fetal "pseudoascites" has been used to refer to a small lucency near the fetal abdominal wall which was a normal anatomical finding. It is thought to be secondary to fat adjacent to the abdominal wall. It must be recognized as normal and not overdiagnosed as fetal ascites. In fetal ascites, bowel loops can be seen floating, the liver can be displaced from the abdominal wall, and fluid can be noted in the hepatorenal angle. Figure 16–285 shows a small amount of ascites (As) displacing the liver away from the abdominal wall. This is slightly more pronounced than what is seen in pseudoascites. There is also evidence of a small amount of fluid on the other side of the abdomen beneath the abdominal wall. Figure 16–286 is another example of ascites in which the liver appears to float away from the abdominal wall, along with some fluid in the hepatorenal angle. The appearance is similar to what is seen in the adult. Figure 16–287 is an example of prominent fetal ascites in which the liver is displaced from the abdominal wall by sonolucent fluid. The umbilical vessels traverse the ascitic fluid on their way to the liver. Figure 16–288 shows severe ascites. The ascitic fluid is displacing the fetal bowel (Bo) centrally. The appearance resembles that of severe ascites in the adult, in which bowel loops float within the ascitic fluid.

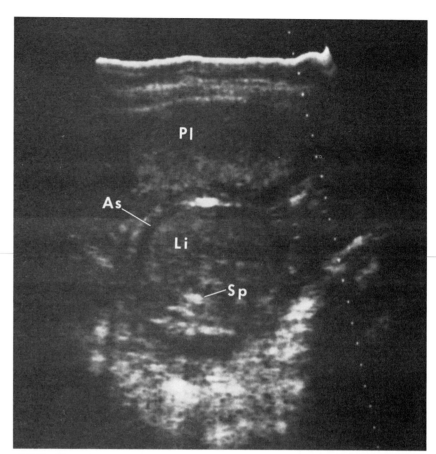

**FIG 16–285.**

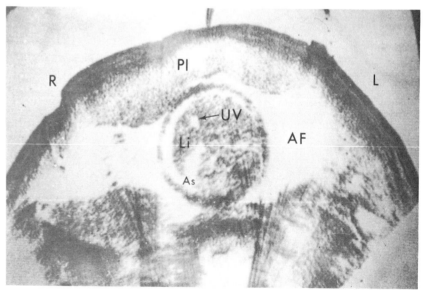

**FIG 16–286.**

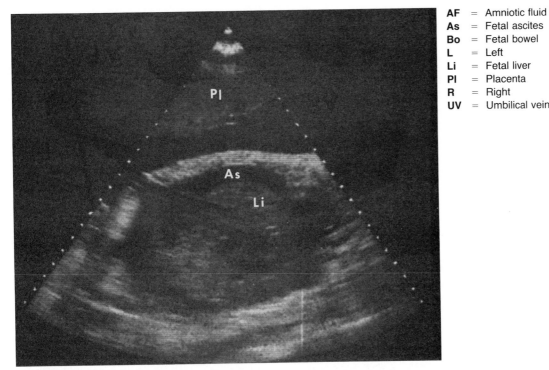

**AF** = Amniotic fluid
**As** = Fetal ascites
**Bo** = Fetal bowel
**L** = Left
**Li** = Fetal liver
**Pl** = Placenta
**R** = Right
**UV** = Umbilical vein

FIG 16–287.

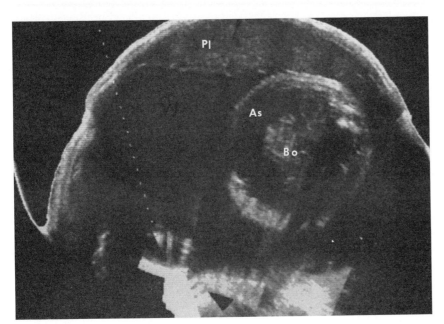

FIG 16–288.

## Fetal Edema

The double ring sign in fetal edema is caused by soft tissue edema displacing the skin echo away from the fetal skull and abdominal wall echoes. Figure 16–289 shows an example of the double ring sign about the fetal skull. The high-amplitude echoes of the fetal head (H) are separated by approximately 6–7 mm from the linear echo of the fetal skin (arrowheads). The distance between the fetal skin and the fetal skull is much greater than normal and is filled with edematous sonolucent fluid representing fetal edema.

A double ring sign may also be found over the fetal thoracic and abdomen. In Figure 16–290, the fetal body (B) is situated in the center of a large concentric ring (arrowheads) which is displaced away from the abdominal wall. The amount of edema in this case is approximately 1–1.5 cm in greatest thickness. This is an example of the double ring sign about the fetal body secondary to fetal edema.

False positive double ring signs may occur. It is important to be aware of these possibilities so that fetal edema is not incorrectly diagnosed. Fetal edema is a serious ultrasound finding and mandates close scrutiny of the fetus for the remainder of the pregnancy. Figure 16–291 shows a partial double ring sign around the fetal skull. The high-amplitude echoes surrounding the fetal skull (arrowheads) are removed from the calvarial echoes of the fetal head (H). The distance is greater than anticipated. However, in this instance the appearance is not caused by fetal edema. Rather, the maternal urinary bladder (arrowheads) in this scan is located just anterior to the fetal skull, giving the false appearance of fetal edema. It is important to recognize such normal anatomical variants so that the diagnosis of fetal edema is not made incorrectly. I have occasionally seen cases of mild polyhydramnios in which a double ring sign of the fetal head may be mistakenly interpreted as fetal edema. An example is shown in Figure 16–292. Note the concentric surrounding echo (arrowheads) slightly

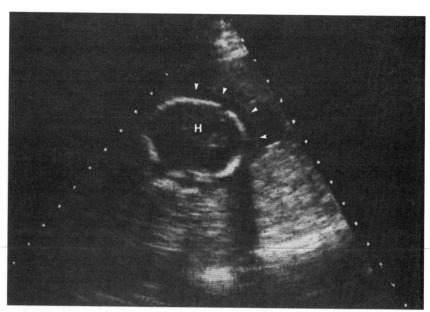

FIG 16–289.

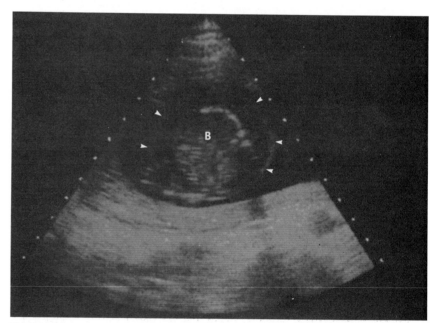

FIG 16–290.

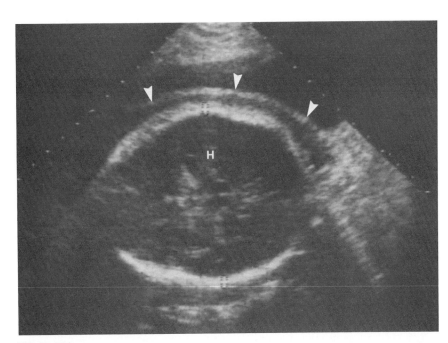

**FIG 16–291.**

displaced away from the fetal skull. This appearance could be considered secondary to represent fetal edema. Instead, it represented normal fetal hair floating in amniotic fluid in the presence of polyhydramnios. I have seen this in several instances and followed these babies to term. On visiting them in the neonatal nursery one finds no evidence of edema, but there is a full head of hair. So be aware of the possibility of a false double ring sign when mild polyhydramnios is present.

**Arrowheads** = Double ring sign
**B** = Fetal body
**H** = Fetal head

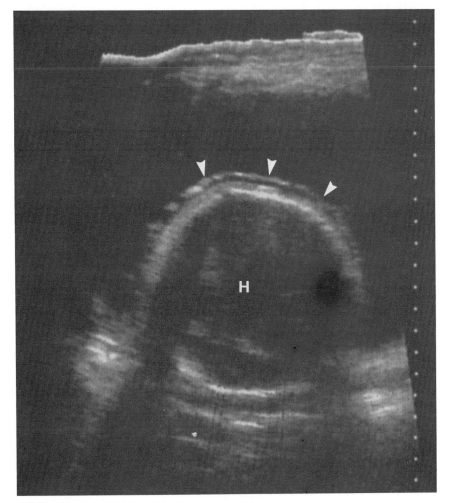

**FIG 16–292.**

## Cystic Hygroma

Another cause of elevated AFP levels is cystic hygroma, a collection of lymph often associated with a large mass about the fetal neck, head, or upper thorax. It may be an isolated lesion but often is associated with Turner's syndrome. Figure 16–293 is a transverse scan of the uterus in which we see a large fluid-filled mass (M) adjacent to the fetal trunk (FT). Initially, this may be thought to be amniotic fluid. However, the mass remained in one location and was surrounded by a capsular wall. It represented a large cystic hygroma.

Often a cystic hygroma is found in close association with the fetal neck or head. In Figure 16–294 a single fluid-filled mass is present adjacent to the fetal head (FH). Amniotic fluid (AF) surrounds the fluid-filled mass (M). To distinguish cystic hygroma from an encephalocele or a meningocele, it is important to evaluate the fetal osseous structures in the region. The occipital bone of the fetus was examined closely and no breaks were identified. The cervical spine was also without any osseous abnormalities. It is necessary to evaluate these structures by ultrasound to distinguish a cystic hygroma from a neural tube defect.

Figure 16–295 illustrates the difficulty of distinguishing between neural tube defect and cystic hygroma. The cystic hygroma (arrowhead) was quite small and situated in the region of the fetal neck. The fetus was only 16 weeks old, and fetal anatomy was difficult to delineate. No definite break was identified in the fetal calvarium or fetal spine. Therefore the diagnosis of cystic hygroma was made. After an elevated AFP Level was found in the mother, the cystic mass was identified in the fetal neck. The distinction between cystic hygroma and neural tube defect was made with ultrasound.

In Figure 16–296 a large cystic hygroma (M) is located in the posterior aspect of the fetal neck. The was initially thought to represent the maternal urinary bladder because of its fluid-filled nature. However, close scrutiny of the scan revealed the mother's

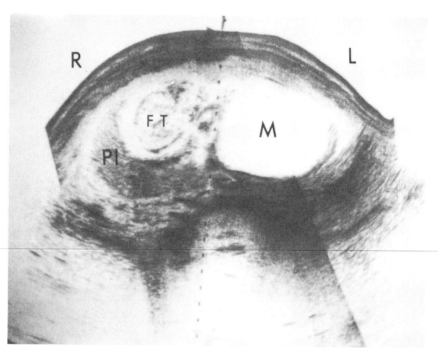

FIG 16–293.

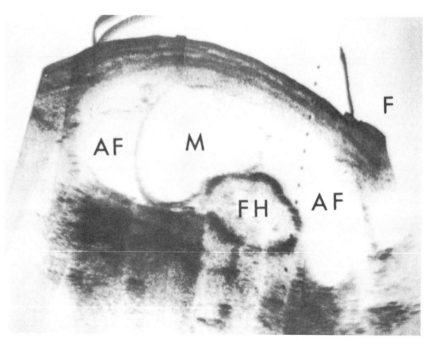

FIG 16–294.

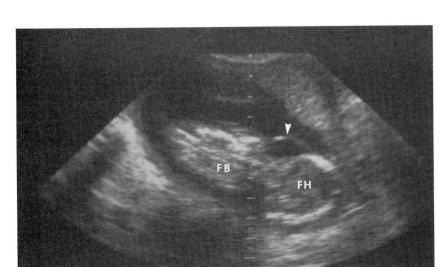

FIG 16–295.

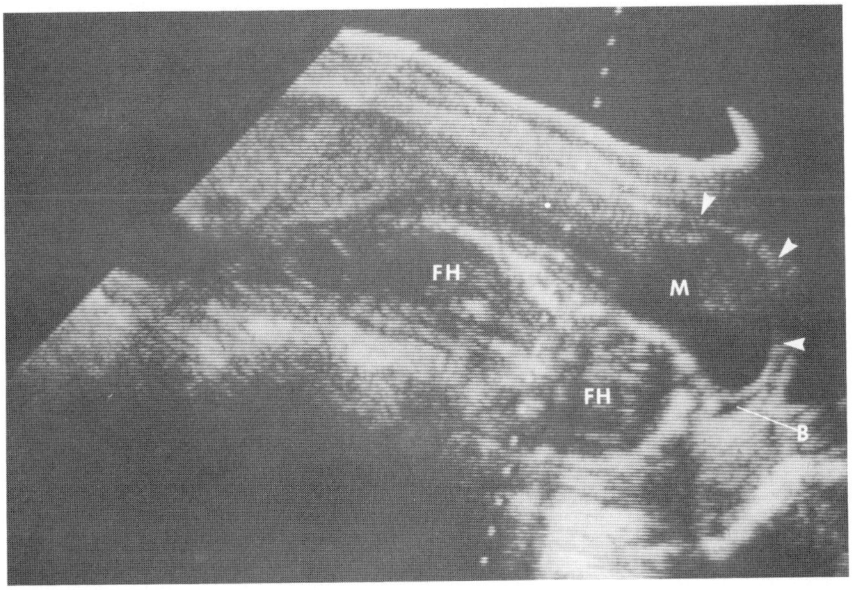

bladder to be markedly compressed (B). This was fortunate because the mass would have been missed. Note the flattening of the posterior aspect of the fetal head (FH) due to pressure from the cystic hygroma (arrowheads). Follow-up scans indicated that the maternal bladder increased in size, confirming the diagnosis of an intra-uterine cystic mass.

| Arrowheads | = | Cystic hygroma |
| --- | --- | --- |
| **AF** | = | Amniotic fluid |
| **B** | = | Maternal bladder |
| **F** | = | Foot |
| **FB** | = | Fetal body |
| **FH** | = | Fetal head |
| **FT** | = | Fetal trunk |
| **L** | = | Left |
| **M** | = | Cystic hygroma |
| **Pl** | = | Placenta |
| **R** | = | Right |

FIG 16–296.

## Cystic Hygroma

An ultrasound examination is extremely helpful in determining the possible cause of elevated AFP levels. When cystic masses are identified in the region of the fetal head and neck, the possibility of cystic hygroma and Turner's syndrome should be considered. If spinal and calvarial abnormalities are ruled out, then these possibilities become more likely. Amniotic fluid determinations will confirm the diagnosis of Turner's syndrome. Figures 16–297 and 16–298 are scans of the head and neck of a fetus which had large cystic hygromas about the neck along with fetal edema. A double ring sign (arrowheads) is present about the head and neck. The fetal neck (N) in Figure 16–298 is surrounded by two fluid-filled areas bilaterally and then by a double ring sign of edema. The fluid areas bilaterally represent large cystic hygromas. The double ring sign is caused by fetal edema.

Figures 16–299 and 16–300 are scans of another fetus that had a large cystic hygroma along with edema. Figure 16–299, a scan near the fetal head (H), shows a large multiloculated mass arising from the soft tissues posteriorly (H). This is a cystic hygroma. Examination of the osseous structures about the region did not reveal any break. Therefore, the diagnosis of cystic hygroma was made. Figure 16–300, a transverse scan about the fetal neck, reveals a large double ring sign (arrowhead), indicating fetal edema. The fetal neck (N) is surrounded by two fluid areas that are secondary to cystic hygromas. The appearance is similar to that in Figure 16–298.

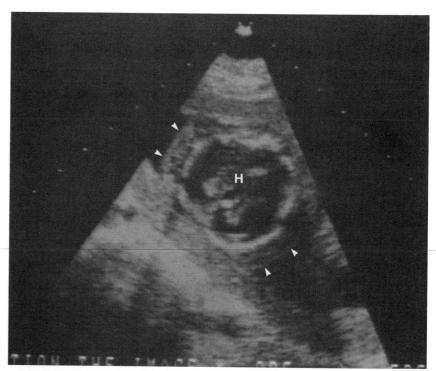

**FIG 16–297.**

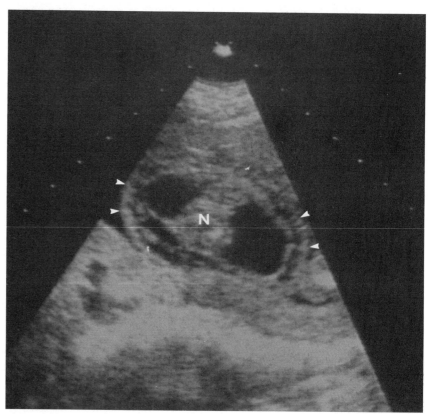

**FIG 16–298.**

Arrowheads = Fetal edema
H = Fetal head
M = Cystic hygroma
N = Fetal neck

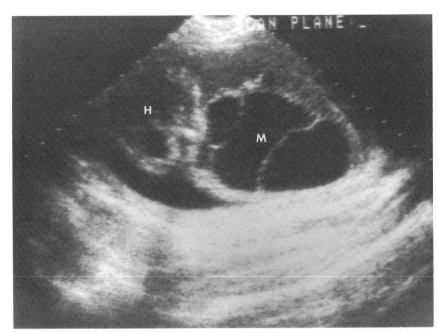

**FIG 16–299.**

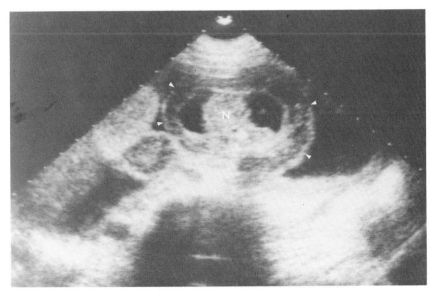

**FIG 16–300.**

## Hydrothorax

Occasionally fluid may be identified within the fetal thorax, either contained within cystic masses or moving freely in the pleural space. To determine whether fluid is in the pleural space, efforts must be made to identify the fetal lung. Figures 16–301 and 16–302 are coronal and transverse scans of a fetus in which large bilateral pleural fluid collections (Fl) are present. The diagnosis of fluid in the pleural space is made by identifying the fetal lung (arrowheads) floating within the pleural fluid. The fluid appears to be contained within an anatomical space rather than a cystic mass. Note the pointed appearance to the fetal lungs in Figure 16–301. This is typical of the appearance of compressed lung floating in fluid. The liver (Li) is situated inferior to the right pleural effusion in Figure 16–301. The left pleural effusion demonstrates the collapsed lung displaced medially. A transverse scan of the same fetus (Fig 16–302) demonstrates the fetal heart anteriorly and the main component of the pleural fluid situated posteriorly. Both fetal lungs are compressed by the large fluid collection.

Figure 16–303 is from a case in which a large fluid collection was noted during examination of the fetal abdomen. The initial transverse scans suggest that the fluid present to the left of the liver is secondary to an abdominal fluid collection. However, an important clue is the region of compressed echogenic lung (arrowhead). A coronal scan of the fetus (Fig 16–304) indicates that the fluid collection is not in the abdomen but in the fetal thorax. This left hydrothorax was so massive that it inverted the left hemidiaphragm, as is shown in Figure 16–304. The left pleural effusion (Fl) is situated in the fetal thorax but the diaphragm has been inverted so that the fluid collection appears to be adjacent to the fetal liver (Li). The echogenic region noted within the pleural fluid (arrowhead) represents a compressed left fetal lung.

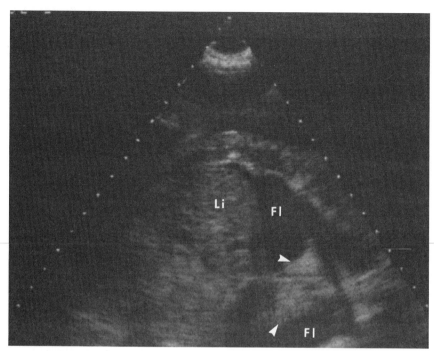

FIG 16–301.

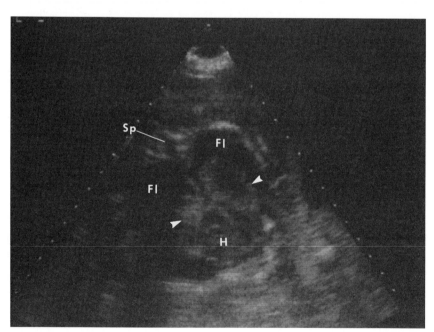

FIG 16–302.

| | | |
|---|---|---|
| **Arrowheads** | = | Compressed fetal lungs |
| **Fl** | = | Pleural fluid |
| **H** | = | Fetal heart |
| **Li** | = | Fetal liver |
| **Sp** | = | Fetal spine |

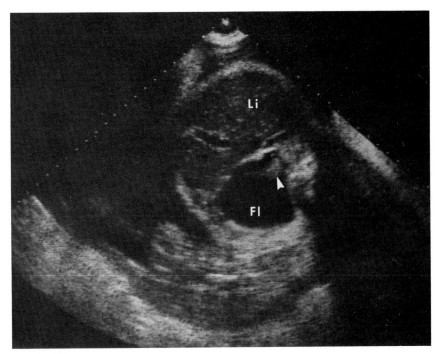

FIG 16–303.

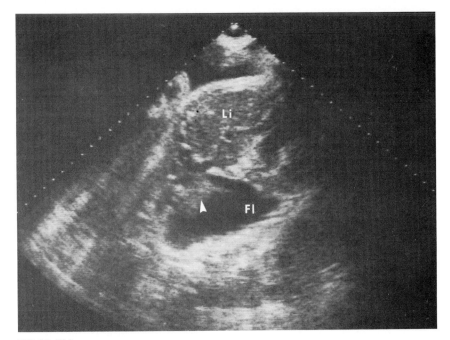

FIG 16–304.

## Thorax Abnormalities

Examination of the fetal thorax may reveal abnormalities in contour or within the thorax itself. Figure 16–305 is a scan from study performed because of suspected omphalocele. On examination of the fetus, the abdominal wall was found to be intact. Instead, a solid mass originating in the right hemithorax was identified. The fetal ribs were distorted. The findings indicated a soft tissue tumor in the region of the right hemithorax. The fetal abdomen and kidney on the right side were within normal limits. The infant was found to have a soft tissue sarcoma of the right hemithorax.

Figure 16–306 shows an echogenic mass in the fetal thorax, cephalad to the liver. The right lung was identified cephalad to the mass and had a normal echogenic appearance. The mass was found to be an echogenic area in the fetal lung on the right side that corresponded to the right lower lobe. The findings are consistent with pulmonary sequestration.

Figure 16–307 is a transverse scan of another fetus in which an extremely large multiloculated cystic mass is present in the right hemithorax. The mass displaces the heart and mediastinum to the left side. Very little normal lung was identified in the left hemithorax. A rim of echogenic tissue is seen around the cystic mass, representing residual right lung. The findings indicate cystic adenomatoid malformation of the right lung.

Figure 16–308 is a longitudinal midline scan in which there is disproportion in the size of the fetal thorax (T) and fetal abdomen (A). The disproportion persisted on numerous scans. It represents deformity of the fetal thorax secondary to thanatophoric dwarfism. This is a lethal abnormality that affects not only the long bones but also the thorax. The discrepancy in size between fetal thorax and fetal abdomen is best evaluated on a longitudinal scan.

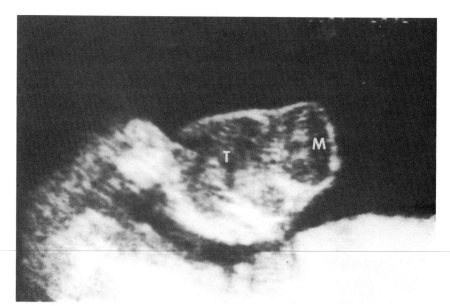

FIG 16–305.

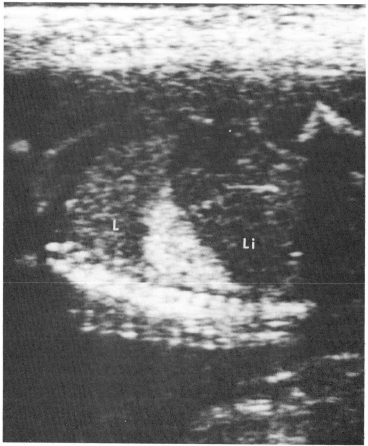

FIG 16–306.

A = Fetal abdomen
C = Cystic lung mass
H = Fetal heart
L = Fetal lung
Li = Fetal liver
M = Soft tissue hemisphere mass
Sp = Fetal spine
T = Fetal thorax

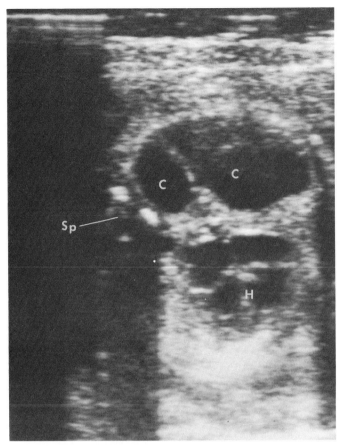

FIG 16–307.

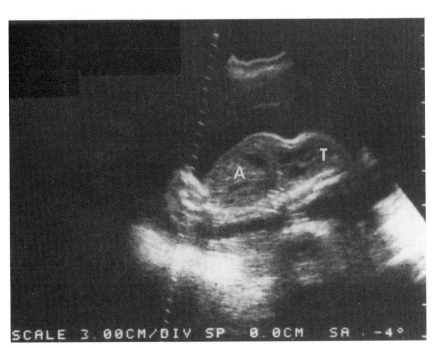

FIG 16–308.

## Fetal Cardiac Ultrasound

## Greggory R. DeVore, M.D.

Fetal hydrops was noted on routine examination of a 29-year-old woman at 19 weeks' gestation. Examination of the fetal heart revealed ventricular disproportion, with the right ventricle appearing larger than the left (Fig 16–309). The diagrams show a normal four-chamber view of the heart (top) and a fetal heart with ventricular disproportion (bottom). The large arrowheads on the scan outline the right atrium and ventricle; smaller arrowheads outline the smaller left atrium and left ventricle, documenting ventricular disporportion. M-mode measurements of the right ventricle showed it to be normal compared to the biparietal diameter. However, the left ventricle was well below the 5% confidence limit. The overall size of the heart was also below the 5% confidence limit. The right-to-left ventricular ratio was abnormal, as is noted in Figure 16–311 (points labeled 1). The diagnosis of hypoplastic left ventricle with a hypoplastic aortic root was made and confirmed at autopsy.

Figure 16–310 consists of diagrams and corresponding images from a 25-year-old woman evaluated at 33 weeks' gestation. Evaluation of a four-chamber view revealed ventricular disproportion. The left ventricle was small, at the 5% confidence limit. The short-axis view revealed the pulmonic outflow tract to be larger than the aortic outflow tract. However, the aortic root dimension was normal. After delivery, when the infant was 24 hours old, cardiac catheterization was performed and revealed coarctation of the aorta. The relative cardiac dimensions are plotted as points labeled 2 in Figure 16–311.

Figure 16–311 is a graph of the cardiac dimensions of the two cases just described.

Figure 16–312 shows the scan of a 29-year-old woman at 26 weeks' gestation. Fetal hydrops was noted. An echogenic mass was identified that originated within the interventricular septum and infiltrated the right ventricular cavity. Diagram A represents a

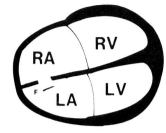
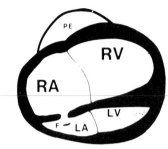
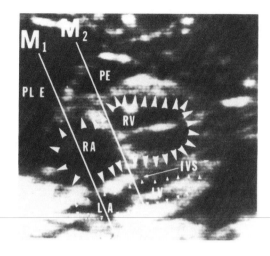

FIG 16–309.

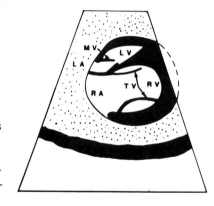
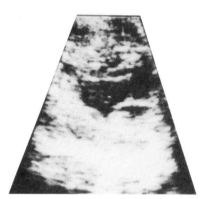

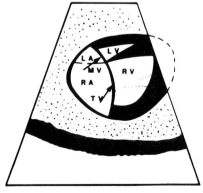
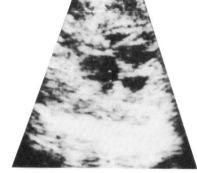

FIG 16–310.

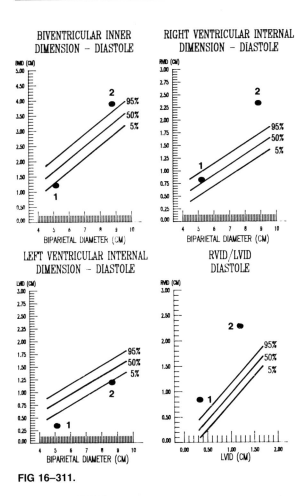

FIG 16–311.

normal four-chamber view of the heart; the abnormal view is shown just beneath it. The large mass in the interventricular septum turned out to be a rhabdomyoma. The fetal heart rate was 98 beats per minute. At 30 weeks' gestation, the fetus died. Autopsy confirmed the presence of a rhabdomyoma of the interventicular septum.

SOURCE: The illustration and discussion are provided by Greggory R. Devore, M.D.

| F   | = | Foramen ovale |
|-----|---|---------------|
| **IVS** | = | Interventricular septum |
| **LA** | = | Left atrium |
| **LV** | = | Left ventricle |
| **MV** | = | Mitral valve |
| **PE** | = | Pericardial effusion |
| **PLE** | = | Pleural effusion |
| **R** | = | Rhadomyoma |
| **RA** | = | Right atrium |
| **RV** | = | Right ventricle |
| **TV** | = | Tricuspid valve |

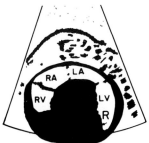

NORMAL

RHABDOMYOMA

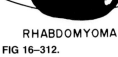

FIG 16–312.

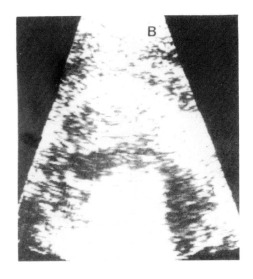

## Fetal Cardiac Ultrasound

A 31-year-old woman was evaluated at 21 weeks' gestation because a previous pregnancy had resulted in a child with transposition of the great vessels. Real-time examination of the aortic outflow tract revealed that it originated from the left ventricle (Fig 16–313). Further examination of the aortic outflow tract revealed brachiocephalic vessels originating from the arch. With the transducer directed parallel to the fetal spine, a short-axis view of the heart was obtained that showed the aortic root in the center with the pulmonary outflow tract draping over it (Fig 16–314). With medial rotation of the transducer bifurcation of the pulmonary arteries was demonstrated (Fig 16–314). With lateral rotation of the transducer the ductus arteriosus and the descending aorta were demonstrated (Fig 16–315). Findings were normal—the fetus did not have transposition of the great vessels.

Figure 16–316 is the scan of a 24-year-old woman who was referred at 30 weeks' gestation because of a fetal cardiac rate of 65 beats/min. The four-chamber view of the heart revealed absence of a large portion of the interventricular and interatrial septa. Also in Figure 16–316 are a diagram of a normal four-chamber view and a diagram of the atrioventricular canal defect seen in this fetus. The best method for imaging the interventricular and interatrial septum is to direct the transducer beam tangential to the septa. If the beam is directed perpendicular to the septa, it is more difficult to identify abnormal anatomy.

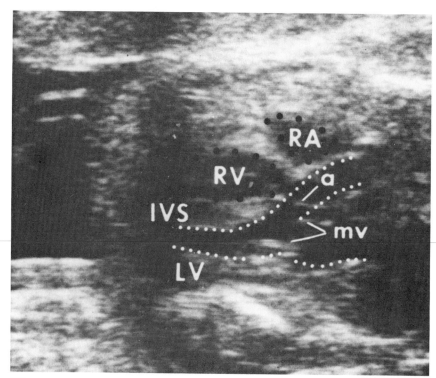

FIG 16–313.

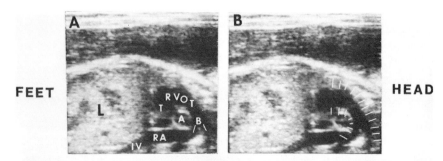

FEET    SAGITTAL PLANE    HEAD

FIG 16–314.

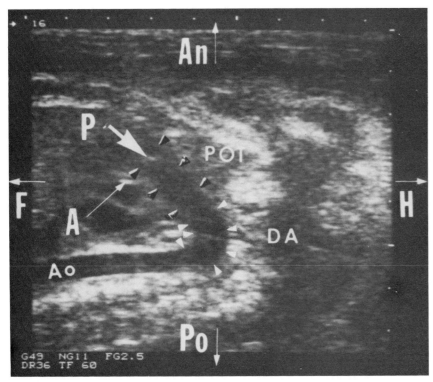

**FIG 16–315.**

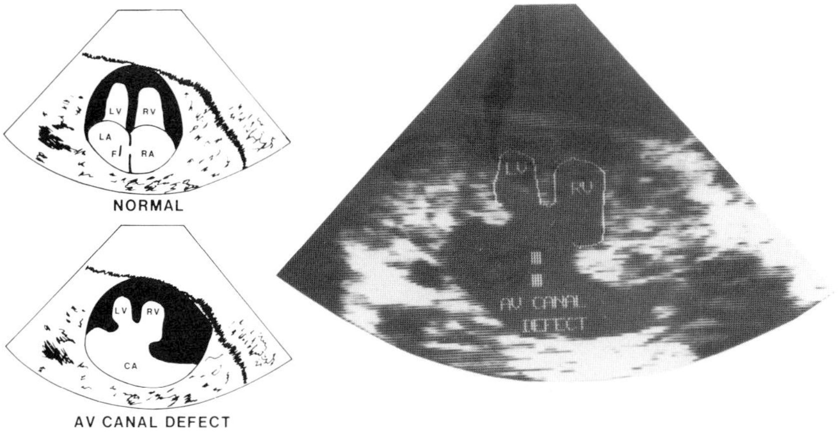

SOURCE: The cases and discussion are provided courtesy of Greggory R. Devore, M.D.

| **White dots** | = | Left ventricular inflow and outflow tracts |
| **Black dots** | = | Right ventricular and right atrial chambers |
| **A** | = | Aorta |
| **a** | = | Aortic valve |
| **Ao** | = | Descending aorta |
| **An** | = | Anterior |
| **B** | = | Bifurcation of the pulmonary artery |
| **CA** | = | Common atrium |
| **DA** | = | Ductus arteriosus outlined by arrows |
| **F** | = | Foramen ovale |
| **IV** | = | Inferior vena cava |
| **IVS** | = | Interventricular septum |
| **L** | = | Liver |
| **LA** | = | Left atrium |
| **LV** | = | Left ventricle |
| **MV** | = | Mitral valve |
| **P** | = | Pulmonary valve |
| **Po** | = | Posterior |
| **POT** | = | Pulmonary outflow tract |
| **RA** | = | Right atrium |
| **RV** | = | Right ventricle |
| **RVOT** | = | Right ventricular outflow tract |
| **T** | = | Tricuspid valve |

NORMAL

AV CANAL DEFECT

**FIG 16–316.**

## Fetal Cardiac Ultrasound

A 32-year-old woman underwent ultra-sound examination at 36 weeks' ges-tation because of spontaneous brady-cardia ascultated in the physician's office. Real-time examination of the fetus disclosed marked ventricular dis-proportion, with the right ventricle ap-pearing larger than the left. M-mode measurements of the ventricles dem-onstrated a dilated right ventricle above the 95% confidence limit. A small left ventricle below the 5% con-fidence limit was also identified, along with a biventricular inner dimension at the 5% confidence limit. Real-time ex-amination (Fig 16–317) and M-mode evaluation of the aortic route (Fig 16–318) disclosed it to be below the 5% confidence limit (Fig 16–319). The newborn survived for 36 hours before dying of a hypoplastic left ventricle. The ultrasound findings were con-firmed at autopsy.

Figure 16–320 is a graph of aortic root measurements in the fetus of a 24-year-old woman who underwent ul-trasound examination because of a fe-tal heart rate of 100 beats/min. Real-time examination of the fetal heart re-vealed a ventricular septal defect with an overriding aorta. The aorta ap-peared to be large on the real-time examination; the large size was con-firmed with M-mode measurements of the aortic root dimension (Fig 16–320). The diagnosis of tetralogy of Fallot was entertained and confirmed following birth.

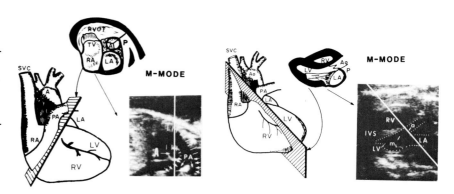

**SHORT AXIS**          **LEFT PARASTERNAL**

FIG 16–317.

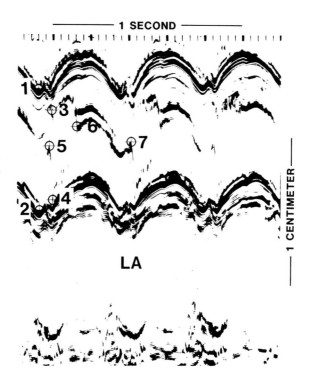

**AORTIC ROOT DIMENSION 1-2**
**AORTIC VALVE EXCURSION 3-4**
**LEFT VENTRICULAR EJECTION TIME 5-6**
**HEART RATE 5-7**

FIG 16–318.

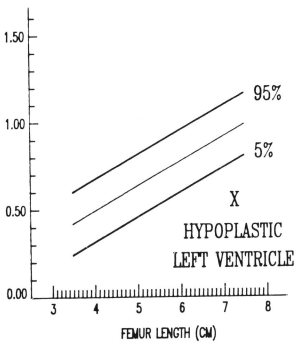

FIG 16–319.

SOURCE: The cases and discussion are provided courtesy of Greggory R. Devore, M.D.

| | | |
|---|---|---|
| **A** | = | Aorta |
| **a** | = | Aorta |
| **LA** | = | Left atrium |
| **LV** | = | Left ventricle |
| **m** | = | Mitral valve |
| **PA** | = | Pulmonary artery |
| **RA** | = | Right atrium |
| **RV** | = | Right ventricle |
| **1 and 2** | = | Aortic root dimension |
| **3 and 4** | = | Aortic valve excursion |
| **5 and 6** | = | Left ventricular ejection time |
| **5 and 7** | = | Heart rate |

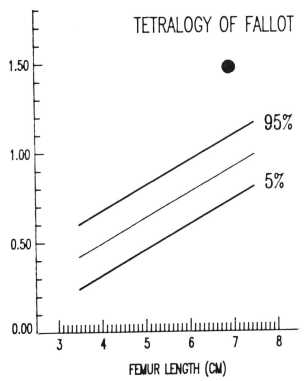

FIG 16–320.

## Intrauterine Growth Retardation; Triploidy

### Dennis A. Sarti, M.D.

During examination of the fetus, the relative size of the fetal head and fetal body should always be evaluated. Occasionally a fetus will be encountered with a disproportionately small body relative to the size of head. If this occurs in the third trimester, the possibility of intrauterine growth retardation (IUGR) should be considered. IUGR can be manifested by a small body size relative to head size. However, the head and body may decrease in growth rate proportionately, so a disproportionate relationship will not always be identified. Figures 16–321 and 16–322 are longitudinal and transverse scans of a pregnancy in the late second trimester. The most important finding is the lack of amniotic fluid (F). A common finding in IUGR is an extremely small volume of amniotic fluid for the time of pregnancy. The placenta is also highly echogenic, compatible with grade III. The longitudinal scan in Figure 16–321 shows a large fetal head relative to fetal body (FB) size. The findings are compatible with IUGR.

Figure 16–323 is a transverse scan of the uterus in another case of IUGR. The fetal head (FH) is much larger than the fetal body (FB). Almost no amniotic fluid is identified.

When disproportion in size of the fetal body and fetal head occurs in the mid-second trimester, the possibility of triploidy should be considered. Usually IUGR will not be detected this early. However, several cases of triploidy (69 chromosomes) have been characterized by a small fetal body relative to the size of the fetal head. Figure 16–324 is the scan of a 20-week pregnancy in which the fetal body (FB) and fetal head (FH) are disproportionate in size. The patient had an elective abortion. Triploidy was detected in the fetus.

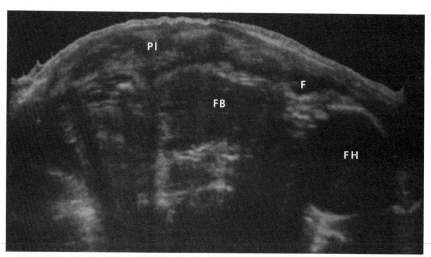

**FIG 16–321.**

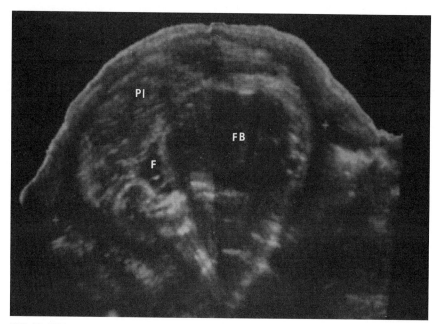

**FIG 16–322.**

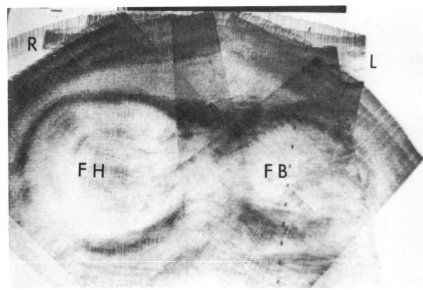

**F** = Amniotic fluid
**FB** = Fetal body
**FC** = Falx cerebri
**FH** = Fetal head
**FS** = Fetal spine
**PI** = Grade III placenta
**R** = Right

**FIG 16–323.**

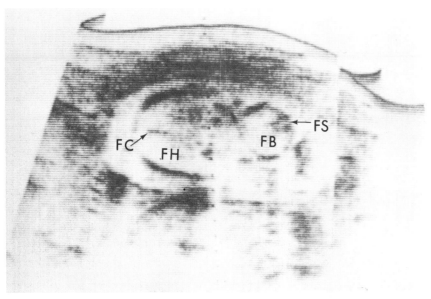

**FIG 16–324.**

## Fetal Death

If there is any question as to fetal viability, it is important to perform a Doppler or real-time examination in an effort to detect fetal cardiac activity. Several signs, however, give evidence of fetal death on a routine examination. The most common sign is fetal edema about the head or the body. Although this is not automatically consistent with fetal death, it is highly suspicious. Fetal edema and congestive heart failure may be seen in the fetus. Figures 16–325 and 16–326 are examples of fetal edema registering as a double ring sign around the fetal head. Edema is usually seen entirely around the fetal head. Mistakes can be made when the fetus is in close contact with the urinary bladder which will give a false double ring sign.

Another sign of fetal death is evidence of collapse of the normal contour of the fetal head. Figure 16–327 is an example of distortion of the fetal head. Marked straightening (arrows) of the fetal contour, which is markedly abnormal, is noted. When we see abnormality of the fetus skull, a Doppler or real-time examination should be performed. Figure 16–328 is an example of the overlapping of the skull bones, another sign of fetal death. Ultrasound visualization of overlapping of the fetal skull has the same significance as the x-ray finding of an overlapping skull. Both indicate fetal death.

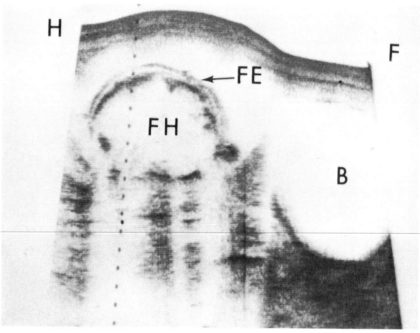

FIG 16–325.

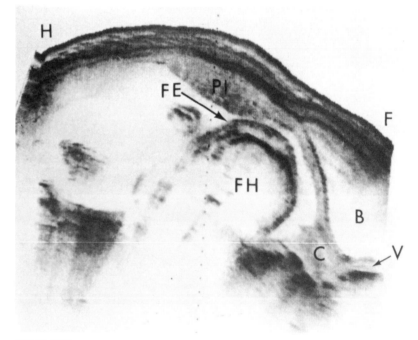

FIG 16–326.

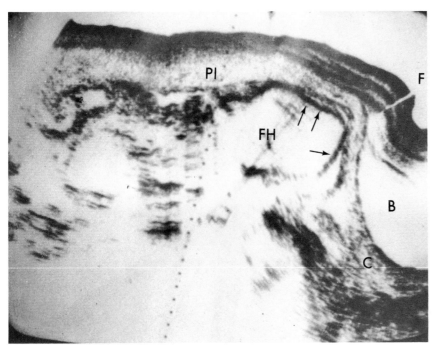

| Arrows | = | Distortion of fetal skull (Fig 16–327) |
| Arrows | = | Overlapping skull echoes (Fig 16–328) |
| B | = | Urinary bladder |
| C | = | Cervix |
| F | = | Foot |
| FC | = | Falx cerebri |
| FE | = | Fetal edema |
| FH | = | Fetal head |
| H | = | Head |
| PI | = | Placenta |
| V | = | Vagina |

FIG 16–327.

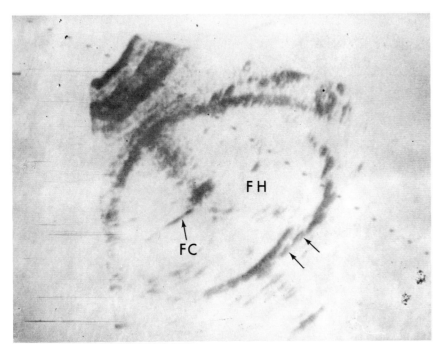

FIG 16–328.

## Fetal Death

Another indication of fetal death is the empty fetal thorax sign. When the fetal thorax is markedly distorted, this should be considered. Figures 16–329 and 16–330 are scans of a twin pregnancy. One of the twins is no longer viable. Here we see the empty thorax sign. The normal echo pattern of the fetal thorax is not seen. Instead, the thorax appears more lucent with coarser echoes within it. There is a marked distortion of the contour of the fetal thorax compared with normal fetal body seen in Figure 16–330. The normal circular to oval structure of the fetal thorax is lost. We are seeing evidence of degeneration of the fetus with collapse of the fetal thorax, similar to collapse of the fetal skull.

Figure 16–331 is an example of distortion of the fetal spine (arrows). Normally the fetal spine is fairly straight on longitudinal scan. Marked distortion and angulation of the fetal spine, however, are present. This ultrasound finding corresponds to the marked angulation in fetal death on x-ray. We again see evidence of fetal degeneration when this marked anatomical distortion takes place. Figure 16–332 is an example of collapse of the fetal head and the fetal body. We see severe oligohydramnios along with marked difficulty in visualizing the normal fetal structures.

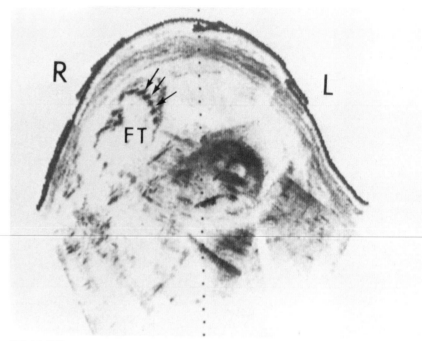

FIG 16–329.

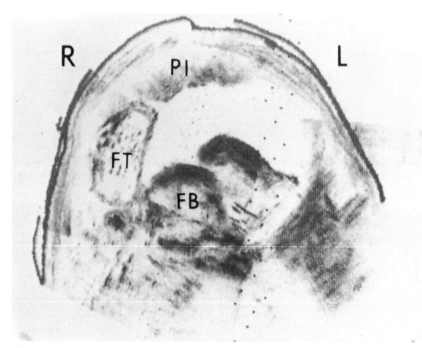

FIG 16–330.

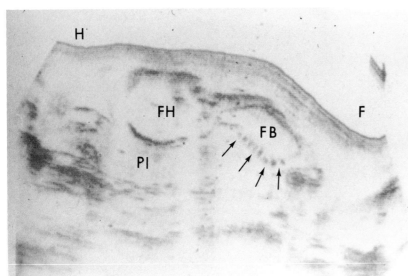

FIG 16–331.

FIG 16–332.

## Fetal Death

Separation of the amnion from the chorion may be visualized in fetal death. In early pregnancy the amnion and chorion are not intact. The amnion can be seen as a sharp linear echo in close proximity with the chorion. However, by approximately 16 weeks, the amnion and chorion are adjacent to each other and no fluid is seen between them. If the fetus dies, fluid can collect in the chorionic space. The amnion can be noted to separate from the chorion, as seen in Figures 16–333 and 16–334. This finding initially may be confused with a large mass around the fetus, such as a cystic hygroma.

One sign of fetal death has been called the empty thorax sign. Figures 16–335 and 16–336 are transverse and longitudinal scans of the fetal abdomen in which we have the equivalent of the empty fetal abdominal sign. No normal anatomical structures are identified in the fetal abdomen (A). There is an irregular, uneven echo pattern with scattered high-amplitude echoes present throughout the fetal abdomen. This disruption of normal tissue planes is secondary to fetal degeneration. An empty fetal abdominal sign is the equivalent of the empty fetal thorax sign. It basically represents degeneration of normal tissue.

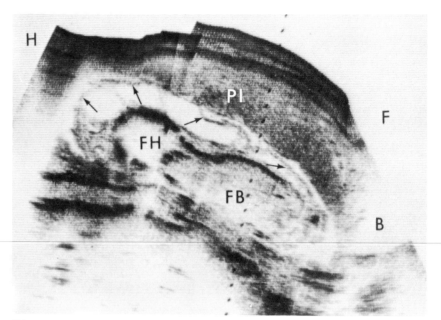

FIG 16–333.

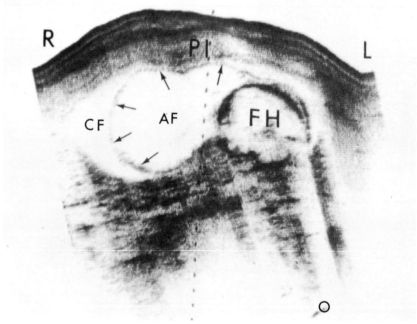

FIG 16–334.

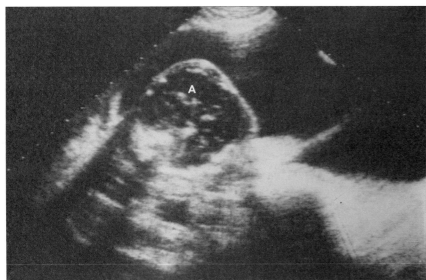

**FIG 16–335.**

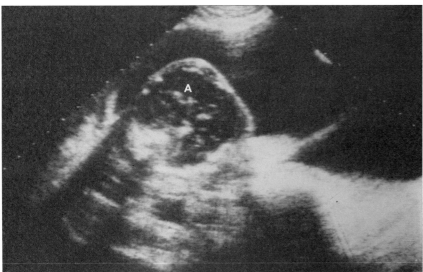

**FIG 16–336.**

A = Abnormal fetal abdomen
AF = Amniotic fluid
Arrows = Amnion
B = Urinary bladder
CF = Chorionic fluid
F = Foot
FB = Fetal body
FH = Fetal head
H = Head
L = Left
Pl = Placenta
R = Right

## Degenerating Placenta and Fetus

A hydatidiform mole can easily be mistaken for a degenerating pregnancy. Figures 16–337 and 16–338 are examples of early degeneration of the placenta (arrows). Numerous sonolucent structures are seen within the placental tissue. This is highly suggestive of a hydatidiform mole. In Figure 16–337, however, enough amniotic fluid is present that there is no difficulty distinguishing this as a pregnancy rather than a molar pregnancy. Figure 16–338 is a transverse scan with some remaining fetal echoes. When severe placental and fetal degeneration occurs, this picture can often be confused with a hydatidiform mole.

Figures 16–339 and 16–340 are scans of a degenerating pregnancy with some confusion as to whether or not we are dealing with a molar pregnancy. The longitudinal scan (Fig 16–339) demonstrates numerous strong echoes (arrows) throughout the uterus. A molar pregnancy usually has a fairly even echo pattern to it, more consistent with placental tissue. A degenerating pregnancy, as in this case, tends to have a coarser echogenic appearance. Figure 16–340 is a scan of the same case. Several sonolucent areas (arrows) are dispersed throughout the uterus. We are usually able to determine a degenerating pregnancy because of the coarseness and unevenness of the echo pattern. A molar pregnancy has a rather even speckled appearance to it. Because of the spectrum, however, overlap of the two entities is possible. In some instances, distinguishing between the two can be quite difficult.

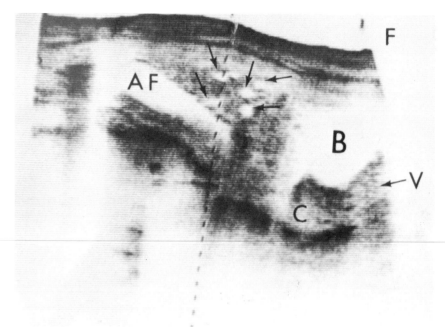

FIG 16–337.

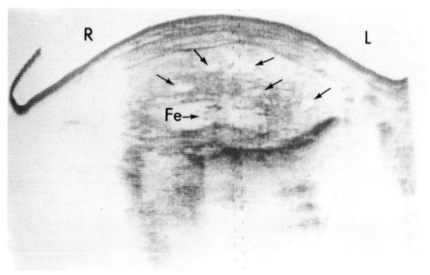

FIG 16–338.

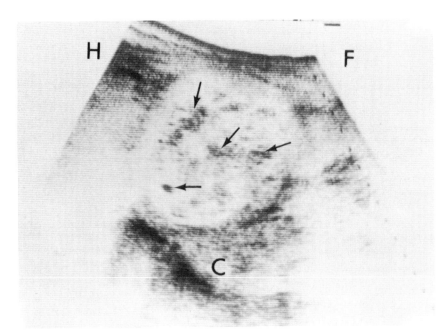

FIG 16–339.

**Arrows** = Degenerating placenta
**AF** = Amniotic fluid
**B** = Urinary bladder
**C** = Cervix
**F** = Foot
**Fe** = Fetus
**H** = Head
**L** = Left
**R** = Right
**Sp** = Spine
**V** = Vagina

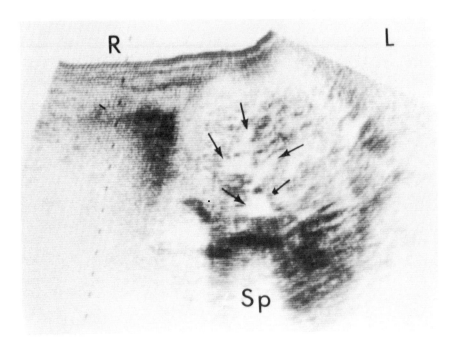

FIG 16–340.

## Incompetent Cervix

The incompetent cervix is clinically described as a painless, bloodless, dilatation of the endocervical canal, usually occurring during the second trimester of pregnancy. Ultrasound can easily depict fluid in the endocervical canal and therefore confirm the diagnosis of incompetent cervix. Figure 16–341 is a longitudinal scan showing the normal appearance of the endocervical canal. The endocervical canal appears as a strong linear echo in the midportion of the myometrial echoes of the cervix. The normal length of the endocervical canal varies from approximately 2.5 to 6 cm. There should be no evidence of fluid in the endocervical canal during the course of a normal pregnancy. When examining a patient for incompetent cervix, it is important to have the bladder well filled. Overdistention of the bladder, however, may actually lead to collapse of an incompetent cervix.

Figure 16–342 is an example of a longitudinal scan in a patient with incompetent cervix and an overdistended bladder. The urinary bladder is markedly distended and actually compressing the cervix. The patient was asked to partially void to relieve bladder pressure. Figure 16–343 is a scan of the same patient after partial bladder emptying. The fluid in the endocervical canal confirms the diagnosis of an incompetent cervix.

We now routinely examine a patient suspected of having an incompetent cervix with a full urinary bladder and again after partial bladder emptying. If the bladder is markedly overdistended, it may cause closure of an incompetent cervix. Figure 16–344 is a transverse scan through an incompetent cervix with fluid in the endocervical canal.

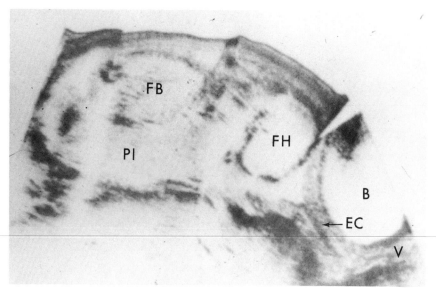

FIG 16–341.

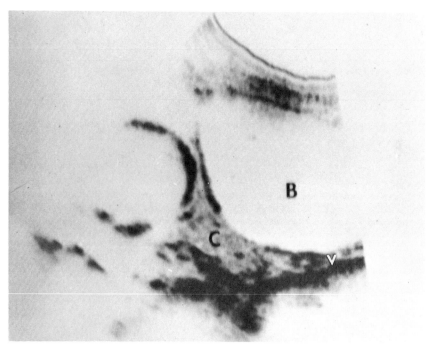

FIG 16–342.

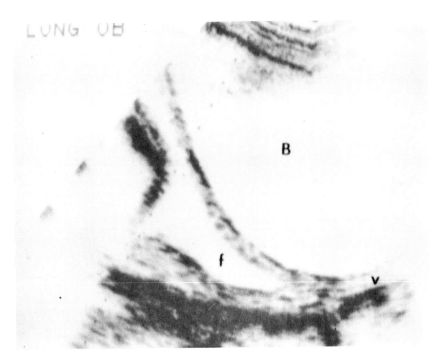

B  = Urinary bladder
C  = Cervix
EC = Normal endocervical canal
f  = Fluid in the endocervical canal,
     secondary to incompetent cervix
FB = Fetal body
FH = Fetal head
Pl = Placenta
V  = Vagina
v  = Vagina

FIG 16–343.

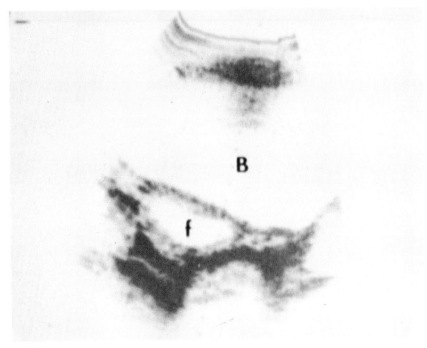

FIG 16–344.

## Incompetent Cervix

Figure 16–345 is another example of incompetent cervix with amniotic fluid in the endocervical canal. The amniotic fluid is visualized almost to the external os. When examining a patient for incompetent cervix, it is important to align the transducer parallel to the long axis of the endocervical canal. This is best determined on the transverse scans by marking the right and left borders of the cervix on the patient's skin. Longitudinal scans are then begun parallel to the long axis of the cervix.

Figure 16–346 is an example of incompetent cervix in a twin pregnancy. A cephalic fetus with the fetal head near the internal os is seen. Amniotic fluid is noted in the endocervical canal, again nearly completely to the external os. A second fetus is noted in the breech position in the fundal region of the uterus.

Figures 16–347 and 16–348 are examples of another case of incompetent cervix. There is markedly severe dilatation of the endocervical canal by amniotic fluid. This patient had marked bulging membranes; this is easily visualized on the ultrasound examination. Amniotic fluid is seen actually bulging into the proximal vagina.

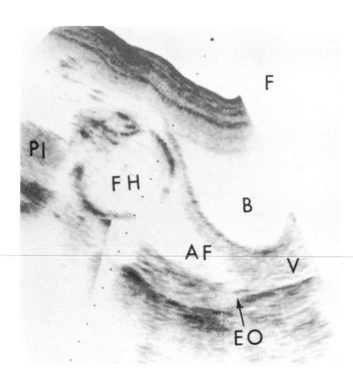

**FIG 16–345.**

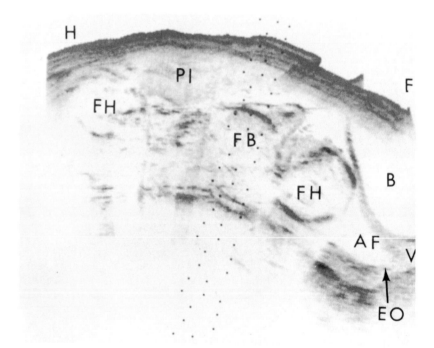

**FIG 16–346.**

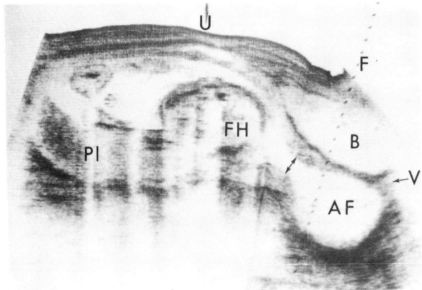

FIG 16–347.

| | | |
|---|---|---|
| **AF** | = | Amniotic fluid |
| **B** | = | Urinary bladder |
| **EO** | = | External os |
| **F** | = | Foot |
| **FB** | = | Fetal body |
| **FH** | = | Fetal head |
| **H** | = | Head |
| **L** | = | Left |
| **PI** | = | Placenta |
| **R** | = | Right |
| **U** | = | Umbilical level |
| **V** | = | Vagina |

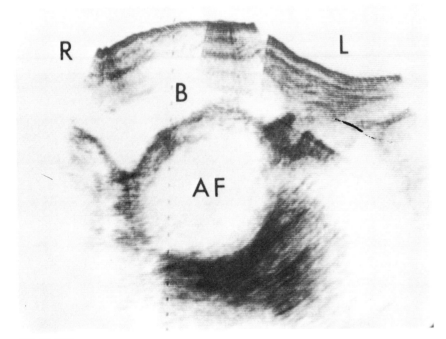

FIG 16–348.

## Incompetent Cervix

If incompetent cervix is suspected, serially examinations at 4–7 day intervals are suggested. The reason for
the short intervals is that incompetent
cervix can develop quite rapidly. Close
examination at short intervals is necessary to detect incompetent cervix
before it develops. Figure 16–349 is a
scan of a patient at 17½ weeks. The
bladder is not overly distended. The
cervix is well seen. The internal os
(arrow) is noted to be closed. The
overall length of the cervix was approximately 3 cm.

Figure 16–350 is the same patient
12 days later. There is the suggestion
of some fluid in the internal canal. The
woman was rescanned with the bladder partially emptied (Fig 16–351). A
large amount of fluid is now seen in
the endocervical canal (EC). The partial bladder emptying revealed the
presence of incompetent cervix. Over
the 12-day interval, incompetent cervix
developed all the way to the external
os.

Occasionally, on examination of the
endocervical canal and cervical region, some fluid will be identified in
the vagina. Figure 16–352 is an example with vaginal fluid (F). Most of
the time this represents reflux of urine
from the urinary bladder. However, it
may be secondary to hemorrhage or
leaking of amniotic fluid. In this instance, there was rupture of membranes with decreased amniotic fluid
noted in the pregnancy and fluid present in the vagina.

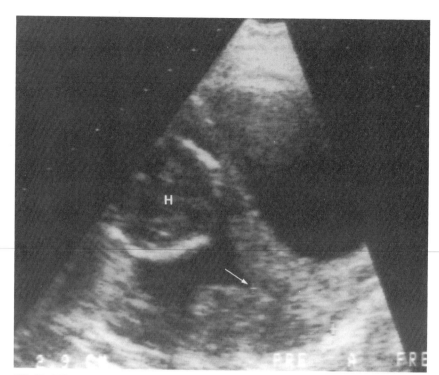

**FIG 16–349.**

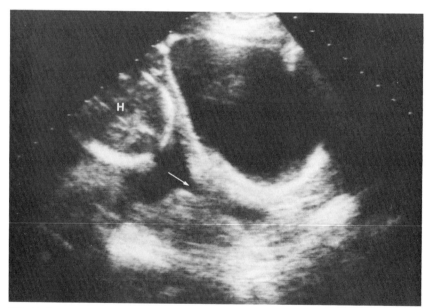

**FIG 16–350.**

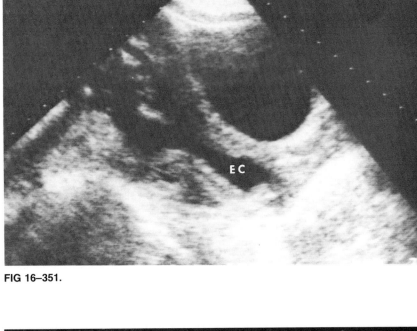

Arrow = Internal cervical os
EC = Endocervical canal with fluid
FB = Fetal body
FI = Fluid in the vagina
H = Fetal head

**FIG 16–351.**

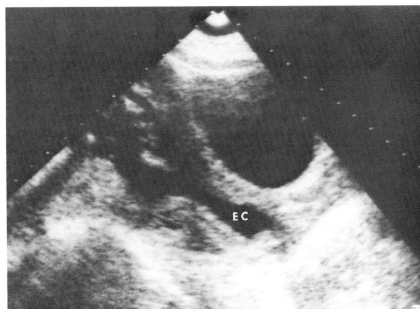

**FIG 16–352.**

# 17.
# Pediatric Ultrasound

Hooshang Kangarloo, M.D.
Jack O. Haller, M.D.

## 17a.
## ULTRASONOGRAPHY OF THE HEPATOBILIARY TRACT, LIVER, AND DIAPHRAGM

Hooshang Kangarloo, M.D.

### Ultrasonography of the Hepatobiliary Tract

Ultrasonography is a major diagnostic modality used in the screening and evaluation of pediatric hepatic diseases. Parenchymal hepatic disease, whether focal or generalized, can alter the normal homogeneous acoustical properties of the liver and allow a finite differential diagnosis. If the liver is secondarily involved, or infected by disease of adjacent structures such as the extrahepatic biliary system, pancreas, or any mass lesion, this may also be evaluated. Assessment of the biliary and portal venous system is a routine part of each examination. The ultrasound examination of all hepatic lesions in children is beyond the scope of this book. However, two areas require attention: liver cysts and liver tumors. Liver cysts may be congenital or acquired. Congenital cysts are of two types. One is solitary, which is rare, and the second is polycystic disease. Polycystic disease is an embryologic maldevelopment analogous to and associated with (in 50% of patients) polycystic disease of the kidneys. Acquired cystic lesions are secondary to hydatid disease, amebic abscess, or pyogenic abscess.

### Liver Tumors

In children, neoplasms involving the liver are usually metastatic, particularly if the lesions arise from neuroblastoma or Hodgkin's disease. Primary neoplasms, benign or malignant, can arise from the liver parenchyma, the bowel ducts, blood vessels, or connective tissues. Hemangiomas may be capillary or cavernous and are the most common benign tumors of the liver. They should be considered as simple vascular hamartomas rather than true neoplasms and may be associated with extrahepatic hemangiomas in some instances. In infancy, hemangioma may present as an abdominal mass and may be associated with anemia, ascites, jaundice, and high output congestive heart failure. These lesions can be solitary or multicentric.

The majority of primary liver tumors in children are malignant. There are two distinct forms of carcinoma of the liver: hepatoblastoma and hepatoma. They both present in most patients as an abdominal mass in an otherwise well child. Hepatoblastoma is more common in the pediatric age group and occurs during the first 3 years of life; it may be present at birth. Hepatomas tend to occur after 5–6 years of age and may complicate other hepatic diseases.

Ultrasonography is an excellent method for evaluating biliary tract dilation. Two entities are particularly important in pediatric patients: ductal ectasia and choledochal cysts. There are two forms of ductal ectasia. The first is more common and is characterized by intrahepatic biliary dilation with associated periportal fibrosis. This entity is properly termed congenital hepatic fibrosis with biliary ectasia. This disease has a poor prognosis, with cirrhosis noted at birth. The second form, Caroli's disease, is less common and is characterized by segmental intrahepatic dilation without associated periportal fibrosis. Caroli's disease is usually not diagnosed until adult life, when biliary calculi may form within the dilated segment and cause biliary obstruction.

Choledochal cyst is a congenital cystic dilation of any segment of the extrahepatic biliary ducts, usually involving the major portion of the common bile duct. Dilation of intrahepatic bile ducts may also be associated. It is more common in females and in Japanese. The majority of patients are diagnosed before they reach 10 years of age. The pathogenesis of this disease, although not well understood, is probably related to the anomalous insertion of the common bile duct into the proximal portion of the pancreatic duct. This anomalous insertion allows reflux of pancreatic enzymes into the biliary ducts, causing inflammation and subsequent fibrosis, which leads to segmental narrowing and proximal dilation. Neonates and infants have symptoms of obstructive jaundice, and older children have a typical triad of jaundice, abdominal pain, and a palpable abdominal mass.

Choledochal cysts can be divided into two major types, and each type in turn may be subdivided. Type 1 is concentric dilation of the common bile duct; this accounts for the majority of choledochal cysts (about 90%). Type 2 is excentric dilation of the common bile duct (bile duct diverticulum). Type 1a is concentric dilation of the common bile duct without intrahepatic biliary dilation, and type 1b is concentric dilation of the common bile duct with intrahepatic biliary dilation. Type 2a is excentric dilation of the common bile duct without intrahepatic biliary dilation.

## Diaphragm; Juxtadiaphragmatic Space

Visualization of the diaphragm by conventional methods such as plain film radiography, fluoroscopy, double exposure technique, and pneumoperitography is well known. However, visualization of the diaphragm on ultrasonography generally obviates the need for more invasive techniques. Patients are examined in the supine or decubitus position. The transducer is placed on the abdomen immediately inferior to the anterior costal margin or in the intracostal space. Using real-time technique, diaphragmatic movement is assessed during inspiration and expiration.

The juxtadiaphragmatic areas are also easily evaluated on ultrasonography. If a juxtadiaphragmatic abnormality is suspected on an abdominal or chest roentgenogram, ultrasonography is helpful in suggesting the proper diagnosis or in indicating what specific tests or procedures are necessary to make the diagnosis. It will also aid in differentiating the origin of a juxtadiaphragmatic lesion (e.g., liver, heart, lung, or diaphragm) and may suggest a histologic diagnosis by depicting the internal architecture of the lesion. The examination is individually tailored to a specific clinical problem. In general, perpendicular views of the region of interest are obtained using the liver or spleen as a sonographic window.

## Ultrasonography of the Adrenal Gland

Ultrasonography is the modality of choice for evaluation of the adrenal glands in infants and children. The examination requires neither ionizing radiation nor sedation and if necessary it can be performed with portable equipment. The flexibility of the technique, permitting visualization of the gland in transverse, longitudinal, and oblique sections, yields details of internal architecture unobtainable with other noninvasive or even invasive imaging modalities.

In order to fully appreciate the sonographic appearance of normal glands in infants and children, it is first necessary to understand the development of the gland. Each adrenal gland consists of a cortical portion derived from celomic epithelium and a medullary portion composed of cells derived from the neural crest. The celomic epithelium forms a grooved ridge that develops into the fetal cortex. During the seventh and eighth weeks of embryonic life, a cluster of neural cells migrating along the adrenal vein invades the cortex, thus establishing the primordium of the adrenal medulla.

At birth the adrenal cortex consists primarily of an actively secreting inner zone, the fetal cortex, surrounded by a thin outer zone, the adult cortex. The adrenal medulla in the full-term infant is represented by clumps of cells linked together by vascular sinusoids near the hilum of the gland which stretches peripherally a short distant into the gland. In neonates the adrenal cortex is relatively large and hypoechoic with convex borders. The adrenal medulla is seen as linear echogenic structures. During the first 3–5 months of life, the inner zone of the fetal cortex atrophies and is replaced by abundant fibrous connective tissue. This results in a relative increase in the echogenicity of the gland, but the convexity of the border is maintained. Although striking in its extent up to 1 year of age, the fibrous tissue in turn completely disappears by 3 years. Meanwhile, the adult cortex differentiates into the three zones of the adult gland. In children older than 1 year the disappearance of the fibrous tissue coincides with the return to a hypoechoic appearance and a change in the contour of the gland from convex to straight or concave. In older children, unlike neonates, convex borders should be considered abnormal.

### Adrenal Pathology

Adrenal lesions may arise from the cortex or medulla and may be functional or nonfunctional. Adrenal hyperplasia causes bilateral enlargement of the glands with convex borders. Adrenal adenoma arising from the cortex causes enlargement of the cortical portion of the gland, leading to an egg-like appearance. Medullary lesions such as pheochromocytoma cause enlargement of the base of the gland with sparing of the apex (apical sign). It is important to remember that about one third of affected children with pheochromocytoma have multiple tumors.

Among nonfunctioning adrenal lesions the most common is the hemorrhagic adrenal cyst seen in neonates. Fifteen percent of cysts are bilateral and, depending on the time of hemorrhage, lesions may be totally sonolucent or contain echogenic material. Follow-up examinations will demonstrate a decrease in the size of the hemorrhagic cyst, differentiating it from cystic neuroblastomas.

### Neuroblastoma

Neuroblastoma is the most common solid tumor of infancy and childhood and accounts for about one half of neonatal malignant tumors. Seventy-five percent of neuroblastomas arise from the abdomen and 40% of these are adrenal in origin. Neuroblastoma may also occur in the thorax (15%), pelvis (4%), and neck (4%). Tumors of unknown origin account for 2%. Most neuroblastomas present in the first 5 years of life, with a peak at ages 1–2½ years. Clinically, neuroblastomas most commonly present as an abdominal mass, usually found by the mother or pediatrician on routine examination. Ultrasonography plays a major role in diagnosing and staging neuroblastoma. Careful sonographic examination will reveal the extent of the lesion and whether there is contralateral involvement. Visualization of the great vessels and celiac axis is important for staging of the disease as well as to determine the effect of therapy during follow-up examinations.

### Urinary Tract Dilation

The term hydronephrosis is technically incorrect, but it is used radiologically to indicate abnormal dilation of the renal pelvis and calyces. Similarly, "hydroureter" indicates abnormal dilation of the ureter. The compound term, hydroureteronephrosis, notes the combination of two conditions. Although the most common cause of dilation of the renal calyces, pelvis, or ureter is some type of obstruction, dilation can occur without obstruction. Therefore, it is important to distinguish between obstructive and nonobstructive dilation. Surgery can potentially correct the former condition; however, it has limited usefulness, if indicated at all, in the later condition.

Since obstructive or nonobstructive urinary tract dilation may appear identical on excretory urography and ultrasonography, two tests are now being used to determine whether or not an obstruction is present. The first is the Whitaker test, which is a measurement of urine flow rate through a suspected obstruction, and the second is diuretic-augmented urography, which entails the intravenous injection of Lasix following excretory urography and observing washout of the contrast agent. Urinary tract obstruction has a number of renal as well as extrarenal complications. These include renal parenchyma atrophy, renal cystic dysplasia, and pulmonary hypoplasia. Anemia, polycythemia, and hypertension may also result from obstructive uropathy.

Sonographic examinations are performed with the

patient in the prone, supine, or lateral decubitus position. Transverse and longitudinal scans of both kidneys are obtained. In neonates the renal pyramids are prominent and the renal cortex is more echogenic than in older children. The perisinus fat is not developed. As the child grows the pyramids become less prominent, and at about 10–12 years of age one can visualize the perisinus fat. Small fluid areas within this renal sinus complex generally represent a normal renal pelvis rather than hydronephrosis. With mild hydronephrosis these dense, central echos are separated by small ovoid or elongated lucencies. With more severe hydronephrosis these sonolucencies become larger and may coalesce. In the most severe form the major portion of the kidney is replaced by a sonolucent sac. Ultrasonography is an excellent screening procedure in suspected cases of hydronephrosis as it has only a 2% false negative rate. However, there is a 26% false positive rate. Therefore, patients with an abnormality detected by ultrasonography may require follow-up excretory urography.

*Pelvoureteric Junction Obstruction*

This is the most common congenital obstruction of the urinary tract. Conditions necessary for the development of pelvoureteric junction obstruction are a renal pelvis and an anatomic pelvoureteric junction. Both of these are absent in the upper moiety of a duplex kidney so that for practical purposes, if a pelvoureteric junction obstruction occurs in a duplex kidney, it will involve the lower pole moiety. A few cases of pelvoureteric junction obstruction involving the upper pole moiety have been reported but have not been anatomically explained. Pelvoureteric junction obstruction of the lower pole moiety may mimic Wilms' tumor in the early phase of an excretory urogram. But ultrasonography can easily differentiate between a hydronephrotic sac and a solid Wilms' tumor. In infants under 1 year of age pelvoureteric junction obstruction is often bilateral, more frequent in males, and often associated with other significant anomalies of the urinary tract and other organs. These associations are usually not present in older infants and children. The most common clinical presentation of pelvoureteric junction obstruction is a palpable abdominal mass or abdominal enlargement. However, there may be diverse clinical manifestations.

*Distal Ureteral Obstruction*

It is imperative to differentiate obstructive from nonobstructive causes (such as reflux) of ureteral dilation. One must remember, however, that these two conditions may coexist, which necessitates careful fluoroscopic examination of the distal part of the ureter on voiding cystourethrography. The primary megaureter, which is usually seen in male infants, commonly involves the left side and is bilateral in 20% of patients. Genitourinary anomalies (such as agenesis of the kidney) and anomalies of other organ systems are commonly associated. A simple ureterocele usually presents in an infant or young child as a unilateral flank mass. A ureterocele is often associated with ectopic insertion of a ureter. This often involves the ureter draining the upper pole moiety of a duplex collecting system and is more common in females. About 50% of patients have a duplicated collecting system on the opposite side. In males, an ectopic ureterocele can occur without duplication and may be associated with a posterior urethral valve. Ultrasonography is highly accurate in diagnosing this condition. Sonograms of the abdomen will demonstrate the hydronephrotic upper pole and the dilated ureter. Scans of the pelvis with a distended bladder will reveal an ectopic ureterocele beneath the bladder mucosa.

Urinary tract dilation may be secondary to reflux without evidence of obstruction. One should also remember that urinary tract infection is one of the most common abnormalities of the urinary tract in children. Ultrasonography is the procedure of choice in screening children with a history of urinary tract infection, but it does not replace the need for voiding cystourethrography.

**Echogenic Kidney**

Increased renal echogenicity on ultrasonography is seen in various pathologic conditions. Correlation of renal size with the pattern and distribution of increased echogenicity and with the patient's age and clinical data will limit the differential diagnosis and suggest appropriate radiographic follow-up studies, thereby eliminating unnecessary procedures. In older children and adults, the renal cortex has a homogeneous echo texture that is less echogenic than the adjacent hepatic and splenic parenchyma. In normal neonates and young infants the renal cortex may be as echogenic as the liver. The medullary pyramids are hypoechoic areas regularly arranged around the central echogenic renal sinus.

Renal parenchymal disease often results in increased echogenicity of the kidneys, with renal parenchymal echoes greater than those of the liver and spleen in neonates and young children and equal to or greater than those of the liver and spleen in older children. Increased echogenicity of the kidneys has been described in many diverse conditions, including acute and chronic glomerulonephritis, hypertensive nephropathy, diabetic nephrosclerosis, acute tubular necrosis, leukemia, renal artery stenosis, nephrotic syndrome, renal dysplasia, nephrocalcinosis, Wilms' tumor, angiomyolipoma, and multilocular cyst. The reason for the development of echogenicity is not clear in all cases. In those with nephrocalcinosis it is due to the position of calcium within the tissue, and associated acoustic shadowing may be seen. Enlarged kidneys with increased echogenicity occur in patients with infantile polycystic disease and in some stages of renal vein thrombosis. However, infantile polycystic disease has a characteristic appearance with bilateral course linear echoes due to the reflection of the sound beam at tissue interfaces between dilated tubules. In contrast, renal vein thrombosis, which may be unilateral or bilateral, has a diffuse, finely echogenic pattern that is relatively uniform. In patients with Wilms' tumor increased echogenicity of the kidney is most likely the result of an inflammatory reaction and at times actual calcification. In patients with Burkitt's lymphoma increased echogenicity is most likely secondary to uric acid nephropathy. In our experience, lymphomatous involvement of the kidneys without associated uric acid nephropathy is characterized hypoechoic areas. In patients with chronic renal failure increased echogenicity is thought to be the result of an increased amount of collagen in the kidney or calcific deposits in the parenchyma. Renal dysplasia demonstrates increased echogenicity that is partly due to the consequences of chronic renal failure and is partly related to malformation of the kidneys. Premature infants who are on long-term Lasix treatment to control pulmonary edema may develop nephrocalcinosis. In these infants the kidneys are generally normal in size, and calcifications may be either unilateral or bilateral.

The causes of increased echogenicity are numerous. Observation of the size and pattern of echogen-

icity demonstrated on ultrasonography, together with pertinent clinical information, can suggest a specific etiology for increased echogenicity, and further diagnostic procedures can be suggested from the initial sonographic findings.

## Cystic Diseases of the Kidney

Numerous classifications have been proposed to define and encompass cystic diseases of the kidney. Microdissection studies are the basis for this classification and provide valuable information about the pathogenesis of renal cystic diseases. Well-accepted entities such as the dysplasias and polycystic diseases are grouped respectively. Those entities with an unknown or poorly understood pathogenesis are grouped according to their anatomic location, e.g., cortex or medulla. The remaining unusual intrarenal cystic lesions are grouped under a miscellaneous category, which includes renal cysts associated with inflammatory, neoplastic, and traumatic lesions of the kidneys.

Several diagnostic modalities are now available for evaluation of renal diseases. Ultrasonography has become a very useful screening modality for these diseases. Computed tomography (CT) nuclear scintigraphy, and angiography will be discussed in their appropriate contexts as they apply to specific diseases.

### Renal Dysplasia

The kidneys require a normal progression and branching of the ureteric bud and ampullae (the expanded forward portion of the dividing tubule) to properly induce metanephrogenic blastema to form nephrons. If this process is disturbed, maldevelopment will result. The following terms and definitions are offered to avoid confusion. *Plasia* originates from the Greek "plassein," meaning "to form." *Dysplasia* denotes abnormal formation. (Severe dysplasia is called aplasia.)

### Multicystic Kidney

The basic defect in the pathogenesis of a multicystic kidney is abnormal development of the advancing ureteric bud. This causes abnormal induction of the nephrogenic tissue, with subsequent formation of primitive, dysplastic tissues. This maldevelopment occurs very early in embryonic life, resulting in atresia of the ureter, pelvis, or both. There are two forms of multicystic kidney: pelviinfundibular atresia and hydronephrotic atresia.

In the more common form, the atresia involves the pelviinfundibular region. As a result, the subsequent growth and branching of the ureteral bud are markedly altered. This severe renal disorganization is seen pathologically as a "cluster of grapes" with no resemblance to a normal kidney. Central cores of solid tissue with recognizable dysplastic elements are surrounded by many cysts, ranging from a few millimeters to several centimeters in diameter. There is almost always an associated severe stenosis or atresia of the ureter. These cysts may or may not intercommunicate, depending on whether the proximal portion of the pelvis is present or obliterated.

In the hydronephrotic form of multicystic kidney, the atretic process involves only the ureter. The cysts in this form represent the dilated pelvicalyceal system, and they communicate via the dilated renal pelvis.

If one accepts the theory of an intrauterine obstruction as the major cause for development of a multicystic kidney, it is possible to explain focal and segmental forms of the disease: the focal form resulting in scattered areas of dysplasia secondary to collecting-duct obstruction, and the segmental form resulting in dysplasia of one moiety of a duplex collecting system.

Most multicystic kidneys manifest clinically as an abdominal mass in a healthy neonate, infant, or child. In fact, a multicystic kidney is the most common cause of an abdominal mass in a neonate. Rarely, the mass is undetected until adult life and is discovered incidentally during a urologic examination for an unrelated condition. In the adult, calcification may be seen in the walls of the cysts; this does not occur in children. No familial tendency has been described.

Up to one third of patients with a multicystic kidney have some form of obstructive uropathy involving the contralateral kidney. Therefore, it is essential to evaluate the urinary system with ultrasonography and excretory urography.

Ultrasonography usually demonstrates a large mass with multiple cystic areas of varying sizes separated by echogenic septa. There is no identifiable renal parenchyma or pelvicalyceal system, i.e., a well-defined ellipsoid and relatively sonolucent band of ho-

mogeneous echogenicity surrounding a linear, central, more echogenic band.

The flank mass may be identified on the scout film of the abdomen. During the total-body opacification phase of the excretory urography, opacification of the cyst walls may be seen as a result of their vascular supply. Subsequently, during the early excretory phase, faint, thin, curvilinear densities (termed "calyceal crescent") appear as a result of stasis of the contrast material in compressed collecting tubules that lie adjacent to the cysts. On delayed films, irregular "puddled" opacification may be seen in the small or medium-sized cystic spaces, probably due to tubular reabsorption of water and therefore concentration of the contrast material. The renal artery is either very hypoplastic or absent. The bladder is normal.

## MULTIPLE CYSTS ASSOCIATED WITH LOWER URINARY TRACT OBSTRUCTION

In children with congenital urinary outlet obstruction, the kidneys usually have small cortical cysts as well as renal dysplasia. These renal cysts are probably the result of increased pressure on the ampullae during fetal development of the kidney. The most common cause in males is a posterior urethral valve. Other less common causes are an ectopic ureterocele or, rarely, urethral atresia. Patients present with advanced renal failure, bilateral flank masses (the hydronephrotic kidneys), and a lower abdominal mass (the dilated bladder).

Ultrasonography and excretory urography will demonstrate bilateral hydroureteronephrosis and a dilated, trabeculated bladder. The pelvicalyceal systems, although markedly dilated, are normally formed and communicate with the ureters.

The cause for the outlet obstruction is usually identified by a voiding cystourethrogram. With a posterior urethral valve, the prostatic urethra is markedly dilated and the obstruction is at or just below the verumontanum. There is often associated vesicoureteral reflux.

### Polycystic Disease

Polycystic diseases of the kidney are divided into two major categories: polycystic disease in children and adult polycystic disease. It is generally accepted that these two forms are unrelated and represent distinct entities.

## POLYCYSTIC DISEASE OF THE YOUNG (TUBULAR ECTASIA)

Polycystic disease of the young encompasses a spectrum of diseases that has at one end the newborn type. It is best to consider polycystic disease of the young a two-organ disease, with the kidneys and liver involved in all patients. Multiple epithelial hepatic cysts, dilated bile ducts, and periportal fibrosis are invariably present. There is an inverse relationship between the kidney and liver with respect to the degree of involvement by the polycystic disease, depending on the patient's age at the manifestation of the disease. In younger children, the kidneys are more severely involved; in older children the liver is more severely involved. Both types are genetically inherited as an autosomal recessive disease occurring in siblings. There is no crossover between the different types of polycystic disease of the young. Therefore, if the disease presents early in life (the newborn type) and the child dies at an early age, all affected children in that family will do the same. If, in another family, the disease presents later in life (the childhood type), all affected children show this later onset of the disease and survive longer.

Pathologically, the kidneys are enlarged but maintain their reniform shape with a smooth cortical surface and normal fetal lobulation. There are numerous small cysts a few millimeters in diameter scattered throughout the kidney, giving it a spongy appearance. Gross inspection of the sectioned kidney shows dilated tubular channels oriented perpendicular to the cortical surface and extending to it. Most of the cysts represent dilated tubules (tubular ectasia), but some represent dilated nephrons. There is no dysplastic tissue present. There may also be cysts in other organs, such as the ovaries, pancreas, and lungs. The bladder and ureter are normal.

It is theorized that initially the ureteric bud and metanephrogenic blastema develop normally and give rise to normal nephrons. But at some time during the last half of intrauterine life, the proximal collecting tubules develop large saccules and diverticula, and the more terminal tubules become enlarged, leading to Potter's term "tubular gigantism."

The clinical presentation and cause of death depend on the type of polycystic disease of the young. Early in life (newborn type), patients have a protuberant abdomen and bilateral abdominal masses. The infant has a "Potter facies." The most common cause of death in the first few days of life is respiratory failure secondary to pulmonary hypoplasia, congestive heart failure, pneumonia, or pneumothorax. The lungs are hypoplastic as a result of the compressive mechanical pressure exerted on the lungs by the fetal abdominal contents and the uterus (associated maternal oligohydramnios). Following assisted ventilation, the alveoli can easily rupture, leading to pneumothorax. In those patients with adequate pulmonary development who survive the first few days, progressive renal failure develops.

The childhood form of the disease presents somewhat later, at 4 or 5 years of age, with the major symptoms related to periportal fibrosis, i.e., GI tract hemorrhage secondary to esophageal varices or jaundice secondary to severe liver disease. The cause of death is usually related to these complications.

**Roentgenographic Findings.**—Roentgenograms of the abdomen show enlarged kidneys bilaterally. The kidney function depends on the degree of renal involvement by the polycystic disease. In the newborn type, there is very poor renal function and the collecting systems are usually not seen satisfactorily. The nephrographic phase is often prolonged, as long as a week, and shows a radiolucent mottled appearance, which is the result of numerous small cysts. The dilated tubules may be visualized, appearing as a "brush border" perpendicular to the surface of the kidney. The diagnosis is obvious in this form of polycystic disease of the young.

In the childhood type, there is better renal function. Medullary tubular ectasia leads to stasis of the excreted contrast material in the dilated ducts and gives a "brush border" appearance. The pelvicalyceal systems and ureters appear normal. Differentiation from the adult form of polycystic disease presenting in childhood may be difficult by excretory urography. However, the demonstration of periportal fibrosis by ultrasonography or liver biopsy favors the diagnosis of the childhood type of polycystic disease of the young.

**Ultrasonographic Findings.**—The nephromegaly and multiple small uniform cysts, which give the kidney an increased echogenicity, are identified on gray-scale ultrasonography. The normal central echoes of the pelvicalyceal system are not seen. However, the most important aid provided by ultrasonography in this disease is in the evaluation of the liver. The demonstration of liver cysts and/or periportal fibrosis assures the proper diagnosis. The liver cysts appear as simple cysts, but the periportal fibrosis imparts a highly echogenic character to the liver.

## POLYCYSTIC DISEASE OF THE ADULT

The adult form of polycystic disease is clearly a different entity than polycystic disease of the young. Adult polycystic disease is inherited as an autosomal dominant trait and is much more common than polycystic disease of the young.

In most patients, the disease is manifested in the fourth or fifth decade of life. Rarely, the adult form of polycystic disease, pathologically speaking, presents in childhood. There are three clinical presentations that may progress into one another: (1) an asymptomatic presentation, with the diagnosis made only incidentally, (2) a symptomatic presentation with the patient having abdominal pain, hematuria, and hypertension, and (3) a uremic presentation, with progressive renal failure associated with proteinuria. Symptoms are related to the size of the cysts.

Pathologically, any portion of the nephron or collecting tubule may be enlarged and cystic, and therefore cysts are distributed throughout both the cortex and the medulla. The kidneys are bilaterally but often asymmetrically involved. In some instances, kidney involvement may be below the resolution of the diagnostic modality used, e.g., excretory urography, ultrasonography, CT or angiography.

The most frequent complications are infection and calculi (up to 20% of cases) secondary to urinary stasis within the ectatic collecting tubules. Other associated conditions may be present and include hepatic cysts, seen in up to one third of patients but without associated periportal fibrosis or portal hypertension; cysts in other organs, such as the pancreas, lung, spleen, ovaries, testes, thyroid, and uterus; intracranial berry aneurysms, seen in 10%–20% of patients; carcinoma of the kidney; and neurofibromatosis.

**Roentgenographic Findings.**—Roentgenograms of the abdomen show bilateral renal enlargement. Occasionally, calculi, "milk of calcium," or, rarely, arcuate or amorphous calcification may be seen in the kidneys, liver, or spleen. Excretory urography with nephrotomography usually demonstrates multiple lucent masses with distortion of the pelvicalyceal system. Retrograde pyelography shows distortion and displacement of the pelvicalyceal system by the large cysts. Angiography will show stretching of the intrarenal arteries and multiple large and small cysts in the cortex and medulla in the nephrographic phase. Visualization of these small cortical cysts, which give an inhomogenous nephrographic appearance, in addition to the larger cysts, will differentiate this entity from multiple cysts, which yield a homogeneous nephrogram with no evidence of multiple small cortical cysts. Failure to visualize these small cysts does not exclude the diagnosis of adult polycystic disease. The demonstration of diagnosis of polycystic disease.

**Ultrasonographic Findings.**—Ultrasonography will show, in addition to nephromegaly, multiple discrete cysts, larger than the infantile type, distributed throughout the kidney. The normal central echogenic pelvicalyceal system is distorted by the adjacent cysts. Other organs that may also be involved, such as the liver, spleen, ovaries, uterus, pancreas, and bladder, are easily surveyed.

### Renal Cysts of Poorly Understood Origin

## CORTICAL CYSTS

Cystic lesions occurring primarily in the cortex are classified as follows: cysts associated with trisomy syndromes or tuberous sclerosis, simple cysts, and multilocular cysts.

*Cysts associated with the trisomy syndrome* are very small cysts that are seen only histologically and have no clinical or roentgenographic importance.

Although renal masses in patients with tuberous sclerosis are usually hamartomas (angiomyolipomas), renal cysts do occur in this entity and may enlarge to the extent of markedly impairing renal function. Accurate diagnosis is usually accomplished following excretory urography, ultrasonography, and angiography.

*Simple (serous) renal cysts* can be solitary or multiple and are very likely acquired lesions. Although simple cysts are primarily lesions of adults, they can occur in childhood and even in neonates. They contain serous fluid and do not (inherently) communicate with the collecting system, although they may rupture into it.

Excretory urography shows a round radiolucent mass usually bulging from a border of the kidney. Nephrotomography will demonstrate a thin rim surrounding the cyst, and the "beak sign," which is a result of compression of normal renal parenchyma by the slow-growing lesion. Ultrasonography will reveal a round sonolucency without internal echoes, a sharply defined, smooth border, and increased through-transmission.

Since the possibility of a hypovascular cystic Wilms' tumor always exists and true simple cysts are rare in children, a cyst puncture under sonographic or fluoroscopic guidance is necessary for laboratory analysis of the fluid. At the same time, contrast material can be injected into the cyst and the entire wall carefully evaluated by multiple cross-table roentgenograms with the patient in prone, supine, and both decubitus positions. Following these procedures, if there is still suspicion concerning the nature of the lesion, exploratory surgery is indicated to avoid misdiagnosing a cystic Wilms' tumor as a simple cyst.

*Multilocular cysts* are the least common of all congenital cystic lesions of the kidney. The etiology of the lesion is not known. This entity has been classified by some authors as a cystic hamartoma and by others as a benign multilocular cystic nephroma (benign form of Wilms' tumor). It usually manifests in childhood as an asymptomatic abdominal mass discovered during a routine physical examination. It is a unilateral lesion involving only a portion of the kidney and sharply demarcated from the normal remaining renal parenchyma by a fibromuscular capsule. Pathologically, the lesion is composed of multiple loculi varying in size and separated from one another by septi composed of compact fibrous and smooth muscle tissue. There is no communication among the locules or with the renal pelvis.

The excretory urogram identifies the lesion as a sharply demarcated lucent area displacing the pelvicalyceal system. Angiographically, the lesion is relatively avascular, but vessels within the cyst may opacify, simulating a neoplasm.

## MEDULLARY CYSTS

Cystic lesions occurring primarily in the medulla include medullary sponge kidney, medullary cystic disease, pyelogenic cysts, and papillary necrosis (medullary typle).

*Medullary sponge kidney (renal tubular ectasia)* is a developmental abnormality of the kidney limited to the medulla. The disease has no significant familial incidence and is usually discovered in the third or fourth decade of life because of the associated complication of infection, hematuria, or calculus formation.

There have been reports of association of medullary sponge kidney with hemihypertrophy, Ehlers-Danlos syndrome, congenital hypertrophic pyloric stenosis, and Caroli's disease.

Pathologically, the collecting ducts in the renal pyramids are ectatic and associated with small cysts, 1–3 mm in diameter, that communicate with the collecting ducts and may be considered as "offshoots" or segmentally dilated portions of the ducts.

**Roentgenographic Findings.**—Nephrocalcinosis (calcification in the renal pyramids) may be present on abdominal roentgenograms and is seen in up to 50% of patients with medullary sponge kidney. The excretory urogram shows typical streaks (and rounded collections) of opacified urine in the ectatic collecting ducts (and cysts) in the renal pyramids. These roentgenographic findings are present bilaterally in 60%–80% of patients. In the remaining 20%–40% of patients, the roentgenographic abnormalities are limited to one kidney or even to a single pyramid. However, the pathologic changes are present throughout the kidneys bilaterally but are too small to be detected roentgenographically. The tubular ectasia may lead to overall enlargement of the pyramids, with a roentgenographic appearance of papillary hypertrophy manifested by splaying and elongation of the calyces. The kidneys are usually normal in size but may be slightly enlarged and, in the absence of complications, function normally. On the other hand, with loss of renal parenchyma due to infection or obstruction by renal calculi, the kidneys may be small and have decreased function.

It is often difficult on the excretory urogram to differentiate minimal tubular ectasia from the normal pyramidal blush seen with high-dose urography. In those instances in which discrete collections or streaks of contrast material, even though few, can be demonstrated, the diagnosis of medullary sponge kidney is more likely since the normal pyramidal blush tends to be indistinct.

Although ultrasonography may reveal scattered areas of dense echogenicity representing the nephrocalcinosis, and possibly the small cysts, accurate diagnosis will be established by excretory urography.

*Medullary cystic disease (juvenile nephronophthisis)* of the kidney is probably a familial disease, although the mode of genetic transmission is not well defined. A higher incidence is seen in patients with blond or red hair. The disease usually presents in a teenager or young adult and is characterized by anemia, salt wasting, progressive azotemia and polyuria. The patients are invariably normotensive until the terminal stage of the disease, when hypertension may develop. Secondary hyperparathyroidism and renal osteodystrophy are relatively common complications.

Pathologically, the kidneys are small, contain numerous cysts ranging in diameter from less than a millimeter to a few centimeters, and are located predominantly at the corticomedullary junction. Microscopically, there is interstitial fibrosis, periglomerular fibrosis, and proximal tubular dilatation without calcific foci.

*Medullary necrosis:* Renal papillary necrosis is the result of ischemia to portions of the pyramids from whatever cause. Conditions associated with papillary necrosis are diabetes mellitus, long-term phenacetin ingestion, shock, renal trauma, sickle cell anemia or trait, ureteral obstruction, and pyelonephritis.

Papillary necrosis can be divided into three categories: (1) total papillary sloughing, or "papillary necrosis," (2) partial papillary sloughing or "medullary necrosis," and (3) necrosis in situ. The medullary type of renal papillary necrosis is included in the differential diagnosis of renal cystic disease.

*Pyelogenic cyst (calyceal diverticulum):* A pyelogenic cyst is a small cavity in a renal column frequently located medial to the corticomedullary junction. The cyst is connected to the adjacent calyx by an isthmus. The pathogenesis of this lesion is unknown; it may be congenital or acquired.

These cysts are usually asymptomatic; however, complications such as infection and calculus formation may occur. Of all the cystic lesions of the kidney, "milk of calcium" is found most commonly as a calyceal diverticulum. On excretory urography the cyst opacifies after visualization of the pelvicalyceal system. The connecting isthmus may or may not be visualized.

## Bibliography

### HEPATOBILIARY TRACT AND LIVER

Kangarloo H, Sarti DA, Sample WF, et al: Ultrasonographic spectrum of choledochal cysts in children. *Pediatr Radiol* 1980; 9:15–18.

Babbitt DP, Starshak RJ, Clemett AF: Choledochal cyst: A concept of etiology. *AJR* 1973; 119:57.

Behan M, Kazam E: Sonography of the common bile duct: Value of the right anterior oblique view. *AJR* 1978; 130:701.

Conrad MR, Landay MJ, Janes JO: Sonography "parallel channel" sign of biliary tree enlargement in mild to moderate obstructive jaundice. *AJR* 1978; 130:279.

Filly RA, Carlsen EN: Choledochal cyst: Report of a case with specific ultrasonographic findings. *JCU* 1976; 4:7.

Fonkalsrud EW, Boles ET: Choledochal cysts in infancy and childhood. *Surg Gynecol Obstet* 1965; 121:733.

Jona ZJ, Babbitt DP, Starshak RJ, et al: Anatomic observations and etiologic and surgical considerations in choledochal cyst. *J Pediatr Surg* 1979; 14:315.

Kimura K, Ohto M, Ono T, et al: Congenital cystic dilatation of the common bile duct: Relationship to anomalous pancreaticobiliary ductal union. *AJR* 1977; 128:571.

McNulty JG: *Radiology of the Liver.* Philadelphia, WB Saunders Co, 1977, p 178.

Kangarloo H, Sample WF: The liver and spleen, in *Ultrasound of the Pediatric Pelvis and Abdomen.* Chicago, Year Book Medical Publishers, Inc, 1980, p 154.

### DIAPHRAGM; JUXTADIAPHRAGMATIC SPACE

Kangarloo H, Sukov R, Sample WF, et al: Ultrasonographic evaluation of juxtadiaphragmatic masses in children. *Radiology* 1977; 125:785–787.

Kangarloo H, Gold RH, Benson L, et al: Sonography of extrathoracic left-to-right shunts in infants and children. *AJR* 1983; 141:923–926.

Fleischner FG, Robins SA, Abrams M: High renal ectopia and congenital diaphragmatic hernia. *Radiology* 1950; 55:24–26.

Wolfromm G: Situation du rein dans l'eventration diaphragmatique droite. *Mem Acad Chir* 1940; 66:41–47.

Lundius B: Intrathoracic kidney. *AJR* 1975; 125:678–681.

Burke EC, Wenzl JE, Utz DC: The intrathoracic kidney: Report of a case. *Am J Dis Child* 1967; 113:487–490.

Caffey J: *Pediatric X-Ray Diagnosis,* ed 6. Chicago, Year Book Medical Publishers, Inc, 1973, p 443.

Goldberg BB: Suprasternal ultrasonography. *JAMA* 1971; 215:245–250.

Goldberg BB: Mediastinal ultrasonography. *JCU* 1973; 1:114–119.

Maklad NF, Doust BD, Baum JK: Ultrasonic diagnosis of postoperative intra-abdominal abscess. *Radiology* 1974; 113:417–422.

Haber K, Asher WM, Freimanis AK: Echogenic evaluation of diaphragmatic motion in intra-abdominal diseases. *Radiology* 1975; 114:141–144.

Wolson AH: Ultrasonic evaluation of intrathoracic masses. *JCU* 1976; 4:269–273.

de Castro FJ, Schumacher H: Asymptomatic thoracic kidney. *Clin Pediatr* 1969; 8:279–280.

ADRENAL GLAND

Kangarloo H, Diament MJ, Gold RH, et al: Sonography of adrenal glands in neonates and children: Changes in appearance with age. *JCU* 1986; 14:43–47.

Oppenheimer DA, Carroll BA, Yousem S: Sonography of the normal neonatal adrenal gland. *Radiology* 1983; 146:157–160.

Abrams HL, Siegel SS, Adams DF, et al: Computed tomography versus ultrasound of the adrenal gland: A prospective study. *Radiology* 1982; 143:121–128.

Sample WF: A new technique for the evaluation of the adrenal gland with gray scale ultrasonography. *Radiology* 1977; 124:463–469.

Elliot TR, Armour RG: The development of the cortex in the human suprarenal gland and its condition in hemicephaly. *J Pathol Bateriol* 1911; 15:481–488.

Uotila UU: The early embryological development of the fetal and permanent adrenal cortex in man. *Anat Rev* 1940; 76:183–203.

Keene MFL, Hewer EE: Observations of the development of the human suprarenal gland. *J Anat Physiol* 1927; 61:302–324.

Barnhart BJ, Carlson CV, Reynolds JW: Adrenal cortical function in the postmature fetus and newborn infant. *Pediatr Res* 1980; 4:1367–1369.

Kangarloo H, Sample WF: Adrenal gland, in *Ultrasonography of the Pediatric Pelvis and Abdomen*. Chicago, Year Book Medical Publishers, Inc, 1980, p 132.

URINARY TRACT DILATION

Kangarloo H, Gold RH, Fine RN, et al: Urinary tract infection in infants and children evaluated by ultrasound. *Radiology* 1985; 154:367–373.

Garris J, Kangarloo H, Sarti D, et al: The ultrasound spectrum of prune-belly syndrome. *JCU* 1980; 8:117–120.

Chopra A, Telle RL: Hydronephrosis in children: Narrowing the differential diagnosis with ultrasound (abs). *Radiology* 1981; 139:770.

Hoffer FA, Lebowitz RL: Intermittent hydronephrosis: Unique feature of ureteropelvic junction obstruction caused by a crossing renal vessel. *Radiology* 1985; 156:655.

Blane CE, Koff SA, Bowerman RA, et al: Nonobstructive fetal hydronephrosis: Sonographic recognition and therapeutic implications. *Radiology* 1983; 147:95.

Sanders RC, Hartman DS: Sonographic distinction between neonatal multicystic kidney and hydronephrosis. *Radiology* 1984; 151:621.

Sty JR, Starshak RJ: Sonography of pediatric urinary tract abnormalities. *Radiology* 1981; 2:71.

ECHOGENIC KIDNEY

Dietrich RB, Kangarloo H, Boechat MI: The significance of increased echogenicity in the detection and differentiation of pediatric disease. *Int J Pediatr Nephrol* 1985; 6:215–220.

Cook JH, Rosenfield AT, Taylor KJW: Ultrasonic demonstration of intrarenal anatomy. *AJR* 1977; 129:831–835.

Haller JO, Berdon WE, Friedman AP: Increased renal echogenicity: A normal finding in neonates and infants. *Radiology* 1982; 142:173–174.

Rosenfield AT, Taylor KJW, Crade M, et al: Anatomy and pathology of the kidney by gray scale ultrasound. *Radiology* 1978; 218:737–744.

Le Quesne GW: Patterns of ultrasonic abnormality in the renal parenchyma in childhood. *Ann Radiol* 1978; 21:225–230.

Glazer GM, Callen PW, Filly RA: Medullary nephrocalcinosis: Sonography evaluation. *AJR* 1982; 138:55–57.

Hricak H, Cruz C, Eyler WR, et al: Acute post-transplantation renal failure: Differential diagnosis by ultrasound. *Radiology* 1981; 139:441–449.

Hufnagle KG, Khan SN, Penn D, et al: Renal calcification: A complication of long-term furosemide therapy in preterm infants. *Pediatrics* 1982; 70:360–363.

Wilson DA, Wenzel JE, Altshuler GP: Ultrasound demonstration of diffuse cortical nephrocalcinosis in a case of primary hyperoxaluria. *AJR* 1979; 132:659–661.

Brennan JN, Diwan RV, Makker SP, et al: Ultrasonic diagnosis of primary hyperoxaluria in infancy. *Radiology* 1982; 145:147–148.

Rausch HP, Hanefeld F, Kaufmann HJ: Medullary nephrocalcinosis and pancreatic calcifications demonstrated by ultrasound and CT in infants after treatment with ACTH. *Radiology* 1984; 153:105–107.

Foley LC, Luisiri A, Graviss ER, et al: Nephrocalcinosis: Sonographic detection in Cushing syndrome. *AJR* 1982; 139:610–612.

Garel LA, Pariente DM, Gubler MC, et al: The dotted corticomedullary junction: A sonographic indicator of small-vessel disease in hypertensive children. *Radiology* 1984; 152:419–422.

Mitnick JS, Bosniak MA, Hilton S, et al: Cystic renal disease in tuberous sclerosis. *Radiology* 1983; 147:85–87.

Boal DK, Teele RL: The sonography of infantile polycystic kidney disease. *AJR* 1980; 135:575–580.

Rosenfield AT, Zemen RK, Croman JJ, et al: Ultrasound in experimental and clinical renal vein thrombosis. *Radiology* 1980; 137:735–741.

Lam AH, Warren PS: Ultrasonographic diagnosis of neonatal renal venous thrombosis. *Ann Radiol* 1981; 24:7–12.

Rosenberg ER, Trough WS, Kirks DR, et al: Ultrasonic diagnosis of renal vein thrombosis in neonates. *AJR* 1980; 134:35–38.

Krensky AM, Reddish JM, Teele RL: Causes of increased renal echogenicity in pediatric patients. *Pediatrics* 1983; 72:840–846.

### CYSTIC DISEASES OF THE KIDNEY

Kangarloo H, Fine RN: Ultrasonography of cystic renal dysplasia. *Int J Pediatr Nephrol* 1983; 4:205–209.

Kangarloo H, Sample WF (eds): Cystic diseases of the kidney, in *Ultrasound of the Pediatric Abdomen and Pelvis: A Correlative Imaging Approach.* Chicago, Year Book Medical Publishers, Inc, 1980, pp 89–94.

Beck AD: The effect of intra-uterine urinary obstruction upon the development of the fetal kidney. *J Urol* 1971; 105:784–789.

Gwinn JL, Landing BH: Cystic diseases of kidneys in infants and children. *Radiol Clin North Am* 1968; 6:191.

Risdon RA: Renal dysplasia: Part 1. A clinico-pathological study of 76 cases. *J Clin Pathol* 1971; 24:57–71.

Mackie GG: Abnormalities of the ureteral bud. *Urol Clin North Am* 1978; 5:161–174.

Mascatello VJ, Smith EH, Carrera GF, et al: Ultrasonic evaluation of the obstructed duplex kidney. *AJR* 1977; 129:113–120.

Glazer GM, Filly RA, Callen PW: The varied sonographic appearance of the urinary tract in the fetus and newborn with urethral obstruction. *Radiology* 1982; 144:563–568.

Haller JO, Berdon WE, Friedman AP: Normal roentgen variant. Increased renal cortical echogenicity: A normal finding in neonates and infants. *Radiology* 1982; 142:173–174.

Cook JH, Rosenfield AT, Taylor KJW: Ultrasonic demonstration of intrarenal anatomy. *AJR* 1977; 129:831–835.

Felson B, Cussen LJ: The hydronephrotic type of unilateral congenital multicystic disease of the kidney. *Semin Roentgenol* 1975; 10:113–123.

Griscom NT, Vawter GF, Feller FX: Pelvoinfundibular atresia: The usual form of multicystic kidney: 44 unilateral and two bilateral cases. *Semin Roentgenol* 1975; 10:125–131.

Flanagan MJ, Kozak JA: Congenital unilateral multicystic disease of the kidney. *Arch Surg* 1968; 96:893–896.

# 17b.

# PEDIATRIC GASTROINTESTINAL ULTRASOUND

Jack O. Haller, M.D.

## Idiopathic Hypertrophic Pyloric Stenosis

Since Teele and Smith described the use of sonography to diagnose idiopathic hypertrophic pyloric stenosis (IHPS) in 1977, the modality has become a common screening test for children suspected of having this disorder.[1-3] A high-frequency transducer (7.5 MHz or 10 MHz) is best. The infant is placed supine and given a pacifier or lollipop. The right decubitus position can also be utilized since it moves stomach gas away from the pylorus. The thin, hypoechoic gastric muscle layers are followed distally to the gastric outlet. Occasionally the left lateral decubitus position can be used to document the passage of gas through the pylorus.

In IHPS the pylorus becomes thicker and elongated, with concomitant narrowing of the pyloric canal. The diagnosis is usually made on the basis of a typical clinical history and palpation of a pyloric mass. However, the diagnosis is unclear in about 15% of cases. Traditionally this diagnosis has been provided by the upper GI tract series, which usually reveals the string, shoulder, beak, and teat signs. Using ultrasound, one can make the diagnosis reliably when the anteroposterior (AP) diameter is at least 15 mm or more. If the wall thickness of the pylorus is greater than 4 mm, the diagnosis of pyloric stenosis can be suggested.[4] "Normal" is usually defined as 10 mm or less. The shoulder and beak sign seen on x-ray films can often be reproduced on ultrasound.[5] If the sonogram is normal or equivocal, an upper GI series is indicated to rule out other causes of vomiting such as a gastroesophageal reflux or antral web.

## Duplication

Duplications of the GI tract are the result of abnormal development during early fetal life. They may involve any portion of the alimentary tract, but the majority are in the ileum or near the ileocecal junction. Another frequent site is the second portion of the duodenum. Duplications are usually elongated, tubular or spherical, and have been found at all levels from the tongue to the anus. Other names for this abnormality are enteric cyst, gastroenterogenous cyst, giant diverticulum, and inclusion cyst. Neuroenteric cysts are often seen with associated spinal anomalies. When duplications impinge on the intestinal lumen, they may cause obstruction. In most cases, however, no obstruction is present. The mass is usually discovered in an asymptomatic patient less than 1 year old who may or may not be suffering from intestinal hemorrhage. One theory as to the pathogenesis of duplications involves vascular insufficiency to areas of fetal gut and secondary epithelial growth that forms a diverticulum or duplication. These structures may communicate with the GI tract or may be totally separate from it. When the structures are sealed off, secretions may accumulate and subsequently cause distention and possible torsion.

Duplications that are isolated from the GI tract appear as sonolucent cystic masses on sonographic examination.[6, 7] If the duplication communicates with the GI tract, the presence of air or food particles makes a sonographic diagnosis difficult. When bleeding has occurred, there may be a layer of fluid and debris. An echogenic inner rim representing the mucosal lining and its secretions has also been noted. Radiologically and clinically these masses are difficult to differentiate from Meckel's diverticula, since both cause obstruction, hemorrhage, and abdominal pain. Meckel's diverticula more frequently communicate with the GI tract, however. The sonographic finding of a pure cyst favors the diagnosis of a duplication.

## Mesenteric and Omental Cysts

Mesenteric cysts are unusual masses of lymphatic origin and occur most commonly in the leaves of the mesentery of the small bowel. Occasionally they are found in the mesentery of the transverse colon, and rarely in the sigmoid colon. They can become large, especially if hemorrhage occurs. Mesenteric cysts are considered by many to be congenital cysts or benign neoplasms that are most likely related to the lymphatic system. They occur in people of all ages, and their most common manifestation is abdominal distention and frequently abdominal pain. They often present following trauma as a result of hemorrhage and subsequent distention.

There are no consistent diagnostic features of mesenteric cysts. They usually cause displacement of bowel as seen on barium studies. Urography is usually performed to rule out an abnormality of the kidneys. Sonography can identify a cystic abdominal mass in most instances. Renal and hepatic origins of this mass can be excluded by ultrasound. Typically,

mesenteric cysts show septa and can usually be differentiated from ascites, which the mass may mimic on a radiographic examination.[8, 9]

## Intussusception

Intussusceptions are caused when a portion of the bowel invaginates into a more distal segment. The mesentery is often carried along with the invaginated bowel. If this condition is not corrected, either by barium hydrostatic reduction or by surgical intervention, ischemia and eventual infarction of the bowel will result. Classically, patient symptoms include an abdominal mass, pain, and currant jelly stools. When children have this classic triad, sonography is not necessary. Diagnostic and often therapeutic barium enema is the first and only examination that should be performed. These children may have unusual symptoms such as vomiting and a nontender abdominal mass. This has been referred to as "silent intussusception."

The diagnostic workup will be as for an unknown abdominal mass, i.e., sonography, intravenous urography, etc. Recognition by the sonographer of the typical bull's-eye appearance of a tubular mass can often be diagnostic and help guide the management. The bull's-eye appearance is the result of edema of the bowel which is the surrounding zone of low echo production, and the tightly squeezed lumen of the intussusceptum-intussuscipiens complex, which is the central collection of echoes. Care must be taken not to overdiagnose this condition, as routine fecal impaction may at times have the same appearance.[10–12]

Abdominal pain is a frequent complaint of children in the emergency room and pediatrician's office. Many of these children have recurrent abdominal pain that leads to an exhaustive radiographic workup. It may be possible to screen some of these children with sonography to avoid radiation. As real-time scanning becomes more prevalent and sonographic findings are better defined, this will be easier.

## Meckel's Diverticulum

Meckel's diverticulum accounts for 90% of all omphalomesenteric duct abnormalities. Meckel's diverticulum is usually described as a blind sac attached to the antimesenteric border of the distal small bowel not connected to the naval. The diverticulum represents remnants of the vitelline duct, which normally disappears at 6 weeks of embryonic life but may persist into adulthood. In approximately 10% of cases a fibrous cord (the vitelline ligament) persists and connects the apex of the Meckel's diverticulum to the umbilicus. The diverticulum is supplied by remnants of the vitelline vessels that are direct branches of the superior mesenteric vessels. These may form bands connecting the diverticulum directly to the mesentery and may act as central points for volvulus formation.[13–16]

Giant Meckel's diverticula are much larger.[17] There are essentially two types. Type 1 is an elongated lesion with a bulbous tip and of approximately the same caliber as the ileum. Type 2 is usually associated with the "giant" type. The more common type 1 may produce intestinal obstruction due to knotting around the small bowel. This is a condition caused by the great length, mobility, and pear-shaped or knob-like end. Type 2 is rare. The complications caused by type 2 include intestinal obstruction, bleeding, and intussusception. Rarely, type 2 diverticula are the focus of inflammation and abscess formation.[18–20]

It is extremely difficult to demonstrate Meckel's diverticula on ultrasound. Only when these diverticula form a mass due to either volvulus, intussusception, cyst formation, or abscess formation may they be detected. Small noncomplicated Meckel's diverticula have not been detected sonographically to date. Complicated Meckel's diverticula should be considered in the differential diagnosis of cystic masses in the right lower quadrant and masses in the hypochondrium.

## Intramural Hemorrhage

Intramural hemorrhage of the GI tract in children frequently occurs in the retroperitoneal portion of the duodenum as a result of trauma. The resulting intramural mass (hematoma) often causes obstruction, vomiting, and abdominal pain. Other causes of intramural hemorrhage include anticoagulatnt therapy, hemophilia, or Henoch-Schönlein purpura. The sonographic appearance of the hematoma depends on the age of the hemorrhage.[21] Duodenal hematomas that look like cysts are difficult to differentiate from pancreatic pseudocysts on sonography, and the two may

coexist.[22] The pancreas, which is a fixed retroperitoneal structure, is frequently traumatized by the same blow. The sonographic finding of an echogenic mass that is separate from the kidneys, pancreas, and inferior vena cava, in conjunction with the radiographic findings of a duodenal intramural mass with edema of the bowel, suggests the diagnosis of intramural hemorrhage. In many cases surgical intervention may be avoided because the hemorrhage can be watched with sonography.

## Imperforate Anus

There are various forms of imperforate anus, depending on the position of the distal rectal pouch with respect to the puborectalis portion of the levator sling. High lesions do not pass through this sling; low lesions do. The level of the rectal pouch is critical in determining the surgical approach. High lesions are treated with early decompressive colostomy and are approached intra-abdominally, while low lesions can be repaired through a direct perineal exploration. Both are associated with the genitourinary malformation.[23–25]

Radiographic evaluation of the distal rectal pouch is achieved by introducing contrast agent either through the distal loop of the colostomy or direct percutaneous injection of water-soluble contrast agent into the pouch from below.[29] Real-time sector scanning is a relatively new method of evaluating imperforate anus.[30]

The technique consists of locating the pouch on sagittal projections. The sonographer then lubricates a finger of a surgical-gloved hand with ultrasonic coupling agent and slowly oscillates it transversely in a scratching motion traveling outward from the anal dimple. With the opposite hand the transducer is angled caudally and aligned to scan both the pouch and the perineal surface. The finger tip can easily be identified as a markedly echogenic structure moving in and out of the plane of section. The distance between the pouch and the perineal surface can be measured with electronic calibers. The Valsalva maneuver will produce false readings, as this maneuver is known to decrease the pouch-perineum distance.

Longitudinal scans through the perineum can be performed and the distance measured in this projection as well. The kidneys are also routinely examined because of the high incidence of associated anomalies.

The levator sling is the caudal portion of the urogenital diaphragm and thus always lies caudal to the base of the bladder. If the distal rectal pouch is identified above the base of the bladder, a "high" lesion may be suspected. A pouch-perineum distance of 1.5 cm is useful in identifying a lesion terminating below the base of the bladder as "low." A pouch above the base of the bladder and 1.5 cm or more from the perineal surface should be considered high until proved otherwise.

## References

1. Teele RL, Smith EH: Ultrasound in the diagnosis of idiopathic pyloric stenosis. *N Engl J Med* 1977; 269:1149.
2. Strauss S, Itzchak Y, Manor A, et al: Sonography of hypertrophic pyloric stenosis. *AJR* 1981; 136:1057.
3. Blumhagen JD, Coombs JB: Ultrasound in the diagnosis of hypertrophic pyloric stenosis. *JCU* 1978; 6:289.
4. Blumhage JS, Noble HGS: Muscle thickness in hypertrophic pyloric stenosis: Sonographic determination. *AJR* 1983; 140:221.
5. Graif M, Itzchaky, Avigad L, et al: The pylorus in infancy: Overall sonographic assessment. *Pediatric Radiol* 1984; 14:14–17.
6. Kangarloo H, Sample WF, Hansen G, et al: Ultrasonic evaluation of abdominal gastrointestinal tract duplication in children. *Radiology* 1979; 131:191.
7. Teele RL, Hanschke CL, Tapper D: The radiographic and ultrasonographic evaluation of enteric duplication cysts. *Pediatr Radiol* 1980; 10:9.
8. Gordon MD, Sumner TE: Abdominal ultrasonography in a mesenteric cyst presenting as ascites. *Gastroenterology* 1975; 69:761.
9. Haller JO, Schneider M, Kassner EG, et al: Sonographic evaluation of mesenteric and omental masses in children. *AJR* 1976; 130:269.
10. Burke LF, Clark E: Ileocolic intussusception: A case report. *JCU* 1977; 5:346.
11. Ein SH, Stephens CA, Minor A: Painless intussusception. *J Pediatr Surg* 1976; 11:563.
12. Friedman AP, Haller JO, Schneider M, et al: Sonographic appearance of intussusception in children. *Am J Gastroenterol* 1979; 72:92.
13. Langman J: *Medical Embryology. Human Development—Normal and Abnormal,* ed 2. Baltimore, Williams & Wilkins Co, 1969, p 269.
14. Brookes VS: Meckel's diverticulum in children: A report of 43 cases. *Br J Surg* 1954; 42:57–68.
15. McParland FA, Kiesewetter WB: Meckel's diverticulum in childhood. *Surg Gynecol Obstet* 1958; 106:11–14.
16. Seagram CGF, Louch RE, Stephens CA, et al: Meckel's diverticulum: A 10-year review of 218 cases. *Can J Surg* 1968; 11:369–373.
17. Cross VF, Wendth AJ, Phelan JJ, et al: Giant Meckel's diverticulum in a premature infant. *AJR* 1970; 108:591–597.
18. Craft AW, Watson AJ, Scott JES: "Giant Meckel's diverticulum" causing intestinal obstruction in the newborn. *J Pediatr Surg* 1976; 11:1037–1038.
19. Mitchel ML, Field RJ, Ogden WW Jr: Meckel's diverticulum: An analysis of one hundred cases and report of giant diverticulum and of four cases occurring within the same immediate family. *Ann Surg* 1955; 141:819–826.
20. Yates HB: A remarkable Meckel's diverticulum. *Br J Surg* 1930; 17:456–462.
21. Foley LC, Teele RL: Ultrasound of epigastric injuries after blunt trauma. *AJR* 1979; 132:593.
22. Sarti DA: Rapid development and spontaneous regression of pancreatic pseudocysts documented by ultrasound. *Radiology* 1977; 125:789.
23. Kiesewetter WB, Nixon HH: Imperforate anus: 1. Its surgical anatomy. *J Pediatr Surg* 1967; 2:60–68.
24. Schuster SR, Teele RL: An analysis of ultrasound scanning as a guide in determination of "high" or "low" imperforate anus. *J Pediatr Surg* 1979; 14:798–800.
25. Kurlander GJ: Roentgenology of imperforate anus. *AJR* 1967; 100:190–201.
26. Kiesewetter WB, Bill AH, Nixon HH, et al: Imperforate anus. *Arch Surg* 1976; 111:518–525.
27. Wagner ML, Harberg FJ, Kumar APM, et al: The evaluation of imperforate anus utilizing percutaneous injection of water-soluble iodide contrast material. *Pediatr Radiol* 1973; 1:34–40.

28. Stephens FD, Smith ED: *Ano-rectal Malformations in Children.* Chicago, Year Book Medical Publishers, Inc, 1971, pp 212–256.

29. Berdon WE, Baker DH, Santulli TV, et al: The radiologic evaluation of imperforate anus: An approach correlated with current surgical concepts. *Radiology* 1968; 90:466–471.

30. Oppenheimer DA, Carroll BA, Schocat SJ: Sonography of imperforate anus. *Radiology* 1983; 148:127–128.

# 17c.
# PEDIATRIC PELVIC ULTRASOUND

Jack O. Haller, M.D.

## The Pelvis

The use of ultrasound for the evaluation of pelvic pathology in children is now well established,[1,2] and in the past few years repeated studies have yielded a relatively clear-cut set of clinical indications for such an examination (1). This section will review disorders unique to the pediatric pelvis.

The clinical indications for pelvic sonography in children are as follows:

Primary amenorrhea
Secondary amenorrhea
Gonadal dysgenesis
Precocious puberty
Anomalous or ambiguous genitalia
To exclude pelvic mass
Unusual vaginal discharge
To exclude pelvic abscess
Anorectal or renal anomaly

## Technique

The technique of ultrasound examination of the pediatric pelvis is the same as that for the adult. The area is best studied in transverse and longitudinal scans with the patient in the supine position. To fill the bladder, infants and young children are given water, milk, or formula to drink about 1 hour before the examination. Older children receive one or two glasses of water from 1 to 3 hours before the examination. Since the ovary may not have completely descended below the pelvic rim, it may be necessary to overdistend the bladder in girls. Frequently we have resorted to instillation of fluid in the bladder via a Foley catheter, and, rarely, a water enema has been used to further elucidate pelvic pathology. Usually children tolerate this well. Sedation is almost never necessary.

In general, the best compromise between penetration and resolution is provided by a 7-mm-diameter, 5-MHz transducer with a short internal focus in neonates and small infants, and a 13-mm-diameter, 3.5-MHz transducer with a medium internal focus or a 19-mm-diameter, 3.5-MHz transducer with a long internal focus in older children and adolescents. Real-time studies are best achieved with 5- or 3.5-MHz transducers in older children. Sector and phased-array equipment can both be used with virtually equal reliability.

1139

## The Uterus

Late in fetal life, the uterus displays an augmented linear growth in relation to most body dimensions. Immediately after birth uterine length and weight diminish sharply, until the organ assumes essentially the dimensions that it would have attained had its early fetal growth rate remained unchanged. This prenatal growth increment is attributed chiefly to a hormone (probably placental in origin), the loss of which at birth allows the growth rate of the uterus to decline to its typical pattern. The reduction in postnatal uterine length is associated mainly with the cervix rather than the body of the uterus.

Shortly after birth, the length of the uterus is approximately 26 mm. The cervix occupies two thirds to five sevenths of the total uterine length, and the corpus is approximately one half the diameter of the cervix. These proportions change at puberty in the nulliparous young adult. The body of the uterus is about 35 mm long, the cervix about 25 mm long, and the total length approximately 60 mm. During menarche, the rate of uterine growth surpasses that of any other part of the female genitalia. This growth takes place primarily in the corpus, and predominantly in width and thickness.

The above measurements serve as a guide for detecting variations in uterine size. An absent or small uterus may indicate a decreased hormonal state, chromosomal abnormalities, or isolated hypogenesis or agenesis. Similarly, a large uterus may be the result of a primary or secondary neoplasm, hematometria, or a functioning endocrine tumor causing precocious development.

On sonographic examination, the normal pediatric uterus appears as a teardrop-shaped structure with the larger portion representing the premenarchal cervix. The uterus is usually identified by demonstrating continuity between the cervix and the vagina. Occasionally, bright echoes representing the endometrial cavity are noted in the center of the uterus. On longitudinal and transverse scans, both the infantile and pubertal uterus typically produce an indentation on the posterior surface of the bladder. The uterus in older children will be similar to that of the adult, i.e., pear-shaped, and will have the normal variations in tilt. The position of the organ varies with changes in the bladder or rectal distention. The uterus and adnexa are well seen when pelvic fluid is present.

Anomalous development of the uterus is rarely diagnosed in infants and young children. This is because the pediatric uterus is small, the clinical indications for imaging it are few, and meticulous scanning is necessary to make the diagnosis of anomalous development. There are few references in the literature pertaining to the ultrasound evaluation of uterine anomalies. The majority of these refer to the pregnant uterus or immediately post partum, during which time the presence of an abnormality can cause a slow uterine involution in the puerperium.[5, 6] The most common anomaly diagnosed is bicornuate uterus. Uterine anomalies can be detected when there is a high index of suspicion. This occurs when there are associated anomalies of the vertebral column, vagina, urinary tract, anus, and/or rectum. The intimate relationship between the primitive urinary tract and the müllerian duct system accounts for this association.[7, 8]

Anomalies of the uterus are also associated with maternal diethylstilbesterol ingestion.[9] Sonographic detection of these abnormalities has been reported.[10]

### Tumors of the Uterus

The most common malignancy involving the uterus is rhabdomyosarcoma. If often starts in the prostatic remnant in females and invades the uterus, bladder, and eventually the entire pelvis. Sonographically the mass invariably appears moderately echogenic with a heterogeneous distribution. Cystic spaces in the mass representing hemorrhage and necrosis are infrequently seen. Often the mass has spread to adjacent organs and mesentery by the time it is discovered.

## The Ovary

Successful sonographic examination of the pediatric ovary if largely dependent on the exact and careful demonstration of adnexal morphology, combined with an awareness of the various conditions that can occur in the pediatric age group. Although sonography can contribute significantly to the evaluation of a number of pediatric ovarian disorders,[1, 2] in many cases its value is limited. A complete clinical analysis may not be possible on the basis of the sonographic examination alone.

Throughout infancy and childhood innumerable follicles in all stages of development are present. Generally there are more follicles in the early stages of development than are present in an adult. The only thing that distinguishes the follicles of the postpubertal and prepubertal ovary is that periodically, approximately once a month, an adult follicle becomes capable of liberating its ovum and being converted into a corpus luteum. Prior to puberty, the cells of the theca interna occasionally become luteinized, and in certain situations, this luteinization may be extreme, but the granulosa cells become luteinized only after follicle rupture, which never normally occurs until after puberty.[11]

The blood vessels in the ovary of the fetus and young infant are relatively few in number and the medulla of the ovary is small and inconspicuous. Vascularization slowly increases but the vascular supply does not approximate that seen in the adult until the child is 6–8 years of age. At approximately age 7 years, the spiral arteries and tortuous veins in the center of the ovary greatly increase in prominence. These tissues form an identifiable medullary zone that may be distinguished from an outer cortical region. The boundary between the two remains indistinct, however.[12]

By age 12 or 12½ years, the ovary is made up of a central medullary zone of loose connective tissue containing many blood vessels, and a peripheral cortical zone which is divided into two portions, a superficial layer and deep layer. Primordial follicles are fairly evenly distributed near the junction of the two layers of the cortical zone.

At about age 12 or 13 years, ovulation begins. Thereafter, nonprimordial, ova-containing follicles in various stages of development are present everywhere under the surface of the ovary. Primordial follicles, many with antra 7 mm in diameter, may also be present, but their number gradually decreases until none remain. The presence of late-developing primordial follicles is normal, however.

The presence of primordial follicles in adolescense has clinical implications. The sonographic diagnosis of polycystic ovaries is often made erroneously in individuals with late regression of primordial follicles.[10] Similarly, the retention of primordial follicles often leads to painfully enlarged hemorrhagic ovarian cyst. This condition is seen in teenagers and young adults, in whom the ovarian vascular supply is at its maximum.

After age 14 years, most of the primordial follicles have disappeared in the majority of females.[12] The ovary of the 14th year has essentially matured sexually and differs little from that of the adult except that the maturing ovary is peppered with the remains of involuting corpora lutea and corpora albicantia which follow the normal menstrual cycle.

### Sonographic Appearance of the Normal Ovary

In most cases, the ovary has descended into the pelvis at birth and lies along the superior margin of the posterior fold of the broad ligament, which extends laterally from the uterine fold. If the ovary does not completely descend, it may lie anywhere from the inferior border of the kidney to the broad ligament in the pelvic cavity.

The normal ovary most commonly appears as an elongated and symmetrica structure at birth. The shape is quite variable and almost any shape may be normal.[13] The size of the ovary at birth is subject to wide variations. Generally it is 15 mm long, 3 mm wide, and 2.5 mm thick. Although the gland does increase in length throughout childhood, growth involves the thickness and width to a greater extent than the length. It is during puberty (generally between the ages of 13 and 14 years) that the ovary attains its adult size of 24 to 41 mm in length, 15 to 24 mm in width, and 8.5 to 19.4 mm in thickness.[11, 13] The width and thickness of the organ are often affected by the presence of cysts, especially during ovulation. Both primordial and corpus luteal cysts may account for increases in ovarian size.[14] Sample et al. calculated ovarian volume on the basis of a modified prolate ellipsoid formula:

$$V = \frac{x \times y \times z}{2}$$

and found that the volume is less than 1 cm$^3$ in the prepubertal age group and no larger than 6 cm$^3$ in the postpubertal age group.[13] Ovaries larger than this should be followed with sequential sonographic studies to detect possible serious pathology.

Because of variation in ovarian position, the sonographer must often search throughout the pelvis. The ovaries can be found in the posterior cul-de-sac, lateral pelvic wall, and, rarely, above the pelvic brim. Finding the ovarian vessels and establishing the positions of the pelvic musculature and iliac vessels will help. Kratochwill et al.[15] have also suggested examining the ovaries via the vaginal or vesicle route as an alternative method.

## Ovarian Masses

The ovary is the most common site of tumor occurrence in the female genital tract in childhood (Table 17–1).[16–22] Children with ovarian tumors often present with pain, abdominal swelling, or a palpable abdominal mass.

Ultrasound is the most revealing noninvasive method for the detection of pelvic masses (as high as 91% sensitivity).[23] However, the technical dependency of sonographic examination imposes practical limitations. Bladder distention is often difficult to achieve in children, and catheterization or accurate timing of liquid feedings is often necessary to obtain adequate bladder distention. Fluid- and stool-filled bowel may create "pseudolesions," especially if an associated ileus prevents real-time identification of peristalsis.[24] We have used the water enema technique successfully to help with this problem. It is quick, easy, and well tolerated by children.

Single or multiple cysts constitute well over 70% of ovarian masses and are the most common pelvic tumors of childhood and adolescence. Histologically, these usually are follicular retention cysts and are commonly seen in pubertal females. Some have resulted in precocious puberty because of hormonal secretion by the lining cells of the cysts.

A number of features of ovarian cysts are unique to the pediatric age group. Ovarian cysts may be found

**TABLE 17–1.**

**Ovarian Neoplasms Encountered at Sony Downstate Medical Center From 1976 to 1984***

Ovarian cyst
Ovarian teratoma
Teratocarcinoma
Dysgerminoma
Endodermal sinus tumor
Theca cell tumor
Leukemic infiltration
Secondary encroachment from contiguous masses
   Rhabdomyosarcoma
   Teratocarcinoma
   Lymphoma
   Adenocarcinoma, primary unknown
   Leukemia
   Neurofibromatosis

*In order of frequency.

in the fetus. If very large, they may be a cause of dystocia.[25, 26] Fleming and McLeary[27] reported a case of nonimmunologic fetal hydrops complicated by bilateral theca lutein cysts. Ovarian cysts may also undergo torsion or may cause the entire ovary to undergo torsion, resulting in amputation of the ovary.[28, 29] The amputated ovary may appear as a calcified mass that may be freely mobile within the peritoneal space. Reports of an increased incidence of ovarian cysts in children with hypothyroidism and cystic fibrosis[30] have not been corroborated in our experience. Stein-Leventhal syndrome of polycystic disease of the ovaries is often indistinguishable from the normally cystic ovaries of an asymptomatic, normal child.[31] Callen and Marks have cautioned against confusing lymphomatous ovarian masses with cysts.[32] Finally, White and Filly[33] have reported cholesterol crystals that give the appearance of "sludge" in an ovarian cyst.

## Teratoma

Benign ovarian teratomas, which occur most often during the early reproductive years, account for 10%–15% of all ovarian neoplasms. These are uncommon tumors in infants and children and are usually discovered only after they have grown large enough to produce a palpable mass or after undergoing torsion, thereby causing abdominal pain. Fat, calcification, or ossification within the tumor are often noted on plain films of the abdomen. Ovarian teratomas in children are predominantly cystic with small foci of fat, hair, and/or calcium which produce intense echoes.[36, 37] Previously we reported a cyst-within-a-cyst sonographic appearance in many benign ovarian teratomas.[21] These masses have also been described as showing a "tip of the iceberg" sign.[38]

If there is an unusual number of solid nodules or the solid component of the teratoma predominates, one should be highly suspicious that the lesion may have foci of malignant cells. In such instances, malignant ascites, metastatic liver disease, omental or mesenteric involvement, and hydronephrosis should be sought.

## Cystadenoma

Cystadenomas of the ovaries are rare in children under the age of 20. We have encountered two such cases that show the typical septa that help identify this mass. Septa are also seen on sonographic examinations in cystadenomas of the bile duct, pancreas, mesentery, and urachus.[39, 40]

### Dysgerminoma

The most frequent malignant mass that is encountered in the pediatric ovary is the dysgerminoma, which is the ovarian counterpart of seminoma of the testes.[41] Fortunately, it is a low-grade malignancy. The peak incidence of dysgerminoma is seen in patients age 20–40 years, but it may occur in younger patients. Pathologically, the tumor is a solid mass, varying in size from a small nodule up to a size that may occupy a major portion of the abdomen. Hemorrhagic necrosis may be present. Because this tumor is highly radiosensitive, any tissue remaining after surgical extirpation is usually well controlled.

Sonographically, dysgerminoma appears as a solid ovarian mass, but necrosis may render a mixed echogenic-sonolucent appearance.[42] Ascites, retroperitoneal adenopathy, and subhepatic metastases occur in advanced cases and can be readily detected on ultrasound.

### Ovarian Torsion

Torsion of the normal uterine adnexa in children is a rare but important cause of abdominal pain. It is difficult to diagnose because the symptoms and physical findings may be confusing and ascribed to many other abnormalities in the pediatric pelvis. The symptoms include a palpable abdominal mass, leukocytosis with a shift to the left, lower abdominal pain (usually lasting more than 48 hours), anorexia, nausea, vomiting, constipation, or diarrhea. In the premenarchal girl the symptoms are often attributed to appendicitis or other disorders such as gastroenteritis, pyelonephritis, intussusception, or Meckel's diverticulitis.

Torsion of the ovary usually occurs in the first decades of life. The normal adnexae are especially mobile in children, allowing torsion to occur at the mesosalpinx as a result of changes in intra-abdominal pressure or in body position. Torsion may involve the tube, ovary, or both. If the adnexae are to be preserved, the diagnosis must be made early and emergency laparotomy undertaken.

The sonographic appearance reflects the surgical and pathologic findings.[28, 29] Ovarian enlargement and free intrapelvic fluid are the hallmarks of torsion. The torsed ovary and tube display numerous internal echoes with overall enhanced sound transmission that correlates well with the pathologic findings of vascular engorgement and stromal edema. A torsed cyst may contain hemorrhage, indicated by suspended or dependent echogenic material. Sonographically, the appearance may be quite similar to that of a nontorsed, hemorrhagic ovarian cyst. It is only through awareness of the sonographic appearance and clinical suspicion that infarction of the child's ovary may be prevented by means of timely surgery.

## Approach to Evaluating the Pelvic Mass

Pelvic masses can be divided into three categories, based on their sonographic appearances: solid, complex, and cystic (Chart 17–1). Most of the diagnostic difficulty occurs in females. The following discussion is directed toward diagnosis of pelvic masses in the female patient.

### Solid Masses

If the patient has a mass which attenuates the sound beam and is echogenic with relatively few scattered sonolucent areas, we consider it solid and proceed on that line of workup. These children will eventually need surgery to rule out torsion or neoplasia, whether benign or malignant. The most frequent solid tumors encountered are rhabdomyosarcoma, lymphoma, and dysgerminoma. Rhabdomyosarcomas are diffusely echogenic with heterogeneous echoes and increased attenuation. Clear planes of separation between contiguous structures usually cannot be distinguished. Lymphoma has the same echo characteristics as other lymph tissues. It is a poor sound attenuator and is uniformly hypoechoic. Occasionally we have encountered a pelvis that is completely filled with echoes as a result of malignancy extending to both pelvic walls. It is impossible to determine the organ of origin in such cases. CT may be indicated prior to surgery to evaluate the exact extension of the malignancy.

Whenever a malignancy is suspected on the basis of coexisting ascites, invasion of contiguous organs, mesenteric implants, liver metastasis, or urinary obstruction, CT is indicated. It is as useful preoperatively

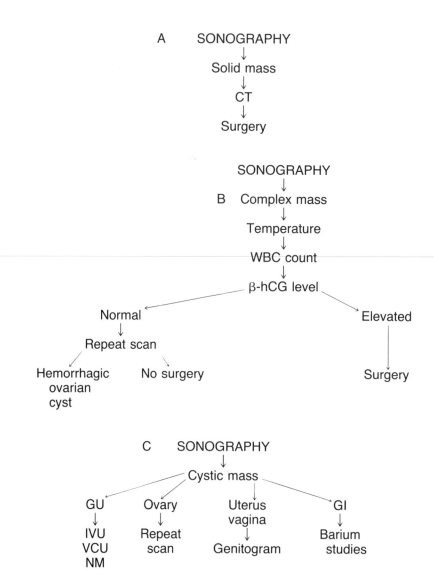

**CHART 17–1.**

as it postoperatively. Torsion, either of normal or abnormal adnexae, usually presents with fever, moderate to severe pain, and an elevated white blood cell (WBC) count. In such cases preoperative CT is not indicated.

*Complex Masses*

The complex ovarian mass is a major area of recent clinical investigation (Table 17–2). If the mass has both cystic and solid components or is septated, the differential diagnosis is long. In girls over 8 years of age, a pregnancy test is the first laboratory investigation obtained. A positive serum β-subunit of hCG, coupled with the sonographic evidence of a complex

adenexal mass, is highly suspicious for the diagnosis of ectopic pregnancy. The patient is treated surgically and no other tests are indicated.

If the pregnancy test is negative, plain films of the abdomen are obtained. If calcium or a tooth is seen the diagnosis of benign cystic teratoma is made. If calcium is not present further clinical information is necessary. The presence of fever and an elevated WBC is pertinent in the diagnosis of any pelvic disorder. Certain conditions such as torsion, tubo-ovarian abscess, and appendiceal abscess will usually present with signs of inflammation. All these conditions require operative intervention.

If a child is not febrile, has a normal WBC count, and the pain diminishes with time, there is no need for immediate surgical intervention. Conservative clinical

**TABLE 17–2.**

**Differential Diagnosis of the Complex Ovarian Mass**[43]

| MASS | HISTORY | PHYSICAL FINDINGS | LAB DATA | SONOGRAPHY |
|---|---|---|---|---|
| Hemorrhagic ovarian cyst | Lower abdominal pain, occasional nausea | None, or may have palpable mass if large enough; fever, if torsion | ↑ WBC if torsion | Variable features:<br>Thick-walled cyst<br>Septated cyst<br>Homogeneous low-level echoes with enhanced transmission.<br>Cyst containing solid components<br>Fluid in cul-de-sac<br>Change in appearance on follow-up study (see Chart 17–1) |
| Benign cystic teratoma | Lower abdominal pain; Nausea, vomiting; severity of pain with torsion | Lower abdominal or pelvic mass; torsion in 25% cases; fever and acute abdomen if with torsion | ↑ WBC if torsion | Complex hyperechoic mass with acoustic shadowing<br>"Tip of the iceberg sign"<br>Solid mass with cystic components<br>Cystic with or without scattered internal echoes<br>Air-fluid level<br>Pelvic radiograph shows calcium in 45%–54% |
| Endometriosis | Chronic pelvic pain during menses, radiating to rectum sacrum, coccyx; dyspareunia; irregular uterine bleeding | Tender, irregular ovarian mass; fixed nodulations behind cervix | . . . | Nonspecific complex ovarian mass<br>Uterus may have small cystic spaces due to coexisting adenomyosis or may be normal<br>Complex echogenic masses in cul-de-sac secondary to endometriosis or fibrotic reaction |
| Ectopic pregnancy | Lower abdominal pain; amenorrhea | Tender pelvic mass | hCG β-subunit positive in 93%–97% of cases | Nonspecific complex adnexal mass<br>Intact gestational sac with fetal structures in adnexae<br>Fetal heart motion on real-time<br>Pseudogestational sac in uterus<br>Stronger uterine echoes in cluster or linear configuration<br>Fluid in cul-de-sac |
| Torsion, normal uterine adnexae | Acute abdominal pain: 50% have had similar episodes with spontaneous recovery in past; nausea and vomiting | Small tender adnexal mass or lower abdominal mass; may have rebound tenderness; fever | ↑ WBC | Predominantly solid ovarian mass with good through-transmission<br>Fluid in cul-de-sac |
| Appendiceal abscess | Right lower quadrant pain; nausea, vomiting | Tender right lower abdominal mass; may have rebound tenderness fever | ↑ WBC | Nonspecific complex adnexal mass<br>Fecalith with shadowing<br>Fluid in cul-de-sac |
| Tubo-ovarian abscess | Lower abdominal pain; vaginal discharge; history of PID | Tender lower abdominal or adnexal mass; fever: purulent cervical drainage | ↑ WBC | Nonspecific complex mass<br>Fluid in cul-de-sac |
| Malignant neoplasm | May have lower abdominal pain which is acute, subacute, or chronic; nausea and vomiting | Lower abdominal mass; fever if torsion; ascites; lymphadenopathy; metastases; | ↑ WBC if torsion | Nonspecific complex ovarian mass<br>Central cystic area of necrosis<br>Uterus may not be identifiable<br>Fluid in cul-de-sac in 50%<br>Ascites, liver, and peritoneal metastases, lymphadenopathy |

Courtesy of Isabel S. Bass M.D., Downstate Medical Center, Brooklyn, New York.

observation with ultrasound repeated in 3–4 days is quite helpful. Hemorrhagic ovarian cysts normally undergo a change in their sonographic characteristics. Classically these blood-filled masses go from poorly attenuating hyperechoic masses through a septated and semicystic stage to eventually an entirely cystic structure. If the mass does not change, then neoplasia, either benign or malignant, should be suspected and surgery recommended.

### Cystic Masses

If the mass is predominantly cystic it is almost invariably benign. The diagnostic thrust is toward discovering the organ of origin, which will dictate the therapeutic approach.

If the mass appears related to the reproductive system and/or urinary tract the workup would follow standard genital urologic workup. A thorough sonographic evaluation of the pelvis and renal fossae is followed by appropriate contrast studies of the organs in question. If the mass is thought to be adnexal, there is usually no hurry for operative intervention. A repeat scan should be performed from 2 weeks to 1 month later.

## Hydrometrocolpos

Hydrocolpos refers to dilatation of the vagina proximal to a congenital obstruction. In hydrometrocolpos both the uterus and the vagina are dilated. Rarely, the obstruction is at the level of the cervix and hydrometria results. The causes include an imperforate hymen and various vaginal lesions ranging from a simple diaphragm to atresia of the vagina, cervix, or both. Most cases of imperforate hymen are not discovered until menarche. Children who have been exposed to a higher level of maternal estrogens may develop a detectable dilatation of the genital tract in the perinatal period.

Infantile hydrometrocolpos usually presents as an abdominal mass. Among palpable midline pelvic and lower abdominal masses in neonatal females, hydrometrocolpos is seen slightly more frequently than ovarian cyst. The condition accounts for about 15% of abdominal masses in newborn girls. Hydrometrocolpos is often accompanied by other severe congenital malformations, such as imperforate anus, urinary tract malformations, and cardiac and skeletal abnormalities. These congenital abnormalities are often a more serious threat to the life and health of the patient than is the hydrometrocolpos itself. A pure imperforate hymen, without cervical or vaginal abnormalities, is not as frequently associated with other congenital anomalies.[44]

The diagnosis of hydrometrocolpos can be made sonographically by identifying numerous internal echoes caused by retained secretions. A normal uterus and vagina will often not be identified.[45, 46] If the hydrometrocolpos patient requires metroplasty or vaginoplasty, ultrasound can be used in follow-up to rule out such postoperative complications as infection or retained secretions. When scanning for a clinically suspected hydrometrocolpos, it is important to examine the urinary tract to rule out congenital anomalies of that organ system as well.[47] Also, radiographs of the spine are indicated.[48]

Following is a list of masses that may be found in the pelvis in children.

> Presacral
>> Sacrococcygeal teratoma
>> Anterior meningocele
>> Neurenteric cysts
>> Chordoma
>> Retrorectal cysts
>> Ectopic kidney
>> Neuroblastoma
>> Ganglioneuroma
>> Neurofibroma
>> Abscess (postraumatic or iatrogenic)
>> Ulcerative colitis
>> Osteomyelitis (sacram)
>> Sacral bone tumors
>> Retroperitoneal sarcomas
> Rectovesical
>> Massive hydroureter
>> Teratoma
>> Diverticulum (bladder)
>> Appendiceal abscess
>> Hydrosalpinx
>> Ovarian cyst
>> Lymphosarcoma
>> Rhabdomyosarcoma
>> Yolk sac carcinoma
>> Hydrometrocolpos
>> Foreign body abscess (from vaginal perforation)

# References

1. Haller JO, Schneider M, Kassner EG, et al: Ultrasonography in pediatric gynecology and obstetrics. *AJR* 1977; 128:423.

2. Kangarloo H, Sarti DA, Sample WF: Ultrasound of the pediatric pelvis. *Semin Ultrasound* 1980; 1:51.

3. Haller JO, Schneider M: *Pediatric Ultrasound.* Chicago, Year Book Medical Publishers, Inc, 1980.

4. Norris HJ, Hertig AT, Abell MR (eds): *The Uterus.* Baltimore, Williams & Wilkins Co, 1973.

5. McArdle CR, Berezin AF: Ultrasound demonstration of uterus subseptus. *JCU* 1980; 8:139.

6. Kurtz AB, Wagner RJ, Rubin CS, et al: Bicornuate uterus: Unilateral pregnancy and pelvic kidney. *JCU* 1980; 8:353.

7. Semmens JP: Congenital anomalies of female genital tract. *Obstet Gynecol* 1962; 19:328.

8. Shenker L, Brickman FE: Bicornuate uterus with incomplete vaginal septum and unilateral renal agenesis. *Radiology* 1979; 133:455.

9. Viscomi GN, Gonzales R, Taylor KJW: Ultrasound detection of uterine abnormalities after diethystilbestrol (DES) exposure. *Radiology* 1980; 136:733.

10. Rennell CL: T-Shaped uterus in diethylstilbestrol (DES) exposure. *AJR* 1979; 132:979.

11. Simkins CS: Development of the human ovary from birth to sexual maturity. *Am J Anat* 1982; 51:465.

12. Potter EL: The ovary in infancy and childhood, in Hugh GG, Smith DE (eds): *The Ovary.* Baltimore, Williams & Wilkins Co, 1963, pp 11–23.

13. Sample WF, Lippe BM, Gyepes MT: Gray scale ultrasonography of the normal female pelvis. *Radiology* 1977; 125:477–483.

14. Hackeloer BJ, Nitschke-Dabelstein S: Ovarian imaging by ultrasound: An attempt to define a reference plane. *JCU* 1980; 8:497–500.

15. Kratochwil A, Urban G, Friedrich F: Ultrasonic tomography of the ovaries. *Ann Chir Gynecol Fenn* 1972; 61:211–214.

16. Cochrane WJ: Ultrasound in gynecology. *Radiol Clin North Am* 1975; 13:457–466.

17. Requard CK, Mehler FA, Wicks JD: Preoperative sonography of malignant ovarian neoplasms. *AJR* 1981; 137:79–82.

18. Goldberg BB, Pollack HM, Capitanio MA, et al: Ultrasonography: An aid in the diagnosis of masses in pediatric patients. *Pediatrics* 1975; 56:421–428.

19. Walsh JW, Rosenfield AT, Jaffe CC, et al: Prospective comparison of ultrasound and computed tomography in the evaluation of gynecologic pelvic masses. *AJR* 1978; 131:955–960.

20. Carter BL, Kahn PC, Wolpert SM, et al: Unusual pelvic masses: A comparison of computed tomography and ultrasonography. *Radiology* 1976; 121:383–390.

21. Haller JO, Fellows RA: The pelvis. *Clin Diagn Ultrasound* 1981; 8:165–185.

22. Neilson OV: Ovarian tumors in children. *Acta Obstet Gynecol Scand* 1968; 4:119–131.

23. Lawson TL, Albarelli JN: Diagnosis of gynecologic pelvic masses by gray scale ultrasonography: Analysis of specificity and accuracy. *AJR* 1977; 128:1003–1006.

24. Lewis E, Zornoza J, Bao-Shan J, et al: Radiologic contributions to the diagnosis and management of gynecologic neoplasms. *Semin Roentgenol* 1982; 17:251–268.

25. Grade M, Gillooly L, Taylor KJW: In utero demonstration of an ovarian cystic mass by ultrasound. *JCU* 1980; 8:251–252.

26. Tabsh KMA: Antenatal sonographic appearance of a fetal ovarian cyst. *J Ultrasound Med* 1982; 1:329–331.

27. Fleming P, McLeary R: Non-immunologic fetal hydrops with theca lutein cysts. *Radiology* 1981; 141:169–170.

28. Farrell TP, Boal DK, Teele RL, et al: Acute torsion of the normal uterine adnexa in children: Sonographic demonstration. *AJR* 1982; 139:1223–1225.

29. Kennedy LA, Pinckney LE, Currarino G: Amputated calcified ovaries in children. *Radiology* 1981; 141:83–86.

30. Riddlesberger MM, Kuhn JP, Munschauer RW: The association of juvenile hypothyroidism and cystic ovaries. *Radiology* 1981; 139:77–80.

31. Swanson M, Sauerberei EE, Cooperberg PL: Medical implications of ultrasonically detected polycystic ovaries. *JCU* 1981; 9:219–222.

32. Callen PW, Marks WM: Lymphomatous masses simulating cysts by ultrasound. *J Can Assoc Radiol* 1979; 30:244–246.

33. White EA, Filly RA: Cholesterol crystals as the

source of both diffuse and layered echoes in a cystic ovarian tumor. *JCU* 1980; 8:241–243.

34. Behan M, Kazam E: The echographic characteristics of fatty tissues and tumors. *Radiology* 1978; 129:143–151.

35. Sandler MA, Silver TM, Karo JJ: Gray-scale ultrasonic features of ovarian teratomas. *Radiology* 1979; 131:705.

36. Siegel MJ, McAlister WH, Shackelford GD: Radiographic findings in ovarian teratomas in children. *AJR* 1978; 131:613.

37. Hyman RA, Von Micsky LI, Finby N: Ovarian teratoma in childhood. *AJR* 1972; 116:673.

38. Fleischer AC, James AE, Millis JB, et al: Differential diagnosis of pelvic masses by gray scale ultrasonography. *AJR* 1978; 131:469–476.

39. Morley P, Barnett E: The ovarian mass, in Sanders RC, James AE (eds): *Ultrasonography in Obstetrics and Gynecology,* ed 2. New York, Appleton-Century-Crofts, 1980, pp 357–385.

40. Goodman JD, Schneider M, Haller JO: Ultrasound demonstration of an infected urachal cyst. *Urol Radiol* 1982; L:245–246.

41. Heald RP: *Adolescent Gynecology.* Baltimore, Williams & Wilkins, 1966, p 73.

42. Schaffer RM, Haller JO, Friedman AP, et al: Sonographic diagnosis of ovarian dysgerminoma in children. *Med Ultrasound* 1982; 6:118–119.

43. Haller JO, Bass IS, Friedman AP: Pelvic mass in girls. *Pediatr Radiol* (in press).

44. Reed MH, Griscom NT: Hydrometrocolpos in infancy. *AJR* 1973; 118:1.

45. Wilson DA, Stacy TM, Smith EI: Ultrasound diagnosis of hydrocolpos and hydrometrocolpos. *Radiology* 1978; 128:451–454.

46. Sailer JF: Hematometra and hematocolpos: Ultrasound findings. *AJR* 1979; 132:1010.

47. Vinstein AL, Franken EA: Unilateral hematocolpos associated with agenesis of the kidney. *Radiology* 1972; 102:625.

48. Vitko RJ, Cass AS, Winter RB: Anomalies of the genitourinary tract associated with congenital scoliosis and congenital kyphosis. *J Urol* 1972; 108:655.

## CASES

### Dennis A. Sarti, M.D.

### Diaphragm

The pediatric diaphragm and the region around the diaphragm can be easily evaluated with real-time ultrasound. Ultrasound examination of the diaphragm is best attempted on the right side thorugh the liver. It is less successful on the left side because of the air-containing stomach and splenic flexure.

Real-time ultrasound evaluation of the hemidiaphragm is extremely helpful when paralysis of the hemidiaphragm is suspected. Figures 17–1 and 17–2 are transverse scans in the subxiphoid region with the transducer angled in a cephalad direction. Figure 17–1 is a scan made at inspiration and Figure 17–2 is a scan made at expiration. Note that in this case the right hemidiaphragm (arrow) changes position with inspiration and expiration, whereas the left hemidiaphragm remains constant in position. This indicates paralysis of the left hemidiaphragm, since it does not move with respiratory motion. In Figure 17–1, obtained during inspiration, the right hemidiaphragm is closer to the transducer. This is often confusing when first visualized. However, the hemidiaphragm moves downward and the dome moves closer to the transducer. Therefore, the hemidiaphragm appears to be closer to the transducer in inspiration (Fig 17–1) and farther from the transducer in expiration (Fig 17–2). Throughout the respiratory cycle, the left hemidiaphragm remains fixed in location. This confirmed the diagnosis of paralysis of the left hemidiaphragm.

Figure 17–3 is a chest film in which a right cardiodiaphragmatic soft tissue mass is identified (arrowhead). If this mass is in contact with the right hemidiaphragm, we can visualize it on ultrasound, as in Figure 17–4. If the mass is above the diaphragm and lung intervenes, we will not be able to see it because of the interposed air. Figure 17–4 is a longitudinal real-time scan in which the rounded echogenic

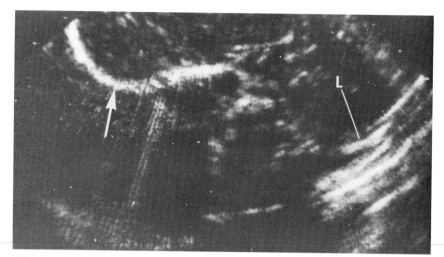

FIG 17–1.

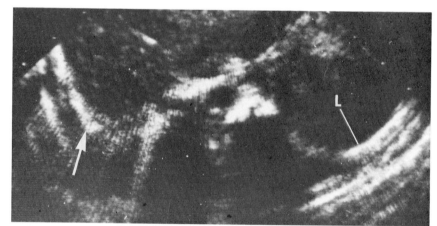

FIG 17–2.

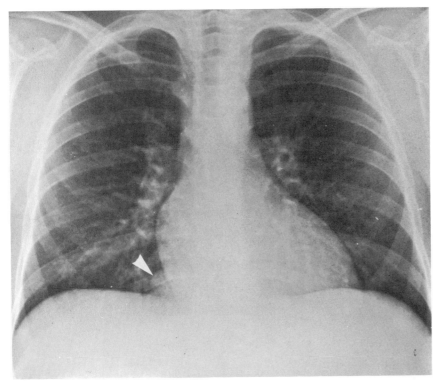

**FIG 17–3.**

mass (arrowhead) can be seen just cephalad to the right hemidiaphragm. This highly echogenic region has some attenuation deep to it. These findings are consistent with fat and led to the correct diagnosis of a lipoma in the region.

**Arrow** = Right hemidiaphragm
**Arrowhead** = Lipoma
**L** = Left hemidiaphragm

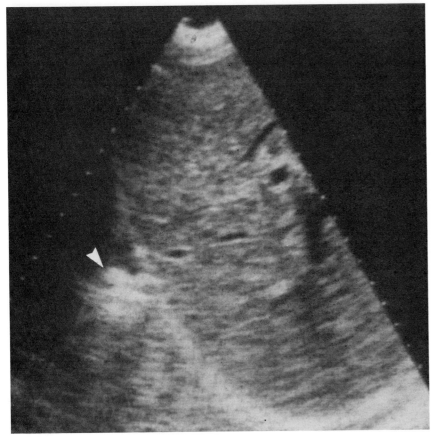

**FIG 17–4.**

## Elevated Hemidiaphragm

Very often elevation of the hemidiaphragm can be correctly evaluated on ultrasound. If the patient's upper abdomen is scanned and the transducer is angled in a cephalad direction, the hemidiaphragm is usually visible. Abdominal pathology can be detected in the subdiaphragmatic region and can lead to the correct diagnosis. Figure 17–5 is a chest radiograph in which the right hemidiaphragm is elevated compared to the left. Figure 17–6 is a longitudinal scan of the right upper quadrant. The right hemidiaphragm is visualized deep to the liver. The liver has a normal echo texture, with no masses identified. There is no subdiaphragmatic mass or fluid collection present. The diaphragm itself has a sharp border and a normal appearance. The diaphragm moved with inspiration and expiration. This constellation of findings is consistent with eventration of the right hemidiaphragm. Since no pathologic entity was identified in the subdiaphragmatic region and the diaphragm moved on real-time examination, the diagnosis of eventration was made.

In Figure 17–7, the chest radiograph of another patient, there is slight elevation of the right hemidiaphragm, not as dramatic as in the previous case. However, a most disturbing finding on the chest film in Figure 17–7 is displacement of the stomach bubble to the left side. A soft tissue mass impinges on the fundal region and lesser curvature of the stomach. This finding, in conjunction with slight elevation of the right hemidiaphragm, indicated the necessity for abdominal ultrasound. Figure 17–8 is a transverse scan of the upper abdomen in the subxiphoid region. The transducer was angled in a cephalad direction. The liver echo texture is markedly abnormal. A large liver mass (arrowheads) is identified in both the right and left lobes of the liver. This mass has echogenic foci along with large sonolucent areas. The mass explained the elevation of the right hemidiaphragm and displacement of the gastric air bubble to the left. The mass was a hepatoblastoma.

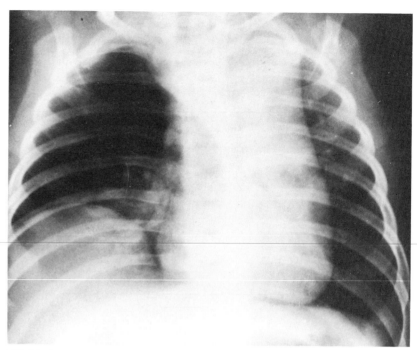

FIG 17–5.

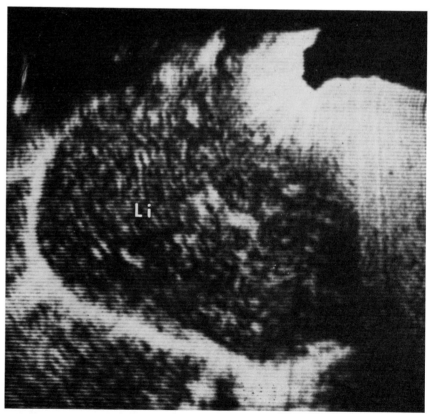

FIG 17–6.

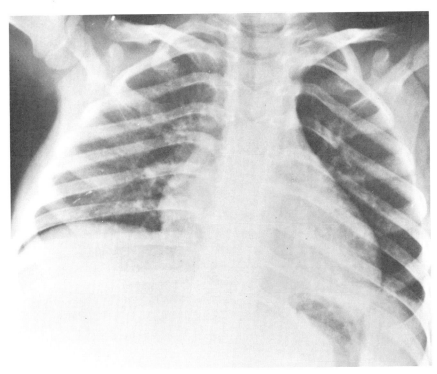

Arrowheads  =  Hepatoblastoma
Li          =  Liver

**FIG 17–7.**

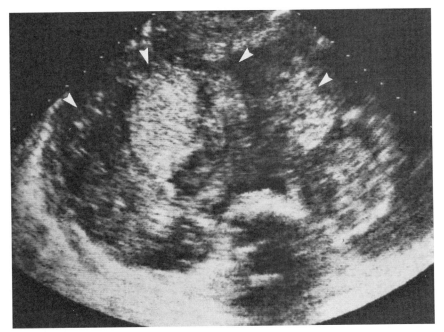

**FIG 17–8.**

## Juxtadiaphragmatic Mass

When a soft tissue mass is in contact with the hemidiaphragm, ultrasound can be used to evaluate the nature of this mass. If the patient is scanned in the subxiphoid or subcostal area and the transducer is angled in a cephalad direction, masses in the thorax can be evaluated. As long as no air intervenes between the mass and the hemidiaphragm, evaluation will be possible. Figure 17–9 is a chest radiograph showing a large soft tissue mass (arrowhead) in the right cardiodiaphragmatic region. This mass is in contact with the right hemidiaphragm, and ultrasound evaluation was possible. Figure 17–10 is a subxiphoid transverse scan made with marked cephalad angulation of the transducer. The liver (Li) is seen anteriorly. A circular sonolucent soft tissue mass (arrowheads) is noted in the posterior aspect of the liver. Figure 17–11 is a longitudinal scan through the plane of the soft tissue mass. The mass (arrowheads) is better evaluated on this longitudinal scan. It has a bull's-eye appearance, which suggests the correct diagnosis. The central echoes suggest the presence of a kidney. The mass was an intrathoracic kidney. After the ultrasound study, intravenous pyelography was performed; an image from this study is shown in Figure 17–12. The left kidney is in normal position. The right kidney (arrowhead) is in a more cephalad position than usual. The findings confirm the diagnosis of an intrathoracic kidney. Ultrasound evaluation of juxtadiaphragmatic masses is extremely helpful in delineating the nature and etiology of such soft tissue masses.

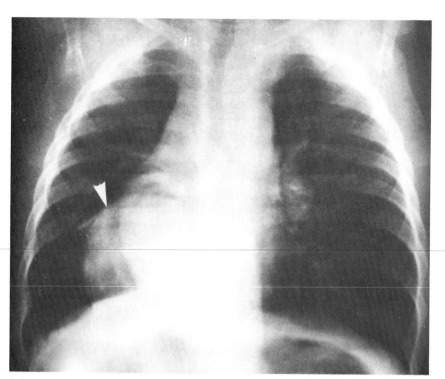

**FIG 17–9.**

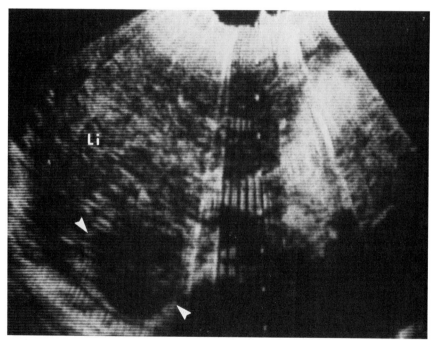

**FIG 17–10.**

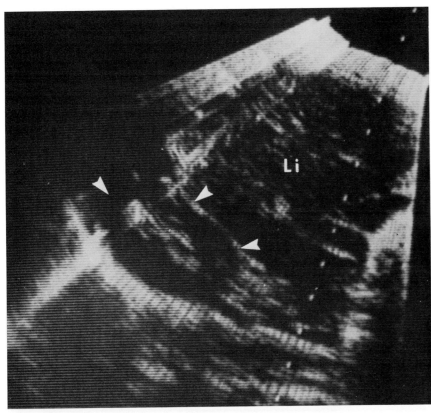

Arrowheads = Intrathoracic kidney
Li        = Liver

**FIG 17–11.**

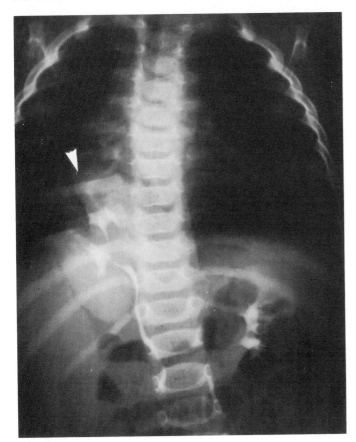

**FIG 17–12.**

## Scimitar Syndrome

Anomalous pulmonary venous return can sometimes be confirmed by ultrasound evaluation of the right upper quadrant. Figure 17–13 is a chest radiograph in which increased density is noted to the right lung field. There is evidence of hypoplasia of the right lung and dextroposition of the heart. An ultrasound scan of the right upper quadrant is shown in Figure 17–14. The liver (Li) is seen anteriorly. The tubular structure deep to the liver represents the inferior vena cava (I). There is a tubular structure arising from the posterior cephalad portion of the inferior vena cava. This structure represents venous drainage from the right lung into the proximal inferior vena cava (arrow). The ultrasound findings suggested the presence of anomalous pulmonary venous return from the right pulmonary vein into the inferior vena cava. This was confirmed on a delayed film obtained during angiocardiography (Fig 17–15). The catheter is in the inferior vena cava and anomalous return of the right lower lobe pulmonary vein is seen draining into the inferior vena cava.

Figure 17–16 will be discussed on the next section, in conjunction with Figures 17–17 through 17–20.

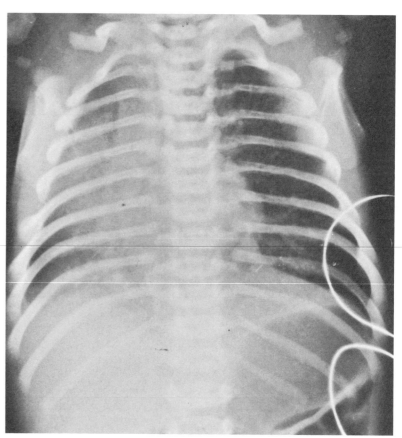

**FIG 17–13.**

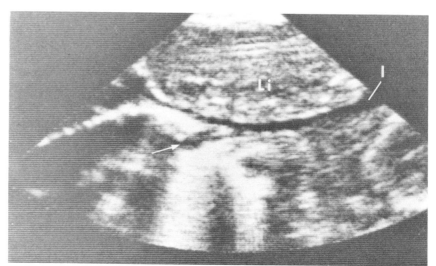

**FIG 17–14.**

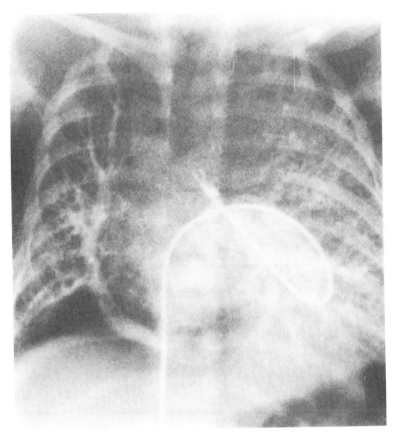

**FIG 17–15.**

| | | |
|---|---|---|
| **Arrowhead** | = | Gallbladder |
| **Arrow** | = | Anomalous pulmonary venous return (Fig 17–14) |
| **Arrow** | = | Dilated common bile duct (Fig 17–16) |
| **Cy** | = | Choledochal cyst |
| **I** | = | Inferior vena cava |
| **Li** | = | Liver |

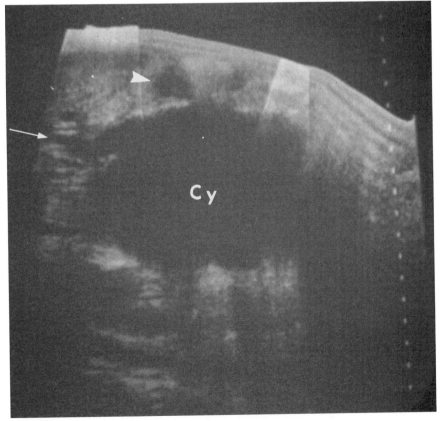

**FIG 17–16.**

## Choledochal Cyst

Choledochal cyst is an uncommon congenital anomaly in which the common bile duct is dilated. Often the patient is first seen as a child and has the classic triad of abdominal pain, jaundice, and a palpable abdominal mass. This triad is not always present. The patient may present only with jaundice. In such cases, the diagnosis of choledochal cyst should always be kept in mind. It is important to attempt to visualize the gallbladder in such cases. A choledochal cyst will often be misinterpreted as the gallbladder.

Figure 17–16, shown on the previous page, is part of the spectrum of cases of choledochal cyst. Figure 17–16 shows a large cystic region in the right upper quadrant. The differential diagnosis of this mass includes a choledochal cyst, pseudocyst of the pancreas, duplication cyst, mesenteric cyst, and hepatic artery aneurysm (in the older patient). The gallbladder is often difficult to visualize. It is seen anterior (arrowhead) to the choledochal cyst. In Figure 17–16 a dilated common bile duct (arrow) is seen emptying into the choledochal cyst. This relationship cannot always be demonstrated.

Figures 17–17 and 17–18 are transverse and longitudinal scans of a pediatric patient with a choledochal cyst (Cy). The cystic region could be misinterpreted as the gallbladder. In Figure 17–17 a small gallbladder (arrowhead) can be seen lateral to the choledochal cyst (Cy). The choledochal cyst is situated lateral to the head of the pancreas, confirming the presence of a dilated common bile duct. In this case there is no evidence of intrahepatic biliary dilatation.

Choledochal cysts may be accompanied by intrahepatic biliary dilatation. Figure 17–19 is a longitudinal scan showing a choledochal cyst (Cy) cephalad to the gallbladder (arrowhead). The gallbladder is filled with biliary sludge. Intrahepatic biliary dilatation is identified, along with a dilated right hepatic duct (HD). Occasionally intrahepatic biliary dilatation is more severe, as is seen in Figure 17–20. In this instance, bile ducts (BD) are seen

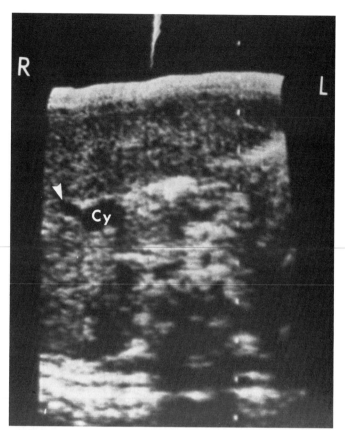

**FIG 17–17.**

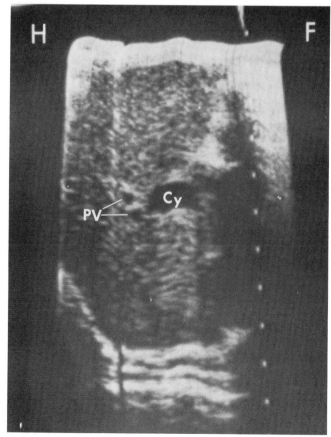

**FIG 17–18.**

within the liver parenchyma. These ducts are not normally visible unless biliary dilatation is present.

| | | |
|---|---|---|
| **Arrow** | = | Common bile duct (Fig 17–16) |
| **Arrowhead** | = | Gallbladder |
| **BD** | = | Dilated intrahepatic biliary tree |
| **Cy** | = | Choledochal cyst |
| **F** | = | Foot |
| **H** | = | Head |
| **HD** | = | Dilated right hepatic duct |
| **L** | = | Left |
| **PV** | = | Portal vein |
| **R** | = | Right |

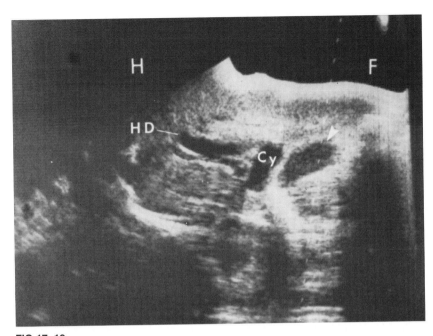

**FIG 17–19.**

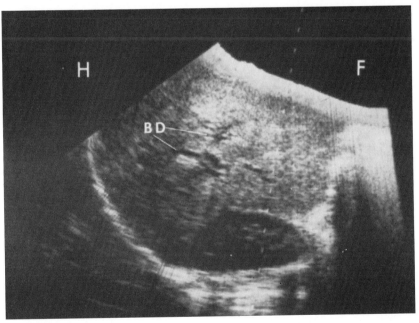

**FIG 17–20.**

## Hepatobiliary Pathology

Liver neoplasms distort the normal liver architecture. Liver neoplasms may be primary or metastatic. Primary liver neoplasms arise from liver parenchyma, bile ducts, blood vessels or connective tissue. The majority of primary liver tumors in children are malignant. Figure 17–21 is a transverse scan of the upper abdomen in which there is diffusely uneven texture pattern to nearly the entire liver (arrowheads). A small portion of relatively normal liver parenchyma is noted in the tip of the left lobe. The mass, a hepatoblastoma, is echogenic centrally with a lucent periphery. Hepatoblastomas are often seen in the first 3 years of life. Figure 17–22 is an angiogram of the same patient which shows diffuse enlargement of the liver by tumor. Note that the vessels drape over the mass.

Figure 17–23, a longitudinal scan of the right upper quadrant, shows the gallbladder in a child with leukemia. The size of the gallbladder was considered to be at the upper limits of normal on this scan. The patient was on chemotherapy. Approximately 2–3 weeks later, another ultrasound scan of the right upper quadrant was obtained (Figure 17–24). The gallbladder wall is now markedly thickened (arrows), to approximately 1 cm. These findings were secondary to acute cholecystitis due to chemotherapy.

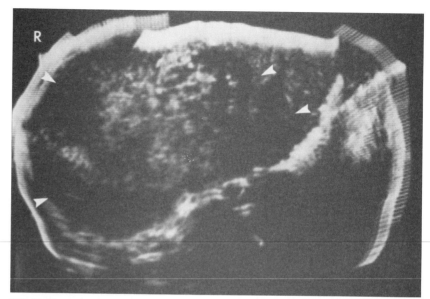

FIG 17–21.

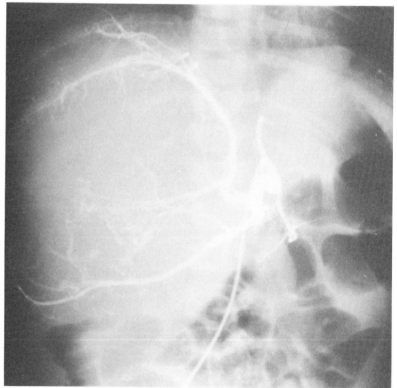

FIG 17–22.

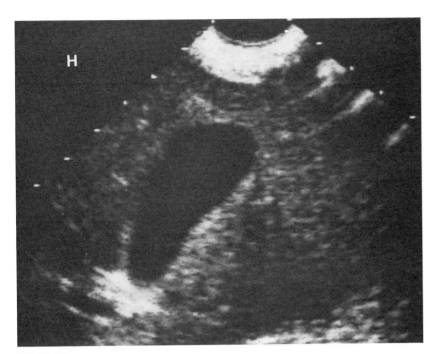

| Arrows | = Gallbladder wall thickening |
|---|---|
| **Arrowheads** | = Hepatoblastoma |
| **H** | = Head |
| **R** | = Right |

FIG 17–23.

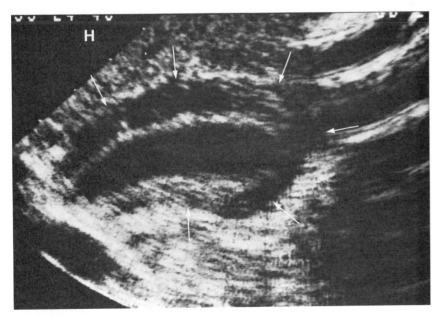

FIG 17–24.

## Hemangiomas

Hemangiomas in the newborn and child have a variety of appearances compared to that seen in the adult. Figure 17–25 is a longitudinal scan of the right upper quadrant in a pediatric patient in which we see a large mass (arrows) with a mixed echo appearance within the liver. The central portion is relatively lucent and the echogenic rim is irregular in appearance. The mass turned out to be a cavernous hemangioma. Occasionally an echogenic rim can be seen around a hemangioma in a newborn. This will suggest the diagnosis of cavernous hemangioma. However, other entities such as liver tumors cannot be excluded on the basis of the ultrasound findings.

Figures 17–26 and 17–27 are upper abdominal images of a pediatric patient with multiple, diffuse hemangiomas throughout the entire liver. The masses are mainly hypoechoic on the ultrasound scan (Fig 17–26). Some have echogenic rims, especially in the region of the left lobe. The CT scan (Fig 17–27) demonstrates the low-density hemangiomas surrounded by echogenic peripheries. The possibility of other diffusely infiltrative processes could not be excluded on the basis of the ultrasound appearance.

Figure 17–28 shows the typical appearance of a hemangioma in the adult. In the adult or older pediatric patient, a hemangioma appears as a well-circumscribed, highly echogenic mass. These hemangiomas are usually single and can be followed by serial examinations to rule out the possibility of metastasis. Usually hemangiomas in the adult are well marginated, as in this case.

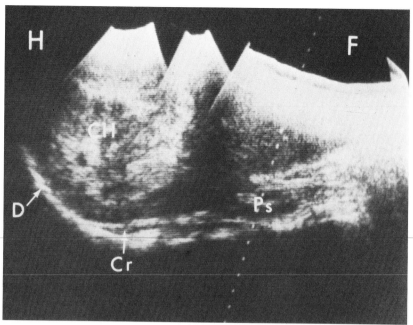

**FIG 17–25.**

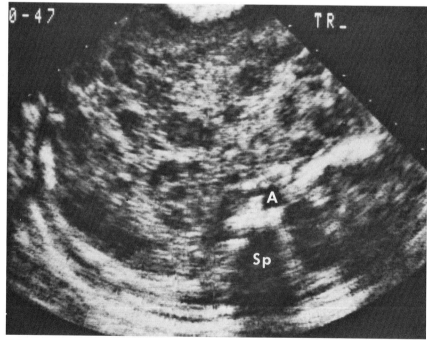

**FIG 17–26.**

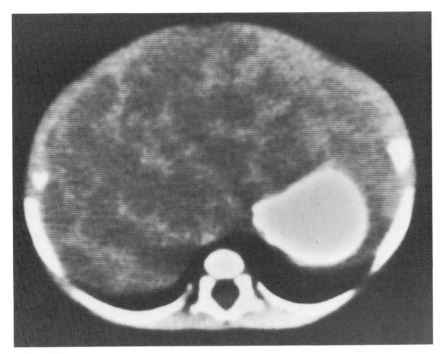

**FIG 17–27.**

A   = Aorta
CH  = Cavernous hemangioma
Cr  = Crus of the diaphragm
D   = Right hemidiaphragm
F   = Foot
H   = Head
He  = Hemangioma
K   = Kidney
Ps  = Psoas muscle
PV  = Portal vein
Sp  = Spine

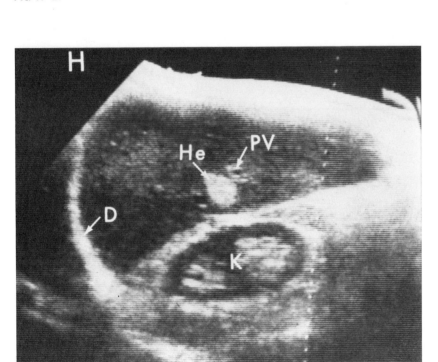

**FIG 17–28.**

## Pyloric Stenosis; Duodenal Hematoma

Infantile hypertrophic pyloric stenosis is more prevalent in males than females. Symptoms usually develop in the first few weeks of life. The initial diagnosis may be suspected on physical examination when a palpable mass is found in the right upper quadrant. Before the development of ultrasound, radiography was used to establish the diagnosis; such a radiograph is shown in Figure 17–30. With modern-day ultrasound equipment, we are able to visualize the hypertrophic muscle of the pylorus. Figures 17–29 and 17–30 are an ultrasound scan and a radiograph of a patient with pyloric stenosis. The antrum of the stomach (An) is seen with fluid and some air. There is a marked increase (arrowheads) in the musculature in the region, confirming the diagnosis of pyloric stenosis. The radiograph in Figure 17–30 shows the small, thin pyloric channel between the antrum of the stomach and the duodenum.

Children are susceptible to numerous traumatic episodes. Ultrasound is often used to diagnose the presence of hematoma. Figure 17–31 is a longitudinal scan of the abdomen of a 4-year-old boy who had recently been punched in the stomach and was experiencing severe abdominal pain. Ultrasound revealed a large sonolucent region just inferior to the liver. This was found to be a duodenal hematoma (He). Because of the ultrasound findings, an upper GI tract series was obtained (Fig 17–32). The third portion of the duodenum is partially obstructed, confirming the ultrasound findings of a duodenal hematoma.

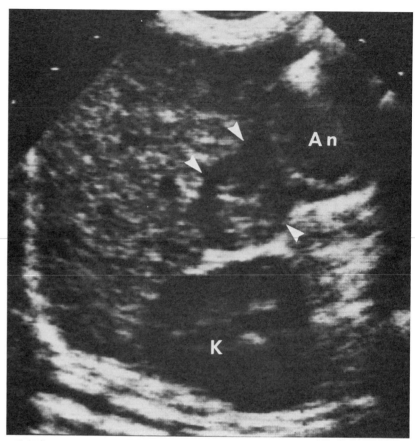

FIG 17–29.

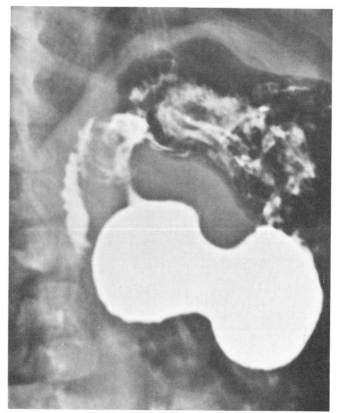

FIG 17–30.

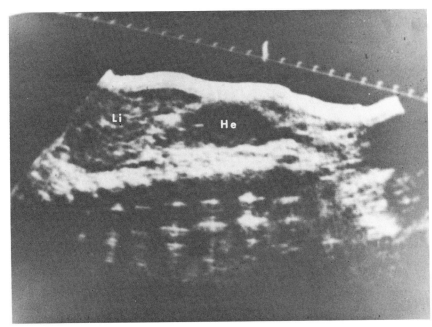

| | | |
|---|---|---|
| **Arrowheads** | = | Pyloric stenosis |
| **An** | = | Antrum of the stomach |
| **He** | = | Duodenal hematoma |
| **K** | = | Kidney |
| **Li** | = | Liver |

**FIG 17–31.**

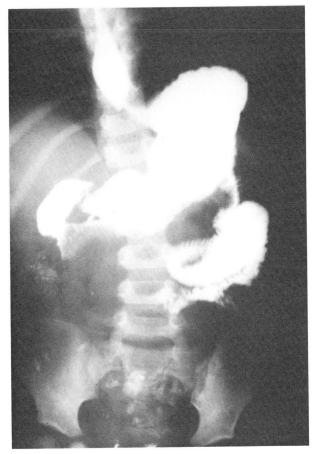

**FIG 17–32.**

## Abdominal Cysts

Duplication cysts of the gastrointestinal (GI) tract are rare congenital anomalies. They may occur anywhere along the alimentary tract. Affected patients often present with a palpable abdominal mass. Other symptoms such as pain or vomiting may be present, depending on the size and location of the cyst. Duplication cysts have a varied ultrasound appearance, depending on their contents. They may be sonolucent with through-transmission if they are fluid filled. If they contain debris or hemorrhage, they will appear as echogenic masses in the abdomen. The differential diagnosis of duplication cysts detected on ultrasound includes choledochal cyst, mesenteric cyst, pancreatic pseudocyst, hematoma, abscess, and necrotic cystic tumors of various abdominal organs.

Figure 17–33 is a longitudinal scan of the right upper quadrant of a 2-year-old boy who has a large sonolucent mass just inferior to the liver and kidney. A mass was palpable in the right upper quadrant mass. This mass could be construed as a gallbladder or a liver cyst. However, the gallbladder was visualized on other scans. The patient was found to have a duplication cyst of the gastric antrum that was mainly fluid filled.

Figure 17–34 is a longitudinal scan through the right abdomen showing large septated cystic mass. Note the abdominal skin line, which indicates the size of the mass. Although the mass is mainly fluid filled, there is a circular echogenicity on the back wall. A small amount of attenuation is present deep to this echogenic region. The mass was found to be a mesenteric cyst containing a calcified blood clot.

Figure 17–35 is a longitudinal scan of the right abdomen in a 3-year-old girl who was admitted for evaluation of a nontender mass on the right side. The ultrasound scan in Figure 17–35 shows a large mass with a cystic and echogenic component. There is a fluid-fluid layer (arrowhead) noted on the posterior wall. The patient had incurred a minor injury to the abdomen in a fall 2 weeks earlier. This mass

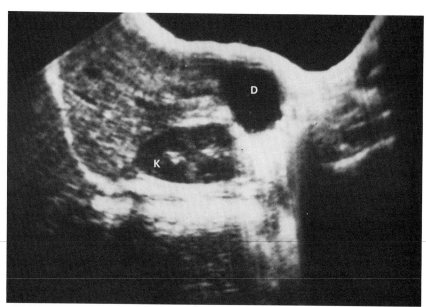

**FIG 17–33.**

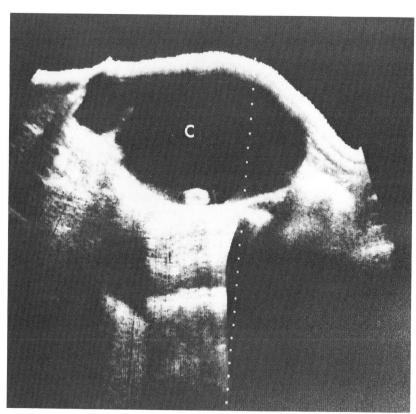

**FIG 17–34.**

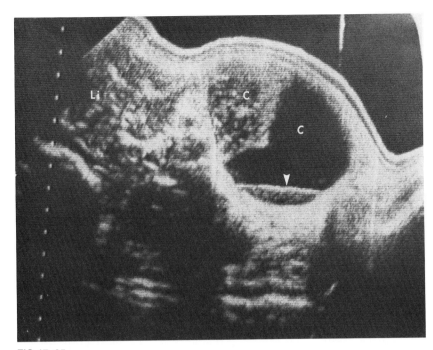

**FIG 17–35.**

was a mesenteric cyst containing some debris and hemorrhage.

Occasionally duplication cysts may be filled with echogenic material. They may or may not communicate with the GI tract. Figure 17–36 is a transverse scan of the abdomen of a young boy. A large mass is present over the mid-abdomen. In this case, numerous echoes are present within the mass. The differential diagnosis would include pancreatic abscess, pseudocyst, hematoma, lymphadenopathy, or other soft tissue masses in the region. The mass turned out to be a duplication cyst of the GI tract that was filled with a large amount of debris, explaining the internal echoes.

| | | |
|---|---|---|
| **Arrowhead** | = | Fluid-fluid layer |
| **A** | = | Aorta |
| **C** | = | Mesenteric cyst |
| **D** | = | Duplication cyst |
| **K** | = | Kidney |
| **Li** | = | Liver |

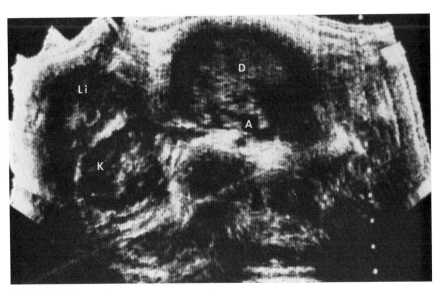

**FIG 17–36.**

## Normal Adrenal Gland

The adrenal gland changes in appearance from birth to approximately 3 years of age. Because of the lucent fetal cortex which eventually atrophies, the ultrasound appearance of the adrenal gland is varied. Figure 17–37 is a longitudinal scan of the right adrenal gland of a newborn. The adrenal cortex is markedly enlarged compared to what is seen in the adult. The adrenal gland is outlined by arrowheads. The central echogenic medullary region (M) stands out quite dramatically against the lucent fetal adrenal cortex. The fetal adrenal cortex atrophies in the first few months of life.

Figure 17–38 is a scan of the fetal adrenal gland (arrowheads) in a neonate several weeks old. The adrenal cortex is still lucent at this stage but smaller in size than in the previous study. The medullary region is represented by the linear echogenicity in the midportion of the adrenal gland.

Figure 17–39 is a scan of the right adrenal gland in a child approximately 5 months old. The previously lucent fetal cortex has atrophied, and the echogenic adult cortex is visible. In this case the fetal adrenal gland is echogenic (arrowheads) in appearance. The lucent band posterior to the adrenal gland represents the crus of the diaphragm.

Figure 17–40 is a scan of the left adrenal gland in a 2-year-old patient. The gland is now hypoechoic and resembles the gland seen in older pediatric patients and adults. The hypoechoic appearance arises from disappearance of the fibrous tissue that was present earlier.

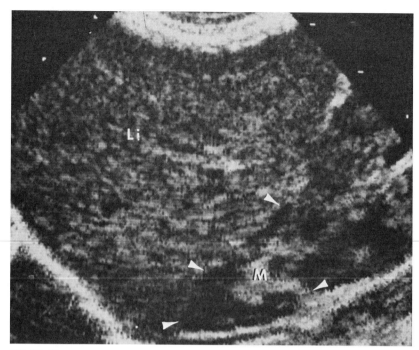

**FIG 17–37.**

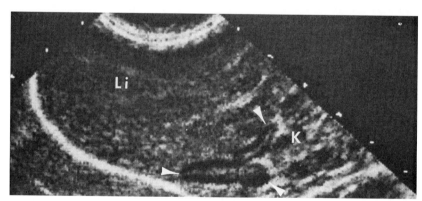

**FIG 17–38.**

**Arrowheads** = Adrenal gland
**A** = Aorta
**K** = Kidney
**Li** = Liver
**S** = Spleen

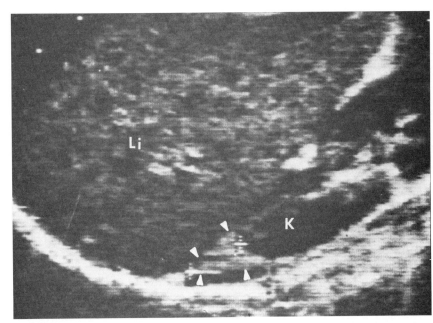

FIG 17–39.

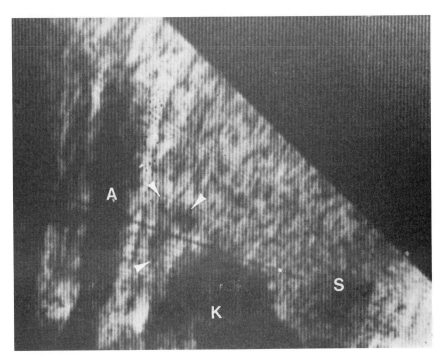

FIG 17–40.

## Benign Adrenal Lesions

Depending on the site of origin, the adrenal gland can enlarge in different directions. Figure 17–41 is a scan of the left adrenal gland in a patient with Cushing's syndrome. In this case adrenal hyperplasia is present. The adrenal borders are prominent and convex bilaterally (arrowheads). Adrenal hyperplasia will cause enlargement of both glands, with convex borders.

Figure 17–42 is a longitudinal scan of the right adrenal gland in a patient with an adrenal adenoma. Adrenal adenomas arise from the cortex. They cause an egg-like enlargement of the cortical portion of the gland. With cortical enlargement, the top portion of the adrenal gland becomes larger than normal.

Figure 17–43 is an example of a pheochromocytoma (arrowheads). This is a medullary lesion that causes enlargement of the base of the gland, sparing the apex. Approximately one third of children with pheochromocytoma have multiple lesions.

A nonfunctioning renal lesion that is commonly seen in infants and children is the hemorrhagic adrenal cyst. This entity has a varied ultrasound appearance, depending on its contents. If the cystic area is mainly fluid filled, it will have a sonolucent appearance. However, this may slowly resolve and give a more echogenic appearance. Figure 17–44 is an example of an adrenal cyst (arrowheads). It may be difficult to separate these from other cystic lesions. Follow-up examinations will demonstrate a decrease in size of a hemorrhagic cyst, differentiating it from cystic neoplasms.

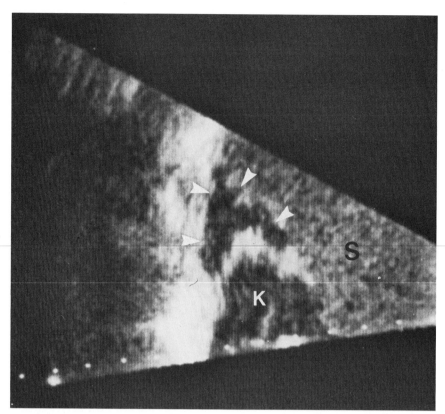

**FIG 17–41.**

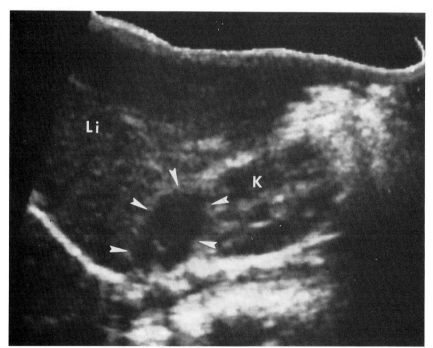

**FIG 17–42.**

**Arrowheads** = Adrenal enlargement
**A** = Aorta
**K** = Kidney
**Li** = Liver
**S** = Spleen

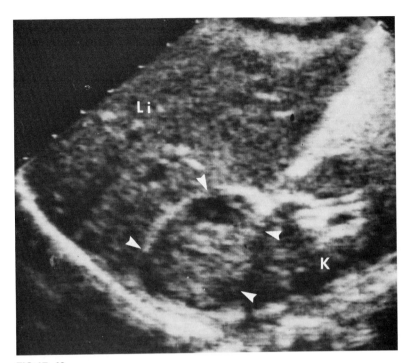

**FIG 17–43.**

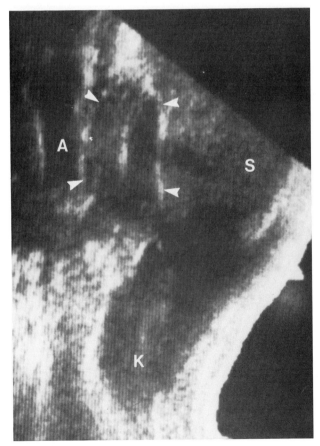

**FIG 17–44.**

## Neuroblastoma

Evaluation of a palpable abdominal mass will often lead to the diagnosis of neuroblastoma. Neuroblastoma is the most common solid tumor of infancy. It may arise from the adrenal gland or other abdominal areas. These lesions usually present as echogenic masses in the suprarenal area. Figure 17–45 is a longitudinal scan of the right upper quadrant in a young patient in which a large mass (M) is seen cephalad to the right kidney. The mass is adrenal in origin and has a large echogenic component. The findings are consistent with neuroblastoma.

Evaluation of the vascular anatomy adjacent to these lesions is quite helpful. Figure 17–46 is a longitudinal scan of the right upper quadrant in a patient who has neuroblastoma (M). The echogenic mass was noted posterior to the inferior vena cava and was displacing this vessel anteriorly.

Neuroblastomas are most often seen in the first 5 years of life. They can be bilateral. Examination of both adrenal regions is necessary when a neuroblastoma is found. Figure 17–47 is a transverse scan of the upper abdomen in the region of the celiac axis. The aorta (A) is well seen. A tubular structure arises from the anterior aorta and bifurcates into a Y shape. This structure represents the celiac axis. Echogenic masses are seen on each side of the celiac axis (M), representing bilateral neuroblastomas.

Wilms' tumors arise from renal parenchyma and must be differentiated from neuroblastoma. Very often they displace the kidney in a cephalad direction, whereas neuroblastoma will displace the kidney in a caudad direction. Figure 17–48 is a coronal scan in which a Wilms' tumor (W) is noted on the inferior aspect of the kidney (K). A small amount of hydronephrosis of the upper pole of the kidney is identified on the scan.

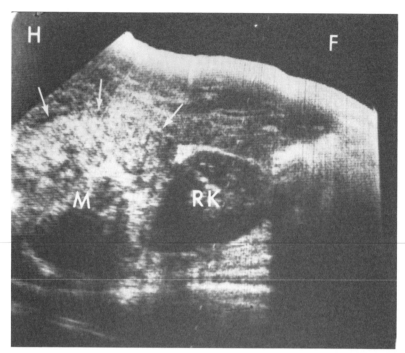

**FIG 17–45.**

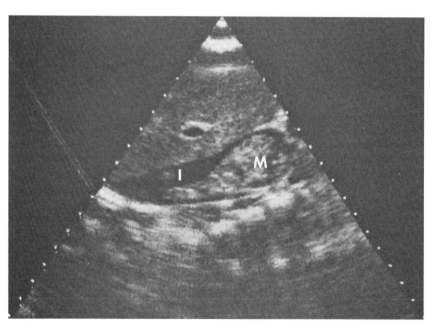

**FIG 17–46.**

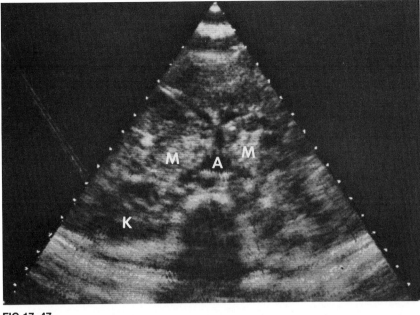

Arrows = Neuroblastoma
A = Aorta
F = Foot
H = Head
I = Inferior vena cava
K = Kidney
N = Neuroblastoma
RK = Right kidney
W = Wilms' tumor

**FIG 17–47.**

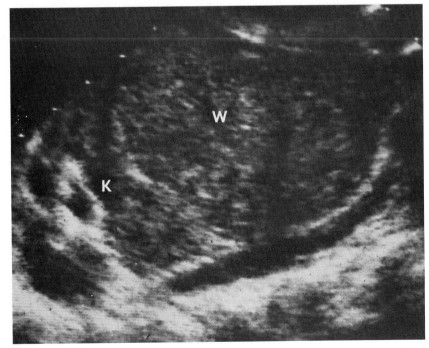

**FIG 17–48.**

## Normal Pediatric Kidneys

Normal kidneys in children appear different from kidneys in adults. The appearance depends on the age of the patient. The neonatal kidney shows little of the sinus echogenicity that is seen in the adult kidney. Figure 17–49 is a longitudinal scan in which numerous sonolucent regions are seen in the kidney. These regions represent the hypoechoic renal pyramids. They stand out quite dramatically in the neonatal period. Figure 17–49 is the scan of a 1-day-old infant. The renal cortex is relatively echogenic in neonates, causing the lucent pyramids to stand out dramatically. These lucent pyramids should not be confused with cystic disease or hydronephrosis.

Figure 17–50 is a longitudinal scan of the right kidney in a 1-month-old infant. Again, the relatively lucent renal pyramids are identified. Note that the renal cortex is echogenic relative to the pyramids.

Figure 17–51 is a longitudinal scan in an 8-year-old patient. By this age, some perisinus fat is noted in the central portion of the kidney. Mild dilatation of the pelvis may be seen; it is a normal anatomic finding.

Figure 17–52 is a longitudinal scan of the left kidney. The left upper pole may have a bulbous appearance. This is a normal anatomic finding and should not be confused with any mass lesion.

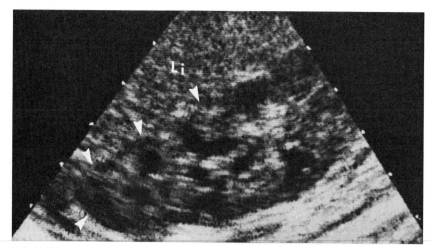

**FIG 17–49.**

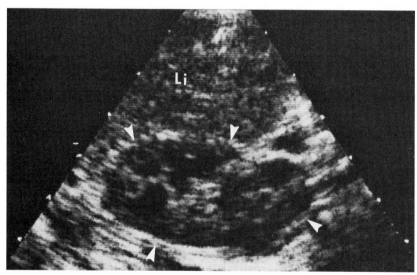

**FIG 17–50.**

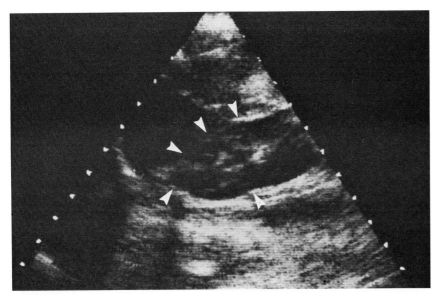

**Arrows** = Bulbous left upper pole
**Arrowheads** = Renal outline
**Li** = Liver

FIG 17–51.

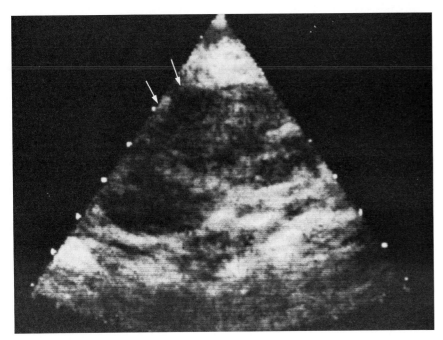

FIG 17–52.

## Urinary Tract Dilation

Dilation of the urinary tract can be visualized on ultrasound in various degrees of severity. Dilation of the urinary tract may be secondary to obstruction, reflux, or infection. Ultrasound cannot distinguish among the various causes of dilation. Figure 17–53 is a longitudinal scan in which a small amount of fluid is noted in the collecting systems. This is suggestive of minimal hydronephrosis. Such a small amount of fluid can also be a normal anatomic variant. This only demonstrates prominent fluid in the renal pelvis. Some patients may have an extra renal pelvis without evidence of any obstruction or dilation.

Figure 17–54 is a longitudinal coronal scan of another patient with definite hydronephrosis (Hy). Not only the renal pelvis but also the infundibula and calyces are dilated. Extensive dilation confirms the presence of hydronephrosis. In Figure 17–55 hydronephrosis is present over the lower pole collecting system but not the upper pole collecting system. The fluid region in the middle and lower portions of the kidney is secondary to a dilated lower pole renal pelvis.

In severe cases of hydronephrosis, very little renal parenchyma will be identified. Figure 17–56 is a longitudinal coronal scan of a kidney in which a large hydronephrotic (Hy) renal pelvis is identified. Peripheral to the renal pelvis are numerous circular sonolucencies (arrows) that represent dilated calyces. Very little renal parenchyma is identified, indicating severe longstanding hydronephrosis.

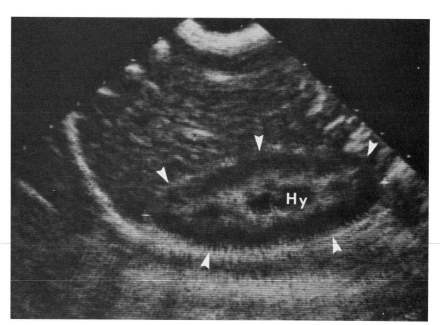

**FIG 17–53.**

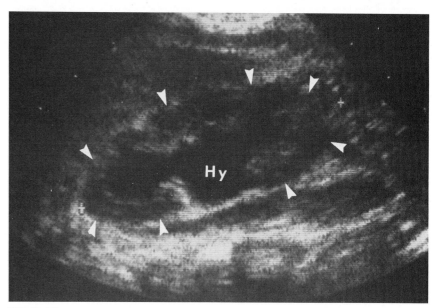

**FIG 17–54.**

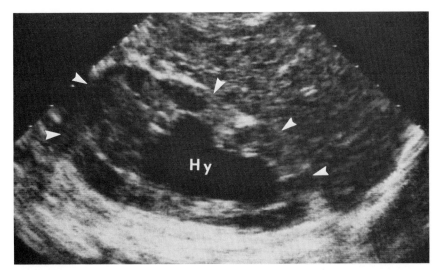

**Arrows** = Dilated calyces
**Arrowhead** = Renal outline
**Hy** = Hydronephrosis

**FIG 17–55.**

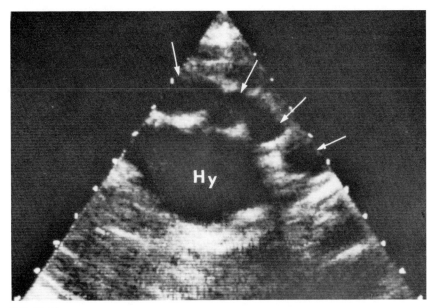

**FIG 17–56.**

## Urinary Tract Dilation

Urinary tract dilation may be secondary to obstruction or reflux. Voiding cystourethrography is necessary to distinguish between the two causes. However, ultrasound can give some important information suggesting the correct diagnosis. Duplication of the renal collecting system may lead to obstruction of the upper pole collecting system secondary to an ectopic ureterocele. Figure 17–57 is a longitudinal scan of the right kidney in which a duplicated upper pole collecting system (DU) is seen as a large sonolucent mass. The central echoes of the lower pole collecting system appear quite normal. Figure 17–58 is a scan of the same patient that was obtained later in the examination. The dilated upper pole collecting system again appears as a large upper pole sonolucent mass. A small amount of fluid is now noted in the lower pole collecting system (arrow). This is secondary to reflux into lower pole collecting system during the study.

Figure 17–59 is a longitudinal scan of a young boy who had a large tortuous ureter (Ur) secondary to prune belly syndrome. This scan shows marked dilation of the ureter. However, very little fluid is noted in the collecting system of the kidney. Other entities such as megaureter can have a similar ultrasound appearance.

Figure 17–60 is a longitudinal coronal scan in which we see dilatation of the ureter (Ur) in association with dilatation of the renal pelvis (P) and the calyces (arrowheads). Such dilatation is secondary to obstruction of the distal ureter at the ureterovesicular junction. Hydronephrosis is present and involves the calyces, renal pelvis, and right ureter.

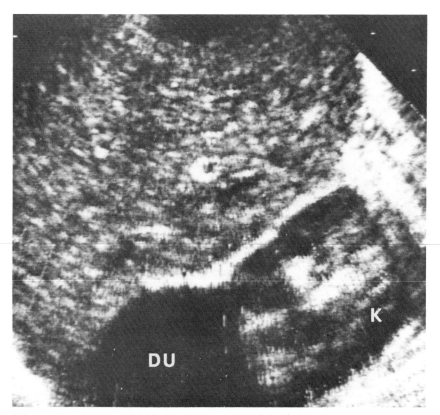

FIG 17–57.

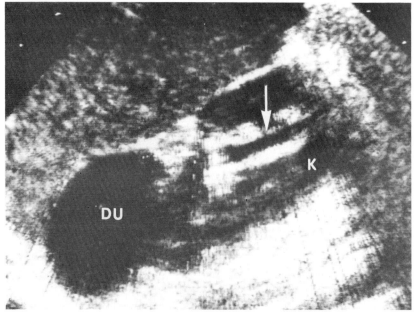

FIG 17–58.

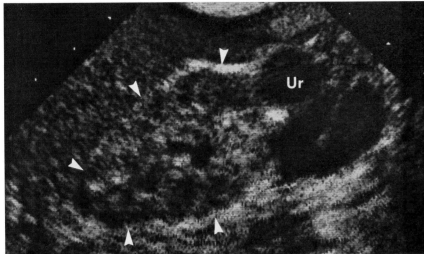

**FIG 17–59.**

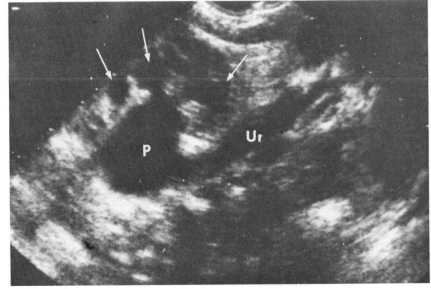

**FIG 17–60.**

| **Arrow** | = | Lower pole reflux (Fig 17–58) |
| **Arrows** | = | Dilated calyces (Fig 17–60) |
| **Arrowheads** | = | Renal outline |
| **DU** | = | Dilated upper pole collecting system |
| **P** | = | Dilated renal pelvis |
| **Ur** | = | Dilated ureter |

## Multicystic Kidney

Multicystic kidney is a common cause of a palpable abdominal mass in the newborn. It may be difficult to distinguish multicystic kidney from hydronephrosis. Multicystic kidney is thought to be secondary to abnormal development of the advancing ureteric bud. Such maldevelopment takes place very early in embryonic life and results in atresia of the ureter, pelvis, or both. When atresia occurs in the renal pelvis, multiple cysts will develop randomly in the renal bed. Figures 17–61 and 17–62 are a transverse prone scan and a longitudinal coronal scan of the right renal fossa. A large multiloculated cystic mass (M) is seen in the region. The mass is secondary to a multicystic kidney on this side. These lucent cystic regions are random in appearance and usually lead to the correct diagnosis of multicystic kidney.

Figures 17–63 and 17–64 are transverse and longitudinal scans of another patient with multicystic kidney. In this case the possibility of hydronephrosis should be considered. When atresia of the ureter occurs, the hydronephrotic form of multicystic kidney may be present. No renal parenchyma is identified in any of the images in Figures 17–61 through 17–64. Such is the case with multicystic kidney.

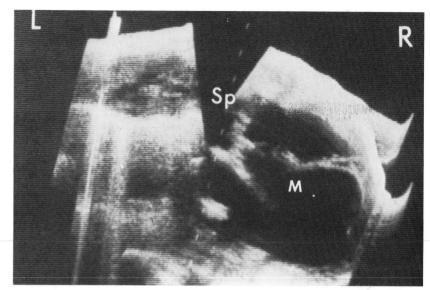

FIG 17–61.

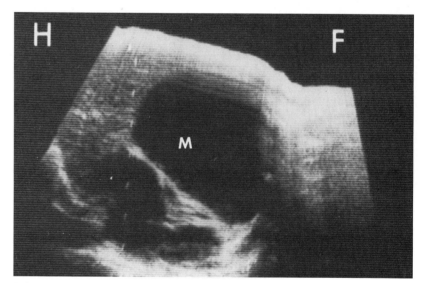

FIG 17–62.

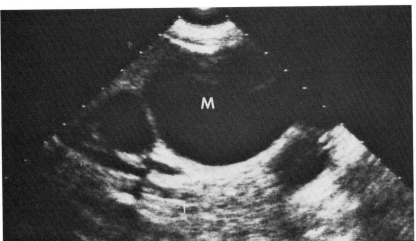

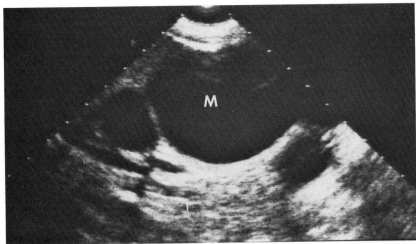

F  = Foot
H  = Head
L  = Left
M  = Multicystic kidney
R  = Right
Sp = Spine

**FIG 17–63.**

**FIG 17–64.**

## Renal Dysplasia

Dysplastic renal disease may involve part of the kidney, all of the kidney, or both kidneys. Figure 17–65 is a longitudinal coronal scan of the left kidney in which there is segmental renal dysplasia. A large cystic mass (M) is identified in the upper pole of the left kidney (K). The mass was secondary to atresia of an upper pole duplex ureter. This resulted in dilatation of the upper pole without communication to the ureter because of atresia. Figure 17–66 is an abdominal film made after injection of contrast agent into the upper pole collecting system. Because of atresia, there was no evidence of drainage of the contrast agent into the upper pole ureter. This is an example of segmental multicystic disease.

Figure 17–67 is a longitudinal scan of the right kidney in a patient with unilateral multicystic disease. Numerous resolvable cysts are seen in the kidney, resulting from atresia of the ureter. The other kidney was normal. Figure 17–68 is a longitudinal scan of another patient with cystic renal dysplasia in association with mild hydronephrosis. The worrisome part of this scan is the increased echogenicity to the renal parenchyma in association with hydronephrosis. This may be mistaken for mild hydronephrosis. However, patients with cystic renal dysplasia usually die soon after birth. The important finding is the increased echogenicity to the renal parenchyma secondary to numerous unresolvable cysts.

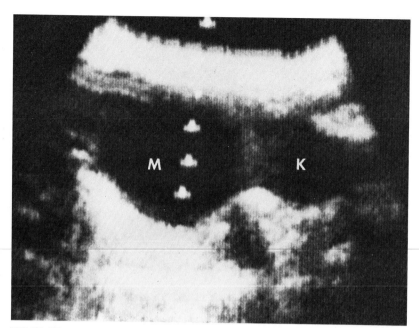

FIG 17–65.

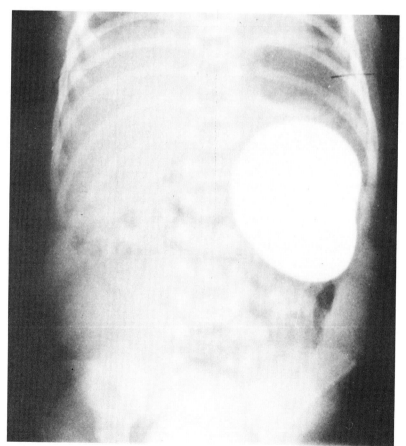

FIG 17–66.

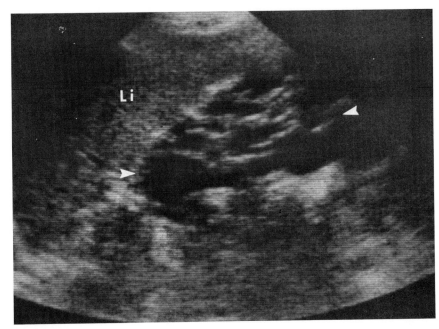

**Arrowheads** = Cystic renal dysplasia
**Hy** = Mild hydronephrosis
**K** = Lower pole of left kidney
**Li** = Liver
**M** = Cystic dysplasia of the left upper pole

**FIG 17–67.**

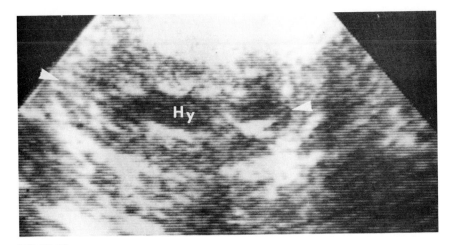

**FIG 17–68.**

## Polycystic Disease

Infantile polycystic disease can be identified in utero, as shown in Figure 17–69. In this scan of a pregnant uterus, both fetal kidneys are visualized (arrowhead). The kidneys are large and highly echogenic. The reason for the increased echogenicity is that the numerous cysts are too small to resolve on ultrasound. The kidneys appear large and highly echogenic because the numerous cyst walls act as reflectors. In this case, oligohydramnios was present in association with the pregnancy. Figure 17–70 is a longitudinal scan of the right kidney in a neonate with infantile polycystic disease. The kidney is markedly enlarged (arrowheads). Increased echogenicity is present throughout the large kidney, compatible with infantile polycystic disease. Examination of the liver did not reveal any cysts in this patient.

Figures 17–71 and 17–72 are longitudinal scans of the right and left kidney in a child with polycystic disease. Note the increased echogenicity of the kidneys, the numerous resolvable cysts, and the well-marginated sonolucent regions in the kidney. In such cases ultrasound reveals increased renal size and multiple discrete resolvable cysts that are larger than the infantile type, illustrated in Figures 17–69 and 17–70. Often other organs are involved in adult polycystic disease. Examination of the liver of this patient did not reveal any abnormalities.

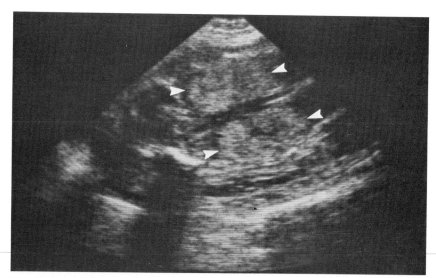

**FIG 17–69.**

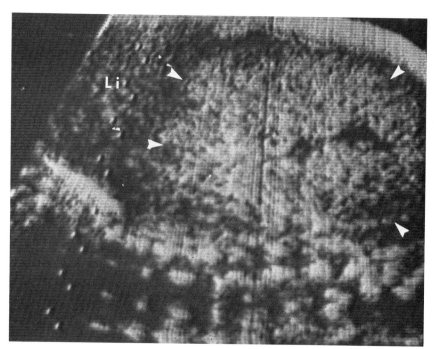

**FIG 17–70.**

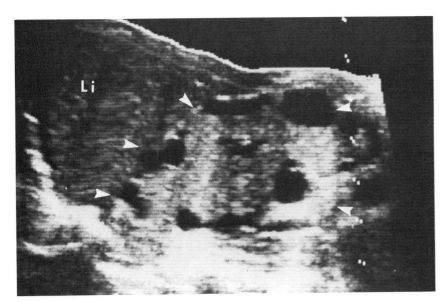

**Arrowheads** = Renal enlargement
**Li** = Liver

**FIG 17–71.**

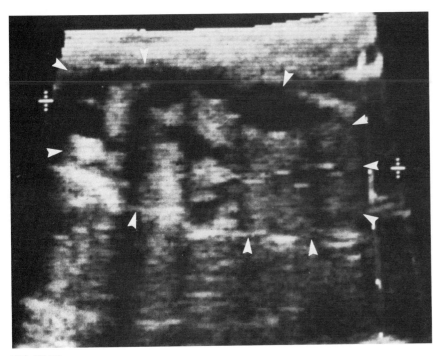

**FIG 17–72.**

## Echogenic Kidneys

In the older child and the adult, the echo amplitude of the renal parenchyma is less than that of the liver and spleen. In the neonate, the renal cortex and liver may be of equal echogenicity, whereas the renal medullary region is quite lucent. When increased echogenicity of the kidneys is identified, the possibility of pathology must always be considered. Figure 17–73 is a coronal scan of the kidney (arrowheads) which shows increased size and echogenicity, secondary to renal vein thrombosis. Renal vein thrombosis may manifest as a large kidney that is lucent or echogenic, depending on the time of insult. In this instance, the kidney appears bulbous and has areas of increased echogenicity.

Increased renal echogenicity may be secondary to numerous conditions. These conditions include glomerulonephritis, hypertensive nephropathy, nephrosclerosis, and numerous other entities. Figure 17–74 is a transverse scan of the right upper quadrant of a young patient. Note the markedly increased echogenicity of the kidneys, secondary to glomerulonephritis. The renal parenchymal echoes are much greater in amplitude than expected. Compare these echoes with the echoes of the liver. In this instance, the renal medullary region is not separated from the cortical area.

Figures 17–75 and 17–76 are scans of two separate patients who have large areas of increased echogenicity in the kidneys. There is the suggestion of some attenuation deep to the echoes, especially in Figure 17–76. These kidneys have the typical appearance of what is seen in nephrocalcinosis.

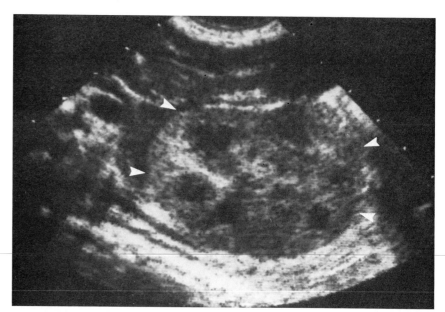

**FIG 17–73.**

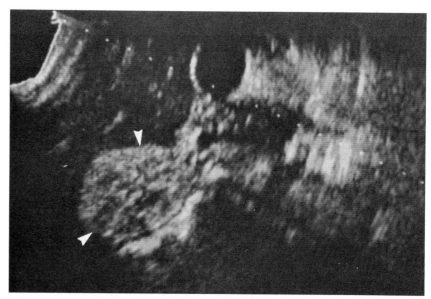

**FIG 17–74.**

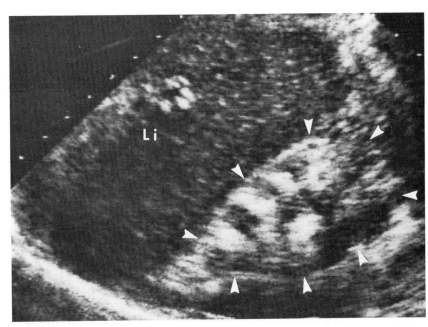

**Arrowheads** = Renal outline
**Li** = Liver

FIG 17–75.

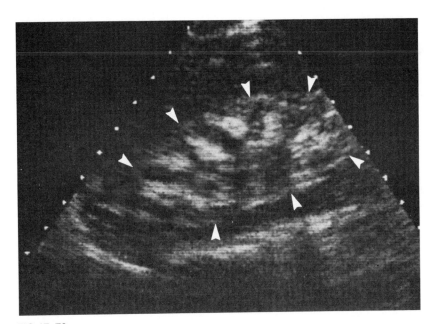

FIG 17–76.

## Wilms' Tumor; Leukemia

Palpable abdominal lesions may appear as solid masses on ultrasound. If they are in the region of the kidney, the possibility of Wilms' tumor must be considered. It is important to attempt to identify the region of the adrenal glands to distinguish Wilms' tumor from neuroblastoma. Figure 17–77 is a transverse scan of the upper abdomen in a patient who had Wilms' tumor (W). The tumor appears as a solid echogenic mass in the renal fossa. No identifiable renal tissue is present. Figure 17–78 is a coronal CT scan demonstrating a solid lesion of the left kidney. The right kidney is normal in size and appearance.

Figure 17–79 is a longitudinal coronal scan in a patient who has leukemia and was undergoing chemotherapy. The patient also developed uric acid nephropathy, manifested by the increased echogenicity of the renal parenchyma. Because of the increased renal echogenicity, it is difficult to identify the renal outline (arrowheads). A small amount of hydronephrosis or extrarenal pelvis is seen and is confirmed on the MR image in Figure 17–80.

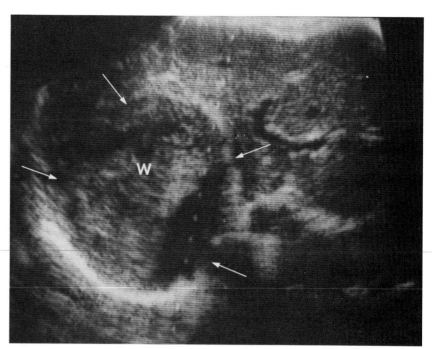

FIG 17–77.

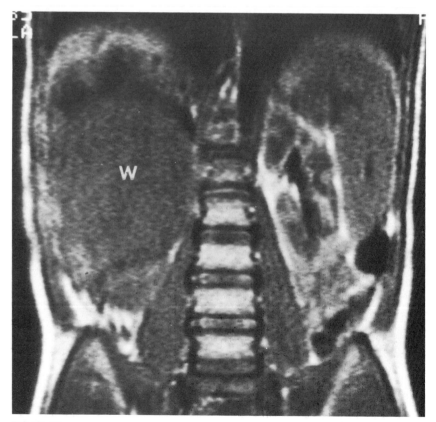

FIG 17–78.

Arrowheads = Renal outline
Arrows = Mild hydronephrosis
W = Wilms' tumor

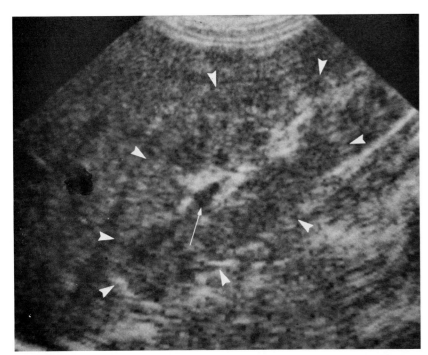

FIG 17–79.

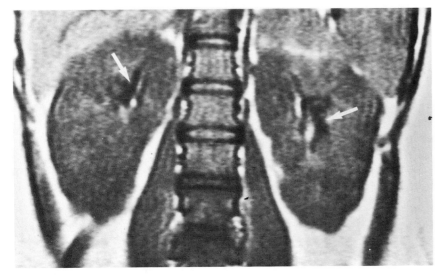

FIG 17–80.

## Pelvic Masses

Ultrasound evaluation of the pediatric pelvis is often similar to that of the adult pelvis. Cystic, solid, and mixed cystic and solid masses can be identified on pelvic ultrasound. Depending on the clinical history and the age of the patient, the ultrasound findings often suggest the correct etiology. Figures 17–81 and 17–82 are longitudinal and transverse scans of the pelvis of a 14-year-old girl. She had not started her menses yet but continually complained of chronic monthly pelvic pain. The ultrasound examination revealed a tubular, relatively sonolucent mass with soft internal echoes. Through-transmission indicated its fluid nature. The mass was seen in the entire length of the suspected uterus and vagina. The patient had distal vaginal atresia. The ultrasound findings confirmed the presence of hydrometrocolpos.

Ovarian masses can be identified on pelvic ultrasound in the pediatric patient. Figure 17–83 is a transverse scan of a 13 year old girl with chronic right lower abdominal pain. The uterus is deviated to the left side. Posterior to the uterus is a circular sonolucent structure with some soft echoes present within it. Through-transmission is present deep to this mass, indicating its fluid nature. The uterus is much more rounded than would be expected for a normal ovary. The patient had a slight elevation of temperature and white blood cell count. At operation torsion of the right ovary was found.

Figure 17–84 is a transverse scan of the pelvis of another patient who had left lower quadrant abdominal pain. The uterus is displaced to the right side by a large mass (arrows). The mass has a mixed ultrasound appearance with sonolucent and echogenic components. Initially, an ectopic pregnancy was suspected. However, no fetal cardiac activity was identified in the echogenic portion. The pregnancy test was also negative. Other possibilities such as a dermoid or cystadenoma would be included in the differential diagnosis. The patient was found to have a hemorrhagic ovarian cyst.

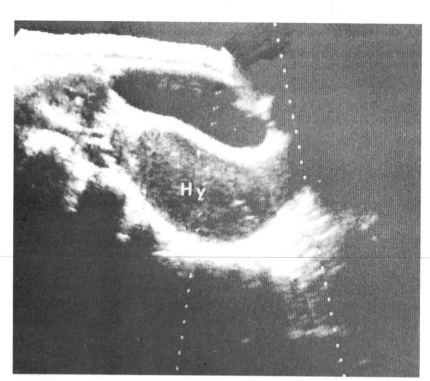

**FIG 17–81.**

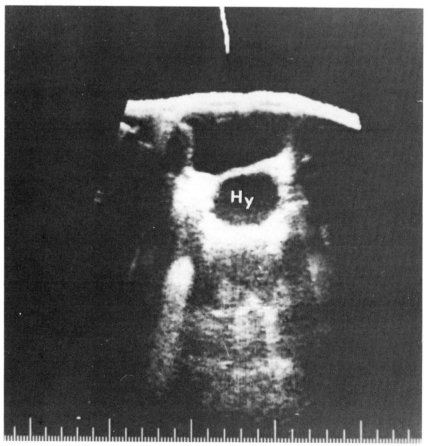

**FIG 17–82.**

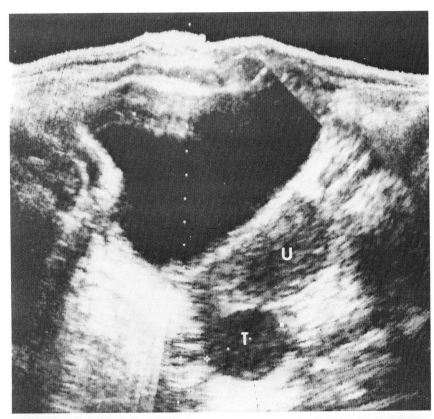

**FIG 17–83.**

Blood clots may form in a hemorrhagic ovarian cyst and simulate the appearance of an ectopic pregnancy. Note the indentation on the posterior urinary bladder wall adjacent to the mass. This is an important ultrasound finding.

**Arrows** = Hemorrhagic ovarian cyst
**Hy** = Hydrometrocolpos
**T** = Ovarian torsion
**U** = Uterus

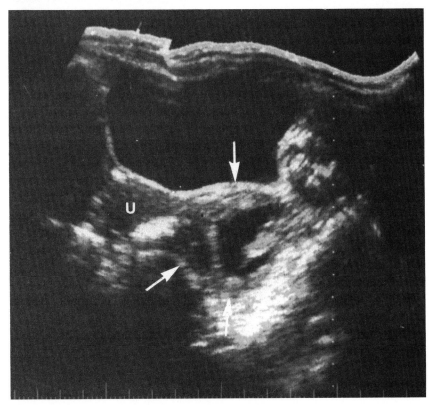

**FIG 17–84.**

## Pelvic Masses

Figure 17–85 is a longitudinal scan of the pelvis of a 13-year-old girl who presented with right lower quadrant pain. She had no fever or elevated white blood cell count. The pain was relatively sudden in onset and quite severe. The ultrasound examination showed the uterus anterior to a relatively echogenic mass. There is enhanced through-transmission deep to the mass. Difficulty delineating the mass from the uterus was noted. A pregnancy test was negative. It was decided to follow the patient serially every 2 days with ultrasound. Early scans revealed some change in the appearance of the mass. A scan obtained approximately 1 week later is shown in Figure 17–86. The mass (M) now has a dramatically different appearance from that seen in Figure 17–85. A sonolucent mass is visualized posterior to the uterus (U). Through-transmission is present, and a sharp posterior border is identified. These findings are secondary to a hemorrhagic ovarian cyst, which undergoes a change in ultrasound appearance. The initial echogenic appearance is secondary to clotted blood. It then went through a septated phase, which is not shown, and finally the more cystic phase shown in Figure 17–86. The cystic appearance is secondary to lysis of the clot. Such a developing spectrum of findings confirms the presence of a hemorrhagic ovarian cyst.

Figure 17–87 is a longitudinal scan of the pelvis of a 12-year-old girl with a palpable pelvic mass, but no other signs or symptoms (no pain, fever, elevated white blood cell count, or vaginal bleeding). This scan is off to the right side. The uterus was normal on the left side. The findings indicate a large echogenic mass in the right adnexal region. The ultrasound appearance suggests a solid ovarian lesion. At operation a dysgerminoma was removed. Dysgerminomas are solid lesions that are seen in the young girl.

Figure 17–88 is a transverse scan of the lower abdomen in a 7-year-old girl who had a palpable pelvic and midabdominal mass. The urinary blad-

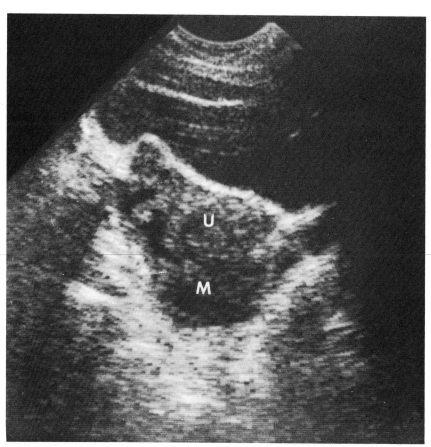

**FIG 17–85.**

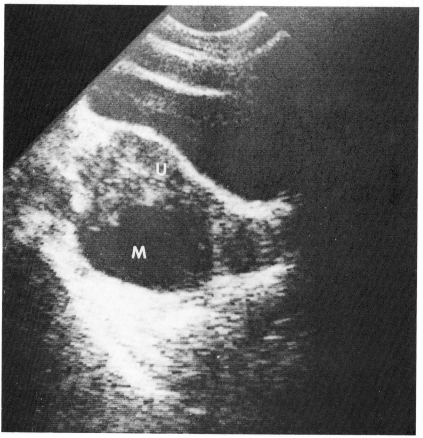

**FIG 17–86.**

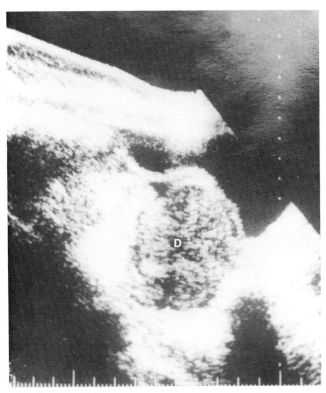

**FIG 17–87.**

der is compressed and displaced anteriorly on the right side (B). A solid mass is noted posterior to the urinary bladder. The mass is quite large and is deforming the abdominal wall contour. At operation a rhabdomyosarcoma was removed.

**B** = Urinary bladder
**D** = Dysgerminoma
**M** = Hemorrhagic cyst
**S** = Rhabdomyosarcoma
**U** = Uterus

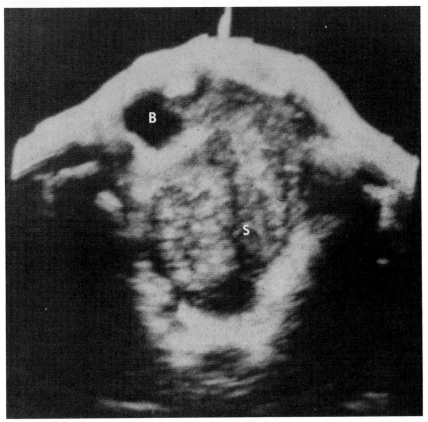

**FIG 17–88.**

## Pelvic Mass

Figures 17–89 and 17–90 are transverse and longitudinal scans of the
pelvis in a four-month-old child who
had urinary retention. The transverse
scan (Figure 17–89) could be misinterpreted as showing the urinary bladder. It is relatively lucent, suggesting
fluid. However, some echoes are
noted within the area on the anterior
wall, indicating its solid nature. The
longitudinal scan in Figure 17–90 indicates that the mass is situated posterior to the urinary bladder. The urinary
bladder (B) is displaced anteriorly.
Figure 17–91 is a cystogram showing
extrinsic pressure on the posterior aspect of the urinary bladder. Figure 17–
92 is a barium enema film showing
contrast in the rectum and demonstrating posterior displacement of the
rectum. The mass was found to be a
sacrococcygeal teratoma. These
masses usually arise from the sacrum
or coccyx. They are composed of multiple cellular elements and have a
mixed ultrasound appearance.

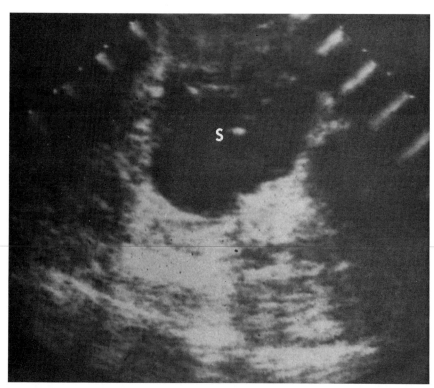

**FIG 17–89.**

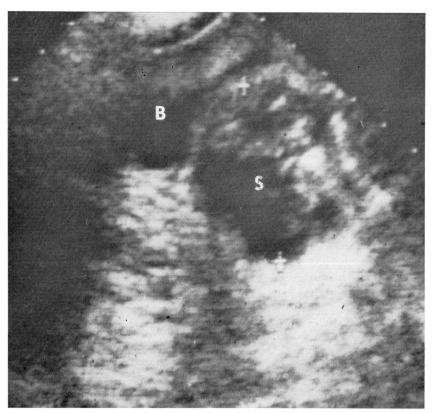

**FIG 17–90.**

B = Urinary bladder
S = Sacrococcygeal teratoma

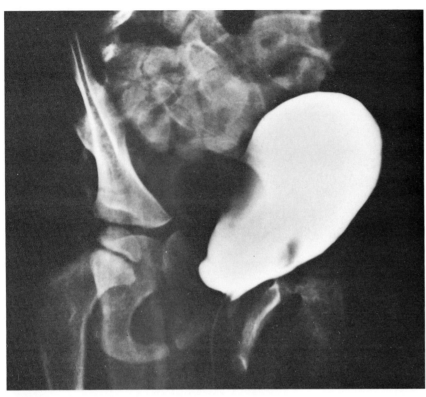

**FIG 17–91.**

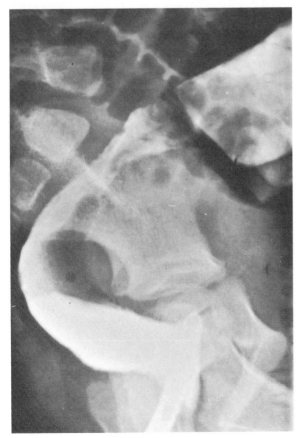

**FIG 17–92.**

## Pelvic Mass

Figure 17–93 is a transverse scan of the pelvis showing a solid mass that contains numerous soft internal echoes. High-amplitude echoes in the midportion of the mass are casting acoustic shadows. A CT scan (Fig 17-94) discloses a soft tissue mass in the right pelvis. CT of the abdomen revealed a para-aortic mass (Fig 17–95). Hydronephrosis of the right kidney is noted. An ultrasound scan of the region (Fig 17–96) shows the relatively lucent mass with numerous internal echoes; the mass is situated anterior to the aorta and inferior vena cava. The patient had Burkitt's lymphoma, which appeared as a large hypoechoic mass on pelvic ultrasound. The patient also had mesenteric adenopathy, as can be seen in Figures 17–95 and 17–96. Evaluation of solid lesions in the pelvis usually does not lead to the correct diagnosis. Solid lesions can be secondary to numerous etiologies. Other details of clinical history and laboratory data are needed before the correct diagnosis can be made.

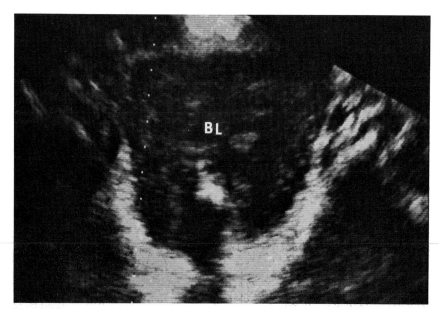

**FIG 17–93.**

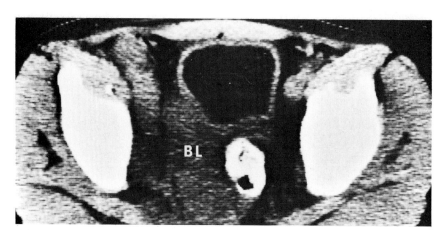

**FIG 17–94.**

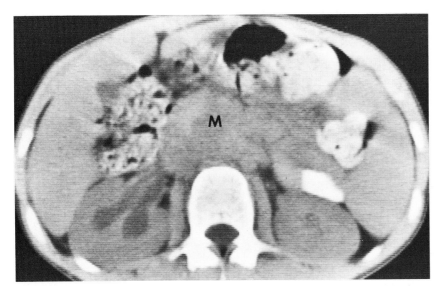

BL  =  Burkitt's lymphoma
M   =  Mesenteric adenopathy

FIG 17–95.

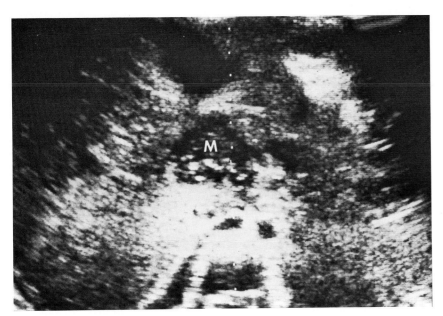

FIG 17–96.

## Turner's Syndrome

In Turner's syndrome, a small uterus may be identified, as is seen in the ultrasound scan shown in Figure 17–97 and the CT scan shown in Figure 17–98. The uterus may be difficult to visualize initially. Evaluation of the adnexal region usually reveals no evidence of ovaries, or extremely small ovaries ("streak ovaries"). Figure 17–99 is an oblique longitudinal scan of the right adnexal region in which an extremely small ovary is identified on that side. Figure 17–100 is an oblique longitudinal scan of the left adnexal area in which no ovary is identified. There are a few lucent streaks in the area that may represent residual gonadal tissue. Most important is lack of visualization of normal-sized ovaries in the presence of a small uterus. If no uterus is visible, other entities such as testicular feminization should be considered.

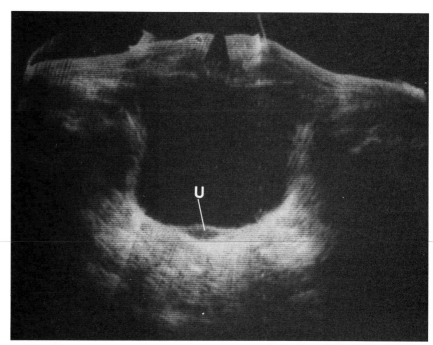

FIG 17–97.

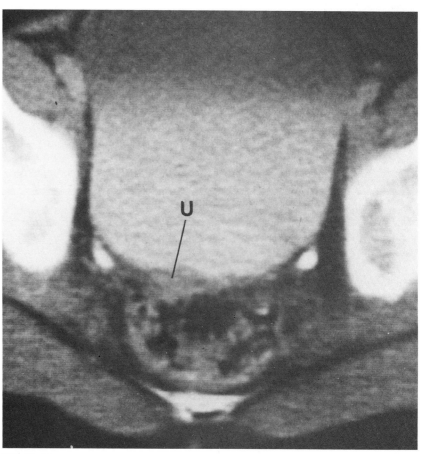

FIG 17–98.

O  =  Small ovary
U  =  Small uterus

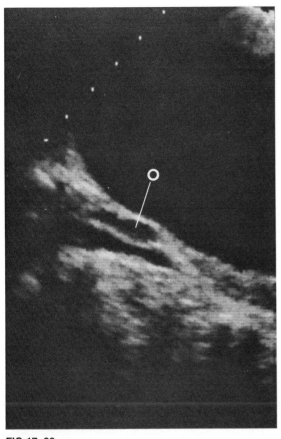

**FIG 17–99.**

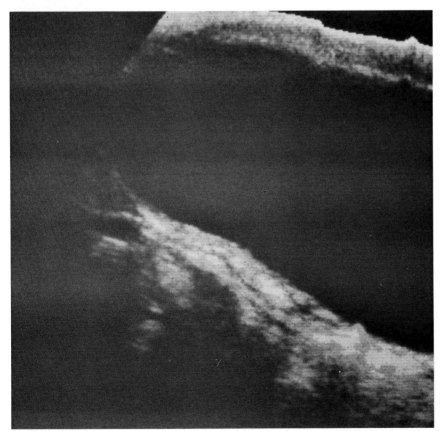

**FIG 17–100.**

# 18.
# Neonatal Brain Ultrasonography

Carol M. Rumack, M.D.
Michael L. Manco-Johnson, M.D.

Neonatal brain ultrasonography has introduced an entirely new area of diagnostic imaging into neonatal medicine and ultrasound. The anterior fontanelle is an acoustic window that allows visualization of the neonatal brain in great detail even in the most critically ill infants. With this knowledge we are beginning to understand the brain sufficiently to evaluate it at all ages in the operating room and through postoperative cranial defects.

## Neonatal Brain Scanning Technique

Preparation of the infant is not necessary for neuroultrasonography but care must be taken to keep the infant warm, the transducer clean, and not to disturb the many life-supporting devices surrounding and attached to the infant. Feeding the infant just before scanning may promote a quick and peaceful study. Sedation is not necessary since all of these studies can be done with real-time ultrasound.

The equipment required for examination of the brain must include both a 5-MHz and 7.5-MHz transducer for good imaging of brain parenchymal detail. A sector scanner with as wide a sector angle as possible is necessary since the fontanelle limits the scanning aperture and even in the operating room one is often working through a relatively small craniotomy. Some of the linear-array scanners give excellent detail but severely limit the field to a narrow center strip of information with the edges determined by the size of the fontanelle. The 7.5-MHz transducer should be used whenever possible since it has a much cleaner near field and results in higher resolution throughout the field of view. The 5-MHz transducer is often necessary in older infants in order to penetrate the far field adequately. Scanning should be performed with the 7.5-MHz transducer first and the 5-MHz transducer later if necessary. This approach will keep the sonographer from missing subdural fluid collections that may be lost in the near field and are a common pathologic finding in the older infant.

The frame rate should be at least 30 frames per second to reduce flicker and loss of information. The triple-loaded transducers that drop to one-third the frame rate for each of the different frequencies cause too great a degradation of the image to be useful in brain imaging.

Both film and videotape are necessary to fully cap-ture all of the detail of the neonatal brain. Complex pathology is often better understood with a continuous sweep through both hemispheres than with multiple static slices. Subtle lesions may be missed and technical artifacts such as those that result from oblique positioning may cause false positive studies when only a few select views are obtained.

Good contact must be maintained with generous amounts of gel. A rocking motion should be used on the fontanelle rather than sliding off the edges onto the bone and losing the edge of the image. Maximum gain settings are necessary for parenchymal detail, particularly in the posterior fossa.

Coronal and sagittal scans are obtained using multiple angulated views. The coronal scan can be centered best by starting at the trigone so that the choroid is symmetric bilaterally. Then multiple slices should be frozen starting behind the trigone, at the trigone, through the bodies of the lateral ventricles, the frontal horns, and as anterior as possible. Sagittal scans should be obtained of both lateral ventricles, the midline, and the brain lateral to the ventricles. Further detail about technique may be obtained from many previous reports.[1, 2]

## Normal Neonatal Brain Anatomy

The neonatal brain is best understood by using the ventricular structures as the basic landmarks. In the *sagittal view,* the lateral view is seen as a thin, lucent, comma-shaped structure in the center of each cerebral hemisphere. The superior part of the comma anteriorly is called the frontal horn and posteriorly the body of the lateral ventricle. As the ventricle curves down around the thickest part of the highly echogenic choroid plexus, it is called the trigone. The trigone continues anteriorly and inferiorly into the temporal horn. From the trigone the ventricle also extends posteriorly into the occipital horn. The choroid plexus extends into the temporal horn but not into the occipital horn. Anteriorly the choroid tapers as it continues to the foramen of Monro and then into the third ventricle.

In the *midline sagittal view,* the corpus collosum forms the roof of the lateral ventricle. It is a long C-shaped structure with two linear echogenic lines above and below it. The superior line is formed by the pericallosal arteries and the inferior line is the top of the septum pellucidum. The genu forms the anterior

curve between the frontal horns and the splenium forms the posterior curve. In the septum pellucidum of most neonates there is a cystic structure called the cavum septi pellucidi anteriorly which often extends posteriorly behind the foramen of Monro into the cavum vergae. This structure closes posteriorly first and disappears by several months of age. The cingulate sulcus carrying the callosal marginal arteries parallels the corpus callosum superiorly and is the first major sulcus seen on ultrasound. The echogenic character of the sulci is caused by the presence of pulsating arteries. Below the cavum septi pellucidi lies the third ventricle which connects to each lateral ventricle via a foramen of Monro. The choroid plexus forms the roof of the third ventricle, and when the ventricle is even slightly enlarged, the massa intermedia can be visualized as well as the anterior and posterior recesses of the third ventricle. The third ventricle connects inferiorly through the aqueduct of Sylvius into the fourth ventricle. The fourth ventricle forms a notch in the cerebellum on the sagittal view. This central portion of the cerebellum is called the vermis and is highly echogenic due to the multiple folds, or folia. The cerebellar hemispheres lie on both sides of the vermis and are visualized below the cerebral cortex at the level of the trigone.

Lateral to the ventricles, the sylvian fissures are defined by the pulsating branches of the middle cerebral arteries and the anterior choroidal artery can be traced to the choroid plexus.

In the *coronal view,* the lateral ventricles are thin, sonolucent, symmetric structures on either side of the midline. The most posterior cuts contain the occipital horns surrounded by the cerebral cortex.

Just anterior to this, at the level of the trigone, lies the thickest portion of the highly echogenic choroid on the floor of the lateral ventricles. The choroid in each ventricle settles toward the dependent side of the head. At this level the cerebellum becomes apparent below the tentorium, which separates it from the cerebral cortex. Laterally the sylvian fissures are highly echogenic due to the multiple branches of the middle cerebral arteries and other arachnoid structures.

Anterior to the trigone lie the bodies of the lateral ventricles, with choroid plexus on the floor, the corpus callosum forming the roof, and the caudate nucleus forming the lateral walls. Between the very thin ventricles lies the septum pellucidum with a cavum vergae if it is still patent. Below the lateral ventricles lie the quadrigeminal cistern between the thalami, then the quadrigeminal plate, the tentorium, and the cerebellar hemispheres. The quadrigeminal cistern is highly echogenic due to multiple arachnoid extensions; its most superior portion forms the cavum vellum interpositum and laterally it extends into the choroidal fissures adjacent to the temporal horns. The inferior border of the cistern is formed by the tentorium and cerebellum. Below this is the cisterna magna. In the center of the cerebellum lies the fourth ventricle, which is seen as a small sonolucent oval area with echogenic choroid often obscuring the central cavity. Careful scanning is required to visualize clearly the fourth ventricle, but this may be particularly important in the evaluation of hydrocephalus.

A slightly more anterior section through the bodies of the lateral ventricles shows the same relationships superiorly but inferiorly the third ventricle with choroid in the roof and thalami on both sides is seen. Beneath the third ventricle, the cerebral penduncles extend toward the cerebellum, fusing in the midline at the level of the pons. Laterally and inferiorly are the cerebellar hemispheres surrounding the fourth ventricle.

The next anterior coronal cut is through the foramen of Monro. The choroid plexus has just exited the lateral ventricles into the third ventricle. Thus the frontal horns do not contain any choroid. The body of the corpus callosum forms the roof of the lateral ventricles just below the bottom of the interhemispheric fissure. Above the corpus callosum lie the pericallosal artery branches in the pericallosal sulci. Between the ventricles is the cavum septi pellucidi. Laterally lie the caudate nuclei and at the surfaces of the brain, the sylvian fissures. Inferiorly the lateral ventricles connect through the foramina of Monro into the third ventricle. The suprasellar cistern lies beneath the hypothalamus at this level.

The most anterior cuts contain only the frontal horns of the lateral ventricles. Beneath the ventricles the internal carotid arteries bifurcate into the anterior and middle cerebral arteries. Due to the angle of the transducer on the fontanelle it may be difficult to image the most anterior cerebral cortex in front of the frontal horns.

*Axial images* are less useful since brain parenchymal detail is obscured by the temporal and parietal bones. However, they may be valuable for comparing the lateral ventricles and cortex for a lateral ventricular ratio and as a comparison with brain computed tomography (CT).

## Intracranial Hemorrhage in Neonates and Infants

Intracranial hemorrhage is highly echogenic on ultrasound in the acute stage. At about 1 week, the echogenicity begins to decrease and a sonolucent area develops centrally as the brain becomes necrotic. Next is the stage of clot retraction, leaving the edges sonolucent and the center more echogenic until the clot is completely necrosed and phagocytized. This phase may take weeks to months, depending on the size of the hematoma. The end result is a subependymal cyst, an area of porencephaly, or an infarct (if it does not connect with the ventricular system).

### Subependymal Germinal Matrix Hemorrhage

Subependymal germinal matrix hemorrhage occurs almost exclusively in premature infants, with an incidence of 40%–60% in infants born at less than 32 weeks' gestation. The incidence of germinal matrix hemorrhage drops to less than 5% for term neonates because the germinal matrix disappears as the brain matures. The germinal matrix is a loosely organized sheet of primitive neural cells that is richly supplied with capillaries and thin-walled veins. Sudden changes in cerebral blood flow occur in the neonate, possibly due to failure of autoregulation. The actual etiology of intracranial hemorrhage is not known but it has been associated with hypertension, hypercapnea, pneumothorax, and patent ductus arteriosus, or a sudden intravascular bolus may rupture arterioles or capillaries. Decreased cerebral blood flow may result from shock, hyperviscosity, hyperventilation, or hydrocephalus, causing ischemic damage which may hemorrhage in this area or just lead to infarction. The germinal matrix lies above the caudate nucleus in the subependymal lining of the floor of the lateral ventricles and in the roof of the third and fourth ventricles. It sweeps from the caudothalamic notch around and inferiorly into the temporal horn.

Subependymal hemorrhage usually occurs in the first 3 days of life but has been reported as late as 2 weeks in association with sudden respiratory distress or abnormal coagulation. The clinical diagnosis of intracranial hemorrhage is difficult and unreliable. *All infants born at less than 32 weeks' gestation should be screened with ultrasound routinely at 5 to 7 days of age* to diagnose the most severe extent of hemorrhage since it may progress and over 90% of cases occur during this period.

Subependymal hemorrhage manifests as a highly echogenic nodule in the region of the caudate nucleus. Care must be taken to obtain symmetric scans so that the very echogenic choroid plexus is not mistaken for a hematoma. There should be a small round choroid in the floor of each lateral ventricle and in the roof of the third (all three are approximately the same size). Choroid is not present in the frontal horn anterior to the foramen of Monro or in the occipital horn. A certain diagnosis can be made if the hematoma is seen in both coronal and sagittal views. Subependymal hemorrhage will frequently enlarge and rupture into the ventricular system, causing intraventricular hemorrhage. It may extend laterally beyond the edge of the ventricle into the brain itself and thus become intraparenchymal hemorrhage.

## Intraventricular Hemorrhage

Intraventricular hemorrhage manifests as highly echogenic material within the ventricle acutely. With resolution there is less and less debris within the ventricles. Because the ventricular system is usually freely communicating, intraventricular hemorrhage from any site may be found in any portion of the ventricular system or in the subarachnoid space. Since the infant is usually supine, blood settles into the occipital horns. When there are large amounts of ventricular blood, it may form a cast of the ventricle obscuring the ventricular margins. Even small amounts of intraventricular hemorrhage can be important if it obstructs the ventricular system, as sometimes occurs, particularly at the level of the aqueduct of Sylvius. This may be the cause for acute development of hydrocephalus which later resolves, presumably as the clot lyses. At about 1 week after intraventricular hemorrhage the ventricles develop very echogenic margins thought to be due to a chemical ventriculitis in response to the blood. Intraventricular hemorrhage most commonly occurs secondary to subependymal hemorrhage in prematures but usually originates in the choroid plexus of term infants. Posthemorrhagic ventricular enlargement develops in about 70% of infants after intraventricular hemorrhage but only about one third of survivors ever require intraventricular shunting. Two thirds have mild to moderate arrested hydrocephalus or return to normal ventricular size.

## Intraparenchymal Hemorrhage

Intraparenchymal hemorrhage usually occurs as an extension of subependymal hemorrhage, but isolated parenchymal hemorrhage may occur with abnormal coagulation and less commonly with arteriovenous malformation or tumor. Unusual types of parenchymal hemorrhage may occur with extension of the hemorrhage into the thalamus from subependymal hemorrhage or from the parietal lobe into the occipital lobe. Cerebellar hemorrhage is relatively rare, but any posterior fossa hematoma is more serious than cerebral hematomas since increased pressure within a confined space may lead to pressure on critical structures within the brain stem. Cerebellar hematomas have had a rather poor prognosis.[3]

Resolution of intraparenchymal hemorrhage usually results in porencephaly and a contralateral hemiparesis, although a few frontal lesions have been clinically silent, as might be expected.

## Periventricular Leukomalacia: Hemorrhagic and Nonhemorrhagic

Periventricular leukomalacia (PVL) is a less frequent cause of hemorrhage or infarction than germinal matrix hemorrhage. The autopsy incidence has been reported at 20%.[4] The present theory is that PVL represents a watershed infarct in the neonatal brain between the branches of the deep penetrating arteries. It occurs most frequently lateral to the frontal horns and in the occipital radiations at the trigone of the lateral ventricles. Secondary hemorrhage occurs in about 25%.[5]

Ultrasound findings include marked echogenicity initially in these areas due to localized edema, infarction, and hemorrhage.[6] With resolution over several weeks, the areas become necrotic, often developing series of small cysts.

Clinical sequelae are more often serious compared to germinal matrix hemorrhage especially as the leukomalacia extends laterally into the motor tracts. Spastic diplegia and sometimes hemiparesis result.

## Extracerebral Hemorrhage

Extracerebral hemorrhage may be difficult to identify at any stage due to the initial transducer artifact. With a 7.5-MHz transducer there is a cleaner near field, but until the fluid is greater than 1 cm thick it may be missed. For this reason, CT is recommended when trauma is the known or suspected etiology. Any infant whose head size increases at an abnormal rate should be evaluated with CT if ultrasound reveals no hydrocephalus. A clue to the ultrasound diagnosis of extracerebral fluid is visualization of the surface sulci of the brain and widening of the interhemispheric fissure. Extracerebral fluid may also cause accentuation of the sulci as the fluid extends along the surface of the brain (either by better through-transmission or by fluid within the sulcus). Extracerebral hematomas are either due to lacerated bridging veins which cause a *subdural hemorrhage* that mimics the surface of the brain or are due to a ruptured artery causing a convexly inward *epidural hematoma* under marked pressure. *Posterior fossa subdural hematomas* are rare but serious. Dissection of the fluid collection within the tentorium has been reported as a cause of acute hydrocephalus due to pressure on the aqueduct. This type of collection has not been described on ultrasound and may be difficult to identify since the cerebellum is normally very echogenic.

*Subarachnoid hemorrhage* can be diagnosed by thickening of the normally echogenic interhemispheric and sylvian fissure acutely and occasionally by filling in of the cisterna magna. Since infants are usually supine it is uncommon to find subarachnoid hemorrhage in the suprasellar cistern. Small amounts of subarachnoid hemorrhage may be difficult to diagnose on ultrasound and may require CT evaluation.

## Congenital Malformations

A short review of brain development may help make congenital malformations of the brain easier to understand.

The brain begins as a neural tube which closes at each end and along the dorsal surface. Then it segments into five basic components, and the first two, forming the prosencephalon, diverticulate or separate into the ophthalmic tracts, the optic tracts, the cerebral hemispheres, the pituitary, and the pineal gland. Neuronal proliferation and migration continue through fetal development, and after birth most of the organization and myelination occurs. Defects in brain development depend on the timing of the insult.

### Disorders of Neural Tube Closure

Failure of neural tube closure most commonly results in a form of dysrhaphism *(anencephaly, encephalocele, or meningomyelocele)* with an opening in the brain or spine. Whenever there is a meningomyelocele there is almost always a Chiari malformation of the brain.

#### CHIARI II MALFORMATION
Chairi II malformation is the most common type. It is present in 85%–95% of meningomyeloceles.[7–9] The fourth ventricle is elongated and compressed due to caudal displacement of the cerebellum into the foramen magnum. The aqueduct is often kinked, with variable amounts of dilatation of the third ventricle. The massa intermedia, which carries fibers between the thalami, is often enlarged. The lateral ventricles are enlarged in a characteristic fashion with very thin, pointed frontal horns and very large occipital horns termed a batwing deformity. The interhemispheric fissure is often widened. Enlargement of the ventricular system often increases after the meningomyelocele is repaired so that evaluation of the severity of hydrocephalus should be done postoperatively.

#### DANDY-WALKER SYNDROME
The Dandy-Walker cyst is an extremely enlarged fourth ventricle caused by atresia of the foramina of Megendie and Luschka with cerebellar vermian dysgenesis. The third and lateral ventricles are also enlarged. Most of the cisterns are obliterated by the pressure of the cyst. Shunting for hydrocephalus via the lateral ventricles will not always decompress the fourth ventricle and a second shunt may be necessary in the posterior fossa. If the cyst is totally separate from the fourth ventricle, the diagnosis is an arachnoid cyst with compression of the cerebellum and resultant hydrocephalus.

#### AGENESIS OF THE CORPUS CALLOSUM
Failure of neural tube closure may leave a longitudinal bundle of fibers on each side of the cerebral cortex that would have formed the corpus callosum. These are termed Probst's bundles and they pass on the superior aspect of the ventricles but are not connected to each other. This is a relatively minor problem clinically but this anomaly is associated with many other major malformations (80%).[10, 11] Typically the third

ventricle is elevated and extends much farther superiorly. The superior and posterior extent of the third ventricle sometimes continues as an interhemispheric cyst. The sulci are radially arrayed from the lateral ventricle instead of parallel to the corpus callosum.

## Disorders of Diverticulation

Disorders of diverticulation include septo-optic dysplasia, in which there is absence of the septum pellucidum, and the various forms of holoprosencephaly. Absence of the opthalamic tracts is not diagnosable on ultrasound, and failure of separation of the optic tracts does not require special imaging in the neonate but may be diagnosed by ultrasound in utero.

### HOLOPROSENCEPHALY

There is a spectrum of holoprosencephaly from a single ventricle in alobar holoprosencephaly to attempted formation of occipital horns in semilobar holoprosencephaly to relatively normal function of the occipital horns in lobar holoprosencephaly.[12] The commonest type is alobar holoprosencephaly, which manifests as a single ventricle with no interhemispheric fissure or midline vessels or falx. The ventricle frequency extends posteriorly into a dorsal cyst. There are no separate temporal, frontal, or occipital horns although there may be the appearance of these because the ventricle drapes over the thalami. The moderately echogenic thalami form their characteristic oval shape but are fused in the midline with absence or only a remnant of the third ventricle. The highly echogenic choroid plexus is fused in the midline and drapes over the surface of the thalami on the floor of the ventricle. The sulci are distorted as they cross the midline and there are often fewer than normal sulci. The cerebellum and brain stem are relatively normal.

## Disorders of Sulcation and Migration

### LISSENCEPHALY

Lissencephaly is a very rare malformation caused by failure of neuronal migration at no later than the fourth fetal month, resulting in a four-layered cortex.[13] Normally the cortex contains six layers. The ventricles are slightly larger and fetal-like; thus the term colpocephaly. Sulcal formation is abnormal because sulci develop with the last two layers, and therefore none or only a few sulci are formed. Sonographic recognition requires careful attention to the sulci. The brain surface will appear smooth with a deep interhemispheric fissure, increased prominence of the subarachnoid spaces, and absence of the sylvian fissures and cingulate sulci. There may be calcification in the midline (roof of the septum pellucidum) or in the basal ganglia.[14] Ventricular enlargement is a common finding. These patients have severe retardation and usually die in the first year of life. Lissencephaly has been reported in siblings and may have a genetic basis.

### SCHIZENCEPHALY

Schizencephaly is a rare anomaly that may be confused with lissencephaly. Although there are large bilateral clefts instead of sylvian fissures, these clefts connect at least on one side to the enlarged ventricles. There is absence of the septum pellucidum and no midline calcification. Porencephaly may be misdiagnosed if the anomalous nature of the brain is not appreciated. Since patients with schizencephaly may live for several years with severe retardation, seizures, cortical blindness, and spastic diplegia, this diagnosis may aid patient management.[15]

## Hydrocephalus

Hydrocephalus is enlargement of the ventricular system when there is an obstruction to flow of cerebrospinal fluid (CSF) and an associated increase in CSF pressure. Ventricular enlargement should be diagnosed if the ventricles are enlarged from a previous destructive process or congenital malformation. If it is not possible to know whether the CSF is under pressure it is probably best to state that it is ventriculomegaly rather than hydrocephalus, so as not to imply obstruction or increased pressure. Premature infants are an exception to this rule because their brain typically compresses against the skull until there is marked enlargement of the ventricular system. If screening for hydrocephalus is not done they will come to medical attention at about 3 weeks of age with an enlarging head and massive ventricles. True hydrocephalus is a common problem with many etiologies (Table 18–1). Ultrasound has proved to be extremely accurate in the determination of ventricular size.[16, 17] The occipital horns may enlarge first, suggesting the onset of ventricular enlargement. Visual-

**TABLE 18–1.**

**Hydrocephalus: Types and Etiologies**

Intraventricular obstructive hydrocephalus
  Foramen of Monro obstruction (lateral ventricles dilated)
    Posthemorrhagic
    Postinfectious (intraventricular septations)
    Tumor or cyst obliterating third ventricle (unilateral, often due
      to brain damage, not obstructive)
  Third ventricular obstruction
    Suprasellar tumor or cyst
  Aqueductal obstruction
    Aqueductal stenosis (congenital, X-linked dominant trait)
    Postintraventricular hemorrhage
    Posterior fossa subdural
    Postinfectious
    Vein of Galen aneurysm
    Quadrigeminal cyst or tumor
    Chiari II malformation (aqueductal kink)
  Fourth ventricular obstruction
    Dandy-Walker syndrome (outlets obstruction)
    Chiari II malformation (4th ventricle compressed)
All ventricles enlarged
  Extraventricular obstructive
    Posthemorrhagic
    Postinfectious
    Achondroplasia
    Absence of arachnoid granulations
  Nonobstructive
    Choroid plexus papilloma
    Superior vena cava obstruction
    Vein of Galen obstruction

ization of the entire ventricular system is the most valid way to diagnose hydrocephalus.

The lateral ventricular ratio may be useful to compare since it changes over time and is abnormal if greater than .34. Care must be taken to be certain that the axial image is symmetric so that the lateral ventricular ratio is valid. Brain mantle is determined by measuring the thickness of the brain from the lateral wall of the ventricle to the inner table of the skull in the parietal region. A poor prognosis has been reported in infants with a skull mantle less than 1 cm.

The level of obstruction is determined by the transition from an enlarged to a normal ventricle along the path of CSF flow. CSF flow begins in the lateral ventricle where it is made by the choroid plexus, moves through the foramina of Monro into the third ventricle, and then moves through the aqueduct of Sylvius into the fourth ventricle. It exits via the lateral foramina of Luschka into the subarachnoid spaces surrounding the brain. It is reabsorbed by the arachnoid granulations on the surface of the brain into the venous system.

## VENTRICULAR PERITONEAL SHUNT PROCEDURES

Ventriculoperitoneal shunting for hydrocephalus is a commonly performed procedure. It is usually considered when the lateral ventricular ratio exceeds .5 in newborns and infants. Posthemorrhagic hydrocephalus may resolve spontaneously or arrest at a mild degree so these infants are often followed up for a longer period without intervention. Most cases of posthemorrhagic hydrocephalus will begin by 2 weeks of age, which is the key time to evaluate for ventricular enlargement. Infants should be followed up until they are at least 6 weeks old, as the degree of enlargement may increase with time.

Intraoperative placement of shunt catheters may be facilitated by the use of real-time ultrasound during the procedure. The most anterior end of the shunt should be in front of the choroid plexus to prevent choroid from entering the shunt tip or sideholes and obstructing the shunt. Intraventricular hemorrhage has been noted during shunting but has not been associated with any complications.

Evaluation of ventricular size can be done with ultrasound after the shunt procedure. The shunt will cause a marked acoustic shadow if it is perpendicular to the beam but it can be fairly subtle if only a small part of the shunt is seen. The sweep on videotape will allow evaluation of the shunt and ventricles more easily.

Shunt complications may be detected, including a trapped fourth ventricle, recurrent obstruction, ventriculitis, meningitis, porencephaly around the shunt tip, and subdural hematomas. Abdominal pseudocyst formation can be detected on abdominal ultrasound.

## Intracranial Infections

### In Utero Infections

The neonates with infections acquired in utero will rarely be diagnosed because of the presence of maternal symptoms but are usually studied for abnormal head size, seizures, or hepatosplenomegaly. The TORCH differential of in utero infections includes toxoplasmosis, rubella, cytomegalovirus, and herpes complex virus. Cytomegalovirus and toxoplasmosis are the most common cause of intracranial calcification, but calcification has been reported in the other viruses. Calcifications may be subtle because there is often no acoustic shadowing, but the calcium is very sharply demarcated compared to hemorrhage. The brain parenchyma will often be highly echogenic with loss of normal sulcal detail. There are often areas of necrosis in the more severe cases.

## Postnatal Infections

Neonatal infections are usually bacterial and are caused most commonly by group *B streptococcus* or *Escherichia coli.* Infections in older infants are usually due to *Hemophilus influenzae.* Meningitis may present with widening of the interhemispheric fissure, echogenic sulci, and subdural effusions. Since the infant has difficulty restricting the infection to the meninges, there are often changes suggesting encephalitis. Diffusely increased brain parenchymal echogenicity may occur due to edema and cerebritis, along with focal areas of increased echogenicity, and abscess. Ventriculitis manifests as debris or septations in the ventricle.[18] Hydrocephalus is a common complication of meningitis, usually obstructing reabsorption due to meningeal scarring, and thus the entire ventricular system is often enlarged. Gyral infarctions may be suggested if a cortical gyrus is more echogenic than the underlying white matter.[19]

## Cerebral Edema and Infarction

Cerebral hypoxia and ischemia may occur secondary to a fetal insult, during delivery, or during the first days of life in a premature infant. Later damage may occur due to shock or asphyxia of any cause, including sudden infant death syndrome. The timing of the insult has a critical effect on the severity of the damage and the development of the infant brain. Blockage of both internal carotid arteries in utero will destroy most of the cerebral cortex and result in hydranencephaly which will manifest as an extremely thin cortex and a relatively normal brain stem and cerebellum. Partial destruction of cortex in utero often leads to porencephaly, which may be present in many destructive processes. Neonatal hypoxic encephalopathy may manifest as intracranial hemorrhage, but results from studies with positron emission scanning have shown that ischemia is often more extensive than the hem-

orrhage. Ultrasound findings in hypoxic encephalopathy are periventricular and parenchymal hyperechogenicity. The ventricles are typically slit-like (94%) with ischemia, but this ventricular appearance can be normal (62%) in controls.[20] Careful attention should be paid to the presence of pulsations in the cerebral arteries for if they are absent for a long period of time, brain death will occur in the area without perfusion. Cerebral edema will present as increased echogenicity either diffusely or surrounding other lesions.[21]

## Tumors, Cysts, and Arteriovenous Malformations

Intracranial tumors are very uncommon in the first 2 years of life.[22] However, they may be detected on routine scanning for other reasons. The most common presentation is as a cause of obstructive hydrocephalus. If there is no cause of hydrocephalus, such as hemorrhage or infection, CT with contrast or a magnetic resonance scan should be performed to exclude a tumor. In the immediate newborn period teratomas are most common; later astrocystomas, medulloblastomas, and ependymomas are most frequent. Hydrocephalus may also be caused by secretion of excessive CSF from a choroid plexus papilloma. Other presentations include unusual types of hemorrhage and failure to thrive. Ultrasound findings almost always include lesions with increased echogenicity and distortion of normal brain architecture.[23] There are often cystic areas within the tumor, and some tumors contain calcification.

Intracranial cysts may be diagnosed when there is a cystic lesion that has mass effect. Lack of mass effect means that the cystic areas is only a normal subarachnoid space such as a large cisterna magna or is an area of infarction or porencephaly. Rarely, an area of porencephaly will show mass effect due to poor communication and thus become a porencephalic cyst. Arachnoid cysts may occur between the brain and dura in any fissure or cistern and are usually an incidental finding. If they occur in certain areas, such as the suprasellar cistern, they may obstruct the ventricular system, causing hydrocephalus. Ventricular cysts may occur if a portion of a ventricle is obstructed. Neoplastic cysts usually have a thick wall, distort brain architecture, and have mass effect. If there is any question about a cystic lesion, a CT or magnetic resonance scan should be performed.

Arteriovenous malformations may manifest as unusually shaped cystic lesions, such as the vein of Galen aneurysm, or as discrete areas of increased echogenicity due to hemangiomas. Doppler examination may be very valuable as a way to exclude a vascular lesion when a cystic area is present.

## References

1. Shuman WP, Rogers JV, Mack LA, et al: Real-time sonographic sector scanning of the neonatal cranium: Technique and normal anatomy. *AJNR* 1981; 2:349–356.
2. Babcock DS, Han BK, Le Quesne GW: B-mode gray-scale ultrasound of the head in the newborn and young infant. *AJR* 1980; 134:457.
3. Scotti G, Flodmark O, Harwood-Nash DC: Posterior fossa hemorrhages in the newborn. *J Comput Assist Tomogr* 1981; 5:68–72.
4. Hill A, Melson GL, Clark B, et al: Hemorrhagic periventricular leukomalacia: Diagnosis by real-time ultrasound and correlation with autopsy findings. *Pediatrics* 1982; 69:282–284.
5. Armstrong D, Norman MG: Periventricular leukomalacia in infants: Complications and sequelae. *Arch Dis Child* 1974; 49:367–375.
6. Chou PP, Horgan JG, Taylor KJW: Neonatal periventricular leukomalacia: Real-time sonographic diagnosis with CT correlation. *AJNR* 1985; 6:383–388.
7. Babcock DS, Han BK: Cranial sonographic findings in myelomeningocoele. *AJNR* 1980; 1:493–499.
8. Naidich TP, Pudlowski RM, Naidich JB, et al: Computed tomographic signs of the Chiari II malformation: III. Ventricles and cisterns. *Radiology* 1980; 134:657–663.
9. Zimmerman RD, Breckbill D, Dennis MW, et al: Cranial CT findings in patients with myelomeningocoele. *AJR* 1979; 132:623–629.
10. Aglas SW, Shkolnik A, Naidich TP: Sonographic recognition of agenesis of the corpus callosum. *AJNR* 1985; 6:369–375.
11. Hermanz-Schulman M, Dohan FC Jr, Jones T, et al: Sonographic appearance of callosal agenesis: Correlation with radiologic and pathologic findings. *AJNR* 1985; 6:361–368.
12. Christensen SL, Rumack CM, Mack LA, et al: Prenatal and neonatal ultrasonic diagnosis of holoprosencephaly. Unpublished manuscript.
13. Daube JR, Chou SM: Lissencephaly: Two cases. *Neurology* 1966; 16:179–191.
14. Ramirez RE: Sonographic recognition of lissencephaly (agyria). *AJNR* 1984; 5:830–831.
15. DiPietro MA, Brody BA, Juban K, Cole FS: Schizencephaly: Rare cerebral malformation demonstrated by sonography. *AJNR* 1984; 5:196–198.
16. Babcock DS, Han BK, LeQuesne GW: B-mode gray-scale ultrasonography of the head in the newborn and young infant. *AJR* 1980; 134:457–468.
17. Rumack CM, Johnson ML: Real-time ultrasound evaluation of the neonatal brain. *Clin Ultrasound* 1982; 10:179–202.
18. Rosenberg HK, Levine RS, Stoltz K, et al: Bacterial meningitis in infants: Sonographic features. *AJNR* 1983; 4:822–825.
19. Babcock DS, Han BK: Sonographic recognition of gyral infarction in meningitis. *AJR* 1985; 144:833–836.
20. Siegel MJ, Shackelford GD, Perlman JM, et al: Hypoxic-ischemic encephalopathy in term infants: Diagnosis and prognosis evaluated by ultrasound. *Radiology* 1984; 152:395–399.
21. Smith SJ, Vogelzang RB, Marzono MI, et al: Brain edema: Ultrasound examination. *Radiology* 1985; 155:379–382.
22. Harwood-Nash DC, Fitz CR: *Neuroradiology in Infants and Children.* St Louis, CV Mosby Co, 1976.
23. Strassburg HM, Sauer M, Weber S, Gilsbach J: Ultrasonographic diagnosis of brain tumors in infancy. *Pediatr Radiol* 1984; 14:284–287.

## Additional Readings

NORMAL NEONATAL ANATOMY
AND ULTRASOUND TECHNIQUE

Ben-ora A, Eddy L, Hatch G, et al: The anterior fontanelle as an acoustic window to the neonatal ventricular system. *JCU* 1980; 8:65.

Dewbury KC, Aluwihare APR: The anterior fontanelle as an ultrasound window for the study of the brain: A preliminary report. *Br J Radiol* 1980; 53:81.

Haber K, Watcher RD, Christenson RC, et al: Ultrasonic evaluation of intracranial pathology in infants: A new technique. *Radiology* 1980; 134:173.

Johnson ML, Mack LA, Rumack CM, et al: B-mode echoencephalography in the normal and high risk infant. *AJR* 1979; 133:375–381.

Johnson ML, Rumack CM: Ultrasonic evaluation of the neonatal brain. *Radiol Clin North Am* 1980; 18:117–131.

Kossoff G, Garrett WJ, Radanaovich G: Ultrasonic atlas of the normal brain of the infant. *Ultrasound Med Biol* 1974; 1:259.

Lipscomb AP, Blackwell RJ, Reynolds EOR, et al: Ultrasound scanning of brain through the anterior fontanelle of newborn infants. *Lancet* 1979; 2:39

Mack LA, Alvord EC Jr: Neonatal cranial ultrasound: Normal appearances. *Semin Ultrasound* 1982; 3:216–230.

Matsui T, Hirano A: *An Atlas of the Human Brain for Computed Tomography.* New York, Igaku-Shoin, 1978.

Pigalas A, Thompson JR, Grube GL: Normal infant brain anatomy: Correlated real-time sonograms and brain specimens. *AJR* 1981; 137:815.

HEMORRHAGE

Babcock DS, Han BK: The accuracy of high resolution, real-time ultrasonography of the head in infancy. *Radiology* 1981; 139:665–676.

Babcock DS, Bove KE, Han BK: Intracranial hemorrhage in premature infants: Sonographic-pathologic correlation. *AJNR* 1982; 3:309–317.

Behrman RE: Serial lumbar punctures and intraventricular hemorrhage (editorial). *J Pediatr* 1980; 97:250.

Blank NK, Strand R, Gilles FH, et al: Posterior fossa subdural hematomas in neonates. *Arch Neurol* 1978; 35:108–111.

Bowerman RA, Donn SM, Silver TM, et al: Natural history of neonatal periventricular/intraventricular hemorrhage and its complications: Sonographic observations. *AJR* 1982; 143:1041–1052.

Briner S, Bodensteiner J: Benign subdural collections of infancy. *Pediatrics* 1981; 67:802–804.

Burstein J, Papile L, Burstein R: Intraventricular hemorrhage and hydrocephalus in premature newborns: A prospective study with CT. *AJR* 1979; 132:631–635.

Burstein J, Papile L, Burstein R: Subependymal ger-

minal matrix and intraventricular hemorrhage in premature infants: Diagnosis by CT. *AJR* 1977; 128:971–976.

Chessells JM, Wigglesworth JS: Coagulation studies in preterm infants with respiratory distress and intracranial hemorrhage. *Arch Dis Child* 1970; 47:564–570.

Deuel RK: Pathophysiology, live. *Pediatrics* 1982; 70:312.

Ennis MG, Kaude JV, Williams JL: Sonographic diagnosis of subarachnoid hemorrhage in premature newborn infants: A retrospective study with histopathologic and CT correlation. *J Ultrasound Med* 1985; 4:183–187.

Fredrich J, Butler NR: Certain causes of neonatal death; II: Intraventricular haemorrhage. *Biol Neonate* 1970; 15:257–290.

Finberg L: The relationship of intravenous infusions and intracranial hemorrhage: A commentary. *J Pediatr* 1977; 91:777.

Fishman MA, Percy AK, Cheek WR, et al: Successful conservative management of cerebellar hematomas in term neonates. *J Pediatr* 1981; 98:466–468.

Flodmark O, Becker LE, Harwood-Nash DC, et al: Correlation between CT and autopsy in premature and full-term neonates that have suffered asphyxia. *Radiology* 1980; 137:93–103.

French B, Dublin AB: Infantile chronic subdural hematoma of the posterior fossa diagnosed by CT. *J Neurosurg* 1977; 47:949–952.

Gilles FH, Shilito J: Infantile hydrocephalus: Retrocerebellar subdural hematoma. *J Pediatr* 1970; 76:529–537.

Goddard-Finegod J, Armstrong D, Zeller RS: Intraventricular hemorrhage following volume expansion after hypovolemic hypotension in the newborn beagle. *J Pediatr* 1982; 100:796–799.

Grant EG, Borts FT, Schellinger D, et al: Real-time ultrasonography of neonatal intraventricular hemorrhage and comparison with CT. *Radiology* 1981; 139:687–691.

Grant EG, Kerner M, Schellinger D, et al: Evolution of porencephalic cysts from intraparenchymal hemorrhage in neonates: Sonographic evidence. *AJR* 1982; 138:467–470.

Grant EG, Schellinger D, Richardson J, et al: Periventricular halo: Normal sonographic finding or neonatal cerebral hemorrhage. *AJR* 1983; 140:793–496.

Grant EG, Schellinger D, Richardson J: Real-time ultrasonography of the posterior fossa. *J Ultrasound Med* 1983; 2:73–87.

Hathaway WE, Mull MM, Pechet GS: Disseminated intravascular coagulation in the newborn. *Pediatrics* 1969; 43:233–240.

Hill A, Taylor DA, Volpe JJ: Treatment of posthemorrhagic hydrocephalus by serial lumbar puncture: Factors that account for success or failure. *Ann Neurol* 1981; 10:284–285.

Hill A, Perlman JM, Volpe JJ: Relationship of pneumothorax to occurrence of IVH in the premature newborn. *Pediatrics* 1982; 69:144–149.

Horbar JD, Walters CL, Phillip AGS, et al: Ultrasound detection of changing ventricular size in post-hemorrhagic hydrocephalus. *Pediatrics* 1980; 66:674–678.

Johnson ML, Rumack CM, Mannes EJ, et al: Detection of neonatal intracranial hemorrhage utilizing static and real-time ultrasound. *JCU* 1981; 9:427–433.

Kempe CH, Silverman FN, Steele BF, et al: The battered-child syndrome. *JAMA* 1962; 181:17–24.

Korobkin R: The relationship between head circumference and the development of communicating hydrocephalus in infants following intraventricular hemorrhage. *Pediatrics* 1975; 56:74–77.

Lazzaru A, Ahmann P, Dykes F, et al: Clinical predictability of intraventricular hemorrhage in preterm infants. *Pediatrics* 1980; 65:30–34.

Levene MJ, Wigglesworth JS, Dubowitz V: Hemorrhagic periventricular leukomalacia in the neonate: A real-time ultrasound study. *Pediatrics* 1983; 71:794–797.

Lipscomb AP, Reynolds EOR, Blackwell RJ, et al: Pneumothorax and cerebral haemorrhage in preterm infants. *Lancet* 1981; 1:414–416.

London PA, Carroll BA, Enzmann DR: Sonography of ventricular size and germinal matrix hemorrhage in premature infants. *AJNR* 1980; 1:295–300.

Lou HC, Lassen NA, Friis-Hansen B: Is arterial hypertension crucial for the development of cerebral hemorrhage in premature infants? *Lancet* 1979; 1:215.

Mack LA, Wright K, Hirsch J, et al: Intracranial hemorrhage in premature infants: Accuracy of sonographic evaluation. *AJR* 1981; 137:245–250.

Martin R, Roessmann U, Fanaroff A: Massive intracerebellar hemorrhage in low birthweight infants. *J Pediatr* 1976; 89:290–293.

Ment LR, Scott DT, Ehrenkranz RA, et al: Neonates < 1250 grams birth weight: Prospective neurodevelopmental evaluation during the first year post term. *Pediatrics* 1982; 70:292–295.

Mori K, Handa H, Itoh M, et al: Benign subdural effusion in infants. *J Comput Assist Tomogr* 1980; 4:466–471.

Newton TH, Gooding CA: Compression of superior sagittal sinus by neonatal calvarial moulding. *Radiology* 1975; 115:635–639.

Pape KE, Wigglesworth JS: *Hemorrhage, Ischemia and the Perinatal Brain.* London, England, Lavenham Press, Ltd, 1979.

Papile L, Burstein J, et al: Relationship of I.V. sodium bircarbonate infusions and cerebral intraventricular hemorrhage. *J Pediatr* 1978; 94:834–836.

Perlman JM, Nelson JS, McAllister WH, et al: Intracerebellar hemorrhage in a premature newborn: Diagnosis by real-time ultrasound. *Pediatrics* 1983; 71:159–162.

Peterson CM, Smith WL, Franken ED: Neonatal intracerebellar hemorrhage: Detection by real-time ultrasound. *Radiology* 1984; 150:391–392.

Robertson WC, Chun RWM, Orrison WW, et al: Benign subdural collections of infancy. *J Pediatr* 1979; 94:382–385.

Roeder JD, Setzer ES, Kaude JV: Ultrasonic detection of perinatal intracerebral hemorrhage. *Pediatrics* 1982; 70:385–386.

Rom S, Serfontein GL, Humphreys RP: Intracerebellar hematoma in the neonate. *J Pediatr* 1978; 93:486–488.

Rumack CM, Guggenheim MA, Rumack BH, et al: Neonatal intracranial hemorrhage and maternal use of aspirin. *Obstet Gynecol* 1981; 58:52s–56s.

Rumack CM, Johnson ML: Ultrasonic evaluation of intracranial hemorrhage in premature infants. *Semin Ultrasound* 1982; 3:209–215.

Rumack CM, Johnson ML: Real-time evaluation of the neonatal brain. *Clin Ultrasound* 1983; 10:179–198.

Rumack CM, Johnson ML: Role of CT and US in neonatal brain imaging. *J Comput Tomogr* 1983; 7:17–29.

Rumack CM, Johnson ML, Johnson JA, et al: Patterns of intracranial hemorrhage resolution: Correlation with clinical prognosis. Presented at the annual meeting of the American Roentgen Ray Society, Atlanta, Georgia, April 1983.

Rumack CM, Manco-Johnson ML, Manco-Johnson MJ, et al: Timing and course of neonatal intracranial hemorrhage using real-time ultrasound. *Radiology* 1985; 154:101–105.

Saubrei EE, Digney M, Harrison PB, et al: Ultrasonic evaluation of neonatal intracranial hemorrhage and its complications. *Radiology* 1981; 139:677–685.

Shankaran S, Slovis TL, Bedard MP, et al: Sonographic classification of intracranial hemorrhage: A prognostic indicator of mortality, morbidity and short term neurologic outcome. *J Pediatr* 1982; 100:469.

Silverboard G, Horder MH, Ahmann PA, et al: Reliability of ultrasound in the diagnosis of intracerebral hemorrhage and post hemorrhagic hydrocephalus: Comparison with CT. *Pediatrics* 1980; 66:507–514.

Simmons MA, Adcock EW, Bard H, et al: Hypernatremia and intracranial hemorrhage in neonates. *N Engl J Med* 1974; 291:6–10.

Slovis TL, Kelly JK, Eisenbrey AB, et al: Detection of extracerebral fluid collections by real-time sector scanning through the anterior fontanelle. *J Ultrasound Med* 1982; 1:41–44.

Slovis TL, Shankaran S, Bedard MP, et al: Intracranial hemorrhage in the hypoxic-ischemic infant: Ultrasound demonstration of unusual complications. *Radiology* 1984; 151:163–169.

Valdes-Dapena MA, Arey JB: The causes of neonatal mortality: An analysis of 501 autopsies on newborn infants. *J Pediatr* 1970; 77:366–375.

Volpe JJ, Pasternak JF, Allan WC: Ventricular dilatation preceding rapid head growth following neonatal intracranial hemorrhage. *Am J Dis Child* 1977; 131:1212.

Volpe JJ: Cerebral blood flow in the newborn infant: Relation to hypoxic-ischemic brain injury and periventricular hemorrhage. *J Pediatr* 1979; 94:170–173.

Volpe JJ: *Neurology of the Newborn.* Philadelphia, WB Saunders Co, 1981.

Volpe JJ, Perlman J, et al: Positron emission tomography (PET) in the assessment of regional cerebral blood flow in the newborn. *Ann Neurol* 1982; 23:225(A).

Wigglesworth JS, Husemeyer RP: Intracranial birth trauma in vaginal breech delivery: The continued importance of injury to occipital bone. *Br J Obstet Gynaecol* 1977; 84:684–691.

Wigglesworth JS, et al: An integrated model for haemorrhagic and ischemic lesions in the newborn brain. *Early Hum Dev* 1978; 2:179–199.

## CONGENITAL MALFORMATIONS

Cayea PD, Balcar I, Alberti O Jr, Jones TB: Prenatal diagnosis of semilobar holoprosencephaly. *AJR* 1984; 142:401–402.

DeMyer W: Classification of cerebral malformations. *Birth Defects* 1971; 7:78–93.

Dublin AB, French BN: Diagnostic image evaluation of hydranencephaly and pictorially similar entities with emphasis on CT. *Radiology* 1980; 137:81–91.

Fitz CR: Midline anomalies of the brain and the spine. *Radiol Clin North Am* 1982; 20:95–104.

Guibert-Tranier F, Piton J, Billerey J, et al: Agenesis of the corpus callosum. *J Neuroradiol* 1982; 9:135–160.

Harwood-Nash DC, Fitz CR: *Neuroradiology in Infants and Children.* St Louis, CV Mosby Co, 1976.

Legge M, Sauerbrei E, McDonald A: Intracranial tuberous sclerosis in infancy. *Radiology* 1984; 153:667–668.

Manelfe D, Sevely A: Neuroradiological study of the holoprosencephalies. *J Neuroradiol* 1982; 9:15–45.

Ohno K, Enomoto T, Imamoto J, et al: Lissencephaly (agyria) on computed tomography. *J Comput Assist Tomogr* 1979; 3:92–95.

Volpe JJ: Neurology of the newborn, in *Major Problems in Clinical Pediatrics.* Philadelphia, WB Saunders Co, 1981.

Warkany J, Lemire RJ, Cohen MM: *Mental Retardation and Congenital Malformations of the Central Nervous System.* Chicago, Year Book Medical Publishers, Inc, 1981.

Williams JL, Faerber EN: Septooptic dysplasia (de Morsier syndrome). *J Ultrasound Med* 1985; 4:265–266.

Yakovlev PI, Wadsworth RC: Schizencephalies: A study of the congenital clefts in the cerebral mantle. *J Neuropathol Exp Neurol* 1946; 5:169–206.

## HYDROCEPHALUS

Garrett WJ, Kossoff G, Jones RFC: Ultrasonic cross-sectional visualization of hydrocephalus in infants. *Neuroradiology* 1975; 8:279–288.

Goldfine SL, Turetz F, Beck R, et al: Cerebrospinal fluid intraperitoneal cyst: An unusual abdominal mass. *AJR* 1978; 130:568–569.

Grant EG, Schellinger D, Borts FT, et al: Real-time sonography of the neonatal and infant head. *AJR* 1981; 136:265–270.

Harwood-Nash DC, Fitz CR: *Neuroradiology in Infants and Children.* St Louis, CV Mosby Co, 1976.

Johnson ML, Rumack CM: B-mode echoencephalography in the normal and high risk infant. *AJR* 1979; 133:375–381.

Johnson ML, Rumack CM: Ultrasonic evaluation of the neonatal brain. *Radiol Clin North Am* 1980; 18:117–132.

Behrman RE: Serial lumbar punctures and IVH (editorial). *J Pediatr* 1980; 97:250.

Dennis M, Fitz CR, Netley CT, et al: The intelligence of hydrocephalic children. *Arch Neurol* 1981; 38:607–615.

Edwards MK, Brown DL, Muller J: Cribside neurosonography: Real-time sonography for intracranial investigation of the neonate. *AJR* 1981; 136:271–276.

Fitz CR: The ventricles and subarachnoid spaces in children, in Lee SH, Rao KCVG (eds): *Cranial Computed Tomography.* New York, McGraw-Hill Book Co, 1983.

Fried AM, Adams WE, Ellis GT, et al: Ventriculoperitoneal shunt function: Evaluation by sonography. *AJR* 1980; 134:967–970.

Knake JE, Chandler WF, McGillicuddy JE, et al: Intraoperative sonography for brain tumor localization and ventricular shunt placement. *AJR* 1982; 139:733–738.

Lee TG, Parsons PM: Ultrasound diagnosis of cerebrospinal fluid abdominal cyst. *Radiology* 1978; 127:220.

McCullough DC, Balzer-Martin LA: Current prognosis in overt neonatal hydrocephalus. *J Neurosurg* 1982; 5:378–383.

Morgan CL, Trought WS, Rothman SJ, et al: Comparison of gray-scale ultrasonography and CT in the evaluation of macrocrania in infants. *Radiology* 1979; 132:119–123.

Murtagh FR, Quencer RM, Poole CA: Cerebrospinal fluid shunt function and hydrocephalus in the pediatric age group. *Radiology* 1979; 132:385–388.

Price HI, Rosenthal SI, Batkitzky S, et al: Abdominal pseudocysts as a complication of ventriculoperitoneal shunt. *Neuroradiology* 1981; 21:273–276.

Rumack CM, Johnson ML, McDonald M, et al: Patterns of intracranial hemorrhage resolution. Presented at the annual meeting of the Society for Pediatric Radiology, New Orleans, May 1982.

Shkolnik A, McLone DG: Intraoperative real-time ultrasonic guidance of ventricular shunt placement in infants. *Radiology* 1982; 141:515–517.

Skolnick ML, Rosenbaum AE, Matzuk T, et al: Detection of dilated cerebral ventricles in infants: A correlative study between US and CT. *Radiology* 1979; 132:119–123.

Slovis T, Kuhns LR: Real-time sonography of the brain through the anterior fontanelle. *AJR* 1981; 136:277–286.

MECHANISMS OF HYDROCEPHALUS

Cubberly DA, Jaffe RB, Nixon GW: Sonographic demonstration of Galenic arteriovenous malformations in the neonate. *AJNR* 1982; 3:435–439.

Eisenberg HM, McComb JG, Lorenzo AV: Cerebrospinal fluid overproduction and hydrocephalus associated with choroid plexus papilloma. *J Neurosurg* 1974; 40:381–385.

Ekbom K, Greitz T, Kugelberg E: Hydrocephalus due to ectasia of the basilar artery. *J Neurol Sci* 1969; 8:465–477.

Ekbom K, Greitz T: Syndrome of hydrocephalus caused by saccular aneurysm of the basilar artery. *Acta Neurochir* 1971; 24:71–77.

Freidman WA, Mickle JP: Hydrocephalus in achondroplasia: A possible mechanism. *Neurosurgery* 1980; 7:150–153.

Gilles FH, Davidson RI: Communicating hydrocephalus associated with deficient dysplastic parasagittal arachnoidal granulations. *J Neurosurg* 1971; 35:421–426.

Greitz T, Ekbom K, Kugelberg E, et al: Occult hydrocephalus due to ectasia of the basilar artery. *Acta Radiol (Diagn)* 1969; 9:310–316.

Hooper R: Hydrocephalus and obstruction of the superior vena cava in infancy: Clinical study of the relationship between cerebrospinal fluid pressure and venous pressure. *Pediatrics* 1961; 28:792–799.

Perlman JM, Nelson JS, McAllister WJ, et al: Intracerebellar hemorrhage in a premature newborn: Diagnosis by real-time US and correlation with autopsy findings. *Pediatrics* 1983; 71:159–162.

Pettorossi VE, DiRocco C, Mancinelli R, et al: Communicating hydrocephalus induced by mechanically increased amplitude of the intraventricular cerebrospinal fluid pulse pressure: Rationale and method. *Exp Neurol* 1978; 59:30–39.

Rosman NP, Shands KN: Hydrocephalus caused by increased intracranial venous pressure: A clinicopathological study. *Ann Neurol* 1978; 3:445–460.

Savolaine ER, Gerber AM: Computerized tomography studies of congenital and acquired cerebral intraventricular membranes. *J Neurosurg* 1981; 54:388–391.

Schultz P, Leeds NE: Intraventricular septations complicating neonatal meningitis. *J Neurosurg* 1973; 38:320–326.

Scotti G, Flodmark D, Hardwood-Nash DC: Posterior fossa hemorrhage in the newborn. *J Comput Assist Tomogr* 1981; 5:68–72.

Steward DR, Johnson DG, Myers GG: Hydrocephalus as a complication of jugular catheterization during total parenteral nutrition. *J Pediatr Surg* 1975; 10:771–777.

Volpe JJ, Pasternak JF, Allan WC: Ventricular dilatation preceding rapid head growth following neonatal intracranial hemorrhage. *Am J Dis Child* 1977; 131:1212.

### INFECTIONS

Carbajal JR, Palacios E, Azar-Ku B, et al: Radiology of cysticercosis of the central nervous system including CT. *Radiology* 1980; 137:397–407.

Cussen LJ, Ryan GB: Hemorrhagic cerebral necrosis in neonatal infants with enterobacterial meningitis. *J Pediatr* 1967; 71:771–776.

Edwards MK, Brown DL, Chua GT: Complicated infantile meningitis: Evaluation by real-time sonography. *AJNR* 1982; 3:431–434.

Diebler C, Dusser A, Dulac O: Congenital toxoplasmosis: Clinical and neuroradiological evaluation of the cerebral lesions. *Neuroradiology* 1985; 27:125–230.

Graham D, Guidi SM, Sanders RC: Sonographic features of in utero periventricular calcification due to cytomegalovirus infection. *Ultrasound Med Biol* 1982; 1:171–172.

Jacobsen PL, Farmer TW: Subdural empyema complicating meningitis in infants: Improved diagnosis. *Neurology* 1982; 31:190–193.

Kotagal S, Tantanasirvongse S, Archer C: Periventricular calcification following neonatal ventriculitis. *J Comput Assist Tomogr* 1981; 5:651–652.

Lee SH: Infectious diseases, in Lee SH, Rao KCVG

(eds): *Cranial Computed Tomography*. New York, McGraw-Hill Book Co, 1981.

Schultz P, Leeds NE: Intraventricular septations complicating neonatal meningitis. *J Neurosurg* 1973; 38:620–626.

Stannard MW, Jimenez JF: Sonographic recognition of multiple cystic encephalomalacia. *AJNR* 1983; 4:1111–1114.

Yamanouchi Y, Soweda K, Tani S, et al: Gyriform calcifications after purulent meningitis. *Neuroradiology* 1980; 20:159–162.

Zee CS, Segall HD, Miller C, et al: Unusual neuroradiological features of intracranial cysticercosis. *Radiology* 1980; 137:397–407.

### INFARCTION AND EDEMA

Chow PP, Horgan JG, Taylor KJW: Neonatal periventricular leukomalacia: Real-time sonographic diagnosis with CT correlation. *AJNR* 1985; 6:383–388.

Delpy DT, Gordon RE, Hope PL, et al: Non-invasive investigation of cerebral ischemia by phosphorous. *Pediatrics* 1982; 70:310.

Flodmark O, Becker LE, Harwood-Nash DC: Correlation between computed tomography and autopsy in premature and full term infants that have suffered perinatal asphyxia. *Radiology* 1980; 137:93–103.

Hill A, Martin DJ, Daneman A, et al: Focal ischemic cerebral injury in the newborn: Diagnosis by ultrasound and correlation with computed tomographic scan. *Pediatrics* 1983; 71:790–793.

Lee TG, Warren BH: Antenatal diagnosis of hydranencephaly by ultrasound: Correlation with ventriculopathy and CT. *JCU* 1977; 5:271–273.

Rumack CM, Johnson ML: Role of CT and ultrasound in neonatal brain imaging. *J Comput Tomogr* 1983; 7:17–29.

Volpe JJ, Perlman J, et al: Positron emission tomography (PET) in the assessment of regional cerebral blood flow in the newborn. *Ann Neurol* 1982; 12:225(A).

### TUMORS, CYSTS, AND ARTERIOVENOUS MALFORMATIONS

Babcock DS: Neonatal Neurosonography. Course No. 810. Presented at the 71st Scientific Assembly and Annual Meeting of the Radiological Society of North America. Chicago, Nov 17–22, 1985.

Cubberly DA, Jaffe RB, Nixon GW: Sonographic demonstration of Galenic arterioventous malformations in the neonate. *AJNR* 1982; 3:435–439.

Fitz CR, Rao KCVG: Primary tumors in children, in *Cranial Computed Tomography*. New York, Mc-Graw-Hill Book Co, 1983, pp 295–343.

Gooding GAW, Edwards MSB, Rabkin AE, et al: Intraoperative real-time ultrasound in the localization of intracranial neoplasms. *Radiology* 1983; 146:459–462.

Grant E, Schellinger D, Richardson J: Real time ultrasonography of the posterior fossa. *J Ultrasound Med* 1983; 2:73–87.

Kaplan HA, Aronson SM, Browder EJ: Vascular malformations of the brain: An anatomical study. *J Neurosurg* 1961; 18:630.

Knake JE, Chandler WF, McGillicuddy JE, et al: Intraoperative sonography for brain tumor localization and ventricular shunt placement. *AJR* 1982; 139:733–738.

Mack LA, Rumack CM, Johnson ML: Ultrasound evaluation of cystic intracranial lesions in the neonate. *Radiology* 1980; 137:451–455.

Mahour GH, Wooley MM, Trivedi SN, et al: Teratomas in infancy and childhood. *Surgery* 1974; 76:309–318.

Maravilla KR, Kirks DR, Maravilla A: CT diagnosis of intracranial cystic abnormalities in children. *Comput Tomog* 1978; 2:221–235.

Martelli A, Scotti G, Harwood-Nash DC, et al: Aneurysms of the vein of Galen in children: CT and angiographic correlations. *Neuroradiology* 1980; 20:123–133.

Masuzawa H, Kamitani H, Sato J, et al: Intraoperative application of sector scanning electronic ultrasound in neurosurgery. *Neurol Med Chir (Tokyo)* 1981; 21:277–285.

Rubin JM, Dohrmann GJ, Greenberg M, et al: Intraoperative sonography of meningiomas. *AJNR* 1982; 3:305–308.

Shkolnik A: B-mode scanning of infant brain: A new approach. Case report. Craniopharyngioma. *JCU* 1975; 3:229–231.

Shkolnik A, McLone DG: Intraoperative real time ultrasonic guidance of ventricular shunt placement in infants. *Radiology* 1982; 144:573–576.

Slovis TL: Real-time ultrasound of the intracranial contents. *Clin Diagn Ultrasound* 1981; 8:13–27.

Slovis TL, Kuhns LR: Real-time sonography of the brain through the anterior fontanelle. *AJR* 1981; 136:277–286.

Taboada D, Froufe A, Alonso A, et al: Congenital medulloblastoma: Report of two cases. *Pediatr Radiol* 1980; 9:5–10.

Tardieu M, Evard P, Lyon G: Progressive expanding congenital porencephalies: A treatable cause of progressive encephalopathy. *Pediatrics* 1981; 68:198–202.

Tsutsumi Y, Andoh Y, Inque N: Ultrasound-guided biopsy for deep-seated brain tumors. *J Neurosurg* 1982; 57:164–167.

## Normal Neonatal Brain

Carol M. Rumack, M.D.
Michael L. Manco-Johnson, M.D.

The normal sagittal scan is obtained by seating a 7.5-MHz transducer on the anterior fontanelle so that it sectors anterior to posterior (Fig 18–1). A midline scan shows the normal corpus callosum forming a long C-shaped structure with two linear echogenic lines above and below it (Fig 18–2). The superior line is formed by the pericallosal arteries (arrows). The inferior line is formed by the septum pellucidum. It is usually only a line because in newborns, the septum contains a cystic structure called the cavum septi pellucidi (P). Initially the cavum extends posteriorly, forming the cavum vergae (V), but it closes from back to front over the first few weeks of life. Below this is a very echogenic structure, the choroid plexus, in the roof of the third ventricle (C). The third ventricle is moderately echogenic because it is so thin that the thalamus superiorly and the hypothalamus inferiorly are averaged into the ventricle. The hypothalamic groove (arrow) is often seen as a lucent line defining these two parts of the brain. The anterior recesses extend into the sella and the posterior recesses extend toward the echogenic quadrigeminal cistern. The fourth ventricle is visualized as a notch in the very echogenic, bean-shaped cerebellar vermis. Below the cerebellum is the cisterna magna. In this normal premature at 28 weeks' gestation no sulci are present.

In Figure 18–3, multiple sulci are evident in a term infant. Paralleling the corpus callosum is the cingulate sulcus (arrowheads), the first sulcus to appear. At term birth, multiple sulci are present throughout the brain. They are quite echogenic because they contain blood vessels. The callosum marginal arteries are in the cingulate sulcus.

The two lateral ventricles (Fig 18–4) are best seen on angled sagittal scans. One ventricle lies in the medial portion of each hemisphere. It forms a

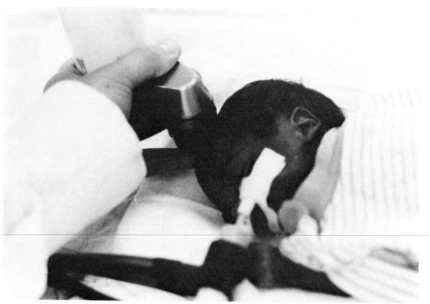

**FIG 18–1.**

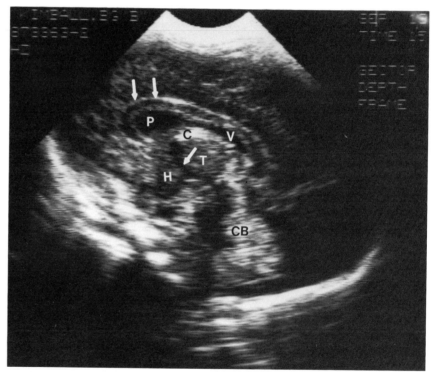

**FIG 18–2.**

larger "C" in the frontal horns anteriorly, the body of the ventricle behind it, followed by the trigone or antrium where the ventricle divides into three parts. The trigone contains the bulk of the very echogenic choroid plexus (C) which tapers anteriorly into the body of the lateral ventricle and then continues through the foramen of Monro into the third ventricle. Then the choroid plexus makes a U-turn along the roof of the third ventricle. The choroid extends inferiorly and anteriorly from the trigone into the temporal horn. The fornix is a thin white line medial to the choroid that curves around thalamus. Below the frontal horn is the head of the caudate nucleus anterior and superior to the thalamus. Multiple sulci may be present, depending on the gestational age of the infant. The infant in Figure 18–4 has a cingulate sulcus and is beginning to develop other sulci near the brain surface.

| | | |
|---|---|---|
| **Arrow** | = | Hypothalamic groove between the thalamus superiorly and the hypothalamus inferiorly |
| **Arrows** | = | Pericallosal arteries on the roof of the corpus callosum |
| **Arrowheads** | = | Cingulate sulcus |
| **B** | = | Body of lateral ventricle |
| **C** | = | Choroid plexus in roof of third ventricle and trigone |
| **CB** | = | Cerebellum containing notch of fourth ventricle |
| **P** | = | Cavum septi pellucidi |
| **V** | = | Cavum vergae |

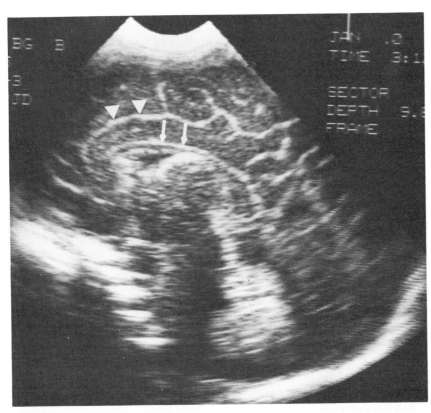

**FIG 18–3.**

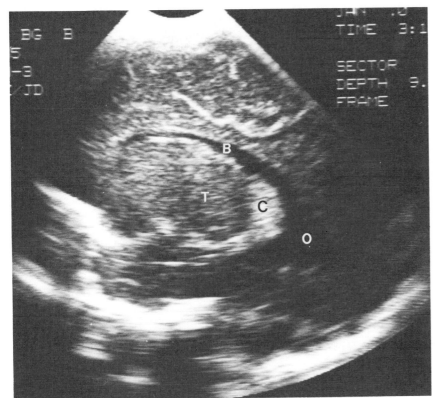

**FIG 18–4.**

## Normal Neonatal Brain

A coronal brain scan is obtained by placing the real-time transducer on the anterior fontanelle such that the beam sweeps from side to side (Fig 18–5). It is easiest to begin posteriorly at the level of the trigone by placing the thickest part of the choroid so that it is symmetric bilaterally (Fig 18–6). The choroid tends to settle toward the dependently placed ventricle. As the transducer is angled anteriorly, the bodies of the lateral ventricle are seen as lucent areas on either side of the midline, with three small, round, very echogenic portions of the choroid arising from the floor of each ventricle and the roof of the third ventricle (Fig 18–7). Superiorly is the inner hemispheric fissure. Inferiorly the tentorium curves across the surface of the cerebellum from each side. The third ventricle is usually seen just as a slit between the thalami if it is visualized at all. The fourth ventricle will sometimes be visualized just above the vermis in the midline. The sylvian fissures (S) form an echogenic Y on both sides where the pulsating middle cerebral arteries divide into multiple branches.

The most anterior coronal section routinely contains frontal horns of the lateral ventricles, which are curved lucent structures on either side of the cystic cavum septi pellucidi (Fig 18–8). The corpus callosum forms the roof of the cavum, and the lateral ventricles, with the cingulate sulcus just above it. Inferiorly, the imaging plane may pass through the foramen of Monro into the third ventricle. If the imaging plane is slightly more anterior, the internal carotid bifurcation will branch in the midline into the two anterior cerebral arteries centrally and the middle cerebral arteries laterally.

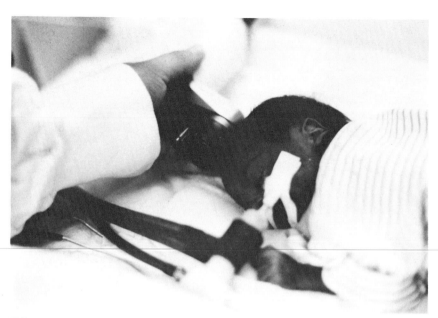

FIG 18–5.

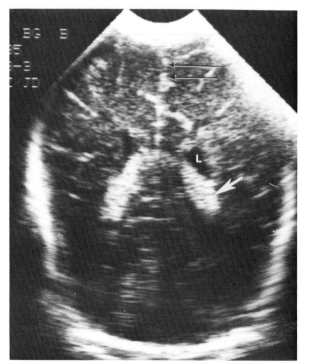

FIG 18–6.

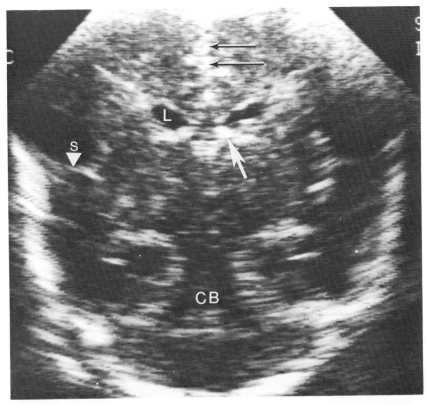

**Arrow** = Choroid in floor of left lateral
*(white)*    ventricle
**Arrows** = Interhemispheric fissure (Fig
*(black)*    19–7)
**CB** = Cerebellum
**L** = Lateral ventricle
**S** = Sylvian fissure

**FIG 18–7.**

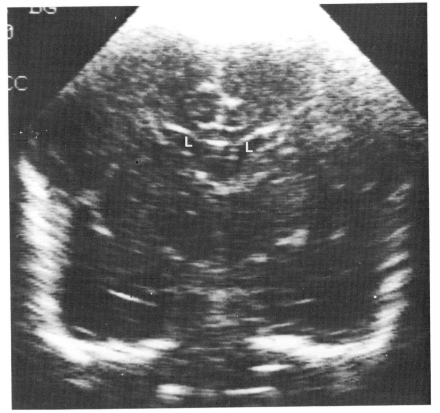

**FIG 18–8.**

## Normal Neonatal Brain and Subependymal Germinal Matrix Hemorrhage

An axial view (Fig 18–9) may be obtained by placing the transducer on the temporal bone about 1 cm above the external auditory meatus. The lateral ventricular ratio is measured from the middle of the midline echo to the lateral ventricular wall over the hemisphere dimension from the midline echo to the inner table of the skull (Fig 18–10). The lateral ventricular ratio is equal to A/B. Reverberation artifacts often obscure visualization of the near hemisphere and near ventricle.

Subependymal germinal matrix hemorrhage typically develops in the caudate nucleus, which lies just inferior and lateral to the lateral ventricles. As it enlarges it may rupture, causing intraventricular hemorrhage (IVH), which may flow throughout the ventricular system and out into the subarachnoid space. Ventricular size will often enlarge after intraventricular hemorrhage. When this is transient, it is probably due to an obstructive clot in the ventricular system. For this reason, all intraventricular hemorrhages are followed to determine if hydrocephalus develops, resolves, or becomes severe enough to require ventriculoperitoneal shunting.

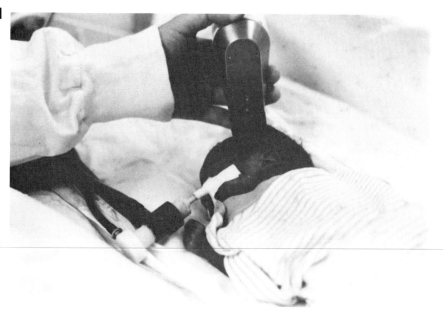

FIG 18–9.

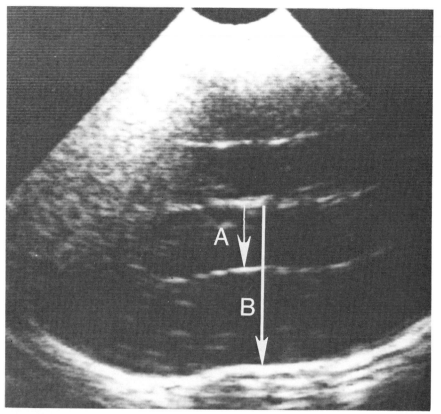

FIG 18–10.

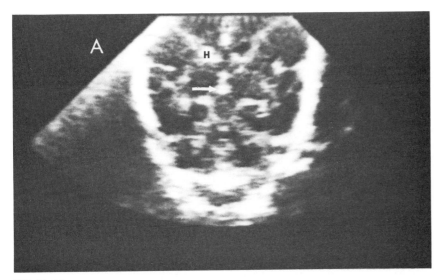

**FIG 18–11.**

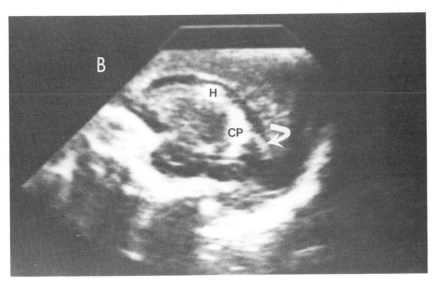

**FIG 18–12.**

SOURCE: Figures 18–11 and 18–12 are reproduced with permission from Rumack CM, Johnson ML: *Perinatal and Infant Brain Imaging: Role of Ultrasound and Computed Tomography.* Chicago, Year Book Medical Publishers, Inc, 1984.

| | | |
|---|---|---|
| **A** | = | Distance from midline ot the lateral wall of the lateral ventricle |
| **Arrow** | = | Blood in the third ventricle |
| **B** | = | Distance from midline to the inner table |
| **CP** | = | Choroid plexus |
| **Curved arrow** | = | IVH clot attached to choroid plexus |
| **H** | = | Hemorrhage in the caudate nucleus |

## Intraventricular Hemorrhage and Intraparenchymal Hemorrhage

Intraventricular hemorrhage develops from rupture of a subependymal hematoma into the ventricle. Initially, it may be difficult to determine whether the clot extends beyond the caudate nucleus. Specific clues to the presence of ventricular hemorrhage include obliteration of the ventricular margins, and echogenic material in the temporal or occipital horns or other parts of the ventricular system (Figs 18–13 and 18–14). Echogenic margins develop along the ventricles about 1 week after the initial hemorrhage due to the chemical ventriculitis evoked by the hemorrhage.

Subependymal hemorrhage may enlarge beyond the caudate nucleus into the brain parenchyma, causing an intraparenchymal hemorrhage (Figs 18–15 and 18–16). A larger hemorrhage often obscures the ventricular margins. In the sagittal view, the occipital and temporal horns are also filled with intraventricular hemorrhage (Fig 18–16). The lateral ventricle is probably already slightly enlarged since the frontal horn is big, but the size of the rest of the ventricle can not be evaluated because of the ventricular hemorrhage. In the coronal view, hemorrhage is seen just lateral to the lateral ventricle at the trigone (Fig 18–15). The choroid plexus blends into the echogenic hemorrhage, indicating that there must be some ventricular hemorrhage at this level.

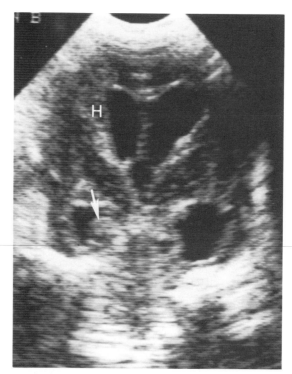

**FIG 18–13.**

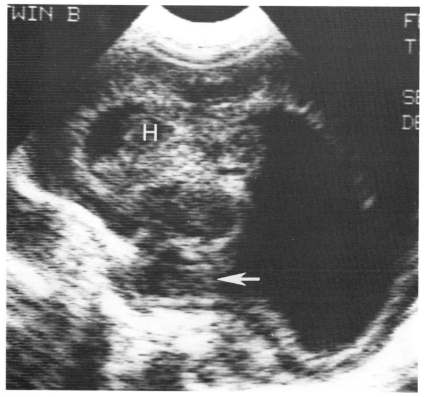

**FIG 18–14.**

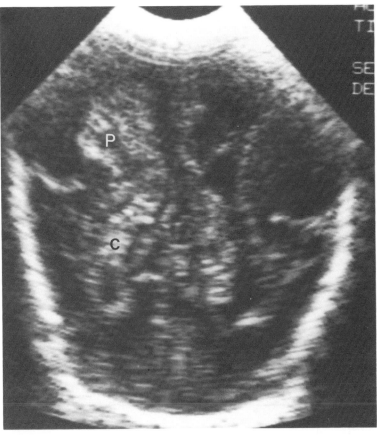

**FIG 18–15.**

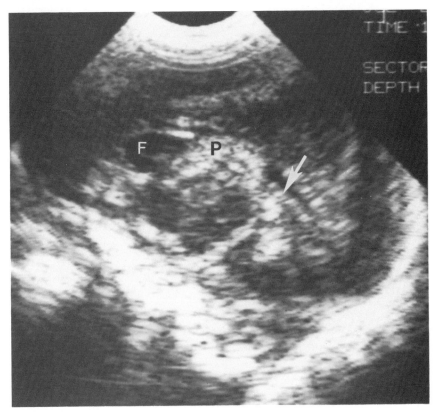

**FIG 18–16.**

Arrow = Echogenic debris (clot) in the temporal horn of the lateral ventricle (Figs 18–13 and 18–14)

Arrow = Intraventricular hemorrhage (Fig 18–16)

C = Choroid plexus
F = Frontal horn
H = Subependymal hematoma extending into the lateral ventricle
P = Intraparenchymal hemorrhage

# Porencephaly; Periventricular Hemorrhage and Infarction

Intraparenchymal hemorrhage typically resolves slowly. It takes about 1 week for the very echogenic hemorrhage to become sonolucent centrally. At about 2–3 weeks, the clot retracts from the edges of the area of hemorrhage (Fig 18–17). Final resolution often takes from 2 to 3 months, resulting in the development of porencephaly (P). If the original clot was fairly large, as in this case, the final appearance is often that of asymmetry of the lateral ventricles due to loss of brain matter along the edge of the affected ventricle. This patient also had hydrocephalus (Fig 18–18) of the extraventricular obstructive type because the entire ventricular system is enlarged, including the third and fourth ventricles (Fig 18–17).

Periventricular infarction, often termed periventricular leukomalacia (PVL), is an uncommon but significant cause of neurologic damage. It appears quite echogenic on ultrasound scans, but pathologic reports indicate that it is more commonly infarction without hemorrhage. CT can be performed to determine if hemorrhage has actually occurred. In this case there is marked echogenicity lateral to the ventricle system. The ventricles are so compressed they can be recognized only by the choroid in the trigone of the lateral ventricle in the coronal view (Fig 18–19). In the sagittal view (Fig 18–20), the imaging plane is just lateral to the ventricular system and reveals extensive involvement of the brain parenchyma in the periventricular region. The more lateral this involvement extends, the more likely it is that the corticospinal tracts are involved, which will result in contralateral hemiparesis. The rest of the brain appears quite echogenic, most likely because of cerebral edema.

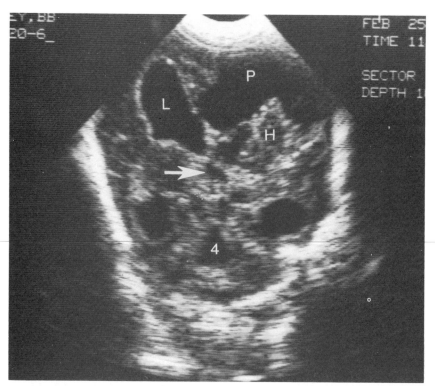

FIG 18–17.

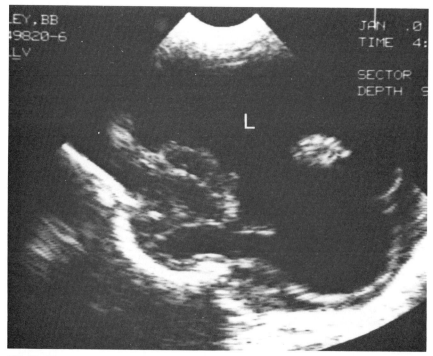

FIG 18–18.

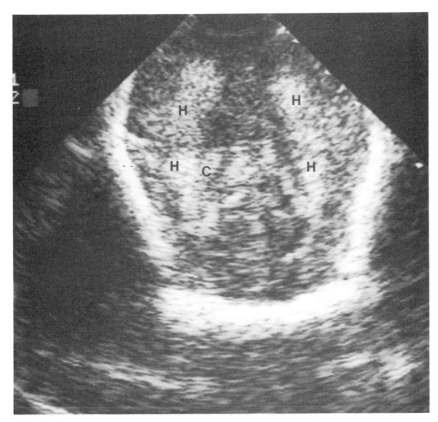

**FIG 18–19.**

SOURCE: Figures 18–19 and 18–20 are reproduced with permission from Rumack CM, Johnson ML: *Perinatal and Infant Brain Imaging: Role of Ultrasound and Computed Tomography.* Chicago, Year Book Medical Publishers, Inc, 1984.

**Arrow** = Third ventricle
**C** = Choroid plexus
**H** = Clot retracted to the bottom of the ventricle (Fig 18–17)
**H** = Periventricular hemorrhage (Figs 18–19, 18–20)
**L** = Body of the right lateral ventricle
**P** = Porencephaly
**4** = Fourth ventricle

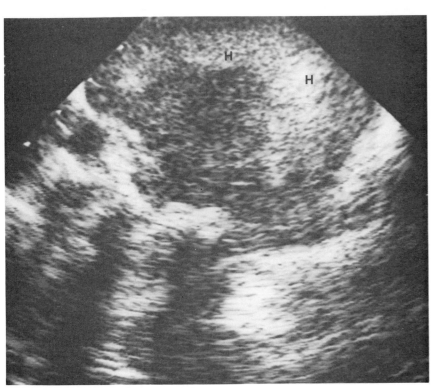

**FIG 18–20.**

## Subarachnoid Hemorrhage and Subdural Hemorrhage

Subarachnoid hemorrhage (SAH) occurs very uncommonly as an isolated lesion. When it does, it is usually in term infants and rarely has any significant sequelae. In the case illustrated here, subependymal hemorrhage and intraventricular hemorrhage fill the temporal horns of the lateral ventricles (Fig 18–21). Subarachnoid hemorrhage has thickened the sylvian fissure and the surface of the tentorium. Usually the cisterna magna is the first site to contain SAH in infants because they are supine and a large amount of SAH is necessary to result in hemorrhage in the sylvian fissure. Figure 18–22 is a CT scan showing the SAH (S) in the right sylvian fissure and layered over the tentorium and vascular structures posteriorly. Intraventricular hemorrhage (V) is also present.

Subdural hemorrhage (SDH) is very echogenic acutely and may blend into the initial transducer artifact. Most subdural hemorrhage is diagnosed in its chronic state for weeks after the initial insult. The subdural fluid must be more than 1 cm thick to be recognized below the initial transducer artifact as fluid between the transducer and the brain. The diagnosis is made by visualizing the surface sulci in the coronal and sagittal views (Figs 18–23 and 18–24). Interhemispheric fissure is often widened by extension of fluid in the fissure.

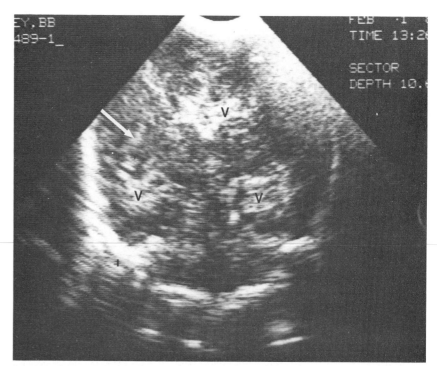

**FIG 18–21.**

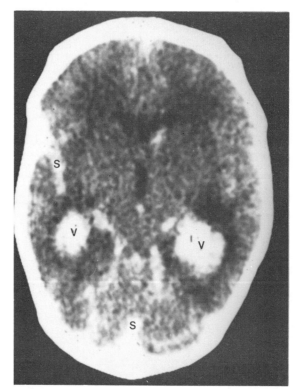

**FIG 18–22.**

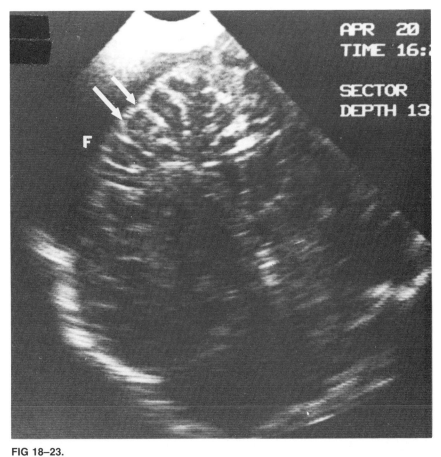

**FIG 18–23.**

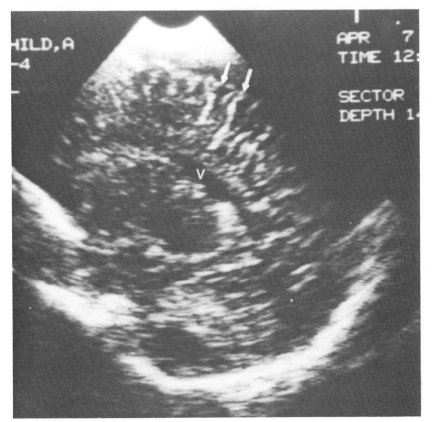

**FIG 18–24.**

SOURCE: Figures 18–21 through 18–24 are reproduced with permission from Rumack CM, Johnson ML: *Perinatal and Infant Brain Imaging: Role of Ultrasound and Computed Tomography.* Chicago, Year Book Medical Publishers, Inc, 1984.

| | |
|---|---|
| **Arrow** | = Sylvian fissure thickened by blood (Fig 18–21) |
| **Arrows** | = Surface sulci of the brain (Figs 18–23, 18–24) |
| **F** | = Subdural fluid |
| **S** | = Blood in the sylvian fissure and cisterna magna |
| **V** | = Intraventricular hemorrhage (Figs 18–21, 18–22) |
| **V** | = Lateral ventricle (Fig 18–24) |

## Chiari II Malformation

The Chiari II malformation typically presents in patients with meningomyeloceles. It may be suggested even in utero by the classic shape of the ventricular system and associated dysplastic findings. The frontal horns are pointed inferiorly and anteriorly and are relatively thin compared to the enlarged occipital horns (Fig 18–25). Hydrocephalus occurs in over 80%–90% of cases and typically becomes more severe after meningomyelocele repair. In the midline, there is usually an enlarged massa intermedia within a dilated ventricle (Fig 18–26). The fourth ventricle is difficult to visualize because it is compressed and displaced inferiorly with the rest of the cerebellum. In a coronal view, the frontal horns are pointed, an interhemispheric fissure is wide, and the massa intermedia fills up a significant part of the third ventricle (Figs 18–27 and 18–28). The tentorial incisura may be quite prominent above the cerebellum, and all of the fissure and cisterns typically are even larger after peritoneal shunting.

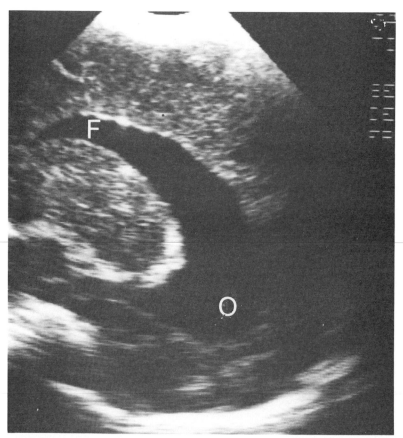

**FIG 18–25.**

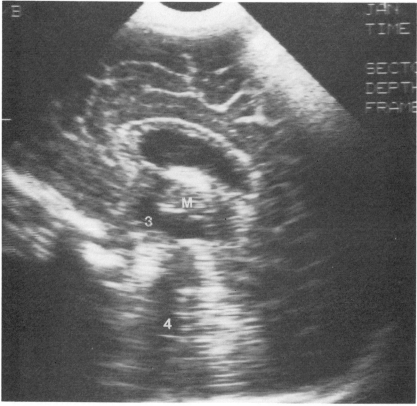

**FIG 18–26.**

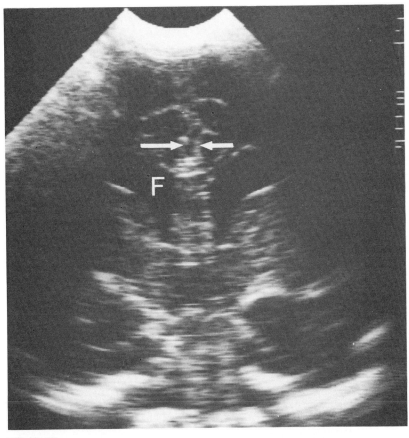

**FIG 18–27.**

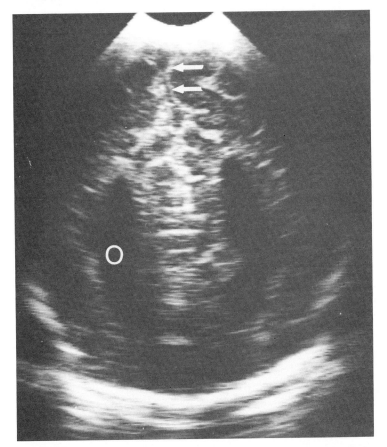

**FIG 18–28.**

| Arrows | = | Interhemispheric fissure |
|---|---|---|
| **F** | = | Frontal horn, anteriorly and inferiorly pointed |
| **M** | = | Massa intermedia |
| **O** | = | Occipital horn |
| **3** | = | Third ventricle |
| **4** | = | Fourth ventricle |

## Dandy-Walker Cyst and Agenesis of the Corpus Callosum

A Dandy-Walker cyst is actually a massively enlarged fourth ventricle associated with hydrocephalus of the entire ventricular system. In a coronal view, the lateral ventricles and third and fourth ventricles are dilated. Note that the septum pellucidum has been torn by the hydrocephalus and the corpus callosum is stretched above the midline of the ventricles (Fig 18–29). A view of the posterior fossa can be obtained when the posterior fontanelle is still open, as is often present in a neonate with massive hydrocephalus. This results in an excellent view of a dilated fourth ventricle and third and lateral ventricles (Fig 18–30). A similar view could be obtained by a steep, posteriorly angled coronal scan from the anterior fontanelle.

In a coronal view in which the corpus callosum is absent, the roof of the third ventricle extends above the level of the lateral ventricles and the floor of the third ventricle is often displaced superiorly from its normal position (Fig 18–31). Posteriorly the third ventricle may extend into a dorsal cyst, which is really a part of the ventricle and does not require shunting. Between the third and lateral ventricles lies the bundles of nerve fibers (Probst's bundles) that were meant to form the corpus callosum. In agenesis of the corpus callosum, the C-shaped corpus callosum is absent in a sagittal view. There is also no cingulate sulcus (Fig 18–32). The sulci are often radially arranged above the third ventricle or even randomly arranged.

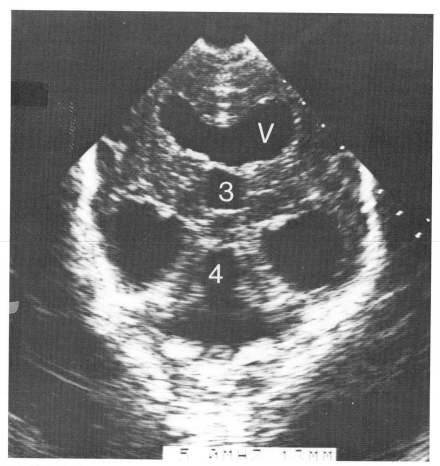

FIG 18–29.

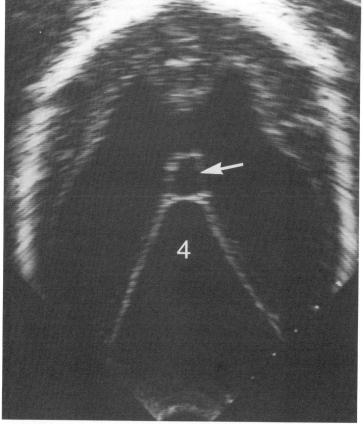

FIG 18–30.

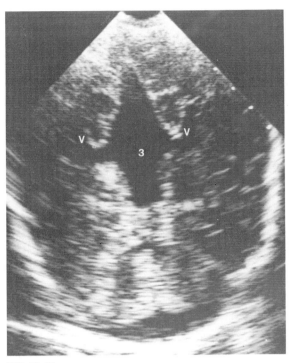

FIG 18–31.

SOURCE: Figures 18–31 and 18–32 are reproduced with permission from Rumack CM, Johnson ML: *Perinatal and Infant Brain Imaging: Role of Ultrasound and Computed Tomography.* Chicago, Year Book Medical Publishers, Inc, 1984.

**Arrow** = Third ventricle
**C** = Dorsal cyst
**V** = Lateral ventricle
**3** = Third ventricle
**4** = Fourth ventricle

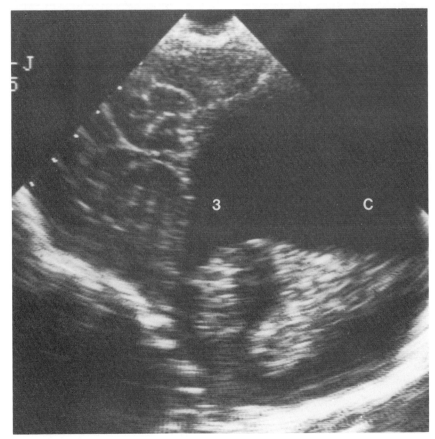

FIG 18–32.

## Alobar Holoporencephaly and Aqueductal Stenosis

Alobar holoporencephaly presents as a single midline ventricle with fused thalami beneath it in the midline. The choroid plexus is fused above the thalamus and drapes laterally and posteriorly (Fig 18–33). No interhemispheric fissure or septum pellucidum is present in the midline due to failure of diverticulation into two ventricles. Often, the single ventricle extends posteriorly into a dorsal cyst. The sulci are randomly arranged, with absence of the corpus callosum (Fig 18–34).

Aqueductal stenosis is an uncommon congenital brain malformation inherited as an autosomal dominant trait. The aqueductal obstruction causes dilatation of the lateral and third ventricles. In this case, the massa intermedia is stretched across the third ventricle (Fig 18–35). In the sagittal view, the lateral ventricle bulges superiorly, stretching the cingulate sulcus. The frontal horns are rounded rather than tapered as would be found if this were a Chiari malformation.

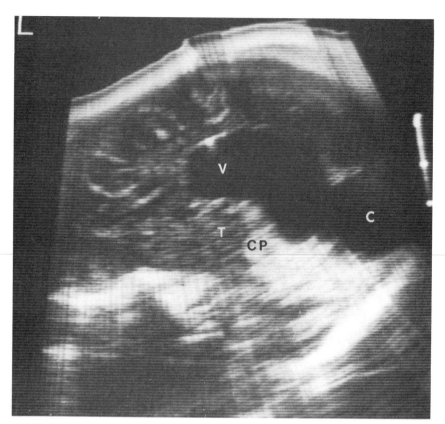

FIG 18–33.

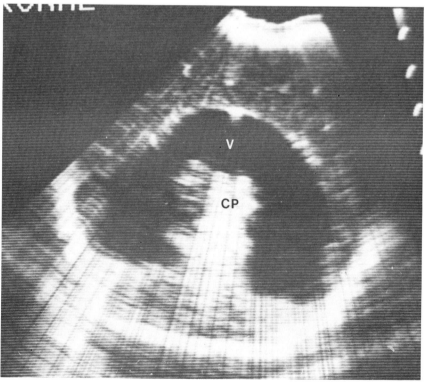

FIG 18–34.

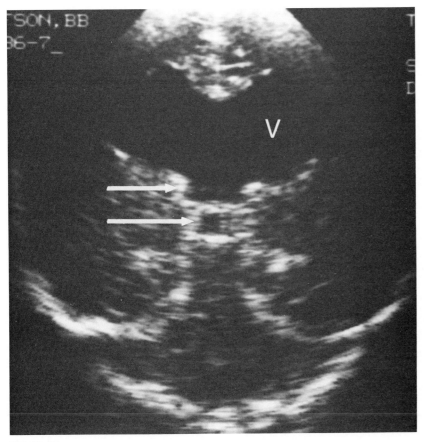

**FIG 18-35.**

SOURCE: Figures 18–33 and 18–34 are reproduced with permission from Rumack CM, Johnson ML: *Perinatal and Infant Brain Imaging: Role of Ultrasound and Computed Tomography.* Chicago, Year Book Medical Publishers, Inc, 1984.

| **Arrows** | = | Third ventricle with thin massa intermedia |
|---|---|---|
| **C** | = | Dorsal cyst |
| **CP** | = | Choroid plexus |
| **T** | = | Thalamus |
| **V** | = | Ventricle (Figs 18–33, 18–34) |
| **V** | = | Lateral ventricles (Figs 18–35, 18–36) |

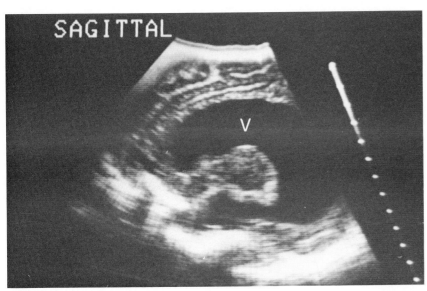

**FIG 18-36.**

## Ventriculitis Post Shunt and Cerebral Edema

Figures 18–37 and 18–38 are coronal and sagittal scans of a neonate who developed hydrocephalus following intraventricular hemorrhage. After shunting, ventriculitis developed secondary to *Staphylococcus aureus* infection. Although there appears to be a shunt in the ventricle, the shunt catheter has already been removed. Echogenic material within the ventricle is due to white cells and bacteria forming an area of pus. The infection has blocked the shunt, resulting in recurrent obstruction and hydrocephalus.

Cerebral edema is caused by diffuse infection or infarction. It is uncommonly diagnosed on ultrasound except in the most extreme cases. Cerebral edema is very echogenic and causes loss of definition of the sulci. Extremely small ventricles may also be present (Fig 18–39). The sylvian fissures are difficult to identify. On rare occasions, cerebral edema is so severe as to cause loss of pulsation in the cerebral vessels. If it is localized, cerebral infarction will occur. If it is diffuse, brain death is likely to occur.

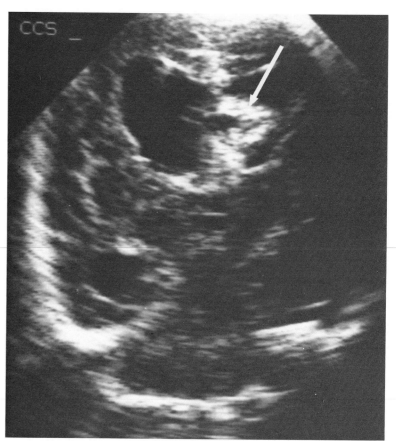

**FIG 18–37.**

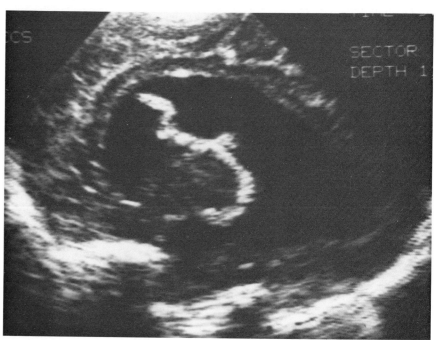

**FIG 18–38.**

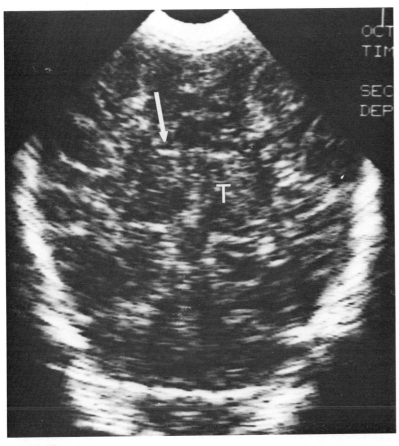

**FIG 18–39.**

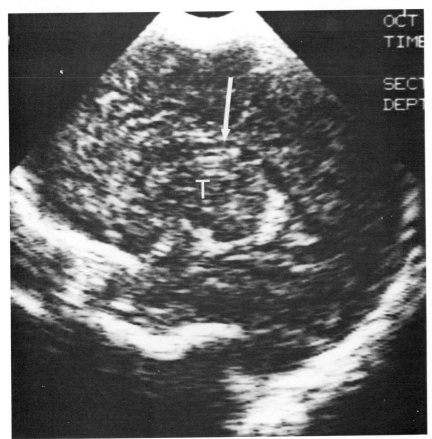

**FIG 18–40.**

**Arrow** = Pus in the ventricule (Fig 18–37)

**Arrow** = Small ventricle compressed by very echogenic, edematous brain (Figs 18–39, 18–40)

**T** = Thalamus

## Cerebral Infection

Cytomegalovirus infection occurs in utero and when first diagnosed may cause only diffusely echogenic brain and thick ventricular margins secondary to active encephalitis. The active phase of encephalitis begins in utero and by birth may have caused calcification. The ventricular margin may be thickened secondary to the infection (Fig 18–41). Ventricular septations may result from ventriculitis of any etiology (Fig 18–42). After months of infection in utero, the neonate will often present on the first day of life with periventricular calcifications secondary to cytomegalovirus (Figs 18–43 and 18–44). The sulci are often obscured secondary to encephalitis. When calcifications are present, they may appear punctate and discrete.

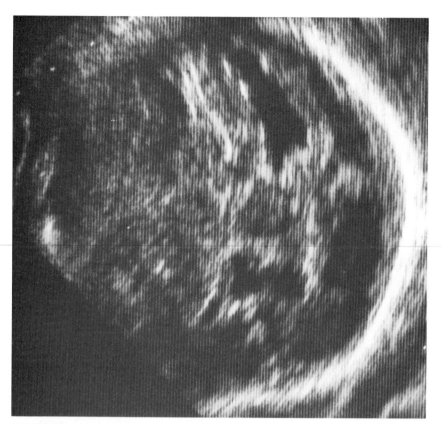

FIG 18–41.

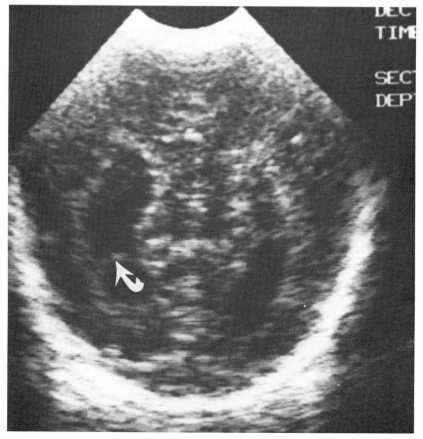

FIG 18–42.

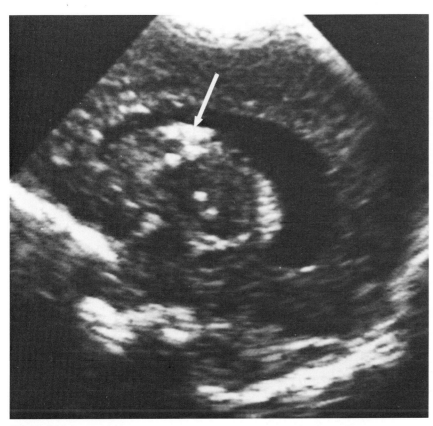

**FIG 18–43.**

**Arrow**        = Calcification in the peri-
                    ventricular region (Figs
                    18–43, 18–44)

**Curved arrow** = Ventricular septation
                    (Fig 18–42)

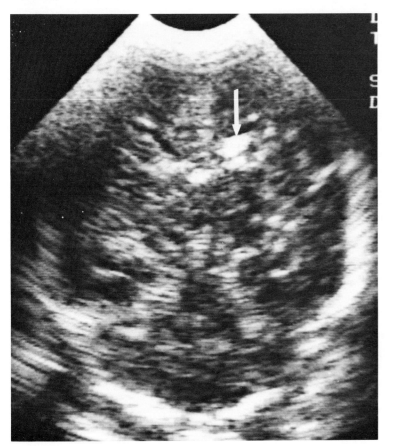

**FIG 18–44.**

## Intracranial Tumor and Arachnoid Cyst

Intracranial tumors have been studied both neonatally and intraoperatively. They most commonly present as echogenic lesions. Figures 18–45 and 18–46 are coronal and sagittal scans showing an echogenic tumor secondary to choroid plexus papilloma (P). Some tumors may have cystic areas or extremely echogenic areas with acoustic shadowing due to calcification. The tumor began within the ventricular system. Like the normal choroid, this tumor is extremely echogenic. It caused hydrocephalus on the basis of excessive cerebrospinal fluid production.

Arachnoid cysts are benign congenital cystic lesions that may present at any time in life. They are usually incidental findings unless they become quite large. If they occur in the contained space of the posterior fossa, hydrocephalus may result. In such instances, the ultasound appearance would be similar to that of a Dandy-Walker cyst, but the cyst would be separate from the fourth ventricle. This infant's cyst was diagnosed in utero and followed up for several months in the neonatal period. There was no change in size of either the cyst or the ventricular system.

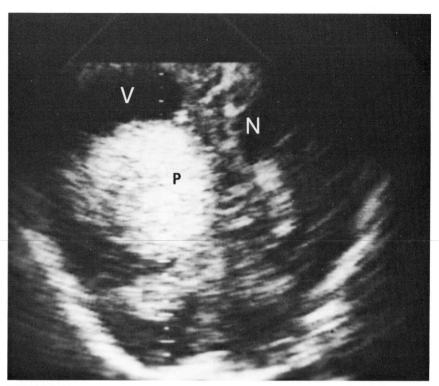

**FIG 18–45.**

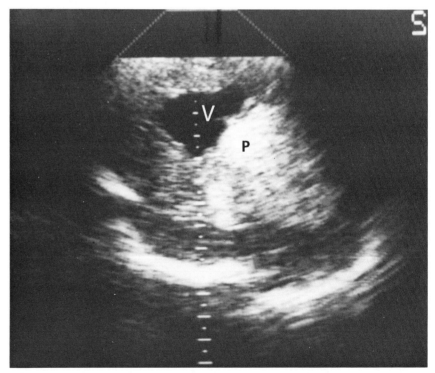

**FIG 18–46.**

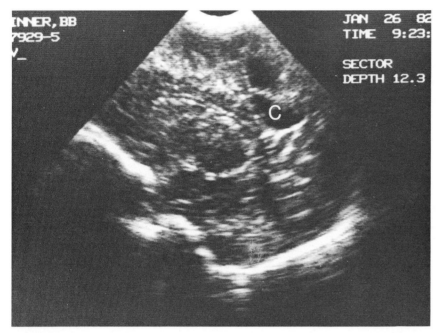

**FIG 18–47.**

SOURCE: Figures 18–45 thorugh 18–48 are reproduced with permission from Rumack CM, Johnson ML: *Perinatal and Infant Brain Imaging: Role of Ultrasound and Computed Tomography.* Chicago, Year Book Medical Publishers, Inc, 1984.

C  =  Arachnoid cyst
N  =  Normal opposite lateral ventricle
P  =  Choroid plexus papilloma
V  =  Dilated lateral ventricle

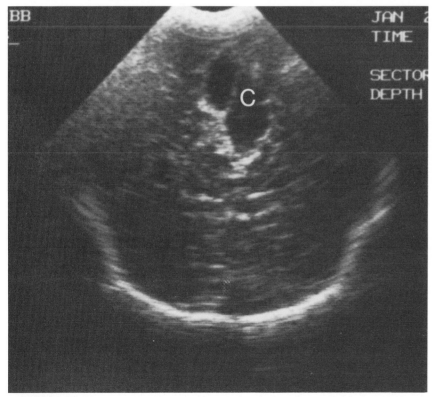

**FIG 18–48.**

## Vein of Galen Aneurysm

A vein of Gale aneurysm arises from multiple arterial feeders which are present from the anterior and posterior cerebral circulation. These feeders steal blood from the cerebral vasculature and result in a greatly dilated vein of Galen. Cardiac failure secondary to the large arteriovenous shunt is a common presenting symptom. Hydrocephalus may also develop since the dilated vein of Galen can obstruct the ventricular system at the level of the third ventricle and aqueduct. Subarachnoid bleeding or intraventricular bleeding may also occur. Figure 18–49 is a coronal scan at the level of the body of the lateral ventricles. The sonolucent structure in the midline is secondary to a vein of Galen aneurysm. A cerebral angiogram (Fig 18–50) shows the arterial feeders to the aneurysm. Figure 18–51 is a sagittal scan showing a large dilated vein of Galen and its posterior continuation into a dilated straight sinus. A sagittal angiogram (Fig 18–52) shows the arterial feeders draining into the aneurysmal vein of Galen and draining sinuses.

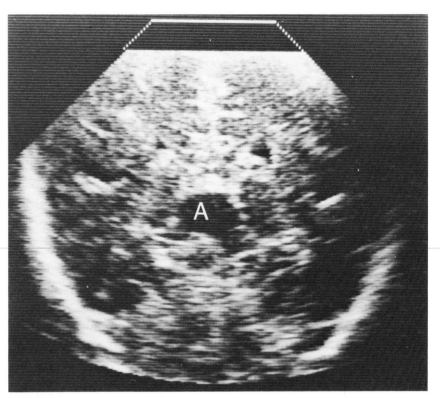

**FIG 18–49.**

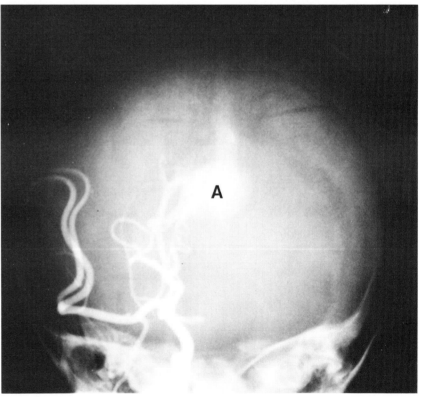

**FIG 18–50.**

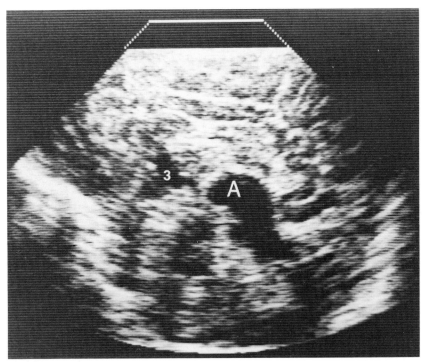

A  =  Vein of Galen aneurysm
3  =  Third ventricle

**FIG 18–51.**

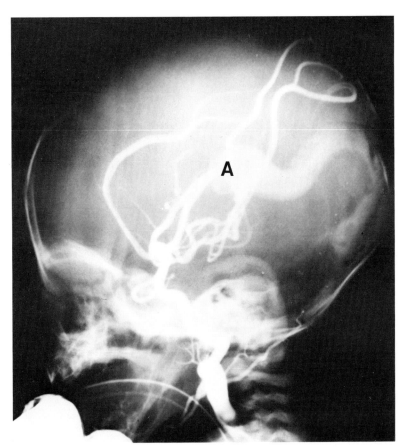

**FIG 18–52.**

# Index